THE SCIENCE
of
HOMOEOPATHIC
THERAPEUTICS

BERNHARD BAEHR, M.D.

TRANSLATED AND ENRICHED WITH NUMEROUS ADDITIONS
from
KAFKA AND OTHER SOURCES
by
CHARLES J. HEMPEL, M.D.

VOLUME I & II

B. JAIN PUBLISHERS (P) LTD.
NEW DELHI

Note from the Publishers

Any information given in this book is not intended to be taken as a replacement for medical advice. Any person with a condition requiring medical attention should consult a qualified practitioner or therapeutist.

THE SCIENCE OF THERAPEUTICS

Reprint Edition: 1996, 2004

No part of this book may be reproduced, stored in a retrieval system or transmitted, in any form or by any means, mechanical, photocopying, recording or otherwise, without any prior written permission of the publisher.

© All rights are reserved with the publisher

Price: Rs. 300.00

Published by Kuldeep Jain for
B. Jain Publishers (P) Ltd.
1921, Street No. 10, Chuna Mandi,
Paharganj, New Delhi 110 055 (INDIA)
Phones: 2358 0800, 2358 1100, 2358 1300, 2358 3100, 5169 8991
Fax: 011-2358 0471, 5169 8993; *Email:* bjain@vsnl.com
Website: **www.bjainbooks.com**

Printed in India by
J.J. Offset Printers
522, FIE, Patpar Ganj, Delhi - 110 092
Phones: 2216 9633, 2215 6128

ISBN: 81-8056-426-2
BOOKCODE: BB-2272

PREFACE.

The work which is here presented to the public is a work of no ordinary merit. It is to take the place of the late Hartmann's Acute and Chronic Diseases; but in point of scientific value and practical usefulness it is as far superior to the former as the present status of Homœopathy is above that of Hartmann's time. Bæhr is a man not only endowed with great scientific accomplishments, but he is likewise a man of large experience.

It is our opinion that this work will be read with pleasure and profit by every physician, and we recommend it to all students of medicine who are anxious to obtain a more elevated perception of Homœopathy.

We have incorporated in this work large sections from Kafka, so that this author is also presented in these two volumes. We have likewise introduced on suitable occasions the new remedies, and have made valuable additions from our Journals and drawn upon our personal records.

It is with infinite pleasure that we commend this highly useful work to our colleagues generally; we have devoted much time and persevering labor to its translation.

Most respectfully,
CHARLES J. HEMPEL, M. D.

Grand Rapids,
March, 1869.

PREFACE.

The work which is here presented to the public is a work of no ordinary merit. It is to take the place of Hempel's Jahr in Acute and Chronic Diseases, for it is point of accuracy and practical usefulness it has no superior to the present state of Homœopathy it shows that of that science that. Such as a work properly executed with great care thus accomplishes the labor is blessing a man of large knowledge.

It is our opinion that this work will be read with pleasure and profit by every physician, and we recommend it to all students of medicine who are anxious to obtain a more elevated knowledge of Homœopathy.

We have incorporated in this work large sections from Jahr's, as that his labor is also preserved in these two volumes. We have likewise inserted in numerous instances the new remedies, and have amplified additions from our own, as drawn upon our personal research.

It is with pleasant pleasure that we commend this highly useful work to our colleagues, upon which we have devoted considerable and persevering labor to its management.

CHARLES J. HEMPEL, M. D.

Grand Rapids,
June, 1859.

CONTENTS OF THE FIRST VOLUME.

Preface.   Page

Introduction .... 1—55
1. The Proving of Drugs on the healthy organism 2
2. The law of Similarity 13
3. Diagnosis of the Natural Disease 28
4. Single Remedies 39
5. Size of Dose 41
6. Preparation, Repetition, etc., of Medecines 48
7. Diet 51

FIRST SECTION.

Diseases of the Brain, the Spinal Cord, and the Nervous System Generally. 57

   A. Diseases of the Brain 57
      Hyperæmia of the Brain and its Membranes 57
      Anæmia of the Brain 65
      Cerebral Apoplexy 70
      Inflammatory Affections of the Brain and its Membranes 86
        1. Meningitis 86
        2. Encephalitis. Cerebritis 94
        3. Tubercular (granular) inflammation of the meninges. Hydrocephalus acutus 99
      Hydrocephalus, [stricte sic dictus.] 109

   B. Diseases of the Spinal Marrow. 110
      Inflammation of the Spinal Cord and its Membranes 110
      Meningitis Cerebro-spinalis, Cerebro-spinal Meningitis, Spotted Fever 130
      Spinal Irritation. Neuralgia Spinalis 135

   C. Diseases of the Nervous System 139
      1. Epilepsy 139
      2. Eclampsia 154
          a. Eclampsia Infantum 154
          b. Eclampsia Parturientium 163
      3. Chorea 170
      4. Catalepsy 177
      5. Tetanus and Trismus 178
      6. Paralysis 183
      7. Hysteria 190
      8. Hypochondria. Hypochondriasis, Spleen 207

Contents of the First Volume.

SECOND SECTION.

Page

Diseases of the Head 218

A. *Diseases of the Scalp* 218
    Cephalæmatoma, Bloody Tumor of the Scalp 218

B. *Diseases of the Cephalic Nerves* 220
    ✓ 1. Cephalalgia, Headache.. 220
        Hemicrania or Megrim 221
    2. Neuralgia Trigemini 227
        Fothergill's Prosopalgia; Tic douloureux; Prosopalgia, Face-ache 227
    3. Spasmus Nervi Facialis. Tic Convulsif. Spasm of the Facial Nerve 234

C. *Diseases of the Eye* 235
    1. Conjunctivitis Catarrhalis 237
    2. Conjunctivitis Blennorhoica 242
        a. Acute Blennorrhœa 242
        b. Chronic Blennorhœa 243
    3. Conjunctivitis Scrofulosa 249

D. *Diseases of the Ear* 257
    1. Otitis Interna 258
        Internal inflammation of the Ear 258
    2. Otitis externa 261

E. *Diseases of the Nose* 263
    1. Coryza, Catarrh, Cold in the Head 263
    2. Inflammation of the Nose, Nasitis 268
    3. Epistaxis, Bleeding at the Nose 269

THIRD SECTION.

Diseases of the Mouth, Fauces and Oesophagus 272
    1. Stomatitis 273
    2. Thrush, Aphthæ of Infants 279
    3. Angina 281
        a. Angina Catarrhalis, Sore Throat 281
        b. Angina Tonsillaris, Tonsillitis, Amygdalitis, Inflammation of the Tonsils. Quinsy 284
    4. Retropharyngeal Abscess.. 294
    5. Diphtheritis, Diphtheria 296
    6. Noma, Cancer Aquaticus.. 307
    7. Glossitis, Inflammation of the Tongue 311
    8. Parotitis 314
        a. Parotitis, Inflammation of the Parotid Gland, Mumps, Angina Parotidea 314
        b. Parotitis Maligna 317
    9. Salivatio, Ptyalism 319

Contents of the First Volume. VII

	Page
10. Scorbutus	322
Scurvy of the Gums	322
11. Ranula	324
12. Oesophagitis, Dysphagia Inflammatoria, Inflammation of the Oesophagus	326
13. Odontalgia, Toothache	328

FOURTH SECTION.

Diseases of the Stomach, Intestines, and Peritonaeum 334

  A. Diseases of the Stomach 334

    1. Catarrhus Ventriculi Acutus. Acute Catarrh of the Stomach 334
    2. Catarrhus Ventriculi Chronicus, Chronic Catarrh of the Stomach 350
    3. Gastritis, Inflammation of the Stomach 361
    4. Ulcus Perforans Ventriculi seu Rotundum. Chronic Ulcer of the Stomach 368
    5. Carcinoma Ventriculi, Cancer of the Stomach 375
    6. Hæmatemesis, Hemorrhage from the Stomach 383
    7. Cardialgia, Spasm of the Stomach 391

  B. Diseases of the Intestinal Canal 404

    1. Catarrhus Intestinalis, Intestinal Catarrh 404
      a. Simple Intestinal Catarrh 406
      b. Cholera Sporadica seu Nostras, Cholerine 408
      c. Catarrhus Intestinalis Chronicus, Chronic Intestinal Catarrh, Chronic Diarrhœa, Cholera Infantum, Summer Complaint 413
      d. Febris Gastrica Catarrhalis, Mucosa et Biliosa; Gastric Fever 422
    2. Enteritis, Inflammation of the Bowels 435
    3. Typhlitis, Perityphlitis, Inflammation of the Cæcum ... 440
      Catarrhal Inflammation of the Rectum, Proctitis 445
      Cellulitis 451
        Inflammation of the Cellular Tissue of the Intestinal Canal 451
    4. Dysenteria, Dysentery 455
      a. Catarrhal Dysentery 455
      b. Dysenteria Epidemica, Dysentery Proper 457
    5. Enteralgia, Colic 468
    6. Stenosis of the Bowels, Occlusion, Obstruction of the Bowels 479
    7. Hemorrhoids, Piles 485
    8. Helminthiasis, Worms 492

  C. Diseases of the Peritoneum 503

    Peritonitis, Inflammation of the Peritoneum 503

FIFTH SECTION.

Diseases of the Liver, Spleen and Pancreas 520
   A. *Diseases of the Liver* 520
      1. Hyperæmia of the Liver 522
      2. Hepatitis, Inflammation of the Liver 528
         a. Hepatitis Acuta, Acute Inflammation of the Liver 529
         b. Perihepatitis, Inflammation of the Capsules of the Liver, Capsular Hepatitis 531
         c. Pylephlebitis, Inflammation of the Vena Porta 532
      3. Hepatitis Chronica, Chronic Inflammatory Affections of the Liver 537
      4. Icterus, Aurigo, Jaundice 554
      5. Colelithiasis, Biliari Calculi 564
      6. Carcinoma Hepatis, Cancer of the Liver 569
   B. *Diseases of the Spleen* 572
      Splenitis, Inflammation of the Spleen 573
   C. *Diseases of the Pancreas* 578

SIXTH SECTION.

Diseases of the Uropoetic System 580
   A. *Diseases of the Kidneys* 580
      1. Nephritis, Inflammation of the Kidneys 586
      2. Morbus Brightii, Bright's Disease of the Kidneys 596
      3. Hemorrhage in the Kidneys 609
      4. Renal Calculi, Gravel 614
      5. Diabetes Mellitus, Melituria, Glycosuria 617
   B. *Diseases of the Bladder* 625
      1. Cystitis, Inflammation of the Bladder 625
      2. Hematuria, Bloody Urine 629
      3. Enuresis Nocturna, Wetting the Bed 631
      4. Cystospasmus, Spasm of the Bladder 632
      5. Cystoplegia, Paralysis of the Bladder 634

INTRODUCTION.

HARTMANN's attempt to apply the doctrines of Homœopathy to special Pathology has, so far, remained solitary and alone in the literature of our school; that is, if we do not include in the list popular publications or such as only refer to one part of Pathology. However strange this may seem to any one who is not familiar with Homœopathy, yet this absence of all pathological treatises after the example of Hartmann, is in perfect accord with the spirit of this doctrine, as we shall show by-and-by. A system of special Therapeutics never was, nor ever will be, a necessary, scientifically founded requisite of our doctrine, but will always depend upon the necessity of mediating between us and our therapeutic antipodes and opponents. In this way they will find it easier to institute clinical experiments with our system of treatment, and to form correct opinions concerning its scientific value. Starting from this stand-point it becomes indispensable, as a preliminary step, not only to explain the general principles of Homœopathy, but likewise to show in what manner this new system of treatment affects the science of Pathology. In this respect our general system of Therapeutics must necessarily differ from that of other therapeutic manuals; our position in the domain of medicine, which is still of a polemic character, compels us to touch certain questions which, though not necessarily included within the range of Therapeutics, yet are of essential importance to ourselves.

Among these questions, the question, What is Homœopathy? What is its aim and object? occupies a prominent place. But few physicians who are not homœopaths, will be able to answer this question satisfactorily. Let us hasten to add that this is in a great measure the fault of the homœopaths themselves. Rashly and improperly the unessential points are made prominent points of doctrine; the essential points are pressed into the background. Under these circumstances, we cannot wonder that our opponents should imitate our example, and, worse still, should charge upon us the most nonsensical fables and absurdities. In many respects,

(1)

Hahnemann, the founder of our doctrine, furnishes them the authority for their conduct; and many of his successors have been but too anxious to multiply the reasons for their justification. In the course of this introduction we shall have an opportunity of laying bare the mistakes that have been committed by our own adherents. First, let us answer the question: What is Homœopathy? It is the doctrine of the effects of drugs upon the animal organism as applied, according to an uniformly valid law, to the doctrine of the morbid changes of the organism. As such, it is not antagonistic to Medicine considered as a scientific whole; on the contrary, it constitutes a necessary completion of this science, inasmuch as the homœopathic system establishes one part of Medicine, which had hitherto been abandoned to the crudest empiricism, upon a scientific basis. Accordingly, it shares with the ancient science of Medicine all the suppositions necessary to a knowledge of pathological changes, and is distinguished from that science only by the mode in which it leads to a knowledge of the remedial agent, and brings this knowledge in union with the curative object. This is accomplished in accordance with two fundamental principles, the principle of proving drugs on the healthy organism and the therapeutic law: *Similia similibus curantur.*

1. The Proving of Drugs on the healthy organism.

In order to perceive very fully and clearly how far this principle exerts an influence upon the arrangement of our Materia Medica, we shall have to examine, in the first place, the manner in which a knowledge of drugs has been obtained hitherto, and is still sought to be obtained.

Casting a retrospective glance at the beginning of Medicine, we have to admit that the first physicians obtained their knowledge of drugs from the people to whom, while using them for their complaints, accidental experience revealed some of their virtues. By partaking of a plant or fruit indiscreetly, vomiting or diarrhœa was caused; the same substance was afterwards employed for the purpose of exciting similar evacuations. In performing such therapeutical experiments, it was likewise found by mere accident that, together with these troubles, certain other affections for which the medicine had not been administered, disappeared simultaneously, on which account the same medicine was afterwards employed for these incidental affections. Thus it was that, gradually, a whole series of facts was collected which were utilized by physicians as a fountain-head of Therapeutics. We need not attempt to show the gaps which must disfigure a knowledge of drug-effects thus obtained; what was particularly injurious was that all that was known of a drug was its relation to some particular morbid condition, without any corresponding knowledge of the kind of action which the drug really exerted. This crude empiricism was not only peculiar to the most remote periods, but it has continued even to the present period, although in a somewhat different form, care being had, by resorting to systematic forms, an adequate nomenclature, and other little artifices, to clothe this empiricism in a more scientific garment. All that was known was a series of exceedingly equivocal facts whose connection was so little ascertained and which very often seemed to contradict each other to such an extent that they gave rise to the most insane hypotheses.

Experiments on the sick organism did not yield any more satisfactory results. The boldness, or, if we did not know that physicians had acted in good faith, we might even say, the want of conscientiousness, with which, even to this day, therapeutic experiments are instituted with substances of whose virtues really nothing is known; the extraordinary perseverance with which these experiments are conducted; the numerous victims that have been sacrificed, ought to have been crowned with better success than the creation of a Materia Medica which is of no use to anybody. This may seem an exaggeration; yet that it is not, can be shown very easily. If the employment of an unknown drug in a given case of disease is to have a definite result, a preliminary knowledge of this case, in every direction, is indispensable. What disease is there which we can diagnose so surely, or, even if this were at all possible, whose course we can predict with so much positive certainty, that this knowledge should enable us to deduce the effects of the drug with mathematical accuracy? And even if we had the means of obtaining this knowledge in single cases; even if we had observed the same effect in a hundred cases, who guarantees to us that the one hundredth case will run the same course? May we not have to consider a variety of circumstances which cannot be determined in advance? For instance, is not one patient more sensitive to medicinal influences than another? Are there not indeterminable idiosyncrasies which we are in the habit of despatching under this name? Does not the influence of the weather, and of other external agents, act an important part? If any one is disposed to deny this, let him read attentively our medical journals.

We will quote a recent example. A French physician hits upon the idea—how he was led to it we are not informed—to employ Ipecacuanha for intermittent fevers; he treats two hundred cases, one hundred and sixty of which with good success. He concludes that this drug is a panacea for intermittent fever, and urges its employment accordingly. Some dozen physicians, imitating his example, suddenly raise a cry against his assertion, not having had any success with Ipecacuanha. Who is right? In our judgment both parties are right, for the reason that Ipecacuanha only cures one class of intermittent fevers. How far is the Materia Medica benefited by this kind of experimentation? The same course is pursued with Arsenic in the same disease, and with other drugs in other diseases. Who is to be believed? The only way to obtain certainty would be to repeat all these experiments. Is there no danger in random experimentations with large doses? Does it not argue a want of conscientiousness to experiment upon patients who expect from us either a mitigation or a cure of their sufferings? Beside the real or apparent curative results, we likewise find such drug-effects recorded as manifested themselves simultaneously with the curative results. Is a deception in regard to these new symptoms or drug-effects much more probable than in regard to the curative results? How are we to decide whether these results were not exclusively due to the peculiar course of the malady or to individual circumstances? It is true that in this manner a number of fixed facts have been obtained, but in proportion to the number of drugs, more particularly as regards single drugs, these facts are too few to enable us to assert that we are fully acquainted with a single drug in every direction of its therapeutic range. Read the article Opium in some of the more important works on Materia Medica. There is scarcely a drug with which experiments have been multiplied as with Opium; yet there is no drug concerning which our Materia Medicas are as full of absurd contradictions as concerning this agent.

The necessity which is becoming more apparent from day to day, of obtaining a more correct knowledge of our drugs before using them in the treatment of disease, has led long ago to experiments upon animals; so far, a vast number of dogs, cats, frogs, etc., have fallen victims to pharmacological investigations. But even in this respect the gain has been inconsiderable. The reasons for this are quite obvious. The organism of the beast differs from that of man in many essential particulars; even the organisms of many classes of animals differ among themselves. A dog frequently bears substances which are decidedly hostile to man; whereas other substances develop violent reactions in the canine organism. This being the case, how is it possible to draw reliable conclusions from experiments on dogs or other animals regarding the human organism? But, supposing even that such a proceeding is not entirely absurd, the profit which it yields is exceedingly small. The animal is unable to indicate subjective sensations according to their form, locality or intensity; we only become acquainted with objective changes. These changes have their value, but even they are generally obtained in an improper manner. They are sought to be obtained rapidly and fully developed by means of large doses of the drug, which, after all, only produce phenomena of the coarsest character. The most we learn is the maximum effect of a drug, nothing of the less marked, and yet so essential, shades of its action. How far do such coarse experiments advance our knowledge of a drug in its capacity as a remedial agent? Only a very little. Moreover, this kind of experimentation exposes us to great deceptions, for most drugs, when administered in large quantities, produce effects very different from those which are produced by continued small doses of the same drug. By what means do we obtain a knowledge of the latter effects which are our sole proper guide in determining the therapeutic uses of a drug? We are far from denying the value of experiments upon animals; but this value is limited, and acquires a certain importance only when judged in connection with other experiments.

The same remarks apply to cases of poisoning observed on human beings. The circumstances which render such accidents less instructive, or ill-adapted for the purposes of a scientific Materia Medica, are the following: In the first place, the poisoning is not under our control. Accident may furnish a number or none at all, within a limited space of time; a hundred may be furnished by a single drug, whereas a hundred other drugs may not furnish one. We possess the history of a large number of cases of poisoning with Arsenic, but of how many cases with Gold? This depends upon the degree of accessibility of a poisonous substance to crime or indiscretion.

Moreover, in every case of poisoning of a human being, the results are necessarily more or less obscure, since we are obliged to employ every means of saving or relieving the patient. What symptoms are, in such cases, chargeable to the poison, what other symptoms to the action of the antidote? These two series of symptoms are very frequently mixed up with a good deal of recklessness. How many cases of poisoning are recorded in our journals, as having been occasioned by a single substance, whereas they were really caused by two or three! How much can we learn from such cases for the benefit of our patients?

Finally, the same objection occurs to us here that has already been mentioned, when speaking of experiments upon animals. Large doses of a poisonous substance only furnish the massive outlines, not the finer shades of a drug-picture.

However, we should commit the most crying injustice against the tendency of our scientific opponents, if we were to assert that they have contented themselves with the above-mentioned partially accidental and partially unreliable means of building up their Materia Medica. This is not the case. Other sources of knowledge have sometimes been sought and employed with an amazing energy and great sagacity. We may mention Chemistry, from which, to this day, the most important yield has been expected for the Materia Medica. Without wishing to lessen the importance of chemical investigations, we must nevertheless confess that Materia Medica is under very slight obligations to Chemistry. It is well to know the constituents of vegetable substances; but to use this knowledge for the purpose of determining approximatively their effects upon the sick, seems a hazardous enterprise, and has never yet led to favorable results. The speculations based upon Chemistry have likewise engendered many errors in theory and practice. We mention the use of Iron in chlorosis. Iron does not always cure chlorosis, and, where it does cure, often entails a disturbed digestion. We admit that Chemistry has shed light upon the nature and connection of a number of facts, but a Materia Medica can never be created by chemical analysis.

As a rich and memorable source of a knowledge of drugs in the domain of ancient Medicine, we have to mention Homœopathy. Not only have many drugs, especially recently, been taken from the store-house of Homœopathy, and applied to the cure of diseases, often, it is true, in a very wrong way, but the very road upon which the homœopath arrives at a knowledge of drugs, has been pursued by old-school physicians. Such a course, it is true, has only been pursued by a few, most systematically by Schroff, of Vienna. This is not the place for a more particular examination of his labors; they contain a great deal that is good, but too little of it when compared to the immensity of his efforts. His effort to obtain a powerful medicinal effect as rapidly as possible, is the cause owing to which his labors have produced such inadequate results. By and by we shall point out the road that has to be pursued by those who are desirous of obtaining a large yield of drug-effects by means of pure experiments; those who take an interest in such matters are invited to contrast our views with Schroff's method of investigation, in order to find out what we censure in his proceedings.

By employing the means and ways above mentioned, the present science of Medicine has been perfected in the course of centuries. Upon examining it more closely we only find the most striking, because most massive and crudest effects of drugs, recorded on its pages; the more delicate shades of the drug-picture are wanting. In accordance with these coarse drug-effects, drugs were divided into classes, the names of which indicated the leading effects of the drugs enumerated in each class. What such classifications, in the gross, amount to, can easily be seen by comparing certain manuals with each other, where the same drug is found recorded under the most diversified heads. How embarrassing it must be for a conscientious physician who wishes to employ a narcotic, and has to hunt it up among thirty or more other drugs, without having a single point of support to lean upon in the selection of his special agent. This is simply a blind-catching process, not a conscious act in accordance with a rational motive.

It is indeed remarkable that modern Medicine which has been so active in investigating physiological and pathological processes, seems to have utterly neglected a corresponding investigation of the curative sphere of drugs. The subtle diagnosis of modern pathologists is certainly not adequately responded to by an exceedingly general random selection of a remedial agent. The defects of the Materia Medica exert even a pernicious reaction upon the diagnosis. To a scientific physician, the diagnosis cannot be sufficiently accurate; but from the moment he abandons the practical side of diagnosis, he becomes content with the vaguest diagnostic generalities, for the reason that they are sufficient to secure the selection of a remedial agent. Thus it is that science and practice have become sharply divided in Medicine, to the detriment of physicians, still more than to that of patients. Quite recently we have heard a Viennese physician exclaim, how strange it was that, in their lectures, Skoda and Oppolzer should despatch a whole lot of drugs against a given case of disease, with the utmost contempt and with a pitiful smile; whereas, at the bedside of patients, they prescribe quantities of these despised drugs. Does the fault rest with the physicians, or with the drugs? Is it because the drugs are powerless, or is it rather because the physicians do not know how to employ them? This latter question we have to answer in the affirmative, for we have the evidence of it in our hands, and shall exhibit it to our readers in the course of this work.

Hahnemann was the first who endeavored consistently and perseveringly to obtain a knowledge of the effects of drugs, and to apply it to practical uses in accordance with a definite law. He found the sources of remedial agents, which had been valid up to his time, either insufficient or deceitful and false, and he set up the doctrine that a knowledge of the true effects of drugs could only be obtained by experimenting upon the human organism, and that these experiments must be instituted upon the healthy organism; since the organism in disease develops and substantiates too many illusory views and perceptions. His extraordinary energy gave birth to the Materia Medica Pura, a work to which the most censorious mania cannot deny the tribute of admiration in spite of the isolated defects with which this noble work is tainted. When did a single human being ever succeed in treading a new path without committing a single mistake, or making a single false step? Let it suffice that so far nobody has ever produced greater results by entering upon a new road of investigation.

Provings upon the healthy constituting the very central point of Homœopathy, which could not exist without them, we shall necessarily have to submit the manner in which such provings are conducted to a more rigorous examination.

In the first place, we have to inquire how the provings are conducted, and, in the second place, how the results of these provings are improved for the benefit of the Materia Medica.

Only such persons are fit for the business of proving who enjoy physical and mental health, and are possessed of a capacity to describe their sensations with clearness and precision. In opposition to this first requisite, it may be said that perfectly healthy individuals are very scarce; an assertion which is certainly not exaggerated. By the term "health" we do not mean to designate the absolute harmony of the physiological processes, but the existing equilibrium of the organic activity of the body. While proving, the bodily functions of the experimenter should not be disturbed in any respect, and, in order to obtain the greatest possible certainty on this point, it may be well to subject the prover to a careful examination. The physicians themselves are always the best provers. If the provings are instituted by other parties, the physician should never cease to exercise strict control in order to prevent unessential symptoms from being assigned a prominent place in the list, or essential symptoms from being described too superficially.

In order that a proving should yield a complete list of symptoms, it has to be conducted by as large a number of individuals as possible, of different ages, sexes, social positions and habits. This condition need not be dwelt upon any further; it is of self-evident necessity. We will add that even children may be included among the list of provers. However, they have to be watched much more carefully, for the reason that they are much less capable of defining the subjective symptoms developed by the drug.

Shortly before, and even during the whole course of the trial, even some time after the last dose of the drug had been taken, the prover should observe a simple and regular conduct. All medicinal substances have to be avoided; likewise every exposure by which the bodily equilibrium might be disturbed, such as excessive bodily or mental exertions, violent emotions, too much or too little sleep, irregular eating or drinking. Such articles of diet which we know to have an injurious influence upon his bodily health, have to be avoided with particular care. If possible, the mode of life which we have to lead during the trial, should be commenced some time previous to the beginning of the trial, so much more since, in order that we might pursue a correct mode of living, habitual dishes or beverages have to be discontinued; otherwise many changes which originate in this very circumstance, might be charged to the action of the drug. It is likewise necessary, before the trial commences, to examine the beats of the heart, the quality of the pulse, the quantity of the urine, as well as the temperament and other peculiarities.

Of the drug to be proved, we must make sure of obtaining a reliable preparation. It is best to employ it in form of a tincture or of triturations with sugar of milk, in case it should not be feasible to take the drug in substance. This mode is preferable for the reason that tinctures and triturations constitute the leading preparations of drugs in homœopathic practice. The dose to be proved, has to vary. A commencement may be made with the smallest doses, even with the thirtieth attenuation, from which we may gradually descend to the stronger and more substantial preparations. The doses should not be repeated in too rapid succession; it is best to first allow all the morbid phenomena of one dose to pass away before a second dose is taken. If no effects are produced, the dose is progressively increased and repeated more frequently. These precautions concerning the dose are of essential importance, for the reason that the susceptibility to medicinal impressions varies exceedingly in different individuals, and it is impossible to determine beforehand how large or feeble the dose should be in order to elicit the smallest possible medicinal symptoms. A good deal depends upon these feeble beginnings; they serve as starting-points in accounting for subsequent more marked phenomena of drug-action. It is a good plan to let every prover take the same preparation of the drug; in order to prevent also in this respect the possibility of a mistake. The best time to take the drug is undoubtedly before breakfast, for the reason that we are better able to observe the symptoms manifesting themselves in the first hours subsequent to taking the drug; and that the medicine is moreover introduced into an empty stomach. However, it is likewise advisable to swallow a dose of the drug some evening before bedtime, in order to observe possible differences of action.

Finally, special rules are required in order to regulate the conduct of the prover, with reference to the medicinal symptoms that may become manifest. Above all things the prover should attentively observe all changes in his feelings, without watching himself on that account with anxious solicitude; what is most particularly to be avoided are fanciful illusions. If the prover is a physician, it is well that he should remain ignorant of the drug he is proving. All changes in the ordinary condition of the patient, even the least and most insignificant, are to be noted down. This should be done as soon as the symptoms are perceived. Accessory circumstances should be carefully recorded. The period of the appearance of the symptoms, their duration, aggravating or ameliorating circumstances, locality and quality of the sensations, etc. These written reports have to be revised by the physician as often as possible, in order that he may have an opportunity of completing defective records by appropriate questions, of clearing up obscure statements, adding objective symptoms, etc. It is more particularly objective symptoms which render a physician's control during the trial indispensable. It is well known how wrongly objective symptoms are sometimes described by lay-provers upon their own persons, such as efflorescences upon the skin, changes of the tongue, alvine discharges, urine; on which account great injury is often done to the provings, since it is precisely these objective symptoms that are the most important, because they do not admit of deception. The physician should moreover accompany the symptoms with annotations referring to circumstances, which either confirm the medicinal symptoms or cast a doubt upon them. If the prover, for instance, is disposed to catarrhal affections of the Schneiderian membrane, and he should be attacked with such an affection during the trial, the physician has to institute inquiries in order to find out whether he has to deal with a medicinal symptom or not; and if a doubt should prevail, he has to mark this symptom with a note of interrogation. As a general rule, the physician should apply to an investigation of the drug-disease all the means of diagnosis that he brings to bear upon an investigation of natural maladies. The changes in the different secretions, especially in the urine, are particularly noteworthy.

A systematic arrangement of the symptoms elicited by such provings constitutes the basis for a full picture of the drug-disease. We say, intentionally, the basis, for an exhaustive proving can never be instituted on a human being, since it is impossible to increase the doses of à drug to the point of poisoning; at any rate it is only with a very small number of drugs that we shall dare to saturate the system, so as to develop their medicinal effects in all their intensity. These provings are to be considered as a basis for the additional reason that, starting from them and by them, it becomes possible for us to apply to practical uses whatever else we may be able to learn of the drug in question through other channels. Experiments upon animals, comparatively valueless, without corresponding provings upon human beings, show us, by the objective symptoms which they develop, how a variety of phenomena in men have to be interpreted, both according to their origin, as well as according to their final course; and conclusions by analogy, from animals to men, can now be made without any great danger of being deceived, since we are now in possession of the most positive points of departure. For these reasons, experiments upon animals are really of decided benefit and importance only to homœopaths.

Starting from the above-mentioned basis, the poisonings of human beings, with which our toxicological treatises are replete, obtain their true value, yea, they become important contributions to our Materia Medica. Poisonings which do not terminate too rapidly in death, and whose characteristic symptoms are not effaced by the intensity of their course, are particularly instructive. Poisons which produce fatal results too rapidly are of but trifling importance even for the toxicologist, inasmuch as their toxical results only denote in almost every case the symptoms of a violent local irritation. In other respects, cases of human poisoning, even if we do not draw any conclusions from analogy or expose ourselves to the danger of deception, as we have to do in making experiments upon animals, furnish us an explanation why the alterations obtained by our provers with small doses should have a definite significance, and why the effects of small doses should, in their turn, shed light in many cases upon the effects of poisonous doses. Of particular value are likewise the material post-mortem changes, which alone render it possible in many cases of a most subtle pathological diagnosis to determine what drug-diagnosis corresponds to it very fully. In cases of poisoning, we should, of course, observe the greatest caution, in order to preserve the distinction between the toxical symptoms and the effects of such antidotes as may have been administered in the case, and the symptoms of a previously existing disease, for which purpose the symptoms elicited by provings on healthy persons will again furnish us a safe standard of comparison. In other respects the relation of the toxical to the pathogenetic symptoms is best ascertained by comparing the toxical symptoms, caused by one of our well-proved drugs, with the symptoms recorded in our Materia Medica. It is but seldom that a symptom will not be found recorded in the latter; on the contrary, it will be found that the toxical symptoms constitute a drug-picture, whose sharp features are reflected by the drug-pictures elicited by our provings in dimmer and more shadowy outlines.

And finally, upon the basis of the pathogenetic series, clinical experience can be made available for the benefit of our Materia Medica, although only conditionally. This experience either consists in the observation of new symptoms not belonging to the disease, which manifest themselves after the administration of the remedial agent, or in the changes which existing morbid symptoms undergo, either for the better or the worse. The former category is of less importance; in many cases it furnishes a valuable confirmation of our provings on healthy persons, and, which is of the utmost importance, makes us acquainted with the doses that have to be employed in order to effect a cure without aggravating the symptoms of the disease. However, the custom of incorporating these new incidental symptoms in the pathogenetic series, and which has been practised in more than one case, should be abandoned. The second category, in so far as it refers to an aggravation of existing morbid phenomena, yields a further basis for the determination of the proper dose which is capable of effecting curative results, without any precursory aggravation of the symptoms. The homœopathic doctrine of dose rests exclusively upon such observations. When reaching the question of dose, we shall again revert to this subject. Our observations concerning the curative action of remedial agents, by confirming the principle in accordance with which the cure was effected, constitute the true system of homœopathic Therapeutics. They show us by the practical result what drug-effects are of real use in determining the curative indication. In a previous paragraph we have already alluded to the deceitful character of clinical observations, and have to apply this remark likewise to observations made in accordance with the principles of Homœopathy. We should add, however, that Homœopathy has done every thing that can possibly be done to diminish uncertainties and to avoid deceptions. If the experience obtained of the effect of a medicine is applied in every case, in accordance with the same principle, the results must necessarily be more homogeneous, than they could be imagined under any other therapeutic proceeding.

It is from the different sources that have been indicated so far that the Homœopathic Materia Medica has obtained its material, and, in accordance with this origin, it alone is justly entitled to the attribute of physiological. Viewed in its integrity, from its origin throughout its whole development, it is a working representative of progress in the domain of Medicine in the presence of the great improvements which have been effected in other departments of this science; ignorance alone can deny it the character of a perfect scientific structure.

Nevertheless, in so far as a want of completeness is a necessary attribute of every science which can never be conceived as a perfect whole, no longer capable of a progressive development, and which, in reality, only becomes a science through an unceasing and systematic struggle after a more perfect form; our Materia Medica is neither a perfectly rounded, nor, in its present shape, a complete and faultless whole. As a closed science it could only be considered in case it should contain every thing that can be used as medicine, a thing that is utterly inconceivable. It would only be a closed and perfect science if every medicinal substance had been so completely and so exhaustively investigated, and determined in the different directions of its therapeutic efficacy, that nothing could be added to the domain of its usefulness. This likewise is inconceivable. Independently of these extreme requisites of completeness, we have to point out defects, which we shall subject to a short discussion in the present place, because an equally suitable opportunity may not present itself at a subsequent stage of our work. It would be unreasonable to entirely omit a consideration of these defects, since it is isolated defects that so readily frighten beginners away from the study of Homœopathy, and furnish points of attack to our opponents. In the following paragraphs, unless special quotations are made, we refer exclusively to Hahnemann's Materia Medica Pura, and to his Chronic Diseases; if we introduce subjects in this discussion with which every one familiar with Homœopathy has been perfectly acquainted for a long time past, our excuse must be that this Introduction is not so much written for the accomplished practitioner, as for those who are only now becoming initiated into our science.

In his Materia Medica, Hahnemann gives us the results of his own provings as well as those of other provers. He only furnishes the final results, saying nothing of the manner in which they were obtained, nothing of the material which has yielded these results. This constitutes the main, perhaps the only defect of his Materia Medica, since all its other defects spring from this one. In the shape in which Hahnemann has left us the results of his great labors, they are like a dense, large forest. Upon first entering it, it seems impossible to find one's way through it; he who is acquainted with the forest, finds his way without any difficulty. The symptoms are pressed into a certain scheme, to accommodate which the symptoms are torn into fragments and numbered without any connection. We are far from censuring this scheme, which, in spite of all the criticisms that have been passed upon it, has after all proved the best possible arrangement; even the splitting of the symptoms for the purpose of accommodating them to this scheme, would do no harm provided Hahnemann had left us the key to it, that is, a record of each single proving that has been made use of in the list of symptoms. This defect is exceedingly grave, and, what is worse, cannot be remedied satisfactorily. Re-provings have helped out in the case of single remedies, and, in many places, very satisfactorily; but to institute a re-proving of every drug that has been proved by Hahnemann, is an enormous task of very difficult solution. It is incomprehensible that Hahnemann, in spite of his accustomed sagacity, should have committed this sin of omission. It seems as though he had fallen into one extreme, in order to avoid the opposite one; he was opposed to every kind of generalizing in Medicine, and, for fear lest he should give rise to it, he omitted reports of his provings, in consequence of which he made it much more difficult for his successors to follow his example. As a matter of course the effects of a drug, in accordance with their importance, their origin and course of manifestation, can only be learned by studying the record of each single proving; by this means a knowledge of drugs is obtained very easily. In this way we become acquainted with the starting-point of drug-diseases, what organs and systems are first acted upon by the drug, and what disturbances of the general organism arise from these beginnings; and, in order to obtain a reliable knowledge of drug-diseases, it is just as important that we should be acquainted with the origin and succession of the morbid changes as in any other natural malady. The defect becomes still more serious in consequence of our remaining unacquainted with the individual condition of the provers, their sex, age, temperament, etc., how long a time the drug required to develop its effects, what quantities it took in order to produce them. The remarks which Hahnemann has added to single symptoms, and which often have the appearance of being snatched from an adventurous fancy, can only be accounted for by a knowledge of the different provings; it was expecting too much that his successors should accept all such statements upon the faith of their master. That Hahnemann did not arrange his Materia Medica without critical judgment is evident from similar remarks, and from his introduction to some of his drugs; nevertheless it was wrong that he should have cut off his successors from the possibility of an independent criticism, and should have placed his work before them with the apodictic authority of an *ipse dixit*. Lastly we are unable to decide what symptoms in the list of Hahnemann's provings belong to the respective drugs as constant and hence characteristic symptoms, since it is only exceptionally that we are told whether a symptom was observed by all the provers, or only by a few, or by one alone. All these defects of the

Materia Medica Pura are still more salient in the Chronic Diseases, where even new ones appear in addition to the former. The circumstance that in this last-mentioned work the medicines were proved almost exclusively with small doses, has occasioned a certain uniformity which cannot possibly be justified in a scientific point of view, and diminishes the number of the objective symptoms, upon which, however, the selection of a remedial agent principally depends. A number of symptoms are moreover taken from observations on the sick; this course might appear justifiable, if all such symptoms had been designated as such. But this has never been done. Nor can we pass silently by the fact that the quotations in both the above-mentioned works are disfigured by great mistakes, erroneous interpretations and defective rendering of the original text.

In spite of these defects, Hahnemann's work remains one of unusual importance and significance. A human work can scarcely be found anywhere that does not bear more or less the imprint of human imperfection. It is the duty of subsequent generations to remedy these defects. Many efforts have been made with occasional success to perfect Hahnemann's work; but a good deal remains yet to be done; only a partial reform has as yet been achieved. We need not show in this place what has already been accomplished, and refer to such works as those of Hirschel, (Die Homœopathie, eine Anleitung zum Selbststudium,) where a correct statement of these new reforms can be found.

Beside the efforts to render Hahnemann's Materia Medica more accessible, and to purge it of all defects, a good deal has been done in the way of proving new drugs, either by individual provers or by Provers' Unions. These new provings have been conducted so as to avoid Hahnemann's faults entirely. This is not the place to discuss these new efforts; we have to consider the results of such efforts rather than their history. These results are found recorded in journals, in essays, and exceptionally in larger works, like Hering's, but at all events in a very scattered form. This scattered mode of publication entails great injury. If any one should ask us where he might obtain a complete Homœopathic Materia Medica, we should not know what to say to him, except giving him the names of a whole list of publications. We do not yet possess a complete collection of provings, on which account the study of our Materia Medica is rendered much more difficult. The labor of collecting all these provings would undoubtedly be a gigantic enterprise; if it has not yet been undertaken, it is undoubtedly because new additions are continually expected. When will the period arrive when our Materia Medica shall be completed?

As long as we are deprived of the means of studying our Materia Medica from original sources, we have to content ourselves with works whose object it is to lay the symptoms elicited by our provings before us in a more concise form, that can be easily looked over and comprehended. Among these works, the following occupy the first rank: Jahr's Symptomen Codex, and Noack and Trink's Materia Medica, both, however, of too remote a date not to omit a multitude of new facts, and being, moreover, adapted to the necessities of the practitioner rather than to those of a mere student. What road had better be pursued in studying Materia Medica cannot well be pointed out more clearly than has been done by Hirschel, in his above-mentioned publication, to which we refer the reader. An example of a model-proving, in accordance with the principles of Homœopathy, is furnished by Watzke in his treatise on Colocynth, in the first volume of the "Oesterreichische Zeitschrift," where the difficulties of producing a complete proving are likewise laid bare. At the same time, this treatise will likewise satisfy any reader of the tendency of true homœopaths to elaborate the science of Pharmacology from a genuinely scientific standpoint.

Having thus far enumerated a variety of defects in our Materia Medica, we now have to show how far, in spite of all these defects, it surpasses the Materia Medica of the dominant School in practical usefulness. The existing material enables us to obtain a thorough knowledge of a large number of drugs; those that are proved less perfectly, give us a tolerable picture of their leading properties. We admit that such a study requires a great deal of labor and perseverance; but by this means we are placed in possession of the great advantage of becoming acquainted with the instruments with which we have to operate in the sick chamber; of learning to examine critically their noxious as well as their saving properties, and of being protected against the possibility of inflicting direct injury where help was expected at our hands. Let us now examine the law according to which we have to prescribe the medicine of whose therapeutic virtues we have acquired a correct knowledge.

Previously, however, we will here record a piece of advice that has been frequently given, but cannot be repeated too often. We have shown that Homœopathy, or rather Materia Medica itself, rests upon the proving of drugs upon healthy individuals; as a matter of course it is the duty of every partisan of this doctrine to complete and perfect it by proving drugs upon himself and others. Those who wish to obtain a knowledge of Homœopathy should regard it as an indispensable condition to prove at least one drug upon themselves. Only he who has made such a proving upon himself is capable of obtaining a complete and familiar knowledge of Materia Medica; a proving upon one's self facilitates a comprehension of the provings of others a great deal. This is an undisputed and an indisputable truth, for whose sake we warmly urge the above-mentioned advice upon every lover of our doctrine.

2. The Law of Similarity.

Before defining this law, we cannot refrain from casting a glance at the laws prevailing in the domain of Medicine, or the rules that have to be observed if we wish to effect the cure of a disease by artificial means. An examination of this kind is necessary in order to comprehend to some extent the position of Homœopathy in opposition to the other methods of cure, and in order to show that the law of similarity alone has claim to a more general validity and completely responds to all scientific demands.

The therapeutic methods of the ancient systems of Medicine can be ranged, without resorting to any forcing process, in the following categories:

1. The disease is cured by removing the cause that produces it. Whenever this method can be pursued, it is undoubtedly the simplest and generally the safest, which, for the matter of that, no physician will neglect. But how small is the number of diseases whose causes we are able to trace with positive certainty! and, among this small number, how few diseases are there the known causes of which we are able to remove! Considering, moreover, that in many cases the disease, even after the cause is removed, still continues to exist as an affection that has acquired an independent existence, we must confess that such causal treatment can never acquire an universal validity.

2. The disease is removed by exciting an artificial condition directly contrary to the natural malady, in other words: *Contraria contrariis curantur.* At first sight, this principle seems to be remarkably applicable to all cases; but a closer examination compels us to admit that it cannot be applied in every case to the treatment of diseases. A disease is a complex of various functional disturbances of the organism; it is only in very few cases that we meet

with diseases confined to only one organ. How can we manage to apply the above-mentioned principle to a complex of phenomena, such as occurs in pneumonia or typhus? Individual symptoms or groups of symptoms can be treated in accordance with such a principle; but their removal does not imply a cure of the whole disease. Constipation can be momentarily removed by a purgative; but this does not secure a cure of the disturbance which engenders the constipation in its course, and keeps it up. Nevertheless, diseases are treated in most cases in accordance with this maxim, but the cure is generally only apparent, for, in the present condition of the Materia Medica, it is next to impossible to find a contrarium for every disease. In the same manner as the authors of Materia Medica have endeavored to range drugs in certain general categories, depending upon a few single massive drug-effects: upon the same basis physicians resort to these categories, for the purpose of conducting a totally symptomatic treatment by opposing these coarse drug-effects to isolated prominent symptoms of the pathological disease. Owing to this gross method of treatment, such irrational generalizations have been introduced in Old-School Therapeutics, as we see them embodied in the history of any case of disease. Thus it is that the maxim "*Contraria contrariis*" is not only defective and insufficient in the treatment of diseases, but it has become decidedly hurtful to pathological science.

3. The disease is sought to be extirpated by alterations excited in non-affected organs or systems by artificial means, the revulsive method. This method of treatment is an imitation of the mode in which Nature herself often seeks to remove diseases. It cannot be denied that a cure is often achieved by pursuing this method; but we are as yet without a guide for such therapeutic imitations, since we are as yet unable to determine, with any thing like certainty, the connection in consequence of which one organ exerts a certain definite influence upon the other. This knowledge has not even been fully acquired with reference to the normal organism; much less are we acquainted with the changes which morbid derangements cause in the relation of one organ or system to another. What is known on this subject are isolated observations which are partially utterly unreliable and certainly illy adapted to founding a law of universal validity. It is the more impossible to pursue such a road to a cure, the more the whole organism is affected by the disease.

4. More recently the more perfect development of organic Chem-

istry has given rise to a new method of treating many morbid conditions medicinally. One or the other organic constituent was either found diminished or increased, and it was supposed that the disease could be counteracted by supplying deficiencies or by removing the excess by neutralization or some other proceeding. It is undoubtedly true that in some cases this method has proved successful, but in most cases this chemical method of treatment was soon found to have no higher value than that of a speculative theory, and that it is not sufficient to introduce the required constituent into the organism, but that, in order to produce a favorable effect, the constituent has to be introduced in such a form and quantity as the organism requires for its special use. It is likewise self-evident that the curative attempts depending upon chemical indications can only be applied to a small number of diseases.

A system of Therapeutics, based upon such doctrines as we have described, would be tolerably perfect, provided the methods mentioned in the preceding numbers should coalesce in such a manner that one of them would help where the others leave us in the lurch. Such a mutually completing process does not, however, take place, and a tolerable number of morbid affections remain against which we have to proceed upon the basis of the purest empiricism, where every species of treatment is no better than a bold attempt at curing without any fixed principles whatsoever, except perhaps a few morbid conditions for which tolerably fixed remedies have been discovered that are designated as specific remedies without any apparent reason. This appellation is erroneous for the reason that these remedies are not specifically curative of a definite species of diseases, which, as specific agents, they should be. For this reason, we declare such a system of Therapeutics defective, without any scientific basis.

In opposition to these vague and defective doctrines, Hahnemann first set up a maxim alike applicable to the treatment of every kind of disease: *Similia similibus curantur*, the law of similarity; in other words, a disease is cured most safely, speedily and easily by a drug which, when acting upon the healthy organism, produces all the symptoms of the disease in their greatest possible similarity.

It is well known that Hahnemann was first led to conceive the possibility of such a law by observing that Cinchona is capable of developing on persons in health all the symptoms of intermittent fever. In order to change a mere possibility into certainty, he commenced to make a trial of all kinds of drugs upon persons in health, and to employ them for purposes of cure in accordance with the maxim he had started. The uniform success obtained by this method of treatment satisfied him that this maxim had all the dignity of a natural law. We, too, might content ourselves with referring to thousands of cures as a proof of the validity of this law, without troubling ourselves about any further explanation. But inasmuch as cures can be disputed, and such testimony is not within everybody's reach, we prefer showing, *a priori*, why such a law must necessarily be of universal applicability.

The literature of Homœopathy is replete with attempts to explain the law of similarity, from Hahnemann down to the present period. We cannot possibly undertake an enumeration of all these different views and opinions, more particularly since they would not possess any essential interest in this place. If anybody desires more special information on this subject, he will find it in the abovementioned work by Hirschel. A brief record of the leading views will be sufficient in this instance; independently of all support derived from experience, the main point is, that the homœopathic law should prove universally valid in practice. Even if Hahnemann could have been reproached, with an appearance of justice, with having abstracted a natural law from a single fact, this reproach can no longer be applied to the Homœopathy of the present day, which might very justly abstract a law from facts of universal and repeated occurrence, even if it were impossible to account for this law by *a priori* arguments.

Hahnemann himself explains the law of similarity by accepting a natural and an artificial disease, the latter of which, being the stronger, annihilates the natural malady, whereas itself is hushed up by the vital forces. This explanation is not satisfactory, more particularly for the reason that it is founded upon hypotheses which cannot possibly be proven. Who can prove the superior force of the medicinal disease, an essential condition upon which Hahnemann's explanation rests? What a hazardous hypothesis to suppose that the natural malady is annihilated by the vital forces, for no better reason than because, after the natural malady is cured, the drug-disease is no longer perceptible! Does it not seem as though this extinction of the drug-disease ought to take place simultaneously with that of the natural malady? It is undoubtedly wrong to base one hypothesis upon a number of others. Hahnemann's view has indeed been abandoned, and has given rise to the most decided opposition. In order to overcome the difficulty that a similar disease is overcome by a similarly acting drug, it was said that a drug occasions in the sick organism opposite effects from what it does in the healthy. This mode of arguing simply substitutes one difficulty for another; such a behavior on the part of the drug can only be accounted for by an entirely wrong conception of the primary and secondary effect of a drug. This designation of primary and secondary has led to many embarrassments, not only in this particular explanation but in Homœopathy generally, by diverting our attention from the conception of drug-action as a morbid process progressing in accordance with an inherent law of necessity, and setting up an arbitrary separation of drug-effects which can never be carried out in practice.

Nor can we admit another view as correct according to which the drug excites the sound portion of an organ against its diseased portion, occasioning by this means an elimination of the disease. This explanation does away with the idea of similarity. For if the effects of the drug and those of the disease are similar throughout their whole course, the medicine must necessarily have affected the same organs and parts of organs as the disease, since without such a supposition the law of similarity cannot be thought of. How does it happen that, in effecting a cure, the medicine suddenly excites the sound parts into action? We know nothing of an action upon the latter. Nevertheless we shall show by-and-by, that, with a slight variation, this explanation has a good deal of probability in its favor.

The supposition of a special predisposition to disease which is hushed up by the medicine, is likewise an unproven or, at any rate, a hazardous hypothesis. How do we understand that by extirpating the predisposition the disease must necessarily be cured?

To account for a cure upon the basis of a chemical neutralization is likewise too hypothetical. If the greatest possible similarity between the disease and the drug-action proves, as it undoubtedly does, their mutual affinity; even if they neutralize each other after the fashion of bodies between which chemical affinity prevails, we shall have to inquire by way of following up the simile, what becomes of the product of neutralization? For the action of two agents upon each other can certainly not result in a nothing. This explanation, like many others, is faulty in this respect that it regards the disease as an entological entity in the organism.

In our opinion, the following explanation comes nearest to the truth, for the reason that the suppositions which it implies are few in number, and the most probably correct. The medicine stimulates certain organs or systems, and, by acting upon sound parts, necessarily produces morbid phenomena, whereas, by acting upon the diseased organ, it produces the stimulation requisite for a cure. This explanation does not imply a contrary action, but the effect remains the same, only that in its union with the morbid action it gives rise to a different product from what it does when acting upon sound tissues. This view likewise renders it possible to account for aggravations occasioned by too large doses.

Our view of accounting for the *modus operandi* of homœopathic agents, leads us to an explanation of the law of similarity, which seems to us, more than any other, to satisfy the demands of logic and the necessary thoroughness in deducing it from known physiological facts. This explanation was originated by Wislicenus, and may be found in his work entitled: "Entwicklung eines wahrhaft physiologischen Heilverfahrens." Leipsic, 1860. In stating the fact that the object of this work is to show the correctness of the law of similarity in a series of logical deductions, we can only mention the chief points of this work in a few concise passages. For this reason many a proposition will necessarily appear disconnected and problematic, because the intermediate links are omitted, and many of our readers may find our short extracts insufficient: So much the more we invite all, in the warmest manner, to read this book. The necessary consequences of the law of similarity, so far as the practical business of the physician is concerned, are moreover so fully developed in this work from the leading maxims of Homœopathy that the book is not only invested with a purely scientific but a directly practical interest. In order to be correctly understood, we have to premise certain statements of physiological facts that constitute an integral portion of our argument.

Health depends in every organic being upon an inherent endeavor to preserve the equilibrium of its organic functions. This endeavor is designated by physiologists as an organic tendency of persistence, or as a physiological antagonism, or as an organic power of reaction. By virtue of this reactive power the organism equalizes the noxious influences acting upon it from without. As long as this equalization is continued regularly and imperceptibly, we call the organism healthy. But if the disturbances are too powerful to be at once and imperceptibly conquered by the reactive force of the organism, in other words to be equalized, we call the organism sick. In proportion as the struggle between these two factors is more or less violent, more or less extensive, we call the disease acute, sub-acute or chronic. The triumph of the reactive power over the disease is designated as a cure, the triumph of the disease leads to death. If the transition to recovery or cure is marked by tumultuous phenomena, we designate it as a crisis; if the process of equalization is gradual, without any violent symptoms, we call it lysis. In so far as the organic reaction is engaged in a struggle with the disease, it is termed the vis medicatrix naturæ. Like any other organic activity, it is based upon the nervous system, without which it cannot exist. But inasmuch as the disease is not a strange something that becomes mixed up with the tissues; inasmuch as it is simply the consequence of a change in the reciprocal relations and functions of organs, disease can likewise not exist without involving the nervous system, a derangement of the nervous functions being the starting-point in every disease. Every disease arises from the action of some external noxa upon the organism, the difference of one noxa from another, together with the peculiarities of the organism, determine the different forms of diseases, and, inasmuch as these two factors may differ from each other in a variety of ways, it follows that there must be a variety of forms of disease. Disease is only recognized by the phenomena it presents to our senses. It is only from these phenomena that we can draw conclusions regarding the morbific agent and the opposing endeavors of the reactive force. Hence it becomes necessary to investigate every trifling circumstance in the picture of the disease in order to obtain a knowledge of its true character, and to use it for the purpose of becoming acquainted with the road which Nature follows in order to free itself from the derangement of its functions, and likewise of obtaining light, by an analysis of the external phenomena, regarding the internal processes which these phenomena reflect. This result can only be obtained if each case of disease is placed before us as a separate individual case; for it is only in this way that we learn to know how far the organism is capable of equalizing the disturbance of its functions by its own unaided efforts, and when it becomes necessary to assist it in this endeavor.

Experience shows that in many cases the organism is capable of throwing off the disease without any external aid, whereas in many other cases the reactive energies of the organism are insufficient and the disease triumphs over the former. It likewise shows that, if the morbific agent acts upon the organism with great intensity, the elimination of the morbific agent takes place slowly and with great difficulty. The desire of accelerating this natural curative process, of facilitating it or bringing it about, induces us to institute a search after remedial agents capable of answering this purpose, and all such remedial agents are called medicines. We have shown in the preceding chapter how we have to proceed in order to obtain a correct and full knowledge of their effects; all we have to do here is to inquire how we have to apply the drugs with whose effects we have become acquainted, to the actual treatment of diseases.

It is an old rule, which cannot be followed too strictly, that a physician should be the servant, not the master of Nature, *minister*, not *magister Naturæ*. If, as such, he means to help the organism, he is under an obligation to examine above all things the road which Nature pursues when endeavoring to free itself from disease; he is bound to try to effect a cure by means of the organic reaction which he has to reinstate into possession of its lost superiority over the morbific agent. Moreover, in order to act with as much directness as possible and to effect a cure as speedily as possible, he has to affect that portion of the nervous system which is the seat of the organic reaction in the present case, likewise in the direction which the curative effort of Nature is disposed to take. But, as the process of every natural cure is governed by an universally valid law, so should the medicinal influence upon the nervous system likewise be regulated by a law of universal and admitted validity. This must be the law of similarity as Wislicenus shows indirectly by his refutation of other methods of treatment, and afterwards directly by the following mode of reasoning: Our drug-provings have shown that a medicine produces a characteristic drug-disease peculiar to itself. If this drug-disease resembles a natural malady in all its essential points, it must necessarily proceed from the same essentially similar processes in the interior of the organism. If, in addition to the natural malady, we excite an essentially similar drug-disease, the former experiences an addition as regards quantity, and likewise an extension as regards quality; for the question is not whether the morbid processes are equal but similar. In the same manner, by adding the medicinal disease, the existing reactive efforts are not simply heightened but qualitatively extended and increased, in consequence of new reactive endeavors characteristic of the medicine having been excited, which, however, are necessarily intimately connected with the existing reaction of the organism.

Experience teaches that the drug-disease, when caused by a moderate quantity of the drug, is easily overcome by the organism which, even after the disappearance of the original disturbance, oscillates in the direction of the opposite medicinal phenomena, which may be regarded as a remnant of the natural curative endeavor directed against the drug. For by this union of the medicinal and natural diseases, the excess of the reactive endeavor of the drug-disease must necessarily go to the credit of the natural disease, since in both the drug-disease and the natural malady the reaction bears upon the same portions of the organism. This cannot take place where the drug-disease and the natural malady are not similar, consequently are deprived of the numerous and essential points of contact existing in case of similarity. From the foregoing remarks we infer that it is only the after-action by the drug which determines the cure, for it alone represents the reactive endeavor of the organism that we have to call into play. In as far as a disease can only continue as long as the organic reaction remains too feeble to control it, and must disappear as soon as the reactive force becomes superior to it, and in as far as we are capable of securing such a superiority by the most similarly acting remedy: just so far the law of similarity precludes the idea of an incurable disease, provided we are able to discover a similarly acting remedial agent. We have it in our power to acquire this knowledge; all we have to do in order to accomplish this object is to continue our provings with persistent energy and correctness, and to unceasingly increase the number of the drugs to be proved. All this shows that the law of similarity necessarily requires the most careful proving of drugs; for it alone enables us to contrast the most comprehensive diagnosis of a natural disease with an equally comprehensive diagnosis of drugs, which, after all, is the main requisite to a cure. The law of similarity invests every apparently insignificant drug-effect with a degree of importance, since it becomes an element in our therapeutic series. On the other hand, the preceding statement regarding the necessity of instituting careful and comprehensive provings likewise argues in favor of the law of similarity, which alone renders it possible to use all the results of our provings for therapeutic purposes.

This explanation of the law of similarity likewise facilitates the explanation of an idea that has heretofore been used very improperly by many physicians: we allude to the expression of specific. If the old system of Medicine applies the term specific to such drugs as had been found to be specially curative against certain morbid processes in a manner that it was beyond the power of analysis or observation to investigate: all that such an appellation accomplishes is to cause us to condemn, *a priori*, every investigation of the causes of therapeutic results as useless; the thing has been given a name, this is all. We know very well that this name has no meaning, and that it does not designate a constant curative effort. There are no specific remedies for entire genera of diseases. If we content ourselves with the definition that a remedy is specific with reference to a certain form of disease; if it exerts under all circumstances a curative influence upon the disease, our previously developed explanation gives us the privilege of applying the term specific to the similarly or rather to the most similarly acting drug. At the same time our explanation shows that there are specific remedies only for individual cases of disease, not for whole categories, and that the so-called specific remedies of the Old School are specific only in so far as they correspond, under the application of the law of similarity, with individual cases in the category. It is only by accepting this explanation of the term specific that Homœopathy can be called the doctrine of specific remedies, the specific curative method.

Speaking of names, we may as well add a few words concerning the term Homœopathy. More recently as well as years ago, attempts have been made to alter this name. It matters not, and we need not inquire whether this name is in strict accord with the rules presiding over the formation of words; but we doubt whether another name can be found indicating the distinction between the homœopathic and other curative methods. The term Homœopathy has become fixed by usage, and will only disappear with the principles of this doctrine. If this name is either erroneously or maliciously associated with notions that have rendered it somewhat odious, we need not concern ourselves about this, provided we endeavor to do the name honor, and do not expect the name to confer honor upon us.

We have already stated in previous paragraphs that an explanation of the law of similarity has only a purely scientific value without influencing the practical treatment of diseases, although it does exert such an influence in many respects. In conclusion, let us now present a point of view which must satisfy every one of the importance of our law without any further demonstration. If we are called upon to treat an affection of a certain organ or system, it is evidently of the first importance that we should find a remedy which acts adequately and definitely upon the diseased organ or system, and more particularly upon the parts where the morbid process is going on. Setting aside the *modus operandi*, the law of similarity alone can reveal to us the existence of such a drug. Considering for the present every kind of treatment as empirical, and imagining ourselves restricted to clinical cases, we must admit that so far we are not acquainted with a single method that leads so surely to the knowledge of a drug exerting a definite action upon a definite locality as the law of similarity based upon physiological provings of drugs. It is with the remedy thus found that we shall have, at all events, to attempt a cure. The correctness of the proceeding may afterwards be deduced from the result, in case opponents should neither be willing nor able to concede this correctness, *a priori*. From this point of view it would seem as though any one who professes to be a physician must consider it as a matter of conscience to try the homœopathic method of treatment.

Let us now consider the consequences resulting, with more particular reference to practice, from the two cardinal maxims that have been discussed in the preceding paragraphs. These consequences are, in the first place, the mode in which the disease has to be diagnosed; and, secondly, the manner in which the remedial agent has to be applied to the treatment of any given case of disease.

3. Diagnosis of the Natural Disease.

Here too we quote as literally as may be Hahnemann's views as he has expressed them in his Organon, in order afterwards to explain what changes they had to undergo in the course of time.

Hahnemann says: "It may readily be supposed that every disease presupposes a change in the interior of the organism. These changes, however, as far as they are revealed by the morbid symptoms, (and these are the only data by which we can be guided in non-surgical diseases,) can only be apprehended by the understanding obscurely and at the risk of being mistaken. The essence of these changes cannot possibly be recognized in its inmost nature, nor can it be recognized at all without fallacious conclusions. The totality of the symptoms is the only aspect of the disease laid open before the eyes of the healing artist; this is the chief part of the disease which he can know and need know for purposes of curing. The physician may be aided in his work by a knowledge of the probable circumstances that induced the acute disease, or by an investigation of the most significant points of interest in the history of a chronic malady, and finally by a study of the constitution of the patient so far as it is amenable to observation, a knowledge of his character, business, mode of living and habits, his social position, age, sexual functions, etc. This externally reflected image of the internal essence of the disease is the chief and only channel through which the disease can indicate the remedy it requires for a cure, the only means of determining the selection of the proper remedial agents. From this truth we infer with absolute certainty that the totality of the symptoms in every individual case of disease is the only indication by means of which the true remedial agent can be found out." We will add to this quotation the manner in which a patient should be examined:

"The individualizing examination of a case of disease, for which I here give only general directions, and of which the examiner may use whatever he may require for a present case, demands of the healing artist nothing but presence of mind and sound senses, attention in observing phenomena, and fidelity in drawing the image of the disease."

"The patient describes the history of his troubles; his family relate his complaints, his conduct, and whatever has come within the range of their observation; the physician sees, hears and notices through his other senses whatever unusual changes have taken place in the patient. He records every thing in the same language in which the patient and his friends have described his trouble. Without saying a word he allows them to finish their statement; he only interrupts them if they lug in unessential trifles, (for such interruptions disturb the mental process of the relator;) all he does is to request slowness of speech in order that he may be able to note down the statemens of the speaker while he utters them."

"With every new statement of the patient or his friends he commences a new paragraph, for the purpose of obtaining a successive list of the symptoms in detached series. In this way he is enabled to make subsequent additions to that which at first seemed to him vague but afterwards was stated more clearly."

"After the parties have said all they intended to say of their own accord, the physician then seeks to obtain more precise definitions of their statements by instituting the following proceeding: He peruses each symptom that has been described to him, and inquires in regard to each symptom in particular: When did this symptom appear? Previous to his taking the present remedy? While he was taking it? Or only a few days after discontinuing it? What kind of pain, what sensation was it, which was experienced at this spot? (These pains and sensations have to be minutely described.)

What was the precise spot? Did the pain occur in isolated, intermittent paroxysms, at different times? Or was it continued, not intermittent? How long did it last? At what time of the day or night and in what position of the body was it worse, or did it intermit entirely? Give an exact statement of this or that symptom or circumstance as it did occur or was felt."

"In this manner the physician elicits a more circumstantial description of every single statement, without, however, suggesting an answer at the same time that the question is asked, so that all the patient would have to do is to either answer yes or no; otherwise he might be induced to state that which is either false or only partially true, or to give an affirmative or negative answer, whichever might seem to suit the views of the questioning physician; all of which would lead to an incorrect delineation of the disease and suggest improper remedies for its cure."

"If, in making these voluntary statements, nothing was said regarding several parts or functions of the body or the condition of the mind, the physician then inquires what has to be stated with respect to these parts and functions, and likewise with reference to his mental and moral condition; but all such inquiries have to be couched in very general terms, so as to compel the respondent to express himself in very definite and precise language."

"After the patient, who is, after all, chiefly to be trusted with respect to his sensations, except in diseases where he naturally seeks to dissimulate, has furnished all proper information to the physician by these voluntary and indirectly suggested statements, and has completed the image of the disease with a tolerable degree of accuracy, the physician, if he should be satisfied that he is not sufficiently informed of the condition of his patient, may then address more special and definite questions to the latter, such as: How often have the bowels been moved? What was the nature of the stools? Did the whitish stool consist of mucus or fæces? Was the evacuation attended with pain or not? What kind of pains and where? All the other symptoms have to be more pointedly examined in a similar manner."

"If the physician has recorded all these statements, he then notes what he himself has observed in his patient, for instance: How the patient has acted during the physician's visit; whether he was peevish, quarrelsome, hasty, whining, etc.; whether he was soporous or wide awake; how he talked; what was the color of his skin, tongue, etc., and inquires how far these conditions differ from what they were in health."

"In chronic diseases an investigation of the above-mentioned and all other morbid symptoms has to be conducted with particular care and circumstantial detail, even to the minutest particulars, partly because in chronic diseases the symptoms are of a more peculiar, strange character, are least like the symptoms of diseases running a rapid course, and, if a cure is to be successful, cannot be noticed with sufficient care, partly because patients become so accustomed to long suffering that they pay little or no attention to lesser, incidental symptoms which, however, are often very significant and characteristic, and even decisive in the selection of a remedial agent. Trifling deviations from the normal equilibrium are even regarded by such patients as a part of their necessary condition, even as a state of health, the true perception of which a suffering of fifteen or twenty years duration has caused to be forgotten; they scarcely imagine that these trifling symptoms, these smaller or greater deviations from a state of health, have any connection with their main affection."

Except a few unessential omissions which we may discuss in subsequent paragraphs, we have here given an outline of Hahnemann's ideas concerning the diagnosis of diseases, and how he intended it should be carried out. We here feel bound to subject his views to a brief critical examination from the present stand-point of medicine. Let no one imagine that, by offering this criticism, we intend an insult to Hahnemann or mean to underrate his labors. If we consider the time when the above-stated rules were laid down; if we consider to what extent, at that time, Medicine was lorded over by speculative theories, we must wonder that Hahnemann, in opposition to the tendency of the age, did not go over to the crassest empiricism. Since then, a good many changes have taken place: in diagnostics the most powerful levers have been set in motion with the greatest success; hence a good deal will have to be modified in Hahnemann's instructions.

The first point we have to examine is the assertion that the physician has only to deal with the externally reflected image of the disease. At Hahnemann's time this proposition seemed perfectly correct. The progress of Medicine has divested it of all such pretensions. Physiology, pathological Anatomy, Chemistry, and even Physics, have furnished us so many points of support by means of which the externally reflected phenomena lead us on the road of rational deductions, very frequently with absolute certainty, to a knowledge of the inner process, that, by neglecting these diagnostic resources, we would commit an equally great wrong as that with which we reproach our opponents for neglecting our diagnosis of drug-effects. With reference to present claims on Homœopathy we have to formulate the above-quoted passage from Hahnemann's instructions far differently, as we shall show by-and-by. In discussing Hahnemann's doctrine of psora, we shall show that he was not so very serious in trying to limit our knowledge of disease to a mechanical delineation of its outward image.

The second point is Hahnemann's assertion that, in examining the patient, the physician requires only presence of mind, sound senses and attention. These requisites may have been entirely sufficient in his time, but in our own time they are utterly insufficient. We assert that, without a knowledge of the above-mentioned collateral sciences, it is impossible to institute a thorough examination of the patient or to obtain an exhaustive diagnosis of his disease. An incoherent juxtaposition of symptoms is not what is required; we have to inquire into their origin, combination, etc.; we should endeavor to have a clear view of the internal pathological process upon which all external symptoms depend, as well as of the laws according to which this process, if there is no interference on our part, will develop itself, and either expand or become extinct. It behooves us, by every known means at our command, to find out what symptoms are the more important and characteristic of the disease, since it is after all upon these symptoms that the determination of the true remedial agent will depend. Where the existing means of diagnosis are not sufficient, it becomes our duty as much as that of any other physician to procure new sources of information or to complete those we have. Hahnemann's proposition must therefore encounter a decided condemnation at our hands.

His doctrine of *psora* shows most conclusively how little importance Hahnemann attached to a rigid adherence to his views of disease, or rather, how deeply sensible he was of the defects of his own teachings. Chronic diseases had driven him, in some measure, into a strait; anxious to solve the knot, he at most made the attempt in cutting, but he failed in accomplishing his purpose. The language in which the deep thinker reveals his invention to the world has a peculiar sound about it; we quote the passage referring to it from the Organon.

"Heretofore syphilis had been known to some extent as a chronic-miasmatic disease, that, unless cured, only becomes extinct in death. Sycosis, which, unless cured, is equally unconquerable by the vital force, was not known as an internal chronic-miasmatic disease, *sui generis;* it was supposed that a cure consisted in destroying the cutaneous excrescences; the internal malady, which continued its course, remained unobserved."

"Of immeasurably greater extent and importance than these two chronic miasms, is the chronic miasm of psora. Whereas the former miasms reveal their internal malady, one by the venereal chancre, the other by cauliflower-excrescences: the psoric miasm, after having infected the whole internal organism, reveals its existence by an intolerable, titillating, voluptuous itching, and by a specific odor. It is this miasm which constitutes the fundamental cause and fountain-head of the numerous, or rather innumerable forms of disease, which, under the names of nervous debility, hysteria, hypochondria, mania, etc., figure in pathological treatises as idiopathic, independent diseases. It took me twelve years to find out the source of an incredible number of chronic affections, to investigate and substantiate this great truth that had remained unknown to our ancestors, as well as to our contemporaries, and, at the same time, to discover the anti-psoric remedial agents which, together, will in most respects prove a match for this hydra-headed monster of disease in its diversified forms and manifestations."

This quotation may suffice, since everybody may learn from it what Hahnemann intended to accomplish. By contrasting this quotation with the above-mentioned propositions, their contradiction must appear self-evident to everybody. In these propositions we are told that the phenomenal image of the internal disease is our only object of cure, and that after its extirpation, health must remain; whereas, in the above quotation, the opposite is presented to us as the truth, moreover with a feeling of ostentation, and as the fruit of a persistent labor of twelve years. Hahnemann sets up the boldest and most unfounded hypothesis in order to get over a difficulty which he had prepared for himself. Practice soon showed that Hahnemann's view of diagnosis of disease caused practitioners who sought to cure chronic diseases of every kind, to stumble upon difficulties; that something more was required than the possession of sound senses and a practised hand; that it was necessary to investigate the internal nature of the malady, especially in cases that had but a few symptoms: all these difficulties were to be remedied by the authoritative assumption of a secret morbific agent, for which purpose the itch, whose true nature was still enveloped in mystery at Hahnemann's time, proved a welcome expedient. We should scarcely deem it worth our while to pursue this subject any farther, except to show Hahnemann's inconsistencies, if psora did not continue to play an important part with many homœopaths, not by any means to the advantage of our doctrine. Our own opinion of the itch will be stated when we come to treat of this disease. In this place we will simply ask the question why the itch, after all its morbid manifestations are removed, should still continue in the organism as a disease, and why, upon the same principle, a flea-bite, which likewise causes an efflorescence upon the skin, should not continue to flourish as a secret malady? Does an explanation of the peculiar processes of chronic diseases render the supposition of the existence of a secret agent at all necessary? This we cannot believe; and, in order to substantiate our belief, we fall back upon our explanation of the law of similarity.

Consequently we accept the proposition that, in a therapeutic point of view, disease is an aggregate of the sensually perceptible morbid symptoms, and that, where no symptoms are seen, a disease does not exist. To these sensually perceptible symptoms belong the results obtained by means of auscultation and percussion, or by any other means of physical diagnosis, as well as by the aid of Chemistry. Besides we should endeavor, by means of this external knowledge, to determine the internal processes upon which the perceptible phenomena depend as their generating cause. That this is not possible in all cases, and never will be altogether, is a defect with which all human knowledge is tainted. So far as it is possible, we are bound to initiate our reason into the internal processes of disease. Speaking of individual affections, we have shown that it is owing to the light which pathological Anatomy has shed upon internal changes, that we have become enabled, in many diseases, to pursue the correct road to a cure, to prove which we refer the reader to our chapters on apoplexy, acute hydrocephalus, affections of the spinal cord, as illustrations of our statement. Accordingly we give it as our opinion, that, together with Hahnemann's requisites, an exhaustive diagnosis of disease implies an intelligent knowledge of the physiological connection of the individual phenomena.

Introduction.

This is not favoring hypothesis; Physiology rests upon facts to which alone it is indebted for its very existence. The physiological connection of the symptoms is the means of arriving at a diagnosis of chronic diseases, without having to lug in invisible, impalpable, incomprehensible morbific agents; this connection not only demands an investigation of the present malady, but likewise, and as an absolute condition of success, a consideration of previous diseases, of peculiar conditions in life, habits, abnormal mental phenomena and characteristics, of all causative, favorable or unfavorable, ameliorating or aggravating circumstances, peculiar local conditions, etc. Nobody will probably wish to deny that such a deeper investigation of the malady must be of great value in practice. If Hartmann informs us in his introduction that the modern science of diagnostics avails the homœopath only in so far as it enables him to arrive at a speedier and more certain cognition of diseases, but is of no avail in the treatment of diseases, since no definite plan of cure can be suggested by it, until provers apply these modern diagnostic contrivances in their provings, and mark the internal changes caused by the drug: he contradicts himself to some extent, since he does not accept the proposition that the sensually perceptible phenomena constitute the sole image of the disease. Besides, he errs if he insists upon a corresponding drug-proving, before such diagnostic resources can be made available for purposes of cure. We admit that it would be desirable, and that it is necessary to a complete elaboration of our Materia Medica, that our modern diagnostic contrivances should be applied to our drug-provings, but we cannot admit for all that, that our present Materia Medica is not adequate to an exhaustive diagnosis of the natural disease. For in the drug-disease we lay no less stress upon the physiological connection of the symptoms than in the natural disease. In the drug-disease, likewise, we have to possess a lucid apprehension of the relative value and significance of the symptoms, of their origin, succession, final tendency, in short, of all the circumstances a knowledge of which we have to acquire in the case of a natural disease. Though a good deal may still be wanting, yet such a want should not deter us from doing our duty as far as possible. It is very probable that we may make many mistakes, but it is likewise certain, that by pursuing the road we have pointed out, we shall err much less frequently than those who strictly adhere to Hahnemann's course. Errors committed by following our own plan have this advantage, that we acquire a lucid perception of the defects in our Materia Medica so far as the what and the wherefore are concerned, whereas Hahnemann's method leads but too easily to a perfect stagnation in the investigation of drug-effects. The history of Homœopathy has shown this to our perfect satisfaction.

As regards the diagnosis of disease, the following proposition is the only one that we can recognize as correct: Investigate by all possible means and contrivances all the changes developed by the disease with reference to their cause, form, origin, course, connection, and succession; in a like manner investigate the symptoms and changes of the drug-disease, and you will be in possession of the two conditions necessary to achieve a cure by remedial agents. The less perfectly these two conditions are fulfilled, the less sure can we be of effecting a cure.

It is readily seen that this proposition includes all covering of symptoms, but in addition requires something else. It cannot be denied that in the present condition of our remedial resources it may often happen that we shall have to select a remedy exclusively according to the similarity of symptoms without any knowledge of their connection or origin, and that such a course will likewise lead to favorable results. However, it would be a mistake, if from a few favorable results of this kind we would draw conclusions regarding all possible cases of disease, and jump at the inference that we must treat diseases exclusively upon the basis of symptomatic similarity; for where a disease manifests itself only with a few morbid phenomena, the selection of the remedial agent can be depended upon as certain and infallible, if the symptoms are strongly marked and characteristic; not otherwise. Covering the symptoms can only lead to a cure by way of exception, not as a rule; in addition to the uncertainty involved in the selection of a remedial agent, such a proceeding is, moreover, highly unscientific.

Our demands relative to a complete and practically reliable diagnosis of disease can only be satisfied in accordance with our previous statements, if the diagnosis remains purely individual, in other words, confines itself to the case in hand, without regard to other similar cases that may have occurred before, or without regard to a general similarity with other cases of the same category. Therapeutically speaking, the homœopath knows of no categories of diseases, of no classifications based upon individual phenomena were they ever so essential, of no names such as are used in Pathology for the purpose of attaching to them equally general therapeutic rules.

Introduction.

Generalizing is the enemy of every correct treatment, more particularly when conducted in accordance with the principles of Homœopathy. It would be going too far if we would condemn all pathological forms. So far as the study of disease is concerned, great benefit is derived by starting from the general phenomena and combining with them the more special symptoms which are peculiar to the individual case. Pathology, for instance, reveals to us the characteristic symptoms peculiar to all cases of pneumonia, but not by any means the symptoms by which one case is distinguished from another, and which are of the utmost importance in practice. The fact pneumonia suggests to us a whole series of drugs, all of which may be useful in this disease; but it does not, at the same time, inform us what remedy may be the best in the present case. Our Therapeutics cannot, therefore, either be united with, or applied to the commonly received Pathology. As it enjoins upon us a rigorously individual diagnosis and selection of remedial agents, so should a manual of Therapeutics, rigorously speaking, occupy itself with individual cases of disease; it should really be a collection of single cases, and yet, in spite of all its completeness, it would even then be only fragmentary, and would, moreover, be such a bulky and unmanageable fragment, that nobody might feel anxious to wade through it. Such a work could not possibly be perfected by one man; it would have to engage for a long time the energies of a number of co-laborers, and even then it would not answer the demands of a really scientific work. Inasmuch as with an exhaustive diagnosis of disease, and a complete knowledge of drug-effects, we are placed in possession of all the requisites of Therapeutics, we might really do without any special system of this science. Up to this time we have not yet reached this point. We are neither in possession of the means to complete our investigations of disease, nor are we thoroughly acquainted with the effects of drugs. This last point we have endeavored to explain in a former paragraph; the former does not require any further argument to demonstrate its correctness. This fragmentary knowledge compels us to avail ourselves in many cases of disease of such knowledge of the action of drugs as we have obtained from their clinical use; consequently, it is this kind of knowledge that has to constitute the chief contents of a manual of homœopathic Therapeutics, for the reason that it completes the knowledge in which we are as yet deficient.

At this stage another difficulty meets us that cannot be overcome. A knowledge of practical results can only be obtained from a collection of complete, carefully recorded cases of disease, which we have to search for in the literature of our School. In surveying the whole field of our literature we cannot help confessing that it contains but very little material available for our purpose, more particularly if we consider that a sure conclusion can only be drawn from a large number of homogeneous facts. Upon the whole, all cases of disease recorded in our literature show, with not very numerous exceptions, a want of complete diagnosis, and, for this reason, cannot safely be depended upon, more especially in morbid conditions which, without a rigorous diagnosis, would lead to the most momentous misapprehensions. By way of example we mention the following three conditions which are very different and yet so often resemble each other symptomatically: meningitis, acute hydrocephalus, and typhus. In the sequel we have never failed to direct the reader's attention to such defects.

In conclusion we have to explain the points of view starting from which this work has been composed. The object of the work, to serve beginners in Homœopathy as a guide in the treatment of diseases, rendered it necessary to follow up a strictly pathological system, and to range, in parallel series with the pathological categories, a whole number of remedies that occupy the first rank in the treatment of diseases. To those who may consider the number too small, we have to reply that too much material confuses the beginner, without doing much good to those who are thoroughly conversant with Homœopathy. In order to satisfy the claims of Medicine regarding diagnosis, we have deemed it necessary to describe diseases as completely and accurately as possible, so much more as, in this respect, Homœopathy is as yet guilty of many sins of omission. Most likely many will blame us for having done too much in this direction. The therapeutic chapter contains but seldom a list of individual symptoms; such lists are only furnished in cases where the symptoms seemed to have a special value, or where a splitting of the symptoms in the Materia Medica might have given rise to a wrong apprehension of their import. In mentioning single remedies, their relation to the disease in point has been described in a very general manner, to which we have added various items that are not found in the Materia Medica and which have been derived from the *usu in morbis*. By this means we believe we have made it impossible for any one to imagine that the statements made in any given case of disease are sufficient for practical treatment. What we intended to accomplish was, to furnish a guide to a knowledge of the Materia Medica, on which account we have indulged in as few special indications as possible, in order that everybody should be obliged to study the special symptoms in the Materia Medica, which is really the true Therapeutics of Homœopathy. In order to facilitate such a study by means of a comparative arrangement of the materials, we have endeavored, instead of adopting the classification of other writers, and more particularly the confused and confusing classification of Hartmann, to follow the plan of the Materia Medica and to adapt to it our arrangement of particular diseases. In this way a comparison of the different drugs among each other bearing upon one and the same anatomical locality, is very much facilitated. As to the dose, it has been mentioned only now and then in the special part of this work. We shall discuss our views concerning this subject in this introduction, in order afterwards to avoid giving offence, on this account, in view of the great divergency of opinions on this subject.

4. Single Remedies.

Next to the two leading maxims of Homœopathy, this subject is undoubtedly the most important. We generalize as follows: Every drug must be administered without the admixture of any other medicinal substance. If Hahnemann had done nothing further than to start the previously expressed proposition, more particularly at such a time as he lived in, he would not only deserve our gratitude, but likewise our admiration. It is undoubtedly this law which has exerted the greatest influence upon Medicine generally. In proof of this it is well known that apothecaries have heaped upon Hahnemann their bitterest curses for introducing this reform.

We do not consider it necessary either to defend or to explain this law any further. This law is an inevitable consequence of the law of similarity. We might be answered that mixed drugs might be proved and employed accordingly. In reply to such an objection we suggest that it would be improper to prove mixtures, whereas so many single drugs still remain unproved, and to employ mixtures where single remedies are sufficiently curative. And then, definite mixtures that have been proved would be like single remedies, since they would have to be prescribed in every case in the same identical combination. So far as we are concerned, we regard medicinal mixtures with a great deal of disfavor; we believe that we do not assert too much, if we maintain that the mixing of drugs has been the main reason why Old-School Therapeutics has not progressed or been improved. We even go so far as to assert that every physician who has an eye to practical results, must become a homœopath from the moment he binds himself as by a law never again to prescribe a mixture of drugs. It is only by pursuing this course that he will be able to obtain results from which he can draw conclusions for himself and others, and upon which he can erect the edifice of experience.

It is impossible to comprehend that even homœopaths could have sinned against the doctrine of a single remedy; alas, it has been done, and is even done at the present time in two different ways.

In the first place two homœopathic medicines have been mixed together with a view of obtaining in this manner a simillimum, one part of the symptoms being arbitrarily separated from the other part in order to decide upon the proper remedies. We need hardly show that this proceeding is contrary to the laws of our system of treatment; it has but few apologists.

The custom of administering two remedies in alternation is much more common and widespread, especially with our English colleagues. Much may be said in its favor, still more against it; nor do we share Hartmann's opinion when he calls the alternation of drugs an improvement in our system of Therapeutics. The method of alternating drugs can be excused under certain circumstances, but can never be defended as scientific. We very frequently meet with cases where it is difficult to at once hit upon the right remedy on account of the inherent difficulty of establishing a correct diagnosis; nevertheless the imminence of the danger may require prompt help. In such a case the use of two drugs in rapid alternation may be excused until our diagnosis is satisfactorily cleared up. Croup may serve as an example. As soon as our diagnosis is perfectly certain, there is no further reason to excuse the alternate employment of drugs; after this it becomes a mistake that weighs so much more heavily, since it renders our observations obscure and unreliable. In cases where we have to depend upon written reports for a selection of drugs, we may be excused for employing two drugs in alternation, but only until we obtain a correct knowledge of the disease.

What we have said shows that the alternate use of drugs is either a forced or self-indulgent palliation of a want of knowledge either of the drugs or of the diseases, or is even a matter of convenience. As a general rule we shall find that homœopaths who are equally well versed in Materia Medica and Pathology do not favor an alternation of drugs. We more especially warn beginners against adopting this custom; it will render their path much more difficult since they cannot place any reliance upon an experience derived from such a source.

5. Size of Dose.

No subject has been discussed by homœopaths with more inveterate and even bitter persistence, and no subject has furnished our opponents so many opportunities for scientific and unscientific attacks as this subject of the size of the dose. In setting up this subject as the fifth cardinal maxim of Homœopathy, we may at the same time indicate thereby the rank which this maxim holds in relation to its four predecessors.

We omit quoting Hahnemann, whose teachings concerning the size of the dose have never acquired any general validity, and are, moreover, couched in language that would require a commentary for its proper elucidation. We will briefly state that Hahnemann, observing that the employment of large doses of similarly acting drugs aggravated the disease for which the medicine was prescribed, diminished the size of his doses more and more, by which means he was led to the discovery that a quantitative diminution of the drug did not necessarily involve a corresponding diminution of its curative power. Starting from the idea of a so-called homœopathic aggravation, he finally hit upon a dose which would be sufficiently powerful for curative purposes, but too weak to occasion any medicinal aggravations. For all that it was a mistake to announce the thirtieth potency as a normal dose, as we shall shortly endeavor to show.

The question of dose is a purely practical question, whose solution can only be approximated and achieved by thousands of experiments; for the action of a medicinal substance upon the human organism is not regulated by a uniform law, but depends upon a number of accessory circumstances. We cannot expect ever to derive the same effect from the same dose, either among sick or healthy individuals. These modifying circumstances are of three different kinds, according as they are founded in different degrees of susceptibility to medicinal impressions, or in differences of the morbid conditions, or of the remedial agents.

The difference in individual susceptibility to medicinal impressions is shown by every proving that is instituted on different individuals, and likewise by the number, be it ever so small, of observations on the sick. We cannot form an *a priori* judgment regarding the degree of susceptibility, even if experience should have satisfied us that certain points may be regarded as fixed. Experience has shown that children, nervous and irritable natures, and men who live as nearly as possible in accordance with the laws of Nature, and with strictness and regularity, are more susceptible to medicinal action than those who pursue an opposite course; that the susceptibility decreases in proportion as the general reactive energies of the organism diminish, in consequence of the persistent use of large quantities of medicinal substances, etc.

Daily experience likewise points to the fact that the size of the dose depends upon the peculiar character of the pathological process. We see that affections of the nervous system do not require such large doses of medicine as affections of the circulatory organs; that contagious or miasmatic diseases require larger doses, etc.

Everybody may likewise see that different drugs, when administered in the same dose, do not manifest the same degree of intensity of action. A grain of Arsenic, of course with reference to the effects peculiar to this poison, acts more powerfully than a grain of the Nitrate of Potash or of Mercury; a drop of Belladonna more powerfully than a grain of Chamomile.

Looking at the subject from these three points of view, a normal dose, be it small or large, is an assertion that cannot be proved--a mere theory that can never be substantiated by practice. If many of our homœopaths still continue to adhere to a normal dose, we have to regret so much tenacity as a damaging mistake, as a direct violation of the spirit of Homœopathy. Upon the same principle that Homœopathy demands the strictest process of individualization in diagnosing a disease; that it even insists upon a rigorous individualization of drug-effects: upon this same principle it likewise demands as a strictly logical consequence, that the dose shall be rigorously individualized in every case by adapting it to the nature and the special circumstances of the case in hand. To meet these requirements we have an universally valid law in Homœopathy, which we shall discuss more particularly in the subsequent paragraphs.

Every cure which a physician is expected to perform is to be conducted in accordance with the principle: Tutò, citò et jucundè curare. In other words: Every conscientious physician will see to it, without impairing the certainty and rapidity of the cure, that, in addition to the existing complaints, the medicine employed in the case, shall not cause additional sufferings to the patient. By prescribing a tolerably large dose of a drug in accordance with the law of similarity, we shall almost always develop a more or less considerable exacerbation of the symptoms, the so-called homœopathic aggravation. Everybody can easily satisfy himself that such an aggravation is not an imagination or vague theory; on the other hand, it is certainly an imagination, if many homœopathic physicians profess to see an aggravation after every dose below the ominous thirtieth potency, remaining in this respect much too literally the faithful followers of Hahnemann. The fear of a homœopathic aggravation led Hahnemann to the great mistake of setting up the thirtieth potency as the normal dose. It is certain that the observations of his successors have not confirmed the statements of their teacher. Now, inasmuch as a homœopathic aggravation—although if it does not manifest itself with too much violence, it is generally a proof of the correctness of our choice of the true remedy in the case—yet is not altogether in accordance with the requirement of "jucunde curare," we are bound to avoid the aggravation by lessening the dose, and to continue this lessening process until we reach a point where the fullest possible curative action of the drug is no longer followed by an aggravation of the symptoms, even if this course should lead us to the thirtieth and even higher potencies.

Beside the homœopathic aggravation, we observe from large doses purely medicinal effects, that is to say, effects that are caused by the medicine outside of the range of the natural pathological symptoms. This medicinal aggravation only sets in after proportionally large doses, whereas the homœopathic aggravation may occur after very small doses. That such an aggravation may sometimes be excited by very small doses, in individuals endowed with an extraordinary sensitiveness to medicinal action, is a welcome proof of their efficacy. We have treated a very sensitive lady, in whom the sixth attenuation of Mercury always excited profuse, though short-lasting ptyalism, accompanied with a metallic taste. The patient, of course, never knew what medicine she was taking. Evidently a purely medicinal aggravation is more than any other opposed to the "jucunde curare," and should, therefore, be avoided with the greatest care.

According to what we have said, the dose should be determined in accordance with the following rule: The dose should be of a size not to develop any medicinal symptoms while the healing process is going on, nor, if possible, any homœopathic aggravation. We use the term "if possible," because it is impossible to avoid a homœopathic aggravation in every case, which, after all, deserves our attention only in case it should set in with much violence.

It must be evident to every one that the rule which we have expressed regarding the dose, cannot be applied without any further thought in every disease, since both the homœopathic and the medicinal aggravations depend upon the above-mentioned relative conditions of the patient, the disease, and the medicine. Practical observation has suggested a few more or less definite and fixed rules bearing upon this subject, which we shall at once proceed to point out.

Previously, however, we will briefly explain how it is possible that such small doses as are employed in homœopathic practice, do at all manifest any curative virtue. Regarding this point a whole legion of explanations has been furnished, which we could not possibly discuss without being carried too far. We avoid such a discussion so much more readily as all explanations of this point never lead to any convincing result. We have already stated in a previous chapter that the small doses of Homœopathy have been suggested by the purest empiricism, and we here add that it is only the practical experiment that can furnish evidence of their efficacy. If any one cannot or will not believe in the efficacy of these small doses—and we do not blame any one for it—let him try them in practice, and obtain practical evidence concerning a subject that seems incredible to his abstract understanding. In view of the tendency now prevailing to observe the course of diseases without the use of drugs, we deem it much more natural and conscientious to find out with how little medicine cures can be effected than to determine how much medicine a patient can bear without being injured or killed by it. If, with reference to the question of dose, the old system of Medicine is in direct opposition to Homœopathy, no unprejudiced person can doubt to what party the palm of discretion and conscientiousness should be adjudged. We know that most diseases terminate in recovery even without our aid;—if this be so, is it not a piece of unscrupulous boldness to operate with large doses of powerful drugs?—We homœopaths are entitled to backing up our mode of administering drugs by the experience of thousands of cases and practitioners; but who is justified, without instituting a final trial, in arrogating to himself an apodictic judgment concerning things which he rejects for no better reason than because he is unable to comprehend them with his purely human imperfect understanding? The actual experiment establishes the belief in small doses much better than a purely theoretical explanation. Are the small doses of Homœopathy the sole thing in Nature which surpasses our comprehension? Should we deny results for no better reason than because we marvel at the road upon which they have been reached?—As we have stated, it is useless to undertake to argue against those who are not willing to believe; we prefer repeating to them Hahnemann's words: "Imitate my example, but imitate it correctly!" We pity those whom mere prejudice prevents from trying small doses; they do not injure Homœopathy, only themselves and the patients who confide themselves into their hands.

In other respects, general propositions are best attached to each of the following truths which experience alone has taught us:

1st—Every medicine which is administered in accordance with the law of similarity, has to be administered in proportionally small doses.

In order that this proposition should be clearly understood, we have to determine in the first place what we understand by large and small doses. The term small can only be understood with reference to the doses that are generally employed in Medicine; hence we might state the case in this way, that medicines prescribed according to the law of similarity can never be given in the same quantity as the same medicines are prescribed according to any other law of cure. If small is to be understood with reference to Homœopathy, the rule then is worded in this wise: The dose should never be large enough to develop either a medicinal or homœopathic aggravation. The proportionate smallness of our doses is founded in the totally different views that guide us in the use of drugs. What we intend to accomplish by means of the drug is to excite the reaction, not to divert the reaction from its natural course. Inasmuch as we intend to excite this reaction within the limits of the parts affected by disease, we do not prescribe the medicine in such a large dose that, in addition to the existing symptoms of the disease, it is able to develop its own inherent drug-effects; this would envelop other organs and symptoms within the range of the pathological process. That only small doses are necessary to excite the reaction, is not only taught us by practice, but we are led to such a conclusion *a priori*, since a diseased organ is much more sensitive to the action of an artificial stimulus than the same organ in health.

2d—The limit up to which the dose of a remedy prescribed in

accordance with the law of similarity can be diminished, without being divested of its curative power, has not yet been fixed up to this time.

Hahnemann had decided in favor of the thirtieth potency as the dose sufficient in all cases; finding even this dose too strong in some cases, he was led to the notorious custom of causing patients to smell of the prescribed drug. Most of his successors have decided in favor of the lower potencies, employing the thirtieth potency only in exceptional cases. Another not altogether insignificant party has carried the potentizing process much higher than Hahnemann. If the partisans of the high potencies profess to have obtained brilliant curative results from the two thousandth or even the ten thousandth potency, those who think differently are certainly not authorized to deny these results without further proof; it is just as rash to brand such curative results as absurd, as it would be rash on the part of the high potentialists to reject as improper the more material doses of their opponents. We admit that high potencies exert a curative influence. But there is no evidence that they act better than the lower potencies up to the thirtieth. It is certain that a remedy in a lower potency, which is unable to overcome a disease, will not overcome it any more if given in a higher. Inasmuch as no one can pretend having seen the thirtieth potency produce a homœopathic, much less a medicinal, aggravation, which must necessarily determine the degree beyond which a medicine need not be attenuated, we cannot comprehend why the immense labor of manufacturing high potencies should be undertaken. Since they do not yield any advantages worth mentioning, this innovation, which carries the "mysticism" of Homœopathy to the utmost extreme, had better be abandoned. For this reason, we can neither invite nor encourage the trial with high potencies. On the other hand, if we adhere to Hahnemann's scale up to the thirtieth as the normal series, we deem it inconsistent and unscientific for any one to use the first numbers of this scale and to reject the higher numbers *nolens volens* as absurd. The practical trial being alone capable of deciding, every one should satisfy himself by actual experiments whether high or low potencies are preferable. This is the only way of arriving at a final and conclusive result. It may suffice in this place to say that we consider it proven that the thirtieth potency is still capable of effecting decidedly curative results.

3d—We consider it an established fact that the lower potencies show a more rapid, momentarily more intense, but less persistent, effect than the higher potencies, which develop their effects more slowly and gradually, but more persistently; and that, for this reason, the lower potencies are more suitable where rapid aid is required—the higher potencies, on the contrary, where the effect can be awaited without any great hurry.

We have purposely avoided lugging in, in this proposition, the idea of acute and chronic diseases. Such a separation is always more or less impractical, since we shall always have transition-forms which it might be very difficult to classify, so much the more as the question of dose would have to be settled in accordance with such a classification. Moreover we have acute affections where higher potencies may be more useful than lower, and, *vice versa*, there are chronic affections where lower potencies will prove more beneficial than higher. The former class, for instance, comprehends all diseases running a definite course, such as typhus, contagious exanthems, or such chronic affections as frequently show an acute exacerbation of the symptoms. It is our opinion that in selecting a drug we should be guided by the urgency of the reaction to be obtained, and we prefer this more general definition to special rules which it is impossible to furnish for all cases; in pursuing this course we shall of course be guilty of many sins of omission.

4th—The more similar the chosen remedy to the disease, the more surely may we expect curative results even from the smallest dose.

This proposition is easily explained by what we have said before in explanation of the law of similarity; it likewise accounts for a fact which is common to all homœopathic practitioners: that is, the more familiar they have become with the Materia Medica, the more correct their knowledge of the curative virtues of our drugs, the more habitually they prescribe smaller doses. This shows that in selecting a drug, its similarity to the natural disease is the first and most important condition, and that the quantity of the dose plays an entirely subordinate part.

5th—In determining the dose, the peculiar nature of the drug demands special consideration.

In a previous section already we have shown that this point is somewhat essential. We have many medicinal substances that do not display their therapeutic power until they have been comminuted. This number includes all inorganic substances that are insoluble either in water or alcohol. These it is which the process of trituration has first to convert into remedial agents; it is therefore impossible that such drugs, when prescribed in material doses, should manifest any curative power. In the case of soluble inorganic and of vegetable substances we have likewise to consider the intensity of the effect. Corrosive Sublimate, for instance, or Phosphorus, Nux vomica or Ignatia can never be given in as large a dose as Chamomile or Sambucus, comparatively large quantities of which can be administered without any injurious effect. In this place we cannot well classify drugs with reference to these inherent differences of medicinal power, and therefore refer the reader to the Materia Medica.

6th—The peculiar nature of the sick individual requires to be carefully considered in the selection of a drug.

This point has likewise been alluded to before; here we add the following to our previous remarks. It is always difficult, when taking charge of a new patient, to determine *a priori* the degree of reaction against medicinal impressions he may be endowed with. In such cases we have to proceed with a great deal of caution, the more so the younger the patient. It is only a protracted observation of individual peculiarities that can afford us a more or less certain basis for a correct judgment.

We believe that the foregoing general propositions have exhausted the question of dose as far as this is possible in the present position of our science. We have intentionally omitted every thing that might convey the suspicion of party-prédilections. We deem it just as wrong on the part of those who prefer the lower potencies to deny the efficacy of the higher, as on the part of those who prefer the higher potencies to condemn the lower as though they only produced toxical results. The former generally pronounce judgment without having made sufficient trials, the latter condemn under the influence of a pitiable one-sidedness. It is therefore fortunate that the dispute about doses which was formerly carried on with so much foolish zeal and repulsive vehemence, has yielded to a temporary armistice. Let both parties first gather up good material, after which they may wage a war of annihilation.

6. Preparation, Repetition, etc., of Medicines.

Under this head we range various points of subordinate importance, which, however, with reference to practice, cannot remain unnoticed.

In his instructions for the preparation of the different medicines we likewise are led to admire Hahnemann's great practical tact.

Introduction. 49

He considered it a physician's duty to prepare all his own medicines, and, in order to do this, the preparation of drugs had to be a very simple affair. Hahnemann's rules in this respect have undergone but few alterations, indeed only such as have been suggested by our superior knowledge, particularly of inorganic substances or by a difference in our views concerning doses. Particulars may be found in Jahr and Gruner's Homœopathic Pharmacopœa, (New York: Wm. Radde.) The following are the general rules to be followed in the preparation of drugs.

Organic substances in as fresh a condition as they can be obtained, are extracted by means of concentrated alcohol. This yields us the mother-tincture. One drop of this tincture shaken up with nine drops of alcohol, gives the first attenuation, (potency or dilution;) one drop of this first attenuation diluted in a similar manner, gives the second attenuation, and so on. This is the decimal scale which is now in almost general use. Hahnemann followed the centesimal scale, where one drop of the tincture is shaken up with ninety-nine drops of alcohol. Many prefer this scale as superior, doubtless without any sufficient reason. The decimal scale yields evidently a more exact, a more uniform attenuation of the drug, and the differences of the single numbers of the series are of less consequence. The centesimal scale is more suited for one who always uses the same potency in his treatment of diseases.

Inorganic substances are best attenuated by trituration. To this end one grain of the chemically pure and, if possible, amorphous substance is rubbed up for one hour in a mortar with nine grains of sugar of milk. This yields the first trituration, one grain of which, rubbed up in the same manner with nine grains of sugar of milk, yields the second trituration, etc. The triturating process is usually continued only up to the third or sixth potency, after which liquid attenuations are prepared by mixing one grain of the triturated substance with ninety-nine grains of diluted alcohol. Some drugs have been triturated up to much higher numbers; this practice has not been generally applied to all drugs.

Organic substances, that can only be imperfectly extracted by alcohol or not at all, have likewise been triturated; likewise such vegetable substances as can only be obtained dry. Soluble, inorganic substances, on the contrary, are prepared in a liquid form at the outset.

For convenience sake—and it is asserted on account of their better preservation—small globules of sugar have been moistened with a few drops of an attenuation, which are afterwards allowed to dry again. These globules are excellently adapted to pocket-cases; however, there is no reason why they should be preferred to the liquid form.

Medicines may be administered to the sick in form of drops or powder, or in the shape of globules, or dissolved in distilled water. There are no fixed rules with regard to this point.

These statements show at once how simple and yet how bulky such a preparation of our drugs must be. Inasmuch as it is impossible to exercise any control over the intrinsic value of the attenuations, it is evident, that they either have to be prepared by the physician himself, or by a reliable apothecary. From this dilemma the bitterest struggles have arisen for Homœopathy, for it involves the necessity of self-dispensation for every physician who cannot avail himself of the services of a reliable apothecary. This is not the place for an elaborate discussion of this subject; let it suffice that we deem it of the utmost importance and advantage for every physician to dispense his medicines to the patient directly, even if he should have a reliable pharmacy to fall back upon.

As regards the repetition of drugs, Hahnemann advises not to repeat the dose until the former has exhausted its action. This sounds simple enough, but is of very difficult application in practice. At all events, in chronic affections nothing is lost by waiting a reasonable length of time; in acute affections, on the contrary, such waiting is very often out of place, and would only be admissible if we could always be sure of the simillimum, and in possession of sure signs by which we could decide when the medicine ceases to act. Let every one ask himself whether he can be certain of this in a given case; we do not believe it, and look upon Hahnemann's rule as a correct theory that cannot be carried out in practice. Nor was Hahnemann quite as indisposed to repeat the dose as it might seem; if he prescribes a tablespoonful of the same solution in frequent doses, this too is a repetition of the medicine. As a general rule all practical homœopathic physicians act upon the principle of repeating the dose the more frequently the more intense the disease. In violent attacks of croup or cholera, for instance, the medicine may be repeated every ten minutes; it is even well to do so. In affections which, although acute and very intense, run a definite and more extended course, a less frequent repetition of the dose is perfectly appropriate. In chronic affections where no great changes take place, one or two doses a week generally advance the cure more than frequently repeated doses.

Frequent changes of medicines are contrary to the spirit of Homœopathy. In acute affections where the life of the patient is in imminent danger, it may be both necessary and pardonable to resort to a rapid change of medicine, since, after all, we are not mathematically certain of having chosen the right remedy; in affections running a less rapid course our best plan is to select a remedy with great care and afterwards to give it a fair trial by continuing it for some time. We should always keep in mind what we intend to accomplish with our remedies; this will induce us to persevere in the proper use of one drug. What we intend to accomplish is to assist the organic reaction and to enable it to restore the equilibrium of the disturbed functions by a normal process; we do not intend to expel the disease from the organism by violent means. This has to be considered more particularly where the disease has developed morbid products of some magnitude, or has produced other material alterations. A pneumonic exudation, an apoplectic effusion, a considerable deposition of pus, etc., cannot possibly be removed within twenty-four hours; it might even be injurious to the organism if it should develop such an extraordinary reactive activity. If we desire to proceed truly physiologically in such cases, we must not indulge in frequent changes of medicines.

7. Diet.

The so-called homœopathic diet such as it was insisted upon in former times, has not been of particular advantage to Homœopathy. In the first place it has deterred a number from adopting homœopathic treatment; the fear of the rigid homœopathic diet is still haunting the public mind; in the next place it has furnished the opponents of Homœopathy a handle they are even now making use of for the purpose of denying the efficacy of our drugs. Experience has shown that these two disadvantages are not by any means counter-balanced by adequate gains. It is perfectly absurd to attempt to furnish stereotyped rules of diet, as is sought to be accomplished by our notorious diet-papers. As we allow Physiology full swing, in all other medicinal injunctions, so we should in diet which should likewise be rigorously adapted to the necessities of individual cases.

This kind of dietetic individualization requires us to consider the circumstances in which the present generation lives. If we would change our mode of living even approximatively to a natural system, we should change our whole surroundings, our occupations, our mental and bodily labor. Such a dietetic Utopia is and will remain a religious desire the fulfilment of which is not even looked for by those who entertain it. Habit is a wicked tyrant and yet so amiable that, in spite of our better judgment, we are unable to shake off his yoke. What wine-bibber would want to renounce his wine? what woman her coffee? what smoker his cigar? Before opposing such habits, we had better inquire first how far they are an obstacle to a cure, and whether it is not possible to attain our object in spite of them. In most cases we shall certainly be able to do so. The so-called obnoxious habits are not hurtful or at least equally hurtful for everybody; with many they constitute a necessity resulting from the conditions of life. Persons who are constantly occupied mentally, and whose nervous system is bad, require coffee as a stimulant; if they are deprived of it, they feel quite sick. For a state of mental and bodily depression, wine is a perfect panacea; physicians know this perfectly well by their own personal experience. What shall we say of tobacco? Are we not compelled to put up with it, unless we wish to make tobacconists as well as druggists our mortal enemies? Many habits can easily be put off, but it is best not too suddenly. Among them we range for instance the use of a number of spices, a want of exercise, too warm clothing. Such habits have to be changed, but very cautiously; as regards other habits, they had better be left unchanged at the beginning of the treatment. Our remedies act in spite of them, and, we believe just as well, unless the habit should happen to antidote the medicine, such as coffee the vomic nut.

Our advice therefore is, do not prescribe a set diet, and do not prohibit too many things in order to secure a more perfect obedience to our positive demands; this may not seem very consistent, but of what avail is all consistency against a secretly sinning patient?

In treating of the different diseases, we have generally indicated the proper diet, and cannot indulge in any further details in this place. We repeat, Physiology gives us sufficient hints what rules we ought to adopt in regard to diet, and likewise points out the reasons why we cannot deem a strictly homœopathic diet necessary to the successful action of our remedial agents.

The maxims of Homœopathy which have been discussed so far, show that in the treatment of diseases this science pursues an entirely different road from that pursued by the Old School. Let us now briefly inquire whether under certain circumstances it may not be necessary or possible that Homœopathy should approximate to or coalesce with other curative methods, and what, in general, is the relation of each curative method to Homœopathy.

We hear it said very frequently that more recently the views of homœopaths and non-homœopaths approximate to each other more and more. This can be admitted with great propriety, since all physicians simplify their prescriptions more and more, and, some of them at least, diminish their doses. Homœopathy cannot make any concessions if it means to remain what it is. Hence it is absurd to suppose that a physician can treat a patient homœopathically at one time or by some other method at some other time. A physician who pursues this course is either a mere beginner in Homœopathy or a common impostor. We do not mean to assert that we alone are able to achieve a cure; we admit that a cure may be wrought in some other way; what we claim for Homœopathy is, that it achieves at least as much as any other curative method, and in most cases assuredly more. Hence we are not under the necessity of seeking help elsewhere; all we require to do is to use earnestly and consistently what we possess. Of course our opponents will never admit this, but what matters it?

As regards surgery, it stands to reason that necessary surgical operations are likewise indispensable to homœopaths; yet it cannot be denied that the number of necessary operations has been very much circumscribed by Homœopathy. There are very many affections which it is not necessary to treat surgically, since they can be managed just as well and better by internal means; such are various kinds of swellings, incarcerated hernia. Nor will we have to decline the use of external, indifferent auxiliary appliances. Cold and warm fomentations, compresses, etc., are indifferent things in a medicinal point of view, but of sufficient importance for the alleviation of many sufferings to deserve the consideration of homœopathic practitioners. These auxiliary means are likewise very frequently used by us homœopaths differently from what is generally the case.

Balneo-therapeutics promises in time to become a curative means of great importance. For the present we are confined with few exceptions to the narrowest empiricism, and it would be desirable if homœopathic physicians were less anxious to subject their patients to a cure whose indications and results are so uncertain. In this matter fashion has unfortunately enforced her behests and has caused many a one to forget that a medicine should not be employed before we are well acquainted with its physiological effects. As regards artificial mineral waters, all we can say is that they belong in the category of medicinal mixtures, consequently are in diametrical opposition to the spirit of Homœopathy

Of particular importance to homœopaths is the hydropathic system of treatment. Its successes are sufficiently striking to excite universal attention. It would be well if physicians could only learn from this method of treatment that it is not always and perhaps never necessary to attack diseases with an excessive quantity of substances that are inimical to the body, and that these diseases are removed much more easily by careful nursing and an awakening of the reactive energies of the organism. Watercure treatment aims in general at what Homœopathy seeks to accomplish by more special means, leading the organic reaction back to its normal condition. For this reason we regard the former treatment as of special importance to Homœopathy, cold water being the only truly constitutional remedy which is not antagonistic to any of our medicines. Our literature furnishes abundant evidence that the value and importance of water as a curative agent have been recognized and appreciated by homœopaths at a very early period. However, we would warn our readers against imitating the extravagances of the modern hydro-therapeutic treatment.

Equally important to a homœopath as the watercure treatment is the movement-cure. If we cannot hesitate to admit that gymnastic exercises are of incalculable importance to the preservation of the normal condition of the body, we must infer from this as a necessary consequence that methodical exercises must exert a powerful influence upon the restoration of the physiological equilibrium. In employing this treatment we have likewise to caution the patient against excesses, especially in diseases that do not admit of an increased acceleration of the circulation. Gymnastic exercises do not merely feed the muscular powers, but likewise exert an all-powerful influence upon the nervous system generally as well as upon digestion. The Swedish movement-cure possesses the undoubted advantage of rigidly circumscribing the mechanical treatment within proper limits, and concentrating its effect upon definite and separate portions of the muscular system.

The treatment by electricity is still so recent that it is as yet impossible to decide for what affections it may prove useful. The experiments which are as yet being made with electricity are more or less empirical; even if it is not otherwise directly antagonistic to Homœopathy, yet so far it is too little founded upon a rational basis to enable homœopathic practitioners to derive positive advantages for their patients from the electro-therapeutic treatment.

We have endeavored to show by this short survey that there are many remedial methods which, though not borrowed from Homœopathy, yet are not contrary to it in any shape or manner. We repeat, however, that no homœopath should ever avail himself of any remedial agent the use of which cannot be justified upon the principles of Homœopathy. Every therapeutic experiment is justified before the tribunal of reason, which is founded upon a knowledge of the remedial agent, and is instituted with all the precautions necessary to render it a standard rule, be the dose otherwise ever so large or ever so small. Experiments without a principle should always be repudiated with becoming energy.

FIRST SECTION.

Diseases of the Brain, the Spinal Cord, and the Nervous System Generally.

A. DISEASES OF THE BRAIN.

Hyperæmia of the Brain and its Membranes.

EVEN up to a recent period, doubts have been entertained whether a true hyperæmia of the contents of the skull is possible or not, and a number of reasons were well calculated to favor such doubts. Recent physiological experiments, however, have shown satisfactorily that the volume of blood within the skull may differ, and we will refrain from taking sides in this purely pathological question, except so far as to pronounce in favor of the opinion according to which hyperæmia of the brain is not only possible but likewise of frequent occurrence.

By hyperæmia of the brain we understand a condition of this organ where the cerebral vessels contain more blood than the normal quantity. This abnormal increase of the volume of blood may be occasioned by three different causes. In the first place, the flow of blood from the brain being normal, a larger quantity of blood returns to the brain. In the next place, the flow of blood from the brain may be abnormally diminished, whereas it may be returned in a normal quantity. Finally, the cause may be located in the brain itself, the cerebral parenchyma may become atrophied or softened, or the capillaries of the brain may become enlarged.

Hyperæmia of the brain is either confined to a limited locality, or extends throughout the whole organ. It will scarcely ever be found possible to establish, during the life of the patient, a sure diagnosis regarding the special seat and the extent of the hyperæmia, for the reason that congestions of limited extent frequently excite much more striking symptoms than more extensive congestions. So far as Therapeutics is concerned, such a diagnosis is scarcely ever of much importance. Even a post-mortem inspection does not always show hyperæmia with absolute certainty, since a sanguineous engorgement is often supposed to exist where there is not any, and, on the other hand, localized or apparently not very marked stagnations are often overlooked. In this respect the meningeal membranes are very apt to lead one into error. On the contrary, the post-mortem signs become much more apparent in consequence of a frequent recurrence of the congestion, since this causes a dilatation of the vessels. By this means the vessels of the meningeal membranes are made to look like varicose veins, having a strongly marked serpentine course, while the substance of the brain, on its cut surface, exhibits more or less numerous bloody points, and even assumes a reddish tint. It often happens that the most unmistakable signs of a high degree of cerebral hyperæmia have been present during life, without any corresponding alterations being discovered after death.

The most important terminations of cerebral hyperæmia, which impart to it a higher significance in practice, are: Sudden death from paralysis of the brain in consequence of excessive pressure of the blood; dilatation of the vessels, especially the capillaries, by which the tendency to congestion is increased; exudation and extravasation.

The causes of cerebral hyperæmia are various and important in a practical point of view, since in most cases they determine the selection of the suitable remedy. These causes are of two kinds, causes which affect the brain directly, and indirect causes, by which, through the operation of influences that are partially unknown to us, the brain becomes involved in an affection more or less remote from the brain. Among the direct causes affecting the brain, the most prominent are: Concussions of the head by a fall, blow, etc., continued, persevering and excessive mental exertions, emotional excitement, exposure to excessive heat of the sun (insolation, coup-de-soleil) or to artificial heat, likewise to excessive cold, more particularly if the influence of cold is suddenly succeeded by the action of intense heat. In the second category we may range, according to circumstances, almost all kinds of febrile affections, since almost all of them may be associated with cerebral hyperæmia; in this place we will content ourselves with mentioning pathological processes where cerebral congestions are almost always present; they are: Erysipelas of the face, angina, parotitis, inflammatory affections of the eyes and ears, irregularities of the teething process.

Hyperæmia of the Brain and its Membranes. 59

Among the more or less chronic affections that may be mentioned in this connection as causal circumstances, the most prominent in the list of those that impede the flow of blood from the brain are: Defects of the right heart, emphysema, tumors on the neck; in the list of those that occasion a general increase in the impulse of the circulation: Anomalies of the left ventricle, suppression of habitual losses of blood, (menses, piles.) In this last category we likewise range, without doing any great violence to the natural order, the cerebral hyperæmias occasioned by the abuse of alcohol or of other narcotic substances, such as Opium. Without doubt, there likewise exists a tendency to cerebral congestions, in which case they may take place without having been excited by any perceptible pathological alteration. This tendency is identical with the so-called apoplectic habitus, but cannot be recognized with any certainty, *a priori*, by definite diagnostic signs, but has to be determined in most cases, *a posteriori*, by the actual fact; it is a certain fact that it is not alone indicated by a thickset frame and a short, thick neck. On the other hand, the idea of a probable occurrence of cerebral hyperæmia suggests itself, *a priori*, in the case of individuals who, while consuming quantities of nourishing food, do not take bodily exercise in a corresponding ratio, and in whom this mode of living develops a condition that may be justly termed plethora. We have already stated in a former paragraph that the frequent repetition of attacks of hyperæmia leads to a dilatation of the vessels, which increases the disposition to renewed attacks.

Generally speaking, the prognosis in this affection is favorable, since a fatal result need not be apprehended unless some other complicating affection should supervene. In one respect it depends upon the age of the patient. Whereas, in persons of middle age, the danger is not very serious; it is, on the contrary, much greater in the case of children and old people. In the case of children, death takes place very frequently in consequence of the cerebral paralysis occasioned by the hyperæmia; in old people, the vessels are generally so fragile that they readily tear, and their contents become effused upon the brain. The apparent violence of the hyperæmia is no adequate criterium of the danger caused by it. On the other hand, the more frequently the congestion occurs, the more dangerous it becomes. Where it depends upon pre-existing derangements, the prognosis depends almost exclusively upon the character of these derangements.

The symptoms by which hyperæmia manifests itself vary probably according as one or the other locality of the brain is the seat of the affection, and according as the pressure upon the brain is more or less violent.

The head feels heavy, confused, or as if encircled by a tight band; the headache, which is scarcely ever wanting, is almost always throbbing, and is aggravated by stooping, unusual exercise and every mental effort. Buzzing in the ears, sensitiveness of the eyes, even seeing of sparks and obscuration of sight, are generally present. Vertigo is seldom wanting; if arising from anæmia, a characteristic sign of this kind of vertigo is to become aggravated by stooping, but more especially by looking up, by which, for that matter, any other complaint in the head is made worse. Generally the patient feels drowsy, without, however, being able to sleep, or else the sleep is anxious, disturbed, full of dreams. The patient feels very languid, and his gait is rendered insecure by a want of firmness of the lower limbs. The pulse may continue normal, and, if the congestion sets in as an idiopathic disease, febrile phenomena are entirely absent.

This mildest form is combined in other cases with a prevailing disturbance in the emotive sphere, characterized by constant restlessness and gloomy ideas; sleep is disturbed by anxious dreams, which, in the more violent cases, do not even entirely disappear while the patient is awake; they even assume the character of hallucinations, and, if the trouble continues without being checked, a permanent mental derangement will not unfrequently result. Palpitation of the heart, ill-humor, distrust, total indisposition to work, fitful mood, are almost always present. This form of hyperæmia mostly befalls individuals who, while indulging in good cheer, take little bodily exercise, but perform a large amount of mental labor. The foregoing symptoms are almost characteristic of hyperæmia consequent upon suppression of certain forms of hæmorrhage.

The trouble is much more dangerous if it sets in as an acute affection, and, although very violent at first, continues to increase in intensity until it terminates in death. In such cases the face looks dark-red, the eyes are injected, the vessels of the head and neck pulsate violently, the pupils are almost always contracted, the organs of all the senses are very sensitive, the headache is maddening. Furibond delirium is apt to supervene. This type is most prominent in hyperæmia occasioned by sunstroke, and, not unfrequently, is an accompaniment of mental derangement.

Not very unfrequently the above-described symptoms are suddenly succeeded by all the signs of apoplexy, regarding which the diagnosis cannot be established with any positive certainty until the proportionally rapid course and the sudden disappearance of the symptoms of paralysis have satisfied one that no extravasation of blood can have taken place, since the fluid could not have been reabsorbed so soon. In this category belong most likely all the cases that are said to have been cured so rapidly. Cerebral hyperæmia may likewise, though erroneously, be supposed to exist during an epileptic attack; here the course of the attack alone gives us perfect certainty concerning its true nature.

Among children hyperæmia is an almost habitual accompaniment of all febrile affections, and not unfrequently conceals the symptoms of the true primary affection, for the reason that the course of the hyperæmia is marked by the more violent symptoms. In every considerable congestion convulsions of one or the other kind almost always supervene; they are accompanied by drowsiness even to sopor, delirium, excessive restlessness and anxiety, and vomiting is almost always present. However threatening such a condition may seem at first sight in almost every case, yet it passes off speedily and without leaving a trace behind, so that the hyperæmia seldom lasts longer than thirty-six hours, and generally abates already after the lapse of twelve hours.

Treatment.

Belladonna.—Among all the remedies of our Materia Medica there is not one which, in its physiological action upon the organism, reproduces the image of cerebral hyperæmia in all its degrees and forms as completely as Belladonna. It is of importance to refer to the many evidences of Belladonna-poisoning where a post-mortem examination reveals a more or less considerable sanguineous engorgement in the vessels of the brain. If nowhere else, it is certainly in cerebral hyperæmia that Belladonna is calculated to show the correctness of the homœopathic method of cure, since, in most, especially uncomplicated cases of this affection it affords relief with wonderful rapidity. It would be useless to detail, in this place, a list of the principal symptoms of this drug, for the reason that their vast number and physiological differences render it necessary that the provings of this drug should be subjected to a special and most careful study. However, it may be of importance to place a few more general points of view more prominently before the reader. As regards temperaments, the sanguine temperament is more especially adapted to our drug. Plethoric constitutions, disposed to rush of blood, together with a nervous system, endowed with a high degree of sensitiveness, likewise childhood and the female organism, constitute the more special sphere of action for Belladonna. The greater the tendency to cerebral congestions, and the more frequently the patient has been attacked by them, the more Belladonna will be found suitable. Hence, it will be found particularly useful in the more important periods of development of the body, during dentition and the period of pubescence, but likewise during the critical period. The more the congestion sets in like an independent disease, the more surely it will yield to Belladonna; by which proposition is not to be understood that, if the congestion depends upon other primary affections, such as angina or scarlatina, for which Belladonna is the truly homœopathic remedy, such affections impair the homœopathicity of our drug to the symptomatic congestion. Having thus indicated, in a few leading traits, the general views that determine the selection of Belladonna as the remedial agent in the case, we do not mean to convey the impression that other temperaments and constitutions are not likewise accessible to the action of Belladonna; such a teaching would be in direct antagonism to the experience of our practitioners. Among the special symptoms, we quote more particularly the delirium which, in the case of Belladonna, is generally furibond, and the characteristic excessive sensitiveness of the organs of sense. Contraction of the pupils does not counter-indicate Belladonna, dilatation of the pupils not being a constant effect of this drug, although much more common than the opposite. Pallor of the face, or even deficient redness, are more reliable counter-indications. Where there is doubt whether Aconite or Belladonna should be given, I have always found that a disposition to perspire constitutes, cæteris paribus, a valuable indication in favor of the latter drug.

Aconite, in its action upon the organism, is so closely related to *Belladonna* that it is sometimes very difficult to choose between the two agents. I have just now indicated a distinctive sign, that has never deceived me. Practically, we have found that a genuine hyperæmia of the brain does not constitute the true field for the action of Aconite. The case is different where the cerebral hyperæmia is a mere symptom of a disturbance of some other organ; in such a case. the hyperæmia does not contra-indicate Aconite, among whose symptoms those of cerebral congestion hold a prominent place. According to Hartmann, Aconite is the best remedy for cerebral congestions that have been caused by violent emotions, such as fright or mortified feelings. This somewhat specific effect may be accounted for by the fact that in such conditions the action of the heart is peculiarly excited, and that Aconite, as we shall show more particularly by-and-by, exerts a remarkably calming influence upon cardiac excitement.

Hyoscyamus and Stramonium, in their relation to the brain, are closely related to both Belladonna and Aconite, especially the former; we think that it will be sufficient to merely indicate them in this place.

Opium is a more important remedy than either of the two last-mentioned drugs, and its action upon the brain is much more correctly delineated. Judging from the scantiness of our clinical records, it would almost seem as if very little use were made of it in congestion of the brain; yet it deserves special commendation, as any one may see, even from a superficial survey of its pathogenesis. The following symptoms constitute characteristic indications for the employment of this drug: Continual sopor, with insensibility of all the senses; dark redness of the face, with paleness and coldness of the rest of the body; slow pulse, slow respiratory movements, stertorous breathing. Such phenomena indeed do not often occur in simple hyperæmia of the brain; they occur more generally in hyperæmia constituting the commencement of more intense affections of the brain.

We must not forget to mention two drugs whose employment as therapeutic agents is limited, in consequence of their being so commonly used as articles of daily consumption, but which acquire importance from the fact that their habitual use is very apt to induce cerebral congestions. These drugs are coffee and tobacco. The effects of coffee upon the brain are much better known than those of tobacco; nevertheless, the use of tobacco causes, in many individuals, the most obstinate congestions, from which they can only be freed by renouncing their habit, which is supposed to be harmless. This may, likewise, show the necessity that, in the presence of habitual congestions, which we are called upon to remove, the use of such agents should be strictly forbidden. For such congestions as are very apt to attack sensitive individuals, in consequence of some joyful event and which generally last some time, Hartmann recommends a few dessert-spoonfuls of ordinary coffee, provided the patient is not an habitual coffee-drinker, in which case *Coffea cruda* should be given. However, it may be doubtful whether *Coffea cruda* has any effect upon coffee-drinkers any more than a drop of *Tabacum* has any effect upon habitual smokers.

Nux Vomica.—This agent will scarcely be suitable in simple hyperæmia, but is important in such hyperæmias as are caused by a sedentary mode of life, excessive mental labor, and more especially by the frequent use of spirituous beverages. In such cases, the selection of the remedial agent will depend upon the digestive derangements with which such patients are always afflicted. It is only at the commencement of the trouble that Nux will render good service; whereas, if the cerebral affection manifests itself at a later period, as a more independent disease, *Sulphur* and *Natrum muriaticum* will prove more efficient aids, to which remedies we therefore direct the reader's particular attention.

Arnica is admitted to be the best remedy for hyperæmia consequent upon concussion of the brain by a fall, blow, etc., or by other mechanical impressions. So far as the wounded locality is concerned, it may be well to apply Arnica externally, but this will not be of any special benefit to the congestion.

[After exhibiting Belladonna for twenty-four to thirty-six hours, giving a dose of the third attenuation every half hour or hour, without any perceptible improvement, Kafka resorts to the *Sulphate of Atropine*, third trituration, giving it in the same manner as Belladonna. If this agent produces no favorable result within twenty-four or thirty-six hours; if the patients start or cry out frequently and suddenly during their slumber; if they are tormented by a variety of frightful optical illusions, which cause anxiety and trembling; if symptoms of incipient compression of the brain, such as sopor, apathy, slight reaction to light and sound, etc., begin to show themselves, and the determination of blood to the head still continues, Kafka has seen happy results from *Apis* 3, in solution, giving a dose every hour or two hours; and, if an active delirium predominates, attended with sleeplessness, restlessness, disposition to escape, violent throbbing of the carotids, great heat in the head, *Glonoin* 3, in the same dose and form, is recommended by this author. Apis is particularly recommended when symptoms of cerebral depression prevail; Glonoin, on the contrary, for symptoms of cerebral exaltation.

Veratrum viride is one of the most powerful remedies for cerebral hyperæmia. It is extensively used by American physicians for this condition, both in private and hospital practice. The symptoms

Hyperæmia of the Brain and its Membranes.

which call for Veratrum viride are almost the same as those that indicate Belladonna: fulness and heaviness of the head, violent headache, heat and throbbing in the head, violent throbbing of the carotids, sensitiveness to sound and light, flushed countenance, heaviness, and a tingling or prickling sensation in the lower limbs, and the preliminary symptoms of apoplexy generally. Regarding the dose, it is the general experience of our physicians that a comparatively large dose, say a few drops of the strongest tincture, in half a tumbler of water, is necessary to develop its therapeutic effects.

Gelsemnium Sempervirens, or the Yellow Jessamine, is appropriate in hyperæmia during dentition.

In hyperæmia from sunstroke, applications of ice to the head, and frictions with ice along the spine and extremities, are indispensable to reawaken the paralyzed reaction of the organism, after which Aconite, Gelseminum or Belladonna may have to be given. H.]

Among the other remedies the following deserve particular attention: *Agaricus, Baryta, Ignatia, Rhus tox., Staphysagria* and *Veratrum*.

Regarding the general conduct of such patients, we shall offer but few remarks, since the diet is easily agreed upon. The local application of cold of course affords momentary relief to the patient, but if the cold is applied too energetically and persistently, it may prove hurtful rather than useful; the case is the same in this respect as with the general or local sanguineous depletions. If the application of cold affords great relief to the patient, he may apply for a short time cold-water compresses which, however, should never be left too long, and should be renewed quite frequently. If the patient is not confined to his bed, derivation by the application of warmth to the feet should never be attempted. Foot-baths are decidedly out of place. As a matter of course, the stomach should not be overcrowded with food, for the reason that even in the normal condition of the organism, the digestive process is attended with a certain degree of congestion. On this account it is highly important that, where there is a tendency to congestion, a horizontal position or sleeping immediately after a meal should be strictly avoided.

Anæmia of the Brain.

In treating of this affection we shall pursue the same course as in hyperæmia of the brain, and, without discussing the admissibility of the hypothesis of a diminished flow of blood to the brain, we shall take this for granted as a fact. In most cases cerebral anæmia is not such a separate affection as to require a separate chapter. This, however, may find its excuse in the great importance that attaches to it in consequence of the ease with which it is confounded with other affections, and of the dangerous consequences based upon a correspondingly erroneous treatment.

Cerebral anæmia either consists in a diminished volume of blood in the brain, or in a supply of blood to the brain destitute of red globules. In the former case it is caused by constriction or compression of the arteries through which the blood courses toward the brain, and by any other circumstances in consequence of which the space within the skull is narrowed; in the second case all the causes of anæmia come into play, whereas the deficiency of blood consequent upon sanguineous losses will have to be counted in both categories, since it is not only the quantitative decrease of the volume of blood, but likewise, and perhaps still more, the qualitative alteration of the blood that determines the anæmia. And finally there is no doubt that circumstances with which we are not yet perfectly acquainted, probably changes of a spasmodic nature, may induce a sudden decrease of the volume of blood in the brain, a lesser degree of which we may very frequently observe in consequence of powerful mental excitement.

The symptoms of cerebral anæmia differ a good deal according as it develops itself more or less rapidly. In the former case we have the most perfect image of syncope: consciousness, the sensus communis, voluntary muscular movements are suspended, most generally amid slight convulsions, and both the breathing and the pulse are slower. This condition is most prominently seen during metrorrhagia in confinement. Evidently such accidents are attended with great danger to life.—If the anæmia sets in more slowly, the sinking of the cerebral activity is always preceded by symptoms of stimulation which are almost always similar to the phenomena of hyperæmia. Here as well as in hyperæmia we have violent headache, great irritability of the organs of sense, buzzing in the ears, obscuration of sight, vertigo, and it is only from the course and the etiology of these phenomena that we obtain light regarding their probable cause. At a subsequent and more or less remote period symptoms of paralysis supervene. Such conditions are most readily misapprehended in the case of children, where they often set in in consequence of exhausting diarrhœa. They are likewise very apt to deceive when they occur in the further course of morbid processes involving a rapid loss of animal fluids, in which case they are but too easily mistaken for an entirely new and more recent affection of the brain. It is characteristic of most cases of anæmia that the symptoms either abate or disappear in the horizontal position, and that the inhibition of food or stimulating substances causes an improvement.—That syncope is generally determined by a suddenly arising anæmia of the brain, and not, as is generally supposed, by a semi-paralysis of the heart, results even from the great resemblance of syncope to anæmic phenomena, and is moreover confirmed by the fact that the same remedies are applicable in either case.

The course and duration of this disorder depend of course upon the determining pathological processes, upon which the prognosis likewise depends. What is certain is that the appearance of phenomena of cerebral anæmia is always a very bad symptom, especially in the case of children.

Treatment. Inasmuch as in subsequent chapters we shall have to revert more than once to cerebral anæmia, and more particularly in the general chapter on Anæmia where this subject is more specially treated of, we should have to indulge in useless repetitions, if we would furnish particular descriptions of every variety and modification of cerebral anæmia. For this reason we refer the reader to that chapter, contenting ourselves in this place with mentioning the most prominent remedies for anæmia of the brain when manifesting itself as an independent, and more particularly in the form of an acute disease.

Ammonium carbonicum. Notwithstanding its decisive action upon the brain, this remedy has not yet been employed to any very great extent in affections of this organ, more particularly for the reason that its cerebral symptoms have been falsely interpreted. These symptoms resemble in a very high degree those of hyperæmia, whereas a comparison of all the phenomena shows most emphatically that they characterize a condition of anæmia. As far as we know, no special accessory indications have as yet been enumerated for this agent which, at all events, is deserving of special consideration.

Camphora. This medicine shows a great contrast between exaltation and depression of the cerebral functions, the last-named condition being the most permanent symptom. Even a superficial view of the pathogenesis of this drug must satisfy everybody that it is remarkably suitable for anæmia. The effect of Camphor setting in and passing away again very rapidly, we shall have to depend upon it more commonly in cases where anæmia takes the form of syncope, more particularly when consequent upon sanguineous losses. An essential condition for its employment is that the organic reaction should not yet be extinct; on the contrary, that it should still be very active. It being known that the action of this medicine is of short duration, the doses should be given in rapid succession.

Ipecacuanha, as a cerebral remedy, is particularly suitable for children and after rapid losses of animal fluids, if symptoms of convulsion are present, together with more or less complete coma. In hæmorrhages it is likewise recommended by a number of practitioners; hence such accidents would not counter-indicate the use of this agent.

Secale cornutum deserves particular notice in the metrorrhagia of parturient females, and the resulting anæmic phenomena; here it acts in a twofold direction, against the hæmorrhage itself and, as is shown by a comparison of its physiological effects, against the symptoms emanating from the brain and the spinal marrow; upon both these organs it acts in a very marked manner.

Cuprum is only suitable in cases where the whole process is developed gradually, and is more especially characterized by spasmodic phenomena. It would hardly be applicable in cases of genuine anæmia; in general, excessive losses of animal fluids do not come within its range.

Other remedies deserving special consideration in this disorder are: *Arsenicum, Calcarea carbonica, Colchicum, Digitalis, Tartarus emeticus, Veratrum, Zincum, Silicea.* Some of these remedies have been mentioned as suitable for hyperæmia, a circumstance that may seem singular. This is in the first place partly owing to the fact that the pathogenesis of such drugs is not sufficiently distinct, and, in the second place, to this other fact that the same drug may manifest its action in two opposite directions, like Arsenic for instance, which not only occasions extraordinary symptoms of reaction, but likewise a complete prostration of all vital energies. In both these directions Arsenic can be used with great effect, which is likewise true of other medicines the successful application of which, in a variety of different pathological processes, shows that the whole series of pathogenetic phenomena, even the so-called phenomena of alternation, may serve as guides in selecting a remedy. In simple syncope medicinal interference will scarcely ever have to be resorted to, except where its frequent recurrence is owing to the existence of some other affection against which the treatment will have to be directed in such a case. A perfectly horizontal position is the simplest remedy against syncope, by which the attack is always considerably shortened; at the same time this may serve as evidence that the abnormal distribution of the blood is most generally the cause of syncope.

— — This is the most appropriate place to speak of a condition which is of importance to a practitioner for the reason that it is exceedingly troublesome and sometimes obstinate: it is vertigo. It is not our intention to give a list of the different kinds of vertigo and the numerous causes from which it may arise; we will confine ourselves to the vertigo about which old people so frequently complain, and which most generally seems such an isolated symptom that it is difficult to decide what causes occasion it. Under all circumstances it is a certain fact that it only emanates from the brain; but whether it is caused by hyperæmia or anæmia, is often as difficult to decide as it is on the other hand essential to do so, since such a decision exerts a most important influence upon the selection of the most efficient remedial agent. In order to arrive at such a decision, the most trifling symptoms are to be observed with the utmost care, and the circumstances under which the vertigo makes its appearance are to be considered with the most scrupulous attention. This course will show that the trouble arises from cerebral anæmia much more frequently than from hyperæmia. In such a case the former results from a defective condition of the cerebral arteries, in consequence of which the supply of blood is impeded, and the cerebral parenchyma is deprived of its proper nourishment, owing to which it may even become atrophied. This explains that anæmia may cause attacks of cerebral congestion, since atrophy of one portion of the brain deprives the other portion of the power to offer a normal resistance to the afflux of the blood. We will here mention a few of the distinctive diagnostic signs. The hyperæmic vertigo is seldom present early in the morning, is made worse by eating a little more than usual, particularly after the use of such stimulants as wine, coffee, etc.; it abates by persevering exercise, patients have to sit in a half-recumbent position; mental labor and excitement aggravate the vertigo, open air diminishes it, and it is generally accompanied by a slight headache. Anæmic vertigo, on the contrary, generally makes its appearance in the morning, is caused, or at any rate increased by exercise, particularly in the open air, is improved by the use of food and stimulants and likewise by exciting mental labor, and very soon disappears in a quiet recumbent position; it is very seldom attended with headache, nor need the patient exhibit any pallor of countenance. The remedies for hyperæmic vertigo are generally the same as those that have been mentioned for cerebral hyperæmia. At the head of the list we have *Belladonna*, which alone will remove it in most cases, beside which we have *Arnica*, *Nux vomica* and *Lachesis*. For anæmic vertigo the best remedies are: *Silicea*, *Baryta carbonica*, *Graphites*;—*Lycopodium*, *Ambra* and *Fluoris acidum* likewise deserve our attention.—After what we have stated it is self-evident that a suitable diet is a matter of course. In hyperæmic vertigo all overloading of the stomach and the use of stimulating substances have to be strictly forbidden, and habitual exercise has to be enjoined; while in anæmic vertigo a nourishing diet, the use of moderate quantities of wine, and mental and bodily rest are indispensable.—The fear of an apoplectic attack which is fully justified during the presence of hyperæmic vertigo, could only lead to false measures during the presence of anæmic vertigo, the employment of which would entail so much more injury as the apprehensive solicitude of the patient, which is already very troublesome, would be uselessly increased by such a proceeding.

[**Aconite** is suitable for hyperæmic vertigo, with nausea; the patients have sallow, dark complexions, or are plethoric individuals with flushed faces. *Digitalis* is excellent in vertigo, with slow, intermittent and irregular pulse. H.]

Cerebral Apoplexy.

We apply this name to a condition of the brain where, in consequence of some cause or other, an extravasation of blood takes place from the cerebral vessels into the substance of the brain. That such an extravasation can only take place from the arteries or capillaries, will not be doubted by any one who takes the laws of the circulatory process into consideration. The influences occasioning the apoplectic extravasation must always be of such a nature as to bring about an overpowering impulse of the sanguineous current over the resistance of the walls of the arteries, since it is only in this manner that the rupture of the blood-vessel is possible. In this respect we have to consider four points of view.—The structure of the blood-vessel may have become altered in consequence of its walls having lost their elasticity and having become brittle by the atheromatous process. In the next place the cerebral substance surrounding the vessel may have become altered in its consistence, so that the counter-pressure exerted by the brain may have become diminished or partially suspended, and resistance against the current of the blood is exclusively confined to the walls of the blood-vessel. This condition of things takes place in softening of the brain, and in apoplectic effusions undergoing the process of resorption. An entirely analogous condition exists in the atrophy of the brain peculiar to persons of an advanced age, and may constitute as frequent a cause of apoplexy as the atheromatous process. A third cause is the inherent weakness of the walls of the vessels that cannot be recognized by any peculiar diagnostic signs, and in consequence of which the vessel is lacerated by the violent impulse of the sanguineous current. Finally as a fourth cause may be viewed an alteration in the blood itself, this fluid becoming so thin that its principal constituents penetrate the walls of the vessels. This arrangement is most distinctly noticed in purpura where the petechiæ form upon the skin without any laceration of the vessels. Even if this last-mentioned form of extravasation does not constitute apoplexy in the rigorous acceptation of the term, yet, for the sake of analogy, this seemed the most suitable place to mention it.

The extravasation at times takes place from one, at other times from several, at times from smaller, at other times from larger vessels, is more or less considerable, and sets in with more or less suddenness. The quantity of effused blood generally, but not always, corresponds to the size of the blood-vessel. In accordance with these circumstances we distinguish two kinds of apoplectic effusion. The first kind is capillary apoplexy where the blood is effused from the finest vessels. In this form the apoplectic centres are generally present in larger number, are very small like ecchymoses, and scattered over a large surface. If they are so closely crowded together that they seem to constitute a single apoplectic locality, they form an apoplectic focus. The second kind of apoplexy is termed the apoplectic insultus, where a considerable quantity of blood is effused into the cerebral parenchyma from one or more larger vessels. The larger the vessel which pours out the blood, the more rapid the hæmorrhage, which is checked in proportion as the brain is capable of resisting the effusion of the blood. More blood is poured out where the brain is atrophied, or its volume had become lessened by contracting cicatrices remaining after former apoplexies; whereas, with a normal size of the cerebral mass, the flow of blood is arrested much more speedily. The hæmorrhage may likewise take place by fits and starts, so that a large coagulum may be gradually formed by the blood discharged from a vessel of proportionally small size. The changes which the cerebral mass undergoes in consequence of the extravasated blood, do not differ in degree merely. If the apoplectic coagulum is small, the fibres of the brain may retain their normal structure, and are only pressed asunder by the blood; in such a case a complete restoration of the affected portion of the brain may be considered certain as soon as the coagulum has been absorbed. But the more considerable and the more sudden the apoplectic attack, the more the affected portion of the brain becomes more or less completely disorganized, so that the cerebral fibres project into the coagulum as so many shapeless shreds or are mixed up with it in the form of a shapeless pap, (so-called red softening of the brain.) Such apoplectic coagula are surrounded by a more or less extensive infiltration of blood and ichor. If death does not take place immediately or very soon after the apoplectic effusion, the effused fluid undergoes certain definite changes. Either —and this is of more frequent occurrence—the blood is gradually absorbed except its solid constituents, the apoplectic coagulum becomes smaller and finally forms only a cicatrix of a yellowish or brownish tint, several of which are often seen in the same individual in different stages of development. Or else the portion of brain surrounding the effused blood reacts so powerfully that it becomes inflamed, and the exudation proceeding from it confines the blood as within a capsule. In such a case, likewise, a gradual metamorphosis of the blood takes place, leading to the formation of a cyst filled with a clear serous liquid. As a third possible result which is of the least frequent occurrence, it may happen that the irritating action of the extravasated blood develops an inflammation which, instead of leading to the formation of a cyst, causes suppuration, in which case all such causative influences come into play as will hereafter be mentioned when we come to treat of encephalitis. Death either takes place in consequence of the pressure exerted by the extravasated blood upon the brain, or, even if the pressure is proportionally slight, in consequence of paralysis of such portions of the brain as are absolutely necessary to the preservation of the vital functions. Although apoplexy may take place in any portion of the larger as well as the smaller brain, yet it occurs most frequently in the large brain, and here again more particularly on the confines between the white and gray substance.

As causes of cerebral apoplexy we may regard, in a general sense, the same as those that have been mentioned under cerebral hyperæmia; in addition to which another very frequent cause is the change caused in the texture of the cerebral vessels by the atheromatous process. From the circumstance that apoplexy is not of sufficient occurrence to justify the belief in epidemic apoplexy, we are authorized to draw the conclusion that atmospheric influences favor such accidents; however, it is not, by any means, certain what kind of atmospheric impressions are favorable to apoplexy, although we are pretty well satisfied that a low range of the barometer is a marked indication of the presence of such influences. Hence it has been observed that most apoplexies take place about the time of the equinoxes. Since cerebral hæmorrhages may take place in every age, no age can be regarded as exempt from such dangers, though small children are very seldom attacked. It occurs most frequently in persons beyond the age of fifty, and its occurrence becomes more frequent in proportion as they advance in years beyond this period. This is naturally owing to the above-mentioned changes in the vessels of the brain, and in the cerebral mass itself.

We have purposely devoted more space to the pathological portion of this section than the object of this work required. We have done this for the purpose of opposing Hartmann's own peculiar views, (vol. II., page 311, &c.) In accordance with the formerly prevailing views about apoplexy, he adopts four kinds of this disease, *apoplexia sanguinea, nervosa, serosa,* and *gastrica,* starting at times from the cause and, at other times, from the effect as a principle of classification, whereas the pathological process in the brain is, after all, the same.—That nervous apoplexy is possible, may be admitted, though not in Hartmann's sense, but we need not care from what cause it arises,—(it is said to have been observed to take place in consequence of crushing mental emotions;)—since, on account of the suddenness of the fatal result, it can never become an object of cure. The other divisions are equally valueless in a therapeutic point of view, especially when the treatment is conducted in accordance with homœopathic principles, since under this treatment the determination of the pathological process in the brain implies an examination of all the exciting and co-operating circumstances with a view of selecting the proper remedy. If we would enumerate corresponding categories, they would be almost endless.

The symptoms by which an attack of apoplexy manifests itself differ a good deal. In many cases the attack is preceded by well-marked precursory symptoms of various kinds, very much like the symptoms denoting cerebral hyperæmia. Very frequently abnormal precursory symptoms are entirely absent, unless we mean to regard, as such, symptoms that are peculiar to the age of the affected person. If the hæmorrhage sets in suddenly, the activity of the brain is suddenly paralyzed, the patient falls down without uttering a sound, is unconscious, insensible, partially or totally paralyzed, so that stool and urine pass off involuntarily; the breathing is stertorous, slow, the expirations are characterized by the blowing movements of the mouth; the pulse is at times full, hard, and slow, at times so feeble that it can scarcely be felt; the pupils are at times dilated, at others contracted, sometimes quite normal, the eyes are staring and glassy; speech is suspended, and one corner of the mouth is drawn down paralyzed. Not unfrequently there is vomiting; the face may neither be flushed nor hotter than usual.—If the extravasation is proceeding slowly, the patients first complain of headache, or even only of a disagreeable sensation in the head, they feel languid and indisposed to any thing, they sometimes have to vomit. They are not yet deprived of the power of motion. Soon, however, according as the extravasation is more or less extensive, symptoms of paralysis set in, with which all the above-described symptoms may become associated. How long it may take before the attack is complete, has been shown me even a short time ago. It was the case of a man who experienced the first symptoms early in the morning; about noon he called at my office, after having walked a long distance. One arm was already semi-paralyzed, and it was late in the night when the whole of one side became paralyzed.—If the quantity of effused blood is small, the symptoms often consist only in paralysis of one side of the body, especially of the tongue or of one arm; or the brain is deprived of the faculty of performing a certain function of the mind, so that the patient has to stutter or is unable to find single words or his memory is lost. These changes often happen to old people who often retire in the evening in good health, and wake in the morning partially paralyzed.

If the patient was not struck with death at the outset, the attack runs a very slow course, such as must necessarily be expected considering the nature of the pathological process. Small effusions are re-absorbed without leaving any perceptible derangements, and the symptoms of paralysis which they had superinduced often disappear again with surprising rapidity. If the effusion of blood is considerable, the paralysis can only disappear partially, for the reason that the destruction of the fibres of the brain causes an unavoidably incurable paralysis; months may elapse before the cure reaches its highest point. As a general rule, it is at the commencement that the progress in the improvement is most distinct, and continues so, as long as those portions of the brain which surround the coagulum, continue to divest themselves of their infiltration, which takes place in a proportionally rapid manner.

At the commencement of the attack, it is very difficult to give a satisfactory prognos's. Although it is true, as a general rule, that the danger to life is greater in proportion as the paralysis extends, beside involving the mental functions, over a larger portion of the body, and that it is greatest if the respiratory and circulatory organs are involved in the paralysis, yet it not unfrequently happens that patients who seem to have been struck beyond all chances of recovery, recover their consciousness and a proportional restoration of the bodily functions, whereas other cases of much more favorable appearance terminate fatally. If the patients live through the first twenty-four or forty-eight hours without any increase of the symptoms, their restoration may be expected so much more certainly. Frequent recurrences of an apoplectic attack render the prognosis of each following attack more dubious; patients who have been attacked once, have constantly to be on their guard against a recurrence of the attack.

Treatment. Before giving a more circumstantial account of the remedies that may be advantageously employed in apoplexy, it behooves us in the first place to answer the question what effect we expect of the remedies prescribed and what expectations we may entertain of their curative action.—Apoplexy of itself is no disease in the same sense as the idea of disease is generally conceived; it is only the last link, at least in the larger number of cases, of a chain of pathological alterations that are made manifest by the preliminary stage. It is only in a very small number of cases that these preliminary symptoms come within the range of professional observation, for the reason that they generally seem unimportant, often last only a short time, and still more frequently are of such a nature that even the physician is unable to recognize them with positive certainty as the precursory symptoms of apoplexy. Most generally the physician is sent for when the apoplectic effusion is in full tide of progress or has even reached its limits. In the former case we have to determine whether the causes of the attack are still in operation, with a view of meeting them and arresting the continuance of the hæmorrhage. In the second case our inquiries have to be confined to what remedies will bring about the absorption of the extravasated blood in order to free the brain from this pressure. It is of the utmost importance that this result should be reached as soon as possible, inasmuch as the probability that the disabled parts of the brain will again resume their functional activity, depends in a great measure upon the speed with which their deliverance from the abnormal pressure is accomplished; if this should take place too slowly, we have to apprehend atrophy of these parts, and the number of the paralyzed parts remains much larger than if the extravasated blood had been reabsorbed more speedily. This is one of those cases where the existing symptoms are not sufficient to determine the proper remedial agent, but where the internal process with whose nature we are acquainted from analogous cases, must necessarily serve as our guide. For this reason it is perfectly useless to undertake to cure paralysis of years' standing, that had remained after apoplexy; such paralysis is, and will always remain incurable, since we cannot well expect to replace material tissues that are lost, by internal treatment.

Although discussions about the results of other methods of treatment are not within the province of this work, yet we cannot refrain from offering a few words of comment upon the favorite remedy in apoplexy, local or general sanguineous depletion. Although in latter years important authorities among our therapeutic opponents have pronounced against blood-letting in apoplexy, yet this expedient is still so generally resorted to by physicians and so devoutly worshipped by laymen that genuine courage is required to criticize. And yet it can be shown *a priori* that its effect can only be injurious; in no case its employment has as yet resulted in an undeniable cure, whereas, on the contrary, it is highly probable,— we have not the means of saying absolutely certain,—that depletion does not diminish the apoplectic extravasation and subsequently facilitates a more rapid resorption.—In one respect the effect of every sanguineous depletion is of short duration, since the impulse of the current of blood is depressed only for a few hours. Viewed from this point, blood-letting may seem an excellent remedy for an apoplectic effusion of blood. But in another respect the loss of blood causes a decrease of the solid constituents of the blood, without occasioning a corresponding decrease of the fluid constituents whose loss is repaired very rapidly. Hence the fluidity of the blood increases, and the blood not only exudes or extravasates much more easily, but it loses the faculty of coagulating and arresting the hæmorrhage by the formation of clots in proportion as more blood is drawn off by the artificial depletion. Even if the process of extravasation should still be going on, the usefulness of depletion is, to say the least, counter-balanced, if not outweighed, by the previously mentioned disadvantages. If this were not so, why should not sanguineous depletions have been resorted to for the purpose of arresting other hæmorrhages, from the uterus, for instance; in a case of this kind the ancient theory of blood-letting might either easily be confirmed or else demonstrated as mischievous and absurd. Even if in some or even many cases the patient experience a momentary relief, a short suspension of the hæmorrhagic process, this apparently favorable result is abundantly neutralized by the usually considerable reaction succeeding the brief period of rest. The same thing takes place here as in pneumonia, where the depletion, generally speaking, is likewise followed by an abatement of the symptoms, which is very soon succeeded by a so much more considerable aggravation. Resorting to such evanescent expedients implies not only a deception of one's own judgment, but likewise a disappointment of the poor patient's expectations. But, we will ask in conclusion, does not blood-letting favor the resorption of the extravasated blood? To effect resorption a certain amount of vascular activity is undoubtedly required. That resorption is not favored by a loss of animal fluids; that it is effected most rapidly in the normal condition of the organism; that it becomes slower and more insufficient in proportion as the patient is more enfeebled: is noticed in so many cases more immediately accessible to observation, that we may conclude with certainty the action of the brain is similarly affected. Under all circumstances the whole body is weakened by a loss of blood which depresses vascular activity and acts in opposition to the very conditions upon which a rapid resorption depends.— The reasons we have mentioned seem to us sufficient to reject a resort to sanguineous depletion in every case of apoplexy. Even if we were willing to concede to blood-letting in this affection an appearance of usefulness or even of active aid, after all it would only be against the hyperæmia that accompanies and as it were occasions the apoplectic attack. Where the apoplexy is an accomplished fact, blood-letting seems to us like a crime. All the previously mentioned reasons derive a higher significance from the circumstance that the individuals who are struck with apoplexy are generally very far advanced in years, in whom the functional equilibrium, if once disturbed, is restored much more slowly than in young people.

We have already stated that the preliminary stage generally presents the symptoms of a more or less violent cerebral hyperæmia, on which account we may content ourselves with referring for the treatment of this stage to our statements concerning the treatment of hyperæmia. The other functional derangements with which the preliminary symptoms may be complicated, present such a great variety that it is impossible to furnish even an approximative enumeration of all imaginable cases; in such cases which rank undoubtedly among the more serious, the study of the Materia Medica itself can alone come to our aid. The remedies mentioned under hyperæmia have such an extensive range of action that it is only in rare cases that one of them will not be found available; in order to be convinced of this fact, all that we shall have to do, will be to institute a careful comparison of the special symptoms. If, in the following paragraph, we repeat some of the remedies that have been mentioned for hyperæmia, it is because in every case of apoplexy it may still be necessary to first act against the hyperæmia that may continue to exist; it is less important to aim at a resorption of the fluid that has already become effused than to prevent a further spread of the extravasation.

Belladonna. There is scarcely one case of apoplexy where this remedy is not suitable and sometimes has a magic effect. What we have stated above regarding the constitutions that are a suitable sphere of action for Belladonna points to apoplexy. But inasmuch as the symptoms of hyperæmia are much more characteristic of Belladonna than the subsequent symptoms of apoplexy, it will be found more particularly indicated in cases where the apoplectic effusion is still attended with violent symptoms of congestion. Belladonna is more particularly indicated by the following symptoms: red and injected conjunctiva; sparkling, glistening eyes; greatly dilated pupils; diplopia; excessive restlessness of the extremities; great anxiety; illusions of the senses. It is not likely that this remedy will have any direct influence over the extravasated blood itself, and will therefore have to be given within the first twelve hours of the attack. But inasmuch as, according to our previous remarks, the extravasated blood may, according to circumstances, excite a powerful inflammatory reaction, Belladonna will, although rarely, come into play even in the further course of the attack. In this last-named condition it competes with

Aconite, which we do not think possesses any special power in hyperæmia or apoplexy, but which is in its place, and preferable to

Belladonna, if a process of exudative inflammation should have to be overcome. This alone shows that it is only in a few cases of apoplexy that Aconite will be found indicated.

Of **Coffea**, Hartmann says that it deserves especial notice in cases of apoplexy that have been caused in very sensitive individuals by a variety of violent emotions. According to this author the effect of Coffea is evanescent and only palliative. This remedy is particularly suitable in cases characterized by extreme irritability of the organs of sense and of the nervous system generally, sad and whining mood, sleeplessness on account of excessive mental and bodily excitement, frequent flashes of heat in the face, anxiety and a headache as if the brain had been bruised, or vertigo, with a sensation of heaviness in the head, excessive sensitiveness of hearing on the days preceding the attack.

Opium is undoubtedly a remedy of particular importance in most cases of apoplexy. We do not think that the characteristic indications for this remedy in apoplexy can be given with more precision than by copying the essential parts of Hartmann's own statement: " Opium corresponds to all those forms of apoplexy whose symptoms resemble those that we notice in drunkards. This drug is of great use were it for no other reason than because in apoplexy the vital force is so much depressed that even the most appropriate remedies do not excite any organic reaction and hence remain without any effect whatever. Opium possesses the important and peculiar faculty of supplying this deficiency of reactive power in very many cases and rousing the vital forces from their lethargic condition. In order to attain this object a single small dose is often sufficient; sometimes more than one dose is required. Since Opium has a limited sphere of action and seems to exert a beneficial influence only in cases of recent origin, it is evident that its exhibition in apoplexy must not be delayed too long if we expect to derive benefit from its employment. The following symptoms are in every case characteristic indications for its use: Comatose sopor, with stertorous and rattling breathing, and depression of the lower jaw; impossibility to rouse the patient; or he can at most only be roused enough to cause him to gaze around unconsciously without answering a single question; the face is flushed, bluish-red, bloated; the patient moans, groans, moves his lips continually as if he were talking; the pulse is large and slow, the breathing oppressed and anxious; the face is covered with a profuse and cold sweat; the head feels heavy; if the patient attempts to raise it, it immediately sinks back upon the pillow; the temporal arteries pulsate strongly and visibly."

In real apoplexy **Hyoscyamus** may not often be found suitable; Hartmann mentions as a characteristic sign of this drug: suddenness of the attack, the patient falls down at once with a violent cry, followed by convulsive motions, and rattling and snoring. The patient looks wild and livid.

Laurocerasus. Without contradiction no poisonous agent, in its physiological as well as toxical effects, exhibits so much similarity to apoplexy as this one. In the lesser grades of poisoning with Laurocerasus a very marked hyperæmia of the brain is one of the most constant phenomena; in the higher grades this hyperæmia increases until paralysis results from it. A post-mortem examination almost always shows a copious extravasation of blood in the cranium. There is scarcely a more characteristic image of apoplexy to be found anywhere. Nevertheless, our literature does not furnish any evidence that this drug is used much in apoplexy, certainly much less frequently than it ought to be. Special characteristic indications are nowhere to be found. In Hartmann's recommendation that the drug should be used if the attack sets in suddenly, without any precursory symptoms, and the patient is struck down suddenly as if dead, there is scarcely any thing characteristic to be seen; moreover such cases are very rare, nor do we see why the signs of cerebral congestion that necessarily precede the extinction of nervous activity, should be entirely overlooked in such cases. The effects of *Prussic acid*, on the contrary, give us the image of a peculiar form of apoplexy; we subjoin a description of these effects for the reason that this knowledge will facilitate a determination of the cases where this remedy will prove suitable. As soon as the poison is swallowed the individual experiences a sensation of excessive and unconquerable muscular debility, vertigo, stupefaction, inability to stand. The pupils become dilated, the visual power is extinct, the patient is seized with violent anguish and palpitation of the heart. The skin becomes cold, moist, insensible, the pulse can scarcely be felt. At this stage convulsions frequently set in, the more readily, it would seem, the smaller the quantity of the poison that had been swallowed; these convulsions affect more particularly the muscles of the face or represent peculiar rotatory movements of the trunk; trismus is almost always present, in some rare cases opisthotonos. Very frequently, however, all convulsive symptoms are absent, and the poisoned individual is struck down as by the hand of death a few seconds after the poison had been swallowed, and without uttering a cry. This concise picture contains a few symptoms that are undoubtedly calculated to determine the choice of this agent; they are the following: palpitations of the heart while the pulse is almost imperceptible; a cold and moist skin, trismus, convulsions of the facial muscles. Coma consequent upon poisoning with Prussic acid has this peculiarity that it completely resembles a deep, very quiet sleep. By these symptoms it would seem we might easily decide where this drug is suitable or not in a case of apoplexy.

Nux vomica. If we include this drug in the list of remedies for apoplexy, it is not because we place much reliance upon it in this affection, but in order to satisfy the numerous recommendations of other practitioners. Except the paralytic depression of the lower jaw, no symptom is indicated that would justify the selection of this agent. Its being suitable to wine-bibbers and coffee-drinkers is probably mere theory. Considering the totality of its toxicological effects they do not point to apoplexy, but, on the contrary, to simple hyperæmia.

The following drugs are likewise worthy of mention in this place: *Ipecacuanha*, *Cocculus*, *Veratrum* and *Phosphorus*. For a chronic disposition to apoplexy, with danger of a frequent recurrence of the attack, Kafka likewise recommends Glonoin.

We shall now turn to the remedies that have to be employed against the apoplectic effusion in order to effect or rather accelerate its resorption, or to oppose the excessive reaction of the organism. Many who are as yet unacquainted with the practical results of Homœopathy, will scarcely be willing to admit, on account of all sorts of theoretical reasons, that the resorption of the extravasated blood can be affected at all by such small doses of internal remedies. We shall not attempt to refute their theoretical arguments by other theories, but we claim the full right to refer to our practical results. It is true that in apoplexy these results can scarcely ever be presented as incontrovertible facts, since opponents can fall back upon the expedient of attributing all such cures to the healing powers of Nature. But if in other cases of exudation, the existence of which can be demonstrated by physical investigation, the effused fluid has been re-absorbed under the influence of small doses of internally administered medicines, we have a right to conclude from analogy that, in a case of apoplectic extravasation, the internal employment of medicines is not only founded in reason, but must likewise lead to successful results.

Among all the medicines belonging to this category, Arnica occupies the first rank. Even in the Old-School Materia Medica it is recommended as an excellent remedy for apoplexy. To a homœopathic physician its physiological effects reveal its important action upon the brain, since these effects contain all the signs of violent congestion; moreover we are justified in concluding from what we witness of the action of Arnica in injuries complicated with external sanguineous extravasations, that this agent possesses an extraordinary power of determining the re-absorption of the extravasated blood. It is most suitable for individuals not too far advanced in age, with a full habit and vigorous frame, and it is rather important, if we wish to secure a favorable result from this drug, that its employment should not be delayed beyond the period when the process of extravasation in the brain may be considered terminated. The presence of slight febrile reaction constitutes an additional indication for Arnica in persons of that description. As a matter of course no immediate improvement can be expected after its employment, hence it will be well to continue its use for some time before other remedies are resorted to

Sulphur comes into play in apoplexy where the action of Arnica terminates. This statement defines very exactly the relative position of Sulphur in the list of remedies for such an accident. Hence it is applicable in the subsequent stages of the apoplectic effusion. Its employment in apoplexy is sufficiently justified by its extraordinary effects in other depositions of long standing. The remedies that compete with *Sulphur*, and are of special importance in cases where, from reasons that we are unable to account for, this agent remains without effect, are *Silicea* and *Baryta carbonica*. The latter is particularly suitable for old people. Hartmann relates a brilliant instance where Baryta caused a great improvement in the organs of speech.

Iodium is not indicated in simple, uncomplicated apoplexy; at any rate it yields the palm to the other remedies that have already been mentioned. If the reaction becomes so marked that it has to be regarded as depending upon an inflammation of those parts of the brain that surround the extravasated coagulum, *Sulphur* comes into play. We shall revert to this subject when speaking of meningitis to which we refer. These remarks likewise apply to *Mercurius*.

None of the remedies that we have named are capable of healing an apoplectic attack where a good deal of blood has become extravasated and a portion of the brain is destroyed, so that the functions of the brain will be completely restored. Isolated symptoms of paralysis will remain, the removal of which we may pronounce a very questionable task, but which, especially in cases of somewhat recent standing, we ought not to give up without trying all proper means of effecting a cure. In many cases we have often succeeded, contrary to our expectations, in removing such derangements either totally or at least partially. The medicines upon which we shall have to depend in such cases have not so much any immediate connection with apoplexy as with the subsequently remaining paralysis.

Causticum here occupies very properly the first rank. Although this drug has been regarded with suspicion, especially in former times, and although many homœopaths continue to regard its action as questionable and problematical when judged from a purely theoretical stand-point, yet its practical results are so surprising that this fact alone compels us to believe in its efficiency. In cases of paralysis belonging to this range, *Causticum*, even after every other drug has been tried in vain, will still show good results which, it is true, are often enough confined only to a very slight improvement. It is most suitable in paralysis of the extremities, especially when complicated with muscular contraction; it is less suitable in paralysis of the organs of the head, such as the tongue, pharynx, eyelids. Among the derangements of the mental functions it is an inability to select the proper words, for which this remedy may be prescribed.

Zincum is particularly indicated in cases where the senses remain disturbed after the attack; complete paralysis does not come within the therapeutic range of this drug; it is even doubtful whether any thing can be done for the hemiplegia when manifested by constant involuntary movements.

Cuprum. Everybody knows how constantly paralysis is present in poisoning with copper. It has this peculiarity that the motor power is extinct and the paralyzed part grows thinner, while the nerves of sensation preserve their normal functional power. Copper does not affect the functions of the senses in the least, the mental functions remain undisturbed; total or partial paralysis of the tongue, on the other hand, occurs very frequently, and shows itself by a stuttering or deficient speech. In accordance with these indications it will be found easy to determine the cases where copper is indicated. We may add that violent, almost unyielding contractions or chorea-like paroxysms and automatic movements constitute additional indications for the use of this agent.

Plumbum is still more characteristic in its effects than the previously mentioned drug. We believe that we can do no better than to give a connected list of the principal symptoms of lead-poisoning, by which means they will become much more comprehensible than by a perusal of their scattered record in our ordinary treatises on pathogenesis. We have obtained the symptoms from various cases of poisoning which are described with marked accuracy in some of our journals. We have: hypochondriac, peevish, indifferent, desponding, apathetic mood; the consciousness is blunted, dull, not wanting altogether; loss of memory, complete absence of volition; the speech is impeded and interrupted; single syllables are omitted, or the patient is unable to combine syllables which he had spelt, into words; mimic spasms of the mouth and face when speaking; trembling of the tongue when it is put out; semiparalysis of the buccinator muscles and of the velum palatinum, which manifests itself by violent snoring;—sleeplessness, fear of death; the organs of the senses are torpid and insensible, the eyes are principally affected; the eyelids droop as if paralyzed; the pupils are almost constantly and considerably dilated; all objects seem smaller and farther removed from the focus of vision; they may be seen as through a gauze; diplopia; the pulse is always slow, fifty to sixty in the minute; sometimes it feels even hard and tense like a wire; all the muscles may be paralyzed; in partial paralysis the left side is more frequently attacked, a phenomenon that may be connected with the marked heart-symptoms caused by lead;—the paralysis affects equally the motor and the sentient nerves, is often attended with violent pains in the paralyzed parts, likewise with considerable contractions of the paralyzed parts, especially of the extensor muscles which feel hard as wood; in other cases the spasms are tonic which, if they reach their full development, run into completely epileptic convulsions. The muscles of the affected parts become atrophied. If the paralysis is not complete, the patient's gait is unsteady, with particular tendency to fall forward. Even the respiratory muscles seem to be susceptible to the poisoning action of lead, on which account such individuals are often attacked with a high degree of dyspnœa. The sphincters are scarcely ever paralyzed; if they should be, death is imminent. This description of the essential features of lead-poisoning not only shows very fully and clearly where lead comes into play after an attack of apoplexy, but it likewise shows the characteristic differences between a poisoning by lead and one by copper. Lead might suggest itself at the very outset of an apoplectic attack, if we merely look at the symptoms without considering the mode and manner of their origin; this poison never acts instantaneously, or in every case with a certain degree of rapidity; on the contrary, a long time intervenes between the commencement of the intoxication and the fatal termination, from which we infer that the medicinal action must likewise be very slow. This may likewise serve as a hint that the drug should not be discontinued too soon.

If we deviate in this instance from our purpose to omit all remarks concerning doses, and allow a suggestion bearing upon this point to slip in, we have to justify this exceptional proceeding by the importance of the subject. The last-named medicines act much better in paralysis when given in high than when given in low potencies. If one of them has not effected any thing in the lower preparations and still seems indicated by the symptoms, it should by all means be tried in the higher potencies and in less frequent repetitions before it is dismissed as not suitable. We have seen too many cases where good results were not obtained until this change was made, to justify our urgent advice.

The following remedies may likewise be added to the present list: *Argentum, Graphites, Rhus toxicodendron, Anacardium.*

Regarding dietetic and other rules, it seems hardly necessary to offer any suggestions. We would warn, however, against the diet being too severely restricted in every case of apoplexy. Though this should undoubtedly be done in the case of well-fed or perhaps too well-fed individuals, yet apoplexy may likewise befal persons with impoverished constitutions; in their case it would certainly be wrong if we were to deprive the body of the diet which it requires in order to restore the normal equilibrium of its functions. As we have previously contended against sanguineous depletions, we here contend against applications of cold water or ice. In simple congestion these applications refresh the patient a good deal, and certainly do not do the least harm; but in a case of apoplexy we deem such applications both useless and hurtful, so much the more the older and feebler the affected individual, and the greater the difficulty of restoring the lost warmth.

Inflammatory Affections of the Brain and its Membranes.

The phenomena of most of the inflammatory affections of the brain resemble each other so much in all their general characteristics that it is sometimes impossible to point out, during the lifetime of the patient, the precise locality of the brain that is the seat of the affection. We may dispense with the almost useless trouble to specify the particular processes, so much more as it is of no particular use in practice. Viewed from this point we shall discuss only three kinds of the inflammatory processes as being distinguished from each other by essential characteristics: meningitis, a partial inflammation of the cerebral substance, and granular meningitis.

1. Meningitis.

This species of inflammatory affection of the brain is by far the most frequent; it is seated in the pia mater, but most generally the arachnoid and even the brain become involved in the pathological process. Regarding its origin, it is scarcely ever a genuine primary, more frequently a secondary affection. In the former case the causative circumstances which we have mentioned already as causes of cerebral hyperæmia, are likewise applicable to meningitis, more especially the poisoning by alcohol and excessive mental exertions, nor ought we to omit mentioning sexual excesses as an exciting cause. Very often no opportunity is given for ascertaining the particular causes of the inflammation. It may set in in the form of a secondary affection as a continuation and complication of other pathological processes within the cranium, for instance of inflammatory affections of the ears, or it may constitute a continuation of a neighboring inflammation to the brain, as in erysipelas, or it may exist as a complication of the inflammation of other important organs, as in pneumonia, more particularly if the serous membranes of these organs are the seat of the inflammation, (pleuritis, pericarditis, etc.,) or finally it may set in suddenly as a most serious complication during the period of convalescence or, at any rate, during the decrease of some important disease of the general organism. This is most frequently observed during the course of acute exanthems from whose sudden disappearance we are too easily disposed to derive the opinion that the inflammation has a metastatic origin, to which subject we shall refer more fully when treating of the exanthemata. We may likewise mention that in France an epidemic meningitis has been observed, the more immediate cause of which is still enveloped in obscurity.

In almost all cases the seat of meningitis is the convex portion of the brain, scarcely ever the base, which, however, may become involved in the inflammatory process in a more or less intense degree. The pia mater is found injected in various degrees of intensity and extent, the arachnoid is covered with a layer of exsudation, and the subarachnoideal space is filled with an exuded substance, most generally of the consistence of jelly. If the brain is involved in the inflammation, the cortical substance is alone affected. In chronic meningitis the pia mater is found dim, thickened, adhering more or less firmly to the brain; the subarachnoideal space contains a small quantity of a badly colored exuded material.

Symptoms and Course.—The symptoms of incipient meningitis differ according as it sets in as a primary or secondary affection. In the former case the disease often commences like other inflammations of important organs, with a violent chill, which is very speedily succeeded by a great increase of temperature, or the attack may be preceded by a precursory stage where, beside a general feeling of sickness, disturbed appearance of the countenance and violent headache, no other local symptoms are yet present. As soon as the disease has reached its full development, the most striking symptom is an unusual increase of the temperature and an equally unusual frequency of the pulse, as high as 160 beats in the minute. The headache increases to an almost intolerable degree of intensity, the organs of the senses are extremely sensitive to external stimuli, the eyes more particularly are sensitive to the light, touching the skin even causes pain. The face shows a peculiar expression of anxiety and tension, the look is restless and confused, the conjunctiva is strikingly injected. Sleep is restless, disturbed by frightful dreams from which the patients are frequently roused with a loud cry; or else the patients are completely deprived of all sleep, and during the few moments of slumber they may sink into, the observer is struck by a constant motion of their hands. There is consciousness, but it is confuse, and the patients are apt to give uncertain, tardy answers. If there is sleeplessness, delirium of a light character often sets in during the waking state of the patient. Respiration is very irregular, at times strikingly hurried, at other times unusually calm. At this stage the pupils are generally contracted. Vomiting is not unfrequent. In this condition, which has few characteristic symptoms peculiar to it and sometimes seems so little threatening that no apprehension is felt regarding a change for the worse in the next stage of the disease, the patients continue sometimes one, and at times even eight days, when all at once the more dangerous symptoms break out, usually attended with short-lasting convulsions, a prominent feature of which is a contraction of the cervical muscles. The delirium now becomes more continuous, at times furibond, at others more muttering, consciousness disappears more and more, the patient's look becomes staring and fixed. Paroxysms of clonic as well as tonic spasms set in. In proportion as the other threatening symptoms increase, the pulse does not increase in frequency, on the contrary it becomes slower, sometimes irregular and intermittent, the cutaneous temperature becomes unequal, hands and feet are often icy-cold while the rest of the body feels burning-hot. The patient sometimes falls very suddenly into a deep sopor from which he wakes only for a few brief moments half-conscious or delirious; the features sink as if collapsed. The headache evidently still continues, the patients grasp at their heads, which now begin to feel cold whereas their bodies continue hot. At this stage the pulse almost always becomes slower, either resuming its normal frequency or sinking even below it; the irregularity of the respiration likewise becomes a very prominent symptom. Symptoms of paralysis sometimes make their appearance, occasionally with rigid contraction of single bundles of muscles; whereas the bowels are obstinately confined, the urine passes off involuntarily. While these threatening symptoms develop themselves, an apparent improvement sometimes takes place which is, however, deceptive. Death ensues during the sopor, sometimes after a previous acceleration of the pulse and the respiration, scarcely ever beyond the third week. If the disease runs a favorable course, the improvement commences with a deep sleep during which the pulse and the respiration have to improve if this sleep is to be regarded as a favorable prognostic. In such a case the patient wakes restored to consciousness which, however, is not entirely free; in general, recovery from this disease takes place very gradually. The diagnosis of this disease is not, by any means, absolutely reliable. In the first stages it is easily confounded with simple hyperæmia or acute anæmia. This, however, would only be of importance in regard to anæmia, whereas in hyperæmia the treatment is pretty nearly the same as in the first stages of meningitis. It is much more important, however, if meningitis is confounded with typhus. That such a mistake can be easily made and for a long time, has been shown us by the case of our own child, which the many physicians who saw it, diagnosed as meningitis, whereas the true character of the affection was only revealed during the period of convalescence, when everybody who had nursed the child had a more or less violent attack of abdominal typhus. The only symptom which induced us to adhere to our opinion that the child had typhus was a diarrhœa that lasted a fortnight. Whatever favorable an opinion we may entertain of a purely symptomatic treatment, we certainly shall have to investigate the real origin of the symptoms, since it cannot be regarded with indifference whether we treat a case of typhus or meningitis even if the symptoms should be ever so similar. Of the other affections that may be confounded with meningitis, we mention uræmia and an acute attack of tuberculosis. It is likewise difficult to establish a sure diagnosis in cases where meningitis sets in from the start as a complication of inflammations of important organs, such as the lungs, pleura or pericardium. In such a case the inflammation of the brain is very readily overlooked in consequence of the absorbing interest excited by the inflammation of the other organs.

As a secondary affection the disease sets in very gradually; the patient at most complains of headache, after which the symptoms of exudation break out quite suddenly, the patient becoming dull, indifferent, the features collapse, a light delirium sets in, the extremities become less movable, the pulse decreases in frequency. Death ensues amid a continual increase of the sopor and the paralytic phenomena.

The prognosis in this affection is always very dubious, generally very unfavorable, the more so the more marked and extensive are the symptoms of paralysis. Nevertheless we know that, under homœopathic treatment, a cure is still possible in every stage of the disease; whereas physicians of other Schools declare that, in the stage of exudation, recovery is so little possible that; where it is supposed to have been accomplished, it is almost certain that some other affection had been mistaken for meningitis. Statistical evidence in meningitis and diseases of the brain generally, is very little reliable, since an absolutely certain diagnosis can only be established in very few or fatal cases. In homœopathic statistics a number of cases would undoubtedly be impugned as incorrect: is this not done by our opponents even in regard to cases whose diagnosis has become a thing of absolute certainty to every educated physician? On the other hand it cannot be denied that in our literature many cases are described as meningitis which, in reality, are simple hyperæmia of the brain; all we have to do, in order to be satisfied on this score, is to compare Rückert's short extracts, (Klinische Erfahrungen, vol. I., page 105, etc.) If all these cases had been cases of incipient meningitis, it would imply that we possess much more efficient remedies for meningitis than we do for other inflammations whose diagnosis we are able to watch and establish at every step with perfect certainty. Why do we scarcely ever hear of pneumonia cut short? Is it more difficult to cut such an inflammation short? It is undoubtedly proper to treat all such lucky and successful cures to a good dose of scepticism.

Treatment.

Belladonna is one of the medicines that is most frequently resorted to at the commencement of a supposed meningitis. In Rückert's above-mentioned work, *loco cit.*, we find the reports of a number of strikingly successful and rapid cures which excite in our minds most particular doubts. An attentive comparison will show that in those cases only the remedy acted in a marked manner where a sure diagnosis was not yet possible, whereas in inflammations that had progressed to a higher degree, the improvement was either slower or else was not at all due to the sole action of Belladonna. A number of reasons prompt us to believe that Belladonna is no remedy for meningitis, or, at any rate, that we possess better remedies for this disease. This opinion is confirmed by the results of postmortem examinations in cases of poisoning with Belladonna, where we indeed find a high degree of hyperæmia, but never a trace of exudation; it is likewise a known fact that the lighter cases of poisoning with Belladonna, having no fatal termination, recover in a proportionally short period of time in spite of the severest cerebral symptoms. Nevertheless, in spite of all opposing arguments, the symptoms of incipient meningitis will first and foremost point to *Belladonna*, and almost any one who is familiarly acquainted with the Materia Medica, will first exhibit this remedy without laying particular stress on a precise diagnosis. That the Belladonna enables us to establish such a diagnosis, may be asserted without fear of contradiction. This medicine exerts so positively a curative influence upon hyperæmia when simulating meningitis, that, where it does not cure, it at least causes an improvement within at most twenty-four hours with so much certainty, that to most cases we may apply the rule: where, in apparently inflammatory conditions of the brain, *Belladonna* is not succeeded by, at least, a striking improvement within twenty-four hours, no hyperæmia is present; in such a case it should be discontinued, and some other remedy should be given in its stead. Another symptom which counter-indicates *Belladonna* to some extent, is an extraordinary frequency of the pulse, which is very seldom present in hyperæmia of the brain.

Aconitum. At the commencement of meningitis this remedy is almost as important a remedy as Belladonna at the commencement of hyperæmia. It is almost always suitable to the previously expressed conditions, where Belladonna seemed indicated, but had no curative effect, namely in the initial stage of meningitis; if meningitis can be arrested in its course by any one remedy, it is by Aconite. Corresponding as it does to the whole process of the inflammation, the improvement caused by Aconite cannot be as rapid and complete as the improvement caused by Belladonna in hyperæmia. This remedy is in its place as long as no symptoms of exudation have made their appearance. As soon as the pulse becomes slower and the intensity of the general symptoms increases; as soon as the first symptoms of paralysis set in, Aconite is no longer indicated.

Opium. In so far as this drug is recommended as a remedy for meningitis, we have to apply to it the remarks which we have offered in a previous paragraph concerning Belladonna. At a later stage of the disease, when sopor sets in, it frequently acts very favorably against this condition, and, when given as an intercurrent remedy, it paves the way for other medicines, as has been observed more fully when speaking of apoplexy.

Rhus toxicodendron. In simple primary meningitis a case will never occur where this medicine is indicated; on the other hand it may prove indispensable in erysipelas of the face which sometimes develops itself as a secondary disease in the course of meningitis, if this disease assumes a typhoid character and is attended with unusually violent symptoms. In such cases *Apis* may have to be considered. However, our clinical experience with this agent is as yet insufficient to enable us to furnish more particular indications for its use.

Arnica. Meningitis is more frequently than is generally believed a consequence of slight injuries or mechanical concussion of the head. Arnica not only meets this general indication in most cases most fully, but the symptoms of the drug represent most perfectly the image of meningitis, both in the congestive and exudative stage. The absence of all signs of reaction contra-indicates this agent most decidedly.

[Concussion of the brain may result from a very slight mechanical injury, and the symptoms of meningitis caused by the injury may not develop themselves until two or three weeks after the accident had happened.

A lady standing by the mantel-piece, dropped a match. She stooped to pick it up, and on raising her head rather suddenly, she knocked it against the sharp edge of the mantel-piece. Concussion ensued which developed meningitis four weeks after the accident occurred. The case terminated fatally in the hands of the late distinguished Valentine Mott.

A boy of twelve years while running after his sister, stumbled against the mantel-piece. Concussion of the brain took place which resulted in meningitis about a fortnight after the occurrence of the accident. It was a bad case, but the patient recovered in a fortnight in my hands. H.]

Bryonia. The pathogenesis of Bryonia embodies a characteristic image of meningitis. Moreover we know from practical experience that Bryonia is a capital remedy in all serous inflammations, hence also in meningitis. As a general rule the selection of this drug is determined by the period when Aconite ceases to be indicated; in other words, when symptoms of incipient exudation are beginning to set in. At a later stage of the disease, its favorable action becomes doubtful, more particularly when all symptoms of reaction which constitute essential indications for the use of this drug have become effaced by paralysis of the affected organ. The most important indications are: a livid, flushed face, a high temperature of the body together with readily breaking out, copious sweats, nausea, with desire to vomit, and obstinate constipation, with distention of the abdomen; scanty and painful secretion of urine.

Helleborus niger is one of the most important remedies if the meningeal exudation may be considered as having reached its climax. Although we do not altogether agree with Wahle's sanguine recommendation who promises good results from the use of this drug even in a few hours; on the other hand, if success is still possible, no other medicine is more likely to achieve it than Helleborus niger. The proper period for its application has arrived if reaction has almost entirely ceased and the symptoms of paralysis are more or less completely developed.

Sulphur has been exhibited with success in many cases. Its employment is governed by general considerations of analogy rather than by its physiological action upon the tissues. It will only be found appropriate as a means of assisting the delaying resorption of the exuded fluid, hence in the stage of paralysis after it has continued for a time without any perceptible change. As a matter of course no certain result ought to be expected in the presence of such an unfavorable prognosis; but the important and practically ascertained action of Sulphur upon the absorbent system in other organs (we mention more especially pneumonia and peritonitis) furnishes sufficiently adequate reasons for its employment in the exudative stage of meningitis.

Of the other remedies that belong to this category, we mention as particularly noteworthy: *Hyoscyamus, Stramonium, Digitalis, Iodium, Mercurius, Tartarus stibiatus, Zincum*. In the order in which these remedies have been mentioned they will very generally be found to constitute the successive series in which their use may be required in the management of a case.

[In the place of Iodium, Kafka recommends the *Iodide of Potassium* as better adapted to effect the resorption of the exuded fluid, and to ameliorate the constitutional diathesis. If Belladonna does not effect a speedy improvement, he generally recommends the *Sulphate of Atropine* 3 to be given in solution, a spoonful every hour or two hours. H.]

As regards the management of such patients in other respects, we must not omit to notice several important points. With reference to sanguineous depletions we refer the reader to what we have stated in this respect in our remarks concerning apoplexy; we have to condemn them likewise as hurtful and therefore useless in the management of meningitis. The effect of cold applications to the head is at all events very uncertain; with some patients they disagree very decidedly. If such applications are to be resorted to at all, it has to be done with a good deal of discretion. In the stage of exudation when the vital activity of the organism is depressed to a dangerously low degree, it is certainly a hazardous proceeding to continue the application of external cold. At the commencement of the disease when the fever is high, the patients refuse of themselves every thing except fresh water. Abundant draughts of this beverage should be given the patient during the whole course of the disease. If the vital turgescence is lowered, we need not fear to administer milk and water, and beef-broth; these things are even imperatively necessary. It is likewise proper and pleasant to the patient that the action of the skin should be stimulated by frequently and cautiously used cold ablutions followed by friction of the moistened surface. During convalescence the utmost caution has to be used in eating and drinking as well as in regard to mental labor. In the case of children it is well to converse with them as little as possible, (a precaution which is unfortunately too often neglected;) to keep all objects and persons that might excite the patients, away from them. Adults had better be kept strictly isolated.

2. Encephalitis. Cerebritis.

Inflammation of the substance of the brain never extends over the whole brain, but is always confined to single localities. It occurs proportionally very rarely. It may occur in every age, but is most frequently met with in persons of middle age. It is not always possible to determine its causes with absolute certainty; the most frequent causes are: mechanical injuries, (which often seem trifling,) the irritation caused by extravasated fluid, tumors, diseases of the skull-bones, (especially of the mastoid process,) morbid conditions, with decomposition of the blood. The inflammation may be located anywhere in the brain, but it occurs chiefly along the boundary between the white and gray substance. Encephalitis commences with exudation between the fibres of the brain, sometimes confined to a very small space and at other times extending over a space of the size of a hen's egg. Owing to the peculiar structure of the brain, an exudation of this kind results in softening and disorganization of its fibres; red softening of the brain sets in, which afterwards, through resorption, assumes a more yellow color. Or else, in consequence of influences which it is difficult to account for, the exuded fluid changes to pus and an abscess forms in the brain. Such an abscess may have various terminations: it may become circumscribed and a gradual resorption may take place, or it may penetrate into the ventricles or work up to the surface of the brain, thus causing meningitis and speedy death. The abscess generally results from an injury, but need not necessarily correspond to the locality of the injury. Lastly encephalitis may terminate in the formation of a cyst in consequence of the definitely circumscribed localization of the inflammatory process. The destruction of the walls of the vessels permeating the inflamed portion of the brain may likewise readily lead to apoplectic extravasations.

Symptoms. The phenomena of encephalitis are remarkably

vague and uncertain. There are numerous cases where the first symptom of the disease indicates a meningitis breaking out suddenly and running a rapid course; or where death takes place quite suddenly in consequence of effusion into the ventricles, or apoplectic extravasation. In such cases the inflammation is not necessarily confined to a limited space, but may be quite extensive, showing in a most striking manner that large portions of the brain may become disorganized without its functions being correspondingly or even to any considerable extent impaired. But even in cases where encephalitis sets in with a whole series of symptoms, they are not sufficiently definite at the first outbreak of the disease to enable us to establish a positive diagnosis upon such an uncertain foundation. All we can do is to conjecture with more or less certainty the character of the disease from the few circumstances that may be positively known to us. In such cases the phenomena of a gradually, never tumultuously increasing pressure on the brain become manifest, such as: headache generally violent and continued, and attended with vertigo; disposition to fainting fits; deep disturbance of the emotive sphere; heaviness in the limbs and an unsteady gait without any decided symptoms of paralysis; sensitiveness of the organs of sense; wandering pains in the extremities. These symptoms are very speedily followed by more general symptoms of depression, the organs of sense become duller, the extremities lose their sensibility, the paralysis of the motor system of nerves becomes more apparent. The mental functions are almost always impaired, and from the very commencement of the disease exhibit characteristic signs of depression: the patients are apathetic, drowsy, think slowly, the memory is weaker, the speech is interfered with, and is either heavy or is no longer serviceable as a means of distinct utterance. In the further course of the disease it often happens that the patient is troubled with vomiting, syncope, epileptiform convulsions; the pupils become dilated, the pulse and the respiration become slower; according as one or the other portion of the brain is affected, paralytic conditions of very limited extent may supervene. If the disease runs a slow course, with occasional momentary periods of distinctly perceptible ameliorations, the morbid process may continue for months before the increasing paralysis or the supervention of other affections terminates the patient's sufferings. Complete recovery can only take place in the first period of the disease; a partial recovery takes place when consequent upon the formation of a cyst or the localization of the abscess within a definite capsule, the phenomena of paralysis depending upon the disorganized portion of the brain, of course remaining unchanged. In a number of cases the symptoms of paralysis are so little perceptible that the cure may be considered complete and that the evidence of a previously existing inflammation can only be traced to the cicatrix which a subsequent post-mortem examination of the brain may reveal. As has already been stated, in many cases it is impossible, and in other cases difficult to diagnose encephalitis; hence it may not be unprofitable to enumerate some of the leading diagnostic signs of this disease. The gradual development of the symptoms of pressure on the brain precludes the idea of apoplexy as well as of meningitis, except perhaps chronic meningitis, from which, however, encephalitis is distinguished by the presence of striking symptoms of partial paralytic conditions Tumors in the brain are the least easy to diagnose, which likewise are very frequently attended by symptoms of a gradually increasing compression of that organ. The uncertainties attending a case of this kind are more or less cleared up by the fact that the paralytic symptoms of encephalitis are characterized by more or less marked remissions which are entirely absent in the case of tumors.

The prognosis is doubtful in every case, the chances being decidedly rather against the patient than in his favor. If the patient recovers, the recovery is generally only partial. The position of the physician in such cases becomes still more complicated by the circumstance that the malady runs such an extraordinarily protracted course.

Treatment. We cannot unfortunately point to any cases of encephalitis in our literature calculated to shed light on the treatment of this disease. Hence we have to confine ourselves to a few cases in our own practice all of which terminated fatally; it is true they were intrusted to our care only after the disease had been progressing for some time towards its final termination. As a rule the patients should be kept free from all violent excitement; such signs of congestion as may manifest themselves have to be counteracted at once by appropriate remedies. The diet has to be regulated with as much strictness as possible. The most suitable remedies for this affection almost all belong to the category of inorganic medicines. It is only at the beginning of the disease, more particularly if it can be traced to external injuries as their primary cause, that *Arnica* is the most appropriate remedy. Other remedies which, however, we mention, without any further particular indications for the reason that their useful effect in this disease is very questionable, are: *Mercurius, Iodium, Cuprum, Sulphur, Zincum*, and more especially *Plumbum*. Iodium has obtained some reputation in chronic affections of the brain even in the hands of our therapeutic opponents who, on the other hand, very frequently furnish us material for toxicological observations. I have been treating for years a young man who had been afflicted with constitutional syphilis. After having been treated both internally and externally with a quantity of mercurial preparations, his physicians decided to subject him to a rigid course of Iodine treatment. I was unable to ascertain how large a quantity of Iodine-preparations he had used. After the treatment had lasted about a fortnight, he was attacked with violent headache and some fever. Continuing the Iodine by direction of his physician, he lost in a few days almost suddenly all consciousness, and his left lower extremity became paralyzed. This case offers a striking picture of partial encephalitis. We may observe that in this case the paralysis still continues in the form of hemiplegia. We beg leave to refer to *Plumbum* among the remedies for apoplexy; to the indications we have furnished in that paragraph we here add the following post-mortem appearances: head and brain hyperæmic; in the left hemisphere, at the base of the middle lobe, a prominence of the size of a hen's egg and of a yellowish color, is perceived, very soft to the feel and surrounded by dark-red places. An investigation revealed within the swelling four smaller nuclei of a yellowish softening, separated from each other by normal cerebral substance that merged into the softening without any definite boundary. This abscess had formed in the space of several years in consequence of gradual poisoning.

This is an appropriate place to mention a pathological process which is closely related to, or rather identical with, encephalitis: we allude to yellow softening of the brain properly speaking. Its origin is as yet enveloped in great obscurity. It generally occurs only in individuals of an advanced age, and looks very much like the spontaneous death of the cerebral substance; in rare cases it is met with in young subjects of a cachectic habit of body. It may exist in the brain as an isolated affection, or side by side with a distinct inflammatory softening or apoplectic effusions, with which, however, it has no immediate connection. It is principally met with in the large brain. The phenomena which the yellow softening develops are almost identical with those of encephalitis. The curability of this disease is very questionable; the remedies that may be employed against it are the same that have been indicated in the previous paragraph.

[In encephalitis, when the symptoms of cerebral hyperæmia still predominate and the disorganizing metamorphosis is progressing, Kafka has been for some years in the habit of employing *Glonoin* 1 to 2, with the best success, giving children six to eight drops of the second attenuation in half a tumbler of water, of which solution they take a teaspoonful every two hours. To adults he gives one or two drops of the first or second attenuation on sugar of milk two or three times a day. The effect is truly surprising; in twenty-four or forty-eight hours the turgescence, heat in the head and the engorgement of the vessels diminish much more promptly and safely than could be accomplished by means of sanguineous depletions, cold applications or the use of purgatives. This treatment secures moreover the incalculable advantage that the strength of the patient is spared in the fullest measure, and the disease is enabled to institute its retrograde metamorphosis without being arrested in its course.

Kafka relates the following case, which we reproduce as worthy of note. A man, sixty-five years old, who had had an apoplectic attack two years previous, in consequence of which his left side remained paralyzed, was, at the time we undertook his treatment, in a condition of cerebral hyperæmia, so that his relatives apprehended momentarily and very properly another apoplectic attack. Side by side with the symptoms of cerebral hyperæmia, (see this chapter,) those of cerebral softening, with progressive increase of the morbid phenomena, likewise co-existed. We prescribed *Glonoin* 1, two doses a day, with the most marked success; the congestive phenomena disappeared entirely. The patient being robust and corpulent, *Iodium* 2 was exhibited in two daily doses. Until the end of March, 1865, the patient who had first come to us in December, 1864, remained in a condition of tolerable ease and comfort; the hyperæmia of the brain did not return, and the speech, sensibility and motor-powers of the patient improved very strikingly. At that period a death took place in the family which made a deep impression upon the patient; the hyperæmia returned and was immediately followed by convulsions. They were of a clonic nature. While the face and the extremities were thus convulsed, *the patient uttered a roaring cry.* The consciousness remained unimpaired.

When asked why he roared so horribly, he answered that the roaring was involuntary and that he could not help it. Our explanation of this phenomenon was that the roaring was a violent expulsion of air produced by a spasmodic contraction of the diaphragm or a sudden and spasmodic compression or contraction of the bronchia. For the convulsions with cerebral hyperæmia we prescribed *Belladonna* 3, and, no improvement having taken place in forty-eight hours, *Atropinum sulph.* 3, likewise without any result. Looking into Dr. Clotar Mueller's Repertory, we found, page 18, art. " Clonic convulsions attended with cries," *Arsenicum* mentioned as a chief remedy verified by clinical experience. After giving a few doses of this drug, one every hour, the spasms as well as the cries ceased, nor have they so far occurred again, end of August, 1865. H.]

3. Tubercular (granular) inflammation of the meninges. Hydrocephalus acutus.

This disease is one of the most important affections of the brain, partly on account of its relative frequency and partly on account of its extraordinary tendency to a fatal termination. It is only recently that a more correct discrimination between tubercular and simple meningitis has become possible, whereas formerly by tubercular meningitis was simply understood an inflammation of the brain attended with profuse exudation. The difference, however, is not merely founded in the granular character of the disease, but these two forms of meningitis differ even with regard to their locality, a difference that accounts very fully and satisfactorily for many distinctions in their symptomatic manifestations.

Granular meningitis is more particularly located at the base of the brain; only in rare cases the convex portion of the brain becomes involved. As in simple meningitis we find in the subarachnoideal space an exudation of a jellylike consistence; in the pia mater we see the millet-sized yellowish-white granulations which sometimes occur in simple miliary tuberculosis without exudation. The ventricles contain a more or less copious quantity of exuded serum, in consequence of which these cavities not only become very much distended, but the adjoining parts become softened to an extraordinary degree. It is this circumstance which has led to the designation of acute hydrocephalus.

Granular meningitis is very rarely an entirely primary affection, but most generally constitutes a partial manifestation of a more general tubercular process, especially of pulmonary tuberculosis; or it is a sequel of previous affections, more particularly of measles, typhus and whooping-cough, after which diseases the tubercular inflammation at the base of the brain frequently develops itself as the first symptom of constitutional tuberculosis. It chiefly invades the infantile organism between the ages of two and ten years, very rarely older children or adults. It may be inferred from these remarks that perfectly healthy children are scarcely ever attacked by this disease as a primary malady, although the presence of tubercles may sometimes remain hidden until they are revealed by a post-mortem examination. Either the children exhibit at a previous period more or less prominent symptoms of a scrofulous taint; or they are delicate subjects, the offspring of tuberculous parents, stunted in their bodily development, but endowed with a good deal of mental quickness, and distinguished by a precocious intellect. This precocity is very apt to induce parents to stimulate the mental powers prematurely, and thus, by this continued stimulation of the brain, to hasten the outbreak of this malignant disease. As in simple meningitis, so in this disease, external injuries, a fall, blow, etc., may, if the organism is otherwise endowed with the necessary constitutional predisposition, constitute the proximate causes of an actual manifestation of the malady; at any rate it will often be remarked that the change observed in the conduct of the patient prior to the outbreak of the disease dates from the time when some external force had exerted upon the skull only a slightly disturbing impression. Very frequently, however, all perceptible causes to which the disease might be attributed are wanting, and the outbreak takes place with an unexpected suddenness.

Symptoms. The disease scarcely ever begins without any morbid phenomena, in a manner that would justify one in conjecturing an affection of the brain at all with any thing like positive certainty. For a longer or shorter period the outbreak of the disease is preceded by precursory symptoms which not unfrequently are so slight that they are often overlooked even by the nearest relatives who afterwards are reminded of them when the more violent symptoms begin to develop themselves. However, inasmuch as it is necessary, for a timely correctness of the diagnosis, that the preliminary stage of the disease should be accurately known, the physician should never content himself with a general denial of all morbid symptoms by the relatives, but should institute minute inquiries into all the particular circumstances of the case. The children who have hitherto been of a bright and playful disposition, seem changed, avoid play, become taciturn and, contrary to their former habit, sit by themselves in some remote corner, their sleep is restless, and they are tormented by many anxious dreams. If their intelligence is sufficiently matured, they complain of headache at an early stage of the disease, although not all the time. There is no marked fever, the appetite vanishes, or, in rare cases, is occasionally very much increased, and an incipient loss of flesh cannot be overlooked. The complexion is not all at once altered, pallor of the countenance generally predominates. Even at this period an unsteadiness in the gait of children becomes noticeable; they incline to fall more readily than before, (which is regarded by the parents as accidental,) and are indisposed to walk any considerable distance. Very frequently the beginning of these phenomena dates from a fall or from some violent emotion. The patients sometimes remain in this condition for weeks without any more dangerous symptoms supervening.

If we consider these symptoms as the preliminary stage, the real first stage of the disease most generally sets in with the first paroxysms of vomiting. This does not occur as a consequence of indigestion, or in a quiet posture of the body, or soon after a meal, but particularly when rising from a recumbent position, walking about or while the children are carried round. During the attack the abdominal walls exhibit almost constantly a peculiar tension and depression. At this stage the headache greatly increases in intensity; the higher organs of sense become abnormally sensitive, sometimes to a high degree; slight convulsions set in, the patient starts frequently as if frightened, is very nervous and excited, the mind seems to dwell on one idea which the patient utters to himself repeatedly; the sleep becomes restless, with frequent gritting of the teeth; the patient is tormented by frightful dreams from which he wakes with a piercing cry without being able to free himself at once from the disturbing phantasm. The pupils now are generally contracted, the pulse is accelerated or at times quicker, at other times slower; other prominent febrile symptoms are wanting. The face is usually pallid, or else pallor and flushes suddenly alternate; the expression of the countenance is peculiarly altered, it is an expression of suffering. The bowels are confined, the urine is scanty, saturated and generally turbid. The peculiar cry, however, the nature of which cannot possibly be misapprehended, is not by any means a characteristic symptom of tubercular meningitis, but is likewise peculiar to other affections of the brain. It may be heard, for instance, in cases of simple hyperæmia; and in the case of typhus, of which mention was made in our chapter on meningitis, this cry was as characteristic and occurred as frequently as it is possible to do in the most marked case of tubercular meningitis. It seems to be extorted from the patient by the paroxysmal exacerbations of the headache. Contractions of the posterior cervical muscles which cause the peculiar boring with the head into the pillow, generally initiate the second stage and henceforth continue to the end.

After the first stage has lasted for a few days, the second stage generally commences with convulsions of various degrees of intensity, at times partial, at other times general, and scarcely ever entirely wanting; these convulsions are followed immediately by symptoms of incipient paralysis. Consciousness vanishes more and more; the children no longer complain of pain, but grasp very frequently at the head, from which it is evident that they experience an intense pain in that region; they are generally restless, and the peculiar cry continues unabated. The vomiting ceases almost entirely in most cases. The eyes become completely insensible to intense light, and the little patients no longer hear even if spoken to in the loudest tone of voice. The pupils become dilated, generally unequally, and squinting sets in. On one side the extremities are often rigidly contracted, while on the other side they are completely paralyzed. The pulse generally becomes slower than natural, and even falls below sixty beats; on the other hand, however, it often retains a frequency of one hundred and twenty beats, and even higher. It may likewise assume an intermittent character, but this is not a characteristic symptom. Respiration is always unequal, at times very feeble and inaudible, and then again a deep sighing moan is heard. The coma becomes more and more persistent, there is no longer a trace of lucid intervals; the eyes either remain open or are only half closed, the upper lid being evidently paralyzed. Convulsions continue to set in in paroxysms of more or less intensity, generally on one side. The urine is discharged involuntarily, the bowels remain confined. This stage continues variously, sometimes only a few days, and at other times several weeks. We frequently observe during this stage striking remissions of single symptoms, which, however, have no favorable meaning; they may even take place with a certain typical regularity; or a striking improvement in the condition of the patient may delude us for a time, for it will soon enough be superseded by a change for the worse.

The last stage lasts seldom longer than forty-eight hours. It commences about the time when the pulse rises to an extraordinary number of beats, even one hundred and eighty and upwards; at the same time the number of respirations increases considerably, whereas the temperature of the skin decreases and a profuse perspiration breaks out. The paralysis has now reached the highest degree; it is only now and then that the possibility of motion is made manifest by short paroxysms of convulsions. The remarkable changes in the pulse and respiration are evidently consequences of incipient paralysis of the vagus. The breathing becomes rattling, during which death relieves the patient. Recovery may take place in every stage of the disease; in the last stage, however, after the pulse has risen in frequency, the chances of recovery are undoubtedly very slim. It can scarcely be said that the patient ever recovers entirely, for the reason that the disease scarcely ever attacks perfectly sound individuals and is generally complicated with tubercular deposits in other organs. Health can therefore at most be restored only to what it was previous to the attack. Very frequently isolated symptoms of paralysis remain, owing probably to the circumstance that the effused fluid in the ventricles is not completely re-absorbed. Even if the disease runs a course ever so favorable it must be expected to break out again sooner or later after it has once taken hold on the organism.

The diagnosis of acute hydrocephalus is undoubtedly a ticklish point. Even from simple meningitis the tubercular form cannot always be readily distinguished, particularly in the first and even in the second stage. The affection is not by any means recognizable by absolutely characteristic symptoms, on which account great importance is to be attached to the preliminary stage, which scarcely ever has a longer duration in simple meningitis. As a matter of course a correctly discriminating diagnosis in these two forms of meningitis is of the utmost importance. The tubercular process in granular meningitis has to be managed very differently from simple inflammation of the meninges. As regards other affections of the brain, they will scarcely ever be confounded with tubercular meningitis. The possibility of this disease being confounded with typhus has already been alluded to in the chapter on simple meningitis.

Under all circumstances the prognosis is involved in a great deal of uncertainty and doubt, so much more as it is very questionable whether, what was supposed to be a cure of tubercular meningitis in the first stage, was not rather a case of simple meningitis or even only of cerebral hyperæmia. However, even though we should have to eliminate a number of cases reported in our books as cases of tubercular meningitis, on account of their questionable character, a sufficient number of cases undoubtedly remain to substantiate the fact that this generally fatal disease can be cured with homœopathic remedies. The sooner the suitable remedies are employed against the disease, the better the prospect of effecting a cure; the more generally and completely the symptoms of paralysis have become manifest, the more questionable will be the final result. Where the pulse has risen to the above-mentioned frequency, recovery can scarcely be expected.

Treatment. The management of this disease is without doubt one of the sorest trials to the feeling physician. If he succeeds in effecting a cure, he is haunted by the thought that he has been mistaken in his diagnosis; if the patient dies, the fatal result simply tends to corroborate his bitter conviction that the disease is in its very nature an incurable malady. The distressing condition of the patient may continue for months without a ray of hope shining athwart the gloom of the sick-chamber; night and day the physician's mind is filled with anxious thoughts concerning the little patient, all imaginable drugs have been tried, and yet the case runs onward towards a fatal termination. The painfulness of the situation is increased by the circumstance that children who are attacked with tubercular meningitis have become an object of intense parental affection on account of their bright intellect and sensitive disposition. Assuredly this is a situation where the physician has it in his power to show that he is such in the noblest acceptation of the term. Under these circumstances we cannot sufficiently guard against an untoward influence which is apt to creep in and complicate the case. The frequent visits both friendly and professional, which it may be necessary to make, but too frequently tempt the attending physician to change the medicine, a proceeding that entails more injury in this affection than perhaps in any other. Inasmuch as the nature of the morbid process renders it impossible for any remedy to effect a rapid and decided change in the symptoms, we should be loth to abandon a remedy if it does not effect a striking improvement in the first twelve or twenty-four hours. Such an improper change of medicine has not only the immediate but likewise the general disadvantage of depriving us of the opportunity of acquiring certainty regarding the action of our drugs and that this lack of positive experience leaves us as ill-advised in all subsequent cases of this kind as in the former.

We may likewise just as well observe at the outset that it will be found extremely difficult to select a remedial agent in all such cases in strict accordance with the symptoms, and that such a purely symptomatic selection would afford very little probability for a successful treatment. On the contrary, in selecting our remedy it is of paramount importance not only that the peculiar nature of the exudation and the pathologico-anatomical alterations should be kept in view, but that our selection should be made with special reference to such pathological products and changes. This is likewise conceded by Hartmann, who does not exactly favor this mode of selecting a remedy. Hence if, in the subsequent paragraphs, we leave medicines that had been recommended in other affections of the brain, unnoticed, it is simply because a more general mode of reasoning has satisfied us that they are out of place in this disease. Definite indications for the treatment of each special stage of this disease have likewise been deemed inappropriate by us, and we prefer considering each medicine separately in its relation to the general features of the disease.

Bryonia alba. We have already made mention of this drug in speaking of simple meningitis, and we likewise enumerate it among the remedies for granular meningitis for the reason that we have witnessed the most striking effects from its use in other forms of the tubercular disease. It is in all respects adapted to the preliminary stage, more so perhaps than to the more fully developed disease. The precursory symptoms undoubtedly point to the fact that the exudative process has already set in, and it is for this period that we have likewise recommended Bryonia in simple meningitis. In order to do justice to the symptoms we call to mind the resemblance of the preliminary stage to an incipient typhus where Bryonia is very frequently the only prominently indicated remedy. In our opinion the therapeutic efficacy of the drug is bounded by the first manifestation of the paralytic symptoms.

Arnica montana. This drug shows likewise in every respect a striking correspondence with incipient granular meningitis, except that the characteristic disposition to vomit is not found in the pathogenesis of this agent. It is preferable to Bryonia in cases primarily originating in mechanical causes and where the febrile symptoms are more marked. Arnica, however, is not, as in simple meningitis, endowed with a specific influence over the tubercular exudation.

Veratrum album corresponds in every respect to the symptoms of the primary stage of this disease. Among the characteristic indications we note more particularly: great inequality in the distribution of animal heat; vomiting and great increase of the cephalic distress when raising the head; proportionate ease in a recumbent posture; the least motion causes nausea and vomiting; considerable unsteadiness of the extremities; rigidity of the posterior cervical muscles; disposition to convulsive movements; peculiar alteration of the features and pallor of the countenance, or else flushes on one cheek only. This characteristic combination of symptoms will scarcely be met with as fully in the pathogenesis of any other drug. Our literature exhibits only a few cases confirmatory of the good effects of Veratrum album in this disease.

Digitalis purpurea is likewise one of the most important remedies in acute hydrocephalus. This remedy is not so much indicated by its symptomatic similarity to the disease as by the circumstance that it develops the most characteristic symptoms of acute hydrocephalus even in the same successive series as the disease itself. Hence this remedy will appear suitable in every stage of the disease, from the precursory symptoms to the paralysis of the vagus. For a detailed statement of the gradually increasing action of Digitalis in this disease, we refer to the Materia Medica, contenting ourselves in this place with furnishing a series of the most characteristic indications: mental depression, interrupted by short periods of excitement; predominant sensation of coldness irrespective of the character of the pulse, with heat and pallor of the face; vomiting at every movement of the body; coma, with twitchings and convulsions; the pupils are either dilated or contracted; rapid emaciation, without any correspondingly profuse abnormal evacuations; increase of all the symptoms when abandoning the horizontal posture; semi-lateral twitchings, especially in the face; continued constipation and diminished secretion of urine. To these highly characteristic symptoms we have to add the character of the pulse. After small or even larger doses the pulse appears at first accelerated, small and feeble; after large doses, or after the drug has continued to act for some time, the pulse becomes abnormally slow, or, after the organism has been thoroughly impregnated with the action of the drug, the pulse becomes so rapid that it can scarcely be counted, and is moreover, if not intermittent, at least continually irregular. No other drug has this characteristic peculiarity of the pulse in granular meningitis as fully as Digitalis. As regards the tubercular diathesis generally, we know that Digitalis is extremely efficacious in scrofulous as well as in tubercular affections, and that it possesses a special affinity to the lymphatic system; and that its physiological effects likewise embody very fully the symptoms of pulmonary phthisis in the first and second stage of the disease. And lastly we must not omit to state that Digitalis is one of our best remedies for acute serous effusions to which this disease is indebted for its name of acute hydrocephalus; whereas, on the contrary, its curative action in chronic dropsies still continues doubtful and exceedingly uncertain.

Zincum is recommended by Hartmann very urgently in the irritative stage, with the assertion that he has often seen a decided improvement set in in twelve or twenty-four hours after its first employment. We are perfectly certain that these cases where such a rapid improvement was noticed, were not cases of tubercular meningitis; on the other hand we do not doubt that Zincum may be adapted to the preliminary stages of the disease; of the symptoms which characterize any of its subsequent stages as prominent symptoms, only a few are found in the pathogenetic series of Zincum; it is much more suitable in simple meningitis, although even in this disease we do not regard it as one of the leading remedies.

Iodium will scarcely ever be selected in this disease on account of its symptomatic similarity, although it has a few symptoms that might serve as starting-points in our selection of the drug. It is when judging by analogy, that the choice of this agent will appear much more justifiable. No one can doubt its extraordinary efficacy in scrofulous affections; of its importance as a remedy for phthisis we shall speak when treating of this disease. Coupling these general indications with the symptoms of the drug, we shall obtain sufficient reasons for its practical application.

Cuprum is one of the most noteworthy remedies in granular meningitis. It will scarcely ever be indicated in the first stages of the disease, but will be found so much more applicable in the stage of decided exudation when convulsions have begun to set in. This is one of the few remedies that cause great irregularity of the pulse which may likewise, like the pulse of Digitalis, fall considerably below the normal standard. This circumstance alone is calculated to direct our attention to this agent whose pathogenetic symptoms do not by any means contra-indicate its use.

If one of the remedies we have named has effected an improvement, but if some of the functions of the brain continue to remain disturbed, it is advisable to continue the drug that had effected the favorable change, in less frequent doses until the remaining symptoms of the disease are removed or until the appearance of other new and striking symptoms renders a change of medicine imperative. Owing to the diversity of the symptoms that may manifest themselves, it is impossible to determine *a priori* what this new medicine may be.

Among the remedies which, in addition to those above described, may still be required, we mention: *Mercurius, Helleborus, Plumbum*. Beside these, other medicines have been urged upon the Profession, probably without any adequate reason, since the cases where these medicines are recommended are not distinguished by very accurate diagnostic statements. At all events we would most likely fall back upon the following series of drugs: *Pulsatilla, Belladonna, Aconitum, Stramonium, Hyoscyamus, Opium, Cina, Artemisia, Rhus toxicodendron*. As regards the last-named drug, it probably owes its recommendation by Hartmann and others to its successful employment in typhus which, as we have stated before, is so easily confounded with granular meningitis. So far as the dose is concerned, our best observers unite in affirming that frequently repeated doses of low attenuations are preferable in this disease.

[In the place of Iodium, Kafka often substitutes the *Iodide of Potassium*, especially if a constitutional tubercular diathesis lies at the foundation of the cerebral disease. *Glonoin, Apis* and *Atropin* are likewise recommended, for the particular indications of which we refer the reader to our chapter on simple meningitis. H.]

It is scarcely necessary to allude to any dietetic rules during the management of the disease, since the patients, in their almost uninterrupted state of unconsciousness, are scarcely able to swallow during the whole course of the disease. As long as deglutition is possible, it would of course be ill-advised to refuse the patients strengthening nourishment; on the contrary, it is of the utmost importance to sustain the struggling vitality by means of broth and milk diluted with water. Fresh water is the best beverage to quench the thirst which torments the patients, although they may not manifest it by any perceptible signs. External applications cannot be of any possible use in this affection, nor can they afford any relief. During convalescence the digestive process has to be nursed with the utmost care, and the physical and mental wants of the patient generally have to be attended to with unrelenting discretion, since we ought to be well aware that the fundamental cause of the trouble, the tubercular deposit, is still present, and, even if no relapse is caused by imprudences, will sooner or later break out again as an actual disease in some other organ. In the case of such individuals a dose of *Calcarea carbonica* or *phosphorica* given from time to time for a certain period of time, may accomplish a great deal of good. Above all things, mental exertions, excessive study, excitements of the fancy are strictly to be avoided; children who are often the most eager to learn, should be kept away from their books, if necessary by main force.

Hydrocephalus, (stricte sic dictus.)

In a general sense we understand by hydrocephalus every abnormal accumulation of fluid in the cavity of the skull. It may either be acquired or congenital.

Acquired hydrocephalus is always seated in the ventricles; it is seldom an idiopathic affection, but is generally symptomatic of some other constitutional affection. It becomes an important symptom when the disease sets in as chief complication of granular meningitis; or when it develops itself so rapidly that it acts like apoplexy and speedily terminates fatally, (serous apoplexy.) The diagnosis of this disease is always very uncertain; its symptoms are the same as those of granular meningitis. It scarcely ever necessitates a special treatment, nor is this feasible. If therapeutic means should have to be used, the remedies that have been mentioned for tubercular meningitis will have to be resorted to.

Congenital hydrocephalus is likewise seated in the ventricles. It commences already before the child is born, but may increase after birth. The quantity of the accumulated serum may be very large, and hence the skull may acquire an extraordinary volume. Its effects upon the child are sometimes imperceptible, at other times very decided; the mental functions of the brain are mostly involved; it is only in very fully developed cases that the motor system is affected, a more or less complete paralysis setting in. The life of the patient is not absolutely threatened; it may even be admitted that hydrocephalic children who have got over the period of infancy, have pretty nearly escaped the most imminent danger of death. However, they always remain weakly, irritable and unusually disposed to frequent and malignant diseases. Hydrocephalus is a curable disease, but such a cure is mostly spontaneous, taking place in proportion as the bodily development progresses. A cure may indeed be facilitated by artificial means, but not by medicines.

A main point is to bring up such children with great care, to accustom them to light and nourishing food and to active exercise, and not to excite their mental faculties prematurely by a forced development. Among medicines we may select *Calcarea carbonica* and *Arsenicum*, but in small and rarely repeated doses. Bandaging the head with strips of adhesive plaster, which has been recommended by some pathologists, has seldom been of any use, but has very frequently been attended with the most dangerous consequences, either in consequence of the violent compression exerting a dangerous pressure upon the brain, or even in consequence of the activity of the vessels of the pericranium being materially interfered with. Judging by analogy, it is indeed not only possible but even probable that a cautious use of this method of treatment may be followed by favorable results.

B. DISEASES OF THE SPINAL MARROW.

The spinal marrow is essentially liable to all the morbid processes that occur in the brain, the structure of both these organs being essentially the same. All these processes may be found described, theoretically rather than practically, in pathological manuals, without it being possible to establish a proper diagnosis at the sick-bed and to initiate a treatment based upon it. For this reason we are not disposed to furnish a detailed description of the manifold pathological conditions of the spinal cord, and shall treat only of two of the best known and most important of them, inflammation of the spinal cord and spinal irritation. Most of the other conditions can be attached to the former as accessories.

Inflammation of the Spinal Cord and its Membranes.

This disease is one of the rarer sort, but is very likely considered so because it is not always properly diagnosed and is often mistaken for another affection. The inflammation may be seated exclusively in the meninges, but if the spinal cord itself is inflamed, the accompanying meningitis is never wanting. The course of the disease is either chronic or acute. The acute form extends mostly over a larger surface, depositing an exudation in the subarachnoideal space, and rarely invading the spinal marrow. The chronic form leads to thickening of the membranes and a more or less copious accumulation of serum in the vertebral canal. Inflammation of the substance of the cord leads very speedily, as in the case of the brain, to softening and disorganization of the fibres of the spinal marrow, likewise to the formation of an abscess; it is generally not very extensive, but always results in an inflammatory affection of the meninges.

If we may believe what is said regarding the causes of spinal meningitis, they are manifold. Among the most certain causes we enumerate: mechanical injuries, a shock, blow, fracture of the vertebræ; affections of the vertebræ, especially spondylarthrocace; apoplectic extravasations; extension of inflammatory affections of the brain to the spinal cord. Less certain causes are: acute exanthems; suppression of hæmorrhages; sexual excesses. In many cases, however, the inflammation seems to arise quite spontaneously.

Symptoms. The symptoms of meningitis spinalis are almost the same as those of myelitis; slight differences will be pointed out. In most cases the disease begins with a chill like all other inflammations of more important organs. The chill recurs quite frequently in paroxysms of shivering. At the same time the patient experiences a local pain at some spot in the vertebral column, which can be pointed out with definiteness; the pain is aggravated by pressure, and is increased to a most violent and even intolerable degree of intensity by moving, and especially by rotating the spinal column. These symptoms are attended with a not inconsiderable fever. As a general rule, the patient complains of pains at the very beginning of the attack; very often these pains constitute the first manifestation of the disease. Very soon the first symptoms of incipient paralysis supervene, consisting in the first place of painful contractions, or twitchings of the correspondingly involved bundles of muscles, or even of tetanic convulsions, after which the paralytic symptoms increase to paraplegia with more or less rapidity. A certain degree of anæsthesia is scarcely ever wanting, commencing with a sensation of pithiness or numbness and gradually increasing in intensity. According as one or the other portion of the cord is inflamed, the symptoms exhibit considerable differences. If the superior portion of the cord is involved, as a matter of course the parts to which nerves are given off by the more deep-seated portion of the cord become paralyzed. Paralysis of the respiratory muscles is particularly inconvenient and dangerous, since an accident of this kind may speedily terminate fatally. If the lumbar portion is the seat of the disease, violent paroxysms of colic are experienced by the patient. The bladder and rectum are almost always more or less paralyzed. Very peculiar, although not of constant occurrence, are the convulsive shocks in the paralyzed parts, which bear a great resemblance to the reflex-movements consequent upon poisoning with Strychnine. In cases where the disease does not run a too rapid course, all these symptoms exhibit distinct remissions and exacerbations. If the cord is alone affected, the consciousness remains undisturbed; the patients are, however, unusually excited, and are either deprived of all sleep or else their sleep is very restless. The disease may terminate fatally very speedily, especially when seated near the brain, but may likewise last weeks before the patient dies of exhaustion. Recovery from this disease is scarcely ever complete, especially if the substance of the marrow itself is involved, in which case various paralytic symptoms always remain behind. It may likewise pass into the chronic form. Before treating of this form, we will describe the symptoms by which meningitis is distinguished from myelitis. In meningitis the pain spreads over a larger surface and is very much aggravated by motion, whereas in myelitis the locality of the pain is circumscribed within very narrow limits, and the pain itself is essentially increased only by pressure. In meningitis the fever is more violent. In myelitis paralysis sets in rapidly and totally, whereas in meningitis it develops itself gradually.

As has been said, the chronic form may develop itself out of the acute. If it arises without any previous acute attack, the pains are less violent, and there are no febrile symptoms. These pains are scarcely ever as severe at the place where the inflammation is seated as in the corresponding parts of the periphery, especially in the lower extremities, and at the commencement of the disease resemble altogether rheumatic pains. The paralysis sets in so slightly that it is scarcely perceived, and its increase is just as gradual. Here likewise as in the acute form, anæsthesia is never altogether wanting. As the disease progresses, the bladder becomes paralyzed. This accident, together with the gangrenous destruction of the dorsal integuments, most commonly results in a fatal termination. Chronic myelitis differs somewhat in its phenomena, especially if, as is generally the case, the meninges are not involved. The local pain as well as the pain at the periphery, is less violent, sometimes quite dull and undefined, only slightly aggravated by pressure and motion. The patient experiences a peculiar sensation as if his body were encased in a tight hoop round about. This pathological process is always accompanied by a higher or less degree of anæsthesia.

Inflammation of the Spinal Cord and its Membranes. 113

Convulsive twitchings need not necessarily be present. The paralysis of the motor sphere commences as a vague feeling of heaviness in the extremities, by which the process of walking is very much interfered with. The gait exhibits a peculiar unsteadiness. The patient raises his foot high from the ground, throws it far out, then sets it down as if it had the appearance of falling down, and sets it down a good deal farther back than he seemed disposed to do when first throwing the foot forward; sometimes the foot is set down outside the straight line. It is a peculiar feature of this disease that the patients are unable to walk with their eyes closed. Amid a gradually increasing waste of the tissues the patients die, as in chronic meningitis, of cystitis and gangrenous destruction of the dorsal integuments. Complete recovery is rare; all that can be accomplished in most cases is a partial improvement or even a mere arrest of the disease.

In acute spinal meningitis the prognosis, so far as a fatal termination is concerned, depends more particularly upon the seat of the affection; the nearer to the brain the paralytic phenomena make their appearance, the more rapidly the disease terminates fatally. Under any circumstances the physician has to be very guarded in his promises to effect a complete cure, since partial paralysis is apt to remain in most cases. A good deal is gained in many cases if we succeed in changing the acute to the chronic form of the disease. Simple meningitis justifies the hope of much more satisfactory results than myelitis. In the chronic form the prognosis is particularly dubious after the disease has lasted for some time and the paralysis is complete.

Treatment. The proper selection of drugs in this disease is just as much involved in obscurity as the certain diagnosis of the pathological process itself. Our literature contains only a very small number of cases; in Rückert's Collection we find only a single case of chronic myelitis. This paucity is certainly not owing to the small number of cases—or else the author of this work must have been very fortunate in not having had any more cases to treat— but rather to the circumstance that the therapeutic results have been very unfavorable, and that unsuccessful cases from which a good deal, however, might be learned, are but too seldom published to the world. This affords an additional inducement to lay before the reader a case that came under our observation in the course of last summer, and which, although the patient resided in a distant locality, took such a characteristic turn that there is no reasonable ground left for misapprehension. A farmer, 60 years old, who had hitherto enjoyed the most robust health, was attacked with dysentery in the month of August. To make sure of the diagnosis, he had kept some shreds of mucous membrane which he had passed with the stool. He had taken some domestic remedy, after which the evacuations ceased and obstinate constipation took place. On the fourth day after the cessation of the discharges we first visited the patient, who, at first sight, did not seem to be suffering much. He complained of violent pains in the left lower extremity, which resembled ischias, extended from the tuber ischii to the knee, increased in paroxysms, and were made worse by the warmth of the bed. The patient was restless, had no sleep, the pulse was normal, there were no febrile symptoms. We gave him *Colocynthis*. Two days after the exhibition of this drug the patient reported his pain and whole condition worse. This written report induced us to administer *Belladonna*. No improvement resulting, we visited the patient a second time five days after our first visit. The disease now presented a very different form. The patient was lying partially turned over on his left side. He felt the pains in both lower extremities, not very acutely except in paroxysms; there were twitchings of single muscles or of the whole extremity; violent, but sometimes remitting pains in the lumbar region, the lumbar vertebræ, however, not being very sensitive to pressure. During the night these pains increased to a fearful degree of intensity. Tingling formication in the skin from the pelvis to the feet; the lower extremities felt very cold to the patient. Paralysis of the bladder; the sphincter of the rectum was unable to prevent the emission of flatus. For the last thirty-six hours the lower extremities had been paralyzed so that he was unable to stand without support; if he tried to put on his shoes, he put the foot forward beyond the place where the shoe stood; he was unable to walk except by hanging on to two persons, one on each side. Some fever. Stool normal. Appetite scanty. Almost complete insomnia, with the following characteristic peculiarity. If, late in the evening, the patient did not drink a small portion of not very strong coffee, he remained perfectly sleepless. On walking after having slept a few hours, he was unable to fall asleep again unless he partook of a little more coffee, which acted almost immediately like an opiate. He had tried for some nights to sleep without taking any coffee, but had remained sleepless until he took coffee. We prescribed *Mercurius* third trituration, requesting him at the same time to continue the coffee, the soporific effect of which seemed to act so beneficially upon the patient; at the same time, however, suggesting the propriety of trying every now and then to sleep without the previous use of this beverage. The patient continued the remedy for nine days, after which we visited him again. He was now able to move his legs off the bed alone and rapidly, introduced his feet into his slippers at once and without missing, and walked across the floor six times by means of a cane upon which he, however, leaned only by way of precaution. The pains had abated quite considerably, the anæsthesia had almost entirely disappeared, the bladder and rectum were no longer paralyzed. The coffee had continued its good effect during the whole of this period, but had no longer been required for the last two days. We now prescribed *Veratrum album*. The improvement continued and the patient recovered perfectly. His disease affords undoubtedly a perfect picture of myelitis. About the same time a second no less marked case of chronic myelitis came under my treatment. The affected locality was between the shoulder-blades. So far the treatment, having now lasted five months, has been unsuccessful, but the distress has not increased. Perhaps we may be able to furnish further details concerning this case before this work leaves the hands of the printer.

Among the remedies which may have to be used in this disease, the first place should undoubtedly be assigned to *Mercurius*. So far as we know, this remedy has not as yet been used to any great extent in this disease. We should think, however, that a single case like that of our farmer, ought to entitle this drug to the most careful consideration in this disease, so much more as other remedies, to our knowledge at least, have not as yet been used with any great success in this affection. The mere inspection of persons whose organisms have been impregnated with Mercury shows, even in the absence of all pathogenetic symptoms in our Materia Medica, that this agent must have some specific affinity to the spinal cord. But we do find all the characteristic symptoms of spinal meningitis enumerated in our Materia Medica; if the drug-picture of this disease should be judged incomplete, we can easily complete the list of symptoms from the many reports of chronic mercurial poisoning which may be found scattered in great abundance through our treatises on toxicology. They show that among the toxicological effects of Mercury we may find recorded all the different phases of paralysis of the lower extremities, of the bladder, rectum, with disposition to the peculiar convulsive shocks; violent pains in the spinal cord aggravated by motion; the restlessness and sleeplessness which is equally characteristic of Mercurius as of myelitis; and finally the anæsthesia of the skin. In the case of our farmer the aggravation at night, while lying in bed, was eminently indicative of Mercurius

[We think Bæhr is mistaken regarding the fact that this farmer was cured by *Mercurius* or *Veratrum*. The domestic remedy which this farmer had taken undoubtedly contained Opium, as all such domestic preparations for dysentery do, and the checking of his dysentery by Opium was tantamount to a case of poisoning with Opium. Or, if we please, the case presented a case of Opium-meningitis. This is the reason why coffee, as the antidote to this Opium-poisoning, acted so beneficially. It is coffee which, in this case, effected the cure. Neither Mercurius nor Veratrum had any thing to do with it. The true remedial agents in this case would have been remedies that antidote the action of Opium, namely, *Aconite* and *Belladonna*. If Aconite had been administered alone, or Aconite and Belladonna in alternation, a cure would have been effected in a much shorter space of time. H.]

Secale cornutum. There is scarcely a medicine which has such characteristic symptoms of myelitis, more particularly of the utter extinction of the functional activity of the cord, as Secale. We have the convulsive twitchings and shocks, painful contractions, tetanic phenomena, complete paralysis side by side with continued and even increased reflex action, violent pains in the back, especially in the sacral region, the most complete anæsthesia, paralysis of the bladder and rectum, and lastly the peculiar tendency to gangrenous disorganization which in myelitis is represented by the gangrenous bedsores. Unfortunately we have no post-mortem appearances of individuals that have died of ergotism. This remedy is not only suitable in the acute, but likewise, and perhaps still more specifically, in the chronic form of this disease.

Iodium is recommended as a remedy for affections of the spinal marrow, probably for the reason that it antidotes Mercury, which so often produces them. Its effect seems to be concentrated upon the brain, on which account it arrests the paralytic symptoms in the extremities. Iodium has not yet been known to produce anæsthesia.

Nux omica. So many of the symptoms of myelitis are contained in the pathogenesis of Nux that it almost seems as though this medicine ought to be the main remedy for that affection. It has been urgently recommended by a number of practitioners. It is, however, very doubtful whether such a recommendation will be corroborated by clinical facts. There are few medicines of which we possess as many toxicologico-physiological experiments, as of Nux vomica, more particularly its alkaloid, Strychnine; but in not one of them do we see any form of myelitis, although a strongly marked, venous hyperæmia of the meningeal membranes is mentioned in most of them. This circumstance is undoubtedly striking. Nux vomica has not so much a paralytic condition at the periphery, as violent tetanic contractions; instead of anæsthesia it has rather excessive hyperæsthesia with increased reflex action, which latter phenomenon is rather the exception than the rule in myelitis. Hence it is our opinion that Nux vomica is rather adapted to non-material affections of the spinal cord and that, among the inflammatory affections of this organ, it is at most suitable in spinal meningitis before the disease has progressed to the stage of actual exudation.

Rhus toxicodendron is at all events a noteworthy remedy in myelitis. Although it is possible to derive the pathogenetic symptoms pointing to paralysis from the decomposition of the blood which is peculiar to Rhus, this point of view does not justify a one-sided application of Rhus as a therapeutic agent in this disease. In the first stages of myelitis the slight fever would rather counter-indicate Rhus, except perhaps in cases where the affection is occasioned by an acute exanthem. On the other hand the stage of complete paraplegia will be found much more adapted to Rhus, both in chronic as well as in acute cases. For myelitis caused by exanthems, Hartmann recommends *Dulcamara* as a specific remedy; only the symptoms which he enumerates, as symptoms of myelitis, do not seem to be the disease of which he supposes them to be characteristic indications.

Veratrum album is one of the most suitable remedies in this disease, and is especially adapted to the symptoms of the second stage. In the above-mentioned case of our farmer it helped very decidedly to bring about a favorable termination. Whether it will prove suitable in chronic cases, will have to be verified by practical experiments.

Plumbum has evidently as marked an action upon the spinal marrow as we have shown it to have upon the brain in our article on encephalitis. It is to be regretted that the poisonous action of Plumbum upon the spinal cord has not been ascertained by post-mortem examinations, which would have revealed with positive certainty the portion of the cord that is morbidly affected by this agent. The known effects of Lead upon the brain justify us to conclude by a process of reasoning from analogy, that it is the marrow itself which is invaded and destroyed; otherwise the paralytic phenomena would not be so completely developed. Owing to the slowness of its action the drug is not adapted to acute cases; in chronic cases a characteristic feature of the paralysis for which Lead is indicated, would be the speedy emaciation of the paralyzed parts which are at the same time violently and painfully contracted. Colicky pains proceeding from the spinal cord would likewise point to *Plumbum* as a leading remedy.

Cuprum. If it is generally difficult to discriminate between the effects of Copper and Lead, this discrimination is so much more difficult with special reference to the spinal cord. It is admitted that among the symptoms of Copper the paralytic symptoms are less clearly defined and that the spasmodic symptoms prevail, whereas in the case of Lead the opposite effects are observed. Both these medicines act decidedly in the same direction, with this difference, that Cuprum is more suitable at the beginning, and Plumbum at the termination of the series. Hence Plumbum may have to succeed Cuprum with tolerable certainty, whereas the reverse will scarcely ever be the case.

Cocculus is another exceedingly praiseworthy remedy, especially at the commencement of myelitis. If we were to select a remedy according to the locality of the disease, Cocculus would be more adapted to inflammation of the lumbar portion of the cord, less to such portions as are nearer the brain; however it still remains difficult to determine whether Cocculus does not, like Nux vomica, rather modify the functional activity of the marrow without causing any material alterations.

We must not omit to make mention of a few other remedies which have either been urgently recommended by physicians or which, at any rate, seem suitable. As regards *Belladonna* and *Aconite*, it is our belief that their employment involves a loss of time without producing any curative results. In myelitis the reaction is never sufficiently violent to oblige us to control the febrile symptoms by means of either of these two drugs. Neither has a marked affinity to the spinal marrow. *Ignatia* occupies pretty much the same position in this affection as Nux vomica. *Phosphorus* is said to be excellent where the inflammation has been superinduced by sexual excesses. *Sulphur* may be thought of in cases where the disease has been arrested and where we desire to act upon the remaining exudation in the spinal canal with a view of improving the paralytic symptoms. Sulphur is here a very important remedy, as is shown by the good effects of Sulphur baths in paralytic conditions remaining as consequences of myelitis. We are acquainted with a lady who is nearly sixty years old and has been suffering for the last ten years with chronic meningitis. The disease seems to exacerbate once or twice in the course of a year, is seated in the lower thoracic portion of the medulla, but does not seem to affect the substance of the medulla very deeply, since the paralytic symptoms are not very distinct, except in the arms; moreover, as is often noticed in spinal hemiplegia, we observe in her case a general increase of her *embonpoint*, except on the paralyzed parts. Every summer this lady uses weak artificial Sulphur baths with decided benefit; even the paralysis of the arms improves every summer very visibly. We have likewise treated in the same place an employé of a company, whose lower extremities had been completely paralyzed for two years, in consequence of myelitis of the lumbar portion of the cord, and who had been using for some time various remedies, among others *Sulphur*, without any further benefit than that he was enabled to move about on two crutches with great difficulty. He was sent by his employers to the Sulphur springs at Eilsen, where he remained for some three months, after which lapse of time he was able to walk with a cane. His recovery is not complete. Cases of this kind show that Sulphur has a decidedly curative action in myelitis, where it may possibly be much more efficacious when used in the form of baths than when taken internally. *Calcarea carbonica* deserves attention, if the inflammation is caused by diseases of the vertebræ, not so much because this medicine has a direct action upon the cord as because it acts in opposition to the causative disturbance. Among the springs which undoubtedly exert an influence upon spinal paralysis, we have to mention Gastein, Pfeffers and Wildbad; of course they should not be used until the inflammatory symptoms have entirely disappeared. They doubtless afford the most help in cases depending upon sexual excesses as their primary causes.

[We do not think that Bæhr's condemnation of Aconite in this disease is justified by experience. In the acute form of meningitis we have succeeded with Aconite alone in effecting a perfect cure in a comparatively short space of time. But we neither give high nor middle potencies in this disease, but a few drops of the tincture or no higher than the first decimal attenuation of the root in ten or twelve tablespoonfuls of water, of which mixture the patient is given one or two teaspoonfuls every half hour or hour until an incipient improvement renders it desirable to lengthen the intervals. If the spine is very hot, tender to the touch, with throbbing, stinging or lancinating pains, we do not hesitate to apply to the spine linen or flannel compresses soaked with a solution of a teaspoonful of the first decimal attenuation of Aconite root in half a pint of water.

Gelseminum causes hyperæmia of the spinal cord and has been used with good success by our physicians in congestive and inflammatory affections of the spinal cord. The consciousness is not much impaired. There is either general or partial paralysis. The patient shows a remarkable tendency to close his eyelids. The pulse is feeble and the temperature of the body very much depressed.

Veratrum viride is administered with more or less special reference to the condition of the pulse. If the pulse is rather full and bounding, of more than ordinary frequency, or else feeble and rapid, and the patient complains of fulness and pain in the head, feels very much prostrated, and the extremities feel numb, twitch and are threatened with paralysis; or if the spinal congestion is attended with a general typhoid state of the system, drowsiness, indistinct consciousness, restlessness, Veratrum viride will induce a very speedy and favorable reaction, if given in quantities of two or three drops of the strongest tincture in ten tablespoonfuls of water, a good teaspoonful at a dose every half hour or hour until an improvement sets in. It is often desirable to alternate Veratrum viride with *Belladonna*.

Kafka, in his "Homœopathische Therapie," has an interesting chapter on inflammation of the vertebræ (spondylitis) which we have deemed it advisable to transcribe literally for the benefit of the American reader.

"Chronic myelitis as occurring in the course of spondylarthrocace has been for years an object of our most careful observations and therapeutic investigations. The results which we have obtained, being exceedingly favorable, we feel induced to communicate the important facts that we have been able to gather up in this domain of medical science.

Inflammation of the vertebræ, (spondylitis,) in consequence of which the meninges of the spinal marrow and the marrow itself participate in the inflammation, is always attended with swelling and softening of one or two, or in exceedingly rare cases, of several vertebræ. Without experiencing any pain or any feeling of illness, children who seem perfectly healthy, or else scrofulous, rickety or tuberculous children, are attacked with a crick in the spinal column arising from softening of one or more bodies of the vertebræ, the body of the softened vertebra being no longer capable of carrying the superimposed weight of the trunk, and, having to succumb to the law of gravitation, becoming displaced to such an extent that its spinous process is turned upwards and forms a prominence which causes the vertebral column to appear curved so as to form an obtuse angle at that point.

The immediate consequence of this curvature and swelling of the vertebræ is a pressure upon the spinal marrow, which becomes much more marked if exudations take place between the transverse processes and between the tendinous structures of the vertebral column, by which exudations the spinal marrow is compressed on all sides.

If one of the lumbar vertebræ is affected, the children experience at once a gradually increasing weakness in the lower extremities; they are unable to walk a long distance or for any length of time; they find it difficult to stand, get easily tired, prefer sitting or lying down, their gait becomes dragging, labored, they do not seem to make the least headway. Finally the lower extremities become partially paralyzed and lose their sensibility.

If one of the thoracic vertebræ is the seat of the inflammation, the above-mentioned symptoms develop themselves more slowly, but, on the other hand, become associated with pressure in the epigastrium, dyspepsia, flatulence, constipation, difficulty of urinating, etc., according as the different abdominal viscera are in anatomical and physiological dependence upon the inflamed portion of the spinal marrow; lastly we have paraplegia together with paralysis of the sphincters of the rectum and bladder.

If the cervical portion of the vertebral column is inflamed, the curvature is in most cases located between the first and second cervical, or between the last cervical and the first thoracic vertebræ; in the former case the head, deprived of its point of support, leans over obliquely to the right or left side, in the latter case the head sinks down between the shoulders, and it is only with great difficulty and a visible effort that it can be maintained erect. In either case the curvature is accompanied by great difficulty of breathing, or by coldness, weakness and paralytic phenomena in the upper extremities. The dyspnœa often increases to a high degree, and is attended with cyanosis, extensive bronchial catarrh and nocturnal cough. If the articulation of the atlas is invaded by the inflammation, we observe dysphagia, dyspnœa, hoarseness and a constant rigidity of the nape of the neck, without any signs of morbid affection of the larynx, trachea or lungs.

We have introduced this pathological statement in order to understand the connection of the symptoms as they appear before us.

If we are fortunate enough to be intrusted with the management of spondylitis at the very outset of the attack, we have it in our power to arrest it very speedily and thus to prevent the further progress of myelitis and meningitis spinalis. Even if the inflammation of the vertebræ has continued for a time and a considerable amount of fluid has become exuded, *but no abscess has yet formed*, if the children are so feeble that they are unable to walk, but have to lie down for the most part of the time, or if they have become dyspeptic, bloated, peevish and sullen; or if the dyspnœa, cyanosis and a wide-spread bronchial catarrh have already set in, we still may effect a decided improvement by the exhibition of *Phosphorus* 3, two or three doses a day. In a few days already the children become more cheerful and active, the weakness of the lower extremities begins to yield; very soon, sometimes already in five or six days, they begin to sit up or attempt to creep about on the floor; the appetite returns, the abdomen loses its bloat, the cough diminishes very strikingly, the cyanosis disappears, the dyspnœa becomes less, and in at most a fortnight the children begin to walk, their posture becomes more and more erect, and every symptom of disease and feeling of illness gradually disappears. Only the vertebral curvature remains; but upon examining the vertebræ more closely, we find that their sensitiveness to pressure gradually decreases, the swelling of the vertebræ and their surroundings becomes less and the phenomena of compression of the spinal marrow disappear entirely. In the most fortunate cases, of which we might mention quite a number, we have never seen the angle of curvature become less obtuse owing to the circumstance that the vertebræ which had become compressed in consequence of the softening of their substance, are no longer able to return to their normal size.

If the improvement goes on very slowly and we have to continue the use of Phosphorus for a long time, it is advisable, after having used this drug for a fortnight, to discontinue its employment for a week, or to administer *Natrum muriaticum* 6, in two daily doses as an intercurrent remedy, after which period the Phosphorus may be resumed until all morbid symptoms have entirely disappeared.

In a former chapter we have directed the attention of the reader to these two remedies in interstitial distention and swelling of the bones, especially the vertebræ, and, after an experience of many years, we are prepared to affirm their efficacy in these diseases. Even if the knee, tarsal and elbow-joints were the seat of these affections, we have derived good results from the use of Phosphorus and Natrum muriaticum.

Both these remedies correspond to the scrofulous as well as to the rhachitic and tuberculous diathesis; only, if such conditions are present, the remedies have to be administered at long intervals, alternating them at most only every week.

As soon as abscesses form, which generally break out at the above designated localities and are attended with shiverings or slight creeping chills, or with an increase of the febrile symptoms, but may likewise develop themselves without any other perceptible morbid phenomena, the curative range of the above-mentioned two remedies is closed; for now we have to deal with soft exudations passing through a purulent or ichorous metamorphosis; these changes require a corresponding change of remedies.

As long as the abscesses are small and not very tense, we give at once *Silicea* 6, two doses a day, ordering at the same time, especially if the patients are weak, pale and emaciated, a nourishing and strengthening meat-diet, and a refreshing beverage. If the season is favorable, we send the patients to the mountains or to a region of country with plenty of woods and meadows. Under this management the abscesses, in favorable cases, become smaller and softer, a gradual absorption may even take place, and a complete disappearance of the paralytic conditions, of the anæsthesia and the spasmodic symptoms, may be the result. In order to obtain it, however, this kind of management has often to be continued for weeks and even months, more particularly in cases where one of the above-mentioned diatheses is present. In such cases, after having continued the exhibition of Silicea for a fortnight, we are in the habit of giving *Sulphur* 6, one or two doses daily, as an intercurrent remedy, or we discontinue all medication for a few days, after which we resume the use of Silicea.

Both remedies correspond perfectly to the above-mentioned constitutional anomalies, and their employment is often crowned with the happiest results.

In less fortunate cases resorption may likewise take place without it being necessary to open the abscess; the subsequent improvement, however, is not perfect; the extremities remain affected with a paralytic weakness, the sensibility of the parts returns only partially, and there frequently remain spasmodic contractions of the muscles, from which phenomena it is evident that the pressure on the spinal marrow has not entirely ceased, or even that structural changes have already taken place in this organ. In such cases we resort to *electricity by induction*, which is sometimes capable of determining a further improvement of the morbid process that had become arrested at a certain point.

If the abscesses are large and tense; if they do not show the least tendency to discharge on the outside; if the patients are at the same time anæmic, feeble, emaciated, cachectic, etc., we open the abscesses with a bistouri, taking care that they do not discharge too rapidly and that no air penetrates into their cavity.

The entrance of atmospheric air into the cavity of the abscess causes the formation of coagula on the inner walls of the abscess, in consequence of which it becomes lined with a membrane resembling mucous membrane, by which the healing of the abscess is impeded.

If the discharge is yellow and inodorous, we give *Silicea* 6 very persistently in order to act upon the carious disorganization which the suppurative process may have initiated on the exterior portions of the vertebræ. This remedy, in conjunction with a strengthening diet, is in many cases sufficient to effect a complete cure of the caries.

If the pus is ichorous and has a fetid odor, we first try to correct the quality of the secretion by means of *Sulphur* 6, giving two doses a day; as soon as this object is accomplished, we give *Silicea*. As a matter of course we never lose sight of the duty of nourishing up our patient by substantial and readily assimilated nutriment in order to make up for the loss of strength and vital fluids entailed by the profuse ichorous discharge.

We have succeeded in curing cases of a far advanced caries of the vertebræ by the persistent use of these two remedies, which we are very fond of administering in alternation.

It is not very long ago that surgeons were very much indisposed to plunge their lancets into a so-called cold abscess, for the reason that they were apprehensive of an unfavorable termination, most generally of the supervention of hectic fever. No later than the year 1850, we had the greatest difficulty in persuading our honored friend, Professor Pitha, to plunge his lancet into a large and cold abscess in the lumbar region, which was connected with spondylitis and accompanied by a high degree of anæmia, emaciation and debility. The quantity of the discharged pus amounted to at least four or five pounds; it was of a very thin, fluid consistence and without any bad odor. By giving two doses of *Silicea* every day, during periods of eight days, allowing an interval of three days between each two successive periods, the assimilative powers of the patient, a girl of six years, were so much improved that she gained rapidly from day to day in weight, strength and external appearance, and she soon was able to boast of a perfect recovery. The curvature of course remained unaltered, her gait as well as her general posture, movements and feelings were almost normal. The patient is now a married lady and has enjoyed good health ever since her previous sickness.

We are now treating a boy of six years who, two years ago, was attacked with inflammation of the second and third thoracic vertebræ, in consequence of which he became afflicted with dyspnœa and cyanosis to the highest degree. A catarrhal râle was heard in both lungs, the respiration was short and superficial, only with great effort the patient coughed up a serous-frothy sputum. Upon examining the thorax it was found to be affected with a rickety mal formation, both the anterior costal spaces below the nipples were pressed in, the sternum bulged out a great deal, and the chest itself was very flat and narrow. In consequence of this deformity the posterior and upper portion of the lungs was evidently compressed, for at the apex of the scapulæ there was bronchial respiration without any dulness of percussion or consonant râles in the corresponding localities. The boy was the child of perfectly healthy and opulent parents and is said to have enjoyed good health until the present sickness set in. His former physicians, supposing that the lungs had become incurably œdematous, had given up all hopes of his recovery.

We gave him *Phosphorus* 3 in solution, a dose every hour, ordered the little patient to be kept perfectly quiet and free from all excitement, and gave him four times a day a weak broth, without salt and stirred up with a little ground rice or flour. Already on the third day symptoms of improvement set in; the dyspnœa became less, the expectoration was thrown off much more easily, the mucous râle decreased, the cyanotic symptoms disappeared more and more. In proportion as the bronchia became disembarrassed, the bronchial respiration decreased, the digestion became more active, and in about three weeks the patient was able to leave his bed and to maintain a more erect posture. His gait became more steady, but the bent in the vertebral column and the swelling of the vertebræ remained unchanged. The painfulness of the vertebræ to pressure likewise decreased very sensibly, and the trunk was moved in every direction, without pain or trouble. After the symptoms of spondylitis had been almost entirely removed, and with a view of modifying the constitutional anomaly, we put the patient for some time on *Silicea* 6, after which the patient, to our own and the parents' joy, developed within a short space of time, both mentally and physically, to great advantage. This apparent improvement continued for nine months. At this time the protruding vertebræ became again inflamed owing to frictions with oil, kneading and squeezing, which the parents had permitted to be done to prevent the boy from remaining a cripple. The consequence of this return of inflammation was paralysis of the lower extremities, with simultaneous loss of sensibility, continual spasmodic stretching of the muscles and occasional muscular twitchings. Stool and urine were passed involuntarily. There was dyspnœa, evening and night-fever, sleeplessness and a high degree of morose temper. For this intense degree of spondylo-myelitis we again prescribed *Phosphorus*, and ordered absolute rest. The general condition of the patient soon began to mend; almost every morbid symptom had disappeared at the end of four weeks, only the paralysis and the phenomena incidental to this condition obstinately resisted Phosphorus as well as the subsequent employment of *Mercurius solubilis* 3, *Iodide of Potassium* 1, *Plumbum* 6, *Arsenicum* 3, *Nux vomica* 3, *Strychnine* 3. Even the douche had no effect. Electricity by induction diminished the anæsthesia and the spasms of the extensor muscles. During this time the exudation softened and an abscess formed. After *Silicea* 6 the abscess grew smaller and softer, and showed signs of incipient re-absorption. As the exudation became softer, the sensibility in the lower extremities increased more and more. Afterwards when the abscess became more tense and larger, and the Silicea had been continued together with a strengthening diet and an invigorating country-air, the first voluntary motion took place in the month of July of the same year. After opening the abscess, which discharged a fine healthy pus, the mobility of the lower extremities increased more and more. The supervention of a chronic intestinal catarrh which yielded to *Phosphorus* 3, caused a high degree of emaciation and debility; these symptoms were soon, however, controlled by a nourishing diet and the use of ale. At the present time the boy is able to walk without support, and is generally doing finely. We have stated this case *in extenso* in order to show that, under a suitable management, even a high degree of myelitis can be reduced in intensity and improve very greatly.

If we desire to effect a speedy and complete cure of spondylitis, it is necessary that the patient should be kept in a state of *absolute rest*. The most suitable position is on the stomach, with the extremities extended and the head raised.

Where absolute rest is not enjoined, we have often seen relapses ensue, and the spondylitis spread further and further in consequence of this neglect.

If the tuberculous disposition is hereditary, or the exudation assumes a tubercular character, the spondylitis frequently terminates fatally. The inflammation is very apt to set in again, evening or night-fever occurs every day, with profuse sweats, emaciation, pallor of the integuments and colliquative diarrhœa. The abscesses discharge an ichorous, badly smelling fluid, decubitus sets in and the patients die of tubercular caries of the vertebræ.

If the tubercular diathesis is noticed in season, *Phosphorus, Calcarea, Natrum muriaticum, Silicea, Iodium* or *Sulphur*, together with a suitable diet and good country-air, are capable of ameliorating the constitutional disposition so as to give a favorable turn to the disease. Hence it is of importance that in a case of spondylitis, no matter what its character, the physician should institute careful inquiries into the hereditary or constitutional tubercular disposition.

Cod-liver oil has been of use to us in the treatment of this disease. To improve the tubercular, rhachitic or scrofulous constitution, we have employed with good effect saline springs and sea-bathing; or, if a high degree of anæmia prevails, the use of chalybeate springs is highly to be recommended.

Paralytic conditions and consequent ailments are treated in the same manner as the paralytic conditions consequent upon meningitis spinalis.

If we have reason to suspect that the myelitis is occasioned by the presence of a syphilitic exostosis, an energetic anti-syphilitic treatment will have to be instituted." H.]

In conclusion, we will offer a few general remarks concerning the treatment. We are not often called to treat a case of myelitis when the disease first breaks out; most generally the patients have already been tortured with sanguineous depletions and other losses of vital fluids before a homœopathic treatment is determined upon. In such cases a main question will always be how far we may encourage the hope of a favorable result in the patient's mind, and we think that our promises in this respect can never be too guarded. Sometimes we succeed in effecting an improvement even in old cases; but very often all medicinal action remains ineffectual; if the paralysis has been of long continuance it will probably always be impossible to effect a complete cure. In the former series of cases an improvement is undoubtedly effected by the gradual resorption of the meningeal exudation which exists side by side with the disorganization of the spinal marrow. A result of this kind alone is sufficient to constitute an essential improvement for the patient. In chronic meningitis a more or less copious accumulation of serum takes place in the meningeal space, the resorption of which is succeeded by the disappearance of a variety of paralytic symptoms. Hence it is our duty in all cases to at least make the attempt of improving the patient's condition, only we should be cautious in promising a cure of the paralysis when superinduced by the destruction of the medulla. Regarding sanguineous depletions we offer the same condemnatory remarks that have already been recorded in our article on apoplexy. Whether a patient afflicted with myelitis should remain in an exclusively horizontal posture, had better be decided by the patient himself, who is the best judge whether motion is hurtful or beneficial to him. It is certainly never productive of absolute mischief, whereas a forced recumbent position may entail great disadvantages. In chronic cases the hope of recovery is in a great measure based upon a methodical, cautious use of the paralyzed parts, as has been, for a long time already, shown by the beneficial results obtained by the movement-cure. In conclusion we will mention a method of treatment the pernicious influence of which in this disease we have had occasion not long ago to witness in the case of a lady: we mean the cold-water treatment. Under certain circumstances it may be useful even in myelitis, but certainly not very often. The cause undoubtedly is, that in a case of myelitis the skin is in a measure deprived of its properties of sensibility and irritability, and hence unable to develop the degree of reaction necessary to experience the blissful effects of cold water.

On this account an excess of warmth is withdrawn from the organism, without this loss being repaired by a corresponding supply of vital warmth. In the case of the above-mentioned lady the cutaneous anæsthesia has undoubtedly become aggravated since the application of cold water.

This is a suitable place for mentioning an affection whose symptoms bear a great resemblance to the chronic inflammatory processes in the spinal marrow: we allude to tabes dorsualis. So far the pathologico-anatomical results of this affection have not by any means been distinctly defined. In many cases, it is true, atrophy of single portions of the cord is met with, but it is not clearly defined, whereas in other cases the atrophy is either entirely absent, or, at any rate, does not come within the ken of our observation. The most correct definition of tabes dorsualis is undoubtedly to regard it as a gradually increasing paralysis of the spinal marrow. The causes of such a paralysis are not by any means clearly defined, and it is undoubtedly wrong to regard sexual excesses as the most common of them. It is undoubtedly true that they constitute a very frequent cause of the disease; but excessive exertions of the back generally may likewise superinduce a wasting and paralysis of the spinal marrow. It is not probable that paralysis of the spinal marrow is the consequence of inflammatory conditions of that organ; the paralysis runs almost always a painless course, and the cadaver exhibits no traces of an inflammatory exudation. The disease attacks principally men of middle age. The symptoms resemble a good deal those of chronic myelitis. The disease does not commence with pain, but with signs of weakness in the muscles of the lower extremities, such as: restlessness, feeling of weariness from the least exertion, tendency to drop to sleep; these symptoms are accompanied by a peculiar, but seldom painful feeling of emptiness in the spine. At an early period of the disease the condition of the genital organs becomes altered. They are not primarily debilitated, on the contrary, they are easily excited; erections and seminal emissions are very frequent, but they have not the normal vigor, more particularly during sexual intercourse, when this want of vigor is particularly apparent. In the further course of the disease the paralysis increases, spreads to the bladder and rectum, until, after the lapse of years, the paralysis of both the motor and sentient spheres of the lower extremities becomes complete. At this stage, portions of the marrow nearer the brain become involved, even the brain becomes affected, vision becomes disturbed, the memory is weakened, apathy and even complete stupor set in.

According to most physicians the treatment of this disease is almost always unsuccessful; most authors assert that it is unsuccessful in every case. If taken at the outset it might perhaps be possible to effect a cure; but at the beginning the affection is not considered so very dangerous, or the patient has no proper conception of the nature of his disease, and neglects, or does not persevere in, the proper treatment. If medicines are to be used, we have to select them among the number of those that have been recommended for myelitis, to which may be added *Silicea*, *Causticum*, *Aluminium metallicum*. The condition of the sexual organs points to *Phosphorus*, but it is questionable whether the exhibition of this agent will be attended with good results. At a later stage of the disease the main point is to maintain the strength of the patient and to see to it that it is not crushed down by excessive exertion. The duration of the disease for years, and the unsuccessful administration of remedies, drive such patients from one physician to another; they generally apply to any one who promises them a cure and drains their pockets as well as their constitutions. This circumstance alone renders a cure impossible, even if it might otherwise be attempted with a chance of success.

[Meningitis Cerebro-spinalis, Cerebro-spinal Meningitis, Spotted Fever.

Professor Felix Niemeyer has recently published an interesting memoir on this epidemic under the title: "Cerebro-spinal Meningitis according to observations instituted in the Grand-duchy of Baden," Berlin, 1865, in which the following concise and characteristic picture of the disease is offered: "Without any other precursory symptoms the patient is at once attacked with a chill attended with violent headache and vomiting. The headache speedily increases in intensity, the patient becomes exceedingly restless, tosses about, the pupils remain contracted, the sensual consciousness remains unembarrassed. The pulse rises to eighty or one hundred beats, the temperature of the body remains moderate, the respirations increase to thirty or forty per minute. Already at the end of the first or on the second day, much less frequently at a later period, we notice that the head is somewhat drawn backwards; the patient continues to complain of violent headache and the pain spreads from the head to the posterior cervical region and to the back. The restlessness becomes excessive, the thoughts of the patient become confused, the pupils remain contracted, the abdomen caves in, the bowels are constipated. The frequency of the pulsations and respirations now increases to about one hundred and twenty of the former and upwards of seventy of the latter per minute; the bodily temperature continues moderately low, increasing perhaps to 39° R., and upwards. In the course of the third and fourth day the tetanic spasms of the posterior cervical and dorsal muscles become more and more prominent, and are sometimes attended with lock-jaw. Opisthotonus supervenes with an extraordinary degree of intensity; the consciousness is gone, but the patient still continues to toss about in the bed, the pupils still remain contracted, the bowels constipated, the abdomen sunken, the urine is discharged involuntarily or else the bladder remains distended and the urine has to be drawn off with the catheter. The patient now lapses into a profound sopor, the moaning respiration is accompanied by a râle, and death takes place with the phenomena of an acute œdema of the lungs.

This picture of the disease is sometimes modified by the occurrence of a short preliminary stage which is marked by slight pains in the head and back; or by the breaking out of herpetic vesicles or of scattered, dark-colored roseola-spots on the first, second or third day of the disease; or else the above-described symptoms develop themselves in a much shorter period, which circumstance constitutes one of the most important modifications of the disease, so that the consciousness vanishes even on the first day of the attack and a violent tetanic spasm of the posterior cervical and dorsal muscles begins; or finally the disease may set in with such terrible violence that a fatal termination is reached even on the first or second day."

Further on, Niemeyer writes: "This cursory picture of cerebro-spinal meningitis and of the general course of the disease applies indeed to most, but not by any means to all cases of the epidemic. This picture does not comprehend phenomena that occur in a variety of cases, such as: deafness on one or both ears, diplopia, ptosis of the upper eyelid, softening and destruction of the cornea, and finally paralysis of the facial nerve, and of the extremities either on both or only on one side of the body."

These last-mentioned phenomena are attributed by Niemeyer to the exudation resulting from the intense inflammation at the base of the brain where the exuded fluid exerts a pressure upon the adjoining portions of the brain and nervous trunks; whereas in sporadic meningitis the exudation takes place for the most part on the convex portions of the hemispheres.

This epidemic has visited several parts of our own country and, under allœopathic treatment, has proved a murderous scourge. The States of New Jersey, New York, Pennsylvania, Vermont, Massachusetts, Ohio, Maine, Michigan, Virginia, and the District of Columbia, have been visited by this fell destroyer. In the November number of the North American Journal of Homœopathy an interesting article on this disease is published by Doctor Bushrod W. James, of Philadelphia. He professes to have treated a considerable number of cases with very uniform success, losing only one case in about sixty, which seems to us claiming a great deal, whereas under allœopathic treatment the mortality was about fifty cases out of every hundred. In the Philadelphia epidemic prostration seems to have been a very prominent symptom. It sometimes set in with such a sudden violence that persons who were afflicted with heart-disease dropped down dead in the street in consequence of the sudden shock. This happened in a number of cases. Many persons died twenty-four or forty-eight hours after being seized with the chill. Operatives over-tasked in the factories of Manayunk near Philadelphia would very often die in fourteen or sixteen hours from the chill. The general features of the disease seem to have been: vertigo with headache; diarrhœa, sometimes of a prostrating and colliquative character; in other cases diarrhœa alternating with constipation; moderate fever, flashes of heat mingled with creeping chills; piercing pains through the head; soreness and stiffness of the upper portion of the spine, with aching pains in the spine, formication; soreness and sensitiveness of the skin; severe muscular pains; numbness of the limbs, with partial paralysis; spasmodic twitchings of the muscular system, sometimes amounting to tetanic convulsions with lock-jaw; the consciousness was not much affected, except when the disease was at its height, when a more or less active delirium and finally coma set in; in the cases that we have treated the conjunctiva was more or less congested and the hearing was impaired. The pulse had a moderate frequency, averaging about one hundred per minute; the tongue remained moist and, in the course of the disease, became covered with a dark brownish fur; the respiration was somewhat accelerated and interrupted by moaning inspirations; during the tetanic spasms the expirations had a hissing sound, the air seeming to be forced out with an effort; the skin had a peculiar bluish pallor in this disease owing to the general turgescence of the venous system; the spots which have given to this disease its name broke out on different parts of the body, generally on the chest, abdomen, and thighs. Sometimes the skin had a mottled appearance, or the spots looked like measle-spots, or had a rose-colored tint.

Doctor James regards cerebro-spinal meningitis as a very changeable and deceptive disease; "one hour the patient will seem quite well, and the next the most alarming symptoms may be present." In the few cases which we have treated in Michigan, this feature of the disease has never come under our observation.

An admirable monograph on this disease has been published by Professor Alfred Stillé, of Philadelphia, which has been very favorably noticed by Professor A. Flint in the January number, 1868, of the American Journal of the Medical Sciences. Doctor Stillé has observed about one hundred and twenty cases of the disease in the Philadelphia Hospital. He rejects the name "Spotted fever." According to Stillé the disease is both a blood-disease and an inflammation of the cerebro-spinal membranes combined. "The inflammatory element and the septic element are both necessary to constitute the disease; either may be in excess and overshadow the other. According to the relative predominance of one or the other, the disease assumes more of a typhoid, or more of an inflammatory type, and it is this diversity in its physiognomy which has led to such opposite doctrines in regard to its nature and its nosological affinities." The cases treated exhibit a striking uniformity of symptoms: headache, nausea, vomiting, diarrhœa or constipation, thirst, hyperæsthesia of the abdomen or of the cutaneous surfaces generally, more or less active delirium, comatose stupor, congestion of the conjunctiva, tenderness of the spine, opisthotonos, subsultus tendinum, severe muscular pains, insatiable thirst, tongue covered with a whitish or brown fur, or sometimes glazed, erythematous and petechial eruptions. Deafness and partial paralysis sometimes remained for some time as sequelæ of the disease.

As regards treatment, Dr. James professes to have derived the most beneficial results from the use of deodorized alcohol of the strength of ninety-five per cent. He seems to have resorted to this stimulant at the onset in every case as soon as the nature of the disease was ascertained. His mode of administering the alcohol was to add two teaspoonfuls of it to two, four, six or eight teaspoonfuls of water, according to the nature of the case, and to give a teaspoonful of this solution every half hour until there was a decided abatement in the symptoms. In cases threatening immediate dissolution, the dose was increased for a brief period. On the other hand, Dr. Stillé objects to this indiscriminate use of the alcoholic stimulant. "On the whole," writes this author, "we regard alcohol as a medicine which ought not to be included in the ordinary and systematic treatment of epidemic meningitis, but as a cordial to be held in reserve against those signs of failure in the power of the nervous system, which call for its administration in diseases of whatever name."

The remedies employed in this disease were:

Aconite, Gelseminum, Belladonna, and **Veratrum viride,** during the congestive stage, when the congestive and inflammatory symptoms predominated. The Aconite has proved less useful in our hands than Gelseminum and Veratrum viride, both of which medicines we did not hesitate to alternate with Belladonna or Hyoscyamus, if the inflammatory and typhoid symptoms seemed to co-exist.

Belladonna and **Hyoscyamus** were relied on if a more or less active delirium had set in, the patient was inclined to sleep, the conjunctiva was found congested, the pupils were alternately contracted or dilated, or one pupil contracted and the other dilated; subsultus tendinum, opisthotonic spasms.

Bryonia and **Rhus toxicodendron** were used with more or less benefit when the inflammatory condition seemed to give way to typhoid phenomena: subsultus, lock-jaw, incipient loss of consciousness, sopor with expression of deep suffering in the countenance; symptoms of paralysis, difficulty of protruding the tongue, the corners of the mouth are drawn down; the muscular pains are very severe. It is very difficult to determine well-defined lines of demarcation between the respective spheres of action of these different drugs. Owing to the uncertain character of the symptoms, we have found ourselves compelled to give many of these remedies in alternation, for instance: Aconite and Bryonia, or Bryonia and Belladonna, or Veratrum viride and Belladonna, or Aconite and Gelseminum, or Rhus tox. and Hyoscyamus, or Hyoscyamus and Arsenicum.

Arsenicum, 2d or 3d decimal trituration, was given when the septic symptoms, foul discharges from the bowels, signs of decomposition of the blood, malignant looking petechiæ, etc., indicated its use.

Calomel was given if the diarrhœa and the hyperæsthesia of the abdomen seemed to require the use of this agent.

Cuprum aceticum seemed to relieve the paralytic symptoms and the mental hebetude which sometimes remained as sequelæ of severe attacks of the disease.

Opium was resorted to as a last resort, if the coma and the paralytic symptoms did not yield to Belladonna or Hyoscyamus, or showed a tendency to become more inveterate.

Relapses in this disease were difficult to manage and, as a general rule, proved fatal. At any rate, this has been our experience in this part of our country. H.]

Spinal Irritation. Neuralgia Spinalis.

For a long time this affection has given rise to a good deal of discussion, and a number of writings have been published on the subject *pro* and *con*, until more recently physicians have adopted the general conclusion not to regard this disease as an independent pathological process, but as a symptomatic manifestation of a more general affection. By spinal irritation we understand a condition where a more or less extensive portion of the vertebral column is abnormally sensitive to pressure, and where all sorts of disturbances are manifested in the sentient and motor sphere of the nerves proceeding from the affected portion of the cord. In this affection no material changes of the spinal marrow or its envelopes have as yet been discovered; and it is probably for this reason that the affection has been designated as a neuralgia, by which means the vagueness of the genuine pathological conception has indeed become more pointed and conspicuous. In many cases partial hyperæmia may be the cause of the phenomena; in other cases the cause undoubtedly resides outside of the vertebral canal, the marrow becoming secondarily irritated and sensitive. On this account we see spinal irritation accompany a number of febrile as well as non-febrile affections. Very seldom we may be able to trace the phenomena of spinal irritation to a sensitiveness of the vertebræ as their primary cause. The disease is mostly limited to the female sex between the age of pubescence and the climacteric period; in the male organism the disease is not only seen much less frequently, but is generally much less extensive and prominent. All kinds of influences have been assigned as causes of this trouble; we shall not attempt to enumerate the whole list of them here, and content ourselves with mentioning the following as the main causes of the disease: all kinds of excessive exertions affecting more specially the spinal marrow, more particularly all sexual excesses; continued losses of vital fluids, excessive nursing, leucorrhœa, exhausting diseases.

According to the locality of the disease, the symptoms of spinal irritation differ so greatly that it is impossible to describe the whole series so as to meet every case. As a general rule the symptoms are located within the domain of the nerves proceeding from the affected portion of the marrow. If the upper portion of the medulla is affected, the pains are principally located about the head, and may even lead us to suspect a cerebral disease, for we do not unfrequently observe illusions of the senses, amaurosis, deafness, even delirium. An affection of the lower thoracic portion of the spine, where the stomach becomes predominantly involved, is likewise of great importance. In a case of this kind, as in all other cases of spinal irritation, it is interesting to inquire whether the affection of the stomach or of other organs is not rather the primary, and the irritation of the spinal marrow the secondary trouble. This distinction is all the more important since the irritation of the spine not unfrequently develops symptoms that completely simulate one or the other severe affections of the diseased organ. The irritation almost always runs a slow chronic course, the duration of which is numbered by years. Usually, however, the symptoms remit, the remissions being characterized by a regular type to such a degree that a subsequent exacerbation may be regarded as an entirely new disease. Indeed it is impossible to determine with perfect certainty the degree of connection between a simple irritation of the spine and other affections, more particularly paralytic conditions, emanating from the spinal marrow. The frequent occurrence of spinal irritation in the case of hypochondriac individuals very often leads to an increase of the mental disturbance until actual dementia results from the spinal disease.

Regarding the treatment we cannot do better than to transcribe Hartmann's own words, vol. II., pages 378 and 379: "The reader comprehends without my reminding him of it that no specific treatment can be indicated for the multitude of symptoms which I have described as diagnostic signs of spinal irritation, and which represent more or less independent groups of diseases to which I have applied generic names. Homœopathy cannot and should not be guided in the selection of her remedies by the essence of the disease of which we have a very imperfect knowledge in the present case; otherwise she might tumble into a vague and unsatisfactory mode of generalizing which is decidedly antagonistic to the spirit of her teachings. I do not see how such a method can be considered consistent with homœopathic principles; what would it avail if I were to indicate here a number of medicines every one of which has been found useful for this or that symptom of spinal irritation? It would not be any the less necessary to take a careful record of the totality of the symptoms and to contrast them with the medicine to be chosen. For what purpose, then, have I here introduced such a general description of the symptoms of spinal irritation? For no other purpose than to enable the reader to obtain a correct comprehension of the morbid symptoms presented to his view, and to decide with more certainty whether a remedy had been selected in perfect accord with these externally or phenomenally reflected manifestations of the internal disease. There is no contradiction in these statements, as might be supposed by older homœopaths who have remained ignorant of the modern tendency of medicine and have given an erroneous interpretation to Hahnemann's teachings in this respect, and who would fain excommunicate me on this account from the pale of orthodoxy. I think I have correctly apprehended Hahnemann's meaning, when he says: it is only the externally reflected image of the disease which shows the physician what is to be cured; profound thinker as he was, he knew very well what he ought to think of each single symptom; the subjective symptoms were as valuable to him as the objective; in his mind a generic image of the disease was involuntarily called up side by side with the special symptoms of the case; this is shown by his Chronic Diseases and by his later provings, in the preface to which he takes pains to direct attention to the general character of each special drug. Unconsciously perhaps he meant to convey the doctrine that it was necessary not only to acquire a correct knowledge of the specific symptoms but likewise of the general therapeutic sphere of a drug. May not this consciousness of the absolute necessity of possessing a general knowledge of the curative range of a drug have been awakened in his mind by the conviction that, in order to obtain a complete image of the generic disease, a full record had in the first place to be instituted of all its special symptoms? I cannot conceive of any other meaning; otherwise there would be no special use in looking at the physiological effects of a drug in any other aspect than that which is most strikingly perceived by the senses, unless it was found necessary, with a view of benefiting therapeutics, to bring Physiology into harmony with Pathology and thus to restore the faded glory of a purely symptomatic treatment. A great deal more might be said on this subject, if the size and object of this work admitted of more enlarged developments."

Spinal irritation is not a morbid process encompassed within definite boundaries, hence there can be no treatment assigned to it. But it is important to correctly apprehend its true character as a partial manifestation of other affections, and to consider its symptomatic appearances with the utmost care, with a view of selecting the right remedy. In the few cases where spinal irritation seems to be the primary affection, it will always be found difficult to select the appropriate remedy; this difficulty will likewise exist where the irritation simulates a more deep-seated affection. But it is strictly impossible to indicate *a priori* remedies for affections of such a general character. Nor is it feasible to seek remedies for spinal irritation that are generally applicable, since, after all, it is questionable whether the same treatment would apply no matter whether the cervical or the lumbar portion of the spine constitutes the seat of the irritation. Hartmann has taken pains to furnish, after the fashion of a Repertory, a series of remedies corresponding more particularly to the symptoms of the back; he takes care, however, to preface this series with the remark that he does not attach any great practical value to it; indeed, the most superficial inspection of this list shows that the symptoms mentioned in this series bear very little resemblance to the symptoms of spinal irritation. For such investigations a Repertory is the best thing to use, and will be the more available the more incoherently the single symptoms present themselves. Only one form of spinal irritation may be mentioned in this place, because it generally appears with the same symptoms: we allude to spinal irritation caused by onanism. The patients generally complain of a pain in the lumbar portion of the spine; it is a peculiar burning pain, is principally excited by unexpected motion, violent exertions and long continuance of the back in the same posture. The mind is generally very much involved. The sensitiveness of the vertebræ is sometimes very great. The remedies indicated in this affection are, in the first place, *Nux vomica* and *Sulphur*. Both these remedies are so specifically antagonistic to this vice that, if they do not help, it may with certainty be affirmed that the medulla is already affected with a more deep-seated disorder.

[The remedies which we have more generally employed for spinal irritation are the tincture of *Aconite* root, *Gelseminum*, *Arsenicum*, *Phosphorus*, *Sulphur*. For the stinging and boring, gnawing and wrenching pains, and for the great heat and tenderness in the spinal region, we have found compresses moistened with a solution of Aconite, one teaspoonful to half a tumbler of water, and applied to the back by means of bandages, very beneficial. H.]

C. DISEASES OF THE NERVOUS SYSTEM.

1. Epilepsy.

By epilepsy we understand spasmodic attacks which occur in paroxysms, are separated from each other by free intervals, and are accompanied by a complete suspension of the consciousness, sensibility and the power of voluntary motion. The pathological changes accompanying this disease remain enveloped in perfect obscurity in spite of all investigations and the frequent occurrence of the paroxysms. We may consider it as proven that the medulla oblongata is the starting-point of these very peculiar nervous paroxysms; but we have no certain knowledge of the changes taking place in the medulla or of the manner in which other derangements affect this organ.

Epilepsy is a disease of frequent occurrence and has a very chronic course. Its causes are manifold, some of which are indeed as yet questionable, others, on the contrary, are definitely known, although the nature of the connection between these causes and the disease is still involved in obscurity and doubt. One of the leading causes of the disease is its hereditary character. Our statistics have shown that a large number of our epileptic patients are either born of epileptic parents, or of parents afflicted with other spasmodic affections, and that, in transmitting the disease, the mother exerts a more powerful influence than the father. Nor does it often happen that the disease skips a generation altogether. Females seem to be more disposed to epilepsy than males; it is more particularly the transition forms between epileptic and other convulsive affections that occur among females in a larger number than among males. The disease is seldom traceable as congenital, breaks out most frequently between the tenth and twentieth year, almost as frequently between the fifth and tenth year, rarely at an earlier age, and uniformly decreasing in intensity as patients advance in age. As regards constitution it is difficult to lay down definite rules, but it must appear self-evident that individuals who are endowed with a very sensitive nervous system are particularly predisposed to the disease. Whether a scrofulous and rhachitic diathesis entails a similar predisposition is questionable; whether the lower classes are likewise more predisposed to epilepsy than the higher, or whether abstemiousness from all sexual enjoyments favors the disease, is likewise a matter of doubt.

Although cases of epilepsy occur that can be traced to an affection of some particular organ, yet in most cases the convulsive paroxysms can be traced with more or less certainty to abnormal conditions of one or the other organ as their starting-point. It is, however, a mistake to base upon these organic differences a classification of the epileptic convulsions into thoracic, uterine, etc., for the simple reason that the form of the convulsions is not modified by their local origin. However, no proof is required to satisfy the homœopath of the importance of ascertaining with positive certainty what organ is primarily affected; and what is the nature of the affection; is not the individualization of every case of disease one of the first requirements of Homœopathy? Hence it cannot be deemed superfluous, if we state here the main facts that have become known to us in this direction, to which we would add the advice that in every case of epilepsy the possible existence of other morbid conditions be carefully inquired into, and that a simple diagnosis of the epileptic paroxysm be not deemed sufficient. Every one of the various affections of the brain may develop epilepsy, but this disease cannot be traced to any of them as its regular or prevailing cause. The structural changes revealed after the death of epileptic individuals may have been antecedent to, as well as consequent upon epilepsy. This remark is especially applicable to hypertrophy of the brain, which has often been noticed in postmortem examinations. It is well known that long-lasting epilepsy affects the brain, from which we may infer that it must gradually produce structural changes in this organ, which a post-mortem investigation does not fail to reveal to us and which we are too apt to regard as the primary cause of the disease. It is to adventitious growths in the brain that the origin of epileptic convulsions can be traced with most certainty. Among psychical influences, fright holds the first rank, not only as the primary cause of the first attack, but likewise as the cause of subsequent paroxysms. It is said to cause one-third of all epileptic attacks; we have numerous opportunities of witnessing its extraordinary influence upon epileptic patients. All violent emotions, more particularly the sight of epileptic individuals during an attack, act, if not with the same intensity, at least with an unmistakable force. Epilepsy is likewise often traceable with positive directness to mechanical impressions on the brain caused by a blow, fall, or other violent injuries, or even the causes which may lead to cerebral hyperæmia, excessive heat or cold, insolation, may likewise cause epilepsy. Tracing the disease to affections of the thoracic organs is more uncertain. The frequently mentioned hypertrophy of the heart may both be cause and consequence of the disease. Very frequently and positively, epilepsy may depend upon affections of the abdominal organs. We distinguish helminthiasis, uterine affections, amenorrhœa, nocturnal emissions, sexual excitement, onanism. The last-mentioned cause is certainly much more frequent than is generally supposed; it is indisputable that the most obstinate cases of epilepsy are occasioned by this vice. Other evident causes of epilepsy are injuries of single nerves, pressure upon nerves by cicatrices, tumors or neuromata; epilepsy has been cured by cutting the affected nerve. Lastly we mention chronic intoxications with alcohol or lead as causes of epilepsy.

Symptoms. Epileptic attacks show a great variety of symptoms. It is this very circumstance that compels us to define the pathognomonic signs of the disease in such general terms. For the most part, however, we can distinguish three distinct stages, the first or last of which, and still less frequently both together, are scarcely ever entirely wanting.

The precursory stage is the least clearly defined. The prodromata may consist of general phenomena emanating from one or the other portion of the nervous system or else involving the whole of it. These prodromata are a general restlessness, palpitation of the heart, a peculiar anxiety, pallor of the face, great depression of spirits or else excitement of the mind which may increase to complete derangement of the faculties. Such phenomena may precede for days the real attack, and very often the patients understand perfectly well the meaning of such phenomena. Much more frequently, however, such precursory symptoms are of short duration. They have been designated as the aura epileptica, because the patients describe the sensation of the approaching attack as a warm or cold breath moving from the periphery, especially from the lower extremities, upwards. The aura is likewise described as a sensation of formication, a simple feeling of coldness or heat, as an ascending ball, or else it consists in simple vomiting. As soon as the peculiar sensation reaches a certain definite point, the paroxysm breaks out. In one, this point is the pit of the stomach, in others the neck, heart, or the head itself. As a general rule, the aura does not last longer than a few minutes, and is frequently so short that it passes off with the rapidity of lightning. It may be stated with a certain degree of emphasis that the origin of the aura, as felt by the patient, does not by any means, not even with any degree of probability, indicate the organ which produces the disease. This remark likewise applies to the cases where psychical emotions take the place of the aura.

The second stage is that of the spasm. In almost all cases of fully developed epilepsy, the spasm sets in with a cry. At the same time as this cry is uttered, the patients fall down without consciousness, so that they are entirely unable to guard against injuries which generally happen to them sooner or later in consequence of the fall. This point becomes important when we are called upon to unmask feigned cases of this disease. It is only when the aura lasts for some time that the patient may find it possible to reach a place of safety before the attack overtakes him. In most cases the cry is at first followed by a tetanic rigidity of the whole body, during which the trunk as well as the extremities are stretched out, the head is drawn backwards or sideways, the mouth is tightly closed. The eyes are fixed, the look staring, the respiration arrested in consequence of the spasm of the respiratory muscles. The face now begins to bloat, turns blue and the veins become turgid with blood. After the rigidity has lasted a few moments, (it is never entirely absent,) the convulsions change to clonic spasms which are sometimes ushered in by violent shocks. The whole muscular system is now powerfully shaken. The face becomes distorted, the eyes are alternately closed and opened, the lower jaw is moved to and fro; at one time the mouth is opened, at other times it is closed again, sometimes with an extraordinary force, during which teeth are sometimes broken and the tongue is injured. A frothy sputum which is sometimes mixed with blood oozing from the bitten tongue is seen forcing its way between the closed lips. The head and even the whole trunk are tossed to and fro. The extremities are stretched out, twisted and bent with terrible violence; at the same time the thumb is mostly clenched and even the toes are flexed. The former symptom is regarded by many, although improperly, as a characteristic sign of epilepsy; for this symptom likewise occurs in many other convulsive attacks, whereas it may be entirely wanting in well-defined cases of epilepsy. The convulsions are not always equally violent during the whole of the attack; there are short remissions which, however, do not point to a cessation of the attack. In consequence of the respiratory muscles being very much involved in the attack, the respiration is greatly interfered with, even in the absence of all spasmodic closing of the glottis; the inspirations are unequal and forced, and in making an effort to overcome the contraction of the glottis, the patient sometimes utters an anxious cry. The pulse is generally smaller and more rapid. Very frequently stool and urine are discharged involuntarily. Erections and even ejaculation of the semen sometimes take place. The consciousness and sensibility are entirely suspended, to such a degree that the patient remains unconscious even of the most frightful pains. It has happened that by falling against hot stoves or the like, the patients were frightfully burnt. This stage seldom lasts beyond a quarter of an hour, and is sometimes limited only to a few minutes. Very seldom the attack ceases with a sudden cessation of the convulsions; they abate very gradually, and the paroxysm terminates in most cases by a deep expiration.

This stage passes into the third stage, that of sopor, through a scarcely perceptible transition. After the convulsions cease, the expression of the countenance becomes calm, the complexion pales, the inspirations become full and deep. In most cases this abatement passes into a sopor from which the patients wake after an interval of longer or shorter duration without being aware that they have passed through a paroxysm of convulsions. In very few cases the consciousness returns immediately after the attack; still less frequently the cessation of the convulsions is succeeded by a return of a perfect feeling of health. Generally the patients feel exhausted, with a dull and confused feeling in the head, unsteadiness of gait, headache, sometimes vomiting, and usually an extraordinary desire to sleep. A quiet sleep, even ever so short-lasting, generally puts a stop to all unpleasant after-feelings, and, until the supervention of the next attack, the patient is generally quite well. Not every attack, however, ends so free from all unpleasant consequences; nervous derangements often remain which are worse than the attack itself. Distinct symptoms of dementia, such as an excess of good humor, or else a dulness of perception, errors of language, fixed ideas, even a raging mania, or else an impaired memory, amaurosis, partial paralysis, sometimes remain after the attack, often for a long period; in inveterate cases they never disappear altogether.

In the previous paragraph we have offered a picture of a fully developed paroxysm of epilepsy. This picture, however, does not cover all epileptic attacks. Affections of this class show transitions from other spasms to epileptic paroxysms, and from incomplete to complete paroxysms, in which cases the diagnosis is determined by the loss of consciousness. Such incomplete attacks frequently consist only in a momentary loss of consciousness, during which the eye stares and the face turns pale without the patient falling down or a single spasm becoming visible. The attack is more complete if it begins with vertigo which obliges the patient to sit down or causes him to stagger and fall, in which case slight twitchings of the facial muscles and trembling of the hands take the place of the convulsions. In a few minutes the consciousness returns, and the patient almost immediately feels well again. We have known a patient whose attacks always came on while he was sitting at his writing-desk, the consciousness vanished without vertigo, and an extremely fantastical and pleasant dreaminess set in, which lasted at most half a minute or a whole minute, after which he was able to resume his writing at the very word or letter where he had left off. He never was able to describe his reveries; all he knew was that he felt extremely happy and elated. If such incomplete attacks are neglected and remain uncured, they often pass gradually, or even quite suddenly, into severer forms, on which account they have to be watched with the greatest care. Inasmuch as no single paroxysm of epileptic convulsions, were it otherwise ever so complete, justifies the diagnosis of epilepsy, but may be set down as a paroxysm of eclampsia, of which we shall treat in a subsequent paragraph, we deem it incumbent to devote a few remarks to the intervals between the paroxysms. These intervals are of indefinite duration. It is rarely the case that epileptic convulsions set in at definite periods, (more particularly about the time when the catamenia are expected;) most generally the return of the paroxysms takes place irregularly, and every new exciting cause may upset the established order. The free intervals may last for years. Sometimes, instead of a single paroxysm, a number of paroxysms may take place in rapid succession, after which the free interval begins. Such groups of paroxysms generally imply a deep-seated character of the affection. In most cases the intervals are quite free from morbid symptoms, unless the attack leaves derangements which disappear either slowly or not at all.

Epilepsy always runs a chronic course, provided always the convulsions are not the expression of some organic affection superinducing a rapid dissolution. The patients may live to an advanced age, nevertheless in the course of the disease derangements result, which do not disappear again with the outbreak of the paroxysms, on the contrary, increase in proportion as the paroxysms become more frequent and violent. The mental condition must necessarily be affected by the disease, were it for no other reason than because there is something horrible in such attacks to every beholder. The mere thought of the horrible nature of this disease may excite in some individuals aversion to company, irritability of temper, melancholy, etc., without these symptoms depending in the least upon structural alterations in the brain. Such alterations are never absent in the severer forms of the disease. Gradually the patients lose their memory, the intellect and judgment become impaired, the countenance assumes a peculiar expression of dejection of spirits and subsequently of mental hebetude. We have already stated that partial paralysis sometimes remains after an attack either momentarily or even permanently. The frequent and excessive excitement of the sexual system is a very striking concomitant of the disease. It not unfrequently happens that an increase of the morbid phenomena during the intervals is attended with a decrease of the frequency of the paroxysms.

There are properly speaking but two terminations of the disease, either recovery or other forms of disease. Death very seldom results as the direct consequence of a single paroxysm, but only in consequence of the organic changes that may have been developed by the disease. Complete recovery is unfortunately a less frequent termination than one is apt to suppose. Recovery can only be regarded as certain in cases where the frequently returning paroxysms either cease suddenly or become gradually less frequent and intense. Numerous deplorable instances show that even in such cases a peculiar disposition to relapses remains; it is more particularly violent emotions that give rise to new attacks. Even a partial recovery may be considered a great success, if the paroxysms, for instance, occur less frequently or with less violence, or without any abnormal phenomena during the intervals. There is no doubt that epilepsy may get well spontaneously; a spontaneous recovery may take place gradually, or may be superinduced all at once by the supervention of some acute disease, or may be consequent upon the shock caused by some startling event, or upon the disappearance of the derangements that had caused the paroxysms, such as retention of the menses, helminthiasis. Epilepsy may run into a variety of other diseases, but these changes are mostly confined to paralytic conditions of the central organs of the nervous system, among which we likewise number mental derangements, idiocy, imbecility.

The prognosis is from the very start very dubious; in no case can a cure be promised with perfect certainty. A good deal depends upon the age when the paroxysms first break out. Persons of middle age are the most difficult to cure; next to these the greatest difficulty is experienced at the age of pubescence. The exciting causes likewise exert an influence; if these can be removed, a cure becomes much more probable. The worst cases are those that have been caused by a long-continued practice of self-abuse; epilepsy excites the sexual system with a disturbing violence, and onanism of itself is apt to superinduce changes in the functions of the brain and spinal marrow. The more recent the disease; the less important the derangements in the intervals between the paroxysms, the more promising the prospect of a cure.

Treatment. Hartmann has the following in his introductory remarks: "Although the homœopathic treatment of this disease has obtained proportionally fortunate results, yet a great deal remains to be done to make our treatment a perfect success, as I can affirm from personal experience. Even if I were to accuse myself of my want of success,—which I do not feel disposed to do, since the treatment of epilepsy affords us an abundance of time to consult our books and select the appropriate remedy in accordance with all the individual symptoms of the case,—we may safely assert that two-thirds of the cases of inveterate epilepsy are beyond the reach of the specific method of treatment; unfounded assertions to the contrary cannot shake my convictions on this point. Epilepsies depending upon internal causes may generally be considered incurable, and even such as are consequent upon violent emotions present great difficulties to the practitioner, for the reason that a certain predisposition undoubtedly exists in individuals thus attacked. I do not care to decide whether the many reports of cured cases of epilepsy were really the disease; many of these cases were nothing more than violent spasmodic paroxysms, and could not be regarded as epilepsy for the simple reason that the truly pathognomonic signs were wanting, namely loss of consciousness and loss of sensibility at the very outbreak of the convulsions. It is well to know that an anti-epileptic treatment offers many difficulties even to us homœopaths, and that a successful cure of an inveterate case of epilepsy is just as rare under homœopathic as under any other form of treatment, and that it should be more or less attributed in every case to the fortunate occurrence of accessory circumstances." We have deemed it indispensable to transcribe this judgment of an experienced practitioner in order to meet at the onset the belief that we possess in our Materia Medica a number of approved remedies against epilepsy, and that we have it in our power to treat this disease with comparative certainty of success.

In treating epileptic patients we always have to keep in view three points: the causal indication, the treatment of the special paroxysm, and of the disease generally.

The causal indication is a subject of great importance, even under homœopathic treatment. In most cases the diagnosis of the exciting cause is unfortunately either impossible or very unsafe. In cases where the attacks can be traced to disturbances of particular organs, we have in the first place to aim at remedying them. If the attacks are caused by the pressure of cicatrices upon adjoining nerves, the cause can only be removed by the knife. Cures may likewise be effected by dividing the main nervous trunk of the affected organ, provided the operation is feasible. This result has been satisfactorily demonstrated in cases of epilepsy depending upon degeneration of the testes. Menstrual derangements, helminthiasis, excessive nocturnal emissions, have to be cured before a cure of epilepsy can be thought of. However, even if such derangements have been removed, the stoppage of the convulsions does not necessarily follow; hidden influences may render the convulsions a permanent disease. This result may be expected with the more certainty the longer, the more frequently and more violently the paroxysms have already taken place. Moreover we should not forget that we often fancy we can trace the cause of the disease to functional derangements which really are mere complications of the convulsions without having any causal connection with them.

The treatment of the paroxysm itself is not within the range of mere medicines. Where the aura is distinctly marked and the circumstances otherwise permit the thing to be done, we may try to ward off the attack by applying a ligature to the extremity involved. It is said that in many cases this proceeding has been attended with success. In other respects, we should constantly bear in mind that the patient has to be protected in every possible manner against injuries; he should, for instance, not be allowed to go out alone, and, during the paroxysm, he should be placed so that he cannot injure himself. This precaution is so much more necessary as it has happened that patients have inflicted fatal injuries upon themselves during the attack. That this may readily take place is evident from the violence with which epileptic patients are thrown down, and from the terrible agitation of the muscular system, in consequence of which fractures may occur in spite of the greatest care with which the patient is placed.

So far as the medicinal treatment of epilepsy is concerned, it offers, as has already been said, great difficulties, for the reason that we have not yet succeeded in assigning definitely specific remedies to corresponding forms of the disease. The cause of this is that, although it is certainly true that a large number of epileptic patients have been treated homœopathically with perfect success, cures of epilepsy are scarcely ever what might be termed typical cures, and hence cannot be given to the public. Another cause is, that it is equally difficult to build up the categories of epileptic convulsions with well-defined discriminating distinctions, and that, with a few exceptions, our remedies do not enable us to construct correspondingly accurate diagnostic series. It is certainly wrong to place the symptoms of the actual paroxysm in the foreground. Of course they are essential; but it is equally true that phenomena occurring between the paroxysms deserve a much more attentive consideration. The case is with epilepsy as with intermittent fever which is treated much more successfully with remedies chosen in accordance with the symptoms that characterize the apyrexia. This rule mainly coincides with what we have said previously regarding the causal indication. Where functional derangements of some particular organ prevail, they should constitute the main object of our treatment, no matter whether convulsions are present or not. Only after the local derangements have been removed, a special treatment can be instituted against the epileptic paroxysms unless they should have previously disappeared together with the local trouble. The greatest difficulty in selecting a remedy is undoubtedly experienced in cases that seem to be of an idiopathic nature, and where the intervals do not show the least symptom of bodily ailment. In the following paragraphs we will mention every remedy that has been recommended for epilepsy with more or less reason; however, it will be impossible to mention every remedy that may have to be employed for the different local derangements which constitute so many exciting causes of epilepsy; for a knowledge of these remedies we refer the reader to the chapters where these pathological processes are more specially described.

Cuprum is one of the few remedies of which we know positively that poisonous doses cause epileptic paroxysms. This circumstance has led to the frequent use of Copper in epilepsy. A great many cures have been effected with this agent. In cases of idiopathic epilepsy this remedy is one of the first that will have to be used; on which account, however, it may not be any the less suitable in complicated cases. In this latter class of cases the accessory symptoms will be found to constitute valuable and characteristic indications for the use of Copper. It is more particularly when the epileptic paroxysms break out in the night, that Copper is supposed to possess specific curative powers, although, as we have said before, such statements are unfortunately not confirmed by a sufficient number of clinical observations. Whether *Cuprum metallicum* is preferable to *Cuprum aceticum* is still an open question. The latter preparation is undoubtedly more effective in the lower attenuations, whereas the former had better be used in the higher potencies, and less frequently. In the treatment of epilepsy it seems generally better to employ the higher attenuations in less frequently repeated doses. We make this remark here once and forever in order to avoid unnecessary repetitions.

Plumbum is very nearly related to Copper, both in its general therapeutic character as with regard to the convulsive symptoms. Hartmann says that Plumbum seems to suit epilepsies emanating from the splanchnic system of nerves, whence they radiate over the sentient and motor nerves of the spinal system and finally reach the brain and the senses. According to this statement, Plumbum is particularly adapted to epileptic attacks with a well-defined aura, or to attacks where paralytic conditions, entire or partial loss of consciousness, remain for some time after the attack. These general statements do not, however, show what special cases of epilepsy do more particularly come within the curative range of Plumbum; we shall have to content ourselves with the general knowledge that this remedy is adapted to epilepsy. More special indications will not be expected, for the reason that the peculiar nature of the disease does not admit of any; hence the remedies for epilepsy will always have to be employed with more or less uncertainty as regards their strict homœopathicity. Plumbum acts very slowly as we have already stated when speaking of encephalitis; on the other hand its action lasts much longer and is much more penetrating. On this account alone, even if for no other reason, Plumbum is more particularly suitable to cases of long duration, even if structural changes have already been superinduced in the brain.

Calcarea carbonica is highly prized by Hartmann as a remedy for epilepsy. However, he is evidently embarrassed in endeavoring to justify the selection of this drug. He bases it more particularly upon the general therapeutic character of the drug and its action in persons with a scrofulous diathesis and sensitive nervous system, for the two symptoms which he mentions as characteristic scarcely account for its use upon homœopathic principles. The influence of scrofulosis upon epilepsy has not yet been definitely ascertained; at any rate this influence is not very marked, any more than that of a sensitive constitution. Hartmann has informed us what is to be thought of the *usus in morbis* as applied to the treatment of epilepsy. There is no difficulty in admitting that Calcarea will do good service in the case of children, especially of scrofulous children; or that, by the removal of complications, it may exert a beneficial effect on the course of epilepsy; but it will be found to have very little direct influence over the epileptic paroxysm generally, and in uncomplicated cases we shall have to use it with a good deal of diffidence.

Hartmann applies almost the same remarks to *Causticum*. We coincide with him in opinion in this respect; would however call attention to the fact that some cases of epilepsy have undoubtedly been cured with this agent, on which account, owing to the paucity of our anti-epileptic agents, it deserves some notice at our hands.

Belladonna has among its pathogenetic symptoms the whole series of the phenomena which characterize an epileptic paroxysm, on which account it deserves to be ranked with Cuprum and Plumbum. A careful examination of its pathogenesis reveals, however, some very essential differences. The epileptic Belladonna-convulsions are the consequences of an intense intoxication of the organism; while running their course they may recur several times, but never in the form of a chronic affection, as is the case with Cuprum and Plumbum. Hence the Belladonna-convulsions, as we indeed know from experience, correspond rather to eclampsia, which has been very properly designated as acute epilepsy. We do not mean to imply that Belladonna should never be used in the treatment of epilepsy. There are plenty of cases where it is difficult to distinguish between epilepsy and eclampsia, and where the further course of the disease has to shed light upon the nature of the existing attack, although even in such a case we are often left in the dark. In all such doubtful cases Belladonna will undoubtedly often be selected and will be found efficient. A special indication for Belladonna are the cerebral congestions occurring during and between the paroxysms.

Cicuta virosa undoubtedly reflects by its pathogenetic effects a faithful picture of epilepsy, but very little is said of its curative virtues in this disease. Hartmann recommends it for the following symptoms: Strange movements of the head and trunk, lock-jaw, a bloated and bluish countenance or cadaverous pallor of the face, protrusion of the eyes, vomiting, a weak and scarcely perceptible pulse, scarcely perceptible and intermittent respiration. The attack is preceded by: Strange feeling in the head, extreme sensitiveness of the eyes to the light, delirium while walking about, slow pulse. There is no aura, properly speaking; the attack is succeeded by insensibility, more or less complete lethargy, the patient lies in a state of stupor. In other respects, special indications for Cicuta are the prevalence of venous congestion, especially of the abdominal viscera; convulsions occurring in confinement or during the act of parturition, although they belong more properly to the category of eclampsia.

Opium has among its effects the characteristic symptoms of epileptic convulsions, for which it is indeed recommended by many practitioners, more particularly for convulsions which occur at night while the patient is asleep. However, according to all the information which we possess concerning this remedy, it does not seem adapted to deep-seated, chronic forms of epilepsy. It has been recommended from theory rather than from practical observations. Otherwise we know that Opium-eating, when continued for years, very frequently causes epilepsy which is most generally preceded by an intense derangement of the mental functions, and that for this reason Opium deserves particular notice in cases where, as is so often the case, the convulsions take place in the case of insane persons as complications of the mental disease.

Secale cornutum has, in our opinion, been rather slighted as a remedy for epilepsy The toxicological effects of this remedy are so striking that scarcely any other can compete with it as an antiepileptic agent. The Secale-convulsions with or without consciousness hold a high rank among its pathogenetic indications. It is difficult to understand why such a remedy is not much more frequently employed than others which are not near as homœopathic to the disease. Unfortunately we are without any more specific indications in the use of this drug; all we can do is to recommend it for sudden and rapidly recurring paroxysms, with rapid sinking of strength and paralysis of the spinal nerves.

Of other medicines among whose pathogenetic symptoms we have convulsions with loss of consciousness and which have been used with partial success against epilepsy, we mention: *Agaricus, Cocculus, Hyoscyamus, Stramonium, Lycopodium, Acidum nitricum, Ranunculus bulbosus.*

The number of remedies that are used for the accompanying ailments of epilepsy, rather than for the disease itself, is so large that an accidental omission of one or the other of them will have to be excused. They will be mentioned when treating of the functional derangements of the different organs. Some among the following list owe their employment entirely to the crassest empiricism; although we are not disposed to deny their efficacy on this account, yet they certainly do not deserve to be placed in the front rank as homœopathic anti-epileptic agents. These remedies are: *Arsenicum, Artemisia, Argentum nitricum, Cina, Digitalis purpurea, Ignatia amara, Indigo, Ipecacuanha, Lachesis, Nux vomica, Pulsatilla, Stannum, Sulphur, Veratrum album, Zincum, Rana bufo.*

Some of these remedies enjoy such high repute, as anti-epileptic agents, that it is necessary to mention them more in detail.

Ignatia and **Nux vomica** are among the most prominent. However, the convulsions caused by these medicines are not attended with loss of consciousness, nor are these convulsions in other respects strikingly similar to epileptic spasms; both these medicines occasion only violent reflex-phenomena, whereas in epilepsy the reflex-action is almost completely extinct. Hence these medicines can only be recommended empirically. Hartmann tries to give more definite indications for Nux, but his indications are entirely erroneous; they may indeed apply to convulsions with increased reflex action, but not to epileptic convulsions. Epilepsy may indeed arise from an excess of reflex-action; in such cases these two remedies may be used, if not in the expectation of effecting a cure, at least with a view of palliating the intensity of the paroxysms.

Regarding **Lachesis** Hartmann says that it is regarded as one of the most efficient remedies for epilepsy, provided the recommendations bestowed upon it by its advocates could be implicitly trusted: "The symptoms of the drug, however, are so mixed up, physiology and pathology are thrown together in such a confused mass, that a scientific physician finds it impossible to employ this poison in epilepsy without incurring the reproach of frivolity. We, therefore, content ourselves with hinting at Lachesis in this disease, and refer the practitioner who wishes to make use of it to the original treatise on this agent." These words do not argue much in favor of Lachesis, and are indeed based upon truth. Lachesis has no convulsions with loss of consciousness; what is recorded concerning it, in those forms of epilepsy for which it is deemed suitable, is not obtained by means of a carefully instituted proving on individuals in perfect health, but has been observed on the sick, hence is entirely unreliable.

Digitalis deserves a prominent place in the list of anti-epileptic remedies in all cases caused by onanism or excessive nocturnal emissions. There is scarcely a drug that diminishes and even arrests nocturnal emissions with as much promptitude as this one. We have employed it in many cases, and always with marked success. We are in the habit of giving the alkaloid *Digitalin*, third trituration, one grain every two days. It produces at once a favorable effect in cases of weakness of the sexual organs caused by onanism. The remedies that have likewise to be thought of in such cases are: *Phosphorus, Acidum phosphoricum, China, Nux vomica*.

Artemisia, whose physiological action is still uncertain, owes its reputation to the use that has been made of it in domestic practice; its beneficial results cannot be denied.

Rana bufo has more recently been employed empirically rather than otherwise; but it cannot be denied that this agent has evinced decidedly beneficial effects in epilepsy. A young man whom we had been treating for three weeks, and who, in consequence of practising onanism, had become afflicted with daily paroxysms of epilepsy, received a remedy for this disease from a friend to whom it had been sent by a foreign non-professional correspondent with the assurance that a great many had been cured with it. After the first doses, the paroxysms stopped for three weeks, but then returned again because the patient, as was afterwards found out, continued his miserable practice in spite of all admonitions. We learned afterwards that the powders contained Rana bufo in some attenuated form. Observations of this kind bespeak the most careful consideration for this agent.

[Doctor G. Cook of Buffalo, N. Y., reports the following interesting cure of epilepsy in the Am. Hom. Observer: The patient was a girl of thirteen years of age. She was attacked at intervals of seven, ten and fifteen days, usually at four o'clock in the morning, with spasms. The first admonition her mother had of an impending attack was that the girl straightened out in bed and made the noise peculiar to this disease. The face almost immediately became livid and, unless the temples and face were rubbed during the fit, dark purple spots remained for two or three days. After a few minutes the muscles relaxed, and she went into a comatose sleep in which she remained several hours. Felt languid on awaking; head ached, and had a severe pain always at the pit of the stomach, and sometimes nausea. She ate nothing for twenty-four hours and then felt nearly as well as usual. At fourteen, the catamenia appeared without, however, mitigating or changing the time of the spasms. She was treated allopathically for a whole year without the least benefit. Animal magnetism and the Acetate of Copper relieved at first, but the spasms soon returned with the former violence. The doctor now prescribed *Bromide of Potassium*, two drachms to half a pint of water, a teaspoonful three times daily. Being greatly benefited by this prescription, she was given three-grain doses, three times daily at first, and increased until she took ten grains at one dose, all the time improving. These ten and twelve-grain doses were continued until the patient was entirely cured, in about six months. No ill effects have resulted. The patient has remained well eight months, and is now eighteen years old, and appears to be healthy; her intellect is perfectly sound.

Dr. Benedict, of the Imperial-Royal Society of Physicians at Vienna, cures epilepsy by means of subcutaneous injections of *Curare*, on the neck; he uses solutions of the officinal preparation in the proportion of one to sixty, and injects one-eighth of a grain at a time. The injections are thrown in three times a week, and continued from six to eight weeks or more, as the case may be.

Dr. Goullon reports a case of epilepsy of long standing, cured with *Causticum*, 3d atten., giving the medicine every alternate week. (See All. Hom. Zeit., vol. 69.)

Hydrocyanic acid is undoubtedly homœopathic to epilepsy. H.]

2. Eclampsia.

By this term we understand convulsions with complete or partial loss of consciousness, which can only be distinguished from epilepsy by the general course of the paroxysm. According to the age and condition of the individual we have eclampsia infantum and eclampsia parturientium.

a. *Eclampsia Infantum.*

Although we here class eclampsia among the diseases of the nervous system, yet there is every reason to regard it as a pathological condition arising from some anomaly of the blood, since it affects more particularly the two epochs in human life where the vegetative sphere is very peculiarly circumstanced, namely childhood, and pregnancy or rather the period of confinement; and otherwise breaks out only where the mass of blood is altered by the intensity of the morbid process, intoxications, etc.

Eclampsia occurs most frequently at an age when epilepsy is least frequent, namely during the first months of infancy until the fourth year. As a general rule, feeble, impoverished children incline most to this disease; nevertheless it is likewise quite frequently met with in well-fed children with apparently robust constitutions. A hereditary disposition cannot be denied, in so far, for instance, as children of the same parents may all of them be subject to convulsions, without either father or mother being afflicted with them; and likewise in so far as parents afflicted with the disease may transmit it to their offspring. Eclampsia is likewise said to be favored by hereditary syphilis. What is more probable, however, is that the disposition to eclampsia is acquired. This view is sustained by the more frequent occurrence of the disease among the poorer classes in the country, who manage their new-born babes in the most outrageous manner, and feed the children, after they are once weaned, indiscriminately with all kinds of proper and improper articles of diet. More special, etiological causes are: mental excitement of the mother or nurse; the partaking of noxious substances by either, such as spirits, narcotics which are also given to the child in order to keep it quiet. Exciting causes on the part of the child are: morbid condition of the stomach and of the digestive organs generally; dentition; febrile diseases where, however, the convulsions are of no greater significance than is, in the case of adults, the chill at the commencement of serious diseases; cerebral diseases, more particularly cerebral anæmia; helminthiasis.

Symptoms and Course of the disease: Eclampsia sets in without any premonitory symptoms only in cases where it constitutes the first symptom of the invasion of some acute disease. As an idiopathic disease it is almost always preceded by preliminary symptoms. These are: ill-humor, a whining mood, obstinacy, indisposition to play, sudden starting when touched ever so lightly without expecting it; sleeplessness or restless sleep, during which the lids are not entirely closed, with a peculiar twist of the mouth, (risus sardonicus,) gritting of the teeth; change of color from the least cause; crying out without any apparent cause; sudden relinquishing of the nipple; uneasy, unequal breathing; sometimes a peculiar livid color around the mouth and eyes, and pointed appearance of the nose and chin.

After these premonitory symptoms have lasted for a time which cannot be accurately defined, the actual paroxysm breaks out with the same suddenness as an epileptic attack, only with this difference that the patient utters no cry. Otherwise the attack has all the characteristic features of an epileptic paroxysm. At the beginning the convulsions are generally for some time tonic, after which they become clonic, and, in less frequent cases, affect only one side. The features become distorted, the eyes stare, generally squinting strongly upwards; the body is tossed to and fro, nevertheless the extremities are not as rigid as they are during an epileptic attack. The respiration is very much impeded, spasm of the glottis is not unfrequently present, the abdomen becomes distended. The face either looks blue-red and bloated, with considerable turgescence of the vessels, or else it is pale and sunken; the bodily temperature is rather decreased than raised. During the height of the convulsion the consciousness and sensibility are completely extinct. Usually the paroxysm ends with a deep, moaning inspiration, after having lasted a few minutes or even a number of hours, and the patients sink into a deep sleep from which they wake in apparent health.

The paroxysm does not always reach such a fearful degree of intensity; eclampsia as well as epilepsy has a series of gradations, the attack being sometimes marked only by partial convulsive movements of the muscles, a staring look with some squinting, risus sardonicus, etc. The consciousness remains either entirely undisturbed, or is only partially interfered with. Sometimes the attacks consist in a comatose sopor which lasts for hours, with the almost characteristic half-closing of the eyelids, and a few convulsive twitchings taking the place of the convulsions; even the face may retain its normal expression and color.

A single paroxysm is scarcely ever the end of the trouble. In the first place there generally remains a disposition to relapses, and in the second place several paroxysms usually follow one after the other, the intervals between the paroxysms being of indefinite duration, and the intensity of the attack varying in degree, sometimes increasing, at others decreasing in violence. The intervals are not always free from morbid symptoms, but the phenomena which we have designated as the preliminary stage sometimes continue more or less until the next attack sets in. Altogether the whole duration of the attack is very indefinite.

Eclampsia may terminate in recovery, partial recovery or death. The former may take place after any paroxysm, sometimes quite unexpectedly, so that a child may be found playing about in the morning which, the day previous, was still the victim of terrible convulsions. In partial recovery some of the symptoms of the attack remain either permanently or disappear only gradually. In such cases it is a question whether such permanently remaining consequences of the attack do not rather originate in some cerebral disease which was likewise the primary cause of the attack. Among such consequences we number paralysis of the muscles of the eyes, less frequently of the muscles of the back, idiocy or only a certain degree of backwardness in the development of the mental faculties, accompanied with an unusual degree of nervous irritability. Death results either during the attack, or else the subsequent coma terminates in death. The only disease into which eclampsia may be transformed is epilepsy, in which case it is, however, always difficult to determine whether the original affection was only eclampsia. It is likewise difficult to draw the line of demarcation between eclampsia and epileptic spasms. Nevertheless it is of essential importance to distinguish with accuracy between eclampsia and epilepsy, both on account of the prognosis as well as the treatment. As a general rule we may take it for granted that, whenever the attack cannot be traced to any definitely exciting cause, the character of the convulsions is that of epilepsy. This rule, however, is not of uniform validity.

The prognosis depends upon many accessory circumstances, and is always rather doubtful. Age is an important consideration; the younger the patients, the more readily they succumb to the attack, more particularly infants at the breast. In hereditary cases the prognosis is decidedly unfavorable. The more rapidly the paroxysms succeed each other, the greater the danger of a fatal termination, more particularly if they continue to increase in intensity, and the subsequent derangements continue for a long time. The more readily the primary disturbance is quieted, the less apprehension need be entertained regarding the final result. Convulsions setting in at the commencement of the invasion of some acute disease, are scarcely ever dangerous. On the contrary, if the convulsions set in during the course of the disease, they almost always justify the most serious apprehensions; they generally mean death. The danger is greatest in the case of robust and corpulent children.

Treatment. As a general rule the treatment of eclampsia is just as uncertain as that of epilepsy, for the reason that we can never be sure whether the paroxysm that had just passed is the end of the disease. A number of paroxysms may succeed each other in rapid succession, in which case, if they stop suddenly, we may feel pretty certain that the disease is cured. On the other hand, the intervals may be of long duration, in which case the certainty of a cure is of course less absolute. On this account it is not enough that the paroxysm should be ended; the subsequent developments of the case will have to be watched for a time, and the same medicine had better be continued for some time longer.

In a case of eclampsia the causal indication deserves a much more attentive consideration than in epilepsy, for the reason that in the former disease it is much easier to trace the latter to its exciting cause. Although not in every case, yet in most cases this cause can be determined with tolerable certainty. The sole exceptions are convulsions depending upon cerebral affections. Here it may be difficult to arrive at a certain knowledge of the cause. Among children, however, such cerebral disturbances seldom manifest themselves for the first time with the first breaking out of the paroxysm; we generally have had opportunities, previous to the occurrence of the convulsions, of obtaining certainty concerning the character and existence of the cerebral disease. In all cases it is of importance to direct our treatment against the exciting cause, so much more as we need not apprehend that the convulsions have become firmly rooted as is the case in epilepsy. In the subsequent paragraphs the reader must not expect to find a record of every remedy that may be indicated by the various exciting causes of eclampsia; their list will be found limited to the most important.

To some extent the prophylactic treatment of eclampsia coincides with our previous remarks. That a prophylactic treatment is possible cannot be denied, for it is a notorious fact that children who are attacked with the disease, are brought up in contravention of all natural rules. It is not only a matter of importance that the child should receive the proper nourishment at the proper time, but that the disposition of the child should be managed with becoming attention from the moment of birth. It often happens that in the first years of the child's existence the mother or nurse is subject to its tyrannical caprice, whereas it is afterwards expected to yield implicit obedience to their behests. How difficult it is to induce a mother to insist upon her will being law from the very first moment of the child's existence. If the child cries, it has to be nursed at once, or has to be rocked or carried about. It is such practices as these that make the child restless and headstrong and have a decidedly injurious effect upon the nervous system. Every child, if otherwise healthy, can easily be accustomed to do without food at night; a little firmness will readily teach it. Our own experience should admonish us that a night's quiet sleep, uninterrupted by the crying for food, must exert a beneficent influence upon the child. During the day, likewise, little children should be allowed to remain in a recumbent posture, for as long as the muscles of the back are not strong enough to support the head, children can only be injured by being carried all the time. As a matter of course it is proper to try to harden the child within reasonable bounds; above all things it should be remembered that the head must not be kept too warm by an excess of covering. The influence of the first management of children cannot well be demonstrated by numbers, but any one who will take the trouble to inquire, whether eclampsia and various other affections do not occur much less frequently in families where children are brought up with a reasonable systematic regularity, will find that our condemnation of the faulty management of early infancy is well founded. As a prophylactic measure it is likewise important that the child's mind should not at once be unnaturally excited as soon as the first dawn of a mental awakening is perceived; on the contrary, the child should be left to its own spontaneous tendencies. It is well known that milk drawn from the breast of a mother or nurse shortly after an immoderate excitement, more particularly anger, has a deleterious influence upon the child; mothers and nurses should never lose sight of this circumstance. Special attention should be devoted to children during the teething period, especially if they have shown a disposition to convulsions at a prior period. The period of dentition acquires additional importance from the circumstance that it generally coincides with the period of weaning, not to mention the prejudices with which the physician has to contend. Lancing the gums is scarcely ever of any use, but may retard the liberation of the tooth in consequence of the formation of cicatrices. We need scarcely add that there are many cases of eclampsia which it is impossible to prevent by treatment.

Before mentioning the remedies for this disease, it may be well to inquire whether it is at all proper to administer remedies during the attack. In general we feel disposed to deny the propriety of this sort of medication, more especially in cases where the convulsions break out suddenly, without any premonitory symptoms. We are not by any means sure of hitting the right remedy, and it is much better not to give any medicine until the attack is over, provided the intensity of the symptoms is not attended with any immediate danger, or we were unacquainted with the primary cause of the convulsions. Hartmann advises to strip the little patients of all clothing, in order to make sure that the convulsions are not excited by tight dresses or the prick of a pin.

Not all the remedies which we shall mention, have among their physiological symptoms convulsions with loss of consciousness. The presence of this symptom which is characteristic of epilepsy, is much less so of eclampsia. Moreover in a case of eclampsia the medicines can be selected much more appropriately in accordance with the accessory symptoms, without paying particular attention to the character of the convulsions which seldom break out as an idiopathic affection.

Belladonna is without doubt the main remedy for eclampsia; most cases will be found to come within the curative range of this drug. It is particularly indicated in the case of robust and corpulent children with unmistakable symptoms of cerebral congestion. In order to show the correspondence existing between this drug and eclampsia, we here mention the symptoms of four children who were poisoned with Belladonna, which will show how constantly the berries of Belladonna produced eclampsia in these cases: Already an hour and a half after eating the berries the children were attacked with the following symptoms: complete stupor and insensibility; exceedingly restless tossing about in the bed, with occasional shrill cries as if the patients were tormented by great anxiety; frequent chorea-like movements of the arms; bright redness of the face; the pupils are dilated; the reflex motions of the lids are entirely suspended; the eyes stare and look glassy, in one case they were in constant, vibrating motion; respiration moaning, sobbing; the lower jaw was firmly pressed against the upper; occasional electrical shocks through the whole body; the head is violently drawn backwards; the urine is voided involuntarily. These symptoms not only are remarkably characteristic of eclampsia, but they occur in almost every case of poisoning with Belladonna, and demonstrate with remarkable accuracy the truth of the principle of similarity as a therapeutic maxim; for it will seldom happen that a second attack of convulsions will occur after the administration of Belladonna.

Hyoscyamus acts very similarly to Belladonna. According to Hartmann the indications for Hyoscyamus are: dark redness and bloat of the face, the abdominal walls are firmly drawn in, the clonic spasms attack now these and then other parts of muscles, and the attack is caused by fright. *Stramonium* is likewise very similar in its action; the turgescence is considerable, clonic and tonic spasms occur in frequent alternation; the increase of temperature affects the whole body rather than the head.

Chamomilla is employed in eclampsia more frequently than seems founded upon scientific accuracy. Hartmann agrees with us in doubting the homœopathicity of this drug to the attack itself; he recommends it for the premonitory symptoms. The question in such cases is, whether the medicine has been of any use. *Cicuta virosa* deserves our attention in eclampsia as much as in epilepsy; the cases where it is indicated are not so much characterized by spasms, as by the circumstance that the children assume all at once a rigid and immovable appearance, which, after a short period, is superseded by a profound prostration lasting some time and attended with a comatose condition.

Opium, as is well known, affects the infantile organism differently from that of full-grown persons. This phenomenon, however, is likewise peculiar to other drugs, such as Belladonna, and has not as yet been accounted for. We are in possession of a considerable number of cases of poisoning among little children, where the following effects of Opium are almost uniformly present; the face, lips and eyelids are swollen, the color of the skin is almost violet, the temperature is depressed, especially at the nose and on the extremities; deep coma with convulsions at rather long intervals which are frequently preceded by vomiting; the respiration is slow and stertorous, the expirations especially are very slow and protracted; the pulse is imperceptible. Attacks of eclampsia with a similar group of symptoms, are not very frequent; the symptoms, taken separately, point to acute anæmia rather than to hyperæmia of the brain, which latter, in the case of adults, is an almost constant effect of Opium, and which has caused us in previous paragraphs to mention this agent among the list of remedies for cerebral diseases. Practical observations have not yet enabled us to determine the cases of eclampsia to which Opium is homœopathic, and we do not consider Hartmann's advice in this respect as of much use. He considers Opium indicated in convulsions arising from fright when attended with fear. They are supposed to commence with trembling of the extremities, which is interrupted by starting of the body and the extremities, attended with a shrill cry; after a while a sort of sopor overwhelms the child, from which it cannot be roused; such paroxysms are said to break out only at night.

Ignatia amara is a much more important remedy for eclampsia than for epilepsy; it is more particularly adapted to cases where the spinal marrow is deeply involved and where the convulsions are chiefly tonic. Such convulsions are frequently met with at the onset of febrile affections; if they are very violent, it is advisable to commence the treatment with Ignatia, and afterwards to give the remedy more particularly adapted to the disease. *Nux vomica* holds the same relation to eclampsia as Ignatia.

The remedies that have been mentioned so far, except perhaps Opium, correspond to convulsions attended with cerebral hyperæmia. These convulsions are undoubtedly the most frequent; but those which are either dependent upon, or complicated with, anæmia, such as frequently occur among children in consequence of losses of animal fluids, are undoubtedly of more importance because more dangerous.

In such cases **Ipecacuanha** deserves the first rank. It is to be exhibited before any other remedy, when the convulsions set in after protracted diarrhœa caused by improper or excessive feeding, or perhaps by the use of too fat nourishment; the face is pallid or livid, the skin is very cool, or is covered with a cold sweat.

Cuprum has already been prominently mentioned as a remedy for convulsions arising from cerebral anæmia. It is one of the most important remedies for this disease even in its most violent and dangerous forms, more particularly if the lethargy continues in the intervals between the paroxysms which follow each other in rapid succession, and if the constitution of the child has become impoverished in consequence of improper or deficient nourishment. Conditions of this kind occur most frequently as malignant complications towards the end of acute or subacute diseases, such as typhus.

Veratrum album is very nearly related to Cuprum; it will prove particularly useful in convulsions caused by rapid losses of vital fluids during an attack of cholera or cholerine, and where the affection sets in in a very acute form. In such cases *Camphor* may prove serviceable.

Platina is likewise recommended by Hartmann as a specific remedy for convulsions arising from anæmia; the consciousness is not suspended; the spasms are rather tonic, trismus may be present. In this place *Arsenicum*, *Stannum* and *Zincum* deserve particular mention. The last-mentioned remedy has been more recently employed with particular success in cases of eclampsia, more especially if it seems to be symptomatic of some cerebral affection.

We would have to add a long list of remedies if we were to enumerate all that have reference to the exciting pathological causes; in order to avoid unnecessary repetitions, it will be more convenient to defer their enumeration until we come to treat of the special functional derangements of the affected organs.

If eclampsia ushers in some acute disease, it is scarcely ever necessary to heed the merely transitory convulsions. It is only in case the convulsions should threaten to become dangerous that a specific treatment has to be pursued. In such a case *Belladonna* and *Ignatia* would be the most indispensable remedies. The case is different when convulsions occur in the course of acute diseases. Under these circumstances they become so threatening that the treatment has to be mainly directed against the convulsions instead of against the general affection.

b. *Eclampsia Parturientium.*

By this term we understand convulsions that are perfectly similar to epilepsy, and which only occur during pregnancy and parturition or shortly after confinement.

This accident is not very frequent, only one case to about four hundred confinements being the general average. At certain periods the disease occurs with more than usual violence without atmospheric or other causes being at the bottom of it. As a general rule, the disease occurs during the ninth month, and even at a later period, scarcely ever before this time, never in the first two or four months. The constitution does not seem to exert a peculiar influence in this disease; robust, plethoric individuals are said to be more readily attacked than others of opposite constitutional tendencies. By far the largest number of patients are to be found among the primiparæ. The disease most frequently occurs about the time when the os tincæ first begins to dilate; next shortly after the expulsion of the fœtus. A variety of circumstances are mentioned as etiological causes of the disease, whereas more recently Frerichs has pointed out Bright's disease of the kidneys as the only cause of the convulsions. This question, however, is not yet decided. It is true that eclampsia most frequently attacks women afflicted with albuminuria; but whether this is a symptom of Bright's disease is questionable, for the reason that, if the patients recover, the symptoms of albuminuria very speedily disappear, which would not be the case if the kidneys were organically diseased. At all events, it is certain that albuminous urine, with œdematous swellings, always augurs badly for parturient females, and very frequently results in the occurrence of convulsions. On the other hand, it is an admitted fact, that these convulsions may occur without the albuminuria and œdema. Proximate causes are: disproportionate dimensions of the sexual organs and the fœtus, rigidity of the uterine fibres, excessive labor-pains, hemorrhage, retention of remnants of the placenta, excessive mental excitement. When occurring during confinement, convulsions generally imply the commencement of an inflammatory uterine affection.

Symptoms. In many cases, but not as a rule, the true paroxysm is preceded by precursory symptoms. The head is heavy and dull, a violent headache is frequently present; the patients show signs of mental hebetude, the memory is impaired; photopsia, even transitory blindness, buzzing in the ears, sensation of some approaching danger, unsteady gait, heaviness of speech, dulness of mien, attended with strikingly glistening eyes, heat about the head, painfulness of the uterine region: these are the leading phenomena from the presence of which the outbreak of convulsions may be prognosticated with a tolerable degree of certainty, more particularly if eclampsia had existed during former confinements, or if the urine contains albumen, cylindrical casts, etc. The precursory stage may last indefinitely from a few minutes to some days. The paroxysm itself is very much like epilepsy, generally, however, the peculiar cry and the falling down, as if the patient were struck by lightning, at the outbreak of the convulsions are wanting, suddenly the patients become quiet and close their eyes. Very soon peculiar muscular movements are seen in the face, the eyelids are rapidly opened and closed, the eyeballs are turned in every direction, the pupils are dilated and become immovable, the muscles of the mouth begin to twitch, the lips are drawn to one side, the tongue is protruded between the teeth. The clonic spasms now extend to the neck which is often stretched with an extraordinary rapidity or bent to one side; then to the arms which first tremble and then are jerked out; the lower extremities are not so much affected and remain rigidly extended, they are only slightly moved to and fro. At every increasing paroxysm the respiration becomes more impeded, it consists of mere sobs, becomes irregular, is even suspended for a short period, the movements of the heart likewise become irregular. In consequence of this interference with the action of the heart and lungs the vessels of the head and neck become turgid. In the midst of these changes the whole body sometimes starts as if struck by some electric shock. After these violent clonic spasms have lasted for some minutes, there is an apparent interval of rest, during which a complete tetanic rigidity prevails with the most diversified contractions of the limbs. For a short time the respiration ceases entirely, the heart works very irregularly, its beats frequently intermit, the skin becomes covered with a cold perspiration, and the discharges from the rectum and bladder are frequently involuntary. This rigidity continues for about half a minute, after which all the phenomena gradually decrease in intensity. The convulsive movements become less frequent, the breathing and the action of the heart become more normal, and lastly a general relaxation takes place with which the patients lapse into a soporous condition. According as the paroxysms are more or less frequent and violent, this stage has a longer or shorter duration, and may even continue for three days. The consciousness gradually returns, and derangements of the senses or mental faculties sometimes remain for some time after the attack. Headache generally lasts longest.

Eclampsia either terminates in complete recovery, or in other diseases, or death. Death seldom takes place during the convulsions, or, if it does, it is caused by cerebral apoplexy; more frequently it occurs during the stage of sopor, likewise in consequence of cerebral apoplexy; or it is caused by acute œdema of the lungs consequent upon the violent interference with the action of the heart and lungs. The affections consequent upon eclampsia generally relate to the functions of the brain: they are mania, idiocy, loss of memory, amaurosis, deafness, or muscular contractions and paralysis. Very frequently puerperal inflammations have resulted after an attack of eclampsia. Complete recovery never takes place suddenly, but more or less gradually.

The effect of the convulsions upon parturition differs according to the period when the accident takes place. If it takes place during pregnancy, uterine contractions are excited by the convulsions and miscarriage takes place. If they take place at the commencement of parturition, the act is considerably delayed in consequence, whereas if they take place towards the end of the act of parturition, the expulsion of the fœtus is considerably hastened in consequence.

If taking place after parturition, the uterine contractions are generally arrested, which may lead to metrorrhagia, retention of fragments of the placenta and consequent inflammatory affections. Parturition influences the convulsions, in so far as they never cease entirely until the uterus has been entirely freed from its contents, and may even continue with less intensity for hours after the birth of the child. The influence upon the fœtus is not necessarily fatal; according to Scanzoni about one-half of the chidren who are born in the midst of convulsions die; the shorter the period between the occurrence of the convulsions and the termination of the act of parturition, the less the danger to the child.

The prognosis is very uncertain. The disease is one of the most dangerous, and becomes so much more dangerous as it may develop equally dangerous diseases. If the convulsions occur at a very early period, the danger to the patient is so much greater. The later they occur, and the greater the chances of a speedy delivery, the better the prospect of a successful issue. Of course the degree of intensity of the convulsions is likewise to be carefully considered in establishing a prognosis.

Treatment. Hartmann introduces his remarks concerning the treatment of this disease with an inquiry whether it is rather a disease of the blood or the nervous system. This point is not yet settled, and, in the present state of our Materia Medica, is of very little importance. We have slightly alluded to it in a previous paragraph. Of far more importance is his advice not to leave a patient who had been attacked with convulsions, until the action of the heart and lungs has resumed its normal character, and, by this means, to prevent any improper interference on the side of the family, and to obtain a satisfactory certainty that the process of parturition is developing normal phenomena.

No remedy responds to this disorder as completely as *Belladonna.* The fact, says Hartmann, that it is repeatedly mentioned in the most diversified forms of disease, should suffice to satisfy beginning practitioners of Homœopathy of the importance of this medicine; and to invite them to study its physiological effects with an increasing care and accuracy, until their leading characteristics have become well defined to the general comprehension, and may be relied on as safe guides in the selection of this drug. That the action of Belladonna is similar to a paroxysm of eclampsia and has, moreover, a special affinity to the condition of a parturient female, is not only shown by our Materia Medica, in spite of the incoherent arrange-

Eclampsia Parturientium.

ment of its symptoms, but may likewise be learned from any recognized toxicological treatise. Moreover it is an admitted fact that Belladonna acts more penetratingly upon the organisms of children and women, and is more particularly adapted to the latter class, if the circulation of the blood is prominently active. The curative effects of Belladonna in this disease have been practically illustrated in a number of cases, and we may rely upon this agent with perfect confidence in cases where our Old-School brethren have to resort to the most heroic and most pernicious treatment.

Although both *Hyoscyamus* and *Stramonium* are intimately related to Belladonna in this disease, yet we believe that both these remedies are effectually superseded by the last-named agent. The difference which Hartmann has indicated between these two medicines, does not seem to us founded in fact, and of difficult application in practice. *Aconite* exhibits likewise among its toxicological effects a complete series of the symptoms of eclampsia, more particularly an alternate change from clonic spasms to tetanic rigidity, and may have to be resorted to, more especially if the convulsions set in subsequent to parturition, and will have to be regarded as symptomatic of an inflammatory puerperal disease.

[An admirable medicine in puerperal convulsions is the *Bromide of Potassium* in large doses, which is now beginning to be universally used by American as well as European homœopathic practitioners. It will often prove efficacious where Aconite, Belladonna or any other medicine, seem to be powerless. Some interesting cases of cure of this frightful malady by *Gelseminum sempervirens* have been published by Dr. Douglas, of Milwaukee, in Lodge's Observer. See also Hale's New Remedies, second edition, pages 444 to 448. H.]

Concerning **Opium** Hartmann offers the following remarks which deserve to be transcribed literally: "Opium seems to me, sometimes, like a veiled Goddess; I perceive general outlines, but sharply marked features, pointing to some definite characteristic sphere of action, are entirely wanting. Hahnemann's observation that Opium can only be used with success in recent and shortly-lasting disorders, has only contributed to darken, instead of clearing up, the clouds hanging over the curative sphere of Opium. We can hardly suppose that physicians have been wrapt for thousands of years in a maze of illusions concerning Opium, without ever dreaming that this agent has a very equivocal therapeutic action! And what brilliant cures have not been accomplished by means of Opium! No, indeed! Hahnemann's assertions regarding

Opium are of the same paradoxical character as so many other views, opinions and notions of his, that had not yet become settled in his mind, and which he either favored or rejected according as they agreed or disagreed with his purposes; if he was unable to loosen the Gordian knot, he cut it with an authoritative assertion. Opium fared similarly in his hands; his provings of this agent did not develop any symptoms of pain, and hence he decreed: Opium does not cure pain! He took many Opium-symptoms from old authors who had observed them in Opium-eaters, and had found that the continued use of this drug develops, even in young people, symptoms that bear a close resemblance to the ailments incident to old age; hence his decree: Opium cures the ailments incident to old age! The long-continued use of Opium causes nervous irritability to such a degree that Opium-eaters start at the least surprise; hence he decreed: Opium removes the bad effects of fright! It is easily seen that morbid conditions of this kind are not obtained by means of regular provings on persons in health, but in consequence of the long-continued and energetic use of the drug, as is the case with a number of others; but then it is wrong to infer that the medicine can only be properly used for a very limited number of symptoms, for the reason that it is only capable of occasioning a small number of ailments which are, moreover, of a very general character. In such cases the medicine, if it is experimented with for a sufficient length of time, will undoubtedly develop a number of fine symptoms that may prove highly valuable in the treatment of diseases. Of course we must not obstinately and foolishly reason in this wise: Because many drugs will cure diseases when administered in high attenuation, therefore all drugs will be capable of accomplishing the same result. By no means; one medicine will cure in small doses whereas other medicines may have to be given in larger quantities. Opium belongs to this latter category. It will scarcely ever prove efficient in the tenth, twentieth or much less in a higher potency, but will almost always have to be given in larger doses, without forfeiting, on this account, its position as a homœopathic agent. Not till I cut myself loose from Hahnemann's decree concerning the normal dose, did I learn to make a correct use of many medicines, and even Opium has enabled me to do a great deal of good with it, which will ever remain inaccessible to those who swear by the words of the Master. In eclampsia, Opium is an admirable remedy in the case of robust parturient females when the attack was, perhaps, excited by a sudden fright or even an unexpected joyful event during the process of parturition. Even if the effects of Opium were only palliative, the medicine would still be of inestimable value, for the reason that the disease only has a few paroxysms which the physician is called upon to hush in order to save two lives; a protracted treatment is anyhow unnecessary inasmuch as the exciting cause of the disease is only of short duration, and the circumstances which favor and feed the pathological process, very soon disappear. I am not able to furnish a list of the special symptoms the presence of which is necessary to justify the use of Opium in this disease; the reader will have to contrast the symptoms of the case with those of the Materia Medica, and will perhaps feel grateful to me for giving him now and then an opportunity of depending upon his own judgment, instead of being held in leading-strings by another whose advice, after all, may be fallible like that of other mortals." To these words of Hartmann we will add the following remarks: Under allopathic treatment *Morphium aceticum* is considered the only reliable remedy for eclampsia, but it is given in such enormous doses—Scanzoni gives one-sixth to one-fourth of a grain every half hour, together with injections of twenty to thirty drops of the tincture of Opium—that it seems almost criminal to pursue such a course of treatment. The disease is, of itself, very apt to superinduce mental derangements, and the medicine may cause a chronic loss of memory. Unfortunately we have no statistical data to show that mental derangements are more readily, more frequently and more permanently caused by the allopathic use of Morphium than by the use of this agent in homœopathic hands. Large doses of this drug should never be given by a homœopath at the commencement of his treatment, they should only be resorted to as a last resort.

Of **Laurocerasus** we have no clinical records as far as we know; if it should be used, it will be necessary to administer it in comparatively large quantities. Of other medicines belonging to the present list, the most important have already been mentioned in the chapter on eclampsia. *Digitalis* may be found useful more particularly if hemorrhages are present; if not indicated at the commencement of the paroxysms, it may be an appropriate remedy for the subsequent derangements.

Of great importance to the successful treatment of eclampsia is the correct management of the process of labor. Scanzoni gives the following advice bearing upon this point: If the convulsions occur during pregnancy without causing labor-pains, artificial delivery is only justified in case the spasms steadily continue to increase in duration and intensity, and the life of both mother and child is threatened. If the parturient woman is already dying, it is better to perform the Cesarean section immediately after her death than to resort to a forced delivery, because the latter jeopardizes the life of the child much more than the former. If, at the onset of the disease, the os tincæ is sufficiently dilated and there are otherwise no counter-indications, the forceps may at once be resorted to; this should, however, be avoided if labor has so far advanced that a few more pains will accomplish the expulsion of the fœtus. If the paroxysms continue after parturition, the placenta should be removed as soon as possible. As regards the sanguineous depletions which are so universally recommended in this disease, we will express our opinion in a few words. Not unfrequently eclampsia is the result of hemorrhages or causes them; how then are we to account for the fact that sanguineous depletions can be of any benefit in this disease? Or what possible explanation of the use of depletions can at all be given in this disease? How can the usefulness of such depletions be maintained when so many other heroic remedies are employed at the same time? The usefulness of a remedial agent cannot be properly contended for until it has produced satisfactory clinical results, without its action being obscured by a combination with other drugs.

As regards the dietetic treatment of eclampsia, it seems to be unnecessary to go into details. Such patients require the same nursing as any other women whose confinement is perfectly free from untoward complications. All excesses of any kind should be carefully avoided.

3. Chorea.

By chorea we understand spasmodic movements of the voluntary muscles taking place contrary to the will of the affected individual. It has different names: Chorea St. Viti, Choreomania, Epilepsia saltatoria, St. Vitus's dance.

Chorea is a disease of the latter years of childhood. It is very seldom seen previous to the sixth year of age, rarely after the fifteenth, it occurs most frequently between the tenth and fourteenth year. Females and individuals with very irritable nervous systems are more particularly inclined to this disease, whereas the bodily constitution otherwise seems to be without any influence over the disease. The etiological causes are involved in obscurity; one fact is well ascertained: the disease occurs most frequently during the second period of dentition and at the age of pubescence. Other exciting causes are: a desire to imitate (in some cases the habit of unusual motions has led to the disease) emotions, especially fright, helminthiasis, onanism. It is frequently met with among individuals with tuberculous constitutions, or with strikingly developed chlorosis.

The classification in chorea minor and major is altogether founded upon the degree of intensity of the morbid phenomena, and is so much more unimportant as the two degrees frequently pass from one into the other. For this reason we have taken no special notice of this classification in the present instance.

Symptoms and Course. A preliminary stage, properly speaking, seldom occurs in chorea; what has been considered as such, generally has already the peculiar character, the involuntary motions of chorea. At first the patients show a certain unsteadiness in their movements, and an unusual hurriedness; these symptoms are accompanied by a certain depression of spirits and irritability of temper, which may, however, result rather from the rebukes which the child receives on account of its apparent carelessness in handling things. It is only after some time that the child's parents become aware of the existence of some nervous disorder. After the symptoms have become more fully developed with a more or less gradually increasing intensity, a real paroxysm suddenly breaks out. It is generally excited more immediately by some violent emotion, fright for instance. The involuntary motions now begin, being either confined to single bundles of muscles or affecting the whole muscular system, in such a manner that the upper extremities are more violently affected than the lower. The face shows every possible contortion, even the eyeballs are rolled about in every direction; the arms and hands are at times flexed, at other times extended; objects can no longer be held firmly, the patient is no longer able to eat alone, or else has to bring the food to his mouth by a very circuitous route; the gait becomes unsteady because the legs can no longer be put down with sufficient steadiness, and even the strength is wanting to keep them straight. Not all the limbs are always affected together; sometimes only those on one side are affected, sometimes only the arms or the face, very rarely the lower extremities alone. A striking feature of the disease is that the movements become so much more violent the more steadily the patient fixes his attention upon them. Eating seems likewise to exert an aggravating influence upon chorea.

If the disease increases in intensity, the spasms which, in a milder degree, are continuous, often occur in paroxysms, and with various but distinct symptoms of impairment of the mental functions, sometimes even with total loss of consciousness. The movements now assume the form of strange leaps, dancing, turning or rolling the body while the patients utter the most varied sounds, sing, laugh and even roar like wild beasts. The intervals between the paroxysms are scarcely ever free from all spasmodic symptoms: on the contrary, the phenomena which we have designated as the milder degree of chorea, continue. If the disease lasts for a length of time, the assimilative functions suffer, and even febrile symptoms make their appearance. Sleep is impaired; on account of the muscular spasms the patient is prevented from falling asleep; during sleep all abnormal movements become suspended. It is peculiar to the disease that even excessive muscular motions do not fatigue the patients. On the other hand they do not unfrequently complain of pains in the joints which generally increase in bed, and, in a measure, are most likely excited by the spasms, but may likewise be felt in parts not affected by the convulsions. A sensation of numbness and formication in the limbs is not caused by the attack itself. Together with the assimilative functions the mental faculties become depressed; the teasing character of the disorder renders the patients exceedingly irritable, dejected and peevish, or even disposed to fits of rage. This is so much more to be deplored as these ebullitions of temper are apt to provoke an attack.

After a gradual increase of the symptoms, the disease reaches its acme, where it remains stationary for a period, lasting a few weeks or even several months, and sometimes terminating in recovery either quite suddenly or only gradually. The cases where the convulsive motions become habitual, are very rare, yet single derangements are very apt to remain, such as partial paralysis, decrease of the mental faculties, general weakness of the limbs. Death is a rare termination of the disease. A great tendency to relapses generally remains, on which account the patients have to be carefully guarded. That injuries, even fractures, may occur during a violent convulsive paroxysm, is self-evident.

According to what we have said, the prognosis is almost always favorable; even if the convulsive movements outlast the genuine chorea-paroxysms, they likewise disappear after a while. Where the convulsions denote the existence of a cerebral disease, the prognosis depends, of course, upon its own nature and importance.

Treatment. Inasmuch as most cases of chorea generally get well of themselves, although the process of recovery may proceed very gradually, it is always advisable not to interfere too busily with violent means. Reports of cures with medicinal agents should be received with a great deal of caution; a great deal of experience is required to determine whether a case of chorea has yielded to the medicines employed, or whether the disease has terminated spontaneously. Hence we shall only furnish very brief indications regarding the drugs that are adapted to this disease.

Cuprum metallicum is one of the leading remedies in this disease. Unless the existing symptoms contraindicate its use very decidedly, this drug will generally deserve our first consideration. This agent has sufficed in our hands to cure most cases of chorea; under its use the disorder continued very rarely longer than three or four weeks. It is, however, more suitable to chorea minor than chorea major; in this latter form of the disease the violent symptoms which characterize the paroxysms, may require some other remedy before Cuprum is employed, until the spasms are mitigated and have assumed the milder form of chorea minor.

Stramonium is more particularly indicated if the whole body is involved in the spasms and the patient is compelled to perform the most grotesque leaps, dancing motions, etc., and at the same time utters the above-described peculiar sounds. According to Hartmann, Stramonium is indicated by the following symptoms: The attack is for some time preceded by formication and a feeling of weight in the extremities, attended with melancholy mood. The disorder inclines to break out about the equinoctial periods, and the convulsions have the characteristic feature of affecting the parts of the body crosswise, for instance the left upper and the right lower extremity, whereas the two other extremities remain unaffected; on the other hand, the muscles of the head and neck are very much agitated. Altogether Stramonium has a number of symptoms that point to chorea. According to Hartmann it has likewise a good effect in the mental derangements remaining after chorea. Here too we cannot forbear to range *Belladonna* and *Hyoscyamus* side by side with Stramonium, only that the last-mentioned drug seems to be more adapted to chorea and the two former to eclampsia. Belladonna is moreover said to deserve more especial consideration if the flexor muscles are particularly affected.

Ignatia amara deserves mention in this affection, probably with more propriety than in any of the previously mentioned diseases. It is more particularly indicated by the following general considerations: The disorder is caused by fright or by some violent mental agitation; the attacks are worse after eating, and abate when the patient lies on the back; the patient is very irritable and peevish. Hartmann is of opinion that many cases of chorea major have been cured with Ignatia with a remarkable rapidity, that were mistaken for epilepsy by the attending physician. The diagnosis, however, is scarcely ever so intricate that the misapprehension could have lasted for a long time; it is more likely that such pretended cures of epilepsy were rather so many cases of eclampsia instead of chorea. At all events the therapeutic value of Ignatia is not impaired by the fact that it is equally curative in affections which resemble each other so closely.

Zincum. We do not understand why Hartmann has not mentioned this drug in his list of chorea-remedies. Zincum enjoys a well-earned reputation against chorea; the cures of this disease which have been effected by the use of Zincum, can all be traced to the homœopathicity of this agent to the chorea-spasms. Homœopathic physicians likewise have employed this agent with success. It is particularly indicated where the convulsions are attended with a deep feeling of illness and the mind is very much depressed. A merely superficial glance at the symptoms of Zincum will at once show that it deserves our attention in chorea, more especially in the minor form, and is pre-eminently suitable in the subsequent morbid changes of the mind.

Beside the above-mentioned remedies the following have likewise been employed or recommended: *Asafœtida, Secale cornutum, Cina, Crocus, Graphites, Rhus tox., Iodium, Pulsatilla, Sulphur, China, Cocculus.* We cannot afford the space to furnish all the particular indications for the use of each of these agents, nor does this seem necessary, since a case will scarcely ever present itself where these remedies may have to be used.

If after the termination of the more violent spasms, convulsive motions of single parts of muscles remain for some time, or if such remnants of the disease are for the first time entrusted to our professional care, the result of our treatment will always be more or less doubtful and uncertain. The remedies which have to be used in such cases, and always at rather protracted intervals, are: *Cuprum*, *Causticum*, *Graphites*, perhaps also *Cocculus*, and *Rhus tox*. A proper hygienic and dietetic regimen should not be lost sight of.

In chorea the selection of the remedial agent is less dependent upon accompanying complications and determining circumstances than in eclampsia and epilepsy, for the simple reason that chorea is a much less important disease. On the other hand it is of great importance to consider existing complications in case of relapses or where relapses are tolerably certain to occur. Three conditions have to be more particularly dwelt upon. First, the age of pubescence and its but too frequent accompaniment: onanism. It is often difficult to exert a controlling influence in this particular, for the reason that we do not always succeed in obtaining a frank confession from the patients. Nevertheless, an absolute cessation of this horrid practice is indispensable to a cure; onanism causes that general irritability of the nerves, and the deficiency of mental energy by which the original disease as well as relapses are excited. Anæmia is another important complication; it occurs but too frequently, even before the age of pubescence, and is undoubtedly prematurely excited by self-abuse, but may likewise owe its existence to other circumstances that will be mentioned in subsequent paragraphs. The third and worst, although not the most frequent complication, is tuberculosis. In a case of chorea we should investigate the existence of tubercles for this additional reason that convulsions very often constitute the first striking symptom of tubercles which it may be possible to cure at such an early age. When giving special indications, we shall mention the remedies that are suitable to such conditions. To the aforesaid three determining causes we may add a fourth, namely a morbid irritability of the nervous system generally. We admit that this may be hereditary; but in most cases it is the result of a faulty education. Premature mental efforts, excitement of the imagination while condemned to a sedentary mode of life, are the great defects of our modern systems of education and the direct causes of the excessive nervousness which has become fashionable among the young ladies of the higher classes and is one of the principal causes of the many weaknesses with which our young women are more than ever afflicted, anæmia, tuberculosis, convulsions, etc. A long chapter might be written on this theme. To what extent a morbid nervousness—not to mention the desire of imitation inherent in all children—predisposes to convulsions, is shown by daily experience without having to quote Bœrhaave as authority for this statement. In one of our young ladies' seminaries for the higher classes, spasmodic attacks, especially during the hours devoted to prayer-meetings, constitute a rule; scarcely ever a case occurs singly, generally several at once.

From what we have said, the measures that will have to be taken in order not only to cure or prevent chorea, but many other ailments attendant upon this disorder, may easily be inferred. Relapses may likewise be prevented by such measures. Premature mental development, or too great a variety of mental labor, or too persistent a strain on the mental faculties, should be prevented not only in the case of older children but likewise of those who have entered upon the period of their second teething. An excessive activity of the fancy should be prevented by every possible means. A proper development of the muscular powers and exercise in the open air should be well attended to. Gymnastic exercises are the best means for this purpose: they not only strengthen the body, but likewise invigorate the mind. Such exercises are not only a preventive means, and excellently adapted to the cure of subsequent ailments, but they likewise render efficient service against the convulsive movements themselves. In France especially they have been variously employed with a great deal of success in the treatment of chorea, sometimes in connection with music, either on account of the influence of the rhythmical measure, or because music has a strikingly beneficial influence over a number of such patients. Gymnastic exercises are particularly advisable in cases where automatic movements of single muscles threaten to remain and to become chronic.

[In recent cases of chorea, *Aconite* and *Gelseminum* are the best remedies that can often be used. A case of chorea of the left arm that had remained after pneumonia of the left lung, the patient, a girl of ten years, having been treated allopathically, yielded at once to a few doses of Aconite. A case of chorea of the upper extremities in a very scrofulous child, and having come on spontaneously, was speedily cured by means of a few doses of the tincture of Aconite in water. A case of the lower extremities brought on by fright, yielded with equal promptitude to the tincture of Aconite.

A terrible case of chorea was cured with Phosphoric acid. The patient was a girl of ten years. For some time she had allowed things to fall out of her hands, cups, plates, etc., which the parents attributed to carelessness, and for which she was duly scolded.

Gradually the spasms began to set in with increasing violence. Every part of the body, from the head to the feet, became affected. The convulsions were frightful to behold. The patient had to be strapped to her bed. She was scarcely able to swallow a drop of liquid. The spasms lasted uninterruptedly day and night. She was utterly unable to articulate a single word. The patient was brought to town from the country, when I had a fair chance to examine her. I had been trying various remedies without success. As soon as the patient had arrived in town, I examined her urine and found it loaded with albumen. She now was placed upon the officinal *Phosphoric acid*, beginning with five-drop doses three times a day, and gradually increasing the dose; after taking the acid for six weeks she was completely restored to health. An improvement in her condition became perceptible already on the second day of this treatment. H.]

4. Catalepsy.

We mention this disease which has remained enveloped in a mysterious obscurity up to this moment, in order not to be accused guilty of a sin of omission. By catalepsy we understand a condition during which the consciousness and the voluntary mobility of the muscles become suspended, though they retain the faculty of passive motion. There are but few well established cases of this affection on record; a most striking case is the one in Skoda's Clinic in the winter of 1851 to 1852, which we had an opportunity of witnessing. It continued for months and was the most interesting phenomenon in the large hospital. A detailed description of this case may be found in the "Zeitschrift der Gesellschaft der Aerzte in Wien," vol. VIII., 1852. A second undeniable case occurred in our own practice; the patient was a lady who had been magnetized. Skoda's case likewise is said to have originated in magnetism.

As an accompaniment of other affections, when it is generally of short duration, we meet the cataleptic condition in epilepsy, eclampsia, hysteria and other diseases of the general nervous system.

It will scarcely ever be necessary to institute a medicinal treatment against this disease; such a treatment must always be uncertain, because it is impossible to determine how soon the cataleptic condition might have terminated spontaneously. Skoda's report of his case embodies everything that was done for the patient, but fruitlessly. Cataleptic patients may be safely left without treatment, for the reason that no case of catalepsy, to our knowledge at least, has as yet terminated fatally. The greatest difficulty in chronic cases is the impossibility to induce patients to swallow; injections and the stomach-pump have to be resorted to.

5. Tetanus and Trismus.

By the term tetanus we designate tonic spasms of the voluntary muscles of more or less extent, without the consciousness being suspended; by the latter term we designate a tonic spasm of the muscles of deglutition.

Tetanus is more particularly a disease of hot climates, but is likewise frequently met with in our own climate, more particularly as trismus and tetanus neonatorum. Its main causes are wounds, especially such as are complicated with contusions, and are located on the extremities or in the face. It is not quite certain whether it is indispensable to the supervention of tetanus, that a nerve should be ligated, torn or involved in a cicatrix. Tetanus may undeniably be caused by sudden and violent exposure to a keen wind and other catarrhal influences. This form of tetanus has been termed rheumatic, in contradistinction to the traumatic form. Tetanic convulsions do not often, like eclampsia, occur at the onset of violent diseases, such as typhus and contagious exanthemata. Robust individuals, and men generally, are more readily attacked by the disease.

Symptoms and Course of the disease. The convulsions are generally preceded by some slight premonitory symptoms, generally of a rheumatic character, on which account they are confounded with rheumatism so much more easily as the patients generally complain of having taken a violent cold. Side by side with slight febrile symptoms the patients complain of stiffness of the nape of the neck, difficulty of deglutition, drawing and tearing pains in the extremities. If there is a wound, it generally assumes a bad look. Either gradually and with paroxysms of rigidity of single muscles, or else suddenly the tetanic convulsion sets in with a violent shock, at times invading the whole body, at other times single localities, particularly the dorsal muscles, the muscles of the jaws, and the extensor muscles of the extremities. In the more violent and more extensive cases not all the muscles are seized at once, generally the spasm progresses from above downwards. The picture of a case of this kind is furnished us with every epileptic paroxysm; in tetanus, however, the face, in consequence of the extraordinary stretching of the muscles, assumes a still more frightful aspect. Owing to the contraction of the dorsal muscles the back is at times bent backwards, (opisthotonos,) or laterally, (pleurothotonos,) or forwards, (emprosthotonos,) or is stretched erect, (orthotonos,) according as one or the other muscular locality, or all the muscles together, are invaded by the tetanic spasm; as a general rule, opisthotonos is the most frequent form. Most usually the posterior cervical muscles first become rigid, after which the trunk and lastly the extremities are seized. In proportion as the phenomena increase in intensity, the respiratory and abdominal muscles, and the muscles of deglutition likewise become involved in the attack; convulsions of the last-named organs render the attack particularly dangerous. In cases which run a rapid course, death takes place by asphyxia, and in cases running a less rapid course, death takes place in consequence of starvation and deficient oxygenation. For the more violent the paroxysms become, the more easily the least motion excites them, so that it becomes utterly impossible for the patient to swallow; even all artificial introduction of food has to be abandoned. From the very beginning of the paroxysm the muscles are perfectly rigid and remain so; nevertheless exacerbations and more or less distinct remissions take place, the latter becoming shorter and more and more incomplete in proportion as the convulsions increase in intensity. The contracted muscles are exceedingly painful, and every new attack often increases this painfulness to an extraordinary degree. Otherwise, so far as the body generally is concerned, no morbid phenomena of any consequence can be perceived. The skin is cool, the pulse is not more rapid, but harder, the patients experience hunger and thirst, alvine evacuations take place, the consciousness remains unimpaired; only sleep is disturbed, the exhausted patients only slumbering now and then for a few moments at a time. As the convulsions increase the pulse becomes more rapid, smaller, intermittent, the symptoms of sopor become more and more prominent, probably in consequence of the stupefying action of the carbonic acid gas which, owing to the impeded respiration, is no longer neutralized by the atmospheric oxygen; the tongue becomes dry. Tetanus most generally terminates in death. It either takes place at the very beginning in consequence of sudden suffocation (spasm of the glottis,) or in consequence of acute œdema of the lungs, or sometimes in consequence of cerebral apoplexy. Or if the disease lasts any time, the patient dies of asphyxia by carbonic acid gas, starvation and thirst. Recovery is always gradual, sometimes taking place with copious sweats; the paroxysms first become shorter, less violent and frequent, and the muscles gradually lose their rigidity. Weeks, however, may pass away before this muscular rigidity disappears entirely, and an equally long period of time sometimes elapses before the patient recovers his strength.

If the disease terminates fatally, it may last from one day to three weeks, but in most cases death takes place on the third day. In traumatic tetanus the prognosis is generally unfavorable.

Tetanus neonatorum is essentially the same disease as traumatic tetanus, from which the former is distinguished only by the peculiar features of infantile age. The cutting and tying of the umbilical cord here takes the place of the wound. That this is really so, cannot be doubted; the accident generally takes place in the first week of the child's existence, and the umbilicus is almost always found in a state of suppuration and discoloration. In the form of trismus the disease is likewise, though seldom, met with among older children.

In the case of children the symptoms vary somewhat from those of adults. In the case of infants likewise the disease seldom begins all at once; in the first place the infants lose their ability to nurse, although the hurried manner in which they seize the nipple, betrays hunger; they have a sick and sunken appearance. Derangements of the digestive functions are not always, but generally present. In a day or so the paroxysm sets in with rigidity of the muscles of deglutition, in consequence of which the lower jaw becomes immovable although not firmly pressed against the upper, from which it remains separated by a narrow interval. The tetanic rigidity now gradually spreads from above downwards, the same as in traumatic tetanus; however, it is frequently mingled with paroxysms of convulsive starts resembling violent electric shocks. At first the attacks are short, with intervals which frequently last for days; but the former keep constantly increasing in duration whereas the latter are as constantly growing shorter. Death takes place more or less rapidly by starvation and impeded respiration. The prognosis is much more unfavorable than in the tetanus of adults.

Treatment. To judge from the paucity of the cases of tetanus which are recorded in our literature, homœopathic practitioners have had but few cases of this disease to treat. We have reports of cases where tetanic symptoms were present, but of genuine tetanus we have only one case recorded by Bethmann in the tenth volume of the "Allg. Hom. Zeitung." If a case should occur in our practice, we should rely upon the curative effects of *Nux vomica* and of such other medicines as contain Strychnine. The similarity of the poisonous effects of Strychnine to tetanus not only extends to muscular rigidity and to the extraordinary increase of reflex action, but even to the most trifling circumstances. The spasms of Nux vomica have distinct intermissions which grow shorter and more indistinct in proportion as the paroxysms occur more frequently and with more violence. The respiration is very much interfered with; the sensibility and the mental functions remain intact. The effects of Nux generally correspond equally fully to single organs and systems. According to these statements Nux vomica must be an excellent remedy in tetanus, if there is any truth in the homœopathic law. We do not deny that there are other remedies homœopathic to tetanus, but many of those which are mentioned in manuals and repertories, are undoubtedly very doubtful. The characteristic phenomena of the disease have to be found in the pathogenesis of the drug, otherwise its choice would not be justifiable; in tetanus these characteristic phenomena are the rigidity of the muscles, the increase of reflex action and the preservation of the consciousness. Now with what right can Opium be recommended as a remedy for tetanus, since the Opium-convulsions, although they may resemble tetanus to some extent, are always attended with loss of consciousness? The same question might be asked in regard to other remedies which have been recommended for tetanus probably for the mere reason that a few tonic spasms are found among their physiological effects. Although we are willing to admit that, at the present time, we are not yet able to get along without drawing conclusions from analogy, yet they should not be too bold. *Arnica* has been mentioned among the remedies for traumatic tetanus, probably for no better reason than because it is traumatic; for, with the exception of the increased sensibility, Arnica has no symptoms corresponding to tetanus. Besides, the wound itself is not the real cause of tetanus, but it is an unknown something which sometimes does not supervene until the wound has lasted for weeks. *Rhus* is said to deserve attention in tetanus caused by a violent cold; isolated phenomena speak indeed in favor of this drug, but they are not characteristic. Among other remedies we have to select those that have a decided influence over the spinal marrow, such as: *Cicuta virosa, Veratrum, Lachesis, Secale cornutum,* [*Aconite,* tincture of the root, and *Bryonia* should not be forgotten. H.]

Tetanus neonatorum is, as we have already mentioned, quite similar, symptomatically, to the tetanus of adults; it is probably a form of traumatic tetanus and therefore requires the same treatment. *Moschus* is particularly recommended for tetanus neonatorum, more especially if the dyspnœa is very great.

Aconite is a drug which hitherto had not been known to cause tetanic phenomena. In the December number, 1860, of the British Journal of Homœopathy we find a case of poisoning by Aconite. After eating a few Aconite-roots, a girl was attacked with tetanus and trismus which gradually decreased in intensity, after which she recovered.

Trismus alone occurs much more frequently than tetanus; it is most frequently met with among small children, seldom among adults. Together with the remedies that have already been mentioned, we direct the reader's attention to *Camphora* and *Belladonna*. With the last-mentioned drug we have effected a rapid cure in the case of a girl, fourteen days old.

We need hardly suggest that, in order to effect a genuine cure, it is necessary to avoid all the circumstances that might possibly excite an attack. Deglutition may have become so much impeded that it may be impossible to introduce medicines by the mouth; in such cases we have to resort to the hypodermic method.

From the British Journal of Homœopathy we transcribe the following extract from the New Sydenham Society's Year-book of Medicine: "Haughton cured three out of five cases of tetanus with Nicotine, one-half to two drops, three to six times a day. It lowers the pulse, and causes an immediate relaxation of the spasms of the muscles of expression, deglutition, respiration, back and abdomen, cessation of delirium, and relief from agonizing pain, profuse perspiration with smell of snuff, tendency to sleep.

Ghesini cured a case of traumatic tetanus by subcutaneous injection of Curare. As much as forty-seven grains of Curare were injected in sixty single and thirty-two double and treble injections. The treatment was commenced on the fifth day, and the patient was convalescent on the seventeenth.

Cannabis indica in large quantities has cured tetanus in the hands of Dr. O'Shaughnessy of Calcutta; he gave it in doses large enough to produce narcotism. [This treatment seems purely palliative or antipathic. H.]

6. Paralysis.

Under this name we comprehend so many different conditions that it is necessary to justify this classification. Paralysis is almost always a consequence of a variety of other affections; nevertheless it is not always possible to recognize the primary affection, so that a paralysis is frequently supposed to be an idiopathic affection when it is in reality something else. We should have been obliged to resort to endless repetitions if we had chosen to treat of paralysis when speaking of the functional derangements which may occasion the attack, and again to describe the disease with reference to its locality. For this reason we have deemed it preferable to devote a special chapter to this class of accidents.

By paralysis generally we understand a suspension of nervous action. It may differ in character according to the number of nervous trunks involved, or according to their characteristic functions and anatomical arrangement. Hence different names have been applied to different kinds of paralysis. By paralysis we understand the complete cessation of both motor and sentient nervous action; if either the sentient or motor nerves are paralyzed, we term this condition incomplete paralysis, or paresis; if only one side of the body is paralyzed, we designate this condition as hemiplegia; whereas by paraplegia we understand a transverse paralysis, of both upper and lower extremities. Besides this, the paralysis may be universal or partial, the last of which is again differently named according as one or the other part is affected, such as blepharoplegia, glossoplegia, &c.

The etiological causes of paralysis are various. The most important are: Suspension of the cerebral activity in consequence of apoplexy, inflammation, softening and other morbid processes of the brain impairing its functions; suspension of the action of the spinal cord by the same causes. There are, however, many other influences to which paralysis may be traced as their direct result. The main causes of this class are: excessive exertions of the parts to which the paralyzed nerve is distributed, in which category we have to number paralysis occasioned by convulsions; continued and excessive pains; interruption of the nervous current from the brain to the periphery by swellings, neuromata, ligatures; a stroke of lightning; rheumatism, hysteria, gout, pregnancy; violent acute diseases, among which contagious and miasmatic diseases occupy the first rank: such as scarlatina, measles, variola, typhus, dysentery; and finally poisoning by vegetable, animal and more particularly inorganic substances.

The symptoms of paralysis may readily be inferred from the functional nature of the organ to which the paralyzed nerves are distributed; we can only meet with difficulties in cases where the paralyzed organ is not directly accessible to our vision.

The prognosis depends upon the nature of the exciting causes and upon the possibility of removing them. Where apoplectic effusions or other pathological processes of the brain or spinal cord constitute the primary disease, recovery is much more uncertain than where paralysis depends upon some cause at the periphery or is a remnant of some acute disorder. That the prognosis is rendered much more doubtful by an advanced age, an enfeebled constitution, and an extension of the paralytic phenomena over a large surface, is a matter of course.

Treatment. Paralytic attacks being almost without an exception secondary affections, it is evident that, in treating them, it is of the utmost importance to investigate the primary affection with the utmost care. There are indeed many cases where every diagnostic inquiry into the causes of an attack leaves us in the dark; these cases are, however, rare, and, whenever they occur, the paralysis generally depends upon a single nervous trunk. Such cases are the most difficult to treat, for the reason that it is exceedingly difficult to select the proper remedy in accordance with symptomatic indications. Inasmuch as diseases of the brain and spinal marrow are the main causes of paralysis, we refer here more especially to the chapter treating of these diseases where the most important remedies have already been mentioned, and we avoid by this means all unnecessary repetitions. In other respects our best course undoubtedly is to mention the remedies appertaining to this category, in a concise series, for which purpose we shall, although not literally, transcribe Hartmann's own arrangement.

Cuprum is one of the most efficient medicines in paralysis. When speaking of apoplexy and the other diseases of the brain, we have treated extensively of Cuprum, and shall here add only a few short remarks. It is not only to the convulsive paroxysms themselves, but likewise to the remaining paralysis that Cuprum is essentially adapted; it likewise deserves attention in paralysis remaining after cholera, typhus, dysentery, etc.

Plumbum has to be ranged next to Cuprum as being most nearly related to it. The last-named remedy is more prominently adapted to paralysis of the motor nerves, sensation is not extinguished, the assimilative process is frequently disturbed, though never in a very high degree, and the paralyzed parts frequently show signs of convulsive twitchings. In the case of Plumbum, on the contrary, both motion and sensation are suspended, the paralyzed parts emaciate very rapidly, and their temperature decreases considerably. With Cuprum the consciousness and the cerebral functions are less disturbed; with Plumbum, on the contrary, always and even violently.

Both agents are specially related to the functions of the tongue and, in paralysis of this organ, they undoubtedly occupy the first rank.

Rhus toxicodendron. Concerning this medicine, Hartmann offers the following remarks: In former times, when the homœopathic Materia Medica was not as well stocked with medicines as it is at the present period, I have made several cures of paralysis of the lower extremities with *Rhus tox.*, even when the paralysis remained after typhus. If I place this remedy in the front rank, it is not because I have a particular preference for it, but because I am anxious to recall this powerful anti-paralytic to the attention of physicians, lest it should be overlooked in the presence of more recently introduced remedial agents whose importance I do not, however, mean to undervalue. Among the primary effects of Rhus, we note a disposition to extinguish organic activity even to the degree of paralysis; a sensation of numbness and a decrease of sensibility in the affected parts constitute chief symptoms of Rhus. Although crampy and contracting sensations, as from shortening of tendons, do not particularly come within the category of paralytic symptoms, yet it cannot be denied that they are to some extent dependent upon a diminished activity of single nervous trunks. This is likewise the case with the bruising and dislocation pains caused by Rhus, and which have often been removed by this agent. It is not always paralytic ailments that we have to combat at the very onset, but it is distressing and gradually increasing drawing pains in the extremities while in a state of rest and the removal of which requires the affected limb to be moved the more vigorously, the longer it had persevered in a state of rest. These pains have the peculiarity of leaving after their disappearance a sort of lameness in the affected part, which, in proportion as the pain lasts longer, becomes more and more intense and permanent, and distinctly points to incipient paralysis. Is not the feeling of weariness and numbness which Rhus causes, a lower degree of momentary paralysis? A leading symptom of Rhus is: lameness in the extremities with stiffness of the joints, worse when rising from a seat; or complete paralysis, hemiplegia as well as paraplegia, with dragging, slow, difficult gait. According to these statements, Rhus is not adapted to paralysis of the central organs, but rather to paralysis at the periphery, and to such as remains after typhus. It is, moreover, particularly useful in rheumatic paralysis, to which the whole series of the pathogenetic symptoms of Rhus corresponds with great accuracy.

Arnica has been extensively mentioned as a remedy for cerebral diseases. It is not only suitable in paralysis depending upon cerebral exudations, but likewise in any other form of paralysis depending upon exudations of any kind.

Causticum is an important remedy which penetrates the organism very deeply, and has been found particularly efficacious in chronic maladies. The reputation of this drug has been somewhat impaired by the circumstance that its primary effects manifest themselves more slowly than those of other long-acting remedies. In paralytic conditions Causticum is at all events one of the most important remedies; its usefulness has been tested on too many occasions to be disputed at this late day. Hartmann has seen the best effects from it in partial paralysis caused by a keen draught of air, and in hemiplegia after suppressed eruptions, attended with striking coldness, especially of the head and feet. After apoplexy he recommends it, when the proper paralytic symptoms are accompanied by frequent congestions of the head, with anxiety, vertigo and a cloudy feeling in the brain. In paralysis of one side of the face, paralysis of the facial nerve, it has been found curative by Hartmann as well as by other physicians. In paralysis of the tongue it is undoubtedly a prominent remedy, although we do not by any means mean to say that every case of this kind can be cured with it. It is well known that this form of paralysis is particularly inaccessible to remedial influences. As a general rule Causticum is more efficient in the paralysis of single nervous trunks than in general paralysis, more efficient in paresis than in complete paralysis, for where Causticum is indicated, the sensibility is generally unimpaired.

According to Hartmann *Cocculus* is most efficient in paralysis of the lower extremities. It starts from the small of the back, and is supposed by the patient to be owing to a cold. As a general rule it is recent cases that are particularly suitable to Cocculus, especially when the paralysis is accompanied by violent pain in the paralyzed parts, or when symptoms of spasm show themselves in these parts. Paralysis of the tongue, face and pharynx is likewise adapted to the curative action of Cocculus.

Sulphur. If we do not reproduce Hartmann's statements regarding the action of Sulphur in this disease, it is because his views and our own do not agree. This is not the proper place to discuss the question of latent psora; enough has been said on this point, and very uselessly. We are not one of the believers in the psora-theory, which we simply regard as a convenient means of getting over difficulties that we do not know how to solve, and over which we glide with vague generalities. It might be very difficult to show what practical benefit has been derived from this theory. Whether a partisan or an opponent of this theory, Sulphur will prove eminently useful in the hands of either, and not simply because it facilitates the action of remedial agents employed after Sulphur. This agent corresponds more particularly to paralysis based upon material changes. In this respect it acts similarly to Arnica, with this difference, that Arnica is more particularly indicated in recent, and Sulphur in more chronic cases. In paralysis remaining after acute diseases, Sulphur will likewise prove curative, probably for the reason that it exerts a favorable influence over exudations, as in typhus, that had not yet been absorbed.

Baryta carbonica is undoubtedly one of the most distinguished remedies for paralysis after apoplexy, and for paralysis of old people, where a want of steadiness, a feeling of debility in the whole body, giving way of the knees and pain in the lumbar portion of the spine had been complained of for some time previous. This agent is well known as a remedy for the ailments incident to old age, and this reputation of our drug has likewise been verified in the paralytic conditions of old people; on this account, however, it is not excluded as a remedy for paralysis of young people; we refer more particularly to paralysis of the tongue, which is seldom cured without the use of this agent. (Hartmann.)

Secale cornutum is a remedy of some importance in paralysis; its sphere of action is, moreover, more distinctly defined than that of many other drugs. All sorts of spasms come within the category of morbid conditions to which this agent may be adapted. It is well known that long-continued or frequently-returning spasms of the same parts often lead to paralytic conditions and even actual paralysis of single limbs, where art has to interfere even though the spasms should have entirely ceased. It is to these forms of paralysis that Secale corresponds; if the lower extremities are the seat of the disorder, involuntary discharges of the fæces and urine are frequently present, and the paralyzed parts emaciate very rapidly. (Hartmann.)

Aluminium metallicum is still of too recent use to admit of definite indications of its use in the treatment of diseases. Bœnninghausen's recommendation, which he backs up with clinical results, may suffice to claim our attention to this new agent. A drug which is useful in tabes dorsualis, in genuine progressive spinal paralysis, must certainly possess a prominent effect upon the nervous system; our stock of remedies for paralysis being anyhow limited, Aluminium is so much the more to be thought of as a remedial agent in this class of disorders.

Dulcamara seems to have been a favorite remedy with Hartmann. He says in reference to Dulcamara: It is certain that this remedy is used much too little by modern homœopaths, and that it is even ignored by many of them as an useless medicine. Nevertheless it has the same medicinal virtues now that it manifested in such a striking degree at a former period, and its curative virtues become so much more manifest, the more familiar we become with the use of this agent. How many paralytic attacks are caused by exposure to intense cold or to wet, or even to the suppression of scrofulous eruptions, where a latent psora is evidently the fruitful soil in which the susceptibility to paralytic attacks is rooted. It is this class of paralytic attacks where Dulcamara constitutes a real specific, and where it will almost always be found curative in alternation with *Sulphur*. For this reason it is adapted to almost every form of paralysis, as its symptoms show. Moreover we find Dulcamara useful for paralysis of the arm, with icy coldness, as if the patient had been struck with apoplexy; paralysis of the upper and lower extremities; paralysis of the tongue and bladder, where Dulcamara is of prominent importance.

Arsenicum, Mercurius and even **Iodium**, after a long-continued use, cause paralytic symptoms, as we know to our perfect satisfaction from a number of cases of poisoning; however, we are not able to specify the particular indications by which we might be guided in the use of these remedies, and we have to content ourselves with the general knowledge that these three medicines exert a powerful influence over the nervous system, and hence may prove powerful auxiliaries in the treatment of paralysis.

Other medicines that may be classed in the category of anti-paralytic agents are: *Oleander, Stannum, Colchicum* (for rheumatic paralysis), *Lachesis, Cantharides* (for paralysis of the bladder), *Anacardium, Zincum, Veratrum album, Staphysagria, Silicea, Phosphorus, Natrum muriaticum, Stramonium,* etc.

For the sake of having a cursory view of the different remedies adapted to the different forms of paralysis, we here subjoin their list: Paralysis of the tongue: *Baryta, Cuprum, Plumbum, Stramonium, Dulcamara, Acidum muriaticum, Cocculus, Belladonna, Causticum.* For paralysis of the facial nerve: *Causticum, Cocculus.* For paralysis of the pharynx: *Cantharides, Stramonium, Belladonna.* For paralysis of the bladder: *Belladonna, Dulcamara, Cantharides, Lycopodium, Natrum muriaticum.* For paralysis of the rectum: *Lycopodium, Ruta graveolens.*

Paralytic attacks caused by poisoning require the employment of suitable antidotes, and subsequently remaining ailments have to be treated with smaller doses. The most frequent kinds of paralysis from this source are: Paralysis caused by Mercury: *Stramonium* (Hartmann), *Acidum, nitricum, Staphysagria, Sulphur.* Paralysis caused by Arsenic: *China, Ferrum, Graphites.* Paralysis by lead: *Opium, Cuprum.*

[It is beyond our comprehension why homœopathic practitioners who are acquainted with the pathogenesis of *Aconite,* and with pathology, do not assign to this agent a prominent rank among the remedies for paralysis. We have cured with it time and again the most violent attacks of paralysis of internal organs as well as of the extremities. The causes are various: Violent emotions, a sudden fright, exposure to keen winds, humidity, draughts of air, etc. The symptoms which indicate Aconite, are: a full and slow pulse, or sometimes an accelerated and small, thready pulse; numbness, a pricking sensation; sense of coldness in the part, or the opposite sensation of increase of temperature, with heaviness and aching pains in the part; sensation as if the part were swollen. The symptoms of course vary according as one or the other organ is affected. We have: paralytic ischuria caused by exposure to a current of air, wet or by suppression of the perspiration; paralysis of the rectum and anus; paralysis of the tongue, with a pricking sensation and a sensation as if the tongue were swollen, increase of temperature in the tongue; paralysis of the optic nerve with intense pain as if caused by pressure; paralysis of the face, of the œsophagus, etc. Very many attacks of this kind, if caused suddenly by exposure to rheumatic influences, yield to the use of Aconite in a very short period of time. In some cases we use the tincture, a few drops in half a tumbler of water, in other cases we have got along with attenuations. We recommend these observations to the careful consideration of practitioners. H.]

As regards dietetic and other measures in the management of paralytic patients, we find it impossible, in view of the great differences prevailing among the different forms of paralysis and their various degrees of intensity, to furnish specific directions; we will content ourselves with indicating one auxiliary agent which has an important bearing upon the treatment of paralysis, namely the movement-cure. Cautious, moderate, as far as possible active, or even passive movements of the paralyzed parts have effected an improvement even in inveterate and desperate cases. It seems as though the paralyzed nerve remained in a state of inaction simply because it is deprived of an unusual stimulus to action, which the movement-cure is to supply. Hence this cure is much more useful in chronic paralytic conditions than in those of recent origin. In spite of the sanguine expectations of its friends, electricity has accomplished much less in the treatment of paralysis than the movement-cure. This lack of success may in a measure result from an imperfect use of this agent, but an imperfect use cannot be the only cause of a want of success. The disappointment in the use of the electric current is in a great measure owing to the impatience of the practitioner as well as of the patient. Great effects are expected already after a few days' treatment, whereas it often requires weeks before a favorable change can be expected. An interesting case of this kind may be read in "Hirschel's Zeitschrift," 1861, Nov. 15th, where magnetism was likewise used with effect. The electric current should never be used with too much force which is always more hurtful than useful. The current should only be felt as a slightly unpleasant sensation, but should never be received as a shock.

7. Hysteria.

It is not only difficult but almost impossible to furnish a satisfactory and sufficiently comprehensive definition of hysteria. The most diversified phenomena are ranged under this name, and a rigorous definition of the term hysteria is subject to so many different individual views and opinions that it seems impossible to generalize them, except in the most comprehensive series. Considering the term hysteria from this general point of view we understand by it a modification of the nervous functions which is almost exclusively peculiar to the female sex, the motor as well as the sentient nerves, the psychical as well as the vegetative activity of the female organism are involved in this modification, sometimes with, at other times without any material changes.

Hysteria is a disease of the full-grown woman. Hence it manifests itself between the periods of pubescence and a change of life; it may outlast the latter period, but is scarcely ever distinctly manifested previous to the former. Men, too, are said to be liable to attacks of hysteria. This, however, is questionable for the reason that the term hysteria is not defined with absolute precision. Hysteric symptoms in the case of a man do not justify the term hysteria, the true definition of which has been more obscured by the fact that men also have been supposed amenable to the Protean forms of this disease.

The etiology of hysteria is not as yet clear. Many material changes which are regarded as causes of hysteria, may just as well be consequences as causes of hysteria; it would be strange if so many different etiological influences should be capable of producing the same disorder. What is an undeniable fact, is that the trouble is rooted in the sexual sphere of woman, for this circumstance is proven by the fact that it breaks out exclusively among full-grown females; but what changes are necessary to the production of hysteria, can only be pointed out with partial positiveness. The most frequent causes seem to be ulcerations of the os tincæ, and displacements of the uterus, likewise pathological changes of the ovaries. There is much less confusion in determining the mental than the material causes of hysteria, or in tracing this disorder to a mingling of both. Onanism, abstemiousness, or an excessive irritation by sexual intercourse, may cause hysteria. Among the mental causes we number all those that impress a wrong direction upon the psychical life of woman, and more particularly feed her fancy to excess, as is unfortunately the case by our modern systems of education, which favor all sorts of fantastical and morbid tastes and extravagances. We should be carried too far if we would investigate this point to the bottom; moreover every physician has abundant opportunities to satisfy himself of the correctness of our remarks. We find hysteria very generally complicated with another affection, which is likewise almost exclusively to be attributed to the wrong education and faulty mode of life of the female sex—we mean chlorosis; we would not, however, assume the responsibility of asserting that chlorosis is the cause of hysteria. That hysteria may likewise be favored by unusual mental occupations, even of a serious or scientific kind, is shown in the case of female teachers. Besides these more or less gradually penetrating psychical influences, hysteria may likewise be caused by the action of some sudden and violent mental excitement, especially when of a depressing character.

Symptoms and course. A satisfactory definition of hysteria is perhaps less difficult than to furnish a general view of its various phenomenal manifestations, for the reason that in a case of hysteria every organ may be apparently, not actually, implicated in the abnormal process, and hence the picture of the disease must vary a good deal. Moreover hysteria complicates and modifies every acute and chronic affection, whose form it often changes to such a degree that the affection is no longer recognizable. Hence it is of the utmost importance to determine whether a woman is afflicted with hysteria; for this knowledge gives us the clue to most of her troubles.

The more general diagnostic signs of hysteria are best studied with reference to the nervous sphere where these signs are located. The mental activity is always and generally very strikingly altered. In the lower degrees of hysteria we meet with a capricious and very fitful demeanor, attended with an unusual sensitiveness to sometimes trifling mental impressions, even mere notions. This sensitiveness, however, is usually more felt towards unpleasant things, and gradually develops a disposition to habitual melancholy and dejection of spirits. Being constantly preoccupied with herself and exposed to the jests and gibes of those near her, the patient simulates an artificial cheerfulness with a consistency and firmness that often seem incredible, and in spite of the most agonizing distress. In the higher grades of hysteria we meet with all sorts of mental conditions that may very properly be ranged in the category of mental derangements, and are sometimes characterized by a peculiar irritability of temper, at other times by extreme depression. The power of volition is sometimes so completely gone that the most serious mental alienation may be apprehended. We have known an hysteric lady who could not make up her mind to anything, not even to go to bed; she frequently remained standing in her chemise for three or four hours in a room without fire, although the cold was intense. This absence of will-power is very marked in hysteric spasms, which can often be arrested by no other means than by exciting this power. We are acquainted with a lady who was frequently attacked with spasms, likewise during her first pregnancy and shortly before her confinement. The child died of eclampsia shortly after birth. We urged upon the mother the conviction that she would never give birth to a healthy child unless she made every effort to suppress the spasms. This advice proved so effectual that the spasms have ceased ever since, and that, whenever a recurrence of the spasms was threatened, they were instantly subdued by the husband reminding her of our advice. It would be wrong, however, if on this account, we were to consider hysteric spasms as pure dissimulation. This is not so; there is simply a lack of internal energy to suppress the convulsive motions. That this psychical sensitiveness likewise extends to the views about men and things, is a matter of course; this manifests itself in excessive inclinations or disinclinations, and frequently gives rise to the most extraordinary idiosyncrasies. Next to the moral disposition, the sensibility is generally altered most strangely. This change assumes more prominently the character of an excessive sensitiveness, which, in common parlance, we are apt to designate as nervousness or nervous debility, and which may affect the whole nervous system. The organs of sense are sometimes extremely sensitive to the most trifling impressions, which would remain unnoticed by persons in health; at other times the perception of external impressions is the opposite of what it would be in a normal condition and *vice versa*, so that the most offensive odors, for instance, seem pleasant, and agreeable odors are repulsive. This nervous irritability sometimes manifests itself in the form of neuralgia, such as megrim, clavus hystericus, pains in the joints, cardialgia, spinal irritation; or it is perceived as a peculiar sensation of pain, while such organs as the lungs, heart, bowels, etc., whose action remains unperceived by persons in a state of health, fulfil their functions in a normal manner. The patients often carry their complaints to such a degree that it is only through the most minute investigation, and the complete absence of all objective pathological changes, that we can satisfy ourselves of the utter absence of some intense organic affection. Derangements in the motor sphere generally assume the form of spasms. They either consist in local convulsions, or they resemble epilepsy, catalepsy or tetanus so closely that even the most practised eye may be deceived for a time. A chief sign for a correct diagnosis is the continuance of the consciousness. Beside the extremities, other parts may be attacked by clonic spasms, such as the pharynx, the diaphragm; the frequently occurring laughing or weeping spasms belong in this category. Paralytic conditions are less frequent; they may assume a variety of forms. That they have not a very deep significance, is shown by the fact that they shift about or disappear quite suddenly, or that the paralyzed nerves show a normal susceptibility to the electric current. However, even after we have by such means ascertained that the paralysis is neither caused nor supported by a more deep-seated affection, it is not on that account removed with any more ease, and often resists every possible therapeutic means with the most obstinate perseverance. These nervous derangements are attended with a peculiarly characteristic condition of the bladder. Most hysteric females void the urine very often, it is generally colorless; a diminished secretion of urine is much less frequent.

All the above-mentioned functional disturbances, except perhaps those of a lighter grade, do not continue permanently, they are very apt to break out in the form of paroxysms, which are excited by influences that it is difficult to trace, most generally, however, of a psychical nature, and the intensity and duration of which are undefinable. Not unfrequently these paroxysms appear periodically, they may even be preceded by certain precursory symptoms, otherwise they are without any fixed rule, and set in quite unexpectedly.

Hartmann gives a cursory view of hysterical local affections which is not unessential to a comprehension of the general character of the disease, and which we therefore transcribe in this place. We would, however, premise that such abstract statements do not constitute the rule, and that the local hysteric disorder is most generally attended with partial manifestations of one or the other derangements.

Hysteria cephalica consists in hemicrania, clavus, sensation of coldness at the occiput, sopor and coma, symptoms of inflammatory cerebral affections, delirium, obstinate sleeplessness.

Hysteria of the mind: Frequent repetition of certain syllables, words, phrases, melodies; nymphomania.

Hysteria of the spinal marrow: Drawing pain through the whole spine, attended with pain in the extremities, formication, muscular contractions, cramps in the calves, paralytic conditions, neuralgic affections of the pectoral and intercostal nerves and articulations. The pains are scarcely ever seated, but always wandering.

Hysteria uterina: The patients complain of pain, tension in the hypogastric and pubic region, frequently with drawing pains in the loins and small of the back, along the course of the round and broad ligaments; they feel as if the uterus were forcibly lifted from the bottom of the small into the larger pelvis. Sometimes these pains are of a colicky nature, at other times they are accompanied with a sensation as if a ball were rising. The sexual instinct is either violently excited or else very much depressed. Menstrual derangements are very frequently present; the catamenia are at times scanty, at other times profuse, generally irregular, the blood flowing by fits and starts, and often attended with leucorrhœa. The hysteric paroxysms are most violent at the time of the menses, and at the commencement occur at very regular intervals. In proportion as the catamenial irregularities increase, the paroxysms cease to be connected with the appearance of the menstrual flow.

Hysteria of the bladder, hysteria vesicalis: The patients are attacked with violent contracting, sometimes burning pains in the lumbar region, following the course of the ureters through the whole pelvis, in the region of the bladder, without sensitiveness to hard, external pressure, by which circumstance the disease is distinguished from nephritis and cystitis. These pains are accompanied by violent urging to urinate, the emission of urine being either suppressed or intensely painful. The voided urine is clear and liquid as water.

Hysteric affections of the bowels, (*colica hysterica*)*:* It consists in spasms generally proceeding from the cœcum or from the sigmoid flexure, the patients experiencing a sensation as if a ball in that region were continually augmenting in size. The pain is like a most violent colicky pain, burning, tearing and stabbing as if the bowel were torn to pieces. The patient utters a piercing cry when any one attempts to touch her, whereas she bears a strong pressure if, during the examination, her attention is directed to some other object. There is borborygmus, tympanitis, sometimes an enormous distension of the transverse colon, with oppressive anxiety, shortness of breathing, vomiting, &c. There is no trace of fever.

Hysteric affection of the stomach: The patients complain of a pain in the stomach which is at times constrictive, burning, or spasmodic, and is attended with oppression, nausea, vomiting, dread of contact, and yet the patient bears violent pressure. In this list belongs the sensitiveness of patients to large doses of the drug, so that even Canstatt observes that a cure can only be effected by truly infinitesimal quantities.

Asthma hystericum: Sometimes hysteric patients are afflicted with violent oppression of breathing, anxiety as if they would suffocate, stitching pains in the chest; nevertheless they are able to draw a long breath, as evidence that there is no trouble with the lungs. Sometimes there is cough, and then again it is missing; it is generally dry, sometimes barking like whooping-cough. In many cases the respiratory process is carried on by means of the abdominal muscles; in other cases the breathing is panting, anxious, the patients have to sit up erect in their beds. Physical signs and fever are wanting.

Hysteric affection of the larynx: The patients have a loud, dry, almost barking cough coming on in paroxysms and being more especially excited by emotions and nervous agitation, also attended with spasm of the rima glottidis and a croupy respiration. Another form is hoarseness and aphonia. This form breaks out suddenly and disappears as suddenly, sometimes after having lasted for years. Sometimes, after a violent mental excitement, the patient speaks again in her natural tone of voice, whereas shortly before she was only able to speak in a whisper. In this category we have to range the sounds of beasts, like the barking of dogs, &c., which are sometimes emitted by hysteric patients in involuntary paroxysms.

Hysteric affection of the heart: Hysteric women are in the habit of complaining of palpitation of the heart, and oppressive anxiety in the region of the heart. The palpitation can be seen externally, and not unfrequently it becomes so violent that it would seem as though the ribs would break. It generally comes on periodically, but without any regular intervals.

The hysteric ball, globus hystericus, one of the best known hysteric symptoms, consists in a constrictive sensation in the throat as if a ball were lodged there; eructations sometimes afford relief.

This enumeration of the local forms of hysteria does not by any means exhaust the multitudinous forms of this disease; however it contains its most important and most usual forms very completely.

The course of the disease is always very chronic; it is only in rare cases that hysteric symptoms show themselves only about the time of the menses or during pregnancy, which disappear again with the menses or the termination of pregnancy.

The most noteworthy terminations are: Transformation of the

hysteric convulsions in real epilepsy, and of the mental irregularities in permanent dementia. Paralytic conditions remain much less frequently.

The prognosis is generally doubtful, and even unfavorable, because we are not able to completely eradicate the defects of education in the mental range, and the necessarily long duration of the treatment fatigues both physicians and patients. The more nearly the disease resembles a mental disorder, the less the prospect of relieving the patient. A long continuance of the disease likewise diminishes the chances of recovery. The prognosis is likewise complicated by the advanced age of the patient, for the reason that the prospect of putting off the pernicious habits and prejudices of youth becomes dimmer with every additional year. Where pregnancy is accompanied by hysteric, convulsive symptoms, the danger of a miscarriage is not slight; and the appearance of such symptoms during confinement frequently leads to lasting and generally incurable mental derangements. The nearer the paroxysms resemble those of epilepsy, the more readily they assume the form of the latter more formidable disease. Where the disease can be traced to definite causes, the chances of a cure depend in a great measure upon the nature of these causes.

Treatment. Following Hartmann's example we introduce this paragraph with Schœnlein's words: "The treatment of hysteria is one of the most difficult tasks, not merely on account of the difficulties inherent in the diagnosis and on account of the protracted course of the disease, but likewise on account of mental complications. The patience of the physician is sometimes tried to the utmost; for, whereas he may be satisfied that the disease is of not much importance, he has to lend a willing ear to the everlasting lamentations of his patient, and has to listen to hundredfold repetitions without showing the least signs of impatience; for the patients are so sensitive, that if the physician should betray the least indifference to their sufferings, and only listen to their statements with a half-closed ear, his credit is instantly lost. If a physician wishes to treat hysteric females, he has to show them the greatest compassion, has to listen patiently to their complaints, and should never appear indifferent or out of humor if he does not wish to be discharged."

The treatment of hysteric patients has to be looked at from a variety of points of view, so much more as it is almost impossible to confine ourselves in our treatment to separate local affections, and to pursue a special treatment for each of them. Again, we ask the question which we have already presented on a former occasion, whether it is possible to treat hysteric patients exclusively in accordance with symptomatic similarities; what becomes with such a supposition of the various derangements of organs which are simulated by hysteria?

According to what we have said in the chapter on the etiology of hysteria, the determination of the specific cause is a subject of great importance. Where the disease is founded upon sexual derangements, a cure is impossible until these derangements are cured; if they are incurable, hysteria itself will likewise remain an incurable malady. Where we have to suspect abuse of the sexual organs, we shall find ourselves in a very ticklish situation, more particularly if our patient is unmarried, in which case a frank and full confession is very much impeded by the sensitiveness of the patient, which outweighs all other considerations of recovery. In such cases a cure, unless the exciting cause can be removed, is likewise not to be thought of. Sometimes, however, we are able to attain, by a circuitous route, the end that would forever be beyond our reach, if we sought to attain it by a direct road. If hysteria depends upon chlorosis, a successful treatment may be more readily expected than otherwise; only we must not forget that chlorosis likewise may be occasioned by some of the above-mentioned hidden causes, in which case it can likewise be removed, but with more difficulty.

Medicinally the disease can be treated with a large number of medicines, of which it would be impossible to furnish a complete list, so much more as their action has not been confirmed by experience. This chapter is so fully treated by Hartmann, that with the exception of trivial changes, we here transcribe his remarks contained in the second volume of his Treatise on Therapeutics, page 500, etc.

Nux moschata responds to hysteric spasms with great debility. It is particularly suitable for females who show a fitfulness of mood, characterized by a rapid transition from extreme sadness to excessive cheerfulness. It is indicated where, previous to the paroxysm, the least labor is followed by lassitude and a sensation as if syncope would set in. It may likewise be found suitable where the disease succeeds fever and ague or typhus accompanied by spinal irritation; likewise in cases depending upon derangements of the sexual sphere, where the menses appear too late or are too scanty, where they are preceded by pain in the small of the back as if a stick lying transversely across the back would be pressed out, together with headache, lassitude, cardialgia with waterbrash, pain in the liver; where the menstrual blood is thicker and darker than usual, whereas, at the time when the catamenia ought to have appeared, leucorrhœa took their place.

Valeriana deserves our serious attention in hysteric paroxysms where the nerves are morbidly excited, with sensation of lassitude and extreme susceptibility of all the senses. This drug has not like the former medicine, a fitful mood, but the disposition is rather of a fearful and desponding cast. Though the symptom of an ascending ball is not found in the pathogenesis of this drug, yet another symptom of equal importance, namely the sensation of warmth suddenly ascending from the epigastrium, with oppression of breathing, takes the place of the hysteric ball. The symptom is attended with nausea as if the patient would vomit, which arises in the umbilical region and ascends to the pharynx, attended with a sensation as if a thread were hanging from the pharynx down the œsophagus, with a good deal of ptyalism and vomiting.

Concerning **Viola odorata**, which some have vaunted as a remedy for hysterical paroxysms, not much can be said. The recommendation of this agent seems to be based upon the peculiar idiosyncrasy of hysteric patients according to which offensive odors are pleasant to their nostrils, and who find the delicious odor of violets less agreeable than the pungent smell of burnt feathers. The disposition to weep without knowing why, the excessive susceptibility to emotional excitement, the continued affection of the chest, the painful dyspnœa, the difficult and painful inspirations and expirations attended with an apprehensive anxiety and mingled with violent palpitation of the heart, may perhaps be suitable indications for the use of Viola.

Secale cornutum, which has already been mentioned in other spasmodic affections, is so much more specifically suitable to hysteria as this disorder is very generally dependent upon disturbances in the female sexual system. At any rate it occupies the first rank against such paroxysms of hysteria as occur during the act of parturition or during confinement. The phenomena of the emotive sphere and of the general sensorium deserve special attention in selecting this drug.

Aurum is one of the few remedies which, beside acting with a penetrating energy, exerts an extraordinary influence over the mind and spirit, almost always in the same direction. Religious melancholy, grief at one's fate which one had caused by one's own indiscretions, great anxiety and apprehension proceeding from the heart, shyness and dread of men, are so significant as therapeutic indications that they alone justify the selection of gold in hysteria as a remedial agent. At all events Aurum. is rather a remedy for hysteria generally as for certain separate local symptoms or paroxysms.

Pulsatilla should be so well known to everybody that it ought only to be necessary here to mention it merely by name. Its prominent relation to the sexual organs, more particularly to the menstrual functions and to mental operations, stamp it indisputably as a remedy for hysteria; the local symptoms are, moreover, of such a nature that their paroxysmal character points to the selection of this drug, especially where the stomach, heart or uterus are prominently affected.

Moschus has from time immemorial been employed in nervous and more especially in hysteric conditions, very frequently with remarkable success. The following symptoms are characteristic indications for its choice: hysteric patients frequently complain of painfulness in the whole body without defining more particularly the locality of the pain; when asked where they suffer pain, they feel it more keenly; with tears in their eyes they complain of weariness all over, with a feeling of malaise as if they would faint; spasmodic paroxysms which resemble hysteric paroxysms, are relieved by Moschus, such as: sudden rush of blood to the head, with staring eyes and spasm in the mouth, followed by a hurried and confused talking, and by death-like paleness with excessive sweat over the whole head; or else sudden staring eyes with pallor of the face, heaviness of the head, pressure in the nape of the neck, coldness of the body, nausea, afterwards obscuration of sight, contraction of the pupils, loss of equilibrium, with rigidity and extension of the hand; sudden vanishing of the senses with slight pressure on the vertex, anxiety, palpitation of the heart, stupefying headache, or as if a nail had been stuck into the head; oppression at the stomach and pit of the stomach, with anxiety proceeding from this region; violent sexual excitement, with intolerable titillation; choking constriction of the larynx. These and many other symptoms assign to this drug a high rank among anti-hysteric agents.

Conium maculatum is often suitable in the hysteric paroxysms of unmarried females whose trouble emanates directly from the sexual sphere. They complain of violent itching of the genitals and in the interior of the sexual organs, with pain as if the uterus were being pressed down, stitches in the vagina; the menses are either suppressed or, if they make their appearance, they are too scanty; the patients are troubled with a smarting, excoriating leucorrhœa, attended with a frequently recurring contracting pain in the abdomen like labor-pains. A characteristic indication for this drug is a feeling of pressure in the pharynx ascending from the pit of the stomach, as if a round ball were ascending from this region. The patient is of a gloomy and melancholy turn of mind; she is dissatisfied with herself and with everything around her. The paroxysms consist of a disposition to weep when alone, scintillations, indistinct vision, lassitude in all the limbs, with a dull headache, or the patients complain of weariness and chilliness, obliging them to lie down, with headache and violent palpitation of the heart, and a pain at every pulsation as if a knife were thrust through the occiput, the beats of the heart being at times strong, at others rapid, and then again unsteady and wavering.

Cocculus has often rendered good service when the patients complained, among other distresses, of frequently recurring singultus, a choking contraction in the pharynx with oppression of breathing and an irritation inducing cough; the menses are delayed and finally set in with cramps, anxiety, oppression on the chest, cramps in the chest, attacks of nausea even unto fainting, and twitching of the extremities.

Natrum muriaticum. "I have often been tempted to believe that many hysteric patients possess the power to obtain a sort of internal perception of their distress, and, by means of this state of clairvoyance and divination, prescribe for themselves such medicines as may lead to their recovery. It is true they do not possess a clear consciousness of their actions, but they are impelled by a sort of intuition to add a little more salt to the food which they usually relish without it: to use quantities of vinegar, to devour greedily chalk or lime. The same thing is true with the so-called idiosyncrasies of hysteric females which gives them such a strong desire for Asafœtida, Musk and other drugs having a strong and, to normal organs of smell, disagreeable odor. Whether these views are merely hypothetical, it is a curious fact that it is precisely these abnormal desires which furnish us the most indubitable indications of the most certain remedy in the case before us. At any rate, I have seemed to make this observation more especially with regard to Natrum muriaticum, and I have found the choice of this remedy confirmed by contrasting its pathogenetic symptoms with those of hysteria. However, I do not wish to be misunderstood as though I meant to recommend the use of salt only in cases where the abuse of this agent by the patients led me to suggest it. Not at all; this empirical use of salt would constitute a slim basis upon which its recommendation as a remedy for hysteria could stand, and which might plunge us into a maze of deceptions. Salt is recommended by its own internal wealth of symptoms, the complex of which responds most fully to the diversified shades of hysteria." So far we transcribe Hartmann's views, which are undoubtedly hypothetical; but, on the other hand, may stimulate us to devote more serious attention to the management of hysterical idiosyncrasies. Natrum muriaticum does not, like Gold, directly affect the mind and spirit, but involves these spheres in so much more intense sympathetic suffering with other organs whose functions are deranged. Its main effect upon the brain and nervous system is depressing, without, however, any further signs of irritation; at any rate, if any are present, they are insignificant and evanescent. The whole series of its symptoms would seem to indicate salt in hypochondria rather than in hysteria; but both affections resemble each other so closely that the same remedies are applicable to both. Special indications are: Frequent recurrence of the nervous paroxysms during the day and vanishing of the same as soon as sweat breaks out; deathlike paleness or a yellowish-gray color of the face, and general debility; a drawing sensation from the left shoulder towards the head, with pressing in the temples as though the head would burst, with pain in the brain as if sore and bruised; continued nausea as if vomiting would take place; desire to lie down, and chilliness with heat in the face; frequent paroxysms of syncope; feeling in various parts of the body as if they had gone to sleep; vivid, fantastical dreams during a light sleep; desponding and melancholy mood; whining melancholy, want of firmness, wavering disposition; absence of mind; clavus in the left side of the brain, delaying and more and more decreasing catamenia.

Asafœtida is particularly adapted to hysteric paroxysms where the hysteric ball is very sharply defined, with the following symptoms: She complains of pressure in the œsophagus, with constriction of the throat as if a foreign body were rising in the throat which obliges her to swallow quite frequently; this pressure mostly emanates from the stomach up the œsophagus, with sensation as if a foreign body were ascending; nausea and feeling of fulness in the pit of the stomach; compressive sensation in the abdomen.

Sepia is one of the most important remedies not only for females generally, but in hysteria in particular. It is particularly suitable for weakly subjects with a fine, sensitive, delicate skin; there is no appearance of weakness externally, since the rotundity of the patient's form is rather beyond the normal size, and the color of the face, aside from a frequent and rapid change, is rather bright-red than pale, with a yellowish-dark circle around the eyes; there is great disposition to excited feelings. More specially characteristic are the phenomena which Sepia causes in the sphere of the emotions: there is constant sadness and depression of spirits; the mood never changes; there is great disposition to start; trifling causes induce vehement ebullitions of temper; dread of company. These ailments are ameliorated when pleasant impressions act upon the patient. In addition to this, Sepia has striking relations to the female organs of generation, for further details concerning which we refer to the Materia Medica. Specially adapted is Sepia to hysteric paralytic conditions of short duration and frequently shifting from one place to another. Beside these more general indications, Sepia has likewise phenomena in most organs, which recommend it for local hysteric affections; it will be found so much more suitable the more the disorder is centred in the digestive organs.

Magnesia muriatica is, according to Hartmann, very nearly related to the female organs and to the abdominal viscera. More particular indications are: Disposition to take cold, frequently recurring pain, as if bruised, through the whole body; general feeling of illness, fainting fits at dinner, with anxious feeling, nausea, pallor of the countenance, green and red light before the eyes, trembling of the whole body, with subsequent eructations which afford relief; spasms proceeding from the uterus; pains in the small of the back, and leucorrhœa, both of which symptoms grow worse in proportion as the catamenia delay more and diminish in quantity, moreover they break out periodically and the cramp-pains spread over the whole abdomen and down the lower extremities.

Beside the above-mentioned remedies, Hartmann mentions *Calcarea carbonica* and *Nitri acidum*, with which he professes to have obtained brilliant results, with the former especially if the convulsions bear such a great resemblance to epilepsy that it was difficult to diagnose between them.

In addition to these leading remedies for hysteria in general, there are many other medicines which had better be mentioned as referring to local symptoms without any further special indications.

For hysteric affections of the head: *Valeriana* for a stitching or pressive pain in the forehead and orbits, alternating with a condition of sopor; *Belladonna* for a periodical nervous headache; *Mercurius* for a nightly, stitching, boring or tearing headache; *Hepar* and *China* for a nocturnal headache; for hemicrania more particularly *Nux vomica*, *Sepia*, *Colocynthis*, *Verbascum;* for clavus hystericus: *Coffea*, *Ignatia*, *Platina*, *Bryonia*, *Veratrum album*, (when the head is cold,) *Aconite* and *Belladonna* when the pain increases to a maddening degree of intensity; for the sleeplessness which is frequently an attendant on headache, *China*, *Silicea*, *Hepar*, *Coffea;* for the opposite sopor: *Opium*, *Tartarus emeticus*, *Hyoscyamus*.

Of the hysteric derangements of the psychical sphere, we mention the most important: nymphomania. The main remedies for this disease are: *Platina*, *Phosphorus*, *Belladonna* (when occuring during confinement), *Veratrum* and *Cantharides*.

Hysteric spinal irritation does not, properly speaking, exist separately, and it might therefore be very difficult to indicate remedies for this condition, for the reason that their selection would mostly depend upon the accessory phenomena co-existing with the spinal irritation.

Hysteric uterine affections almost always accompany or even cause the whole malady; for this reason all the remedies that have been mentioned for hysteria, are likewise applicable in this class of diseases. Also we recommend *Causticum* for delaying menses, with violent colicky pains as if the bowels were torn, with a tearing and bruising sensation in the small of the back and in the back, especially during motion, oppression and fulness in the abdomen with disposition to belch up wind, &c.; she has to loosen her clothes. *Phosphorus* when the menses are either retarded or entirely suppressed, with severe cutting colicky pains in the right side and toward the small of the back, pain in the back as if bruised, vomiting, palpitation of the heart, anxiety. *Stannum* for uterine spasms like a frequent pressing deep in the hypogastrium, aggravated by external pressure and accompanied by a constant yellowish and very debilitating leucorrhœa. In very rare cases only these spasms are isolated, on the contrary the adjoining organs are likewise suffering, even the stomach and diaphragm are involved in the distress which the patient always describes as emanating from the womb. The prevailing sensation is a crampy-tensive pain below and above the umbilicus, rather towards the small of the back, which is alleviated and dispersed by expanding the trunk, stretching the arms, and pressing the abdomen against a broad and firm object. *Stramonium* is suitable when the menstrual flow is excessive, attended with spasms, and more particularly when the flow is attended with hysteric derangements of the moral or mental sphere.

Where the phenomena are principally located in the uropoïétic range, *Sepia* is particularly suitable. Beside Sepia we have: *Belladonna, Zincum, Cantharides, Lycopodium.*

Asthma hystericum occurs rarely, scarcely ever separately, but generally as a symptom of the general paroxysm; the remedies for this form of asthma are: *Ignatia, Pulsatilla, Cuprum, Veratrum* and *Ipecacuanha.*

For the palpitation of the heart with anxiety, to which hysteric females are so frequently subject, without the accompaniment of material changes, *Aconite* is the best remedy, and in the case of debilitated and perhaps anæmic individuals: *China.*

[**Aconite** is more frequently required in the different forms of hysteria, than many physicians are willing to admit. It may perhaps afford a palliative relief only, but even this is of inestimable value to the patient. The hemicrania, clavus, the various constrictive spasms, the sensation as if a current of air or a ball were ascending in the throat or from the uterus, the various illusions of sight, hearing and smell with which hysteric women are afflicted, the oppression of breathing, and the extraordinary depression of spirits, the fitfulness of mood, the forebodings of evil and a variety of pains which characterize hysteria, are very frequently relieved with a few doses of Aconite more promptly and permanently than by means of any other drug.

Cimicifuga racemosa or the black cohosh will prove an excellent remedy in hysteria depending upon menstrual suppression; it may be necessary to prescribe the medicine in tolerably large doses. H.]

The selection of the right remedy being so very difficult in hysteria, it behooves us to direct our attention at a very early period of the disease to other accessory remedial means. A chief rank among these extra-medicinal means is occupied by
treatment of the patient, which should never be neglected, since hysteria can be numbered among the diseases of the mind with the same propriety as among the material or bodily diseases. Although it is necessary, on the one hand, not to contradict hysteric women, yet, on the other hand, it is sometimes indispensable to show them

firmness and determination. The physician has to try with a good deal of caution which course of conduct is best adapted to the case. If it is a difficult task for a physician to regulate his conduct toward a patient, it is still more difficult for him to obtain the proper influence over the mind and temper of the patients and to win their confidence as well as their conscientious willingness to follow the instructions of their physician with scrupulous punctuality. The want of confidence is the cliff on which all attempts to cure the distress, strand but too often. Hysteric women scarcely ever possess the faculty of determined volition; if they once have been brought to will a thing firmly, the cure is half accomplished. For this purpose we have to resort to various accessory means of treatment, cold water, for instance, in order to counteract the disposition of such patients to indulge in effeminate habits and modes of living. It is not always possible to order a rigid cold-water treatment, although it might be the very best thing for this class of patients; we may have to content ourselves with systematic cold ablutions of the trunk or the whole body. Even these effect a rapid and decided change. In other cases a sojourn in a mountainous region, with a good deal of active exercise, affords striking advantages, or sea-bathing may be resorted to with equal success. Patients who have been in the habit of indulging in all kinds of luxuries, should be sent to springs where simplicity and frugality have not yet been superseded by the pernicious habits of a luxurious civilization. The occupation of the patient should likewise be regulated with a great deal of care. Hysteric women generally prefer a kind of work that leaves to their fancy full swing, a purely mechanical or rather automatic occupation, such as sewing, knitting, crocheting, &c. In such cases we must insist upon such labor being performed by them as will tax their bodily strength in an unusual although not fatiguing manner. It is likewise well to select suitable reading matter for them, and to discard novels and the like from their presence.

Our remarks concerning the etiological causes of hysteria lead us to infer that there must be a prophylactic treatment of this disease, which is of particular importance, and indeed more easy of execution in cases where the physician, in his capacity of medical adviser of a family, has an opportunity of watching the development of the young girls entrusted to his professional care. For more detailed remarks bearing upon this point we refer to what we have said in our chapter on chorea. Where the proper equilibrium between mind and body is kept up, hysteria need not be apprehended; unfortunately only a small number of our young ladies enjoy this salutary advantage. The antagonism between the demands of a teacher and those of a rational system of development, is often very great. Is this the fault of the teacher, or rather that of the physician?

8. Hypochondria. Hypochondriasis, Spleen.

If hysteria is to be considered a mental rather than a bodily disease, this is much more the case in regard to hypochondria, where all signs of material changes are decidedly wanting; but inasmuch as it frequently exists as a complication of other affections, this has seemed the most suitable place to treat of this disease.

By hypochondria we understand a morbid alteration of the mental condition, in consequence of which the patient only cares for, and is only busy with himself, overruled by a peculiar feeling of illness of a high and remarkably striking degree of intensity, without any, or at least without any corresponding objectively perceptible abnormal alterations of functions. Hence hypochondria may be designated as a morbidly developed egotism.

Hypochondria is almost exclusively an affection of male adults, which is scarcely ever noticed before the age of eighteen or twenty years. It is either an idiopathic disease, in which case it is designated as hypochondria sine materia, or else it exists as a complication of other abnormal conditions of the organism: hypochondria cum materia. Its etiology is rather obscure, because we are unable to account for the fact that the same etiological influence which, in one, causes hypochondria, has not the effect in others even under otherwise similar circumstances. In some cases there may prevail an hereditary disposition, in other cases there is no sign of it. The following causes have been established with tolerable certainty: Depressing moral and mental impressions; continued, one-sided and exciting mental occupations; homesickness; grief and care; hazardous speculations; in general, all kinds of influences which keep up a continual irritation of the nervous system and, as a consequence, depress its energy. Of somatic influences the most important are: Sedentary mode of life, sexual excesses, self-abuse, gastric derangements, abnormal conditions of the sexual organs, especially syphilis and disorganizations of the testes. Diseases of this kind lead to the diligent study of medicinal works; though in many cases this mania may already constitute a symptom of a fully developed hypochondria, in other cases, on the contrary, it is the main cause of this abnormal condition of the mind. Besides these causes hypochondria, like hysteria, is frequently the result of intense and exhausting general diseases of the organism. There are, however, hypochondriacs who lead a very active life in the open air, and whose disorder cannot be traced to any of the above-mentioned causes. Comparing all the circumstances that bear upon this disease, it seems proper to regard the sexual system as its most probable starting-point. If the disease cannot always be traced to this cause, it may be owing to the imperfect reports of the patients, or to their intentional omissions and deceptions.

Symptoms. Inasmuch as it would be very difficult to draw a complete picture of hypochondria, the Protean forms of which would require a multitude of different delineations, we prefer adopting Hartmann's method, who divides the symptoms of hypochondria in three groups, those of the mind, those of the digestive apparatus, and those that involve the nervous system generally.

The psychical symptoms are the following: Ill-humor, especially during the period of digestion; depression of spirits, sadness, discouragement, intense and almost exclusive preoccupation, with morbid sensations, which are interpreted by the patients as some dangerous disease which day after day assumes a new form; extravagant and self-satisfying description of their own sufferings, delight in reading medicinal writings, and inexhaustible acuteness in hunting up reports of cases that are very much like their own; an exceedingly egotistical contemplation of everything concerning themselves; tyrannical demand that those who are with the patient should sympathize with his distress, unusual irritability of temper, melancholy, distrust, taciturn mood, dread of death, darkness of his prospects; although he suffers, yet he is not averse to living; lastly, inability to do any work, even to live, from sheer distrust in his own strength, and from dread of personal injury These constitute the most essential phenomena in the moral sphere of the hypochondriac. Sometimes the mental dejection is relieved by lucid intervals of cheerfulness, even of an unusual flow of good spirits, but only for a short time. The phases of the moon seem to exert a decided influence upon the hypochondriac; his condition is decidedly worse during an increasing moon. Sometimes these moral symptoms constitute the whole of the disease, or the disease remains stationary at this degree sometimes for years. In spite of this mental trouble, the desire to work at first does not suffer; it is only after the disease has reached a higher degree of intensity that the patients become more and more indolent, unwilling to work, and apathetic towards their nearest friends. It is a peculiar characteristic of hypochondria, that such patients scarcely ever lose the hope of getting well again, and that this hope impels them to try the most absurd means of treatment.

The symptoms of the digestive range do not necessarily accompany a case of hypochondria, but they are scarcely ever wanting. In spite of a good and generally regular appetite and healthy appearance, these patients indulge in constant lamentations about bad digestion. After, and sometimes even while eating, they feel a tightness and pressure in the abdomen which is sometimes really distended. They are disposed to regard this continual development of gas as the sole foundation of their trouble and its inherent inconveniences. Sometimes there is a perceptible bloat under the short ribs and in the epigastric region, sensation of incarcerated flatulence which causes oppression and anxiety, palpitation of the heart, a mounting of heat to the head, loathing, heart-burn, sour eructations, even vomiting of tenacious and sour phlegm are present, but much less frequently. The distress caused by the flatulence may increase so as to cause serious nervous paroxysms, vertigo, syncope, coldness of the extremities, etc. In spite of all these ailments, the appetite of the patients remains good for a time at least, showing that their digestive functions are not as bad as they would have us believe, although they examine every evacuation with the greatest care, and know of no greater delight than a copious stool. Gradually, however, these at first subjective symptoms change to really objective perceptible derangements of the digestive functions. There would be too much hypothetical boldness in trying to account for this circumstance by the fact, that the patient's thoughts are continually directed to these functions; the supposition that the peculiar anxiety and care about himself which torment the hypochondriac, finally have the same effect upon him as any other long-lasting mental disharmony has upon every organism, is undoubtedly more correct. A distressed and cachectic appearance becomes more and more prominent, and the assimilative functions are evidently impaired. These phenomena are in a measure owing to the patient's improper mode of living, more particularly as regards eating and drinking, and likewise to the enormous quantity and variety of the drugs which these patients, who cannot bear to do without medicine, swallow. The mass of cathartics which they take either to remove or ward off constipation, that is dreaded more by them than anything else, probably constitutes the chief cause of the disturbances in the digestive organs and of the irregular evacuations with which such patients are afflicted; every homœopathic physician knows that cathartics promote rather than prevent constipation, and that it is extremely difficult to induce such patients to relinquish their use.

The symptoms of nervous derangement are varied; part of them have already been mentioned in the preceding paragraph; otherwise every part of the body, every function, may be affected sympathetically, on which account the symptoms assume such multitudinous forms that only the main features of abnormal innervation can be recorded in this place. A sensation of coldness or heat or paroxysmal alternations of both, as in fever; itching here and there, formication, asthma, cough, palpitation of the heart, beating in various parts of the body, especially in the abdomen; hemicrania, vertigo, buzzing in the ears, muscæ volitantes, amblyopia, neuralgia, spasm of the bladder, frequent urging to urinate, congestions, increased secretion of saliva or of the tears, copious sweats, tremor of the limbs, convulsive motions, paralytic symptoms, etc.; these are a few of the symptoms that may present themselves combined and complicated in all sorts of ways. Sensibility is altered in a very peculiar manner, and so morbidly intensified that the least change in external influences, such as alterations of the temperature, atmospheric pressure, electrical tension, trifling deviations from their habitual diet, affects such patients very unpleasantly. They complain of headache; are without sleep, or their sleep is restless and disturbed by heavy dreams; they easily start up from their sleep; do not feel refreshed in the morning, on the contrary, they feel brighter in the evening than in the morning on rising. Like the hysteric patient, the hypochondriac discharges quantities of a watery, clear urine; sometimes, however, it is thick, cloudy, turbid, and causes a good deal of anxiety and care to the patient, who watches all these symptoms with a great deal of solicitude.

As has already been stated, these local symptoms appear in a variety of combinations; but they have the peculiarity of being susceptible of rapid changes and not developing any objective phenomena, although, if the patient were to be believed, such phenomena ought certainly to exist.

Hypochondria always runs a chronic course, no matter how it may have originated. If circumstances favor its development, it may last the whole year; but, as a general rule, it does not occur beyond the age of sixty years. During the course of the disease periods of remission of the symptoms occur; they may even cease entirely. This, however, would not justify the expectation that the disease is cured, for relapses are not by any means unfrequent.

The prognosis is relatively favorable; only in rare cases, and when the disease reaches a high degree of intensity, it becomes dangerous to life. It is unfavorable when the disease is of long duration, and, by its capricious behavior and by the frequent change of its symptoms, causes the physician, as well as the patient, a great deal of trouble and anxiety. It is always difficult to enforce the promise of a favorable turn, for the reason that the patient who to-day had the greatest confidence in his physician, may lose it entirely over night. On this account the prognosis, in the case of fickle patients, is always more doubtful. But where the patient obeys the instructions of his physician with confidence, where there is a possibility of changing the patient's mode of life and removing bad habits, the prospect of a successful termination may be very flattering. The more the assimilative functions have become impaired, the less favorable are the prospects of a cure; this is likewise the case where sexual excesses or onanism are persisted in.

Treatment. Hypochondria belongs to that class of diseases whose character it is very difficult to delineate with perfect accuracy. For this reason the physician should not neglect a single means of obtaining as complete a picture of the disease as possible, and likewise of investigating the exciting causes. The patient would soon know whether the physician proceeds carelessly in making his examination, and would become distrustful if the physician would undertake to console the patient by representing to him the dark and complicated group of his symptoms as nervous and hypochondriac ailments. I consider it as a master-piece of art if a young practitioner knows how to examine a hypochondriac who generally moves in the higher walks of life, in such a manner as to win his confidence and to extort from him a smile of satisfaction by the adroit manner in which satisfactory answers are elicited to the physician's questions. The hypochondriac is distrustful, the reading of medicinal works has given him an overweening confidence in his knowledge, if not of medicine generally but of his own condition; and his questions are often so cunningly devised that it requires a good deal of skill on the part of the physician to answer them with à propos and thus to dissipate his patient's suspicions

If he has succeeded in this, not merely for the time being, but for the patient's permanent good, by a truthful and correct comprehension of the disease, the treatment, were it ever so difficult, will certainly be correspondingly successful, for the patient will adhere to it even if his improvement is but slow. (Hartmann.)

It is evident, from the constant changes which take place in the phenomena of this disease, that it is impossible to fix even approximatively upon a positive treatment of hypochondria in accordance with the principles of Homœopathy. This is much less possible with hypochondria than with hysteria, where local derangements are very often present, which is not the case in the former disease. Hence we can only furnish a very general survey of the remedies for hypochondria, and refer to the Materia Medica for all special cases.

Nux vomica holds the first rank among the anti-hypochondriac remedies. It corresponds most completely to all the symptoms of the digestive apparatus, to their appearance after a meal, to the disposition to gaseous flatulence and to constipation. Other circumstances which are of great moment in hypochondria, lead to the choice of this remedy. The circumstances are: the origin of hypochondria from sedentary habit, deficient exercise with rich living and excessive mental exertions; use of stimulants in order to keep awake at night; moreover the excitability of the temper which induces an ebullition of anger from the least provocation; continual cloudiness of the head, with more or less prominent signs of cerebral congestion, more particularly in the case of patients who are fond of wine and good eating. As a general rule Nux is more adapted to material hypochondria proceeding from derangements of the abdominal organs, much less to digestive derangements which are consequences of hypochondria.

Sulphur is almost equally valuable as the former remedy, with this difference that the kind of hypochondria to which Sulphur is adapted, differs somewhat from that of Nux. It is the immaterial forms of hypochondria, exerting a considerable influence upon the process of assimilation, to which Sulphur corresponds, and the symptoms of which are found with remarkable completeness in the pathogenesis of Sulphur. It is likewise suitable in cases where Nux vomica is suitable, more particularly if luxurious living has given rise to hæmorrhoids, the bowels are very torpid and the functions of the liver are manifestly deranged. Finally it is the main remedy where the improper treatment of syphilis has given rise to hypochondria.

Hypochondria.

Staphysagria has a variety of applications. It is a leading remedy where hypochondria has been caused by onanism, or by syphilis and the abuse of Mercury. It is likewise very efficacious where the disease is caused by long-continued, depressing emotions, more especially long-gnawing grief and chagrin. The symptomatic indications, especially in the digestive range, correspond very fully to hypochondria, above all we have great inconvenience from flatulence. Staphysagria may be distinguished from Nux by differences of complexion, that of Staphysagria being pale, of a yellowish-gray and dingy color, whereas a bright complexion is more characteristic of Nux.

Natrum muriaticum is not even mentioned by Hartmann, yet it is indispensable in the treatment of hypochondria. If Hartmann has found salt so useful in hysteria and was reminded of it by the circumstance that hysteric women are often so extravagantly fond of salt food, we have a right to be amazed that he should not have made mention of this agent from similar reasons in hypochondria. Certain hypochondriacs are exceedingly fond of salt, and, in spite of every effort to the contrary on the part of their physician, they persist in the excessive indulgence of this condiment. They are more particularly such patients as lead a sedentary life and perform a good deal of mental labor, and whose digestion is very weak. Persistent and careful inquiries will satisfy any one that the mania of eating salt is much more universal and deep-rooted than one imagines and that, in such cases, it is kept up by an instinctive desire as well as by the power of habit. A comparison of the symptoms of salt with the symptoms of a more fully developed hypochondria will satisfy us, that the two series are very similar to each other, more particularly when the digestion is very much disturbed, the patient has a distressed and yellowish-gray appearance, and symptoms of debility begin to manifest themselves. Hypochondria remaining after slow and exhausting diseases, especially after fever and ague and typhus, likewise corresponds to the pathogenetic series of salt; in such cases the symptoms seem to indicate *China* with which Natrum muriaticum is in very close affinity.

Conium maculatum is likewise a powerful remedy for hypochondria, more particularly when it seems to proceed from sexual derangements without any excesses having been committed. The patients complain of great weakness of the sexual organs, with an unusual irritability of these parts, they are subject to frequent and exhausting emissions and most generally complain of the discharge of prostatic fluid at stool. Such patients are generally those who in spite of excessive sexual excitement, maintain the strictest abstemiousness on account of their virtuous and unyielding principles. Such individuals sink more readily than other hypochondriacs into a state of melancholy, aversion to labor, loathing of life and idiotic weakness of mind. In most cases we have a derangement of the urinary secretions, and a fixed pain in the lumbar portion of the spinal cord, especially after long-continued exercise.

Phosphorus is likewise a noteworthy remedy in hypochondria, if the disease originates in the sexual sphere, with this difference, that whereas the Conium-hypochondria is caused by extreme abstemiousness, *Phosphorus* corresponds to the hypochondria originating in sexual abuse, more particularly onanism. The symptoms in both forms of hypochondria are pretty much the same, except that in the case of Phosphorus the painfulness of the spinal marrow is much more intense.

Beside Conium and Phosphorus, which corresponds more specifically to hypochondria, whose exciting cause resides in the sexual range, a great many other remedies having a particular affinity to the sexual organs, may likewise be found useful in hypochondria, more especially the following, which are distinguished by their affinity to the emotive sphere: *Agnus castus, Anacardium, Aurum*, and likewise *Clematis*. The last two remedies deserve particular consideration where disorganization or simple swelling of the testes is present, disorders which often give rise to the most obstinate and intense forms of mental derangement, even a disposition to suicide, which symptom is particularly peculiar to Gold, (Aurum.)

Stannum is recommended by Hartmann with so much urgency, that we cannot forbear transcribing his remarks literally. Stannum frequently has a marvellous effect in various spasmodic hypochondriac ailments, which mostly originate in the ganglionic system. By walking about the patient is greatly relieved, whereas his distress returns again in a state of rest, which he would like very much to indulge in, owing to his feeling continually weak and weary, both mentally and physically; this makes him sad and melancholy, and he often feels so discouraged that he could almost weep. If with these symptoms are associated a stupefying, pressing distress in the brain, as if the skull were in a vice, or other abnormal sensations in the brain, illusions of hearing, distress in the stomach, with regular appetite, feeling of emptiness in the abdomen, constipation, exhausting night-sweats, etc., the patient feels in the highest degree miserable, and by exaggerating his ailments, renders life disagreeable to

Hypochondria. 215

those around him. It is to this kind of hypochondria that Stannum will be found to correspond, and where it will always be found effective.

Besides these remedies which are always to be considered first, we direct the attention of the reader to the following: *Zincum, Veratrum album, Calcarea carbonica, China, Pulsatilla, Gratiola, Acidum phosphoricum* and *nitricum*.

More important and effective than all medicines, is the dietetic and psychical treatment of hypochondria. This may be inferred even from the intermediate position which this affection holds between mental and material diseases, sometimes partaking rather of the character of the former, at other times of that of the latter. But even in cases where hypochondria depends upon perceptible material derangements, we cannot help recognizing the existence of some important mental disturbance; otherwise the same material derangement would have to cause hypochondria under any other similar circumstances, which is not the case. Besides these a priori arguments, experience shows that an appropriate psychical treatment of hypochondria is absolutely necessary to the restoration of health. We have already alluded to the influence which the manners and personal appearance of the physician exert over the hypochondriac patient; in this respect the physician cannot be too cautious if he means to preserve his patient's confidence. It is, moreover, important to turn the attention of the patient away from himself, which is sometimes very difficult. It is almost next to impossible to prevail upon the patient to discontinue the reading of medicinal works, and his everlasting conversations with everybody about his ailments. Both these points are of importance. Besides these precautions we should see to it, that our patients indulge as little as possible in a state of rest, and spend their leisure hours in studies that are rather outside of the usual range of their regular avocations, and engage their attention in a more serious manner. All one-sided and monotonous mental labor is decidedly unfavorable to the hypochondriac; a variety of occupations is indispensable to his recovery. On this account we have likewise to regulate the pleasures and recreations of our patient, and vary even these, lest habit should transform into a labor what was designed to be a recreation. In this respect nothing has a better effect than intercourse with individuals of cheerful and lively minds; only they must understand that it is not only not advantageous, but decidedly hurtful to the patients, if we deride their apparent, as well as their real imaginings, by unkind jeers and jests. This deprives the physician, as well as the patient's friend, of all moral influence. The degree of cultivation of the patient is, of course, to be considered in our treatment of his complaint. It is much easier to get along with individuals of less education, than with those who enjoy a high degree of mental refinement. With regard to their morbid sensations, the judgment of the latter is indeed clouded, but in every other respect they remain possessed of their usual acumen; they perceive inconsistencies in the treatment with quick readiness, and every discovery of this kind diminishes their confidence. From these general reasonings we can readily draw inferences regarding the management of particular cases; at all events it would be impossible to meet the requirements of every special case by detailed indications; there are too many ways which lead to the attainment of the main object, namely: to lead the patient's attention away from himself by exciting an interest in external objects.

The dietetic treatment of hypochondria is undoubtedly much less important and efficient than the enforcement of moral rules; for many an hypochondriac who follows with the most minute regularity the dietetic regimen prescribed by the physician, yet remains an hypochondriac. It seems therefore to be proper, that not too high a value should be attached to the mode of living; dietetic rules, if enforced with too much strictness, have a tendency to perpetually remind the patient of his ailments, the very point that is to be avoided; habits prejudicial to health, or irregularities in the mode of living which are evidently hurtful, have, of course, to be discontinued. If the patient had been leading a sedentary life, and had indulged in continued mental efforts, he will have to be reasonably restrained in this regard, and more exercise in the open air will have to be recommended; where the disease seems to have been caused by too good living, a simple and regular diet has to be prescribed, etc. As a general rule, however, hypochondriacs apply for medical treatment when the disease has reached a degree of development, where the most rigorous diet has already been established as a rule, and we have to admit, that it is not by excessive eating or drinking that the hypochondria has been caused. The condition of the skin and the proper attendance to muscular development are, on the contrary, very essential, for these two points are very often neglected. With respect to the condition of the skin, cold water is a panacea, for two reasons: it has a beneficial effect upon the functions of the skin, and the use of cold water stimulates the will-power, which is of no slight importance. The development and expansion of the muscular power imply exercise, but it is not by any means indifferent what kind of exercise is indulged in. An hypochondriac patient, for instance, takes, day after day, his routine walk of miles in length, and yet his hypochondria does not leave him. Walking is certainly not the best kind of exercise, and will be found useful to a certain extent only, in cases where a sedentary mode of life had been pursued. Much better results are obtained by gymnastic exercises that give active play to the abdominal and dorsal muscles. For this purpose we recommend sawing and splitting wood, and occupations in the garden, the good effects of which nobody can deny. If this kind of exercise is not convenient, owing to the circumstances of the patient, gymnastic exercises, fencing, etc., will have to be resorted to. Fencing, particularly, has a beneficial influence over the whole frame, and can be indulged in without making any special arrangements as are required for gymnastic purposes. Journeys on foot in pleasant company are likewise very useful. Riding on horseback affords more active exercise and often suits the wishes of the patient a good deal better than any other bodily movement; driving in a carriage, on the contrary, is decidedly objectionable, since nothing favors preoccupation with one's self more than riding in a comfortable carriage.

One other point has to be mentioned, which sometimes embarrasses the treatment, especially if conducted in accordance with the principles of Homœopathy: this is the complaint of all hypochondriacs about constipation. The habit of taking something for constipation day after day; the opinion that a daily evacuation is of the utmost importance to the general well-being of the patient, give rise to so many queer and even absurd notions in the patient's mind, that an interdiction of the use of all cathartics seems to him like a sentence of death. Nevertheless, such an interdiction is indispensable, and the regulation of the alvine evacuations is sometimes a matter of the greatest difficulty. On this account, were it only to quiet the patient, it is necessary at the commencement of our treatment to order cold-water injections. In the long run, however, we succeed much better if we direct the patient to attempt an evacuation of the bowels every morning after breakfast, no matter whether he experiences a desire for it or not, and not to yield to it, if such a desire should be felt during the day. By this simple means I have removed many an habitual constipation radically, without any medicine, sometimes in a few weeks.

SECOND SECTION.

Diseases of the Head.

A. DISEASES OF THE SCALP.

INASMUCH as it seems more convenient to range most of the affections of this class among the cutaneous diseases, we will content ourselves with here mentioning only one disorder, namely,

Cephalæmatoma, Bloody Tumor of the Scalp.

By this term we designate an effusion of blood under the scalp, sometimes under the aponeurosis, and at other times under the pericranium. This disease is peculiar to new-born infants.

The causes of this tumor are undoubtedly referable to the circumstances under which the act of parturition took place; they are purely mechanical. It may be caused by the application of instruments, or by the pressure exerted upon the skull of the infant by a protracted labor, or by the narrowness of the parts, or a rigidity of the os, and occasioning a rupture of the vessels of the scalp. Such a rupture may result even during a comparatively easy labor, since even a moderate pressure may sometimes cause the laceration of one of the delicate vessels of the scalp. The tumor arises immediately after birth, but may commence so imperceptibly and may increase so slowly that it is seen only a few days after birth, and then gives rise to the opinion that it is not an immediate consequence of the act of parturition. It is generally located on one of the two parietal bones; its size varies, from one inch to three or four inches in diameter; its form is likewise uncertain. The color remains unchanged, fluctuation is distinctly perceptible. Pressure upon the tumor does not give rise to any particular symptoms; pressure with the finger does not leave a trace behind. The sutures of the skull bones form a boundary beyond which the tumor cannot expand, and hence its shape is very often determined by these sutures. The tumor may be raised above the skin to the height of an inch. The health of the child is not affected by the tumor, unless there should be special complications.

In the course of the tumor three changes may arise. The extravasated blood may be simply reabsorbed; this change takes place only if the children are very small, and is completed in a few weeks. Or, perhaps, in consequence of the supervention of a peculiar process of exudation, the tumor may become ossified. The formation of bone commences where the detached pericranium unites with the skull, hence in the circumference of the tumor; it feels like crackling paper, may extend through the whole extent of the tumor, and after resorption of the remaining fluid has taken place, the bone at the diseased spot is found slightly thickened. Or, finally, the extravasation may become surrounded by inflammation, and an abscess may form. It is only this last-mentioned change that can endanger the child's life.

Treatment. To Hartmann's remarks on this subject we add something of our own. Hartmann writes: "If we are sure of the presence of extravasated blood, we make an incision with a lancet at the point where the extravasation seems to be most copious, squeeze the contents out with great caution, insert a small plug of lint into the wound to prevent its healing too rapidly, cover the place with a compress of four thicknesses of linen moistened with a solution of two drops of Arnica in two ounces of water, and give internally a few pellets of *Arnica* 6. By pursuing this course the swelling generally disappears entirely in a few days."

A well-founded objection can be raised against this proceeding. Every bloody extravasation, no matter where it may be located, by the contact with atmospheric air has impressed upon it a tendency to form pus; hence it is not advisable to favor this tendency unless the non-opening of the tumor should be attended with particular danger. A bloody tumor of itself is almost without any danger; it suppurates only after it is opened or in consequence of violent compression; otherwise if left quietly alone, it is reabsorbed. Why should we, for the sake of obtaining a somewhat more rapid cure, allow ourselves to be led to perform an operation that is not without danger? It is much better to be patient for a few moments. And if, after all, we decide to open the tumor, the plug of lint can do no good, for the reason that it promotes the communication with the open air. In our opinion, as long as no suppuration has taken place, the opening of the tumor should be postponed.

A weak solution of Arnica tincture may be applied; this can do no harm. Any kind of compression is improper, both as regards the tumor and likewise the head of the child. If pus forms, we should not open the tumor prematurely, lest the suppuration should be unduly hastened, which is generally the case if the incision is made too soon. Under these circumstances *Mercurius* is the best remedy, and, after the suppuration has lasted for some time, *Silicea*.

Other medicines which may have been recommended for this trouble, need not be recorded in this place. The above-mentioned treatment is sufficient, and such a trifling extravasation is so easily absorbed that we may readily be deceived in mistaking it for medicinal action.

To open the tumor by making a much larger incision, seems to us an unjustifiable proceeding, and a trifling with the life of the child. Suppuration will always follow, and it is impossible to tell what the consequences may be.

B. DISEASES OF THE CEPHALIC NERVES.

1. Cephalalgia, Headache.

Headache is one of the most common accessory symptoms of febrile as well as non-febrile affections. Hence we might adduce a great many forms of headache arising from a variety of causes, without, however, helping the treatment in the least by such a multiplicity of causal distinctions. The headache will disappear as soon as the affection upon which it depends is cured. It is true that it is not always so very easy to find out the causes of headache; it is sometimes very violent when the general affection seems very slight, and seems, on that account, to be more or less an idiopathic condition of distress; but all attempts to point out a therapeutic proceeding for all such cases would be in vain; in such cases the selection of a drug is altogether difficult, and disappoints us very often. For even if we compare the statements of the patient concerning the quality, locality and peculiar character of the pain with ever so much care, the proper remedy is not found, for the reason that we have to shape our treatment in accordance with the subjective statements of the patient. Everybody knows how deceptive the language employed by different patients is, and that one calls pressure what another designates as tension or a feeling of weight. If the headache is simply an accompaniment of other complaints, it is of not so much importance what kind of a headache it is. On this account we have only to discuss one form of cephalalgia, namely,

Hemicrania or Megrim.

By this term we designate a kind of headache which occurs paroxysmally at more or less regular intervals, the paroxysms being of equal duration and intensity, and having the characteristic peculiarity that they only affect one side of the head.

There are various reasons to regard hemicrania as a purely neuralgic affection of the cerebral nerves. It is, indeed, true that it sometimes accompanies other ailments, but it occurs just as often as a separate disease, and cannot be accounted for by any anatomical lesion. It seems, moreover, that only the more delicate nerves of the meningeal membranes, not the nerves of the external integuments of the head, are the seat of this affection, even some twigs of the trigeminus being sometimes involved in the attack.

The causes of megrim vary a great deal. Where it occurs as a complication of other diseases, it may depend upon liver-complaint, gastric derangement, cardiac anomalies, but more particularly on a morbid condition of the sexual organs. As an idiopathic affection, it is only met with in constitutions to which, on account of a prevalence of nervous sensitiveness, we apply the term nervous. Hence it is more prominently met with among persons of the female sex. That it is not always and exclusively dependent upon abnormal sexual functions, is evident from the circumstance that it is sometimes met with even in children. As remote causes, we may regard the various influences which engender an excessive irritability of the nervous system, such as precocious mental development, excess of fancy, excessive mental labor, in short all those defects in the present mode of living of our young women, of which mention has already been made in our remarks on hysteria, of which megrim is very often a mere symptom. Losses of animal fluids and protracted diseases likewise often cause that species of nervousness of which hemicrania is a phenomenal manifestation.

In general the symptoms of hemicrania are very constant and uniform, and mostly vary only in their less essential points. In most cases without any precursory symptoms, much less frequently after a previous feeling of malaise, the patients wake in the morning with a violent and constantly increasing headache. The pain is sometimes described as throbbing, at times as tearing or boring, or as an ache, and is generally confined to a sharply circumscribed locality on one side of the head, usually the left. External pressure affords relief rather than it aggravates the distress. Every mental and physical effort is painful, whereas an agreeable excitement of the mind by conversation or some attractive occupation, affords relief as soon as the patient makes up her mind to give herself up to it. This, however, is a difficult task, on account of the general feeling of lassitude complained of by the patient. As the pain increases, the eyes become affected: they are very sensitive to the light, and there is a copious flow of tears. When the pain is at its height, the patient vomits up a watery phlegm after having experienced nausea for some time previous. It is characteristic of megrim that the pain is very often accompanied by a sensation of hunger, and the attack is sometimes shortened if the patient can make up her mind to eat a great deal. After the vomiting, the patients feel better and want to sleep, and after a sound sleep, they generally wake quite well, only somewhat weary. Such paroxysms sometimes recur in a few days already, sometimes not till months have elapsed; in the case of females they are apt to come on about the catamenial period. The general condition of the system is not always affected by the attacks; in the intervals between the attacks the patients may have the appearance of enjoying good health. Very rarely the pain lasts beyond twelve hours; if it lasts longer, it may continue for thirty-six hours.

The prognosis is not particularly favorable even if we succeed in removing the cause of the difficulty. The younger the patients the more we have a right to expect a complete cure. It always takes a good deal of time to achieve success; very frequently we have to content ourselves with diminishing the frequency and intensity of the paroxysms.

Treatment. It has to be shaped so as to meet various phases of the complaint; it has to be directed against the special attack, against the attack as a part of the general affection, and has likewise to act as a prophylactic against the influences which we are satisfied are the determining causes of the paroxysms.

The treatment of the actual paroxysm presents difficulties, in so far as the selection of the appropriate remedy is rendered doubtful on account of the homogeneous character of the symptoms; and it is, moreover, difficult, in view of the variable intensity of the attack, which it is impossible to determine a priori, to what degree the duration or intensity of the paroxysm had been modified by the medicine that had been taken. In addition to this, the physician is seldom called at the commencement of the attack, but in most cases only after it had reached its climax. Of the many remedies which have been recommended for this disease, we mention only a few more in detail, for the reason that we deem this part of the treatment as the least important.

Coffea. Hartmann begins a paragraph about the treatment of hemicrania, with a remonstrance against the use of coffee. We shall find that, as a general rule, all persons who are tormented with this affection, are passionate lovers of coffee, and in many cases the disease can be traced to this abuse as its cause. Since hemicrania affects more particularly individuals of irritable nerves, it is easily seen why they should be so devoted to coffee; it is a pleasant stimulant for relaxed nerves. This is the reason why we find it so difficult to restrain such patients from the use of coffee, although this deprivation is indispensable to a cure, which is sometimes achieved by it alone. This observation leads us to recommend *Coffea* as an important remedy for hemicrania in the case of persons who do not use coffee as an habitual beverage. They are sometimes marvellously relieved by a few teaspoonfuls of good coffee, so that coffee has become a domestic remedy for megrim. Medicinally it is used as a watery or spirituous extract of the fresh, pulverized bean. The headache which coffee causes, has peculiar features with which we are abundantly acquainted from personal experience. The head feels hot and heavy, in very rare cases the forehead is covered with a cool perspiration; there is weariness and great lassitude; the individual is unable to sleep, is tormented by an anxious restlessness and oppression, and experiences a feeling of uneasy and nervous exhaustion, which is exceedingly distressing. The headache is generally a throbbing pain, and accompanied by the sensation of a dull pressure in one temple. Nausea is generally present, sometimes attended with a feeling of emptiness in the stomach, but does not result in vomiting. Regarding the curative effects of Coffea cruda in hemicrania, when given in small doses for a period of time in succession, we have no observations to offer; so much more frequently we have observed a favorable and almost opium-like effect from a few doses of ordinary coffee in the cases of a number of persons.

Nux vomica. Irrespective of the different headache symptoms which this medicine develops, and which we request the reader to look up in the Materia Medica, a few other circumstances invest this agent with the character of a leading remedy in hemicrania. Among these circumstances we point out, in the first place, the antidotal relation of Nux vomica to coffee and other spirituous beverages; next the peculiarity that exercise and the open air are almost unbearable; and lastly, an extreme irritability of the senses. The selection of Nux is moreover determined by a choleric, sanguine temperament, continued mental exertion, together with want of exercise; disposition to congestions and constipation. It is a violent aching pain that is more particularly influenced by Nux as its curative remedy. Not unfrequently it will be found that the exhibition of Nux is followed by vomiting of a bilious fluid, which is to be regarded as a particularly favorable curative result. In our hands small and seldom repeated doses have never had any marked result. Nux vomica can likewise be administered for this affection when invested with the character of a constitutional morbid disposition, in which case the accessory symptoms have principally to determine its choice.

Ignatia amara is in close affinity with the former medicine in a great many respects. It is more particularly suitable for females with irritable nerves and disposition to convulsions, more particularly in the case of hysterical persons. For Ignatia likewise, a pressing aching pain is a prominent symptom, and, according to Hartmann, the remedy is especially indicated when the patients complain as if a nail were pressed into their brain from without inwards. Whereas a red and turgid face is more particularly adapted to Nux, Ignatia, on the contrary, has pallor of the countenance. A marked disposition to vomit is not characteristic of Ignatia.

Belladonna, in comparison with the previously-named remedies, will be but rarely found suitable in hemicrania; even the peculiar time of day when the headache first breaks out, is opposed to Belladonna. Violent congestions, even to the presence of delirium, have to be present in order to justify the use of Belladonna; moreover excessive irritability of the senses, more particularly of the eyes. The pain is throbbing and stitching, and seems to be excited by every single pulsation. Belladonna will be found more especially suitable in attacks of hemicrania lasting beyond the period of twelve hours.

According to our own frequently repeated observations, *Arsenicum* quiets nervous pains better than any other medicine. Its effect is rapid, and sometimes rivals a powerful dose of Opium. It is characteristic of Arsenic to exert this soothing influence only in the case of pains that become worse towards the approach of night, reach their climax about midnight, and are accompanied by an extraordinary degree of anxious restlessness. Hartmann furnishes the following more particular indications: The pain is throbbing and stupefying, either in the forehead, and more especially above the root of the nose, or above the left eye, and leaves almost always a weakness of the head, and a qualmishness in the pit of the stomach. The pain is, moreover, characterized by other accessory symptoms; for instance: it regularly breaks out after a meal, abates by applying cold water to the part, and is aggravated a great deal by removing the cold water; is most violent in the evening and at night, when it is diminished by walking about, by external warmth, and by pressing the head between the hands; not unfrequently, even if the pain is not very violent, it is attended with a general feeling of lassitude and prostration, obliging the patient to lie down.

Glonoin has been frequently recommended for hemicrania, but in spite of very frequent trials, we have never been able to derive any good from it in this disease.

We now come to the series of drugs which correspond to this affection in its essential or inherent integrality. The most important among them is

Sepia. We advise the reader to look up the headache symptoms of this drug in the Materia Medica; they are very characteristic of Sepia, and, in view of the practical results to which these symptomatic indications have led, they deserve the most careful attention. We are not disposed to indicate particular pains as decisive of the choice of Sepia. The accessory phenomena, which play an important part in the selection of the drug, are much more essential. Sepia is most suitable for the female organism, more particularly for females afflicted with liver-complaint and abdominal congestions. A pale, anæmic and cachectic complexion is no recommendation for our drug; on the contrary it is rather indicated by vivid redness, with variable complexion and a yellowish tint, especially under the eyes. Such individuals are exceedingly sensitive to mental impressions, whether pleasant or of a depressing character, and such impressions very readily provoke a paroxysm of headache. It is more particularly the condition of the sexual organs that has to be considered in the case of Sepia. The menses are irregular, not sufficiently copious, always preceded by local pains and a general feeling of malaise, and generally succeeded by leucorrhœa; the headache generally occurs about the time of the menses. Sepia is so much more indicated if the sexual instinct is abnormally excited, even during the headache. The remedy has to be frequently repeated at long intervals, since we cannot be sure whether another paroxysm may not occur. If the attacks do not occur too rarely, perhaps every fortnight, or about the menstrual period, it is well to give a few doses after every attack, and then patiently to await the result. This single remedy is often sufficient to cure even cases of long standing. We must not omit Hartmann's remarks concerning the exhibition of Sepia in hemicrania; he does not seem to think much of this remedy in hemicrania, but recommends it rather for arthritic headaches, a designation that seems to us rather baseless. He ranges Sepia side by side with Belladonna, recommending the former for the constitutional diathesis and the latter more particularly for the special paroxysm. The pain is stinging, is located in one of the frontal or occipital protuberances; the stitches flash through the brain, where they seem to leave a deep impression even after they have darted through it; the more frequently the stitches are felt, the more the patients complain of heat in the head, which finally gives way to a feeling of dulness, which is attended with great sensitiveness of the scalp. These symptoms likewise occur during an attack of hemicrania, on which account we have recited them in this place.

Platina is related to Sepia by its action upon the sexual sphere, only the symptoms of these two drugs in the genital range differ very essentially. Platina is indicated when the menses are very profuse, are accompanied by colicky pains, either at the commencement or during their whole course, and generally cause marked derangement of the nervous functions. Platina is more particularly adapted to plethoric, animated and very sensitive individuals. The headache which Platina occasions, is characterized by pressure, sometimes as from a dull point, at other times as from a tight bandage, and is seated in the sinciput; it is accompanied or succeeded by a peculiar sensation of numbness. If cardiac anguish and dyspnœa are present, or if the disorder seems to be caused by structural changes of the heart, Platina is so much more in its place.

Spigelia. The headache to which this remedy corresponds, varies greatly in its forms. According to our experience it seems to be most suitable in tearing, rheumatic headache, more particularly if the pains are darting; it is additionally indicated if the facial nerves are involved in the distress and the paroxysms occur periodically or nearly so. The sensation as if the brain were detached, is likewise found among the symptoms of other drugs, but among the remedies for hemicrania this symptom is more prominent in the pathogenesis of Spigelia than that of any other remedy; the pain is considerably aggravated by every somewhat unusual motion of the head, especially by stooping. We must not omit alluding to the relation of this drug to the heart; this may be accounted for by the circumstance that the headache affects more prominently the left side. The complexion is usually pallid; a flushed face may be regarded as a counter-indication to Spigelia.

Silicea corresponds to paroxysms of hemicrania, and of chronic headache, generally, which break out very frequently and maintain a marked periodicity; they are attended with rush of blood to the head and occasion great sensitiveness of the scalp. That the headache affects the integuments of the head, is likewise evidenced by the falling off of the hair and by excessive perspiration on the hairy scalp.

To these most important and most efficient remedies a number of other drugs might be added, the effect of which is in a measure doubtful, or which are adapted only to very particular cases, and the use of which depends more especially upon the general affection of which the headache is a mere symptom. Among this latter category we number all those drugs which are more particularly suitable to the hemicrania of anæmic individuals, such as *Pulsatilla*, *Ferrum*, *China*, *Natrum muriaticum*, *Calcarea carbonica*. We shall give more particular indications concerning the use of these drugs when speaking of anæmia, to which article we refer the reader. Beside these the following series deserves attention: *Colocynthis*, *Capsicum*, *Veratrum album*, *Acidum nitricum*, *Aurum*, *Verbascum*, *Sanguinaria*, *Phosphorus*, *Bryonia*. [*Aconite*, in tolerably high doses, should not be forgotten in this disease. H.]

As regards a prophylactic treatment, it is just as important in this affection as in other previously described affections of the nervous system to which females are especially liable (chorea, hysteria, &c.), and in order to avoid repetitions we refer the reader to what we have already said concerning them.

2. Neuralgia Trigemini.

Fothergill's Prosopalgia; Tic douloureux; Prosopalgia, Face-ache.

Of all nerves, if we except perhaps the ischiadic nerve, the trigeminus becomes most easily the seat of neuralgic pains. This susceptibility can easily be accounted for by the fact that it spreads through parts which are exposed to a variety of external hurtful influences, and further by the course it takes, almost all its ramifications passing through very narrow orifices of the skull bones.

The etiology of prosopalgia is very uncertain; it often happens that no causes whatever can be ascertained in a special case. We may arrive at some approximate certainty regarding the seat of the exciting cause; far-spread neuralgias necessarily owe their existence to some morbid impression upon the main nerve, whereas, if the neuralgia is confined to one branch or to part of a branch, the cause of the neuralgia must be located rather at the periphery. The character of the morbid impression has not yet been revealed even by the most careful pathologico-anatomical investigations; it is only in proportionally rare cases that structural alterations of the bones or tumors pressing upon the nerve have been discovered. As mediate etiological influences we may regard all those conditions that have already been pointed out as causes of hemicrania. We have, moreover, wounds, mechanical impressions generally, abuse of poisonous cosmetics, toothache, abdominal ailments, suppression of habitual bloody discharges, syphilis, arthritis, rheumatic complaints. This form of neuralgia may originate in miasmatic influences and is more or less paroxysmal. Sex has undoubtedly more or less influence, for females are more generally attacked with this form of neuralgia than males. It is likewise a well ascertained fact that it occurs most frequently between the ages of thirty and fifty years. Children do not seem to be liable to this disorder.

The symptoms of this disorder, although the same in essence, yet differ a great deal as respects their location and extent, according as one or the other branch of the main nerve is affected. Prosopalgia almost always comes on in paroxysms separated from each other by irregular, but most generally perfectly free intervals; the painful sensations which continue without intermission, cannot properly be termed neuralgic. The paroxysms either occur in rapid succession, or in groups which are succeeded by a complete remission for a certain period; or else the paroxysms occur only at long intervals. They are very rarely preceded by preliminary symptoms; if such are present, they are altered sensations in the tract of the nerve. The pains set in suddenly, generally with a moderate degree of intensity, which gradually increases. They follow the course of one or more of the larger trunks of the trigeminus, but may likewise be confined to the portion of a larger trunk. The right side is often more prominently affected; among the single branches the superior maxillary, and next to it the ophthalmic branch is more particularly the seat of the pain. When at its acme the pain seems intolerable, jerking, tearing, burning, darting or flashing, so that the patients cry out aloud. It is rarely continuous, in most cases it breaks out in paroxysms. The face is at times pale as in death, at other times it has a bluish appearance and, if the paroxysms last any time, it looks bloated, which bloat sometimes remains permanent if the paroxysms recur frequently. In most cases the motor-nerves participate in the attack, giving rise to twitchings of the muscles, distortion of the features; even more distant parts of the muscular system are convulsively affected, the cause of which, in most cases, is undoubtedly the extreme pain. We need not particularize the manner in which the pains radiate to different parts, since this can easily be inferred from the anatomical distribution of the different branches of the nerve. It is only in special cases that we may find it difficult to arrive at a correct diagnosis of the disorder, namely when the more deeply-coursing twigs of the trigeminus, those, for instance, which provide the eye with functional power, are the seat of the pain. The neuralgia likewise affects the vascularity of the affected organ, the eye, for instance, appears injected, the salivary glands secrete more saliva. During the paroxysms the irritability of the affected nerves becomes extraordinary so that the least irritation (a current of cold air, talking, etc.) provokes a fresh exacerbation. On this account the patients desire to remain absolutely quiet, and to avoid every impression from the outer air.

The duration of a paroxysm, when several attacks follow each other in succession, varies a good deal; so does the duration of the separate attacks. The general paroxysms may not come on again till years have elapsed; the single attacks may only be separated by intervals of a few minutes. Neuralgia depending upon miasmatic influences, returns again after regular intervals, but their total duration is likewise uncertain although, on account of the greater facility with which they are cured, it is shorter than that of other forms of neuralgia.

The prognosis is in so far favorable as life is not directly threatened by an attack of prosopalgia. It happens, however, that excessive and frequently returning neuralgic pains become the cause of suicide; apoplectic attacks are likewise said to have been caused by such violent attacks of neuralgia. In its higher grades the disorder always has a pernicious effect upon the general constitutional condition, the mind is easily affected, and melancholy is the result; but even without such disastrous consequences the nervous system becomes very irritable and the sensitiveness excessive. The possibility of a cure depends upon several circumstances. Where the affection is occasioned by organic changes of structure, such as osseous disorganizations, tumors, etc., there is scarcely any hope of a cure, whereas intermittent neuralgia and a neuralgia that had been caused by a recent cold, is easily cured. The shorter the duration of the paroxysms, the less frequently they occur, the less intense and wide-spread they are, the sooner we may hope to effect a cure.

Treatment. Prosopalgia is one of those affections which is best calculated to substantiate the superiority of the homœopathic method of cure over other modes of treatment. We often cure cases that had been treated fruitlessly for years, by other means, and even, where we do not effect a cure, we at least succeed in moderating the violence and frequency of the attacks. This of itself is often rendering the patient a great service. The peculiar nature of the affection; the mystery in which its causes and the anatomical changes which act as determining causes of the attack, are still involved; frequently oblige us to select a remedy simply in accordance with symptomatic similarities, a course of treatment that often leads to the best results. Of course it is difficult to select the best remedy for an affection that has only subjective symptoms, and we may meet with frequent disappointments. A remedy is much more easily chosen where we can trace with more or less certainty the causal relation of prosopalgia to some other morbid condition or some definite deleterious influence; in such cases a number of remedies necessarily suggest themselves among which a choice is offered. Here too, as in the case of other ailments, of which we have already treated in former chapters, we have to select remedies for the special attack and likewise such as will prevent a recurrence of the paroxysms. For even if, after the exhibition of a suitable remedy, no other attack follows, this result cannot be regarded as the rule, and we have every reason not to anticipate too hastily a radical recovery.

In the following paragraphs we only mention a few remedies more in detail, giving only the names of the balance, the number of which is very large and whose pathogenesis may be looked up in the Materia Medica.

Spigelia deserves, in our opinion, the first place in the list of remedies for prosopalgia. If we were to apply a general designation to the pains for which it is most suited, we should term them rheumatic. The pain is more particularly a violent jerking or tearing pain, is aggravated or excited by dampness, contact or even by motion, is sometimes a periodical pain, and is always attended with a feeling of anxiety at the heart and great restlessness. The face is pale, disfigured, frequently bloated. The pain is more especially felt in the nerves of the forehead, orbit and upper jaw, or it may emanate from the teeth, where Spigelia likewise excites peculiar jerking pains. If Spigelia affords prompt and permanent relief in prosopalgia, it is probably owing to the fact that the kind of neuralgia to which Spigelia responds, is more easily cured than any other form of the disease. In chronic cases its use is questionable but even in such cases, if the symptoms are similar, we may at least obtain relief, if we cannot effect a cure.

Belladonna. The pain is more particularly a violent cutting pain, and involves a great many branches of the trigeminus. It is attended with symptoms of vascular excitement, such as flushed face, injected eyes, lachrymation, great nervousness and restlessness, palpitation of the heart, buzzing in the ears, scintillations before the eyes. The pains break out towards evening, and are most violent towards midnight. Convulsive movements of the facial muscles are likewise present. Every motion or contact of the affected part is exceedingly painful. According to Hartmann, it is particularly the neuralgia of the infraorbitalis for which Belladonna is indicated. As for an exciting cause, we would call attention to prosopalgia, caused by abuse of Mercury, and likewise to a form of prosopalgia which accompanies an inflammatory affection of the face as a coexisting complication; in the Belladonna-prosopalgia, the affected side of the face is sometimes swollen and looks inflamed.

Verbascum, though not one of our very carefully proved drugs, has been successfully used in a number of cases of prosopalgia. The pain to which it corresponds is a stupefying, pressing pain, or a tensive pain, breaks out in short paroxysms, is more particularly seated in the zygomatic bone, is aggravated by pressure, by mastication, and likewise by exposure to cold air, and is accompanied by vertigo and a feeling of fulness in the head, together with great coldness of the rest of the body.

Sepia. As we stated in our remarks about hemicrania, the Sepia pains vary a great deal, and may be studied more fully in the Materia Medica. Sepia is one of the most important remedies for the prosopalgia and the nervous toothache, with which females are so frequently afflicted.

Platina. The pain is characterized by a sensation as if the head were constricted, attended with a peculiar feeling of numbness. It is apt to break out at regular periods; is worse at night, and aggravated by rest. It is frequently accompanied by cardiac anguish and palpitation of the heart.

Mercurius. This remedy has chiefly tearing, less frequently stinging pains; they either set in at night, or else—which is a still more characteristic symptom—they exacerbate at night, and reach their highest degree of intensity about midnight; they are increased by the warmth of the bed and likewise by external cold. The pains are accompanied by great restlessness and by sleeplessness, and very frequently the affected part is swollen and very sensitive. Mercury is particularly in its place when the pains emanate from carious teeth, and thence spread over the whole half of the face as far as the interior of the ears. This condition is more readily developed by catarrhal exposure, but may likewise originate in an inflammatory affection of the nerves. Mercurius is moreover indicated by a disposition to perspire, especially on the affected part.

Mezereum. The pains are less characteristic; it is a stupefying pressure, especially in the region of the upper jaw from without inwards. This medicine is so much better indicated by the accessory symptoms. From the most painfully affected locality the pains spread like violent tearing pains over the face, neck and nape of the neck, break out in sharply defined paroxysms; are aggravated by warmth, especially by the warmth of a room after a walk in the open air; are accompanied by chilliness or by muscular twitches of the affected part, which is very sensitive to the least contact. The evening exacerbations are usually the most violent. In cases of prosopalgia where syphilis had existed previously, or where a good deal of Mercury had been used, Mezereum is worthy of particular consideration.

Arsenicum is one of the most important remedies in this disease, and will be found the more effective the more purely nervous the pains are. The pain is chiefly burning or stinging as from a number of red-hot needles. The paroxysms break out or exacerbate about midnight. The countenance looks distressed and sunken; during the attack the patient is exceedingly restless. For prosopalgia, caused by miasmatic influences, Arsenicum occupies the first rank as a curative agent.

Colocynthis. According to present experience, this remedy is excellent in neuralgia, generally and more particularly in recent cases where catarrhal exposure can be traced as the cause of the trouble. According to Hartmann, it is likewise indicated in cases arising from, or aggravated by, mortified feelings. The Colocynth-prosopalgia is mostly a tearing, tensive, less frequently a burning distress, greatly aggravated by every motion of the facial muscles, ameliorated by perfect rest and external warmth, and generally attended with inflammatory heat and swelling of the affected part.

The remedies which we have mentioned are the most important of those that may have to be administered for prosopalgia. Beside these remedies, the following likewise deserve our consideration: *Aconitum, Stannum, Conium, Thuya, Capsicum, Staphysagria, Veratrum album, Nux vomica, Ignatia, Pulsatilla, Lycopodium, Ferrum, Calcarea.* Prosopalgia being a local affection, it is not so very difficult to consult the Materia Medica in particular cases. If the prosopalgia is occasioned by chlorosis, syphilis, or some other pathological process, the medicines required by the primary affection are likewise required for the prosopalgia. We refer the reader to the chapters where these primary affections are treated of.

If prosopalgia is treated with the lower attenuations, we shall often produce homœopathic aggravations whose occurrence it is impossible to deny. For this reason it is, as a general rule, better to employ the higher attenuations, and not to repeat the dose too often. *Arsenicum* especially requires to be used with a good deal of care; we have seen aggravations occasioned by the sixth attenuation and still more certainly by the sixth trituration. Among individuals who are afflicted with prosopalgia, these aggravations can easily be accounted for by the extreme irritability of their nerves. This, however, is not always the cause of the aggravation, which is known to be occasioned by large doses even in the case of robust individuals. The patient's confidence in his physician is so easily shaken by such an occurrence that it is desirable to avoid it if possible.

[In prosopalgia caused by malarious influences, or occurring with the regularity or in the place of a fever and ague paroxysm, we have scarcely ever been able to get along without Quinine. Say what you please against Quinine, it is one of the most indispensable antidotes to the intermittent type of paroxysms resulting from the influence of malaria. We have so often and so satisfactorily cured intermittent prosopalgia with five or ten grains of Quinine, administered in grain doses every two hours during the apyrexia, that we can recommend its use to homœopathic physicians with all the earnestness of one whose knowledge is based upon the most unimpeachable experience, and we advise our friends not to mind the absurd twaddle of a few antiquated ignoramuses, who would fain confine Homœopathy to the narrow horizon of their own childish folly.

Aconite is another great remedy in Fothergill's prosopalgia; it should be given in high doses, and may be applied externally, first or second attenuation, with great benefit. H.]

3. Spasmus Nervi Facialis. Tic Convulsif. Spasm of the Facial Nerve.

Spasm of the facial nerve is not a very rare occurence, and is in so far of importance, as it may easily become habitual, in which case it is an incurable infirmity. As a symptomatic manifestation of other affections it is met with in prosopalgia, hemicrania, hysteria, chorea, epilepsy, and several other morbid conditions, likewise in helminthiasis. As a mere symptom of other affections it has no particular significance and disappears, together with the main trouble, without leaving a trace behind. On the other hand it occurs rather frequently as an idiopathic affection, and, if lasting for some time, becomes very obstinate. As an idiopathic disease it arises mostly by exposure of the face to keen winds, a current of air, etc., or is caused by some violent emotion. Another cause which cannot be denied, is the habit of making faces; a cause of this kind prevails among young girls rather than boys. Spasms of the facial nerve, arising from such a cause, are just as obstinate as those that may have arisen from any other cause.

As regards the extent of the spasm there is considerable difference, although it is generally confined to one side. At times the spasm is limited to isolated convulsive motions of the eyelids, mouth, alæ nasi; at other times we have tonic contraction of one whole side of the face. The patients are scarcely ever capable of preventing or arresting the spasm by the mere force of the will. The disorder is scarcely ever attended with pain, perhaps only at the commencement of the attack. The course and duration of the attack are uncertain; if it sets in suddenly, the trouble may last for life. If the spasm continues a long time, the face may remain permanently distorted. Such instances occur quite frequently, but escape our more particular notice; many persons retain forever the anxious expression of the countenance, which a deep mental agitation may have caused, even after every trace of the exciting cause had completely vanished.

The **treatment** of this spasm bids fair to have a favorable termination only in recent cases, and is unsuccessful in proportion as the disease has had a longer duration. The best remedies for spasm caused by a cold are: *Rhus tox.*, *Belladonna* and *Ignatia;* the last-named remedy deserves particular consideration, if the spasm is caused by some mental agitation. Beside these remedies we have *Cannabis* and *Veratrum album.* In chronic cases *Zincum* and *Cuprum* may be tried. A better result than from any medical treatment may be obtained from persevering trials to recover the normal control of the facial muscles by regular exercise; this result can always be accomplished to some extent, if not wholly. The favorable action of electricity is still questionable; however, there are sufficient reasons why cautious and persevering experiments with the electric current should be tried. If children are attacked with the spasm in consequence of mimicking other children, the best means of cure is to constantly reprimand them; and if this should prove ineffectual, to inflict corporal punishment immediately after every indulgence of the naughty practice.

[Two admirable remedies for this spasm are *Gelseminum* and *Aconitum napellus*, tincture of the root.]

C. DISEASES OF THE EYE.

Diseases of the eyes, as a general rule, are treated by pathologists as a special department so strictly, that no mention is made of them in therapeutic treatises. This arrangement is undoubtedly correct, in so far as the diseases of the eyes are too important to be dispatched in a few short chapters, and a number of special treatises are at our disposal where these diseases are treated of in a comprehensive manner. In our school, unfortunately, we have no special work devoted to affections of the eyes; and although the absence of such works can easily be accounted for, yet, on the other hand, it is to be regretted, since there is scarcely an organ whose diseases have been investigated as fully and intimately as those of the eyes.

On this account the effects of drugs in diseases of the eyes could be determined with more accuracy than in any other disease. In spite of this, ophthalmic practice has been very much neglected by homœopathic physicians. We are anxious to investigate more fully the reason of this apparent neglect, since by so doing we depart much less from the object of a therapeutic treatise than it might seem at the first glance. Two circumstances it is which we have to notice more prominently. In the first place, the position of the homœopathic physician is of such a nature, that it does not allow him to devote himself exclusively to a special department of medicine. Everybody, who has been engaged in homœopathic practice, knows that this statement is correct. We are still too much upon the defensive towards our professional opponents, to enjoy the privilege of exclusively cultivating a department that requires extraordinary manual dexterity. But even supposing, that this privilege should exist, the homœopathic practitioner will still find it very difficult to conquer for himself the position of an oculist, for the reason that it matters not, in general practice, how many prejudices a physician may have to contend against; but the case is different when a special department only is attended to. A physician of this class has to be pecuniarily independent, in order to be able to maintain his position in a dignified manner. We are still deprived of the only means by which our object could be attained in a different way,—we mean a sufficient number of large hospitals.

But even if all these material obstacles had been removed, an oculist would still have a great many difficulties to contend with, which are inherent in our Materia Medica. We confess without hesitation, that there is no section in our Materia Medica less useful and less adapted to homœopathic treatment, than the symptoms referring to diseases of the eyes. This chapter is much less practical than the symptoms referring to the cutaneous diseases or the morbid changes of the urine; for, in treating the eye, we have to consider a number of important organs, all of which are of essential importance, such as the conjunctiva, sclerotica, cornea, lens crystallina, etc. Our provings do not even contain vague allusions to these various parts, whose organizations and functions differ so greatly from each other. This is the reason, why we cannot boast of great success in our treatment of affections of the eyes; what we consider as an indispensable condition of successful treatment, an accurate determination of pathogenetic and pathological similarity, is wanting in the management of diseases of the eyes. It is strange, that so little has as yet been done to remedy this defect. Yet this is so much more desirable, as diseases of the eyes are regarded with so much interest by the public, and nothing would contribute more to the spread of our doctrines, than numerous brilliant cures of ophthalmic diseases.

Hence, in diseases of the eyes, we have to depend in a great measure upon arguments suggested by analogy, and upon the empirical use of drugs. Nevertheless, in spite of these drawbacks, we effect more numerous and more satisfactory cures with our imperfectly proved drugs than our allopathic opponents are capable of accomplishing with the whole apparatus of their surgical and medicinal appliances.*

We may as well here call attention to a point, which has been discussed on many other occasions, but without any satisfactory completeness. The question namely is, whether in affections of the conjunctiva, for instance, it be not advisable to apply the proper remedies externally. That many medicines act more favorably when locally applied, is evident from the local use of the Sulphate of Zinc, Corrosive Sublimate, red Precipitate, etc. Unfortunately we are not in a position to reason upon the basis of comparative experiments, howsoever easy it would be to institute them, for, even the lower attenuations of any medicine may be applied to the eyes, provided they are made with distilled water instead of alcohol, and the triturations may be locally applied without any modification.

In the following chapters we shall treat only of the main diseases of the eyes, omitting all those which require operations, and likewise those which cannot be correctly diagnosed without the use of the more recently introduced appliances for the recognition of ophthalmic diseases.

1. Conjunctivitis Catarrhalis.

As a simple inflammatory catarrh of the conjunctiva we define a condition of hyperæmia of this membrane attended with the more profuse secretion of a fluid similar to the normal one.

Symptoms. While the patient suddenly experiences a sensa-

---

* We see no reason why the author should feel discouraged regarding the success, which has attended the homœopathic treatment of diseases of the eye. In some of the public ophthalmic Infirmaries of New York homœopathic treatment has been substituted by the authorities in the place of the ordinary allopathic treatment, for the very reason, that the former has been found to be eminently more successful than the latter. H.

tion as if sand were under the eyelid, generally the upper one, the conjunctiva assumes a reddish appearance, single vessels of the conjunctiva, first of the tarsal and afterwards of the transition-portion, becoming injected. In slight cases the catarrhal irritation may not go any further; but if it should increase, the redness may spread to the conjunctiva of the bulbus; the vessels running from the transition-portion of the conjunctiva to the cornea, become engorged and, while the inflammation goes on increasing in intensity, approach more and more closely the margin of the cornea where a small pustule forms, generally near the outer margin. At the same time serum is effused under the conjunctiva which sometimes swells up quite extensively and even gives rise to small ecchymoses. The sensation of a foreign body generally continues for some time, and is accompanied by a violent itching or smarting pain with a peculiar feeling of dryness and heaviness of the lids. The eye becomes sensitive to the light, even complete photophobia sets in, much less frequently dimness of sight and photopsia. At first the secretion of the conjunctiva is rather diminished than increased, after which it becomes more copious, clear as water, and is mixed with mucous flocks, and, on account of the secretion going on continually, excoriates the skin of the face by keeping it moist all the time. It is not quite certain, but probable, that the secretion is contagious. All the symptoms exacerbate at night, less frequently in the morning. Cold, more particularly damp and cold weather intensifies the whole process, and more particularly promotes the serous infiltration of the mucous membrane. Humid warmth, on the contrary, is very pleasant to the eyes, at least in most cases. In violent cases the conjunctiva may swell up to such an extent that pad-shaped protrusions between the lids may prevent their closing. The cornea is scarcely ever involved.

The causes of this catarrhal inflammation are not very certain. Undoubtedly it occurs more frequently at a period when catarrhs prevail generally during the transition-seasons of the year; it may, however, occur without any atmospheric influences prevailing. It is very much disposed to accompany a catarrh of the nasal mucous membrane. An inflammation of the Meibomian glands, so-called styes, may be the cause, a consequence or a complication of catarrhal conjunctivitis; styes may cause the disease, more especially if they are located on the inside of the lids.

The disease may last indefinitely, from a few days to several weeks, if relapses take place; the acute form is very apt to pass into the chronic. Unless culpably mismanaged, the inflammation scarcely ever leaves unpleasant consequences.

Chronic conjunctivitis may develop itself without any previous acute inflammation, in which case it may result from swellings of the lid or from diseased conditions of the Meibomian glands; but as a general rule it arises from the acute form. In chronic conjunctivitis the conjunctiva of the bulbus remains quite free from inflammation, the tarsal and transition-portion of the conjunctiva look dark, even bluish-red, velvety, thickened and bulging out like a pad; the swelling is more prominent along the margin of the lid. The secretion is always more profuse than usual, the secreted fluid is turbid, of a gray-yellowish appearance, tends to agglutinate the lids, gives rise to excoriations both at the borders of the lids and on the cheeks. The subjective symptoms are not very considerable, and are only distinguished in degree from those of the acute form. This form of the disease may run a protracted course. Disastrous results, such as incipient ectropium, only occur as the consequences of very bad management.

Almost every form of conjunctivitis can be ranged in the category, of which we have given a description in the previous chapters; it may, however, be desirable to add a few remarks concerning the forms of conjunctivitis, which used to be described as rheumatic and arthritic, designations of which even Hartmann still makes use. We do not approve of such a classification, because it is of no use practically, and impairs the value of pathology in consequence of the Babylonian confusion which such classifications introduce into the nomenclatures of pathological treatises. If we compare the pathological pictures which Hartmann gives us, we discover scarcely a single essential difference between them, and if the rheumatic form is supposed to be characterized by a peculiar pain, we know very well that such subjective symptoms are too deceptive to be used as a basis for a pathological classification. We know moreover, that such classifications owe their origin to the mixing up of a variety of morbid conditions. Nor are such classifications really important to the homœopathic treatment of the disease, for, it is self-evident, that in selecting a remedy we have to consider every symptom, the exciting causes, former diseases, etc. The best proof against the usefulness of such subdivisions is the impossibility of making them available in practice.

Treatment. Before beginning a strictly medical treatment, we have to examine the eye with the most perfect care in order to ascertain beyond all doubt, whether the foreign body, which the patient imagines is in the eye, be really present. A strict search frequently reveals the presence either of a little hair which has become lodged in the eye, or of an eyelash that has grown inwards and causes the inflammation. Irritating causes of this kind have to be removed before we can expect to effect a cure by the use of medicines.

At the commencement of the inflammation, *Aconite* is the best remedy in almost every case; unless very peculiar complications exist, it alone very often removes the inflammation in a few days. *Belladonna* will be found less frequently curative where the inflammation is still confined to the eyelid, and hence has not yet reached its highest degree of development. It deserves all the more consideration, the more the eyeball itself has become involved in the inflammation, and the more prominently the vessels have become injected in which case there is always a good deal of photophobia. *Euphrasia* may be ranked side by side with Belladonna; additional indications for Euphrasia are pustules near the border of the cornea and the co-existence of a violent nasal catarrh, attended with profuse secretion of mucus. For all that, in spite of the presence of these symptoms, Euphrasia will often disappoint us, as we know from abundant experience. When locally applied, Euphrasia often has a very excellent effect even after its internal administration had proved absolutely useless. If the eye-affection is accompanied by general catarrhal symptoms, we may expect much better and much more certain effects from the use of *Mercurius*. In such cases it has just as good an effect upon the mucous membrane of the eye as in other cases upon that of the nose, and deserves the name of our most efficient remedy for catarrh. It will be found most useful in the case of children. *Hepar sulphuris* is one of our more important remedies for conjunctivitis. At the outset it is less suitable than in the further course of the disease; it acts well after Belladonna, in the more acute cases, where a profuse quantity of thick mucus is secreted. In chronic conjunctivitis Hepar sulphuris may likewise have to be resorted to, although we have better remedies for this form than Hepar. *Euphorbium* is an efficient remedy in the more violent forms of this disease, where the secretion is more purulent; it is particularly indicated by a feeling of great dryness in the eye, in spite of the increased secretion, and by the excoriations which so readily take place in the corners of the eyes. *Rhus tox.* is suitable in simple catarrhal inflammation of the eyes, where a somewhat considerable serous puffing up of the conjunctiva is attended with a comparatively scanty secretion and the pain is very great. It is likewise appropriate to the chronic form. *Sulphur* is not indicated in the acute form of the disease, but it will act with advantage when the passage from the acute to the chronic form has fairly set in and the hyperæmia of the conjunctiva has begun to abate. At this stage *Arsenicum* will be found an excellent remedy, especially when the redness has assumed a dark tint and the margins of the lids show considerable disposition to become excoriated. It acts very beneficially if small quantities of the third or fourth trituration are scattered on the lids. Beside these two, and other remedies that have already been recommended for the chronic form, we have *Iodium*, *Mercurius iodatus*, *Hydrargyrum præcip. rubrum* and *Staphysagria*. With this last-named remedy we have cured several cases of a very obstinate chronic catarrh, with considerable swelling of the lids, after other remedies had entirely failed.

[A favorite remedy for conjunctivitis is *Apis mellifica;* it is used with varying benefit; it will be found, however, that in cases where it is said to have produced striking results, it was generally given in alternation with Aconite. H.]

Inflammation of one or more Meibomian glands, designated by the term hordeolum or stye, is sometimes a mere symptom of catarrhal inflammation, but may likewise exist as an idiopathic disease, especially during the prevalence of keen, damp and cold winds. It is very much disposed to relapses. This disorder is very seldom epidemic, and it is well to check it as soon as possible. For this purpose *Mercurius* is the best remedy, for, under its influence suppuration takes place very rapidly. As regards *Pulsatilla*, we have never seen the good effects from it, which Hartmann professes to have obtained; if, as he thinks, Pulsatilla prevents suppuration, the use of this drug can only have the effect of prolonging the course of the trouble. On the contrary, our best plan is to hasten the suppurative process as much as possible; if the patient is able to keep his room, it is even well to apply warm poultices, and to open the little abscess, taking care, however, to squeeze all the pus out. By this method a return of the difficulty is more effectually prevented than by any other means. If a larger number of glands are involved, the margin of the lid becomes hypertrophied in consequence of the indurated glands which feel like hard lumps; there is, moreover, a constant disposition to inflammatory exacerbations. For this condition *Staphysagria* is an excellent remedy, only we should not expect any immediate results. *Calcarea carbonica* and *Silicea* may likewise be given with advantage.

[For chronic conjunctivitis we likewise recommend *Pulsatilla* and *Phosphorus*, more particularly in the case of individuals with lymphatic temperaments; the former is more adapted to cases with profuse secretion of purulent mucus, the latter to cases where the eye remains dry, except perhaps a slight agglutination of the lids in the morning.

An interesting case of inflammation of the lachrymal sac of the right eye, with swelling of the sac, pain on pressure, burning pain, and flow of tears over the cheek, is reported by Dr. Dudgeon in the 13th volume of the British Journal of Homœopathy; the case was treated with Aconite, Silicea and other medicines, but yielded principally to Silicea. We have cured similar inflammations with Aconite, Pulsatilla and Silicea. H.]

2. Conjunctivitis Blennorrhoica.

Recent works on ophthalmic surgery are filled with so many different opinions and such a confusion of names regarding this disease, that it is next to impossible to exhibit a satisfactory and complete picture of this difficulty; we therefore prefer to adopt Arlt's example of treating of this form of blennorrhœa. We distinguish an acute and a chronic form.

a. *Acute Blennorrhœa.*

It is distinguished from catarrh principally by a plastic exudation into the tissue of the conjunctiva, the slimy-purulent secretion and its decided contagiousness.

Amid the symptoms of a violent catarrh the whole conjunctiva of the lids looks puffed, swollen, and uniformly red, and from the transition-portion of the membrane numerous vessels run towards the cornea; the secretion is not clear, but rather turbid and mixed with firm yellowish flocks, and the lids begin very speedily to swell and feel hotter than usual. The more rapidly these symptoms develop themselves, the greater is the certainty, that we have to deal with a blennorrhœa.

This first stage sometimes passes into the second stage even after the short period of twelve hours; the interstitial puffing of the conjunctiva increases so that the internal margin of the lid is no longer sharply circumscribed, the lid is no longer in contact with the bulbus, and the absorption of the tears is no longer possible. It is particularly the transition-portion of the conjunctiva, that looks swollen and deep-red, likewise the semilunar fold. The conjunctiva bulbi is likewise infiltrated, very much injected and red. The lids are swollen, generally to such a degree that they can no longer be opened. The secretion becomes thick, turbid, creamy, very copious. Photophobia is almost always present, generally there is fever, dulness of the head, and violent tearing or stinging pains in the eye.

In the third stage all the phenomena, of which mention has been made, become worse; the lids are swollen to such an extent, that it is no longer possible to raise them, and the cheek becomes involved in the swelling. The secretion is very copious, purulent or even ichorous. The pains are intense, sometimes unbearable. The infiltration of the conjunctiva bulbi reaches a very high degree, so that the cornea looks as if surrounded with a deep-red wall, it even is partially covered by the swelling. The cornea, which at first retained its lustre, is now invaded by the disease; either it becomes inflamed and is rapidly disorganized, or it loses its epithelium, shows superficial ulcerations or pannus forms, that is to say: an exudation takes place beneath the epithelium, and the vessels look very much injected.

b. *Chronic Blennorrhœa.*

We subjoin here a description of the chronic form of the disease, because, so far as symptoms are concerned, both the chronic and the acute form run a similar course.

In the chronic form, unless other very striking noxious complications are present, the morbid process is confined to the palpebral conjunctiva.

This form commences likewise with the symptoms of a catarrhal conjunctivitis, except that at the very outset the redness of the tarsal portion looks darker and more velvety, and the swelling is more considerable. The patients complain of a feeling of dryness and roughness in the eye, and of an aching or burning pain, together with an increased secretion of tears. After this condition has lasted for a rather indefinite period of time, the second stage sets in, where infiltration of the conjunctiva of both lids is the most essential symptom. The papillary portion looks as if covered with closely crowded little warts, which are soft at first, and sometimes bleed readily, and afterwards assume a cartilaginous hardness, imparting to the conjunctiva an appearance as if cracked. Their color is darkred. The conjunctiva of the bulbus is not involved in this morbid process, except, perhaps, a little injected at the commencement. The swelling of the lids is not very considerable. The secretion is more copious, sometimes clear, with a few flocks floating in it; sometimes turbid, afterwards thick, creamy, and adhering with some firmness.

If at this period specially irritating causes should affect the eye, a general blennorrhœa of the conjunctiva may develop itself, similar to that which we have described when treating of the third stage of the acute form.

Course and Terminations. A retrograde metamorphosis of blennorrhœa may take place in the first as well as in the second stage, and the disease may either terminate or else it may pass into a chronic form; its course may likewise become so rapid that the cornea may be destroyed in thirty-six hours.

If the disease remains stationary in the first stage, it is generally looked upon as simple catarrh, until its true character has become manifest by the infectious nature of its secretion, or the disease has acquired a higher degree of intensity by an additional cold or very impure air.

In the second stage the disease may persevere for years without any decided change; but the passage into the third stage may take place at any moment. The exudation is either re-absorbed, a scar remaining, without, however, the cartilage becoming involved, or else the exudation terminates in a fungoid growth, in consequence of which the lids become everted. The cornea either remains unaffected, or else it is temporarily affected only, and as it were by accident.

In the third stage the disease always runs an acute course, and, if the cornea is invaded, the danger is always very great. The third stage seldom sets in until the other phenomena have reached their climax, and sometimes not till these phenomena have commenced to abate. The cornea softens very suddenly, becomes infiltrated with pus, and under these circumstances generally breaks. Iritis is apt to supervene during the affection of the cornea. Retrograde metamorphosis from the third stage generally takes place without leaving any fungoid growths; sometimes, however, there remains a disorganization of the conjunctiva in the shape of puffed fungoid growths around the cornea, of a loose and flesh-colored appearance, so that it is either partially or totally covered.

Causes. The disease may break out sporadically, but likewise among a large number of individuals at once, who live crowded together. It is principally met with among new-born infants and among adults at the age of pubescence, and after they have attained the age of manhood.

The blennorrhœa of new-born infants may originate in exposure to glaring light, in a cold, in epidemic influences, in contagion by the blennorrhœic secretion from the mother during the act of parturition, although the secretion need not necessarily have had a syphilitic character; simple leucorrhœa may cause blennorrhœa in the case of new-born infants.

In rare cases only blennorrhœa breaks out among adults without any contact with some blennorrhœic secretion; here a purely spontaneous appearance of the disease has to be presupposed, which supposition is favored by the observation, that even a simple catarrh may assume the form of a severe blennorrhœa. As a general rule the blennorrhœa originates in some infection by blennorrhœic secretion, no matter whether it emanates from the eyes or from the genital organs. We may observe that the limpid secretion of the first stage, and the clear secretion of the chronic form, are not contagious. On the other hand, the turbid secretion of the beginning second stage produces blennorrhœa of the first stage, and the purulent, more consistent secretion of the second and third stages, always causes a blennorrhœa, which passes rapidly through the three stages of the disease. The more intense the disease is, from which the contagious matter had emanated, the more suddenly the disease breaks out after the infection, even six or twelve hours after the infectious matter had been communicated at the third stage.

It is self-evident, that the contagion is favored by every circumstance which tends to facilitate it, above all things by the crowding together of a number of individuals in the same room, whence the disorder is so frequently met with among soldiers and in foundling-houses.

The prognosis depends, in the first place, upon the more or less rapid course of the disease; the more rapidly one stage passes into another, the more we have reason to apprehend a disastrous termination. If the quality of the contagious matter can be ascertained, the prognosis can be established with more certainty from such a basis. It is only when the cornea is invaded, that the visual power is threatened with danger. The duration is indefinite, from eight days for the lighter grades of the disease to several years for the chronic form.

Before we enter upon the treatment of this disease, it behooves us to agree upon the nomenclature which other pathologists have adopted. The acute form responds to the ophthalmia gonorrhoica, and in certain respects to panophthalmitis. The chronic form represents granular ophthalmia, ophthalmia militaris, ægyptiaca, contagiosa. Many other names may be recorded in the vast domain of ophthalmic surgery: at all events those which we have named are the best known and those in most general use.

Treatment. After what we have said about the contagiousness of the disease, it must seem a matter of course, that special attention should be paid to prevent the further spread of the disease, if it breaks out in localities where a number of individuals live closely together. Since it has been shown beyond a doubt—more particularly by ingenious apparatuses invented for such a purpose—that atmospheric air may act as a vehicle of the contagion, it is of the utmost importance that the patients should be kept isolated as much as possible. Moreover, the greatest cleanliness should be observed; the eyes cannot be too often bathed, and the secretion removed. The air of the room should be renewed as often as possible, and both the patient and those who are near him must have their attention directed to the facility, with which the disease can be propagated by contagion.

Among the most important remedies after the disease has broken out, Arlt ranks applications of ice. Four to six thicknesses of linen are laid on ice wrung out and afterwards applied to the eye as closely as possible. They have to be continued day and night, and should be changed quite often. Where they cannot be made according to rule, they had better be entirely omitted. There is no doubt that an energetic application of cold can neutralize an existing contagion.

Although in describing the disease we have avoided all details, we cannot well get along without them as soon as we undertake to point out the treatment, for the reason that as yet no remedy has been discovered, that embodies in its pathogenesis the full characteristics of the disease. Hence we have to dwell more particularly on the single stages of the disease, and upon the quality and course of the general affection.

Owing to its rapid course, a blennorrhœa, caused by a very poisonous secretion, opposes great difficulties to the selection of an appropriate remedy, for the reason that no time is allowed to await the full action of the drug. The similarity of the pathological process going on on the conjunctiva to syphilitic gonorrhœa, and the origin of blennorrhœa by syphilitic infection, lead us to the conclusion, that *Mercurius* is the most suitable remedy for the disease. As regards the kind of mercurial preparation that had better be used, we prefer most unhesitatingly the most powerful among them, the *red* or *white Precipitate*, and still more, the *Sublimate*. The last-mentioned offers the great advantage that it readily admits of local application, which, in view of the great danger to which the visual power is exposed by the destructive agency of the contagion, should never be omitted. In order to elicit the best effects of Corrosive Sublimate, it will not be necessary to use a very powerful solution; on the contrary, we have found, that by using a solution of a few grains of the second trituration in water the same favorable change can be effected, without the disadvantages arising from the cauterizing effects of a more powerful solution. This has more especially to be considered in the case of children, for whom it is any how very difficult to hold still, and where a second application is scarcely ever necessary, provided the first application was sufficiently thorough. Of other remedies, *Hepar sulphuris calc.* seems to us the only one worthy of a trial, not so much on account of the phenomena which this drug has elicited on persons in health, as on account of its correspondence to the gonorrhœic infection. By giving other remedies, which might possibly be indicated by the accompanying pains, we shall simply lose a precious time, which we can hardly afford in this disease.

Ophthalmia neonatorum, which is very frequently regarded as gonorrhœic ophthalmia, does not run such a terribly rapid course as the latter in its worst form. For ophthalmia neonatorum the most important remedy is likewise *Mercurius*, more particularly if a syphilitic taint can be traced in the mother. However, since other causes may have occasioned the disease, other remedies should likewise be pointed out, among which Belladonna occupies the first rank. Beside Belladonna, we have *Bryonia* and *Rhus tox.* Hartmann seems to understand by ophthalmia neonatorum every catarrh of new-born children, otherwise we could not account for the remedies which he recommends for the disease. Even *Aconite*, which is such an excellent remedy in other affections of the eyes, cannot possibly be suitable in ophthalmia neonatorum, neither according to its symptoms, nor according to what we know of its effects upon other organs or upon the general organism. We suppose that it is recommended for the exceedingly violent inflammatory process; this, however, would be a very one-sided indication, and the result might not answer our expectations. Moreover, ophthalmia neonatorum should not be treated carelessly as time runs on. If the disease, as is often the case, is the local expression of a general affection of the mucous membranes, only such remedies as are indicated for the general disease can be properly used for the local affection, and the selection of which is determined with much more definiteness by the general condition of the organism than by the symptoms of the eye alone.

For the less acute form of the disease, *Belladonna* will be found most suitable at the commencement to check the inflammatory process. The more, however, the conjunctiva becomes infiltrated, the more slimy and thicker the secretion, the less the remedy is indicated. At this stage of the disease, we have, beside *Mercurius*, *Bryonia* and *Rhus tox*. Bryonia, especially, has a few symptoms that are essential in this disease, namely: considerable swelling of the lids, purulent discharge and dark-red conjunctiva, which is likewise very much puffed up. *Hepar sulphuris* likewise is appropriate for these symptoms.

In the chronic form the diagnosis of the disease will at first have great inconveniences, unless we meet with a number of cases at once and the very fact of its spreading among so many individuals reveals the true nature of the disease. Under such circumstances Mercurius is again the most prominently indicated remedy. It is much more important to determine the medicines that are suitable in the second stage. On looking at the exciting cause, at the peculiar form of the granulations, we cannot help contrasting these granulations with similar symptoms on the mucous membrane of the sexual organs, and regarding the granulations as so many condylomatous growths. It might be somewhat hazardous to exclusively recommend *Thuya* for this form of ophthalmia. Since the symptoms of the drug represent a very strongly marked catarrhal affection of the eyes, it seems less illogical to recommend Thuya, and to try to cure the disease with this remedy. We have given a prominent place to Thuya for the reason that this remedy has several accessory symptoms which do not occur in such a full combination in the pathogenesis of any other drug. Thuya likewise can be applied externally without the least difficulty; such an external application is so much more advisable as the usefulness of Thuja in condylomata is very well known. This is the place to introduce *Sulphur*. It has been so often recommended for the acute stage of blennorrhœa that it seems as though we ought to believe in its good effects in this disease although we have never witnessed them. It is certainly more adapted to the chronic form of blennorrhœa, since Sulphur is generally much more appropriate about the period when, in acute affections, the exudation shows signs of being reabsorbed, but neither before nor during the development of the exudative process. *Acidum nitricum* is reported to have effected a cure of gonorrhœal ophthalmia (see Allg. Hom. Zeit., vol. 19), which invites our attention to this drug, even if it had not otherwise a multitude of corresponding symptoms. Beside these remedies we direct attention to *Graphites, Silicea* and *Staphysagria;* at the same time we are bound to admit that we cannot offer any practical illustrations of the curative virtues of these remedies in the above-mentioned diseases, and that the diagnosis in the few cases that have been reported, is very questionable. This shows that we are without much experience in the treatment of blennorrhœa of the eyes, and this want should excite everybody who has such a case to manage, to publish the details of his treatment as well as its results, no matter whether favorable or otherwise. Even unsuccessful cases may teach others a good deal of wisdom, were it only that they may learn to avoid the mistakes of their predecessors. Our own experience being rather limited, we dare not express ourselves too positively regarding the methods that other practitioners have pursued, although the results obtained by the latter, have likewise not been very brilliant. We must not omit to give publicity to the observation that, in the acute form, the *Nitrate of Silver*, and, in the chronic form, the *Sulphate of Copper* have been found to be the best cauterizing agents.

[In the acute stage of this form of blennorrhœa we use the Nitrate of Silver in the proportion of one grain of the Nitrate to an ounce of water. With this solution we pencil the eye or eyes every four hours thoroughly, taking care to have the camel's-hair pencil washed out in fresh water before it is used for the other eye. This operation is continued for a few days until the suppurative process has ceased. Appropriate internal treatment is attended to at the same time. H.]

3. Conjunctivitis Scrofulosa.

This form of conjunctivitis is more particularly characterized by the circumstance that it only affects the conjunctiva of the bulbus, and that the cornea is generally involved in the inflammatory process. The fact that it is one of the most frequently occurring and most obstinate affections of the eyes, imparts to it a peculiar significance in the eyes of practical physicians, even if they do not make ophthalmic surgery an exclusive branch of practice.

Symptoms. Not unfrequently the beginning of the inflammation is attended with febrile symptoms preceding for a short time the actual disease and, as a general rule, being regarded as the symptoms of a general catarrhal affection, to which they bear indeed a very strong resemblance. All at once, as if a foreign body had suddenly become lodged in the eye, the conjunctiva appears injected, and photophobia and a copious secretion of tears set in, the former symptom becoming so intense that it is almost impossible to obtain a view of the interior of the eye, for the reason that the spasmodic closing of the lids cannot be overcome, even if the children are ever so willing. The appearance of photophobia, however, does not imply that the conjunctiva of the bulbus is already invaded by the inflammation, for this invasion may take place at a later period. The little patients may be seen for weeks, day after day, on the arms of the mother or seated in the corner of a sofa, with their eyelids firmly pressed together in order to prevent the light from penetrating between the eyelids. A forcible opening of the lids is not advisable, for the reason that such a proceeding only tends to favor the disorganizing process, and that any considerable involvement of the cornea need only be suspected, if the margin of the upper lid looks swollen and red, and mucus is secreted. As a general rule the intense pains and the photophobia abate at dusk, when the patients open their eyes spontaneously. This is the best time to obtain a view of the condition of the inner eye, without any forcible means having to be resorted to. This is an important circumstance, for children are very apt to be intimidated by the application of force in examining their eyes. The alterations of the bulbus which may succeed the invasion of photophobia after an indefinite period of time, refer more particularly to the margin of the conjunctiva around the cornea, or to the conjunctiva of the cornea itself. In this locality a small, either vesicular, or pustulous, or papulous exudation arises, surrounded by an areola of a deeper redness, and frequently accompanied by a rose-colored narrow areola around the whole cornea or a portion of its periphery. Two parts are scarcely ever invaded at the same time. Not till a vesicle has formed do the vessels of the conjunctiva running towards this vesicle begin to swell. The swollen vessels form a triangle the point of which is at the vesicle, and the basis lies in the transition-portion of the conjunctiva. If the exudation is situated on the cornea, the vessels run towards it in the shape of a narrow band. The conjunctiva may remain unaffected all this time, or else it may exhibit more or less distinctly marked catarrhal symptoms. If the bulbus is affected, the photophobia does not furnish a sure criterium for the intensity of that affection; the photophobia may be intense and yet the affection of the bulbus may scarcely be perceptible, whereas the most dangerous ulcerations of the cornea may be unattended by scarcely any sign of photophobia. The secretion of tears is generally very profuse and, by keeping the cheek constantly moist, inflame and excoriate it, or cover it with clusters of pustules.

The vesicles, which are never completely filled with a clear, watery fluid, either gradually disappear, or else break, leaving superficial ulcers with a suppurating base. The papulæ form a grayish, vascular covering of the cornea, giving rise to pannus. Pannus may likewise accompany the breaking out of vesicles or pustules.

It is upon these exudative processes and the structural changes resulting from them that the danger to vision in scrofulous ophthalmia depends. If the exudation is located on the margin of the sclerotica or close to the margin of the cornea, vision is not endangered. On the contrary, if the exudative process is located more towards the middle of the cornea, the visual power is always more or less in danger. The best thing that can happen is, when the vesicles or pustules do not burst, in which case, after their re-absorption, they leave a sort of grayish dimness which gradually disappears of itself. The vesicles, after bursting, leave a colorless, superficial ulcer which heals, leaving a somewhat dim, milky spot behind. Nor does pannus, as a general rule, endanger the sight; only it lasts a long time. Ulceration, succeeding the bursting of the pustules, may become very dangerous, if it shows a tendency to attack the cornea very extensively; it may lead to the destruction of this organ and may involve the iris in the disorganizing process. The ulcerative process may lead to cicatrices in the cornea; its laminæ may become infiltrated with pus; a staphyloma may result and finally the cornea may burst, and all the disastrous consequences of this accident may be entailed upon the patient.

The duration of this affection does not follow a definite rule; not unfrequently, after a severe attack had been overcome, another attack takes place, sometimes on the same, and at times on the other eye. Only in rare cases both eyes are attacked at the same time and in the same manner.

In many respects the etiological causes of the disease are not difficult to determine; in some cases, on the contrary, they are involved in a good deal of uncertainty. The most frequent cause of the disease is undoubtedly a scrofulous diathesis; but there are cases where the antecedents of the patient preclude the idea of scrofulosis, and again other cases where the disease commences with a simple inflammation of the eye. As a general rule, scrofula acquires its most marked development between the second and seventh year, although it may break out at any age. Unwholesome, dark, damp dwellings, improper nourishment, excessive quantities of farinaceous food, want of cleanliness, insufficient exercise in the open air, are not only the causes of scrofulosis generally, but likewise the causes of scrofulous ophthalmia specially. Where a disposition to this disease prevails, an outbreak is provoked by mechanical injuries, catarrhal irritations, excessive use of the eyes, etc. The influence of the season is undeniable. This results from the circumstance that the inflammation is apt to return in the same individual at the same period of the year; it is particularly in spring and fall, during the prevalence of cold and damp weather and keen winds, that the disease is apt to break out. Not unfrequently ophthalmia changes about with eruptions in the face or otorrhœa. Howsoever often this phenomenon has been observed, yet it is impossible to account for it. What is certain, however, is that it is wrong to presuppose the existence of a metastatic process, so much more as both these morbid conditions sometimes replace each other for years.

Treatment. It has to be directed against the attack itself, and likewise against the disposition to relapses, in other words against the scrofulous diathesis itself.

In selecting a remedy for this disease, we have to consider the constitutional disposition of the patient, whether it is erethic or of the torpid and scrofulous cast, for the attacks vary accordingly.

In the erethic form, as long as there is violent photophobia without any affection of the cornea, *Belladonna* is to be preferred, more especially if the pains are very acute and febrile symptoms are noticed. If there is photophobia without any corresponding pains or other inflammatory phenomena; if the photophobia is accompanied by a violent spasm of the eyelids, or if, as is often the case, this spasm is the cause of the photophobia, *Conium maculatum* is preferable to Belladonna, but it is indispensable to administer the drug in rather large doses, a few drops of the concentrated tincture, as we can aver from abundant experience. Belladonna, likewise, had better be administered in the lower preparations, the higher ones leaving us frequently in the lurch. If the disorder has reached the stage of exudation near and upon the cornea, *Mercurius* is undoubtedly the best remedy, and more especially the *Sublimate*, which, if possible, should likewise be used externally. Since in scrofulous ophthalmia we cannot expect a sudden effect from any remedy, the exhibition of Mercurius should not be discontinued too soon, for the additional reason that it is likewise an excellent remedy against the ulcerative process. It is still more indicated by a co-existing exanthem, more particularly eczema in the face, with violent itching. The local use has to be managed very cautiously after the ulceration has penetrated the cornea to a certain depth. *Rhus toxicodendron* should not be overlooked. It is true we are not yet in possession of very positive, practically verified clinical indications of this drug; on the other hand, this remedy is certainly recommended by eczematous affections co-existing with ophthalmia, particularly eczema of the ears; marked swelling of the lids and cheeks, and violent pains in the eye with rather scanty secretion. *Graphites*, likewise, should not be forgotten if exanthemata are present, more particularly if the trouble has already lasted for some time.

In the decidedly torpid form of ophthalmia the photophobia is not near as violent as in the erethic form, nor is it as lasting. It will not, therefore, be necessary to resort to Belladonna or Conium. In this form the disposition to the formation of pustules and ulceration of the cornea is more prominent, and may render the exhibition of Mercurius desirable; in general, however, *Hepar sulphuris* will act to better advantage. Hepar sulphuris is undoubtedly one of the most certain remedies in this affection, and is often alone sufficient to remove the disease speedily and completely. With Hartmann we likewise recommend the use of larger doses, second or third trituration. If the inflammation inclines to terminate in suppuration, and the deeper layers of the cornea have become attacked by the disorganizing process, *Sulphur* is undoubtedly appropriate, as it is likewise appropriate in the case of ulcers, the bottom of which remains persistently unclean. This remedy deserves particular attention if the cornea is covered with a firm exudation, or if pannus has formed and the affection evinces a decided disposition to run a protracted course. In this latter case, *Acidum nitricum* is likewise indicated.

Beside the medicines that have already been mentioned, we still have to point out two other remedies that are frequently used in scrofulous ophthalmia. One of them is *Arsenicum*. This remedy has undoubtedly a prominent effect upon the conjunctiva. It is particularly suitable in the chronic forms, where photophobia, excoriation and redness of the lids are constantly present, and where we have frequent exacerbations by a recurrence of the paroxysms. Such exacerbations are met with in thoroughly scrofulous constitutions, for which Arsenic, independently of the ophthalmic affection, has proved an excellent remedy. During the paroxysms the use of this medicine may be somewhat questionable; sometimes the photophobia seems to disappear more rapidly after the use of Arsenic; but then it is difficult to judge of the medicinal effect of a medicine, since a photophobia, which is very distressing one day, frequently disappears without any medicine on the day following. Arsenic is almost more than any other medicine indicated in affections of the cornea running a rapid course, where suppuration and infiltration reach such a high degree in one day that they threaten the destruction of the organ. The second remedy is *Apis mellifica*. We must confess, however, that in spite of the brilliant encomiums of the advocates of the honey-bee, and of the numerous trials we have made with it, we have not yet, in a single case, succeeded in producing with the honey-bee a single favorable effect in scrofulous ophthalmia. Hence our advice is not to experiment with the honey-bee until other well-tried remedies have been used in vain.

Of other remedies belonging to this class, or having been recommended for scrofulous ophthalmia, we note the following: *Pulsatilla, Staphysagria, Silicea, Cannabis, Ferrum, Calcarea carbonica*.

The treatment of the disease as an integral pathological condition requires the same general considerations, that will be mentioned more in detail when we come to treat of scrofulosis generally. Otherwise it is not always necessary to eradicate totally the scrofulous taint in order to prevent the recurrence of new attacks; all we are able to accomplish in many cases is to check the disposition to ophthalmia, whereas in other respects scrofulous phenomena may continue to remain. For a more detailed indication of the necessary remedies and dietetic rules we refer to the section on Scrofulosis; all we need do in this place is to confine ourselves to the special rules referring to the ophthalmic affection.

The intense photophobia, and the painful spasm of the lids caused by it, render the patients so apprehensive of the least ray of light penetrating into the interior of the eye, that they retreat to the darkest corner in the room, or bandage their eyes in order to pro tect them from the light. Neither one nor the other of these proceedings is proper. The former prevents the enjoyment of fresh air, the latter heats the eye. On the contrary, the eye should never be deprived of light altogether, and instead of bandaging the eye, it had better be protected by means of a dark pasteboard screen.

Not merely lay-persons, but even practitioners, sometimes try to assuage the pain by applying cold water compresses to the eye at the very height of the inflammatory process. It is, however, a peculiarity of scrofulous ophthalmia not to bear the application of cold water; at any rate, the inflammation is not moderated by it. It is sufficient to bathe the eyes frequently with warm water; this is likewise the best means of moderating the painful excoriation caused by the constant flow of tears.

As regards nourishment, we might easily be led by the idea that when an inflammation has to be subdued to confine the patient to a spare diet. This would be very wrong; on the contrary, the patient should have nourishing, although easily digested food. An excellent diet is good dried fruit, which does more to meliorate the digestion of scrofulous children than any other highly praised luxuries. It is strange that there is so much opposition to the use of fruit both among physicians and laymen. There is no reason for it. Only good fruit should be given. It will never produce bad effects, even if the digestive organs are ever so weak.

The three kinds of conjunctivitis of which we have treated constitute those ophthalmic affections that are of the utmost importance to the practical physician, because they occur the most frequently, and because he is generally expected to treat them. We have hesitated for a long time whether it was desirable to treat of the affections of the cornea and of the more deep-seated tissues of the eye, and at the same time to state what has been already accomplished in this direction by Homœopathy; but various reasons decided us to omit this part of ophthalmic surgery. The diagnosis of these affections requires all the different instruments peculiar to modern science, and their treatment requires the necessary operative skill, two suppositions which a practical physician can scarcely comply with for want of time. Moreover, we are not as yet in possession of the necessary provings which might enable us to contrast the pathological series with a corresponding pathogenesis. This section would therefore necessarily have remained very imperfect.

However, inasmuch as a physician who is somewhat isolated from other practitioners, may be placed under the necessity of treating affections of the internal eye, we cannot forbear indicating in subsequent paragraphs what has been accomplished by homœopathic treatment.

Inflammation of the cornea is generally a partial manifestation of conjunctivitis. The treatment of the former inflammation coincides with the treatment of conjunctivitis, as we have had occasion to show in former chapters where some particulars in this direction have already been furnished. Where the cornea is primarily affected, the choice of the remedy depends upon the peculiar manner in which the exudative process establishes itself. For pannus the most efficient remedies are: *Hepar sulphuris*, *Euphrasia*, *Baryta carbonica* and *Calcarea carbonica*. For abscesses of the cornea *Mercurius* is the main remedy, so much the more, the more the suppuration is circumscribed within definite limits. For purulent infiltration and threatening rapid disorganization of the cornea *Arsenicum* is the most trustworthy remedy. *Iodium*, *Sulphur*, *Silicea*, deserve our attention in chronic exudative processes. We must never lose sight of the fact that affections of the cornea, corresponding to the peculiar structure of this organ, run a very protracted course and that, on this account, we cannot expect a rapid effect from the medicines we may have to prescribe.

The sclerotica is seldom affected isolatedly. Sclerotitis is generally symptomatic of the so-called rheumatic ophthalmia, and is of importance in so far as it calls our attention to certain remedies which might perhaps not be thought of in simple conjunctivitis. A fine, uniform, rose-colored redness round the margin of the cornea is the characteristic symptom of this affection which is but too easily confounded with conjunctivitis. This phenomenon may likewise constitute one of the symptoms of iritis.

Iritis, like corneitis, is seldom an idiopathic disease, but is generally a symptom of general ophthalmia. As a primary affection it most frequently depends upon syphilis. At the commencement of the disease, when there is no syphilitic taint at the bottom of it, *Belladonna*, and perhaps also *Aconite*, may have to be prescribed, but always only at the commencement of the attack; for owing to the rapid course of the disease, we very soon have to resort to *Mercurius* as the main remedy, which should be exhibited in the form of *Corrosive Sublimate*. In the further course of the disease, when the exudation has come to its end, *Sulphur* and *Iodine* are indicated. Hypopyon does not require special mention, since, as a general rule, it is rapidly reabsorbed.

Cataracts are generally considered incurable by internal remedies. This proposition has been refuted in Homœopathy by a number of successful cures, and we can boldly assert that we have succeeded in controlling this disorder by the use of internal agents. Unfortunately, however, when the proper remedy is to be selected, we are compelled to admit that we have not yet succeeded in determining what remedies are adapted to the different forms of cataract. The main remedies are: *Phosphorus, Pulsatilla, Sulphur, Calcarea carbonica, Lycopodium;* the less certain and less tried remedies are: *Silicea, Cannabis, Euphrasia.* Of course we do not mean to say tha' we can remove every cataract by homœopathic remedies. As a general rule we can only say that the prognosis is so much more favorable the younger the patient, the shorter and the less developed the disorder. In the case of old people, where cataract may be regarded as a gradual dying out of the lens, it would be absurd to suppose that internal treatment is of any use. The prognosis of capsular cataract is more favorable than that of any other form.

By means of the ophthalmoscope the diseases of the retina have latterly been much better appreciated and diagnosed than at any former period. We are as yet unable to indicate therapeutic proceedings adapted to this advance in diagnostic means; in given cases we prefer referring the reader to a good Repertory by means of which the remedy corresponding to the generally subjective symptoms of the patient, can most easily be found.

D. DISEASES OF THE EAR.

As regards diseases of the ears, we are still worse off than in diseases of the eyes. In general the diagnosis is a very difficult one, sometimes impossible; how then shall we be able to select the right remedy? We have to confine ourselves to furnishing a cursory and condensed list of the pathological conditions and remedies, with which a somewhat empirical and not very reliable use at the sick-bed has made us acquainted; for the selection of a remedy in accordance with a symptomatic similarity, is still more deceptive in the case of ear-affections than in other morbid conditions; nevertheless, it happens but too often that we have nothing else to fall back upon than symptomatic similarities. The inflammatory processes in the interior of the ears are among the less frequent diseases, but are of particular importance for the reason that the brain becomes so readily involved in the inflammatory process, especially when it is localized in the inner ear. An inflammation of the outer ear likewise tends powerfully to pass to the inner ear; it is for this reason that we treat these two forms of inflammation of the ears somewhat more in detail.

1. Otitis Interna.
Internal Inflammation of the Ear.

Inflammation of the inner ear is chiefly recognized by the extraordinary pain it causes. The pain is chiefly a tearing, throbbing or burning pain, is very much increased by motion, likewise by chewing, loud noise, contact of the outer parts. Inflammatory earache is one of the most distressing tortures that man can suffer. The excruciating character of this pain accounts for the cerebral irritation which is almost always present in this disease. The fever is very violent, and the pulse hurried and small. The head glows, whereas the extremities are cold as ice; delirium and fainting fits set in, before the brain can be said to sympathize with the distress. The outer ear usually shows signs of inflammation; the meatus auditorius is swollen, sometimes entirely closed, red and very sensitive, and the swelling spreads to the ear and the surrounding soft parts. Otitis is very apt to result in suppuration, and is still more inclined to spread to the brain, more particularly if the cells of the mastoid process are inflamed. It is not certain whether the invasion of the brain takes place more easily when the inflammatory process has reached its height, or after the pus has begun to form. Suppuration supervenes but too frequently during the course of a chronic affection of the bones; hence suppuration of the mastoid process may involve the brain and lead to a fatal termination even after all danger consequent upon inflammation seems to be entirely removed. Otitis may be complicated with a meningitis which runs a very rapid course, and is one of the most dangerous diseases. Its treatment has already been indicated in a former chapter. Otitis may terminate in favorable cases in complete recovery; this result, however, is rare; generally a disturbance of the functions of the ear remains behind, sometimes assuming the form of perfect deafness. If pus forms, it is fortunate if it is discharged externally, even if the tympanum should be greatly injured and chronic otorrhœa should be the result.

The causes of otitis cannot be mentioned with positive certainty.

A cold is said to be one of the chief causes. Whether, as Hartmann imagines, otitis may arise from suppressed itch, is very questionable; it is undoubtedly a convenient thing, after the previous existence of the itch has been ascertained with great trouble, to refer to it all chronic as well as acute ailments, even after years had elapsed between the itch and the subsequent disease. On the contrary it does happen that violent acute and sub-acute cutaneous diseases involve the ear in the pathological process, in which case the outer ear is, of course, first attacked by the inflammation, which thence spreads to the inner. Among the dyscrasia's it is particularly syphilis and scrofulosis by which the ear is attacked.

Treatment. We will first transcribe the following passage from Hartmann, page 551: "My experience in the treatment of otitis with delirium and agonizing pains, with swelling and closing of the outer meatus, swelling of the ear and the adjoining parts, induce me to regard *Pulsatilla* as the specific remedy in this form of otitis. I rejoice at being able to communicate this experience to my colleagues, for, as far as I know, no one before me suspected that Pulsatilla had this specific curative power in otitis. Otitis from internal causes is a comparatively rare occurrence, and this may be the reason why but few homœopathic practitioners may have met with it in their practice, and, for this reason, may not have had an opportunity of employing Pulsatilla in this disease. Lest a physician who may have a case of otitis to treat should be dissuaded from using Pulsatilla on account of the presence of some symptoms in the pathological group which do not occur in the pathogenesis of the drug, I will add that every homœopath undoubtedly knows from Hahnemann's Materia Medica, that Pulsatilla must not be given where excessive thirst and constipation are prominent symptoms; nevertheless, in spite of these symptoms, which are always present in this form of otitis, I have never hesitated to prescribe Pulsatilla, and the success which I have uniformly met with, has satisfied me that the presence of thirst and costiveness in this disease are no counter-indication to Pulsatilla.

"Now although abundant experience has satisfied me that Pulsatilla is the specific remedy in otitis where the external and internal inflammations run a parallel course, both break out simultaneously, and are equally acute and violent, yet there are cases where Pulsatilla is not sufficient, and where *Belladonna* has to be given in its place; this is the case when the internal inflammation is, from the start, more acute than the external, or when the consensual affections of the brain, which are closely bordering on meningitis, such as a feeling of intense pain in the head, delirium and rage, convulsions, fainting-fits, aphonia and the like, are very prominent. In this latter case *Rhus tox.* may prove a valuable drug."

If Hartmann asserts, that with appropriate homœopathic treatment, he has always been able to prevent the inflammation from terminating in suppuration, all we can say is that this result speaks equally well for the superiority of the treatment as for the success of the physician, for not every one can·boast of such favorable results in his practice. Suppuration will sometimes set in, in which case we shall find *Mercurius* the chief remedy. It will be found particularly suitable in cases where syphilitic individuals are attacked with the inflammation, provided they have not already taken Mercury in massive doses; otherwise it is perfectly appropriate. Side by side with Mercurius we have *Hepar sulphuris*, in cases marked by a highly developed scrofulous taint or mercurial-syphilitic poisoning.

In cases running an unfavorable course, the discharge of pus from the outer ear becomes profuse, the pus has a cadaverous odor, is ichorous, and the symptoms of a sudden collapse are very apt to supervene. In such desperate cases *Arsenicum* may sometimes be able to afford relief, and where symptoms of pyæmia have become prevalent, more particularly pyæmia of the lungs, *Phosphorus* is the only remedy from which help may still be expected, provided it is not too late. In a case to which we were called one day previous to the patient's death, after the disease had already lasted four weeks, the pyæmic affection had reached the highest degree of development. The patient unfortunately was already moribund, and medical action was out of the question. If the suppuration has resulted in carious destruction of the ossicula, without any of the terrible symptoms that have just been described, *Lycopodium* sometimes affords help, together with *Sulphur* and *Silicca*.

[An interesting case of otitis interna, with discharge of foul-smelling pus, constant buzzing in the ears, agonizing pains in the ear from the moment the patient, a young lady of thirteen years, retired to rest until the morning, partial deafness, and very painful and considerable swelling of the mastoid process, yielded as if by magic to a single drop of *Mercurius vivus*, 30. The case had been going on for nearly two years, and the symptoms were steadily increasing in violence. The noises in the head were exceedingly distressing, and the sensitiveness of the ear and the adjoining parts intense.

The patient took a single drop of Merc. viv. 30, at bedtime; in about an hour the distress vanished utterly, the young lady slept all night, woke perfectly free from any of the above-mentioned symptoms, and has never been troubled with earache since. The deafness continues to some extent, probably owing to the partial destruction of the tympanum and the ossicula, but otherwise no trace of the otitis or earache is visible. The cure was effected some years ago. H.]

2. Otitis externa.

As we remarked above, an inflammation of the external meatus usually accompanies an inflammation of the internal ear, and, by its presence, always reveals the existence of a higher grade of otitis interna. As an idiopathic affection, disposed, however, to extend to the inner parts of the ear, it is either an inflammation of the cellular tissue in the external meatus, spreading uniformly all around, very painful, but not very dangerous and of short duration, or else it consists in suppuration of one or more glands of the outer meatus auditorius. In such a case a small abscess is seen on one or the other side, more or less deeply in the inner ear. In this form of the inflammation the pain is likewise comparatively very acute, but usually ceases all at once, when at its height, by the bursting of the abscess. This inflammation very frequently accompanies, as a complicating disorder, an inflammation of the parotid gland or of other adjoining parts. Erysipelas likewise does not unfrequently attack the outer ear, and, if it begins at the ear itself, may lead to errors in diagnosis.

For idiopathic otitis, the chief remedies, when the cellular tissue is the seat of the disease, are *Bryonia* and *Pulsatilla ; Mercurius* is principally indicated by the formation of an abscess; likewise *Chamomilla,* which generally, however, has already been abused as a domestic remedy when the physician is called. In the secondary forms the remedies which are adapted to the primary disease, upon which the otitis depends, are alone appropriate.

[We wonder, that *Aconite* is not mentioned by the author as a remedy for otitis, whether internal or external. In rheumatic otitis, with dark redness of the inflamed part, stinging, lancing and throbbing pain in the ear, swelling and great sensitiveness of the outer ear, discharge of blood and purulent serum from the ear, *Aconite-Radix;* a drop of the tincture, or a few drops of the first decimal attenuation, in a small goblet of water, in dessert-spoonful doses every half hour or hour, will be found an indispensable remedy. It sometimes is advantageously given in alternation with *Belladonna.* H.]

As a consequence of otitis, but sometimes from other causes, we frequently meet with a discharge from the ears, which is at times slimy, at others purulent or ichorous, at others again watery or bloody. The slimy discharge is of a catarrhal nature, makes its appearance in the cases of many children, whenever they are attacked with a severe cold, and has no special significance. As a general rule, it very soon yields to a few doses of *Pulsatilla.* The other forms of otorrhœa are symptomatic manifestations of otitis, and require the same treatment as this disease. Injections of lukewarm water have always a good effect, and should never be omitted.

Hardness of hearing may depend upon a variety of causes, by the peculiar nature of which its curability is determined. If it proceeds directly from the auditory nerve, and is the commencement of complete deafness, it is not likely that much can be done for it by internal treatment. If we choose to try it, we may use *Causticum, Petroleum, Platina, Plumbum.* If the deafness is caused by a stoppage of the meatus externus, various obstacles may prevent the free entrance of sound. The most common obstacle is the accumulation of indurated cerumen in front of the tympanum. This is most effectually removed by continued injections of lukewarm water, until the plug is loosened, after which it can readily be grasped with a pair of pincers and drawn out. If an unopened abscess is the cause, which is not often the case, its reabsorption is easily accomplished by frequently dropping lukewarm water into the ear, which has to be retained in it for some time. A polypus in the meatus may, if possible, be twisted or cut off; where this is not possible, the polypus can gradually be caused to shrink, by touching it frequently with the half diluted tincture of Thuya. If the tympanum is injured, a cure is, of course, impossible; in such cases the patients hear often much better by inserting a loose plug of cotton in the ear. This custom is so common with many people, that they are never seen without cotton in their ears. It is a bad habit, which favors more than any other proceeding the formation of little plugs of ear-wax; for, the nuclei of most plugs, which we have removed in large numbers, were found to consist of cotton-fibres. Still more hurtful is the habit of introducing medicinal substances into the ear. We are acquainted with a lady who has been using Camphor in this manner until her tympanum has become perforated in consequence. If little children are hard of hearing, we have to ascertain, in every case, whether they have not inserted some foreign body in their ears.

Just as frequently, as upon changes in the external meatus, does hardness of hearing depend upon stricture or stoppage of the Eustachian tube. Such a defect may easily be caused by a severe catarrh of the nasal fossa, likewise by considerable hypertrophy of the tonsils. Here we have, of course, to employ the remedies that will be mentioned in subsequent chapters, when treating of the affections of the nasal and buccal cavities.

E. DISEASES OF THE NOSE.

1. Coryza, Catarrh, Cold in the Head.

Catarrh of the nasal mucous membrane is one of the most common and most frequently occurring affections, is of very little inherent importance, and is considered as a mere pathological trifle by our therapeutic opponents, not worth the trouble of having anything done for it, although the real cause of this omission is that they really have no remedy for it. It is for this very reason that a catarrh is particularly interesting to us, the same as toothache, for which we have a good many efficient remedies; a lay person is often more astonished at the sudden cure of a catarrh or a toothache, by a few of our little powders, than at the most brilliant cure of a case of pneumonia. He has had catarrh often enough to be thoroughly acquainted with its course; hence he is surprised at seeing it shortened by treatment.

A simple catarrh arises from a cold. Individuals who watch themselves somewhat, know very well that, if they feel chilly from exposing themselves to a current of air after being heated, they will have a catarrh within twelve hours. Severe attacks always commence with a febrile sensation, lassitude, dull headache, especially above the root of the nose. At first the nose is drier than usual, sensitive to cool air, the smell is sometimes remarkably affected; there is a tingling in the nose and a desire to sneeze. If a discharge takes place at the commencement, it is generally very tenacious, yellowish, or almost entirely watery. In most cases the adjoining parts are involved, especially the tonsils, which are slightly reddened, and where a stinging pain is experienced. The larynx is likewise affected, the speech being somewhat hoarse. A peculiar symptom is the remarkable frequency of the pulse, with which some persons become affected at the commencement of a catarrh, and the striking elevation of the temperature. Among children particularly the constitutional symptoms are much more striking than among adults; whereas the latter continue in the enjoyment of a sound sleep, children, on the contrary, spend restless nights. Usually after the lapse of twenty-four hours a copious secretion of mucus takes place, after which the patient feels better and the constitutional symptoms disappear. Within nine days at most, the patient is completely restored to health, unless a relapse should have taken place. This very common form of catarrh scarcely requires to be treated medicinally. Cases may, however, occur, where the secretion remains copious and watery for three or four days, the patient feeling very much indisposed and very anxious to be freed from his complaint. Moreover, in the course of the catarrh, relapses may take place, in consequence of which the febrile exacerbations may increase to such an extent that a catarrh, which was at first quite unimportant, becomes a real torture.

Under favorable circumstances, especially if the patient exposes himself to frequent relapses or is otherwise constitutionally predisposed to the complaint, the acute form passes into the chronic. Generally the chronic form consists in a profuse secretion of mucus, without any other trouble. Frequently, however, the profuse mucous secretion is accompanied by swelling of the mucous membrane and impeded respiration. After a number of relapses the swelling increases to such a degree, that breathing through the nose becomes impossible, which gives rise to a number of ailments: the speech has a nasal twang, the throat hurts in consequence of the dryness induced by breathing exclusively with the mouth open, and sleep is variously disturbed. These difficulties remain even after the mucous secretion has entirely ceased; in that case they are even more unbearable than before. If there is a peculiar predisposition, such as scrofulosis, the internal parts of the nose become inflamed side by side with the catarrhal irritation, and an ulcerative process sets in, which secretes a foul-smelling purulent matter, (ozæna.) A bad smell from the nose may, however, take place, without any ulceration. The structural changes in the mucous membrane frequently give rise to fungoid growths, polypus, etc. We may as well relate here a case of ozæna, which originated in a peculiar manner. On a certain occasion a farmer showed us his little three years old daughter, with the remark that she was always troubled with catarrh, and that the discharge had a very bad smell. An examination showed that the left nostril was stopped up, with a partly whitish and partly blackish-gray substance. On removing it with a pair of pincers it proved to be a bean, which had swelled up very much and had become rotten. The ozæna, which had lasted upwards of six months, ceased at once.

Of the catarrh caused by syphilis we shall treat in the chapters devoted to that disease.

A catarrh is usually very seldom present during other inflammatory affections; if it exists before the latter, it generally disappears as soon as the latter affections break out. This circumstance may have given rise to the story of retrocession of a catarrh, and is of particular importance in croup, where it is so easy, at the commencement of the disease, to make a wrong diagnosis. We can scarcely ever be mistaken if, in cases where the peculiar croupy sound of the cough, and other symptoms of incipient croup are accompanied by catarrh, we diagnose catarrhal croup, and promise a rapid improvement, which scarcely ever fails us. No more frequently, or scarcely ever, will catarrh be met with as an accompaniment of pneumonia.

Catarrh will only have to be treated medicinally, if it is accompanied at the onset by symptoms of severe constitutional disturbance, or the catarrhal phenomena themselves are unusually violent. The symptoms during the first twenty-four hours generally demand *Aconite; Belladonna* may have to be used, if the tonsils are inflamed. If the subsequent symptoms, except their intensity, are like those of a common catarrh, if the discharge is slimy, *Mercurius solubilis* is a distinguished remedy, which will scarcely be surpassed by any other. If the secretion is very copious, the lips and nose become rapidly excoriated, the headache is very violent, and particularly at the root of the nose a burning and stinging pain is felt, and the constitutional symptoms are very prominent and intense, *Arsenicum* acts almost instantaneously. The other medicines belonging to this series will be mentioned in the chapter on Influenza, since they will be found more particularly appropriate, if, beside the nose, the larynx, trachea and lungs are likewise affected. In the case of infants at the breast, a catarrh, even if it runs its ordinary course, becomes a source of distress, because it prevents them from nursing. In such cases *Pulsatilla* may afford more relief than any other remedy; if the catarrh breaks out during the period of dentition, *Chamomilla* may be preferable.

The chronic form of coryza is, under all circumstances, a very obstinate complaint. This is probably owing to the circumstance that such patients do not take the least care of themselves, and that the swelling of the nasal membrane is constantly increased by new relapses. The more the swelling increases, the more difficult it is to cure the complaint. In recent cases *Mercurius* and *Hepar sulphuris* may render good service. In neglected cases *Sulphur* and *Iodium* often afford help; the latter especially deserves attention. *Kali bichromicum* has been praised beyond its due; it is useful only when the coryza is attended with soreness and ulceration of the nose. *Calcarea carbonica* is indispensable in cases depending upon scrofulosis, and where the discharge has a foul odor. In real ozæna *Aurum* is by far the best remedy; we prefer *Aurum muriaticum*, the metallic gold is much less reliable. *Alumen* has likewise been recommended for ozæna.

[In the 22d volume of the British Journal of Homœopathy, the following interesting case of cure of ozæna with the Permanganate of Potash is copied from the Paris Gazette des Hôpitaux: The patient was an English young lady, at school in Paris. Her breath was so offensive, that her presence in the school-room had become unpleasant to her companions. Her approach caused nausea, and in one instance severe vomiting was induced. Cauterization, injections of every description had proved unavailing. Sir I. Olliffe now resorted to injections of the Permanganate of Potash. They were repeated every three hours, and in the course of three weeks the offensive odor had entirely disappeared, and the patient was again able to associate with her companions. Alternate injections of the Permanganate and Chlorate of Potash were continued for some time longer, and the patient remained permanently cured. The Permanganate was likewise used internally, as follows: Thirty-six grains of the Permanganate to five drachms of syrup of orange-blossoms and six ounces of water, a tablespoonful three times a day.]

In view of the obstinacy of chronic coryza and of the bad consequences it may entail, among which loss of smell is one of the most important, it is certainly advisable to devise a course of treatment that shall prevent relapses. One of the most useful means, to accomplish this result, is a gradual hardening of the whole body by means of cold water. Cold water is altogether an important remedial agent in the treatment of catarrh. When drunk at the onset of an acute attack, in considerable quantity, it very soon moderates the most disagreeable sensations; and, in the chronic form, it renders good service when drawn up into the nose several times during the day. This last-mentioned use of water likewise acts as an excellent prophylactic. For catarrh, properly speaking, it is better to draw up tepid instead of cold water; tepid water loosens the tough mucus better than cold. In the chronic form, likewise, cold water is often much less suitable than warm water, which feels much more pleasant. That it has a favorable effect upon existing ulcers, is evident a priori, were it only by cleansing the suppurating surface and preventing the formation of crusts. It is well known that copious draughts of some lukewarm beverage are likewise recommended for catarrh; it is undeniable that it has an excellent effect in catarrhal conditions of the respiratory organs. This management, however, seems so annoying to many persons, that only a few are willing to take this trouble. Of much more importance is the use of water in the epidemic catarrh of the respiratory organs; we shall revert to its use when treating of this disease. An ordinary proceeding in domestic practice is to excite a profuse perspiration. It is undeniable that this proceeding moderates the course of a catarrh, almost without an exception. Nevertheless serious doubts may be entertained against such a course. In the first place, sweat is sought to be excited by medicinal herbs. This conduct is decidedly reprehensible, for the reason that the organism should never be drenched with medicinal decoctions without the most urgent necessity. And, in the second place, the skin is rendered more susceptible to cold, which is much worse than that the first cold should remain uncured. If the skin is to be excited to increased action, the best and least hurtful means to accomplish this, is a moderate vapor-bath; or, if we desire to excite perspiration in the bed, we may drink a glass of warm water with a little syrup.

We have to devote a few remarks to polypi in the nasal fossa. If we except the cancerous growth, there are two distinct kinds of polypi. One is a simple fungoid growth of the nasal mucous membrane, and owes its origin to chronic catarrh; the other is rather an idiopathic growth with vessels and cellular tissue. These excrescences sometimes impede respiration to such an extent, that they have to be removed either by an operation, or by medicinal treatment. That the latter is sometimes adequate to their removal, has been placed beyond all question by numerous successful results. In treating a nasal polypus, we use the following remedies: *Teucrium marum verum*, especially for mucous polypi, to be used internally and externally; as an external application we use the pulverized herb as snuff. *Calcarea carbonica*, in the higher attenuations, is recommended by many authorities, likewise for polypous excrescences of the Schneiderian membrane. We have never been able to obtain any good from its use in this disease. Against sarcomatous polypi we frequently find useful: *Kali bichromicum, Phosphorus* or *Sulphur*. The result of the treatment, however, in such cases, is much less favorable than that of mucous polypi.

2. Inflammation of the Nose, Nasitis.

Inflammation of the Schneiderian membrane generally occurs under the form of a more or less intense catarrh, of which it is very frequently a symptomatic manifestation. The ulcerative process to which attention has been called when treating of catarrh, depends upon this inflammation. The treatment is conducted with the same remedies that have already been indicated in the former chapter.

There is another form of nasitis where single follicles are attacked, in consequence of which abscesses form. This disorder is very painful, and it is desirable that its course should be shortened as much as possible. The best remedy for this purpose is *Mercurius; Hepar Sulphuris* may likewise prove useful. In some cases, if the affection is just beginning, it may be well to commence the treatment with *Belladonna*. The application of a warm fluid does the same good here as in any other abscess.

Inflammations of the nose, which constitute partial manifestations of other constitutional affections, will be spoken of in connection with the latter, where the proper treatment will likewise be explained.

A peculiar inflammation of the nasal mucous membrane, which bears the greatest resemblance to eczema of the external skin, and frequently spreads in the form of an eczematous process to the external nose and to the lips, results in a continual formation of crusts and runs a very slow course, requires for its cure *Mercurius, Kali bichromicum,* or in more chronic cases, *Graphites*. Inasmuch as the cure does not take place very rapidly, it is well not to change the remedy too soon. [A case of phlegmonous nasitis, with a large ulcer at the tip of the nose, was radically cured in five days with the German tincture of Aconite. H.]

3. Epistaxis, Bleeding at the Nose.

Bleeding at the nose is one of the most frequent occurrences; no organ is as easily inclined to bleed as the nose, the cause of which has to be sought in the peculiarly delicate structure of its mucous membrane, in its great vascularity, and in the circumstance that the nose is remarkably exposed to external influences and injuries.

Bleeding at the nose generally sets in unexpectedly without any precursory symptoms, which, when existing, consist of congestion about the head, such as headache, vertigo, buzzing in the ears, etc., or fever. Generally the bleeding takes place only from one nostril, and, as regards quantity, varies from a few coagula, mixed with nasal mucus, to whole pounds. Sometimes it is a scarcely perceptible flow of blood, sometimes a mere dribbling of a few drops, and sometimes, but very seldom, the blood rushes out in torrents. According as the bleeding vessel is located, the blood is poured forth from the external nostrils, or else from the posterior nares into the pharynx. The latter result is apt to occur at night during sleep. On waking, the patient vomits up the blood, or, if it had run into the larynx, it is coughed up, leading both the physician and the patient to suppose that he had an attack of hæmoptoë, so much the more when the other coexisting symptoms render this supposition more or less founded in fact.

The bleeding may continue from a few seconds to whole days. If the single turns follow each other in rapid succession, it may often seem as if the bleeding continued for days.

The causes are various; but if a good deal of blood is lost, it is always desirable to investigate them with accuracy. There undoubtedly is such a thing as a constitutional predisposition to nose-bleed, in consequence of which the vessels are abnormally inclined to fill up and burst. This predisposition may even be hereditary, although it does not show itself in the looks of the individual. Besides this, a marked hyperæmia of the nose, or even of the whole head, is one of the most frequent causes; likewise mechanical impressions, ulcers of the mucous membrane, and finally a peculiar composition of the blood which favors the exudation of the blood, as in typhus, scurvy, anæmia, hæmorrhoidal dyscrasia. The frequent appearance of nose-bleed at a time when the barometer is very low, causes us to adopt the theory that the atmosphere exerts a peculiar pressure, resulting more particularly in the production of congestions about the head.

Although nose-bleed, as we stated above, is, generally speaking, an occurrence of trifling importance, yet, under certain circumstances, it acquires a peculiar significance. In the first place, the quantity of the blood that is lost by one or by a series of successive bleedings, may be so great that the most dangerous symptoms of anæmia may result from such a loss. In the next place, the hemorrhage is dangerous in such conditions as anæmia and typhus, which do not bear any loss of blood. It is undoubtedly wrong to view the nose-bleed in such conditions as a critical endeavor of the organism, although such a view seems justified by a momentary amelioration of single symptoms, especially the congestive head symptoms. Such an improvement is very soon followed by a so much more disagreeable exacerbation. Nature thus points out the value we are to attach to artificial bleedings, and that they at most only palliate the distress at the expense of the general organism. In little children and old people, nose-bleed is always a dangerous occurrence.

In treating this disorder, as a matter of course, the exciting causes are of great importance. Where the symptoms of violent congestion of the head are present, the remedies which we have recommended for cerebral hyperæmia, particularly *Belladonna*, *Aconite*, *Nux vomica*, [also *Gelseminum* and *Veratrum viride*], are especially to be kept in view. At the commencement of a general acute disease, *Bryonia alba* is the best remedy; but it is not here alone that it is useful, but likewise in the bleedings depending upon strongly-marked venous hyperæmia of the brain, and belonging rather in the category of passive hemorrhages. If such bleedings set in without any other accessory symptoms or fever, we give *Crocus* and *China*; the last-named, more particularly, where distinct symptoms of anæmia were already present previous to the hemorrhage. In the subsequent course of acute affections, with decomposition of the blood, *Arsenicum*, *Lachesis* and *Secale cornutum* are mostly to be commended. Hartmann has seen *Moschus* act with quick success in cases where jactitation of the muscles had already set in in consequence of the loss of blood.

As a general rule the above-mentioned remedies will be found sufficient; in particular cases one of the following remedies may have to be chosen: *Conium maculatum*, *Acidum muriaticum* and *sulfuricum*, *Arnica*, *Ferrum* and *Ipecacuanha;* the last-mentioned especially in the case of little children.

If the nose-bleed has become habitual, we should try to extirpate the disposition. If constitutional symptoms are present, we have to proceed against these; if the bleeding is an isolated symptom,

Sulphur, Lycopodium, Acidum nitricum, Ferrum have to be tried. With *Hamamelis virginiana*, which has been so universally recommended, we have never yet obtained the least result.

The employment of medicines externally has two sides. The application of cold water to the nose may sometimes be very useful; on the other hand drawing up cold water in the nose will too readily prevent the necessary formation of thrombus. Hot hand-baths may be tried, but hot foot-baths are more hurtful than useful. In arterial hemorrhage we have often derived benefit from placing a piece of coarse filtering paper under the tongue. We do not know how to account for this result, but we do know that the result has been obtained and that the paper is frequently resorted to in domestic practice.

[*Tanacetum*, our Tansy, often arrests epistaxis, when other remedies fail. H.]

THIRD SECTION.

Diseases of the Mouth, Fauces and Œsophagus.

In no chapter of pathology does such a confusion of nomenclature prevail, as among the diseases of the mouth and pharynx. There are scarcely two authors who use the same names for the same pathological processes occurring in these parts, and it takes considerable trouble to find one's way through this labyrinth. In homœopathic literature the thing is still worse, for the reports of special cases are generally prefaced by an unmeaning diagnosis. What is the use of such reports? They have no other use than to fill our periodicals. In spite of numerous and energetic remonstrances cases are reported in our Journals with the same superficiality as before. At the same time, as this is of very little use to ourselves, our opponents use this weak side in our literature as a point of attack, in order to prove the nothingness and erroneousness of our pretended cures, and in many cases we must admit that they are correct. The fact that reports of cures of the most important pathological processes still continue to be dispatched in a few lines, shows a censurable ignoring of that which is most needful to us. A system of Therapeutics corresponding to the spirit of Homœopathy, can only be built upon a large number of isolated observations. In the present condition of our School this end is still far from being attained, and the demand for an exhaustive system of Therapeutics is not founded in reason. In order to accomplish a work of this kind, all must co-operate, otherwise we cannot expect to succeed;—nor can we succeed unless all work together according to the same plan. Who would undertake to publish the results of our treatment of diseases of the skin, if one reports them under one name, and another under another? The same criticism applies to diseases of the mouth and throat.

We have premised these remarks in order to justify the apparently arbitrary classification we have adopted in the following paragraphs. We found it inconvenient to follow Hartmann's example;

his method of separating the affections of the same organ, presents many disadvantages, and the nomenclature he has adopted, is not at all positively acceptable to science.

1. Stomatitis.

We comprehend under this name all the catarrhal affections of the mouth and fauces, from simple hyperæmia to the formation of erosions, aphthæ.

The hyperæmia of the mucous membrane of the mouth has, in most cases, neither a pathological, much less a therapeutic interest, and is, generally speaking, a mere symptom of some more general disease. In a few rare cases it is, to some extent, an idiopathic affection, shows a tendency to run a chronic course, and torments the patients to such a degree that it becomes necessary to proceed against it. In such cases we find certain places of the mucous membrane, most frequently the arch of the palate and the dorsum of the tongue, covered with spots of various sizes, of a uniform bright, and very seldom of a dark, redness, causing a feeling of intense burning, impeding mastication, and frequently disappearing very suddenly in order to break out again in some other part, and running altogether a very obstinate course. We have observed this not very frequent affection in two female patients, both of whom had cancer of the womb; we have likewise noticed it in three ladies, members of the same family, who otherwise enjoyed perfect health, so that we could not help suspecting a certain degree of contagiousness. In these three persons the disease acted very capriciously; sometimes the parts would remain perfectly sound for weeks, after which period the disease would break out again. There was no ptyalism, nor could the disease be traced to any definite cause; it was perfectly certain that syphilis and hydrargyrosis were not the exciting causes.

The more intense hyperæmia of the mouth and fauces, which is very nearly allied to inflammation, is likewise rarely met with as an idiopathic affection, and is important in a practical point of view only in so far as ulcers are apt to form. It is always accompanied by febrile motions.

A catarrhal affection of the mouth and fauces accompanies the most diversified diseases of the digestive apparatus, as well as of the organs adjoining the mouth, and acquires importance not so much from its inherent dignity as from the fact that by it we determine the condition of other organs. The coating of the tongue, for instance, which depends upon the degree and form of stomatitis, is, undoubtedly, an important diagnostic sign. The main symptoms of catarrh of the mouth are painfulness, which is particularly prominent in the case of little children, altered taste, secretion of a greater or less quantity of tenacious mucus, attended with diminished secretion of saliva, fetid smell from the mouth, sometimes frontal headache. If the fauces are prominently affected, we have the picture of angina catarrhalis, of which we shall treat more fully further on, in the chapter on Angina. The chronic form of catarrhal stomatitis is likewise characterized by an unusual secretion of mucus, altered taste and bad smell from the mouth, which is even perceptible to the patient. Of more importance is the chronic form of catarrh of the fauces, which is a source of great annoyance. It is generally met with among singers, smokers, drinkers, and is, likewise, one of the remote consequences of syphilis. If the affection springs from the last-mentioned cause, it fills the patients with great anxiety, because they are in constant dread of a syphilitic affection in the mouth. It is generally confined to the posterior wall of the pharynx; the tonsils, however, are frequently involved in the morbid process. The affected part shows a somewhat deeper redness, is traversed with distinctly injected, varicose vessels, is more or less swollen, sometimes exhibiting granulations, and at times streaks of swelling, so that the mucous membrane seems divided in regular parallel puffy elevations, between and on top of which streaks of a very tenacious, yellow mucus are seen. This secretion of tenacious mucus is the greatest torture to the patients, for the affection is not painful of itself, but only becomes so when, by the constant efforts made to hawk up the mucus, the mucous membrane of the fauces becomes irritated. This trouble is always very obstinate.

In one category with the catarrhal affection, we may range two processes which generally originate in it, and are of some interest to the physician, namely: the exfoliations and superficial ulcerations of the mucous membrane, and aphthæ.

The former pathological process, sometimes designated as stomatitis or even diphtheritis, occurs both among children and adults; its causes, however, are wrapped in obscurity. The disease begins with the symptoms of acute catarrh or hyperæmia, sometimes with, but generally, without fever. Circumscribed spots are seen on the tongue or mucous lining of the cheeks, red, sensitive, and we soon discover that the epithelium at these spots is abraded. Sometimes the trouble does not progress any further, but generally the abraded spots change to ulcers of the size of split peas, and having an unclean aspect; they heal very slowly. Some ptyalism and fetor from the mouth are generally present. This process which, if occurring but once, lasts from one to two weeks, frequently inclines to relapses, which succeed each other with more or less rapidity, and differ greatly as regards duration and intensity. At this point the disorder becomes very obstinate.

By aphthæ we understand a peculiar vesicular disorganization of the buccal mucous lining. Aphthæ generally set in with the symptoms of acute catarrh of the mouth, seldom without premonitory symptoms, having the appearance of small, watery or whitish vesicles on the lips, tongue or cheeks, surrounded by a narrow, red areola. They soon break, leaving small ulcerations of the epithelium, with a yellow or yellow-gray base, and a vividly red, sharply circumscribed border. With the outbreak of the vesicles, the fever often disappears, and only continues if the eruption, instead of breaking out all at once, makes its appearance in a successive series of crops. The single little ulcer usually heals very rapidly, and it is only under very unfavorable circumstances that more deeply-penetrating ulcerations and diphtheritic membranous formations take the place of the simple aphthæ.

Stomatitis proper, that is, inflammation of the mucous lining of the mouth, and pharyngitis, commences with the symptoms of a violent, more or less extensive hyperæmia, from which, however, it soon differs by the greater swelling of the more especially affected parts, particularly the gums. Every part of the mouth is very painful, not even the softest nourishment can be taken without intense pain; if infants are the victims of this disorder, they refuse the breast very obstinately. In the further course of the disease, the gums look dark-red, with whitish streaks, but, at any rate at the beginning, without any loss of substance. There is no increased secretion of mucus, but profuse ptyalism, with metallic taste and disagreeable odor of the breath. Fever is always present, sometimes to a high degree, and attended with the most threatening cerebral symptoms. After a while the digestion becomes impaired, the deficient nutrition leads to a loss of strength, which is still increased by the fact that the sleep is usually very much disturbed. In the higher grades of the inflammation the salivary glands are always very much inflamed, swollen and painful.

This disorder scarcely ever runs a rapid course; it lasts at least seven days, and may become very much protracted by secondary ulcerations and inflammation of the salivary glands. In this way the lives of little children may be placed in jeopardy, or by an extraordinary increase of the cerebral irritation and the appearance of convulsions. A number of observations in families where several children and adults were attacked by the disease, and where it could not be traced to any dietetic or hygienic irregularities, lead me to believe that it is contagious, if not in every case, at least in its most violent form. It seems as though the more violent morbid processes of the buccal mucous membrane were, like other mucous membranes, possessed of a conditional contagiousness.

The morbid processes of the buccal mucous membrane which we have enumerated so far, occur much more frequently and break out much more readily in the organisms of children than in those of adults. Whether this is owing to the greater delicacy of the infantile mucous membrane, or to deficient nutrition, is not very clear. Most diseases of this class, among infants at any rate, undeniably arise from the circumstance that the mouth is not kept sufficiently clean, whereas, on the other hand, stomatitis often attacks children where the utmost cleanliness is observed. One great cause of the disease is the pernicious habit of giving children the breast much too frequently; not only is the proper digestion interfered with by this pernicious habit, but the mouth cannot be kept clean when it is continually lined with milk. A mother cannot be too careful in this respect; a slight derangement in the functions of the mouth is sometimes sufficient to interfere with the assimilative process and to bring on a condition of things that must inevitably lead to the deterioration of the infantile organism.

Treatment. We have placed these apparently different and yet in many respects homogeneous diseases together, because the remedies which they require are generally the same, and unnecessary repetitions are thus avoided.

Belladonna. What we have said of Belladonna, in speaking of its curative virtues in cerebral hyperæmia, that they afford the most striking illustration of the truth of our therapeutic law, we apply these same remarks to the employment of Belladonna in the various inflammations of the mouth and fauces. Independently of the circumstance that children are most liable to these inflammations and that Belladonna acts most powerfully in the infantile organism, certain abnormal changes in the buccal cavity constitute some of the constant, we might almost say characteristic, pathogenetic symptoms of this drug. It corresponds more particularly to stomatitis proper at the commencement of the disease; likewise to the higher grades of acute catarrh. On the contrary, its usefulness in the exanthematic forms of the catarrhal process is very questionable, although we have frequently seemed to check the formation of aphthæ by its timely use. The more marked the constitutional symptoms, the more specifically is Belladonna indicated. In chronic catarrh it will probably never be of any use.

Mercurius solubilis is as specific in certain forms of stomatitis as Belladonna is in others. Everybody knows how constantly Mercury causes stomatitis, and that this affection runs its course with certain definite phenomena. We would have described mercurial stomatitis when treating of the other forms of this disease, if we had not preferred, owing to the important position of Mercury as a remedial agent in stomatitis, postponing a description of the mercurial form of this disorder until the opportunity of recommending Mercury as a remedial agent should naturally present itself.

Mercurial stomatitis sets in with a more or less extensive hyperæmia of the mucous lining of the mouth, which is generally most marked on the gums of the lower incisors. The simple engorgement is very speedily followed by swelling and sponginess of the gums. The gums are bright-red, separated from the teeth, bleed readily, and are extremely sensitive. The mucous lining of the lips and tongue swells likewise, the latter to such a degree that the tongue is pressed against the teeth, which make indentations in that organ. The posterior parts of the mouth are only attacked in the higher grades of mercurial action, more particularly the corner of the mucous membrane where the upper and lower jaws unite. The more violent the action of the poison, the more marked the swelling and the more intense the redness; the motion of the tongue and jaws is impeded not only because it is painful, but likewise because the tongue and corners of the jaws are very much swollen, so that the jaws can neither be completely closed nor separated. The saliva is secreted in larger quantity, and is mixed with a tenacious, very troublesome phlegm, and the odor of the breath is very foul; the taste is metallic, and is mixed with the same kind of foul taste that responds to the foul odor. During this whole process, sometimes at its commencement and sometimes in its further course, there is a great disposition to the formation of ulcers. The ulcers generally break out first on the gums and on the lower lip. On the gums it is the free margin that is invaded, which frequently causes a considerable retraction of the gums. On the lips we observe flat, not very large, spots, surrounded with red, sharply circumscribed borders, having a yellowish-white base, and being very sensitive, especially when first breaking out. At a later period the tongue likewise shows ulcerated places, mostly only at the margin, as if caused by the friction of the teeth, of irregular shape, and having an unclean base. The most extensive and most destructive ulcerations take place in the corners of the jaws, whence they may spread to the pharynx and nose. The ulceration may even cause permanent adhesions of the jaws.

In the preceding paragraph we have given a description of mercurial stomatitis which does not contain all the symptoms of this disease. These, however, can be supplied from the Materia Medica. In completing our picture of the disease by these additional symptoms, it is, of course, important to arrange every symptom in its right place. At all events, there is no medicine that furnishes such a complete image of the most violent form of stomatitis as Mercury; the resemblance is so great that without an exact investigation of the anamnestic circumstances of the case, we should, in many cases, be unable to decide whether the disease is mercurial or a simple form of stomatitis.

What we have said renders all further indications for the use of Mercurius unnecessary; it is suited to every grade of the disorder, even to ulcerations of the mucous lining and to aphthæ. It is not so certain whether its employment in chronic cases, especially in catarrh of the fauces, will prove equally advantageous. As we said before, this condition is frequently met with among individuals who had contracted syphilis and had been treated with Mercury; in such cases Mercury should not be used. We have better medicines adapted to such individuals.

Borax is not so much adapted to the aphthous form of stomatitis as it is said to be; it is frequently given without any result. On the other hand, it seems to be more effectual against thrush, of which we shall speak by and by.

Of the other remedies which have been administered and recommended in this disease, the most important are: *Nux vomica, Phosphorus, Dulcamara, Acidum nitricum* and *Phosphoricum*. These last-named remedies are, together with Belladonna, the best remedies for mercurial stomatitis. *Acidum nitricum* is particularly efficacious in this affection.

In chronic stomatitis, the appropriate medicines have to be used for a tolerably long period. We recommend *Acidum nitricum, Iodium, Staphysagria, Kali bichromicum.*

Besides the remedies which we have mentioned, a number of other medicines may come into play, when the disease is not an idiopathic affection, but a sequel or complication of other derangements in the organism.

Dietetic precautions are particularly important in the case of infants and children; the measures which have to be adopted in their case necessarily follow from what we have said in the paragraph concerning the etiology of stomatitis. A frequent cleansing of the mouth has a curative and palliative use, not only in the case of children, but likewise in that of adults. Warm water is the best means to cleanse the mouth with. The use of fat food has to be strictly forbidden; after eating fat food, every symptom of the disease becomes aggravated, without even any symptoms of catarrh of the stomach being present.

2. Thrush, Aphthæ of Infants.

If we devote a special chapter to this affection it is in order to show the distinctive difference between it and the disorder which we have just now discussed, and with which thrush is generally considered identical.

Thrush is a disease of the first months of infancy, or else becomes an affection of a threatening import in later years, during the last stages of very acute diseases, such as tuberculosis and typhus. It is characterized by the formation of fungi on the mucous lining of the mouth.

Very rarely in perfectly healthy children, but mostly after the phenomena, which we have designated by the collective name of stomatitis, have existed for a longer or shorter period, scattered white spots make their appearance upon the mucous lining of the mouth, as if cream had been deposited there. They spread with great rapidity, sometimes grow in size quite considerably, and finally may line the whole buccal cavity and extend even into the œsophagus and, under favorable circumstances, into the larynx. The spots consist of a tolerably firm, cheesy mass which is not easily detached and underneath which superficial ulcers form. At first they have a whitish look, which afterwards changes to a yellowish tint. In the course of their development the digestive functions become very deeply disturbed, which is undoubtedly, in a measure, owing to the circumstance that the nutritive functions are very much interfered with by the disturbed digestion or nursing; but likewise to the passage of the fungi into the intestinal canal. Under favorable circumstances the mucous membrane may be left perfectly sound after the superincumbent layers have become detached; on the other hand, if the exciting causes continue, the layers may constantly keep forming anew, and the disorder may thus become very much protracted.

Of itself thrush is not very dangerous to children, except in cases where its outbreak indicates the near approach of death. The danger is less in proportion as treatment almost always succeeds in removing the morbid product and preventing its reproduction. We know for certain that uncleanliness of the mouth is almost always the cause of thrush, although a vitiated, damp air likewise favors the outbreak of this disease, and sickly, weakly children are more liable to it than those whose constitutions are sound.

In accordance with what we have said, the treatment requires, in the first place, that the mouths of the children should be washed after every nursing or feeding; moreover, if the children are brought up by the bottle, both they and their bottles have to be kept clean; if the children nurse, the nipple has to be carefully washed before as well as after nursing, lest the thrush should be communicated to the mother. If possible the dwelling should not be neglected and always be properly ventilated. The mouth need never be cleansed with anything but water. The custom of some nurses to rub the mouth with white sugar, is reprehensible, in so far as white sugar interferes with the digestion, and does not diminish the disposition of the particles of milk remaining in the mouth to become decomposed. It is of importance not to put the children to the breast too often, and not to let them hold their bottle in the mouth by the hour.

That the formation of thrush is not alone owing to the abovementioned causes, but very often to an inherent constitutional disposition, is evident from the fact that thrush will sometimes persist, in spite of the most scrupulous cleanliness. For this reason we cannot always depend upon external treatment, and had better resort to internal treatment from the start. The chief remedy, which is sometimes sufficient without any other drug, is *Borax*, with which the diseased parts may be dusted by means of a camel's-hair pencil. The second trituration may be used. Beside Borax, *Acidum sulphuricum* and *muriaticum* have an excellent effect, the latter more particularly if there are distinct signs of decomposition of the blood. If thrush supervenes during the presence of other morbid derangements of the mouth or the general organism, it is better to proceed against the primary affection exclusively, since the lesser grades of thrush are not, of themselves, a threatening disorder, and the trouble is sufficiently attended to, if its further spread is prevented.

3. Angina.

By this name we understand an inflammatory affection of the posterior parts of the mouth and pharynx. According as it consists only in a catarrhal irritation of the mucous lining or in actual inflammation of the parts, it is distinguished into catarrhal and tonsillary angina, which are two essentially distinct forms of the disease.

a. *Angina Catarrhalis, Sore Throat.*

Angina catarrhalis is synonymous with acute catarrh of the pharynx and the posterior buccal cavity; but we have considered it in this chapter as something separate from the catarrhal process, because the treatment is rather identical with that of angina tonsillaris. The disease usually arises as independent of other affections, less frequently in the course of other catarrhal processes. Its most common cause is a cold; it likewise breaks out as a symptom of scarlatina, less frequently as a symptom of typhus, and sometimes it seems to spread even epidemically. Many individuals have from their youth a peculiar disposition to angina catarrhalis, without showing in their external appearance any signs of a peculiar irritability or weakness; on the contrary, they are persons of healthy-looking and vigorous constitutions.

Symptoms. These vary according as children or adults are affected. In either case the disease usually breaks out suddenly without any premonitory symptoms. The children were quite cheerful the moment previous, and are suddenly attacked with all the symptoms of a very violent fever and marked cerebral congestion. The temperature of the skin is very high, the pulse disproportionately accelerated, that is in comparison with the trifling importance of the pathological process, the children want to lie down, and they sink into a soporous condition from which they are frequently roused by sudden exclamations or anxious fancies, which sometimes continue even after the patients are wide awake, so that they seem really delirious. All these symptoms are worse towards evening and attain their climax about midnight, after which they decrease in intensity. The cerebral symptoms are so intense and, by their form and violence, cause so much anxiety, that it would seem at first sight as though the little patients were attacked with inflammation of the brain; there is but one certain diagnostic sign, which is the copious sweat that is scarcely ever wanting in this disease, and which always breaks out if the patients are covered ever so little, sometimes even if they are not covered at all, and which is never wanting if the patients are sleeping. The appearance of the tongue may be perfectly natural; generally, however, it shows a thin whitish coating at an early stage of the disease. The pupils are at times dilated, at times contracted. If the children are old enough to describe their morbid feelings, they complain much less frequently of pain in the throat than of pain in the pit of the stomach and in the ears. The pain in the latter may increase to a high degree of intensity, and may cause the patients to moan all the time. The apparently threatening intensity of these symptoms in the evening or at night bears no proportion to their striking decrease in the morning, when the children are seen playing about very cheerfully, and perhaps, feeling a little more tired than usual. If left to itself, the disease does not terminate here, but soon after dinner a fever sets in which, however, does not attain the same degree of intensity that the fever had at the first outbreak, and ceases on the third, sometimes not till the seventh day. The appetite is very bad, the bowels constipated, thirst moderate. There is very frequently a peculiar odor from the mouth, which is not so much a foul smell, as rather like that of Phosphorus; and is always more marked in the more violent cases, perhaps because in such cases the stomach is generally very seriously involved.

Angina catarrhalis is undoubtedly one of the most common causes of the cerebral congestions with which children are so often attacked, and is but too seldom recognized as their exciting cause. We are firmly convinced that many cases of supposed meningitis, where the remedial agent effected a complete cure in twelve hours, were nothing more than a catarrhal angina, on which account such an angina is of more practical importance to the physician than it would otherwise deserve. The above-mentioned diagnostic sign has never left us in the lurch, and we deem it so much more important as it is difficult, especially in the case of little children, to undertake an inspection of the throat. In children of six or seven years, marked cerebral congestions do not usually accompany this form of angina, which runs the same course in their case as in the case of adults.

Among older individuals angina catarrhalis generally sets in without any decided febrile symptoms; if they are present, they correspond to the febrile stage of every catarrhal fever, that is to say, they consist of alternate attacks of chills and heat, great lassitude, and rheumatic drawing and tearing in the extremities. At the same time they complain of disagreeable dryness in the throat, and painful deglutition, especially of the saliva, which is generally very tenacious, and secreted in small quantities. Drinking or swallowing solid food is generally much less painful. The fauces, especially at the arch of the palate, appear uniformly red, less frequently dark than bright red; the uvula is involved in the attack, looks swollen and elongated, so that its tip touches the root of the tongue, by which many patients are obliged to swallow all the time, and even causes an inclination to vomit. The tonsils are likewise somewhat swollen.

If the disease is neglected at this first stage, or if the patient takes, perhaps, a second cold, the difficulty of swallowing increases a good deal, even to such an extent that the liquid returns by the nose, and the attempt to swallow solids causes actual paroxysms of suffocation. In such higher grades of the disease, even adults are affected with a very foul breath, the fever assumes a more continuous type, and violent headache, nausea and vomiturition are seldom wanting. On inspecting the mouth we find the whole of the posterior part of this organ dark red, sometimes we notice a few superficial ulcers; the mucous lining is very much swollen, and the tongue thickly coated. In children we have seldom an opportunity of watching these different degrees of the disease; on the contrary, they always feel sickest at the commencement of this pathological process. Amid a gradual decrease of all the symptoms, the patient generally recovers in seven to nine days, provided no untoward accident interferes with the cure. Only in the lighter forms of the disease recovery may take place in three and even in two days.

Angina catarrhalis is a prevailing affection of young people; however, where there is a constitutional disposition to this disease, its attacks continue to a late age; decreasing, however, in intensity. Before the first year it occurs less frequently, between the second and seventh it is one of the most common diseases. Whereas among young people it is very commonly an idiopathic disease;

among individuals between the ages of forty and fifty, on the contrary, it is most generally a mere symptom of some general disorder.

The prognosis is always favorable, especially if the catarrhal angina is the only morbid symptom. Some profess to have seen death result from the convulsions caused by the cerebral hyperæmia; in such cases, however, the cause of death has most likely been ascertained only superficially.

Treatment. In its ordinary form there is no better remedy for this affection than *Belladonna;* when given every two or three hours, not too high, it hushes in twelve to twenty-four hours the most violent pains in the throat, removes the febrile and congestive symptoms, and leaves mostly only a little lassitude and an impaired appetite. This effect of Belladonna is almost constant among children, who are sometimes seen in the morning jumping about bright and cheerful, even if they seemed deathly sick the evening previous.

In older persons, where the angina exists seldom as an idiopathic affection, Belladonna only removes the pain in the throat, whereas the other symptoms which correspond to the catarrhal process, remain unchanged, and require the remedies indicated by them. If Rummel (see Hartmann I., 418) tells us that in catarrhal angina Belladonna, and likewise *Dulcamara,* act better after a dose of *Mercurius,* we have to deny this statement, for the reason that we have seen Belladonna produce its favorable effects without a previous dose of Mercury.

Hartmann quotes also *Pulsatilla* among the medicines belonging to this series. He gives the following symptoms as indicating this drug: the throat is dark-red, some of the vessels being engorged and very prominent; the general disturbance is not very violent, but violent earache and tearing-darting pains in the cervical muscles are generally present.

As in the catarrh of the buccal cavity, so also in this disease may *Mercurius* be an appropriate remedy, especially if the tonsils are ulcerated, which is not unfrequently the case. Such anginas frequently assume an epidemic type of limited extent, in which case they become very obstinate.

b. *Angina Tonsillaris, Tonsillitis, Amygdalitis, Inflammation of the Tonsils. Quinsy.*

We designate by this name the parenchymatous inflammation of the throat, where the tonsils are generally most affected.

This affection is really met with only to the age of forty or fifty years, very seldom at a later period; most frequently between the years of seven and fifteen. Here too we find a disposition to pharyngeal inflammation, the same as in catarrhal angina, without any externally perceptible signs by which such a predisposition might be recognized; for, although we can always assert very positively that amygdalitis always arises from a cold, and we have, therefore, to believe in a certain predisposition to colds in those who are attacked with the disease, yet it is not clear why the same injurious influence makes some persons hoarse, causes a coryza in others, and an angina in a third party. What is certain is that persons who have to use their voice a good deal are more liable to an attack of angina, and are more generally affected with the chronic form. One attack of amygdalitis predisposes in a striking manner to relapses. Such diseases are more frequent in spring and fall than in summer and winter; their frequent appearance in the same locality at certain periods, justifies the inference that this disorder is sometimes epidemic. Damp, gloomy, and badly-ventilated dwellings, are undoubtedly very frequent causes of amygdalitis; we attend families in whom the children are very frequently attacked with this disease, and where, in the absence of any other unfavorable circumstances, the frequency of these attacks can only be accounted for by the unwholesomeness of their habitations. The peculiar relation of syphilis and Mercury to the tonsils, although as yet beyond the bounds of comprehension, is well known; both these causes develop almost constantly a parenchymatous inflammation. In scarlatina we meet with amygdalitis as a characteristic symptom of the disease; in less frequent cases, amygdalitis likewise accompanies other exanthems, least frequently measles.

Symptoms. Acute amygdalitis generally commences like all other acute affections, with a violent chill which is speedily followed by an unusual rise of temperature and increased frequency of the pulse, with violent headache and sometimes violent symptoms of cerebral hyperæmia; so that in the absence of local symptoms which have not yet made their appearance, we are easily led, especially in the case of children, to suspect the invasion of some acute disease. Generally all the morbid symptoms which occur in catarrhal angina make their appearance in this disease, only they are more continuous; the fever, especially, is less remittent, on which account acute tonsillitis is more readily than catarrhal angina, confounded with some violent acute disease, such as meningitis, even in the case of adults. This is particularly owing to the fact that the local throat-symptoms do not make their appearance at once, but not till the fever has lasted already a whole day; in consequence of which we neglect to examine the throat at the onset of the disease. The throat looks generally redder, more so on one side than on the other. The vascular engorgement is very soon followed by a swelling of the tonsils; at first only one tonsil being affected, the other tonsil remaining either unaffected or being attacked subsequently to the former. The more rapidly the inflammatory swelling increases in intensity, and the higher the grade to which the inflammation is carried, the greater the danger of the inflammation terminating in suppuration. The swelling sometimes enlarges to such an enormous size that it is no longer possible to see the posterior wall of the pharynx. As the local symptoms increase, the general condition of the patient becomes more and more unfavorable; the fever remains at its height; deglutition is almost entirely impeded, and yet there is a constant urging to swallow. Speech becomes guttural, sometimes quite impossible; the respiration is more or less impeded according as the posterior nares are involved in the inflammatory process. During perfect rest the pain is not so great, but is excited or aggravated by every motion. The lassitude is continually on the increase, partly owing to the violence of the fever, and partly to the deficient supply of solid, and more particularly of liquid, nourishment. The tongue is lined with a thick, tenacious phlegm, which is exceedingly troublesome to the patient, and seems to cause the urging to swallow, which frequently results in an inclination to vomit. The bowels are constipated, the urinary secretions diminished, and the urine is very thick. In this manner the disease continues about nine days, and sometimes increases to such a degree of intensity that the patient, the day previous to the opening of the abscess, seems to be like one near death. Very seldom the general condition improves during the formation of the pus. As soon as the abscess breaks, the threatening symptoms disappear almost immediately, so that it would seem as though the cerebral hyperæmia, at least towards the end of the process, were in many cases consequent upon the impeded respiration, the same as in croup. That perfect recovery cannot take place at once, must be self-evident to any one who considers how much strength the body has lost by sleeplessness and deficient nourishment.

Not in every case, and, as we shall show more particularly when speaking of the treatment of this disease, scarcely ever under homœopathic treatment, is the course of tonsillitis as acute as we have described. From the most violent fever, with sopor and delirium, to a scarcely perceptible disturbance of the general health, all sorts of degrees of constitutional malaise can be noticed, even though the local affection should be the same. If the inflammation is dispersed, this result does not take place very rapidly ; on the contrary, in such a case the inflammation is very apt to pass into the chronic form, which is much more rarely met with when the inflammatory process terminates in suppuration. But even if the inflammation is dispersed, a febrile condition of the system, lassitude and loss of appetite, continue for some days, whereas the decrease in the inflammatory symptoms ought to lead one to infer that the general wellbeing was much improved. The prognosis is almost always favorable. Only in children the disorder may terminate fatally, either in consequence of cerebral difficulties, or by suffocation, or even, under certain unfavorable circumstances, by mortification of the parts. Among adults this danger need not be apprehended. Anginas initiating or accompanying exanthematic affections, have to be viewed from a different stand-point to that of idiopathic angina ; we shall treat of them in a subsequent chapter when speaking of exanthemata.

The chronic form of amygdalitis arises in most cases out of the acute form, in consequence of the reabsorption of the inflammatory exudation only taking place partially, and the swelling of the tonsil remaining. It seems as though, independently of all constitutional predisposition, such remaining infiltrations superinduced a tendency to relapses. Every new attack increases the swelling, so that an hypertrophy may ensue, by which access to the pharynx may be almost entirely prevented. In the houses to which we have alluded, when speaking of the etiology of this disease, every child has such hypertrophied tonsils, even a girl of two years and a half; and every one of these children has twice a year a more or less violent attack of acute angina. After an abscess, hypertrophies of any size occur much less frequently. Without any previous acute attack, chronic amygdalitis may develop itself almost imperceptibly, in persons who have to exert their vocal organs a good deal, such as ministers, singers, actors ; but acute cases arising from such causes are not near as violent or important as cases arising from the previously mentioned causes. In chronic tonsillitis the swelling looks pale, with prominently engorged vascular ramifications. The surface is rugged, uneven, sometimes traversed by whitish cicatrized streaks. Sometimes the follicles are very much enlarged; they look like dark excavations between the protuberances on the tonsil, or like white points filled with a caseous substance, similar to acne. Ulcerations occur but rarely, and still less frequently for a long period.

It is only exceptionally that the hypertrophy of the tonsils causes trouble to the patients. It is seldom that they experience any pain; nor is the pain ever very acute, unless an acute attack has just taken place. The most common derangement is an altered tone of the voice, as in an acute attack, and a weakness of the vocal organs, in consequence of which the sufferer is easily attacked with hoarseness. In spite of the swelling, which is sometimes very large, the difficulty of swallowing is either trifling, or else there is no difficulty at all. Only in rare cases the patients complain of the swelling, as of a foreign body in the throat. It is a peculiar feature in such cases, that every cold brings on an acute attack of amygdalitis, which is generally, however, confined to some fever with pain in the throat, and some difficulty of deglutition, with moderate redness of the tonsils. By neglecting such attacks, they may recur so often, and in such rapid succession, that the patient's health may remain disturbed for weeks.

The hypertrophy of the tonsils is always a very obstinate difficulty, which it is so much more troublesome to remove, as the patients who feel tolerably well otherwise, do not feel disposed to take medicine. In an advanced age the swelling generally disappears spontaneously.

Treatment. We are justified in regarding the treatment of angina faucium, no matter whether of the catarrhal or parenchymatous type, as one of the most striking evidences of the superiority of the homoeopathic method of cure, for the reason that the disease precludes even the possibility of committing an error of diagnosis, and the affected organ is directly accessible to sight, so that we have it in our power to determine all changes with positive certainty. Our successes in this direction cannot be slurred over on the score of a false diagnosis, and it may be well worth the trouble to briefly compare the different methods of treatment.

It is scarcely to be believed, almost inconceivable, that legions of the most heroic remedies are advised and actually employed for a disorder which, although it may seem to run a threatening course, yet is really unimportant. One praises venesections, to be resorted to in rapid succession, as the best means of shortening a pathological disorder which reaches a spontaneous termination in nine days.

One day is said to be gained by such treatment. To save one day, a dozen or more venesections are recommended, or at least a dozen leeches to the throat. From these violent means of cure, down to common ice-water, every thing is recommended, emetics, purgatives, calomel, etc., local astringents, nitrate of silver, chlore, blisters, cold and warm fomentations. If this apparatus of violent remedies is not replete with the most absurd nonsense, it certainly shows an immense deal of unscrupulous recklessness, for the reason that every physician knows that the disease against which he plants such terrible batteries, beats a spontaneous retreat in a few days. Such heroic interference with the natural course of the disease, cannot, therefore, be justified on the score of necessity, owing to the dangerous character of this disorder, as in the case of internal organs, where an acute inflammation may readily terminate fatally. And after all, the result of such fearful therapeutic havoc is simply to abbreviate the course of the disease for one day, without, however, preventing suppuration, for all therapeutic manuals inform us that suppuration will almost regularly result. The expectant treatment has this advantage, that it does not impregnate the organism with deleterious medicinal substances; however, it likewise is unable to prevent suppuration.

What now is the result of homœopathic treatment? Under this treatment the formation of an abscess is a rare occurrence, especially if the physician is called at the onset; even if suppuration takes place, he will scarcely ever have the patient under treatment nine days. This is a matter of common observation. Or is it mere accident that every homœopath is so fortunate? Of course our opponents would much rather admit, if any thing at all, an unexampled good fortune than an efficacious treatment. An honest critic cannot help testifying to the great superiority of our treatment over any other in this disease. And with how few remedies do we achieve such success. Owing to our perfect knowledge of the positive effects of our drugs in angina, a few only are sufficient to enable us to effect a cure.

As in other purely inflammatory affections of the mouth, so also in angina is *Belladonna* the chief remedy. We have mentioned this remedy so frequently in the gravest disorders, that anybody may infer from this circumstance the necessity of studying its physiological effects, even to their most delicate shades; for we do not possess a medicine that admits of a more diversified application. In angina tonsillaris Belladonna is only suitable at the commencement of the disease, and in a form of angina which can scarcely be distinguished from angina catarrhalis. In general, however, it is scarcely possible in practice to establish a strict difference between these two forms of angina, nor is this essential to successful treatment. The darker the redness of the fauces, the more marked a bluish tint, the more considerable the inflammatory swelling, the less is Belladonna suitable; and even the presence of cerebral symptoms would no longer justify its use. The presence of such symptoms might tempt us to continue the exhibition of Belladonna, for the reason that we attach more importance to the congestive symptoms than they really merit. In many cases Belladonna will suffice to control the disease, and prevent suppuration; this result ought to be obtained, however, in forty-eight hours at the longest, otherwise we cannot depend upon it. In other cases the febrile symptoms disappear, but the tonsils remain red and swollen; in such cases the continued use of Belladonna would only involve a loss of time, for we should miss the favorable moment of preventing exudation. In the acute paroxysms of the chronic form, Belladonna removes with certainty the pain and the vascular engorgement, and in milder attacks suffices to restore the tonsils to their former condition. In view of the certainty with which we can cure an angina, in a comparatively short period, it is to be regretted that a physician is not called to such a case at the very commencement of the attack, when the suitable period for the efficient exhibition of Belladonna is not yet passed. Persons who are liable to attacks of amygdalitis, should be recommended to keep a vial of the proper medicine on hand, with a view of using it as soon as they begin to experience the symptoms of the trouble.

Mercurius will rarely be suitable at the onset of the disease, unless it should be accompanied by violent catarrh of the buccal cavity, or originate in it. Usually, however, the physician is not called till the inflammatory swelling has reached a higher degree, in which case Mercurius is generally indicated. The more particular phenomena which indicate this remedy, are: The whole of the fauces have a deep-red or a bluish-red tint, more particularly the tonsils, which are darker than any other part, and usually show small ulcers, with pseudo-membranous exudations. The saliva is very tenacious and slimy, obliges the patient to swallow frequently, and the buccal cavity exhibits the symptoms of a highly developed catarrh, as we have described it in the chapter on stomatitis. The breath has a peculiar foul odor. The pains are generally less than when Belladonna is indicated, but the general health is worse. All those symptoms are present, of which we can say, with positive certainty, that they precede suppuration. Generally, however, unless the process is too far advanced, we succeed in preventing the formation of an abscess. The most suitable preparation of Mercurius is the Mercurius solubilis in one of the lower triturations, frequently repeated. It should not be given up too soon if no striking improvement sets in all at once, or the disease seems to increase in intensity, for not unfrequently the symptoms threatening suppuration recede, although this result seemed unavoidable.

Hepar sulphuris calcareum is the most important remedy next to Mercurius; that is to say Hepar may be given when an abscess is evidently on the point of forming and we simply desire to hasten the suppurative process and the breaking of the abscess. The abscess is generally seen in one tonsil as a roundish prominence reaching beyond the swelling, having sometimes a dark and sometimes a lighter color. Sometimes, however, it is impossible to determine in the misshapen flabby swelling formed by the tonsils, the exact spot of the abscess, which not unfrequently is located entirely on the side of the pharynx. Sometimes there are several abscesses, each abscess being small. In this case the morbid symptoms continue for a longer period, because the abscesses discharge only little by little. That Hepar exerts an influence over the suppurative process and the emptying of the abscess, is evident from the fact that under its use the disease scarcely ever lasts eight days which is the common duration under any other treatment.

Beside these three remedies, which will be found sufficient in all ordinary cases of amygdalitis, we have a few other medicines which are indicated by special symptoms and which we dare not pass over.

Apis mellifica has more recently been warmly praised for amygdalitis; we confess we are not one of the admirers of Apis in this disease, where we are yet to witness the first unequivocal effect from this agent. Besides the symptoms of Apis, which might possibly be twisted into indications for its use in angina tonsillaris, are not at all characteristically prominent in the American provings, more particularly if we separate the clinical effects which are taken from reports of cures. According to the simple physiological symptoms, Apis is better indicated in simple angina catarrhalis, than in the parenchymatous form. Why should we use such a vaguely defined drug where so many characteristic remedies are at our disposal?

Lachesis deserves attention in the few cases where the fauces exhibit a livid redness. the inflammation has consequently reached a very high grade of intensity and gangrene seems to threaten. When this condition prevails, the constitutional equilibrium is very much disturbed: the respiration is labored, speech is impossible, the cerebral symptoms very marked. The internal swelling is associated with considerable swelling of the outer neck. The face has a very strikingly sick expression, and, instead of a vivid redness, exhibits a yellowish-gray pallor. This form is more frequently met with as an accompaniment of exanthematous fevers than in idiopathic angina.

For **Ignatia amara** we transcribe Hartmann's own indications (I., 419): "The following symptoms of angina are characteristic of Ignatia, as has already been stated by Hahnemann in his remarks on this drug: stinging in the throat between the acts of deglutition; sensation when swallowing as if the patient were swallowing over a bone, with a rolling sound; sensation of a plug or tumor in the throat, only between the acts of deglutition. Ignatia will never prove useful if the stinging is only felt during deglutition, but very certainly when the stinging is felt between the acts of deglutition, or when it passes off by continuing the act of swallowing; of course the other symptoms must likewise correspond to Ignatia. On looking at the buccal cavity the fauces look inflamed and red, the tonsils are swollen and inflamed, covered with small ulcers. Another kind of angina which likewise yields to Ignatia, consists in a painful soreness of the throat, which is only felt during deglutition; or in the sensation when swallowing as if a tumor had formed in the throat which hurts when swallowing. The sensation of a swelling in the throat, with painful soreness during deglutition, is therefore a chief criterium for the use of Ignatia." From these indications we infer that Ignatia must be particularly suitable for the acute paroxysms of chronic amygdalitis, which run their course without reaching a high degree of intensity and without showing any disposition to suppurate.

In the common form of amygdalitis, *Bryonia alba* will scarcely ever or perhaps never be suitable, but may be useful in cases where the tonsils are not very much inflamed, and where the cellular tissue of the throat is invaded, causing apprehensions of internal as well as external suppuration. Such forms generally occur in limited epidemics, they run a very protracted course and involve the whole organism by causing a marked feeling of sickness.

Aconite requires to be mentioned in a few words. It is frequently used at the commencement of angina, more, however, to moderate the fever than to counteract the local process, where it does not seem to be of much use. To persevere in the use of Aconite beyond this point, would imply a loss of precious time, in consequence of which the period when Belladonna manifests such striking effects, slips from us.

Chronic amygdalitis is more or less easily controlled according to the time it has lasted, and to the character of the swelling. If we have to deal with a first attack of angina where the exuded matter had not been completely reabsorbed, *Sulphur* is most usually the most appropriate remedy to promote absorption. If the tonsils have become entirely hypertrophied, we generally require a good deal of time to change this condition; moreover, every new acute attack may totally annihilate the advantages we have gained. The principal remedies in such cases are: *Iodine*, *Baryta carbonica* and *Calcarea*; of course they have to be continued for a long time and in the higher attenuations. Where the swelling of the organs is caused by the patient's mode of living and by excessive use of the throat, medicines will prove totally ineffectual, as long as the causes continue; in such cases, if the swollen tonsils really interfere with speech, they have to be extirpated with the knife.

As regards other particulars connected with the treatment of acute amygdalitis, it seems scarcely necessary to allude to them. The patients being unable to swallow, nothing need be said about diet. The best gargle is tepid water, which is abundantly sufficient to clear the mouth of the troublesome phlegm as far as possible; generally the patients are unable to introduce a fluid into the mouth, much less into the pharynx, far enough to enable it to exert any salutary effect. Cold applications to the neck are much more hurtful than useful, even if they are continued for a long time. Usually the skin remains very active, and the patient perspires profusely; hence why should such applications be resorted to? Where suppuration cannot be prevented, it may of course be hastened by warm poultices. Opening the abscess with a bistoury is much more easily said than done; the patients being scarcely ever able to open their mouth sufficiently to admit a view of the parts.

We will conclude this chapter with a remark, which every homœopathic practitioner has undoubtedly been able to verify in his own practice, namely, that after the homœopathic treatment of angina, relapses are much less frequent than after any other treatment, and that even the disposition to relapses seems to become extinct. This result strikes the patient much more forcibly than the physician who apprehends the reason of this phenomenon, while it is of the utmost consequence to one who had been in the habit of passing through an attack of angina every spring and autumn. A similar result prevails with other affections where relapses occur quite frequently, particularly with erysipelas.

[4. **Retropharyngeal Abscess.**

Kafka has the following concise notice of this abscess:

It is seated in the connective tissue between the pharynx and the anterior side of the vertebral column.

An accumulation of pus on the posterior wall of the pharynx forms a swelling, which, by encroaching upon the pharyngeal space, narrows or totally closes the pharynx.

The abscess either perforates the wall of the pharynx or gravitates downwards, and sometimes finds an outlet into the œsophagus or the thoracic cavity.

Etiology. This abscess either occurs spontaneously from some unknown cause, under the form of a phlegmonous inflammation, or it is the result of a scrofulous or tuberculous, and in some cases even of a syphilitic, inflammation of the vertebræ; one or more vertebræ being swollen and painful, and causing stiffness or curvature of the neck, in consequence of a displacement of the spinous processes. This disease sometimes occurs as a secondary morbid process during the course of typhus, puerperal fever, pyæmia, etc.

Symptoms. During the course of phlegmonous inflammation of the throat, without any simultaneously existing affection of the cervical vertebræ, febrile motions set in, which are sometimes very intense and attended with rather severe difficulties of swallowing. Gradually a swelling is seen on the posterior wall of the pharynx, bulging more and more from behind forwards, and showing signs of fluctuations. If the swelling becomes considerable, the velum and uvula are pressed forward more and more; if the swelling is seated further down, the larynx and the os hyoides are pressed forward, and if seated on one side or the other, it may be discovered at the angle of the lower jaw. The larger the swelling, the greater the difficulty of swallowing and breathing, the speech is altered, there is a hoarse cough, and the hearing is impaired. Little children distort their features when drinking or nursing, they cough some, or the liquids return again by the mouth and nose. If the pharynx is closed by the abscess, the breathing becomes extremely troublesome, the patients become cyanotic, bloated in the face, the eyes protrude from their sockets, the carotids pulsate violently, and there is danger of sudden suffocation.

If the abscess is occasioned by some disease of the cervical vertebræ, they are generally very sensitive, swollen and displaced, the neck is stiff, the cervical muscles are in a state of tension, and the patients incline to hold their necks to one side. In either case, a careful examination of the neck, both on the inner and outer sides, is indispensable.

Course, Terminations, Prognosis. A phlegmonous inflammation always runs an acute course. The retropharyngeal abscess, occasioned by a disease of the cervical vertebræ, runs a chronic course, and sometimes remains hidden for a long time. For this reason, if children find it difficult to swallow, their necks are stiff, and they incline to hold their heads to one side, it is advisable to institute a careful examination of these parts.

The secondary retropharyngeal abscess has the same symptoms as the phlegmonous form, except that many of the symptoms are modified by the character of the primary disease. These abscesses become dangerous by the circumstance that they may break during sleep or a state of partial unconsciousness, and cause danger of suffocation.

In the phlegmonous and secondary form, the abscess always discharges either into the pharynx or the œsophagus.

In spondylarthrocace the pus gravitates downwards into the larynx or the thoracic cavity; in either case the result is attacks of suffocation or fatal inflammation, or else the suppuration continues and causes caries of the vertebræ.

In the phlegmonous form, the prognosis is favorable. If the cervical vertebræ are inflamed and pyæmic abscesses occur, the prognosis is unfavorable.

Treatment. The phlegmonous form requires the same treatment as acute quinsy. If fluctuation is perceived, the abscess should at once be opened; this will afford great relief to the patient, and obviate the danger of suffocation, or of a burrowing of the pus downwards.

If the vertebræ are inflamed, the speedy lancing of the abscess may prevent caries.

To restore the vertebræ to their normal condition, we give *Phosphorus* 6 to 30, or *Natrum mur.* 6 to 30. If caries is present, we give

Silicea 6 to 30, or *Asafœtida* 3 to 6. Country air and a strengthening diet will help to mend the constitution.

To prevent suffocation during sleep, in the case of little children, or while they are lying in a state of unconsciousness, it is of the utmost importance that the abscess should be opened as soon as its condition will admit of it. H.]

5. Diphtheritis, Diphtheria.

The diphtheritic process on the lining membrane of the mouth and fauces is in many respects enveloped in obscurity, whence the great confusion prevailing in its description, and consequently in its nomenclature. Small differences in the totality of the symptoms, or in the course or complications of the disease, have been taken advantage of to establish new species, without any practical advantage; for the study of the pathological alterations characterizing this class of diseases, is rendered very much more difficult by such efforts at systemization. This work being designed as a guide in Therapeutics, we have kept aloof from all minute pathological distinctions, and have ranged these allied processes under the name of diphtheritis, by which we mean all those processes in consequence of which exudations take place upon the lining membrane of the mouth and pharynx, without caring whether they are simply superimposed upon the mucous lining, or constitute alterations of its tissue. Hence we mean all the different processes to which a variety of names have been applied, such as: stomacace, croup of the mucous lining of the mouth and fauces, angina maligna or gangrænosa, or pseudo-membranosa, fegar, garotillo, diphtheria epidemica, etc.

Such a comprehensive arrangement in one series and under one name has this great advantage: that, in the therapeutic chapter, many useless repetitions can be avoided, since the same remedies have to be mentioned for the different forms of the disease.

The formation of membranous exudations upon the lining membrane of the mouth, is a very common occurrence, and may either be without any importance or entail the worst consequences. This prognostic can readily be determined by the character of the causes upon which the exudations depend, on which account the etiology of the disease is of the highest importance. In simple inflammation of the mucous lining, the formation of pseudo-membranes constitutes an unimportant complication; it does not even at all times indicate a remarkably high degree of the inflammatory process.

Membranous layers are likewise observed when the tonsils are very much inflamed. As a somewhat idiopathic affection, this pathological process is seen in croup, where it spreads from the larynx to the fauces under conditions of which we are ignorant, but which seem to depend upon epidemic causes. It seems, moreover, as if there existed some peculiar predisposition for diphtheritic exudations, and as if this predisposition were founded in a peculiar delicacy of the mucous lining, or in such general diseases as generally predispose to abnormal processes of exudation, particularly scrofulosis and tuberculosis. The latter supposition is confirmed by the fact that unwholesome dwellings, deficient food, vitiated air, undoubtedly occasion diphtheritis. Lastly, the disease is the result of epidemic influences; but even under these circumstances, attacks, more particularly, individuals who are exposed to the above-mentioned obnoxious causes. The epidemic form is most likely contagious. Peculiar forms of the diphtheritic process are likewise met with in various exanthematic diseases, more particularly scarlatina, and in several derangements depending upon constitutional poisoning, but we omit them in this place because special mention will be made of them in subsequent chapters.

Symptoms and Course. In drawing a picture of the disease, it matters a great deal whether the pseudo-membranous process appears as an idiopathic or a secondary disorder. In the latter case we suddenly find in the course of other diseases, upon circumscribed spots of the lining membrane, a whitish layer which rapidly thickens, and proves to be a firmly-adhering membrane. This membrane is either detached at an early period, while the affection which causes it decreases at the same time, in which case a mucous membrane is discovered in its place, which is slightly reddened, disposed to bleed, or sometimes, but less frequently, presents a normal appearance; or else the membrane, favored by circumstances adapted to its growth, increases in thickness, becomes discolored, of a grayish-yellow hue, and shows a tendency to become decomposed, and to engender, upon the mucous lining, ulcers which generally remain flat, and only lead to considerable ulcerations when favored by circumstances antagonistic to the patient. These phenomena have been generalized under the name of pharyngeal croup. This designation is, in so far proper as the croupous process upon the mucous membrane of the larynx, is likewise without any tendency to cause more penetrating ulcerations. In opposition to this morbid process, there is a form of diphtheritis which attacks the mucous membrane in its whole thickness, and is characterized by a constant tendency to destroy it. This diphtheritis, properly so-called, has of late years made its appearance as an epidemic in England and America, and has likewise broken out in the north of Germany with such a fearful violence that it has become the terror of both physicians and the public. English and American physicians describe this epidemic form of diphtheritis under the name of diphtheria.

The disease generally commences with unimportant febrile symptoms, and most commonly without any local appearances. Only in a few cases we observe symptoms of a not very intense inflammation of the tonsils. Hence the physician does not always have a chance to observe the course of the disease from the commencement, because neither the patient nor his family are specially disturbed by the morbid phenomena. At first there is slight redness of the fauces, the vessels in one or more places being considerably injected. It is here that, in a few hours only, we discover the first traces of exudation. At the same time the redness increases considerably, without, however, spreading to the anterior portions of the mouth. One or more snow-white membranous patches seem to be laid loosely upon a deep-red, or even bluish-red, or violet base; they have altogether the appearance of a layer of cream spread upon the mucous membrane. As yet the constitutional equilibrium is not very much disturbed; the fever is slight, the pulse not very much accelerated, the skin not very dry, a slight perspiration even breaks out from time to time. Deglutition is not very much impeded, the pains at the affected part of the throat not very acute. Only a general lassitude shows that the local appearances have a much deeper significance than one would suppose. The affection may thus remain unchanged for the first seven days, only the exudation at most invades a few other parts in addition to the former. In the most fortunate cases the membranes become detached at the end of this period, leaving superficial ulcers with shaggy borders, which heal rapidly and leave the patient restored to perfect health.

If the disease does not take this favorable turn, it then assumes a much more formidable form in the second week. The formation of the membranes keeps spreading; they assume a rather dingy-blackish hue. The constitutional disturbance is more marked, the pulse remaining about the same. The prostration increases, yet the patients, even in violent cases, are not always compelled to lie down. Sleep is generally very much disturbed. The pains in the throat are intense, deglutition and speech are very much impeded, the patients often complain of violent earache, which, however, is not constant, but comes in paroxysms. The alvine evacuations are normal, only diminished owing to the lessened quantity of nourishment. This stage likewise lasts a week, and may be followed by recovery; the ulcerative process, however, is much more penetrating than at the end of the first week.

The further progress of the disease in the third week consists in an increase of the constitutional phenomena, but principally in gangrenous destruction of the affected parts in the fauces. There arise deep ulcers of various sizes, with a gray or blackish bottom, with shaggy borders, and having a horrid smell. The loss of substance may be very considerable. The ptyalism is copious and very fetid; the patients look very ill, although they may yet be capable of walking about. The termination in recovery is a very slow process, in so far at least as recovery depends upon the healing of the ulcerated surfaces; for the constitutional symptoms already show a marked improvement, at a period when the ulcers still retain their malignant appearance. The return of the appetite is the most favorable symptom, likewise the decrease of the ptyalism and the fetor from the mouth. It takes several weeks before the ulcerated surfaces are completely healed. It is peculiar to this disease that, as the local symptoms disappear, a more or less universal paralysis sets in. This is not always the case, but very frequently, and it is inexplicable why, as in a case that came under our observation, an apparently trivial, local affection of the throat should be succeeded by paralysis of the arms, and an almost complete paralysis of the lower extremities. This paralysis disappeared very suddenly, after having lasted five weeks, subsequently to a slight attack of catarrhal angina.

In the previous chapter we have furnished the description of an attack of moderate violence, and running a favorable, although very protracted course. This case may be regarded as a fair illustration of most cases of diphtheria. Under certain circumstances, however, of which mention will be made hereafter, the disease offers a very different group of symptoms, which the importance of the subject demands should be faithfully portrayed by us.

In the more violent cases the preliminary stage is very often quite short. The disease sometimes invades the organism so rapidly, and with such extraordinary intensity, that the patient is at once attacked with excessive prostration, a small, filiform pulse, cadaverous pallor, and death takes place as soon as the membranes begin to form. In other cases the affection begins quite suddenly, with vomiting and an intense angina, violent fever, somnolence, stiffness and external swelling of the neck, and extraordinary frequency of the pulse. The speech is peculiarly altered, on account of the more difficult mobility of the tongue. The vomiting consists of a thin, yellowish liquid, and is very often accompanied by a similar diarrhœa. The exudation of the membranes takes place very rapidly, spreading almost simultaneously over the entire buccal and pharyngeal cavity as far as the nose. The swelling of the subjacent parts, and of the external neck, becomes quite considerable, so that it extends like a thick pad around the lower jaw. At the same time the febrile symptoms are not very considerable, even if the fever had run ever so high at the commencement of the outbreak, but the strength decreases very rapidly. As a rule the urine now becomes more or less albuminous, and generally remains so during the whole course of the disease. When the attacks are so violent, the exudative process most commonly spreads to the respiratory organs, where it occasions all the symptoms of true croup, superinduces at an early period suffocative paroxysms and coma, and usually terminates fatally, death being frequently preceded by very violent vomiting. Very seldom consciousness remains undisturbed until the moment of death. After such violent attack death generally ensues in two to four days, so that a gangrenous decomposition of the membranes and a more deeply penetrating ulcerative process is not readily observed in such cases. In the formerly described, more protracted cases, the ulcerative process is usually fully developed, and amenable to observation.

In certain conditions of the system, the affection runs a chronic course, the membranous exudation being frequently detached and renewed again, and at the same time remaining confined within definite localities. In this way the strength of the patient vanishes by degrees, and death is almost always the end of this chronic form of the disease.

If the constitution of the patient is, at the outset, thoroughly tainted with scrofulosis, tuberculosis, and other dyscrasias, the membranes evince from the commencement an extraordinary tendency to decomposition, and death results at an early period, although the extent and intensity of the disease may not yet seem very far advanced. Unfavorable external circumstances, such as damp dwellings, a crowd of persons living together in small rooms, insufficiency of fresh air, likewise exert a deleterious influence, on which account the worst forms of the disease are more frequently met with among the lower than among the higher classes.

The causes of diphtheria, if we except the previously mentioned etiological influences, are enveloped in obscurity. The epidemic propagation of the disease, and its rapid spread in the organism, necessarily lead to the idea of a peculiar virus, whether of a vegetable or animal nature, is not certain. The contagious character of the disease, which no one will be bold enough to dispute, favors the assumption of a specific virus. Considering more particularly the peculiarities of the disease, we are compelled to adopt a general toxication of the blood, for the local process cannot possibly induce such a sudden and extraordinary waste of strength, without any corresponding increase of the secretions; moreover, as we stated above, a great many patients die at the very beginning of the exudative process.

The supposition that diphtheria represents a masked scarlatina, is mostly derived from the circumstance that the fauces are mainly invaded by the diphtheritic process, and from its resemblance to the malignant angina of scarlet fever. The course of diphtheria, however, is very different; moreover, we do not find in diphtheria, as a rule at least, the unusually high elevation of temperature, and the frequency of pulse, which are always present in scarlatina.

Judging by all these various circumstances, diphtheritic angina is a plague whose behavior is, in all respects, similar to that of acute exanthemata and Asiatic cholera. Our first correct reports concerning the disease, date as far back as forty years ago, when the disease was prevalent in France. In England the spread of the disease, until the year 1856, was not very considerable, since which period, however, this plague has overrun the country with extraordinary rapidity, has migrated to Holland, thence in 1863 to the North of Germany, where it overran Ostfriesland, and likewise infected various localities in the interior of the country with its epidemic taint. Peculiar states of the atmosphere and conditions of the soil do not seem to be necessary to further the spread of this epidemic; otherwise how could we account for the fact that Norderney on the North sea, Aurich in Ostfriesland, Scesen on the Hartz, and Muender in the Deister mountains, were visited at the same time. Except Aurich, the above-mentioned localities are the most salubrious in the country. In the city of Hanover we have, so far, only had isolated cases, almost all of which occurred in opulent families.

We have to point out in a few words the difference between croup and diphtheria; so far as treatment is concerned this difference is of the utmost importance. In croup the membrane is apparently of the same character as in diphtheria. The assertion that in croup the exudation is fibrinous and in diphtheria albuminous, is certainly unsupported. But it is an essential characteristic of the diphtheritic exudation, to be constantly tending to a gangrenous decomposition, and to involve the subjacent mucous membrane in the gangrenous process; which is never the case with croup. So far there can be no question of transition-forms between the two processes; where such transition-forms have been supposed to exist, the diagnosis, which, in isolated cases, can only be established with certainty in the further course of the malady, has undoubtedly been premature. Besides all this, the constitutional symptoms are opposed to the croupy character of diphtheria, more particularly the extraordinary, unusually rapid prostration, which mostly terminates fatally, whereas in croup death is caused by the mechanical obstruction of the respiration with its subsequent influences on the composition of the blood. Lastly, croup is almost exclusively a disease of childhood, and has never yet been suspected of being a contagious disease; whereas diphtheria, though it prevails more especially among children, spares no age in particular, and is a plague whose contagiousness cannot well be denied.

The prognosis of diphtheria is always doubtful, for the disease may terminate fatally, no matter what course it may take. If the disease sets in accompanied by symptoms of violent constitutional disturbance, the danger of a fatal termination is very great, since we may almost be sure of a more general spread of the poison. The more rapid the prostration, the more unfavorable the constitutional and domestic conditions of the patient, the more considerable the gangrenous disorganization, and the sooner it takes place, the less the chances of recovery. The extension of the diphtheritic process to the larynx and lungs is almost always fatal. Nor should the protracted and mild course of the disease superinduce a feeling of security, for even then a malignant aspect may supervene. One of the most threatening symptoms is an albuminous deposit in the urine, especially if it is very copious.

As sequelæ of the disease we notice, more particularly, symptoms of paralysis, which may affect the extremities, or the cervical muscles, or even the pharynx; and is very obstinate. Deafness and amaurosis have likewise been noticed as sequelæ of diphtheria.

The cicatrization of the ulcers not unfrequently causes impediments in swallowing, talking and masticating. An unusual constitutional debility, which does not correspond to the grade of intensity of the morbid symptoms, and has the appearance of a general paralysis, sometimes remains for months, even if the appetite is completely restored and the waste of tissue has been repaired.

Owing to the shortness of time that has as yet been vouchsafed to practitioners, in observing the course of the disease and investigating its causes and nature, we have not yet been able to determine the remedies that hold a positive and specifically-homœopathic relationship to the disease. For the present, at least, it seems an established fact, that the selection of remedial agents in this disease cannot be strictly conducted in accordance with the law of symptomatic similarity, for the reason that we are not yet in possession of any proving embodying a full counterpart of this pathological series. All we can do is to mention all the remedies that have been recommended for diphtheria, and leave it to time and more extensive observation to determine which of these remedies are in specific curative rapport with this disease.

Notwithstanding this incompleteness of our curative resources, we can boldly assert that the results obtained under homœopathic treatment, are far more satisfactory than those obtained by allopathic practitioners. Even if we are not as yet in possession of full and accurate statistical tables, yet we know to a certainty that in many epidemics at least fifty patients out of a hundred have died under allopathic treatment, whereas, under similar circumstances, the homœopaths only lost ten per cent.

Before enumerating the different remedies, we cannot forbear subjecting a very common proceeding in this disease, we mean local cauterization, to a brief critical examination. In England this proceeding has been very generally resorted to, even by homœopathic physicians, together with the exhibition of other remedies, and is generally recommended as indispensable. Nobody seems to have derived any real benefit from it, and several weighty authorities reject it as prejudicial. The greatest contradictions are more particularly met with among the different escharotics employed for the purpose of local cauterization. One holds to the exclusive use of the Nitrate of Silver, another rejects this entirely, and relates wonderful effects from Chlorate of Potash or the tincture of Muriate of Iron. It is difficult to obtain light in this confusion; at the same time it is fortunately not very important. We assume *a priori* that cauterization, if not positively hurtful, is at least useless and therefore an unnecessary torture. Diphtheria is not a local affection, but a constitutional disease, a characteristic symptom of which is the exudation in the fauces. Of what use can the destruction of the local symptom possibly be, since the disease continues on its destructive course? With the same propriety Variola pustules might be cauterized. Even if these local cauterizations were of some advantage, which, however, will always be trifling, is it not unreasonable to inflict this torture upon patients who are mostly children? We could never make up our minds to adopt this kind of treatment, and can excuse our English colleagues, only on the ground that they were not yet fully acquainted with the proper remedies for this disease, and therefore sought refuge in this exceedingly deceitful species of polypharmacy.

Moreover, our English colleagues have been in the habit of giving two remedies in alternation, and, by this proceeding, obscuring the specific action of each. Hence their observations only constitute a very scanty foundation for further therapeutic experiments. We call attention to this defect with all becoming emphasis. If the incompleteness of our drug-provings, and the consequent uncertainty of the therapeutic effects of some of our remedies, render the alternate exhibition of two drugs an excusable practice, yet results obtained by such means should not be given to the public, for the simple reason that they cannot be accepted as reliable testimony.

Belladonna has a sphere assigned to it in diphtheria; it is only indicated when the disease sets in with severe febrile motions and marked inflammation of the tonsils. After exudation has commenced, it is no longer in its place.

Mercurius. The pathogenesis of this drug evidently points to it, from the commencement, as a remedy for diphtheria. The results of its employment have not, however, been very favorable. An accurate comparison of its pathogenetic effects with the symptoms of the disease, shows that this could not well be otherwise. Mercury has not the extraordinary and rapid prostration of strength and the complete suppression of cutaneous activity. These are two important and significant symptoms. English physicians have been in the habit of using the stronger mercurial preparations, particularly the *Iodide of Mercury*, much less frequently the *Corrosive Sublimate*. No particularly rapid success has ever been achieved by either of these agents, nor can we boast of better suc-

Diphtheritis, Diphtheria.

cess in our own latitude. It sometimes seems as though the employment of these agents involved an useless waste of time.

Kali bichromicum is generally given in alternation with the Iodide of Mercury by our English colleagues. The symptoms of this drug undoubtedly point to its use in diphtheria, and assign to it an important rank among the remedies for this disease. Striking therapeutic results have not yet been obtained with it.

The same remarks apply to **Bromine**, which is recommended by Black for the more malignant forms of diphtheria. This drug has a characteristic symptom relating to diphtheria, namely: great debility and nervous prostration, remaining for a long time after all other morbid symptoms have disappeared. We have already stated that this symptom is characteristic of diphtheria.

According to Black, **Kali bichromicum** is more particularly suitable, if the exudation is composed of loosely-adhering shreds, *Bromine* being more adapted to firmly-adhering, tenacious membranes. We may inquire, however, to what extent these two indications differ one from the other, since the membranes usually adhere very firmly at the commencement, and afterwards become like loose shreds.

Acidum muriaticum. Most observers praise this remedy more than any other. It is scarcely ever adapted to cases having a rapid and violent course, but so much more to cases without much fever, but with marked lassitude and weariness, and having the appearance of lentescent typhus. The dose should not be too weak; a few drops of the first or second attenuation in distilled water may be given. Children are generally too young to employ a solution of this acid as a gargle. Besides, there may be very little advantage in such a proceeding. The same circumstances which recommend Muriatic acid, likewise argue in favor of *Phosphoric* and *Nitric acid*. The local symptoms of diphtheria are certainly to be found, in an eminent degree, among the pathogenetic symptoms of Nitric acid, and we do not comprehend why the preference has been given to Muriatic acid almost to the exclusion of the former.

The rapid progress of gangrenous disorganization has generally been opposed by *Arsenic*, probably more with regard to the constitutional than to the local phenomena. Symptomatically this remedy is scarcely ever indicated, nor can the employment of *Ammonium carbonicum* be accounted for, unless the cerebral symptoms which sometimes set in justify its use.

Besides the medicines which we have named, we find the following remedies mentioned as adapted to this disease: *Iodium, Capsicum, Argentum nitricum, Kali chloricum, Kali bromatum, Creasotum.* Iodine most likely owes its recommendation to the eminent services it renders in croup; but such a recommendation by analogy is, as we have already stated above, not advisable, since the two processes are essentially distinct. Creasotum has no symptom in its pathological series that points to diphtheria, and has probably been selected only on account of its efficacy against gangrenous disorganizations. Nor is Capsicum homœopathic to this disease.

In opposition to the somewhat contradictory observations furnished by our English colleagues, Baumann's notice, in No. 9 of Vol. 62, of the All. Hom. Zeit., deserves the most attentive consideration. In a series of cases he only gave one remedy from the commencement, and, according to his statement, he obtained by means of it marvellous results. This remedy was *Apis mellifica.* If his experience should be confirmed in other epidemics, we would have made a valuable discovery; we would have obtained additional evidence that mere drug-symptoms do not constitute a criterium for the homœopathicity of a drug. However, the recommendation of this agent emanates from V. Meyer, who has called attention to it in Vol. 59 of the Zeitung, (see page 48.) Baumann gave one drop of the fifteenth attenuation, every two hours, in a little water. We mention this circumstance for the benefit of those who may desire to imitate this experiment, which we trust will be confirmed by numerous trials.

Independently of this last-mentioned remedy, the rest would stand in the following order: At the commencement, *Belladonna.* After the membrane is formed, *Mercurius iodatus,* and afterwards, *Kali bichr.* or *Bromine.* In case of severe gangrenous disorganizations, *Arsenicum* or *Creasotum.* If the disease progresses more slowly after the exhibition of Mercurius, one of the above-mentioned acids. In slight cases, *Kali chloricum.* For the subsequent debility *China* has so far proved the best remedy.

Regarding the patient's diet, we must take care to supply a sufficient quantity of nourishing food, nor need we hesitate to administer small quantities of wine and water. Fresh air and cleanliness are a matter of course; the proper means should likewise be used to prevent contagion. The best local means of cleanliness is fresh water, which cleanses without doing any hurt. The patients need not be confined to their beds, but they must not be permitted to make any exertion.

Against the secondary diphtheritic, or rather croupous, affection of the buccal and pharyngeal cavities it is not necessary to institute a special medicinal proceeding. The primary affection will suggest the proper remedy in such a case. It is only in exceptional cases that the membranous exudation, owing to its copiousness, will have to be considered in the first place.

If the diphtheritic process spreads to the larynx, we indeed obtain all the symptoms of croup, but it would be wrong to employ for this form of the disease, the same remedies that are generally used in the ordinary form of membranous croup.

[American practitioners have used, with much success, the pokeweed, or *Phytolacca decandra;* the *Permanganate* of *Potash*, of which Professor Allen, of the Chicago Hahnemann College, has furnished a very thorough proving, has likewise been recommended. *Lachesis* is recommended by its admirers; some employ it in every stage of the disease; others only when symptoms of gangrene are beginning to set in ; others again rely upon it principally in diphtheritic croup. We have several special treatises on diphtheria, among which the following deserve honorable mention: Ludlam on Diphtheria, Chicago; Helmuth on Diphtheria, St. Louis; and Neidhard on Diphtheria, Philadelphia. H.]

6. Noma, Cancer Aquaticus.

We designate with this name a peculiar gangrenous destruction of the soft parts of the cheeks and mouth. It occurs almost exclusively among children between the ages of two and ten years, and befalls adults more frequently than children at the breast. It attacks exclusively children of unsound constitutions, who live in want and are deprived of the necessary supply of pure air and wholesome nourishment, or are brought up amid the privations of orphan asylums and foundling houses. Noma, properly speaking, is always a secondary affection breaking out after measles, less frequently after some other very acute disease, such as typhus, variola, intermittens, etc. Where it is described as an idiopathic affection, the diagnosis may be regarded as uncertain. The disease is of rare occurrence in practice. Why it only attacks the soft parts of the mouth, has not as yet been satisfactorily accounted for. Hartmann compares this process to pustula maligna. The resemblance between these two diseases is undoubtedly very great.

Symptoms and Course. Without being accompanied by constitutional phenomena, there appears, during the period of convalescence after some acute affection, upon the mucous membrane of the cheek, an aphthous vesicle or whitish-red pimple upon a dark-red, hard base, or without any abnormal surroundings. There is no pain either with or without contact. Very soon the vesicle bursts, or the little pimple scatters, and in its place we discover a more or less deeply-penetrating ulcer, which is speedily covered with a scurf. With the formation of the ulcer, the phenomena in the surrounding parts become more marked; the hardness spreads, the cheek and afterwards the whole face and even the neck, become œdematous. This œdema occurs less frequently, previous to the breaking out of the vesicle. Very soon the ulcer assumes a livid discoloration, which is soon after imparted to the whole of the surrounding mucous membrane. This is transformed into a yellow-gray or blackish pulpous mass, which is sharply separated from the normal parts of the cheek. The gangrenous disorganization continues to spread so rapidly, that, in a few days, not only the cheek, but likewise the eyelids and the maxillary bones, even the integuments of the neck down to the breast, are destroyed. It sometimes only takes three days for this disorganization to reach its climax. The odor from the mouth is extremely fetid, even the saliva has a cadaverous smell. The gangrenous parts are partially covered with a scurf, or in some places they are dirty-looking sores of great depth, even perforating the cheek, with shaggy borders without a sign of reaction. Hemorrhagic effusions are, generally speaking, of rare occurrence, for the reason that the vessels are attacked last. At the commencement of the disease, or even after it has reached a considerable height, the general health is not much disturbed. The children are more languid than usual, have some fever, less appetite, sunken features; but these changes do not by any means correspond to the importance of the local process. Not till the integuments have been reached by the gangrenous process, do the constitutional symptoms assume a threatening aspect. The languor increases to a comatose sopor, whereas the nights are very much disturbed by delirium. The temperature of the skin becomes depressed or irregular, the extremities being cool and the trunk very hot. The pulse continues to increase in frequency, becomes more and more feeble, the thirst is intense. Vomiting and diarrhœa are of less frequent occurrence; it is remarkable that the appetite sometimes remains unimpaired even until shortly before death; a sort of canine hunger even often takes possession of the patients. Death takes place amid signs of perfect collapse with sopor. If the disease shows a disposition to terminate in recovery, which may take place at any stage of its progress, although the chances of recovery lessen in proportion as the gangrenous destruction spreads over a larger surface, the healthy parts become surrounded with a more vivid redness, and a circumscribed inflammation results, within whose boundaries the gangrened patches become detached, leaving a healthy looking ulcer with tendency to granulation. The healing takes place slowly, according as the loss of substance is more or less extensive. The prognosis is generally very bad, the patients being mostly children with such impoverished constitutions that the reactive energies necessary to a cure are almost always wanting.

Regarding the treatment of noma we have no past experience to appeal to. The disorder is of such rare occurrence, and, if it has at all been treated homœpathically, the case has most likely resulted so disastrously, that a case of noma has not yet been reported in our publications. Hence we can only point out the remedies which it may be necessary to employ, if a case should occur in practice. Among the medicines whose pathogenesis is known to us, there is but one that answers to the two characteristic features of noma, the gangrenous destruction with painlessness—we mean *Secale cornutum*. This remedy has been warmly recommended by Hartmann; instead of transcribing the highly-wrought text of his remarks, we refer the reader to the oft-repeated descriptions of ergotism in our Materia Medica and toxicologies. Although Secale, in this disease, seems to have shown a preference for the extremities in developing its gangrenous effects, yet this is no reason why it should not likewise be applicable in noma, since such conclusions from analogy are perfectly proper. A careful comparison of the pathogenetic effects of Secale with the phenomena of noma shows various other accords between the two series of symptoms. Gangrene after Secale is consequent upon a very different constitutional disturbance which disappears as soon as the gangrene breaks out. During the existence and the further development of gangrene the general health is not correspondingly disturbed, but the pulse is feeble, small and frequent. Without pointing out any other special symptomatic similarities, all we can say is that, for the present at least, Secale is our only known remedy for noma.

Among the other medicines that have been recommended for this disease, or seem otherwise indicated, we are not acquainted with any that seems to correspond to the essential characteristics of noma. These medicines are: *Arsenicum, Acidum muriaticum, Iodium, Kali hydriodicum, Mercurius sublimatus, Helleborus niger, Chlore, Carbo vegetabilis, Creasotum.* Whereas various accessory symptoms point to Arsenic, yet it is counter-indicated by the circumstance that the gangrenous destruction of noma goes on without any signs of reaction, whereas the destruction of organic tissue, caused by Arsenic, is attended with the most violent and most painful general and local symptoms. *Carbo vegetabilis* is much more specifically indicated than Arsenic, since the absence of organic reaction is much more marked under Carbo than under Arsenic. However, is such a symptom, in the absence of all other characteristic indications, sufficient to determine the selection of a remedy? Creasotum is not homœopathic to this disease; but other physicians report good effects from it in this disorder, and, in the absence of more specific remedies, it may, undoubtedly, be tried. Doctor Hasbach, in the "Organ for Therapeutics," vol. II, 1853, recommends it as a local remedy for the purpose of promoting or exciting the detaching of the gangrened parts; he paints them with the Creasotum by means of a camel's hair pencil. Whether its internal use produces favorable effects, will have to be decided by further trials.

We must repeat the statement, which we have already made elsewhere, that cauterization is just as improper in noma as we have shown it to be in diphtheria. The affection is no local process, how then can it be removed by local means? Moreover, the strength of the patient being already very much reduced, the effect of a deeply penetrating cauterization should not be esteemed too lightly.

In view of the etiological as well as the special pathological conditions of the patient, the diet should aim at supporting his depressed vitality. A little generous wine is often better than the most nourishing food, which the stomach may be too weak to bear. The fact that the patients, in spite of the fearful havoc they are undergoing, are often tormented by a most devouring hunger to the last, shows that the diet is a matter of the utmost importance. We need scarcely suggest the propriety of seeing to the utmost cleanliness of the patient as well as the sick-room; the ichorous discharge spreads such a pestiferous stench through the room, that ventilation and deodorizing agents have to be resorted to to keep the room sweet. The mouth should likewise be washed out as often as may be necessary, lest the children should swallow the ichor and the gangrened patches.

7. Glossitis, Inflammation of the Tongue.

Although acute glossitis is of tolerably rare occurrence, this cannot be said of the chronic form of this disease, which has, moreover, a peculiar importance on account of certain diagnostic errors connected with it.

The causes of acute glossitis are, in the first place, such deleterious influences as have an immediate action upon the tongue, such as caustics, injuries, burns, stings of insects, drinking very cold water; in the next place, indirectly acting influences, such as the inflammation of adjoining parts, syphilis, suppression of an habitual perspiration of the feet, of piles and the menses. However, there are likewise cases that cannot be traced to the presence of any exciting cause.

Acute glossitis generally sets in without any precursory symptoms; if induced by external irritants, the inflammation develops itself soon after they have begun to act. While a generally very violent fever is present, the tongue becomes painful, its mobility is very much embarrassed, and it swells so rapidly that the swelling sometimes fills the whole cavity of the mouth within the space of twenty-four hours, and even protrudes between the teeth. The tongue has a deep dark-red or even blackish hue, it is very hot and dry. The more the swelling increases, the more acute are the pains, and the more difficult the processes of mastication, deglutition and speech. In the higher grades of glossitis, even respiration is very much embarrassed, both by the tongue itself as well as by a readily supervening œdema of the epiglottis, and even of the larynx. The febrile symptoms are strongly marked, and the symptoms of considerable cerebral hyperæmia are scarcely ever wanting. The inflammation easily terminates fatally, if the respiration is seriously interfered with. Otherwise the inflammatory exudation is gradually dispersed more or less completely, or an abscess forms, after whose discharge a rapid improvement takes place. The disease always runs a very rapid course.

Chronic glossitis either remains after an acute attack, or else it develops itself gradually. In the substance of the tongue, one or more hard places are felt, not elevated above the surface of the tongue, and mostly painless on contact, but otherwise causing now and then dull pains. It is most generally caused by the irritating action of the sharp edges of some of the teeth, and is accordingly most frequently met with in the outer border of the tongue. Chronic glossitis is not very rare, and although patients do not often heed the pain, yet they are very frequently tormented by the apprehension that their trouble might be of a carcinomatous nature. The circumstance of the swelling sometimes continuing for years without any apparent change, finally satisfies the physician that it is not malignant. This conviction is of especial importance, in so far as it often helps to prevent mischievous, or at least useless, surgical operations. The termination of chronic glossitis in an abscess, does not often occur, except where the chronic form is the result of an acute attack, in which case the formation of an abscess is much more common.

Treatment. According to the statement of pathological treatises, acute glossitis is a very dangerous inflammation, which has often terminated fatally. When treated homœopathically, this inflammation becomes a very mild affection for which we possess specific remedies, under whose influence the suppurative process is almost surely prevented.

In most cases of glossitis, more particularly if the disease has an idiopathic character, *Mercurius* is the surest and most suitable remedy. According to Hartmann, it should be exhibited in the second or third trituration, with which he professes to have cut short recent cases that had not yet progressed too far. "I admit," he adds, "that the disease can be cured with a small dose of a higher attenuation; but in a case of so much danger, where experience and a reliable method of treatment have proved perfectly safe, mere theoretical experiments are out of place; so far as I know but few cures of glossitis have been reported by homœopathic physicians in opposition to my own statements." That *Mercurius* is likewise the specific remedy in cases depending upon syphilis, should not be forgotten; only in such cases it is well to administer the more powerful mercurial preparations, the Corrosive Sublimate or the white Precipitate. Although Hartmann's statement, that a cure can be accomplished in a few hours, is somewhat extravagant, yet suppuration will scarcely ever take place after the timely use of this agent. If suppuration has set in, it is best to give *Hepar sulphuris*, without regard to the threatening symptoms which accompany this process. If the inflammation is caused by corrosive substances or a burn, it is speedily and safely removed by *Cantharides*, whereas Mercury would have no effect. Inflammations of the mucous lining of the tongue, with the parenchyma being more or less involved, are generally more readily controlled by *Belladonna* than by Mercury, unless the inflammation should emanate from ulcers in the lining membrane. Under these circumstances *Acidum muriaticum* and *nitricum* may likewise prove serviceable. During the further progress of the inflammation *Arsenicum* may still be resorted to as a last but very efficacious remedy, especially if the general organism seems to be very much prostrated. Where the inflammation had resulted from contusion or a mechanical injury of the tongue, *Arnica* is jumped at by many, in conformity with the general theory that Arnica is indicated by contusions and the like. The symptoms do not point to *Arnica*, nor have we any practical evidence for its appropriateness in such cases. According to Hartmann, *Conium* is the best remedy under such circumstances; indeed the symptoms point to its employment as a suitable agent. We will likewise mention *Apis* and *Lachesis*, which are useful in inflammatory affections of the buccal cavity generally, and more especially in glossitis. There is scarcely a remedy that has such marked symptoms of glossitis as *Apis*. In one case of poisoning the inflammatory swelling was not the result of a sting in the lining membrane, or of the introduction of the poison into the stomach, so that the inflammation might be accounted for upon the ground of local action; but the inflammation occurred after a sting in the temple, showing that the virus has a specific effect upon the tongue. The symptoms of *Lachesis* are not nearly as clearly marked.

In chronic glossitis we have to try *Sulphur* above every other remedy. In recent cases *Conium* is likewise indicated. In protracted cases we may expect aid from *Aurum* and *Iodium*, and likewise from *Silicea*. Where the induration is situated under an ulcer or surrounds it, we have to inquire in the first place whether carious teeth or other mechanical irritants are not the real cause of the trouble; in such a case a cure is obtained by removing them. It sometimes happens that such indurations have become so inveterate, that they continue even after the removal of the cause, in spite of persevering treatment.

[In phlegmonous glossitis, with high fever, hot and dry skin, headache, slight delirium, etc., *Aconite* in the lower preparations of the root will be found an indispensable remedy. A drop of the tincture, or a few drops of the first decimal attenuation, in half a tumblerful of water, the medicine to be repeated every hour or even half hour, will be found the proper dose. H.]

8. Parotitis.

We comprehend under this designation two tolerably distinct conditions which have, however, this in common: that the salivary glands are the seat, or rather the starting-point of the disease. Consequently we shall first describe parotitis proper, or an inflammation of the parotid gland, together with the non-malignant inflammation of the other salivary glands, and afterwards the malignant form of the disease attended with gangrene of the cellular tissue.

a. *Parotitis, Inflammation of the Parotid Gland, Mumps, Angina Parotidea.*

This affection is at times idiopathic, and as such has received the above series of names; at other times it is a secondary disorder, to be regarded as a complication of other diseases. The symptoms differ accordingly.

Idiopathic parotitis is generally preceded for a few days by febrile symptoms. The patients feel languid, sleep is uneasy, the appetite is gone; headache, with a feeling of stiffness in the posterior cervical muscles is scarcely ever absent; a slight catarrhal irritation of the digestive tract is likewise generally present. After these preliminary symptoms have lasted for a short period, sometimes even for several days, the region below the lobule of the ear on one side begins to swell, the swelling spreading very rapidly over the cheek and the submaxillary region; in a short time the face looks very much disfigured by the swelling. The swelling is not very painful even to rather hard pressure; the color of the swelling does not differ from that of the surrounding integuments, except sometimes a slight redness; the swelling is at times of a stony consistence, at times it is soft, and at other times has an uneven feel. The movements of the head, more especially of the jaws, are very much impeded. With the appearance of the swelling, the general symptoms usually improve, the fever abates rapidly, and the patients, in spite of their great disfigurement, feel tolerably well. In most cases the swelling spreads to the other side in one or two days, but here never attains the same size as on the former side. If the swelling runs a normal course, it generally reaches the climax on the fifth day, after which it gradually begins to disperse, so that between the tenth and fourteenth day no trace of the swelling remains visible. With a higher grade of inflammation, or under otherwise unfavorable circumstances, the redness assumes an erythematous character, and suppuration may take place, which, in comparison to the size of the swelling, remains inconsiderable, but protracts the course of the disease very greatly. The swelling takes this course more frequently in the case of adults than in that of children; in the case of the former, an inflammatory hardness of greater or less extent sometimes remains for some time. Only in rare cases, or if the affection assumes a certain degree of malignancy, as it sometimes does in certain epidemics, the brain may become involved in the process. What is more frequently the case is, that the testicles, or the labia majora, swell suddenly, while the swelling of the parotid gland disappears; both swellings may, however, coexist, and the supposition of a metastasis should not be entertained too lightly.

Secondary parotitis occurs in the course of many acute diseases, particularly typhus; in some typhus epidemics it is a constant sequela of the disease, whereas in other epidemics it is entirely absent. The appearance of the swelling is not bound to any definite period of the disease; at times we see it break out at the commencement, at other times during the period of convalescence. It is generally preceded by local pains, increased congestions of the head, even delirium and chilly creepings; its rapid development is seldom attended with abatement of the fever. The further course of the local process is similar to that of the idiopathic disease; the swelling either scatters or else it terminates in violent inflammation with suppuration, which, during a state of great constitutional prostration, may assume a malignant form, with the discharge of ichor. Whereas, in the former case, parotitis always indicates a favorable course of the general disease; the formation of pus, on the contrary, always portends danger, and is at least a disturbing complication. It is difficult to determine *a priori*, of what character the swelling will be; but when parotitis sets in at the acme of the disease, it is always more dangerous than when it occurs at the commencement or during convalescence. Here, too, as in the case of mumps, an induration may be left behind for a long time. In isolated cases of either variety the ear seems to be affected, hardness of hearing and purulent otorrhœa remaining after the disappearance of the swelling.

The etiology of parotitis is involved in obscurity, in so far as we are unable to determine by what atmospheric or other influences the disease is caused. Its epidemic character leads us to adopt the existence of some peculiar miasm, similar to the miasm of typhus, cholera, etc. We know, moreover, that the common epidemic mumps prevail most frequently in the transition-seasons. But it is a mystery why the parotid gland should be invaded in acute diseases of the general organism, in one epidemic quite frequently, in another scarcely ever, or why at one time it should be harmless and at another time a phenomenon portending great danger. This difference accounts for the circumstance why some consider this form of parotitis a dangerous, and others a trifling, disease.

An inflammation of the other salivary glands often accompanies parotitis as an accessory disorder, and may likewise break out in an idiopathic form. Numerous facts lead us to believe that each separate salivary gland may become the seat of an affection like mumps. After very acute diseases we have often noticed stony swellings of the lesser salivary glands of a very obstinate character, and running their course amid a general prostration of strength.

Treatment. In ordinary mumps, which run a very rapid and painless course, it makes very little difference what medicine is given; indeed, the affection might safely be left to take its own course. However, inasmuch as we cannot well know what the final termination of the affection may be, it is best to always give the suitable remedy, since we can rest assured that under its use suppuration will only take place exceptionally. The best remedy is *Mercurius.* The specific action of Mercury upon the salivary glands is well known. It not only increases the secretions of these glands, but likewise causes a real inflammation in the body of the glands which may readily terminate in suppuration, as is often seen in the violent treatment of diseases with large doses of Mercury. No remedy prevents suppuration as certainly as Mercurius. *Belladonna* deserves a preference if the constitutional symptoms are very severe, and the swelling assumes an erysipelatous character. *Rhus toxicodendron* rivals Mercurius in efficacy; for a more accurate description of their distinctive pathogenetic symptoms, we refer the reader to our Materia Medica. We content ourselves with mentioning in this place that Rhus, independently of the symptoms of typhoid parotitis, is more suitable to a kind of mumps where the inflammatory swelling is not very hard, not very red, and not very painful. These three remedies will always prove sufficient in mumps; in typhoid parotitis other remedies will likewise have to be used, for which we refer to our article on typhus. The induration remaining after typhus is often very obstinate, and only yields gradually. In such a case, *Baryta carbonica* is the best remedy, provided it is continued for a sufficient length of time. Besides these remedies, *Co-*

nium, Aurum and *Silicea* may be thought of. The metastasis to the genital organs is best met by *Pulsatilla* [and *Belladonna*. H.]

As regards general hygienic measures, we are decidedly opposed to the abuse of external warmth, of which both physicians and patients are guilty, in the supposition that they will by this means prevent a metastasis. This abuse is of no sort of advantage to the course of the disease; but it is a source of great discomfort to the patients if they are compelled to envelop their heads with a quantity of covering. The headache is always increased by such a proceeding. If suppuration threatens, and the swelling is very painful, lukewarm, moist cataplasms not only afford relief, but they likewise promote the dispersion of the swelling.

b. *Parotitis Maligna.*

We apply this name to a specific inflammation of the cellular tissue surrounding the salivary glands; it is characterized by a tendency to gangrenous disorganization. Synonymous appellations are: Cynanche cellularis maligna, angina externa, metaphlogosis or gangrenous inflammation of the cervical cellular tissue. The reason why we mention this affection in this place is, because the disease always starts from the lesser salivary glands, and seems to have a preference for their locality.

Upon the whole, parotitis maligna is a very rare disease that has so far been chiefly observed in the South of Germany. We know that it makes its appearance more particularly in the fall and winter; attacks chiefly individuals of the lower classes with impoverished, dyscrasic, scrofulous constitutions; and occurs most frequently in low lands, marshy districts, and damp dwellings. The real cause of the disease, on looking at its whole course and essential characteristics, seems to be a peculiar toxication of the blood, such as occurs in typhus and diphtheria. When cynanche maligna was prevalent some time ago, typhus, with tendency to putrid decomposition, was likewise very frequent.

Symptoms and Course. The disease commences at once at the affected part, without any preliminary symptoms. Accompanied by febrile symptoms, consisting of alternate chills and flashes of heat, with general languor and prostration of strength, dulness of the head, loss of appetite and coated tongue; the patient experiences slight difficulties of deglutition, with dull pain in the lower maxilla and teeth, and a feeling of stiffness in the articulation of the lower jaw of the affected side, which is generally the right side. The saliva is secreted in somewhat larger quantity, the buccal cavity shows no abnormal symptoms. While the constitutional symptoms are increasing in intensity, we notice on the third day, and, in violent cases, often in a few hours, a swelling in the region of the submaxillary or sublingual, much less frequently of the parotid gland, which keeps on increasing and spreads over the whole side of the neck. The swelling is of a stony consistence, sharply circumscribed, lies close to the bone, does not feel very hot, is not red, nor very painful to contact. As the swelling increases in size, the process of deglutition becomes more and more difficult and the opening of the mouth almost impossible. The general condition of the patient becomes worse and worse; he has restless nights, his pulse is small and quick and the skin inclines to perspire. All the symptoms increasing in intensity, the disease reaches its acme about the tenth day. The face and neck are terribly disfigured, the swelling occupying the lower part of the face and the submaxillary region as far as behind the ear, sometimes extends even down to the clavicle, and looks like a thick pad laid around the neck. The mouth now can no longer be opened, deglutition has become next to impossible; the voice is rough and without resonance; a quantity of tenacious mucus flows out of the mouth. The fever is intense. If, as is possible, but not very probable, the inflammation should disperse at this period, the difficulty of swallowing decreases in the first place, the swelling diminishes from the periphery towards the centre, the fever moderates, the sleep becomes quieter, the cutaneous transpiration takes place easily and affords a feeling of ease and comfort. The process of reabsorption goes on very slowly.

Generally, however, suppuration takes place at the acme of the disease, with speedy transition into ichorous decomposition and gangrenous destruction. At the same time the fever increases, after which it rapidly assumes an adynamic character. If the pus is evacuated in good season, an immediate improvement may set in, or else the septic character is too far advanced, the ichor is formed again and again, and the symptoms assume the appearance of malignant typhus. The extremities grow cold and the scene ends with delirium, subsultus tendinum, unquenchable thirst, miliary eruptions, paroxysms of dyspnœa and finally paralysis of the lungs. In the case of adults a fatal termination may be reached between the eleventh and twentieth day, children sometimes die as early as the third day

If the disease runs a favorable course, there frequently remains for some time, besides disfiguring cicatrices, and on account of the destruction of considerable portions of the integuments, an induration at the lower jaw, which at times involves a salivary gland, and at other times the periosteum of the jaw-bone.

Beside the gangrenous destruction on the neck, which may not only have invaded the cellular tissue, but likewise the muscles, bones and even the cartilages of the larynx, a post-mortem examination very frequently reveals signs of pulmonary stasis, softening of the spleen, and typhoid degenerations in the bowels. The prognosis is very unfavorable, the disease being one of the most fatal diseases known.

In describing it we have followed almost literally Schweickert's detailed delineation of cynanche maligna in the "Hom. Vierteljahrsschrift," (Hom. Quarterly,) vol. XIII, 1; he proposes the following treatment:

As soon as the inflammatory swelling makes its appearance, warm poultices are applied to it without intermission; as soon as we discover a trace of fluctuation, a deep incision is made in order to secure an outlet to the ichor and to prevent its gravitating downwards. The wound has to be cleansed with water, as often as necessary, and in order to facilitate the discharge of the ichor, a horizontal posture should be maintained. In one case Schweickert gave internally *Aconitum*, *Belladonna*, *Rhus tox.*, *Mercurius*, *Baryta carbonica*, *Silicea*, without the least success. In three other cases he gave *Anthracin* 9th and 30th attenuation, and effected a cure in every instance. These results may perhaps be confirmed by further trials. Somebody has recommended *Bryonia* for this disorder. Why *Arsenicum* was not given in the first-mentioned case, we are unable to say. For the remaining indurations *Aurum muriat. natr.*, and *Silicea* were found the most efficient remedies.

There is a less malignant inflammation of the cellular tissue of the neck, which runs a more subacute course. It arises like the malignant form of this disease and seems to depend upon atmospheric influences. We have treated three cases of it within the last three weeks, the patients belonging to the poorer class. The constitutional symptoms are not very striking, but there is great prostration of strength. Poultices and the internal use of *Mercurius* and *Baryta carb.* effected a cure in every case.

9. Salivatio, Ptyalism.

An increased secretion of saliva is not often an idiopathic affection; it generally is a symptomatic occurrence in the course of some more general disease, and constitutes, moreover, a very unimportant complication. There are cases, however, where salivation is a very serious disorder, and we have deemed it necessary to devote a short chapter to it.

The causes of salivation are either an irritation of the mucous lining of the mouth or of the salivary glands themselves, or it may result from affections of other organs, such as the stomach, pancreas, liver, uterus, or from paralysis of the tongue, the muscles of the mouth and pharynx, or the salivation may be a consequence of the toxical action of Mercury, Iodine, Gold; or finally it may be caused by other general influences, a cold for instance.

Salivation arises gradually, very seldom suddenly; the quantity of the secreted saliva may amount to several pounds a day. At first the saliva contains a good deal of mucus, is tenacious, insipid; but if the secretion increases in quantity, it acquires a sweetish taste and is attended with fetor from the mouth. Ulcerations of the mucous lining of the mouth, catarrhal symptoms of the digestive tract, and febrile motions likewise supervene. Sleep is frequently interrupted by the necessity of swallowing the profusely secreted mucus. The constitutional equilibrium is always considerably interfered with after salivation has lasted for some time, nutrition being very much impaired, not only by the loss of fluids, but likewise by the imperfect admixture of saliva with the food and its consequent imperfect digestion. The affection is scarcely ever painful, but there is the tormenting sensation of a constant afflux of saliva in the mouth. Only exceptionally the salivary glands are painful and swollen. The duration of the disorder varies from a few days to several months and even years, according as it may have been caused by one circumstance or another. Sequelæ are: Catarrhal puffing up of the lining membrane of the mouth, ulceration of this membrane, caries and looseness of the teeth, and, moreover, the phenomena of altered digestion.

Treatment. Ptyalism being generally a symptom of some constitutional derangement, we refer the reader to the chapter where these derangements are treated of, and shall here mention only such medicines as may be required when ptyalism has reached such a degree of intense virulence that the first attention in the treatment of the case has to be devoted to it, or perhaps in the few cases where it occurs as an idiopathic disease. Where it is a mere partial manifestation of a more general constitutional disorder, the remedies for the latter will likewise remove the ptyalism.

The most important remedy for this affection is, under almost all circumstances, *Mercurius*, except where the ptyalism had been caused by the abuse of this drug. Its specific action upon the salivary glands necessarily implies its great efficacy as a curative agent in this disease. It is not only suitable in salivation pure and simple, but likewise in salivation depending upon affections of the mouth, fauces, stomach, liver and pancreas. Recent cases, or such at least as have not yet become inveterate by age, yield more readily to its curative influence. The tenacious and ropy saliva must have a sweetish, metallic, insipid taste, accompanied by a putrid-sweetish odor from the mouth. The best mercurial preparation in such cases is *Mercurius vivus*, lower triturations; next to it *Corrosive Sublimate*.

Iodium is not only valuable against mercurial salivation, but likewise in salivation depending upon other causes; more particularly upon affections of the stomach or pancreas. It is preferable to Mercurius in cases where the assimilative energies have become very much depressed by the protracted duration of the disease.

Acidum nitricum is likewise an excellent remedy for mercurial ptyalism, but, like Iodine, may likewise be applicable in other forms of this disease. The saliva has a marked sweetish taste, is tenacious, although not very copious; the lining membrane is very much affected, the smell from the mouth very bad. *Acidum sulphuricum* has almost the same symptomatic indications as the former acid; indeed, it would be a difficult matter to draw well defined lines of demarcation between the two.

According to Hartmann, *Colchicum* is particularly adapted to ptyalism, caused by suppression of the perspiration, and accompanied by all sorts of rheumatic ailments whose increase is attended with a corresponding increase of the ptyalism. When swallowing the saliva, it causes nausea and a desire to vomit; notwithstanding the quantity of secreted fluid, the patient experiences a troublesome feeling of dryness in the throat.

Dulcamara is likewise urgently recommended by Hartmann, who seems to think a great deal of it in a variety of complaints. Judging by the symptoms we certainly have better remedies; of practical results none are as yet recorded. *Belladonna* is far superior to Dulcamara, both in mercurial and other forms of ptyalism.

Without continuing our list of remedies, we now add a few that deserve particular consideration in cases where ptyalism is a mere symptom; they are: *Nux vomica, Capsicum, Sulphur, Hepar sul-*

phuris, Baryta carb., Staphysagria, Mezereum. Of course this is not the whole list of remedies that may be employed against ptyalism; we must remember that almost every drug in our Materia Medica induces an increased secretion of saliva.

In the rare cases where ptyalism develops consumptive symptoms, *Natrum muriaticum* may deserve attention.

[Rheumatic inflammation of the gums and sublingual glands is not an unfrequent occurrence. In such cases the saliva sometimes flows out of the mouth in a continuous stream. It seems to be mere water, without much taste or bad smell from the mouth. Chilly creepings and slight flushes of fever are likewise present. We have cured such cases in a very few days, sometimes in a single day, by mixing one or two drops of the *Tinctura Aconiti Radicis* in half a goblet of water, giving a dessertspoonful of this solution every half hour or hour, and widening the intervals in proportion as the patient began to improve. H.]

[10. Scorbutus.
Scurvy of the gums.

According to Kafka scurvy of the gums usually commences with a red border along the upper margin of the gums; their indentations between the teeth become bulbous, spongy, and sometimes recede from the teeth; the gums are swollen, spongy, and look bluish. The gums sometimes overhang the teeth in palmated excrescences, or bulge out here and there in thick, spongy, pad-shaped swellings. As the disease progresses in intensity, the swellings on the gums and the gums adjoining the teeth soften, become discolored and ulcerate. In case of improvement, the swellings decrease, the gums again adhere closely to the teeth, recover their firmness and normal color.

Scurvy of the gums is caused by bad and improper nourishment, want of fresh vegetables, fresh water, or by the continued use of salt meat, or by a deficiency of nourishment; or, it may be occasioned by excessive bodily labor, with an insufficient supply of food, by an utter neglect of all bodily exercise; by bad, damp, cold, foul air, marshy emanations, or by continued depressing moral emotions.

Disease of the gums is always the first sign of incipient scurvy, and is not so much caused by an abnormal condition of the blood, as by a peculiar disease of the walls of the capillaries, upon which the hemorrhages, the swellings and the rest of the morbid phenomena depend.

Scurvy of the mouth is exclusively seated in the gums. It is a remarkable fact, that persons who have lost their teeth are not attacked by this disease.

Mastication is painful, sometimes even impossible. At every attempt to masticate, or on pressing upon, or cleaning the gums, or even when talking, the gums bleed more or less. In the further course of the disease, the continued decomposition of the blood and the necrosed tissues, cause a penetrating, repulsive fetor from the mouth; the secretion of mucus and saliva is considerably increased. Necrosis and consequent loss of the gums may cause the roots of the teeth to become denuded, the teeth become loose, and finally fall out.

Course, Terminations, Prognosis. Scurvy of the mouth, if neglected, or if the influences that occcasion it are permitted to continue, is an exceedingly chronic and obstinate disease. This form of scurvy is curable in the majority of cases; if neglected, it may cause considerable destructions of the gums, and the loss of teeth. The prognosis, although generally favorable, yet, in the presence of considerable destructions in the mouth, and a deep involvement of the constitution, may become very dubious.

Treatment. As long as the disease is purely local, the gums bleed, are swollen, loose, bluish, tuberous, a local treatment, with spirituous or astringent washes is sufficient. For this purpose we cause the mouth to be gargled with brandy or vinegar diluted with water. If these means should prove insufficient, we resort to a weak solution of burnt alum, in the proportion of ten grains to six ounces of water, or to a mixture of dilute muriatic or sulphuric acid, in the proportion of ten to twenty drops to six ounces of water. If the gums ulcerate, the fetor becomes excessive, the salivation increases in quantity, and the affection is still confined to the gums, we give *Nitri acidum* 3, internally, and have the mouth gargled with the same acid, as recommended previously; or else we give *Corrosive Sublimate* 3, internally, and for a gargle we prepare a solution of one grain of the sublimate to four ounces of water; *Creasotum* 3, internally and externally, the same as Nitric acid, is likewise excellent. *Nux vomica* 3, internally, and ten drops to eight ounces of water as a gargle, is sometimes very appropriate. *Ammonium carbonicum* used in the same manner, may prove serviceable.

As a matter of course, everything that tends to keep up and develop the scorbutic disease, has to be avoided, and all pernicious influences have to be absolutely removed. The general mode of living in regard to diet, habitation, cleanliness, etc., has to be regulated with strict care and attention. If the disease should progress and develop itself into a general constitutional disease, we shall then have to institute an anti-scorbutic treatment, which will be described in the article on Scurvy. H.]

[11. **Ranula.**

Kafka has treated several cases of this disease internally with perfect success. This swelling may be located in the excretory duct of the submaxillary glands, the Whartonian duct. It is soft, fluctuating, almost transparent. The orifice of the duct is closed, in consequence of which the saliva accumulates, becomes inspissated, and the duct enlarges and finally forms a sacculated swelling. Ranula may likewise constitute a hard and firm swelling under the tongue, either in consequence of calculi stopping up the ducts, or in consequence of the ducts having become inflamed. It is with this latter class of ranulæ that the physician has to deal; the former belong to the domain of surgery.

At the commencement of the disease the patients complain of a pain under the tongue, which is made worse by chewing and talking. Upon examining the mouth at this period, we find the Whartonian ducts swollen, somewhat hard and red. These phenomena increase gradually, both in intensity and extent; sensitive patients commence to experience febrile motions, the slowly increasing swelling becomes more painful, and interferes with the motions of the tongue quite considerably.

Gradually the sublingual cellular tissue becomes infiltrated, and a swelling forms, which, if left to itself, frequently attains to a considerable size, until it fills the larger portion of the buccal cavity, in consequence of which the tongue is pressed upwards towards the fauces, the respiration is impeded, and speech and deglutition become impossible. Or the swelling may form under the chin, and bulge more and more towards the outside, in which case the tongue is much less involved in the pathological process. In either case the pain and constitutional disturbance are very great.

If we do not succeed in effecting a reabsorption of the swelling, chills set in and throbbing pains in the swelling; these symptoms point to the formation of an abscess which will have to be treated by surgical means. The abscess either perforates the anterior side of the neck, or else, which is of more frequent occurrence, the base of the buccal cavity.

Course, Terminations, Prognosis. The course of this swelling is either acute or chronic. In the former case the inflammation sets in suddenly; pain, redness and swelling come on at once, and the dispersion of the swelling or its termination in suppuration likewise occurs at a much earlier period. If the swelling reaches a considerable size, (sometimes it attains the size of a hen's or goose egg,) the pressure of the tongue upon the pharynx and larynx, and consequently hyperæmia of the brain, may result fatally.

In the chronic form the pain is at first imperceptible, so that the patients often wait a long time before sending for a physician. The swelling develops itself very gradually, nor do the single symptoms reach a very high degree of intensity. If suppuration cannot be prevented, the swelling becomes more and more inflamed, and it is at this stage that the previously described threatening disturbances arise, and do not cease until the abscess has either found a natural or artificial outlet. After the swelling has changed to an abscess, dispersion is no longer possible.

On account of the danger that may arise before and during suppuration, the prognosis should be very guarded.

Treatment. In treating ranula, the question is, in the first place, whether the course of the disease is acute or chronic. In the former case, if the pain is intense, and the swelling red, hard and inflamed, we give *Belladonna* 3, in solution, and at the same time apply cold compresses under the chin; or, if the inflammation is intense, we resort to applications of ice. The cold water compresses have to be renewed every five minutes. As a rule, the violent pain abates in a few hours; at the same time the redness decreases, and talking is much less difficult. Under the influence of Belladonna, retrograde metamorphosis progresses very finely for two or three days; about the fifth or sixth day it seems to stop. The redness and pain are indeed much less, but the swelling remains hard, and interferes with mastication and speech. In such a case we give every day three to four doses of *Mercurius solubilis* 2, after which the hardness decreases in a very short time, the swelling becomes smaller and softer, and finally disappears altogether. In three cases that we have treated in this manner, suppuration was entirely prevented. If suppuration sets in, the abscess should be opened as soon as fluctuation is perceived. An incision may be made either in front or at the base of the mouth.

In the chronic form of the swelling we commence the treatment with *Mercurius solubilis* 2 or 3, two or three doses a day. If there is no decrease of the swelling in six or eight days, and the swelling is not any softer, we give *Calcarea* 6, a dose morning and night. In one case this remedy alone effected the complete absorption of the swelling. If no absorption had taken place, we should then have given *Silicea* 6 and *Thuya* 3 or 6.

If no dispersion is brought about by internal treatment, the swelling gradually shows signs of inflammation, which becomes more and more acute until an abscess forms, when surgical means have to be resorted to.

As long as mastication and deglutition are difficult, we feed the patients on milk, soft-boiled eggs without salt, mush, and the like. H.]

12. Œsophagitis, Dysphagia Inflammatoria, Inflammation of the Œsophagus.

An inflammatory affection of the œsophagus may simply constitute an acute catarrh of the mucous lining of the œsophagus, in which case it is accompanied by a catarrhal inflammation of the mouth and fauces, or of the stomach, and is without any importance, or even without any more prominent symptoms than characterize the accompanying affection of the other organs.

In œsophagitis proper, it is not only the mucous membrane that is attacked, but likewise the subjacent tissue; hence the symptoms are much more violent, and seem more marked, for the reason that œsophagitis occurs much more frequently as an idiopathic affection.

The causes of the disease are almost always of a mechanical or chemical nature, foreign bodies, acids, corrosive substances, or excessive heat of the ingesta; without such demonstrable causes the inflammation is of much less frequent occurrence.

Owing to the slight sensibility of the œsophagus, the symptoms, if the attack is not too acute, are not very marked. Patients complain of a dull pain, according as the inflammation is seated near the throat, or between the shoulder-blades; it is much aggravated by every effort at swallowing. Deglutition is more or less interfered with, the food regurgitates, and at intervals a tenacious mucus, which is sometimes streaked with blood, is hawked up with a great effort. In acute cases, however, the pain becomes intense and even intolerable, deglutition is almost impossible, and the least attempt is so painful that the patients do not even dare to gratify their burning thirst. The mucus, which is hawked up with an agonizing distress, is of a purulent character; speech is almost impossible, and the breathing is oppressed even to suffocation; fever is almost always present, and signs of cerebral congestion may occur. If an abscess forms, every symptom increases with the fever until it reaches a most threatening height. The violence of the symptoms abates as soon as the pus is discharged. Where no abscess occurs, the symptoms disappear more slowly and almost imperceptibly.

Œsophagitis acquires particular importance through the consequences which it sometimes entails upon the patient, more particularly stricture. It does not set in at once after the disappearance of the inflammatory process, but develops itself very gradually. At first the patients only experience at times a difficulty of swallowing, or, when attempting to swallow large pieces, they do not seem to descend readily into the stomach, and arrive at their place of destination only after a time, or after drinking a little water. These difficulties increase very gradually, until deglutition has become so difficult that all kinds of solid food are rejected again. With the stricture there generally supervenes a dilatation of that portion of the œsophagus lying between the stricture and the pharynx. In consequence of this alteration, the food remains for some time in the œsophagus before it is rejected.

In treating œsophagitis we have in the first place to inquire into the causes of the disease. Foreign bodies have to be removed without any loss of time. If the trouble has been caused by corrosive substances, a lukewarm, slimy beverage should at once be drank in large quantities; dilute lukewarm milk may likewise be taken. The principal medicines are: *Arnica*, if the injury was produced by foreign bodies, *Cantharides*, if caused by burns, and *Rhus tox.*, if caused by corrosive substances. If the disease cannot be traced to any definite cause, we may give *Mercurius* preceded by a few doses of *Belladonna*. Beside these medicines Hartmann mentions *Cocculus, Sabadilla, Arsenicum, Secale cornutum, Mezereum, Laurocerasus* and *Carbo vegetabilis*. The thirst of the patients is best quenched by little bits of ice in the mouth.

Strictures can only be reached exceptionally by internal remedies, and then only in recent cases. If the stricture is owing to the presence of a cicatrix, no internal treatment is of any avail, any more than in a case of dilatation or cul-de-sac. Only where the stricture is owing to an hypertrophied condition of the mucous lining, the following remedies may be administered with a reasonable hope of relief: *Sulphur, Iodium, Mercurius, Hepar sulphuris* and *Arsenicum*. Considering what excellent effects have been obtained by means of the introduction of a graduated sound, internal treatment should never be exclusively depended upon, but surgical treatment should at once be resorted to.

[Spasmodic dysphagia may yield to Tartar Emetic, Aconite, Nux vomica. H.]

13. Odontalgia, Toothache.

Toothache is such a stumbling-block for authors of therapeutic manuals, that no mention is made of this distressing affection, which is, by tacit consent, assigned to the domain of the dentist. This is natural enough, owing to the fact that the Old School never has had any real remedies for toothache, except perhaps a dose of *Opium*. Common practice, however, is not bound by therapeutic compendia; what is most needed in practice, is often not to be found in printed treatises. This is the case with toothache. With our present mode of living, no pain is more frequently complained of than toothache, and nothing is more urgently demanded by the patient, and at the same time more embarrassing to the truly rational physician, than to find a sure remedy for this complaint. On the other hand there is no derangement more calculated to place the advantages of homœopathic treatment in more brilliant relief than the management of toothache. How many sceptics have been converted into zealous adherents of Homœopathy by the relief from toothache which a few small powders had afforded them as if by magic; for were not the powders taken internally? What homœopathic physician cannot relate a number of such cases?

On this account we cannot conceal our opinion that toothache has a practical significance for the homœopathic physician as well as for his patients. The case is with toothache as with many other isolated morbid phenomena. Homœopathy alone is in possession of a definite method of curing this complaint, and we regard the successful treatment of toothache by homœopathic means as a greater triumph for Homœopathy than the cure of a disease in which the whole organism was involved. The evidence of the cure having been effected by internal treatment, is too striking not to overcome the most inveterate scepticism.

We do not mean to assert that we succeed in curing every case of toothache; we know very well that homœopathic remedies have no magical power and that we may be deceived in the selection of a drug. We certainly can boast of curing at least one-half of all our cases, which is a great deal more than the Old School can brag of.

We need not analyze the causes of toothache. A remedial agent had generally better be chosen in accordance with the symptoms; it is only in a few cases that the remedy will have to be selected from a higher and more universal stand-point. For this reason a Repertory is nowhere more useful than in a case of toothache; we can only regret, however, that a number of remedies have been received among the list of curatives for toothache, which have, indeed, toothache symptoms, but have no specific reference to the teeth. This circumstance diminishes the value of a carefully constructed Repertory, so far as toothache is concerned. The better way would be to construct a Repertory of the few remedies for toothache, from which we have already seen definite curative results. In affections of the stomach we do not make use of every drug that has symptoms of gastric derangement among its pathogenetic effects, but only those which produce derangement of the stomach as a constant result of their pathogenetic action. This remark applies to all affections confined to one definite organ. Those who wish to become acquainted with every medicine that has some sort of toothache among its pathogenetic symptoms, and may possibly cure a case of toothache some time or other, will therefore have to consult a Repertory, whereas in the following paragraphs we only indicate the principal remedies whose curative powers in toothache have been verified by actual observation, and which will be found sufficient to cure most every case of toothache that may be met with in practice.

Mercurius is placed at the head of the list because no remedy has such constant effects upon the teeth as Mercurius. Mercurius is particularly adapted to ailments from carious teeth. The pains are stitching, tearing or boring, are not limited to the point they start from, but radiate to the ear, forehead and even occupy the whole side of the head. They are aggravated by the warmth of the bed, by a horizontal posture, by eating and drinking, and are momentarily relieved by the application of cold water. Their regular period of exacerbation is from evening till midnight, when they sometimes become unbearable without afterwards abating altogether. The contact of warm substances with the tooth increases the pains, whereas warm applications to the cheek relieve them. External cold, a draught of air, etc., are particularly aggravating. At the same time we cannot possibly overlook an inflammatory affection of the surrounding soft parts; the gums are red, swollen, sensitive, the glands are engorged with blood, the secretion of saliva is increased, the constitutional condition is feverish, with disposition to perspiration that affords relief, constant anxiety and restlessness compelling the patient to resort to a frequent change of posture. If the pains last much longer, the gums become spongy, recede from the teeth, bleed readily, and show ulcerated spots, especially at the margins. Moreover we have the symptoms of catarrh of the mouth; abscess at the root of the tongue. The best mercurial preparation is *Mercurius solubilis*, next to which ranks metallic quicksilver.

Belladonna. The pains are very violent, rather throbbing, but sometimes digging or jerking. They break out in paroxysms, are worse towards evening, are aggravated by contact, access of atmospheric air and eating; they abate by the application of cold water and by complete rest. They are attended with marked redness of the gums, erysipelatous redness of the cheeks, but without any marked swelling, with violent congestions of the head, alternate chills and heat, violent thirst, and are apt to assume the character of prosopalgia, by simultaneously invading several branches of the fifth pair, or by migrating to some other region while the toothache ceases or only abates.

Nux vomica in its action upon the teeth is very similar to Belladonna. The pain is drawing, tearing or jerking, mingled with violent, short, keenly-acute stitches or with throbbing pulsations. It attacks the patient at any time of the day, but is most violent early in the morning; the pain is not continuous but consists of detached paroxysms. Warmth neither aggravates nor decreases the pain; rest induces an improvement; mental efforts, chewing, drawing in cold air, coffee and spirituous beverages cause a severe aggravation of the pain. Marked congestive symptoms are generally present, but the pain may be purely nervous, and, as in the case of Belladonna, may shift to other branches of the trigeminus. Swelling, redness and painfulness of the gums do not counter-indicate Nux. A choleric temperament, abuse of coffee or spirits, are a recommendation for its use.

Bryonia is particularly adapted to a toothache to which the appellation of rheumatic is generally applied. Redness, inflammation and swelling of the gums are absent. The prevailing pain is a tearing distress, accompanied by stitches and a sensation of looseness and elongation of the teeth. It sets in or is aggravated in the evening or at night, and is likewise aggravated by warm drinks, warm food, chewing motions, lying upon the non-affected side, whereas it abates by lying upon the affected side, by contact with cold water, or by continued exercise in the open air. The pain shifts easily and readily from one tooth to another, not only in the same row, but likewise from the lower to the upper jaw. Touching the affected tooth is not usually very painful.

Chamomilla corresponds most specifically to the toothache which is most violent at night, more particularly when the person sleeps on a feather-bed. It comes in paroxysms, does not attack any particular tooth; in its milder form the toothache is a formicating, jerking pain, in its more violent form it is a tearing pain, which, in its highest degree of intensity, darts into the ear. It is aggravated by warmth, also by eating and drinking, and by cold water; swelling of the cheeks, profuse secretion of saliva, heat and redness of one cheek, excessive nervousness and restlessness, disposition to weep, and in some cases swelling of the gums, looseness and a feeling as if the teeth were elongated, generally accompany the toothache. (Hartmann.)

Pulsatilla. The pain is tearing, extending throughout one-half of both jaws, less frequently through the whole row of teeth; or else the pain is jerking, lancing, a maddening pain, or as if the nerve were violently put upon the stretch and then suddenly let go again; in no case is it possible to point out a definite tooth where the pain is localized. An aggravation takes place at night, also in the evening, after warm eating or drinking, by the warmth of the bed or in a warm room, or by picking at a tooth. The toothache moderates by contact with cold, especially with cold water; or, in the open air, with sudden aggravation when entering a warm room; it is likewise moderated by the application of vinegar and by sleep. The pain inclines to shoot into the ear, eye and temple, is often accompanied by hemicrania, otalgia, chilliness. The complexion is pale, at any rate it must not be of a vivid redness if Pulsatilla is to be used. Chlorosis, anæmia, pregnancy, are additional indications for Pulsatilla. Pulsatilla is likewise an excellent remedy in toothache preceding or accompanying the menstrual period. The presence of inflammation and swelling is not adapted to this remedy.

Spigelia. We have already spoken in praise of this remedy when on the subject of prosopalgia, and we likewise recommend it for toothache, with the following symptoms: The pain is not seated in one tooth, but in an indefinite number of teeth, especially in the anterior row; the pain is a flashing, not throbbing, pain, darts even into the face, is generally felt only in the day-time, less frequently at night; is aggravated by air, cold water, eating, heat, and abates during rest, or when tepid warmth is applied; it is attended with pallor and bloat of the face, chilliness, palpitation of the heart, neuralgic pain in the face.

Staphysagria affords help when the pain attacks sound as well as carious teeth; it is aggravated by the ingestion of food and drink; it is a tearing pain emanating from a carious tooth, and extending throughout the whole side as far as the pes anserinus, where it excites the most violent pains, which are aggravated by a light touch, but diminished by hard pressure; when the pain is a gnawing pain in a decayed tooth, with a drawing distress in other teeth; it is particularly violent early in the morning, is aggravated by chewing, open air and cold beverage, improved by warmth. The gums bleed easily, are swollen and painful. (Hartmann.)

Rhus toxicodendron is suitable in cases of toothache caused by rheumatic exposure and by getting wet. The prevailing pain is a tearing or jerking pain, or like the pain of a sore; has prevailing evening and night exacerbations; always affects a number of teeth; is aggravated by both warm and cold substances in the mouth, whereas it is often diminished by the application of external warmth; the warmth of the bed is intolerable; the teeth feel as if loose and elongated; indeed, they sometimes really are. Severe exercise affords great relief.

Sepia is more particularly efficient in chronic toothache, especially in the obstinate and violent toothache of pregnant females. It is generally attended with severe congestions, is worse at night, and sometimes intermits entirely in the day-time. Every motion of the mouth, the contact with cold things in the mouth, fresh air, or the passage from the open air into a room, aggravates the pain. The toothache to which Sepia corresponds is, as we have already stated when speaking of prosopalgia, no characteristically definite pain; almost any kind of pain is to be found in the pathogenesis of Sepia. Sepia is still more specifically indicated if the teeth decay very rapidly. There is not much swelling, but a more or less violent prosopalgia is apt to accompany the toothache.

Mezereum is suitable if the pain is characterized by violent burning, stitching or boring. It is worse in the evening and at night, and is aggravated by motion. The pain is apt to occur paroxysmally, with perfectly free intervals between the paroxysms. A general chilliness, with heat about the head, great restlessness, ill-humor, and an extreme sensitiveness of the external parts of the head, accompany the toothache.

One of the most efficacious remedies for toothache, which is seldom mentioned among this class of remedies, is *Arsenicum*. No medicine relieves more surely than Arsenic, a toothache which reaches its climax about midnight or immediately after lying down, and becomes so intense that the patients are unable to describe it, who tormented by anxiety and restlessness, run about, uttering moans and groans. Sleep sometimes sets in after the patients have taken a single dose of the remedy, which sometimes acts with such magic effect that they vow they have been given a dose of Laudanum. If the cheek is swollen, the remedy has no effect. If palpitation of the heart is present, or if the toothache is in relationship with the approach or the appearance of the menses, the good effects of Arsenic are so much more certain.

Beside the above-mentioned remedies, which will generally prove sufficient, the following medicines, although less definitely indicated in affections of the teeth, may likewise render good service: *Aconitum, Baryta, China, Coffea, Hepar sulphuris, Ignatia, Opium, Phosphorus, Platina.*

In conclusion, we beg to protest against the assumption that homœopathic medicines can cure any species of toothache in a short period of time. Where an abscess has already formed, where the root of the tooth is carious, where the periosteum is affected, or where the pain is excited by foreign bodies in the tooth, any remedy is either useless, or a favorable effect can only be obtained very gradually. This remark is intended for malicious opponents or for oversanguine friends. It is an essential requisite to the cure of toothache that the use of coffee should be strictly avoided. If, in order to effect a cure, it should be necessary to remove the tooth, no reasonable physician will waste time with useless attempts at healing the disorder by the administration of internal remedies; the forceps is the only reliable remedy. Nevertheless, we dare assert, that, in the majority of cases, an operation is rendered unnecessary by the timely and proper use of our specific remedies.

[**Aconite** deserves a much higher rank among the remedies for toothache than Bæhr has assigned to it. In congestive toothache, with violent throbbing pain, sensation as if the tooth would be shattered to pieces, excessive soreness and sensitiveness of the tooth, flushed face, sparkling eyes, headache, chilly creepings, alternating with flashes of heat, etc.; a dessertspoonful of a solution of a drop of the tincture of Aconite root in half a tumbler of water will sometimes scatter the pain as if by magic. If the tooth is decayed, a small plug of cotton, soaked with a little tincture of Aconite, inserted into the cavity of the tooth, will sometimes remove or, at least, suspend the pain in an instant, as it were. In many cases of this kind, Aconite is preferable to Belladonna. H.]

FOURTH SECTION.

Diseases of the Stomach, Intestines, and Peritonæum.

A. DISEASES OF THE STOMACH.

1. Catarrhus Ventriculi Acutus. Acute Catarrh of the Stomach. Acute Indigestion. Acute Dyspepsia.

To this morbid condition of the stomach, according as it is more or less intense and complicated with affections of the intestines, liver complaint, etc., such a variety of names have been applied, that it is quite a task to indicate all its synonymes. Nevertheless, this seems indispensable, for the reason that those names are still in use, without, however, possessing any scientific value. In this respect we refer to a subsequent chapter, where the affections of the stomach and intestines are to be treated of under the general designation of gastro-intestinal catarrh, by which arrangement numerous repetitions will be avoided. In this place we will content ourselves with discussing the condition which is often alluded to as gastricism, status gastricus, derangement of the stomach, and, in a higher degree, febris gastrica simplex.

The causes of catarrh of the stomach are of special importance, both as regards prognosis and treatment. We may, therefore, be excused if we dwell upon the etiology of this disease with more than ordinary minuteness.

The boundary line between the normal and abnormal functional activity of the stomach, cannot be definitely drawn, owing more particularly to the physiological incorrectness of our present habits of living. Even ordinary digestion becomes, in some respects, analogous to a morbid process, through the febrile symptoms which we experience after a copious meal. In the case of one person the same phenomena may appear normal, which in other persons might look like morbid appearances, the distinction being determined by their duration. If this does not exceed the duration of the digestive process generally, we do not interpret them as abnormal conditions; such an interpretation is only put upon them, if the disturbance continues until the next meal, or even longer. If a person, after partaking of a large quantity of fat food, is attacked with heartburn, we do not regard this as a disease; but if every time we partake of a little fat, we are attacked with a sour stomach, and the acidity continues, we conclude that there is functional derangement of the stomach. Now, it is well known that the capacity of the stomach to digest certain aliments, and to equalize disturbances, differs greatly in different individuals. Hence so far as catarrh of the stomach and other disturbances of this organ or of the intestines are concerned, we have to infer that there exists an inherent disposition to derangement, the degree of which can only be determined by experience. We need not call attention to the important influence which this inherent disposition exerts in the management of gastric derangements; it is upon a correct knowledge of this disposition that the possibility of preventing the recurrence of functional disturbances depends. This knowledge is of particular importance in the case of little children, in whom inattention to constitutional tendencies results in impoverishment of the organism, whereas a compliance with its inherent demands leads to vigor and health. A constitutional abnormal disposition need not always be congenital, but may be acquired. Catarrh of the stomach, for instance, may become habitual; strength of body and the functional activity of organs may become impaired by bad or deficient nourishment, or even by an excess of dietetic regularity, or the avoidance of stimulants beyond the normal limits established by our recognized and generally adopted mode of living. This last-mentioned point is strikingly illustrated by children who are brought up without the use of mixed food, and whose stomachs consequently become so sensitive, that the least change, which does not disturb children who are brought up with less uniformity in diet, at once causes gastric derangements.

Beside a constitutional disposition, catarrh of the stomach may be caused by overloading the stomach with food, which we have frequent opportunities of witnessing in the case of children. The quality of the food likewise plays an important part, the heavier and more indigestible the food, the more easily the stomach is deranged, even by a small quantity. Even an otherwise readily digested aliment may become indigestible, in consequence of not being sufficiently masticated, and thus being introduced into the stomach in a state where the gastric juice cannot act upon it. The temperature of the food likewise has great influence; we frequently notice this by the effect, upon the stomach, of ices, cold fruit, cold beer. On the other hand, a very high temperature may likewise prove hurtful.

Beside these more normal substances of not unfrequent use, a quantity of other articles which are introduced into the stomach, either as articles of diet or as medicines, may cause catarrh of the stomach. Among the former we place, in the front rank, alcohol in its different forms and degrees; the excessive use of coffee is another cause of catarrh of the stomach. Tea has the same effect as coffee, but not in the same degree. Every smoker knows that tobacco is very apt to cause derangements of the stomach. All these substances have the peculiar effect of retarding digestion; hence the action of such medicinal substances as impede the functions of the intestinal canal, resembles that of large doses of Opium.

Beside these material causes of catarrh of the stomach, we have to mention several important immaterial etiological causes of this disorder. First, depression of cutaneous temperature. Usually this causes catarrh of the respiratory organs; but in many individuals, and more particularly in children, a cause of this kind leads frequently, and even most commonly, to catarrh of the lining membrane of the stomach; or else the respiratory organs and the stomach are both affected with catarrh, and thus it happens that catarrh of the stomach very often accompanies a simple catarrh, angina, bronchial catarrh, etc. In this category belongs the influence exerted by certain epidemic conditions of the atmosphere, etc., so that we may have an epidemic influenza with a normal state of the stomach, whereas, on the other hand, epidemic influenza may be accompanied by the most violent catarrh of the stomach.

In conclusion we call the attention of homœopathic practitioners to an important point. Every febrile affection superinduces a higher or less degree of catarrh of the stomach. Under Old-School treatment this catarrh is generally made worse, and becomes so obstinate that it outlasts the primary disease and is one of the chief causes of a retarded convalescence. This circumstance should not be overlooked, in cases that come to us for treatment, after the disease had been running its course for some time.

Violent mental disturbances or disagreeable emotions of any kind, anger, mortified feeling, etc., are very apt to induce a catarrhal irritation of the stomach.

Symptoms. The phenomena of this affection vary in accordance with the intensity of the local affection and with the individuality of the patient; we will therefore describe the various degrees of the affection in the case of adults and the gastric catarrh of children.

A few hours, perhaps, after one of the above-mentioned disturbing influences has been able to act, a feeling of pressure and heaviness is experienced in the region of the stomach, which the patient fancies is bloated. Local pressure, even of the clothes, is painful and causes anxiety. The appetite is gone, the very thought of food causes a feeling of aversion. In cases where a certain kind of food had caused the disease, a loathing is felt against this very article of diet. These incipient symptoms become very soon associated with phenomena depending upon incomplete or otherwise abnormal digestion and consequent decomposition of the food. On account of a copious development of gas, the epigastrium becomes more or less puffed up, and the sensitiveness of that region increases; the gas which is belched up, is either inodorous or else has a fetid smell; an excess of acid may likewise be secreted in the stomach, and heartburn may arise, with sensation as if a fluid were ascending in the throat. The aversion to food increases even unto loathing, nausea and vomiting, the food being vomited up with mucus and water and with an admixture of acid and, finally, bile. These phenomena of gastric derangement are always accompanied by symptoms of a general constitutional irritation. First, the patients feel unusually languid and depressed, an extreme irritability and ill-humor are accompanied by flying heat alternating with chilly creepings; the head feels heavy and dull, a pressure in the frontal region is particularly annoying (cephalea gastrica); on stooping and moving about rapidly, a feeling of dizziness is experienced, or the sight is obscured. The tongue is lined with mucus, although not in every case; the taste is insipid or slimy, pasty, acid, putrid, and the breath has generally a bad, sulphurous smell. Usually the urine is turbid, mixed with mucous flocks. The bowels may remain constipated during the whole course of the disease; this is more particularly the case when the disease was not caused by dietetic transgressions; where it was induced by improper nourishment, the nausea and vomiting are generally accompanied by soft stool and lastly diarrhœa, which, however, never becomes excessive if the stomach is the only suffering organ.

The slight attack of gastric catarrh sometimes gets well in half a day; it seldom lasts longer than a few days. Whether it lasts a few days, may depend upon the intensity of the attack, and upon the admission of hurtful articles of diet in the course of the disease. Where dietetic precautions are not observed, the acute form may easily run into the chronic form, or the genuine chronic catarrh of the stomach; or the intestines may become involved, giving rise to the gastro-intestinal catarrh of which we shall speak afterwards, or else the complaint may increase to a higher grade of intensity, giving rise to the so-called gastric fever.

Gastric fever, if it is not the result of an increased intensity of common catarrh, usually commences with violent febrile phenomena, alternate chill and violent heat, accelerated pulse, etc. The local symptoms of the stomach are scarcely distinguished from those of the milder form of catarrh, not even as regards intensity: sometimes they are even less marked; the vomiting, for instance, being wanting, the nausea slight, the phenomena of reaction of the stomach against its contents being generally trifling. The constitutional symptoms, on the contrary, are more prominent; the lassitude, for instance, being so great early in the morning, that the patients feel compelled to remain in bed; the legs refuse to support the body. The headache is distressing, the sleep is disturbed and restless, the patients are tormented by a craving for fresh water, the tongue is very much coated, and the taste in the mouth very bad. The disease never terminates in one day; the fever very soon assumes the type of a continuous remittent, with evening exacerbations, increases in intensity, though not regularly, during the first week, and gradually decreases in the second week. Where the stomach is alone affected, and the bowels do not become involved, they sometimes remain constipated for days. The urine is saturated. In violent attacks, with immoderate fever, especially if the patients are young, symptoms of considerable cerebral congestion with delirium, develop themselves. Recovery takes place gradually; convalescence is a slow process, with great tendency to relapses, so that the disease may become protracted for several weeks, and may entail great debility and emaciation.

The acute stomach-catarrh of children offers deviations in the course and consequences of the disease, only in so far as it attacks children who are chiefly confined to milk as an article of diet, consequently children under one year. Although the lighter grade of the disease may be safely considered an entirely unimportant derangement, yet the higher and highest grades constitute the most dangerous diseases of childhood. Before describing the symptoms, we will mention, somewhat in detail, some of the etiological causes of the diseases.

Since this form of catarrh of the stomach only occurs among infants, very seldom, at least, after the first year, we have, as a matter of course, to trace the causes of the disease to faulty nutrition. The great and frequent transgressions of which parents are guilty in this respect, may be inferred from the frequency of this disorder. Where children are simply brought up on milk, the causes may be of two kinds: The milk is either bad, or else the good milk is given the child in improper quantity and form. The milk is bad when it comes from women who are again menstruating, or who are sick, or are laboring under the effects of some severe mental or moral disturbance, or who nurse their children too long. This last circumstance is a main cause of the frequent attacks of illness of children, of one or two years old, among the poorer classes; more particularly of peasant wives, who sometimes nurse their children to the age of three or five years, in order to prevent conception. That this supposition is correct, is evident from the fact that children improve as soon as they are weaned and properly fed with more appropriate nourishment. Cow-milk may likewise be bad food for children who are brought up by hand, more particularly if it comes from a diseased cow or from a cow whose milk is too old. The second point is still more important, for the reason that it occurs more frequently; if we do not dwell upon it more fully, it is because we cannot spare the space for such a disquisition. It is highly improper to feed the child too frequently: as soon as the child stirs, it is put to the breast, or the bottle is given. Now we know that it takes two full hours to digest milk. If the child is fed again before this period has elapsed, the fresh supply is added to the half-digested contents, so that neither portion is properly digested, and the consequences of catarrh of the stomach very soon make their appearance. That this must be so, every adult person may observe on himself; let him take nourishment for a few days every hour or two hours, and he will soon experience symptoms of gastric catarrh. If bad milk is added to the excessive feeding, illness must necessarily result.

Beside the above-mentioned circumstances, want of attention to cleanliness constitutes another cause of sickness. The milk is not fresh enough, or the bottles and nurslings are not kept clean, or the mother forgets to cleanse the nipple before the child is put to it, so that the child draws in the decomposed milk, that may have remained adhering to the nipple, with the fresh milk from the breast; and we know full well that the stomach of the child is not capable of resisting the deleterious influence of this spurious nourishment. It is a peculiarity of some children's stomachs to reject fresh cow-milk, whereas boiled milk agrees with them; yet the reverse is commonly the case.

Where the child is not exclusively fed on milk, the gates are wide open to an attack of sickness. For children who have no teeth, milk is the only proper food, in spite of everything that may be said to the contrary. All slimy, farinaceous or sweetened articles of diet are generally hurtful. If the bad effects are not seen at once, let us watch children that have been brought up on such food, in their second year, and we shall find that their apparent embonpoint is not natural, and that they are troubled with a disposition to derangement of the stomach. Usually, however, this result is observed in the first months after this method of feeding the children has been commenced. The mixed food is assimilated so much the less readily, the younger the child; this truth is so firmly established that it is inconceivable how experienced practitioners can recommend slimy decoctions for children immediately after birth, together with a small quantity of milk, and how they do not even seem to suspect that the sickliness of children with whom this system is pursued results from improper nutrition. Instances of this kind are of daily occurrence. The only food, beside milk, which agrees with the digestive organs of children, is the extract of beef, prepared cold, of which we shall speak more fully when describing the treatment of this affection. If the child, with its stomach preserved in its normal condition by means of adequate nourishment, has arrived at the period of dentition, it has to encounter other dangers in the next following period, which includes two great changes in the infantile development, namely: the cutting of the teeth and the beginning of a mixed diet. The last-mentioned change is either initiated too soon, that is, before at least four teeth are through, which fact is generally a sign that other food besides milk may be introduced into the stomach; or else the transition is too sudden, and we expect the infantile stomach, which has had nothing but milk so far, to digest, the very next day, all kinds of farinaceous food. Such irrational changes beget an impoverished condition of the tissues, and we often see children who had become robust and fleshy at the mother's breast, emaciate shortly after they are weaned.

Ordinary people, so far from noticing this change, do not even suspect its real causes, namely: improper food and disturbed digestion. They even smile if they hear a physician volunteering such statements.

Besides the above-mentioned circumstances in the mode of nutrition to which children are subjected, we will mention another custom which met with a great deal of favor in former times, and which has been the certain cause of a great many cases of catarrh of the stomach—we mean the so-called bibs. The decomposition of the remaining particles of milk which such a bag causes in the mouth, and the almost invariably following derangement of the stomach, show that it is no superfluous precaution to carefully cleanse the bottles, nipples, and the mouth of the child, in order to prevent the decomposed particles of milk from getting into the stomach.

Symptoms. The first morbid symptom generally is vomiting. We know that a certain kind of vomiting is one of the phenomena of health, in a little infant, provided the infant is without fever and grows fat, and unless the milk which is discharged immediately after nursing is not curdled, whereas the milk which is thrown off some time after nursing should be curdled. Where these symptoms are not present, the vomiting has an entirely different significance, and leads us to infer the presence of gastric catarrh. As a general rule, the morbid vomiting takes place some time after nursing, the little patient throwing off milk which is either uncoagulated or only partially curdled, and shows an admixture of mucus after the disease has lasted for a short period. The milk which is thrown off shortly after nursing is less frequently completely curdled, and has a very sour smell. The children do not seem to suffer much at the commencement; they look a little paler and more sunken than usual; their appetite is good, sometimes it seems even better than usual, which, however, may be owing to the circumstance that the children are very thirsty and may want to drink rather than eat; at any rate, they swallow with great avidity small quantities of fresh water, and the mouth is evidently very dry. Very soon the vomiting is followed by increased restlessness; bloating of the region of the stomach, which seems very sensitive; drawing up of the lower extremities, and crying immediately after partaking of food. The skin feels hot and dry, and less elastic. This increase of morbid symptoms is attended with irregularity of the alvine evacuations. They are loose, of irregular color, yellow, green or brown; they contain undigested milky coagula, sometimes of large size, and resembling stirred eggs; their odor is very much changed, at first sometimes sour and afterwards fetid.

Such a slight attack of gastric catarrh sometimes terminates in recovery in a few days, although an unusually rapid emaciation is always a striking symptom. On the contrary, if the disease turns out unfavorably, the most threatening symptoms set in very rapidly. The vomiting occurs less frequently, for the simple reason that much less nourishment is introduced into the stomach, but it has an intensely sour smell, and contains a large quantity of mucus. The diarrhœa increases, assumes a liquid consistence, of a lighter color, so that the main portion of the evacuations is colorless, and only contains a few isolated yellow or greenish cheesy coagula; their odor continues sour, but has a peculiarly disagreeable smell. The evacuations are seldom more consistent, gray or entirely white, but very fetid. With these very violent symptoms in the digestive range, the greater intensity of the constitutional symptoms corresponds. The children sink very rapidly, and their features acquire a peculiar expression of suffering, with the folds in the face deepening more and more. The temperature of the trunk is raised above the normal standard, while the extremities feel cold. The appetite vanishes, the children refuse the breast or bottle, and only draw very feebly, if they touch the bottle at all; on the contrary, they swallow cold water with great avidity; hence they are very thirsty. The restlessness yields to sopor, during which they lie with their eyes half closed, and often squinting. Their ordinary crying ceases, they merely utter plaintive moans, more particularly about the time when they soil their diapers. If the disease has progressed thus far, there is the greatest danger that convulsions and other cerebral symptoms may terminate the patient's life. In case of a favorable turn, the vomiting gradually ceases, the diarrhœic stools become less frequent, have a better color, and the appetite returns. Convalescence progresses very slowly, and relapses are readily brought about by the slightest errors in diet.

The disease is sometimes of very short duration, even in fatal cases, but it may extend beyond several weeks. Gastric catarrhs running a very rapid course are always attended with violent intestinal symptoms, and will be treated of more fully in the chapter on gastro-intestinal catarrh, under the appellation of cholera infantum.

The pathologico-anatomical changes, produced by gastric catarrh in the case of adults, are too unimportant and unessential to require a more special description at our hands. On the contrary it behooves us to add a few remarks on the post-mortem appearances in the case of children. In their case the stomach is often found softened, a change that so far has given rise to many differences of opinion. According to some, gastromalacia is an idiopathic morbid process, observing its own laws, and running its own specific course; according to others, it is a post-mortem appearance, which begins when gastric catarrh assumes its most violent form, and can, therefore, be diagnosed with perfect certainty in some particular cases. The latter supposition is undoubtedly the best founded, and is more especially corroborated by experiments made upon the exsected stomachs of animals. If such stomachs are filled with milk, and are placed for a short period near a warm place, they show all the anatomical signs of gastromalacia. In a similar manner gastromalacia is said to develop itself in an infant, if, shortly before death, milk is introduced into the stomach, and fermentation takes place during the fatal hour. This view is confirmed by the fact that the stomach has been found softened, in the case of children who did not show a single sign of the disease while still alive, and who partook of a little milk shortly before death.

It being of the utmost importance, in a therapeutic point of view, that this disorder should be diagnosed with perfect certainty, we will add a few additional remarks. The lower grades of acute gastric catarrh cannot easily be confounded with other affections, except with gastric fever. This fever but too often has the appearance of typhoid fever, and it is of the utmost importance for a physician, that he should not diagnose falsely at the onset, and in a few days should have to give a different prognosis. The most essential characteristics of typhus are: the breaking out of the disease without any demonstrable exciting causes, especially errors in diet; a higher temperature of the skin, and an increased frequency of the pulse. In the further course of the disease, so many pathognomonic signs turn up, that it is scarcely possible to confound the two diseases. The existence of herpes labialis positively precludes the idea that the disease before us is typhoid fever.

Treatment. Although it may be impossible, in the case of adults, to ward off gastric catarrh by means of an energetic prophylactic treatment, we should not lose sight of it whenever repeated attacks, or other reasons, have satisfied us of the existence of a predisposition to this disease. It is more particularly in the case of persons who are convalescing from an attack of gastric fever, that the greatest caution has to be observed in the use and selection of articles of diet, lest a relapse should take place by the use of inappropriate nourishment. In the case of children the employment of prophylactic means is not only more important, but likewise much more gratifying. By imparting proper instructions to the parents, and exerting a proper control over their management, a physician has it in his power not only to protect the infant from many an attack of illness, but also to save himself a good deal of trouble. The main points have already been stated in the paragraph on the etiology of acute gastric catarrh, and what has not been said in that place, can easily be inferred from the remarks there made.

Before mentioning the remedies belonging to this class, we beg leave to cast a glance at the ordinary method of treating this disease. The most common prescription is an emetic. Is this treatment proper or not? It is known that the stomach has been made sick and irritated by the use of hurtful or too copious quantities of food, and it is undoubtedly natural to jump at the conclusion that the noxious material must be removed, in order to restore the normal condition of the stomach. We sometimes succeed in accomplishing this result. More frequently, however, the emetic adds an additional irritation to that which is already existing, and, instead of abbreviating the affection, its duration, on the contrary, is lengthened, and with the duration its intensity. Hence this method is more or less hazardous, so much more as we are in possession of easier means to reach the same end. The use of tepid water, in case a desire to vomit should be felt, is a much safer emetic than Tartar emetic or Ipecacuanha. Next to the emetic, a purgative is most thought of. Now, we have no purgative that does not more or less irritate the stomach, and after that the intestinal canal; hence the gastric disorder is increased first, after which the intestine, which is so very greatly disposed to sympathize with the condition of the stomach, becomes still more disposed to become involved in the gastric derangement, so that, instead of abbreviating, we, on the contrary, prolong the suffering. In the place of such violent means, Homœopathy possesses remedial resources that act much more rapidly and safely than any others. However, soon after exhibiting the suitable remedy, we often provoke vomiting and diarrhœa; but these are simply critical evacuations, and of good omen. In such cases it will not be necessary to change the medicine.

As regards the selection of the proper remedy, we have already given our reasons why it is a difficult and often deceptive task. In every pathogenesis we find, under the head "Stomach," all the symptoms of catarrh of the stomach, and yet not every medicine of this kind is on that account a remedy for gastric catarrh. As in the case of toothache, experience has had to confirm the practical value of the symptoms, and has thus pointed out a small number of medicines that have reliably curative effects in this disease. Here we have another proof that the superficial selection of a remedy, in accordance with mere symptoms, will often deceive us, and can only lead to good results if the origin and combination of every symptom in the provings have been logically stated. We will first give a cursory view of the chief remedies for gastric catarrh, and shall afterwards endeavor to bring them into homœopathic accord with each form and stage of the disease.

To judge by the success that has been obtained with **Bryonia alba,** this medicine is the leading remedy in this disease. The symptoms having special reference to the stomach, are full of meaning, and are, moreover, supported by corresponding symptoms in other systems and organs. The aggravation of the symptoms by eating, the sensitiveness and bloating of the præcordial region, the painful sensation of swelling in this region, the nausea with disposition to vomit up the ingesta, point more particularly to catarrh of the stomach. Besides these symptoms, the following deserve particular attention: nausea, with feeling of coldness and chills, soon after midnight, followed by vomiting of the ingesta, which, in its turn, is succeeded by vomiting of mucus and bile; sweetish, insipid, pappy and nauseous taste; sensation of hunger, with complete absence of appetite, or even loathing of food. To these symptoms we add the following passage from Hartmann: *Bryonia* is a distinguished remedy in gastric fevers which emanate from a twofold cause, a cold, and mortified feelings. The gastric symptoms are attended with severe feverish heat mingled with chills, lassitude, aggravation of the symptoms at night, irritable nervousness and frontal headache, as if the forehead would split open; constipation and rheumatic distress generally.

Belladonna has no less marked symptoms than Bryonia, the local symptoms, however, being much more violent and the fever more intense. The pain in the stomach is very violent, stinging, cutting, contracting, with prevalence of violent pressure, aggravated by eating any kind of food, with distension of the epigastrium. Great nausea results in difficult vomiting with straining, the patient brings up mucus and bile rather than food. The appetite is gone, the thirst intense, but only for sour and piquant beverages. Characteristic indications for Belladonna are gastric catarrh accompanied by catarrh of the mouth and pharynx, and evidently owe their origin to a severe cold. With such catarrhs the fever is always very acute, the skin, however, is moist in spite of the heat, the head feels dull and tight. Such conditions are mostly met with only in the case of children, for whom this medicine is a real panacea in such affections. The breath has a foul or sulphurous smell.

Ipecacuanha is a chief remedy for gastric catarrh, without fever, or when the fever is very slight, more particularly if the catarrh had originated in overloading the stomach or eating fat food. The stomach symptoms are: feeling of emptiness, pressure, stitches, pinching pains, with bloating of the pit of the stomach. Other characteristic symptoms are: insipid, bitter or rancid taste, as from spoiled oil; no appetite, or only a desire for sweet and delicate things, a symptom which is frequently met with in the case of children; vomiting of the ingesta, afterwards of bile and quantities of mucus, accompanied by diarrhœa. The gastric catarrhs corresponding to Ipecacuanha generally occur in the hot season, it is seldom indicated in gastric catarrhs of the winter-months.

Pulsatilla is in many respects similar to the previously mentioned remedy. It is likewise adapted to gastric catarrhs brought on by eating fat food, but likewise to catarrhs caused by cold fruit, ices, or acid food. There is no fever except chilliness or chilly creepings. A characteristic symptom is the sensation as if the food were lodged undigested above the stomach. The taste is greasy, rancid, bitter or very slimy, the eructations are bilious or acrid; there is no appetite, warm food is especially repulsive. The tongue has a thick white or yellowish coating. Other characteristic symptoms are the complete absence of thirst, and the irritable, whining mood, likewise the aggravation of the symptoms during the hours preceding midnight. According to Hartmann, Pulsatilla is likewise suitable for the subsequent nervousness, prostration, chilliness and loss of appetite, which symptoms sometimes remain after gastric fever.

Nux vomica is particularly adapted to catarrhs arising from the excessive use of spirits or coffee, or from a fit of chagrin. In attacks arising from other causes, it is often suitable at a later period of the catarrh after the fever has entirely disappeared. The stomach symptoms are not very intense. The region of the stomach is somewhat sensitive, but not a great deal, nor does it correspond to the bloat; the sensation of fulness is somewhat troublesome, and the prevailing pain is a severe pressure. The taste is sour or bitter or sulphurous, the tongue is thickly coated. Symptoms of marked prominence, are the continued frontal headache, especially during the morning hours, with sensation as if the brain were loose; and the aversion to bread and milk.

Antimonium crudum is one of the chief remedies for gastric catarrh without fever. It is most suitable if the catarrh is caused by overloading the stomach; the contents of the stomach have been rejected, but great nausea is still remaining. The region of the stomach is not very sensitive, the pain is principally a clawing or pressing pain and comes on in paroxysms. The tongue has a thick whitish coating, the breath has a foul or unpleasantly sweetish odor; the mouth is slimy, the appetite is not entirely gone, or else there is a sensation of hunger with loathing of food; the thirst is tormenting, with eructations without any particular taste. The general condition of the system is unfavorable, the patient feels very languid. The bowels are torpid; there is never any very troublesome diarrhœa.

Acidum phosphoricum is an excellent remedy if the characteristic local symptoms are entirely wanting; there is no fever, but excessive debility with complete loss of appetite. Conditions of this kind sometimes occur somewhat epidemically, having the appearance of typhoid fever.

These remedies will generally suffice to cure any attack of gastric catarrh; of other medicines that may likewise prove serviceable, we will give a cursory list in accordance with Hartmann's example.

In the lower grades of gastric catarrh, it is of importance to be acquainted with the exciting cause, in order to be certain of the specific remedy. If arising from overloading the stomach, hunger is certainly the best remedy. Only gruel should be allowed, and a little black coffee at the commencement, which is apt to result in a critical discharge from the bowels. If there is a marked disposition to vomit, coffee is of no avail, because it makes the vomiting more difficult; a little tepid water had better be drank first, in order to facilitate the vomiting, and afterwards a little coffee may be used. If fat food is the cause, we give *Pulsatilla* or *Ipecacuanha;* after cold fruit or ices, *Arsenicum* or *Pulsatilla;* after a fit of anger or chagrin, *Chamomilla* or *Bryonia;* after spirits or coffee, *Nux vomica;* after mental or bodily efforts immediately after a meal, *Nux vomica;* after continued grief and chagrin, *Ignatia* and *Staphysagria;* in the case of debilitated individuals, *China* is recommended; to anæmic females we give *Ferrum, Pulsatilla* or *Arsenicum.*

The higher grade of gastric catarrh, or the gastric fever proper, seldom follows immediately, as soon as the influence of the exciting cause is perceived; there generally occurs a preliminary gastric derangement, unless, perhaps, some atmospheric or other cause, not amenable to observation, should induce a sudden breaking out of the fever without any special precursory symptoms. Many physicians recommend *Aconite* for the incipient fever, if it is sufficiently marked; but we confess we look upon this use of Aconite as a loss of time. If the fever is violent, which is not often the case in the gastric fever of adults, *Belladonna* does more efficient service than Aconite, more particularly if the region of the stomach is very painful and puffed up. If the fever is not very violent, the local symptoms less prominent, the symptoms of a general constitutional disturbance are threateningly conspicuous, and there is a resemblance to incipient typhus, *Bryonia* will be found the most suitable medicine. *Ipecacuanha* is preferable to Bryonia if the gastric symptoms are very violent, and there is great loathing of food, continued nausea and frequent vomiting, without the tongue being much coated. Beside these two remedies, *Pulsatilla* and *Tartar emetic* may be found suitable at the commencement of the attack. In the subsequent course of the disease, when the urging to vomit has completely disappeared, and there only remains great weakness of the stomach, *Nux vomica* deserves our highest attention; after taking which, the appetite sometimes returns with remarkable rapidity, and convalescence takes place. *Acidum phosphoricum* and *Antimonium crudum* may deserve attention at this period of the disease. For the frequently remaining debility, *China* is the chief remedy; *Ferrum* may likewise do good, especially in the case of chlorotic individuals; so may *Arsenicum*, especially if the debility is accompanied by severe pains in the stomach.

Colocynthis is less a remedy for genuine gastric catarrh, than for a peculiar condition of the stomach that can be traced to a cold as its exciting cause. The appetite is not entirely gone, nor do they greatly complain of nausea or aversion to food; but the region of the stomach is sensitive, and, after eating, the patients complain of raging crampy pain, which can only be moderated by warm applications; there is neither bloat nor belching up of wind. Evidently the pain chiefly resides in the muscular fibres of the stomach, and has very much the character of colic pains. These symptoms yield to Colocynth very soon. Such conditions are generally met with only during the transition-seasons when the air is cold, but the sun is still powerful enough to heat the blood; they likewise occur in summer, in consequence of sudden changes in the weather.

In ordinary cases of infantile gastric catarrh, the above-mentioned remedies are undoubtedly applicable; but it is often difficult to discover the right remedy, for the reason that the patients are too young to explain their distress. For this reason it is well, if no improvement takes place after a time, to frequently change the medicine, for it is more than likely that it is not adapted to the case.

As we said above, the first symptom is vomiting. If vomiting takes place soon after feeding, and the milk is thrown off unchanged, *Ipecacuanha* should be the first remedy given. After *Ipecac*, the normal condition of the stomach will soon return, provided the proper dietetic measures are resorted to in other respects. If the vomiting is excessive, the child seems very sick, and a rapid collapse takes place, *Veratrum album* is preferable to Ipecacuanha; it is likewise indicated by the absence of diarrhœa. If, soon after nursing, the milk is rejected in a curdled state, if it has a sour smell and is, as usual, mixed with a good deal of mucus, *Pulsatilla* is preferable, provided there is little or no diarrhœa; *Chamomilla*, on the contrary, if copious greenish diarrhœic stools are present. *Veratrum* may be suitable in such cases, especially if the evacuations contain only a very trifling admixture of bile. If the vomiting takes place a long time after nursing, and the milk is not decomposed, *Nux vomica* is the very best remedy. This last-mentioned form of vomiting is generally the most dangerous, and is easily succeeded by the most threatening phenomena, so that *Arsenicum* and *Creasotum* may have to be administered. In such a case we have no longer to deal with the simple gastric catarrh, but with the gastro-intestinal catarrh, of which we shall treat in a subsequent paragraph. If the disease sets in in a rather mild form, and the little patients pine away slowly, *Cuprum* is entirely in its place, likewise *China*. If the trouble arises from sickness of the mother or nurse, we have to inquire carefully into the causes and circumstances, and it is well to give the nursing female the same medicine that is taken by the child. If a sudden emotion is the cause, *Ignatia* may be the right remedy; after a violent fit of chagrin, we give *Chamomilla*; after fright and a subdued but violent mortification of the feelings, we give *Opium*; after drinking spirits, *Nux vomica* or *Tartar emetic*; after partaking of other kinds of food or drink, we give the remedies that have been mentioned previously. If the affection threatens to become chronic, we give the medicines that will be mentioned in the next chapter.

As regards the most suitable diet for children, we have also stated all that need be said on the subject, in a former chapter; we will here simply add a description of the method in which the extract of beef should be prepared. Take lean meat from a recently killed ox that is not too young, cut it fine and pour four times its weight of cold water upon it. Stir occasionally and let it draw for three-quarters of an hour or a whole hour, add a very small quantity of kitchen salt, allow the whole to boil up once over a good fire, and sift through a strainer. This extract is well-tasting, strong and adapted to the weakest organs of digestion; according to circumstances it may be mixed with milk, or sweetened with a little sugar, and the little patients may drink of it at least twice a day. The extract has to be made fresh every third day. Any other decoction of meat is averse to the child's taste, or agrees less or not at all with its stomach. This remark is particularly applicable to veal-broth, which is still preferred by many physicians and lay-persons to beef-tea, both for children and debilitated adults, although everybody might easily understand that it is rather indigestible and not very nourishing.

Further remarks on this subject will be deferred to the next chapter in order to avoid unnecessary repetitions.

2. Catarrhus Ventriculi Chronicus, Chronic Catarrh of the Stomach. Dyspepsia.

Both the acute and chronic catarrh of the stomach are very common complaints. Like the acute catarrh, so is the chronic form a very common accompaniment of other diseases, but likewise occurs quite frequently as an idiopathic affection. It is the frequency of its occurrence, together with its great importance, either as a complication or an independent disease, that has induced us to devote a special chapter to its description and treatment.

Chronic catarrh of the stomach often arises from the acute form, in consequence of its not being completely cured, or, by repeated attacks causing a deep-seated alteration of the lining membrane of the stomach, or in consequence of the morbid condition being kept up by improper diet. In this respect all the deleterious influences of which mention was made in the previous chapter, are to be regarded as etiological causes of the disease. Besides these different originating circumstances, the chronic form may likewise arise from the commencement as an independent disease; it may be caused by frequent derangements of the digestive process, in consequence of mental exertion, emotions shortly after a meal, too frequent eating, or by continued depressing affections, and, finally, by the habitual abuse of spirits, more particularly spirits containing a large percentage of alcohol. Chronic catarrh of the stomach likewise occurs as a coexisting complication in a variety of other diseases, such as anæmia, hydræmia, tuberculosis, liver complaint, affections of the spleen, pancreas, heart disease, pulmonary catarrh, etc. The influence of pregnancy upon the stomach likewise occasions, in many instances, a very obstinate and severe catarrh of the stomach.

The symptoms of chronic catarrh of the stomach are very various, on which account it is exceedingly difficult to furnish a complete picture of the disease, including its origin and course; hence it is preferable to treat of each particular phenomenon as a detached manifestation of the ailment.

Among the local symptoms the pain in the epigastrium occupies the first rank, as regards frequency. It is seldom violent and mostly amoun's to a painful sensation of pressure in the region of the stomach, which is either distended in reality, or feels as if it were. The pain is scarcely ever a stinging or burning pain, nor does it break out in distinct paroxysms like cardialgia. It is almost always aggravated or excited by the digestive process, or may likewise be increased by external pressure. It is characteristic of this disorder to be variously excited by various substances. Whereas one person cannot bear rye-bread, another eats fresh bread with perfect impunity. With others meat, milk, beer or cold food, do not agree. Scarcely any one afflicted with chronic gastric catarrh, is able to partake of acrid, sour or fatty substances, without experiencing distressing results. So far it has been impossible, even to chemistry, to account for these differences. To judge by the local pain, a disturbance of the digestive process is evidently the most constant symptom. The food is digested very slowly, sometimes remains in the stomach for days, thereby causing a variety of striking symptoms, among which heartburn and flatulence are most prominent. The latter may exist to an excessive degree, causing a distinct puffing of the epigastrium. The gas is either belched up with a feeling of relief, or else it passes off by the rectum with a great deal of trouble from the flatulence; at times it has no smell and at other times the odor is very fetid. Although the acute catarrh is often attended with vomiting, yet it is seldom present in the chronic form. If vomiting occurs, the ingesta are seldom included; where this is the case, there is every reason to suspect the existence of a very troublesome and dangerous alteration of the coats of the stomach. Most generally the vomiting is slimy, tenacious, ropy, insipid, attended with great straining, and commonly takes place in the morning or after the digestion is accomplished. In other cases it is more like a frothy, liquid saliva, with an occasional admixture of bile or acids from the stomachs, that are constantly brought up with an extremely tormenting effort. The mere ascension of the fluid as far as the pharynx, is much more frequent than actual vomiting; this commonly imparts to the patient a sensation as if a worm were crawling up the œsophagus.

These more local symptoms are never isolated, but are generally accompanied by more or less considerable changes in other organs, or in the constitutional state of the patient. A common companion of chronic gastric catarrh, is the catarrhal affection of the buccal cavity. The tongue is covered with a thick coating, especially at the root, the whole of the mucous lining is swollen, the breath has a disagreeable smell. At the same time the taste is generally insipid, slimy, or is entirely suspended, or perverse; the saliva is secreted in increased quantity. The appetite varies; at times it seems quite normal, at other times it is increased, usually it is less or even extinguished. The patients have, it is true, the sensation of appetite which is sometimes increased even to canine hunger, but all desire to eat has vanished. The increase of appetite is sometimes only apparent, the patients often eat sparingly, finding it impossible to eat larger portions at one time. Almost all such patients are devoured by a desire for sharp or piquant aliments, which, however, are relished only for a short time and are rapidly exchanged for others. The thirst is seldom increased. The stools are either as usual, or less, and, in consequence of the participation of the intestinal canal in the catarrhal process, are lined and permeated with mucus.

Even in the lesser degrees of the disease, headache is seldom wanting; most frequently it is a dull pressure in the forehead, with dulness of the whole head, ill-humor, hypochondriac mood, irritable temper, want of disposition to work, drowsiness in the daytime and sleeplessness at night. If the disease lasts any time and acquires a higher degree of intensity, the assimilative functions become rapidly and severely depressed, the countenance assumes a yellowish-gray hue, the expression is that of suffering and mental and moral disturbance. At this stage the liver and pancreas become readily involved, the urinary secretions become morbidly altered, urates being secreted in more copious quantities.

If left to itself, the course of the disease is, under all circumstances, a very protracted one. Under proper management most cases terminate favorably. If certain deleterious influences continue to affect the stomach, gastric catarrh may, without any other complication, lead to gradual emaciation and death, or certain degenerations of the mucous lining may result, that may finally terminate fatally. Among these, the chronic ulcer of the stomach is the most dangerous, next to which we class hemorrhage from the stomach, and lastly hypertrophy of the mucous membrane. The last-mentioned disorganization leads to stricture of the pylorus and consequent dilatation of the stomach, which usually results fatally, although after a long period. In this case there is constant vomiting, which has the peculiarity of occurring a few hours after eating, when the stomach digestion is entirely completed. The food is vomited up completely digested, with an admixture of water and mucus. The vomiting is exceedingly distressing and occurs at regular intervals. Although this state of things exerts a most deleterious influence upon the assimilative powers of the organism, yet the patients may drag their miserable existence along for eight years and more.

The anatomical changes in this disease, provided it has not run too protracted or too violent a course, usually consist in an insular or unequally distributed puffing of the mucous membrane of the stomach, either of a very pale, or dark-red or gray color. The vessels at these places are injected, varicose and prominent. In violent cases of long duration the other membranes are likewise very much thickened, but not throughout; only in part and most prominently at the pylorus. In such a case the folds of the mucous membrane are more distinct, the single follicles project, so that in some cases they form a shaggy surface. The extensive hypertrophy of the coats causes a stricture of the pylorus, and *vice versa*, the stricture of the pylorus leads to dilatation of the stomach. Superficial erosions and ulcers are frequently met with.

We will treat of the diagnosis of gastric catarrh when we come to treat of the affections with which it is easily confounded.

Treatment. As in the acute form, so in the chronic, the diet plays an important part, since it has to be regulated not only with a view of meeting the cause but, likewise, the characteristics of the disease; hence we prefer devoting a more extended chapter to its claims.

Of course the habitual use of hurtful substances has to be strictly avoided. Spirits containing a good deal of alcohol are to be entirely prohibited, in the case of persons who are made sick by such things. In other cases, on the contrary, the moderate use of good wine, even of rum or cognac, improves and even removes the disease, as is often witnessed among farmers' wives, who use the two last-mentioned beverages as domestic medicines, and sometimes with excellent success. The use of coffee is sometimes the sole cause of the disease; it is more hurtful in the shape of a powerful extract and adulterated with surrogates, than when drank strong and properly filtered. For this reason we see women made sick by the use of coffee much more frequently than men, and country people more frequently than the inhabitants of cities; that this observation is correct, follows from the circumstance that the patients get well as soon as they leave off the use of coffee. The peculiar power of coffee to retard digestion—lay persons generally believe the contrary—renders even the best quality of coffee a prejudicial article of diet to all patients whose digestion is naturally very slow; it is more particularly immediately after a meal that coffee must be avoided, for at such a time it might excite the rising of sour water and increase the pressure. The pleasantly stimulating and thirst-quenching effect of coffee is only momentary and should deceive no one, for the malaise induced by coffee, generally, is not experienced until half an hour or more has elapsed.

Tea has pretty much the same effect as coffee, except that it agrees much better with some, and proves an excellent sedative to others. At all events it is not a reliable beverage, for we are scarcely ever perfectly sure of obtaining it unadulterated and suitably prepared.

Fat is to be avoided, particularly boiled or fried fat, whereas small quantities of raw fat are easily digested. To this class belong all kinds of fat meat, all kinds of baked or farinaceous dishes prepared with fat, all kinds of vegetables boiled with a great deal of fat, and finally the different kinds of fat gravies. All do not comprehend why this kind of food should hurt them, although their own feelings might tell them that it does.

Finally we have to oppose the abuse of spices with all firmness, however such advice may be disliked by patients who love spiced food for the reason that it stimulates their bad appetite.

Next to these articles of diet which are hurtful under all circumstances, the manner in which food is to be eaten, likewise deserves our attention. We cannot enumerate all the bad habits which are indulged in at table, on the contrary we prefer to show how the meal should be partaken of. Above all, the food has to be properly masticated and eaten slowly, nor should it be swallowed when yet very hot. After eating, the stomach must not be pressed upon by an inappropriate posture of the body, nor is a recumbent posture advisable; severe bodily exercise is as prejudicial as hard mental labor; a reclining-sitting posture is the most suitable. A single deviation from these rules is often sufficient to render chronic catarrh of the stomach a permanent disease, and, inasmuch as the physician does not always become acquainted with the dietetic transgressions of his patients, the best rule he can adopt is to give positive instructions regarding the diet to be observed and the manner of eating.

However, it is impossible to indicate positive general rules by which the patient can be bound in all cases. The patient has to find out what agrees with him, and all we can do is to see to it that he does not commit any positive infractions of dietetic rules. We shall scarcely ever be able to determine *a priori* whether the one or the other regime will have a favorable influence upon the patient. What is pleasant to one person, is often repulsive to another. A great deal evidently depends upon our former habits. Whereas simple food agrees much better with a person who has been accustomed to luxurious habits, others require the most invigorating nourishment. One cannot bear milk, whereas another thrives under its use. The same is true with regard to meat, to some it does good whereas it is hurtful to others. This shows that the plan of prescribing fixed dietetic rules is not feasible; and in no affection has the individuality of the patient to be regarded with so much care as in chronic catarrh of the stomach. We will mention, however, a few more general points of view. As a rule, physicians dread to allow the use of fruit in affections of the stomach. These apprehensions and doubts may be well-founded, if the acid of the fruit decomposes, or interferes with the action of certain medicinal substances; or if the stomach has become so sensitive, in consequence of the abuse of drugs, that it cannot bear the most harmless article of nourishment. Under homœopathic treatment such cases never occur, and inasmuch as good fruit is most excellent to regulate digestion, the use of it should be encouraged instead of being forbidden. Fruit is, moreover, very refreshing to the patient. Few persons only do not readily digest it, only we may try to find out in what shape it agrees with them best, fresh or stewed, or dried fruit stewed. In corroboration of these views we refer the reader to the well-known grape-cures. Beer likewise is a beverage, the use of which is sometimes denied and at other times highly praised. The moderate use of ale has often a surprisingly good effect in the case of women; we do not know any good reason why such a beverage should be prohibited. The case is different with beer-drinkers. Inasmuch, however, as beer seldom causes catarrh of the stomach, it is not well that beer-drinkers should be forbidden the use of their favorite beverage at once, without rhyme or reason. There may be differences of opinion regarding the use of ale, but our sweet-beer deserves favorable consideration on the part of all physicians. When not spoiled, it is undoubtedly the best artificial beverage; its use is not only urgently to be recommended in catarrh of the stomach, but likewise in all febrile affections. When used in the latter, it is a good plan to add a little sugar and to allow part of the carbonic acid to escape. This course should likewise be adopted in acute gastric catarrh; beer, however, should not be drank if the patient has to vomit a great deal. If beer does not agree with a person cold, it frequently does the same amount of good if boiled with a little sugar, except that in such a form it is not near so refreshing.

In conclusion we have again to call attention to milk in a few words. We have already shown that a rigorous milk diet is sufficient to cure gastric catarrh. With many it does not agree at all, with others only when recently drawn, others can only use it when boiled. This knowledge has to be acquired by cautious experiments; the patient must not be injured by obstinately insisting upon a preconceived method on the part of his medical adviser. Many experience the greatest amount of comfort from drinking sour milk, but this is less frequently the case. Fresh buttermilk agrees with persons more generally than any other kind of milk. If we desire to institute a milk cure, it is best to begin with buttermilk, if we have a favorable opportunity of obtaining it.

It need scarcely be observed that the balance of the patient's physical conduct must not be neglected, and that every thing concerning it must be regulated in accordance with sound principles of health. Since it cannot be denied that catarrh of the stomach is not only caused, but likewise maintained, by a disposition to take cold, cold ablutions of the trunk, together with a reasonable amount of clothing, are of essential benefit.

In enumerating the medicines belonging to this class, we meet with several difficulties. In the first place, it is impossible to make use of the existing literature with any certainty, for the reason that we find gastric catarrh described under a variety of names, according as one or the other symptom is more prominent, sometimes as vomiting, or at other times as heartburn, or weak stomach, or cardialgia, chronic gastritis, etc. Since all these symptoms may occur without the existence of chronic catarrh of the stomach, we find a reference to our existing literature an uncertain business, so much more as the diagnosis is very often incomplete. The changing forms of the symptomatic combinations, likewise render it difficult to indicate remedies for the main group of symptoms constituting gastric catarrh. Hence, in special cases, the reader will have to institute frequent comparisons with the Materia Medica, which are so much more necessary, as the number of the remedies we shall have to mention is necessarily large.

Nux vomica. We frequently meet in our literature with the statement that Nux is only adapted to nervous affections of the stomach, not to affections with a material basis. Even in the absence of other satisfactory reasons, experience ought to be sufficient to upset views of this kind. For gastric affections arising from the use of spirits, coffee, wine, etc., we scarcely know of a better remedy than Nux vomica; and it is a well known fact, that these substances engender gastric catarrh in its most prominent form. In making this statement we do not mean to deny that Nux vomica is likewise adapted to neuralgia of the stomach, but we must not too hastily assume the existence of pure cardialgia, which is undoubtedly a somewhat rare disease. The stomach-symptoms of Nux are very numerous. This fact shows the characteristic relation of Nux to affections of the stomach, and justifies us in giving prominence to the phenomena in which Nux has evinced a specific curative power. The taste is either bitter or sour, so that the food seems to have an altered taste. Coffee is repulsive, likewise tobacco and rye-bread. The appetite is gone, yet there is a sensation of hunger, which even increases to canine hunger. The symptoms are either excited or made worse by eating. After every meal there are violent, or even painful, bitter or sour eructations. Nausea and a disposition to vomit are not strongly marked; there is not much vomiting, and then only of water and mucus. The region of the stomach is sensitive, especially after a meal, and generally distended. The pains in the stomach are more especially a hard pressure, less frequently tearing or crampy pains. The buccal cavity shows symptoms of an intense catarrh. Stool is hard and retarded. No other pathogenesis contains the symptoms of gastric catarrh more fully than Nux. However, it is more suitable in recent cases without any marked symptoms of material changes. As we have stated before, the remedy is of particular advantage in cases resulting from excessive mental labor and sedentary habits.

Bryonia is, in many respects, closely related to Nux. Both remedies correspond more particularly to chronic catarrh that had developed itself out of an acute attack, and not so much to chronic catarrh setting in gradually and imperceptibly. The prevailing Bryonia-pain is likewise a hard pressure, as from a stone; it sets in soon after eating, is caused by gas in the stomach, and is relieved by frequent eructations. These eructations, however, are not like those of Nux, at times bitter, at other times sour, but having rather a foul and spoiled taste, and are apt to result in the spitting up of food, or in vomiting of the ingesta mixed up with bile and mucus. The taste is a spoiled bitter and pappy taste. Bryonia differs from Nux by exciting a violent and continued desire for copious quantities of cold drinks, and by causing a depression of the temperature.

Antimonium crudum has already been mentioned under acute catarrh; it is especially suitable in cases of protracted or mismanaged acute catarrh, if the tongue has a thick yellow or whitish coating.

Pulsatilla resembles Bryonia in many respects, except that there is great chilliness without thirst, and the symptoms do not show themselves at once, but some time after eating, and are diminished by exercise, whereas exercise aggravates the pains of Bryonia. Pulsatilla deserves particular attention if the stomach symptoms are accompanied by uterine derangements; against the gastric ailments of pregnancy it is utterly powerless.

Cocculus acts similarly to Nux in gastric affections; it is particularly useful if the patient is troubled with flatulence that gives rise to colicky pains.

Beside these remedies we have to mention: *Ipecacuanha*, *Veratrum album*, *Ignatia* and *Staphysagria*, which complete the list of remedies in cases of more recent origin, whereas the following list of remedies is more adapted to more chronic and more deeply-seated cases.

China has several very definite symptoms; the taste is bitter or else it is entirely absent. The local pains are not very violent but continued; the appetite is gone, the stomach is altogether very inactive, so that the food either remains for a long time in the stomach, and causes a feeling of fulness, or it passes off with the stool, either partially or completely undigested. This remedy is particularly suitable for gastric derangements that have remained after severe diseases.

Sepia is more particularly, although not exclusively, adapted to the chronic gastric catarrh of females. The catarrhal symptoms are attended with a variety of nervous pains, especially with painfulness of the back, which sometimes has the appearance of spinal irritation. The appetite is perverse, the patient craves pungent food. There is considerable acid in the stomach, which causes a disagreeable burning some time after eating, especially at night, that can be relieved by eating a little solid food. Sepia sometimes removes very rapidly, or at least mitigates, the gastric complaints of pregnant females. In a certain condition of the system, which we have so far only noticed in females, it affords considerable aid. After the exacerbation of chronic gastric catarrh has lasted a few days, with intolerable burning pains, the renal region, more particularly on the left side, becomes painful, a violent burning pain is felt in this region, and a quantity of saturated, highly-colored urine is discharged, which deposits copious quantities of urates, or else a clear urine, with a copious sandy sediment, loaded with uric acid. After this discharge the pains generally abate, and only return again if the stomach has not yet been fully restored to its normal condition. In this affection the pains are generally very fierce, and may readily be confounded with simple cardialgia, if the changes in the urine are not attended to.

Phosphorus renders excellent service in chronic catarrh of the stomach. Its symptoms are more like those of chronic inflammation than of simple catarrh, in the lesser degrees of which it will scarcely ever be found suitable. Phosphorus likewise has a tendency to the excessive formation of acid, except that the eructations and the vomiting have an oily taste. The pains are intense, and are aggravated by eating. This circumstance, in addition to the other phenomena, points to considerable alterations of the mucous membrane, on which account we employ Phosphorus with success in ulceration and hemorrhage of the stomach.

Lycopodium is one of the most frequently used medicines in chronic catarrh of the stomach. It is not so much adapted to the lower grades of the disorder, nor where the local symptoms are very prominent; it is more particularly in its place where the constitutional equilibrium is very much disturbed and the patient grows thin. The face has a grayish hue and an expression of suffering, so that we are led to suspect the presence of malignant disorganizations of the stomach, under which head we shall again refer to it more especially. Where Lycopodium is suitable in gastric catarrh, we generally have structural changes in the spleen or liver. The symptoms referring to the mental and sensorial range are characteristic, and, therefore, of special importance in determining the selection of Lycopodium.

Arsenicum album is known to us as one of our leading stomach-remedies. In a general sense, it corresponds more especially to an inflammatory affection of the mucous membrane of the stomach, but likewise, as we know from experience, to catarrhal symptoms in their higher grade of development, as we observe them more particularly in the case of drunkards. Characteristic indications are: the local pains are a violent pressure alternating with burning, or a burning distress exclusively; the thirst is intense and tormenting; the taste is bitter, sour or foul; the vomiting is very hard, and attended with excessive pain; the desire to vomit is felt after every meal. Arsenicum is likewise indicated for the peculiar, painless torpor and inaction of the stomach of long duration, and leading to a gradual decay of the tissues. Here, too, we have to point to the condition of the urine, which, after Arsenic, has a larger quantity of uric acid. Violent cardialgic pains are an additional indication for this drug.

The symptomatic indications of **Sulphur** are so numerous that it is difficult to point out the whole list. Almost all of them correspond to chronic catarrh of the stomach and its disastrous consequences. More than all theories does experience confirm the use of Sulphur in chronic gastric catarrh, for it cannot be denied that it has often given a favorable turn to the disease when other remedies had been used in vain. Chronic vomiting is arrested by Sulphur more surely than by many other drugs. Experience has taught us, that large doses of the lower triturations are not near as useful and effective as not very frequently repeated doses of the higher attenuations. We cannot point out a single exception to this rule. The adherents of the fabulous psora-theory, praise Sulphur in all possible diseases; likewise in the gastric complaints of individuals who have had the itch once in their lifetime. A complication with liver affections and piles is an additional indication for Sulphur, as we shall show more fully by and by.

Calcarea Carbonica is scarcely ever indicated in the chronic gastric catarrh of adults. The gastric complaints of chlorotic females are an exception, for in these Calcarea may render good service. In such cases the remedy is more particularly indicated by the following symptoms: A strong desire for acidulated drinks, and a good deal of thirst generally; excessive secretion of acids; perverse longing for very sharp, sour substances; aversion to animal food, with copious use of farinaceous diet; canine hunger, without the least appetite; disposition to diarrhœa. Calcarea is particularly suitable for children under two years; adults require it much less frequently Simple gastric catarrh is very seldom met with in the case of children, for the whole of the intestinal canal very soon becomes involved in the morbid process, on which account we shall have to recur to this drug in our chapter on gastro-intestinal catarrh. Disturbances of the gastric functions, which constitute the imperceptible commencement of gastric catarrh, such as vomiting, loss of appetite, or else an excessive avidity for food, especially farinaceous food; flatulent distension of the abdomen, sour smell from the mouth, disposition to catarrh of the mouth, yield most promptly and safely to Calcarea.

Beside these remedies, the following deserve our attention: *Plumbum*, *Ferrum*, *Cuprum*, *Carbo vegetabilis*, *Iodium*, *Natrum muriaticum*. It would take up too much space if we would write out a complete symptomatology of each of these drugs; moreover, the full pathogenesis of each can be found recorded in the Materia Medica. We wish, however, to mention one remedy of which we have no very extensive provings, but which has already shown its valuable curative powers in practice—we mean the *Sulphate of Atropine*. It is particularly suitable where violent local, intermittent pains are complained of; they are ameliorated by vomiting up mucus with a good deal of straining, or they are momentarily suspended altogether, and are felt principally at night. We have never effected a complete cure with this salt, but have always afforded partial relief, after which the cure was completed with a few doses of Sulphur.

3. Gastritis, Inflammation of the Stomach.

Acute gastritis is a pathological process concerning which the views of pathologists differ as yet a great deal. Some even go so far as to suppose that this inflammation, in so far as it originates spontaneously, is identical with acute catarrh of the stomach. This view rests upon a one-sided comprehension of the post-mortem appearances, without at the same time interpreting them with reference to the morbid symptoms. It cannot be denied that the same post-mortem changes may result from acute catarrh and from gastritis, but their meaning differs according as the generating cause is of a different nature. We must not forget that in dealing with the stomach, we deal with a highly complicated organ and not with a mere mucous membrane. Inasmuch as the phenomena during the lifetime of the patient do not always indicate, with unmistakable accuracy, the tissue where the inflammation is seated, we do not deem it essential to dwell any further upon uncertain differences.

Owing to the different views entertained by pathologists regarding the nature of gastritis, the etiology of this disease must necessarily be involved in a good deal of obscurity. Among its causes we have to mention, in the first place, the various circumstances which have already been alluded to in the chapter on acute catarrh, namely, the introduction of excessively hot or cold articles of diet into the stomach, and violent colds. Besides these causes the stomach may become sympathetically involved in other acute diseases. That excessive moral emotions, especially of a depressing kind, may cause acute gastritis, has been shown by striking examples. Mechanical injuries by foreign bodies, such as glass or needles, are not very unfrequent causes of gastritis. The most frequent causes of this disease are violently-acting poisons, either vegetable or mineral, among which alcohol occupies a prominent rank. And, finally, we may state that cooks, whose abdomens are exposed the whole day to a high degree of radiant heat, are frequently attacked with affections of the stomach, and generally with gastritis.

The symptoms of this disease change according to the degree of the local affection, or the irritability of the individual attacked by the disease. From these symptoms we cannot draw any reliable inferences regarding the actual character of the local changes. In a few cases the inflammatory affection does not develop any marked symptoms, the patient sinks all at once, and a post-mortem examination reveals the phenomena of inflammation, which had resulted in ulceration and perforation. In the milder cases we merely find the symptoms of an acute gastric catarrh, only the sensitiveness of the region of the stomach to external pressure is generally more intense, nor is the pain exclusively a painful pressure; the pulse is likewise more hurried than during the existence of catarrh. In a practical and therapeutic point of view it is, of course, important that the diagnosis should be correct; in some cases, however, this seems impossible, and the only certain diagnostic sign is the appearance of the tongue. In acute catarrh of any intensity, the tongue has a whitish or yellowish coating, whereas in gastritis it is generally clean, dark-red, or more smooth and marked with red spots.

The most violent attacks of gastritis occur after the ingestion of intensely-acting poisons, without any premonitory symptoms and very suddenly. If the disease sets in idiopathically, it is no less violent and begins with a violent chill, which generally ushers in all very acute diseases. The first sure diagnostic sign is a raging pain which seems intolerable, and is generally burning, less frequently a tearing or crampy pain, which at times is limited to a small spot, and at other times extends over the whole region of the stomach. This region is often so sensitive to contact that the weight of the bed-quilt cannot be borne. Very soon it becomes distended. The pain is likewise apt to spread over the abdomen and chest, and the pain caused by the depression of the diaphragm impedes the breathing even to the most violent dyspnœa. In one case which we had to take charge of, after it had been under allopathic treatment, the pain in the stomach became associated with an exceedingly violent, stitching pain in the right side of the chest, which the attending physician interpreted as pleuritis, and consequently treated with leeches applied to the right side of the thorax. A post-mortem examination showed the pleura and lungs perfectly sound. The mistake was the more easily made, as the patient was tormented by a distressing cough, setting in shortly previous to an attack of pain in the right side. As a rule vomiting sets in at the onset, even if no poisoning had taken place, in consequence of which the rest of the food is ejected from the stomach, and afterwards a watery or tenacious and, in the higher grades of the disease, a bloody mucus. The blood and mucus are more particularly thrown up when a corrosive poison has been swallowed. Every ingestion of food or beverage excites the vomiting, so that the patient scarcely dares quench his horrid thirst even by small quantities of water; solid food is not retained at all. The bowels are constipated as a matter of course. The participation of the general organism in the morbid action is first manifested by a more or less intense fever, with a small, feeble but frequent pulse; the urine being at the same time diminished. The pains either continue unabated or increase gradually; the countenance which has an expression of suffering from the start, soon assumes a cadaverous pallor and looks disfigured, the extremities are cool, the skin is covered with a cold sweat. An inexpressible anguish causes an unceasing restlessness, and deprives the patient of all sleep. In proportion as the disease approximates to a fatal termination, the strength sinks with an unusual rapidity, hiccough, fainting fits, delirium, etc., set in, until death terminates the scene. In other cases the patients die suddenly without any alarming symptoms.

This picture of acute gastritis of course admits of certain modifications, if the disease is caused by a poisonous substance; for in such a case the peculiar effects which this poison produces in other organs, have likewise to be considered.

In all somewhat acute cases the disease always runs a rapid course, so that death sometimes sets in in a few hours; sometimes the disorder continues to the fourth week, or it assumes the form of chronic catarrh of the stomach, which has already been described. It is a subject of great importance to know the exact character of the anatomical appearances in this disease. Recovery scarcely ever takes place suddenly, and it is easily disturbed by the least error in diet. Beside the termination in chronic gastritis, the trouble may continue as suppuration of the mucous membrane, together with its consequences, a statement of which will be furnished in a subsequent chapter.

The post-mortem changes do not always strictly correspond to the symptoms observed during the lifetime of the patient. The mucous membrane appears red over a greater or less extent; it is at times of a lighter and at other times of a darker hue; sometimes of unequal thickness, softened or eaten away in some places, or perforated in consequence of a more deeply-penetrating ulcerative process. These changes, of course, differ if they are caused by the action of poisons, but these differences need not be described more minutely in the present instance.

The prognosis is uncertain, especially in cases running a slow course. Acute idiopathic gastritis is one of the most fatal affections, whereas toxical gastritis is much more promising as regards a final cure. A good deal depends upon the conduct of the patient during convalescence, for we need scarcely state that the peculiar structure of the stomach is very favorable to relapses, and that, independently of such considerations, the ulcerative process, if it should have commenced, requires the greatest care.

Treatment. We have already stated that gastritis, in its different degrees of intensity, assumes different forms of symptomatic manifestation. The milder forms often resemble an acute gastric catarrh to such an extent that it is impossible to distinguish one from the other. On this account the remedies mentioned under catarrh of the stomach will likewise have to be used against gastritis. In the more violent forms of this inflammation we have, in the first place, to determine the cause. This, of course, cannot be done when the disease originates spontaneously; but it is perfectly feasible if the inflammation was caused by poison. In such a case, we must not only try to remove the swallowed poison by an emetic, but we may likewise have to employ the stomach-pump or neutralizing antidotes in order to prevent absorption of the poison, and thus render it less dangerous, and perhaps harmless. We omit the mention of the antidotes to the various poisons, for the reason that they can be found fully recorded in any toxicological treatise. We may observe, however, that in every case where vomiting is attended with violent symptoms of gastritis, the vomited substance should be carefully preserved for examination; chemical analysis is the only certain means of making sure of the fact of poisoning in a given case. That which still remains to be done after the first management of the case, which is common to all schools, has been attended to, becomes properly the subject of homœopathic treatment. It is likewise of importance, in a case of poisoning, to consider whether the ingestion of copious quantities of cold water, for which the patients long, on account of the burning distress in their stomachs, may not have a prejudicial effect by promoting the solution of the swallowed poison. Where there is any uncertainty, we give the preference to slimy decoctions, oily substances, milk which is not too much diluted.

Regarding the treatment of gastritis, it would seem that it cannot be very difficult to enumerate a multitude of remedies for this disease. Almost every drug in our Materia Medica has symptoms resembling the symptoms of gastritis; and, according to the law of similarity, must therefore prove curative in this disease. This view, however, is based upon entirely false notions. With most poisons, inflammation of the stomach is not caused by the same property that renders them valuable and useful as remedial agents; but it is generally the consequence of a purely chemical and mechanical action, and, for this reason, without any practical value for homœopathic treatment. In some respects our inability to discriminate between the toxicological and pharmaco-dynamical effects of a poison, interferes very much with a successful homœopathic treatment. In this respect we have to act by the rule, that only such poisonous substances can be regarded as remedial agents as have simulated a state of gastritis, in consequence of the absorption of small doses into the general organism. Following this rule, we can only select a small number among the whole list.

Arsenicum produces, more specifically than any other poison, the symptoms of gastritis, whether by its direct introduction into the stomach, or by its absorption by the skin when applied to this organ in form of an ointment, or by the inhalation of arsenical dust. This statement is corroborated by several very striking observations. One is the case of a young woman living in a room, the walls of which were covered with a green paper containing Arsenic; she passed through the different degrees of gastritis up to the blood-streaked, distressing vomiting. The cause of these toxical symptoms was the more easily accounted for, as the symptoms disappeared on the third day after she had changed her domicile. Here the poisonous dust had been absorbed through the respiratory organs. Cases where the external application of Arsenic in the form of a solution or ointment causes the phenomena of arsenical poisoning, are not very rare. This shows that the stomach-symptoms belong to the most constant and characteristic symptoms of Arsenic, and that we are fully justified in regarding Arsenic as one of our most efficient agents in the treatment of gastritis. Owing to the importance of the remedy, we here range the symptoms in one series: Violent pressure in the stomach; distressing burning in the stomach; extreme sensitiveness of the region of the stomach to the least pressure; swelling of the pit of the stomach; gagging and painful vomiting after every meal, even after drinking liquids, particularly after eating sour substances or rye-bread; unquenchable thirst, with longing for cold drinks, with inability to swallow more than a small quantity at a time; the respiration is embarrassed; horrid anguish and restlessness, the patient has to be in constant motion; retention of stool and urine; coldness of the extremities, with burning heat of the trunk; sweat from sheer anguish; frequent, small, easily compressible pulse; distorted, cadaverous expression of the countenance. This list of the most prominent symptoms may suffice. Strangely enough, our literature does not contain a single cure of gastritis by Arsenic. Some gastric affections, which are reported under the name of cardialgia, do not seem to have been anything else than cardialgia; but it is difficult to establish a correct diagnosis from the reports as furnished in the journals. This gap in our literature may be owing to the circumstance that gastritis resulting from other than toxical causes is a very rare occurrence, and that the lesser grades of gastritis have been reported under other names. According to the above-mentioned symptoms, Arsenic would seem to be adapted only to the most violent forms of gastritis; but a cursory perusal of the pathogenesis of Arsenic in our Materia Medica will suffice to show that this agent is suitable in every form of gastritis, from the mildest to the most violent.

Phosphorus has the symptoms of gastritis neither as completely and prominently, nor as intensely as Arsenic. Beside the burning distress in the stomach, Phosphorus has likewise a cutting pain as a prevalent symptom; the heat of the trunk is very great, the extremities are cold, the patient has frequent attacks of chills, the power of reaction sinks very speedily, and convulsions set in. In a given case, a good deal of attention and careful comparison will be required to establish the difference between Phosphorus and Arsenic.

Belladonna is scarcely ever appropriate in the more advanced stages of gastritis, but is quite in its place at the onset, if the attack is not too violent. If our diagnosis is firmly established, the question is, whether it is not better to give at once the medicine that is the simillinum for the disease from its first outbreak to its final termination. At all events Belladonna is preferable to Aconite. We do not see upon what grounds Aconite is recommended as a remedy for gastritis. The fever is not such as corresponds to the Aconite fever; it is a wrong method to undertake to give a remedy for the whole complex of the symptoms in a strictly local affection. [In *rheumatic gastritis*, with great tenderness of the region of the stomach, distension of this region, a burning and throbbing or stinging and tearing distress in the stomach, raising of blood from the stomach, synochal or even moderate fever preceded by a more or less violent chill or a succession of slight chills, and general constitutional symptoms, such as weariness, expression of distress in the countenance, thirst, constipated bowels, dyspnœa, etc., Aconite is an indispensable remedy, as we can assert from experience. It is particularly the muscular coat which is the seat of the disease. We mix one or two drops of the tincture of the root in half a tumbler of water, and give a dessert-spoonful of this mixture every half-hour or hour, until the patient is better. The attenuations in such cases are either useless or insufficient. H.]

Camphora is not in curative rapport with the whole pathological process of gastritis, but is exhibited with great benefit, if the disease breaks out suddenly with great violence. The attack is very similar to the stage of invasion of Asiatic cholera; the strength seems paralyzed all at once, the circulation stops, and the skin is icy-cold.

The symptoms of **Cantharides** that seem to have reference to gastritis, are very questionable; they are probably the effects of the local action of the poison. What Hartmann relates concerning *Nitrum* is so indefinite, that we hesitate to repeat his remarks.

Many other remedies have single symptoms that seem to belong in this category, but the indications are very imperfect. The most noteworthy among them are: *Bryonia, Digitalis, Mercurius, Mezereum, Tartarus stibiatus,* and *Antimonium crudum.* The two last-named remedies deserve particular consideration in the deceitful and not very intense gastritis of drunkards. Moreover, we refer the reader to the treatment of acute catarrh.

The diet fills an important place in the treatment of this disease. When the disease is at its height, it is not necessary to prohibit any kind of food, for the patients do not desire any; and it is, moreover, impossible for them to eat anything; all they care for are refreshing drinks, and since quantities of fresh water would be out of place, the best method of alleviating the craving for cooling beverages, is to allow a few small pieces of ice to dissolve upon the tongue, and to satisfy the want of something liquid by means of some mild slimy decoction. During convalescence the greatest caution should be observed in regard to the use of solid food, which should be given in very small and gradually increasing quantities.

That an ulcer may not form even at this period, is not certain; moreover, the stomach has become so irritable by the long deprivation of solid food, that if given in too large a quantity, it may either cause a relapse, or at least superinduce a condition resembling acute or chronic catarrh. A gastritis which runs its course without causing much trouble to the patient, likewise requires the most careful management regarding the diet to be observed.

4. Ulcus Perforans Ventriculi seu Rotundum. Chronic Ulcer of the Stomach.

Every mucous membrane, and particularly that of the stomach, inclines to ulcerate. In a subsequent chapter, when treating of hemorrhage from the stomach, we shall speak more fully of ulcerative processes in general. Here we shall simply treat of a peculiar form of ulcer, recognized by unmistakable characteristic symptoms. In order to prevent all misapprehensions, we will commence with the anatomical description of the ulcer.

Ulcus Perforans Ventriculi seu Rotundum.

The perforating ulcer generally occurs as a single ulcer in the stomach; only in rare cases we meet with several together. It is almost exclusively situated near the small curvature, the pylorus, and in the posterior wall of the stomach, very rarely in the fundus of this organ. At first it is a sharply circumscribed hole in the mucous membrane, of the size of two inches in diameter and upwards, without any inflammatory infiltration or coloration of the surrounding parts. In the further course of the ulcer the base, as well as the surrounding parts, may become corroded by the ulcerative process, imparting to it a more oval or even elongated form. If the muscular and afterwards the serous coat become involved in the ulcerative process, the ulceration of these coats never spreads as extensively as that of the mucous coat, so that the profile of the ulcer acquires a flat funnel or terrace-shaped appearance. The ulcer inclines very much to perforate all the coats of the stomach; this, however, takes place slowly, and is preceded by the formation of adhesions, which prevent the escape of the contents of the stomach into the cavity of the abdomen. Where this course does not take place, the perforation with immediately following fatal peritonitis, is the usual termination of this process. The healing of the ulcer takes place by means of a ray-shaped cicatrix, and considerable contraction of the cicatrized part.

These anatomical peculiarities show that the perforating ulcer must depend upon characteristic pathological changes, and that it cannot result from any of the processes which we have described in previous chapters. Among the numerous hypotheses that have been offered in explanation of this very peculiar form of ulcer, the most probable is, undoubtedly, the theory, that the occlusion of an arterial vessel of more or less size had caused the death of a circumscribed piece of mucous membrane, and that consequent absorption and ulceration had been set up by the action of the gastric juice. In this way the round form of the ulcer is most easily accounted for.

The etiology of this process is almost entirely enveloped in obscurity, although this disorganization is by no means a very rare occurrence. Most diseases occur among persons of middle age. Tuberculosis, carcinoma, and other deep-seated affections are frequently met with among individuals affected with this ulcer, but whether they are the cause of the ulcer, and how, is questionable. It is said that much exposure in front of a big fire, during work, often causes the disease.

Symptoms and course. The circumstance that cicatrices of the round ulcer are often met with in persons who have never complained very particularly of gastric derangements, must satisfy us that this ulcer sometimes runs its course without any striking symptoms. It likewise happens that an individual dies of peritonitis consequent upon perforation of the stomach, without any signs of disease of the stomach having been perceived during the lifetime of the patient. We have already shown that gastritis may exist without any striking symptoms. It is difficult to say with what phenomena the round ulcer generally commences; the characteristic pain is the first symptom of which the patient complains, he may at most have experienced slight disturbances of the digestive functions. The pain caused by the ulcer is very peculiar; although spread over a large portion of the region of the stomach, yet the pain seems to be located at a definite spot, and is very much aggravated by external pressure. Beside this pain, which is roused by pressing on the parts, the patient complains of other more intense pains which are either excited or very much aggravated by the ingestion of solid or stimulating food. These pains often seem like cardialgia, with which they are easily confounded, for the reason that they are apt to occur in paroxysms. The patient traces them very positively to the place where the ulcer is located. They are felt during the first two hours of the digestive process, but may last much longer. They are generally burning pains, or cutting as with many knives, seldom lancing as with a single blade, they radiate more particularly toward the back, likewise into the abdomen, are aggravated by external pressure sometimes to an alarming degree, and generally cause a great deal of dyspnœa. In some cases they have complete intermissions, in others they have a remittent type. Not unfrequently the pains occur so perfectly free from other complications that they seem more like an attack of pure neuralgia; generally, however, they are attended with signs of gastric derangement, and increase in intensity in proportion as the characteristic symptoms of the ulcer become more prominent. The appetite is less, the patients complain of distension of the stomach, violent eructations, heartburn, waterbrash. The bowels are torpid, and sometimes obstinately constipated.

This mild commencement of the disorder is sooner or later associated with vomiting. The vomiting is most usually connected with the paroxysms of pain, which it generally winds up and therefore relieves. It is exceedingly distressing, and, as a general rule, causes at least a partial expulsion of the food that had been partaken of last, as mixed with water and mucus, has an acrid-sour taste, and always occurs a few hours after partaking of the food. Sometimes no food is vomited up, but only mucus and sour water. As the ulcerative process spreads, the vomiting is apt to become mixed with blood. If no large vessels are corroded, the vomited material is only streaked with blood; but if an important artery should be destroyed, the hemorrhage is more copious and may even terminate fatally. We have seen several quarts of blood vomited up in twenty-four hours.

Independently of the consequences of such hemorrhages, which of course superinduce hydræmia, the ulcer exerts a depressing influence upon the assimilative functions, which is so much more penetrating, the more considerable are the disturbances caused by the sore.

As we have already stated, the course of the ulcer may be very rapid, provided we do not mistake the date of its origin; more commonly, however, the ulcer runs a chronic course, even for years, with more or less protracted intermissions. These often depend upon the cure of one ulcer, whereas a second attack indicates the formation of a second ulcer.

In the smaller number of cases the termination of the disease is death, which either takes place in consequence of the disturbed nutrition, or hemorrhage, or perforation with consequent rapidly developed peritonitis and sudden death. Recovery may be complete; but if the ulcer was very large, the cicatrized part very much contracted, and the contraction is situated in the region of the pylorus, the consequent encroachment upon the capacity of the stomach may induce more or less important derangements. Sometimes perforation may take place quite suddenly even after complete recovery seemed to have been achieved; the reason is that when penetrating to the subjacent tissues, the disturbances caused by the ulcer are less striking than when the ulcer spreads superficially. Hence the prognosis is pretty uncertain; as a general rule not very bad, but in case of frequent hemorrhages, very doubtful at all events.

If a majority of the above-mentioned symptoms are present, the diagnosis of ulcer of the stomach is not very difficult; in other cases, on the contrary, where the symptoms are not very striking, a diagnosis cannot be made with certainty. It is more especially of importance where carcinomatous degenerations are suspected, or where the symptoms justify the suspicion that cardialgia is the character of the existing disturbance. We shall revert to these distinctions in a subsequent paragraph.

Treatment. This is another of those pathological processes, concerning whose treatment our literature has nothing to show, and where again the fact is demonstrated, that the report of a case, without any special diagnosis, is of no use to us. Many of the cases reported as cardialgia, undoubtedly come under the category of perforating ulcer, likewise some of our reported cures of carcinoma of the stomach; more particularly the latter, for the reason that the cure of a real carcinoma is, if not questionable, at any rate very uncertain and doubtful. As far as a rigorous discrimination is concerned, the most necessary points of comparison are wanting.

In looking at the symptoms in our Materia Medica, we meet with considerable difficulties in selecting a remedy, namely the absence of objective phenomena and of such as have been confirmed by post-mortem examinations. On the other hand some of our provings are so characteristic that the selection of a suitable remedy cannot be very difficult in all cases. Moreover the slowness of this pathological process and the comparative absence of immediate danger, enable us to devote a reasonable amount of time to a careful comparison of the pathogenetic with the pathological symptoms, and to cautiously institute therapeutic experiments. In searching for a simillimum we must not forget that, although the round ulcer is characteristeric of the pathological process of which we are treating, yet it alone does not constitute this process, but forms the terminal solution of a whole series of morbid developments; and that therefore a medicine may be specifically homœopathic to an affection, of which we are not as yet able to demonstrate the round ulcer as the final pathological result. In selecting our remedy it is likewise important to remember that ulcer of the stomach is a very chronic affection, which is best treated with medicines that have a slow, deeply-penetrating, continued action. In our chapter on hemorrhage of the stomach, we shall have to mention the remedies that are in homœopathic rapport with perforating ulcer, and therefore refer the reader to that chapter.

Atropine. It may seem strange that we should open the list with a remedy of which we have no full provings, but the striking results that have been obtained with this remedy, in perforating ulcer, compel us to confer this distinction upon Atropine. We know from experience that no medicine is better calculated to subdue the frightful cardialgic pain of ulcer of the stomach than the Sulphate of Atropine. At the same time we know that this medicine alone is not sufficient for a complete removal of the difficulty, for all it accomplishes is to effect a temporary palliation of the distress. Hence the medicine can only be administered as an intercurrent remedy. The fourth trituration is most advisable; the third is still apt to develop medicinal symptoms. The improvement caused by Atropine is best continued by *Sulphur*, giving a dose of a higher potency at prolonged intervals. Atropine generally arrests the vomiting.

Baryta carbonica possesses among its pathogenesis all the symptoms that characterize ulcer of the stomach. In Hahnemann's record we find: Ulcerative pain or a feeling of soreness in the stomach after external pressure, or when drawing breath; a painful writhing sensation in the stomach when swallowing a morsel of food, as though the food had to be forced through a stricture and came in contact with sore places. These, in connection with other symptoms, must necessarily suggest Baryta to us as a specific remedy. Our own practical observations have confirmed these expectations. But a curative action only took place if no vomiting was present, or only vomiting of a small quantity of mucus, and if the cardialgic pains did not occur in distinctly separate paroxysms, but were rather of a remittent type.

Carbo vegetabilis is more important than Baryta, although the local symptoms may be less distinct. At any rate, they are sufficiently distinct to show its homœopathicity to ulcer of the stomach. It is a distinctive symptom of Carbo not only to excite the pains by eating, but they are likewise felt when the stomach is empty, especially when the stomach is very sour; but it is likewise appropriate in cases where this symptom is wanting, and where no other reason exists to account for this exceptional circumstance. In many regions of country, vegetable charcoal is a much employed domestic remedy for cardialgia, though the vomiting, which is never absent, shows that the name is wrongly applied. We are acquainted with a gentleman who was cured of a gastric affection that evidently depended upon perforating ulcer, and had continued with uninterrupted violence for three years, by means of the pulverized young shoots of the common poplar. We are unable to decide whether the poplar has any curative virtues inherent in it, or whether the charcoal alone exerts the curative influence. It is certain that our own charcoal likewise has an excellent effect.

Argentum nitricum, although its pathogenesis is not yet very thorough, yet has been variously exhibited in affections of the stomach, and has been found more particularly useful in the complaints arising from perforating ulcer. This likewise corresponds to what Hartmann has stated regarding its employment in cardialgia. We transcribe his remarks literally: "My experience with Argentum nitricum is as follows: I have only had occasion to make use of it in the case of females; menstrual irregularities have always constituted my chief guide, more especially premature and profuse menses, developing an impoverishment of the constitution and consequent nervous irritability. The violent, spasmodic pains in the stomach, obliging the patient to bend double, do not intermit with any degree of regularity, but occur early in the morning as well as in the afternoon and evening, or even at night, attended with violent retching, resulting in the expulsion of a fluid having an acrid, sour, or bitter taste like bile, and having a yellowish-green color, and of a tenacious consistence." This is not a true picture of cardialgia. Otherwise Arg. nitr. acts just as well upon the stomachs of male as upon those of female patients. Hartmann recommends the first three decimal-triturations. Everybody can easily convince himself that Arg. nitr. in the higher potencies is entirely powerless, or that it acts, at any rate, with much less efficacy than in the lower.

Beside these most prominent and most important remedies, the following deserve particular consideration: *Arsenicum, Phosphorus, Plumbum, Natrum muriat., China, Secale cornutum, Veratrum, Calcarea carb.* and *Lachesis.* Of these, *Arsenicum,* as well as *Phosphorus,* have already been mentioned in the chapter on gastritis, where they are much more appropriate than in the chapter on ulcer of the stomach, especially Phosphorus. As regards *Arsenic,* we can show such a number of fine results that it deserves to be classed in the foremost rank among the remedies for perforating ulcer, except that the symptoms will not always be found to correspond with the pathological phenomena. Arsenic is particularly indicated, together with *China* and *Calcarea carb.*, where the ulcer is consequent upon previous emaciating morbid processes or occurs with them simultaneously; for instance, after intermittent fever or in anæmic individuals. *Natrum muriaticum* likewise deserves our attention under such circumstances.

Concerning the appropriate diet, we have only a few remarks to offer. Of course the stomach has to be managed with great delicacy; overloading the stomach, or indigestible substances, stimulating and irritating articles of diet, or such as cause an excessive secretion of gastric acid, such as fat, are to be strictly avoided. We do not mean to say that it would be a good plan to restrict the patient to a scanty and poor diet; this neither advances the cure nor helps the patient. We have to see to it, that the strength is upheld by a light, nourishing diet, since marasmus is too apt to set in.

The slow course of the disease and the inability to effect a rapid cure, should teach us not to change our remedies too frequently; hence it is best to exhibit them at rather long intervals. The frequent and violent attacks of cardialgia are apt to induce us to pursue the contrary course, in order to afford speedy relief to the patient; but these kind intentions do not lead to any good results.

5. Carcinoma Ventriculi, Cancer of the Stomach.

We should have placed this form of cancerous disease in the category of carcinoma, if the importance of this pathological process, and the facility with which it is confounded with other pathological processes of the stomach, did not bespeak for it more particular consideration.

The etiology of cancer of the stomach, belongs, in most cases, to the domain of hypothesis; all sorts of causes are accused of the disease, but with what right is questionable. It is admitted that this affection seldom occurs before the fortieth, and scarely ever before the thirtieth year, and that it is more frequently met with among men than women. There is no doubt that this form of carcinoma, as well as any other form, is hereditary. Moreover, we have to repeat the causes which we have assigned to chronic catarrh of the stomach, more particularly the habitual abuse of strong alcoholic beverages. Want and poverty, continued grief, constant care and mental depression, tend to develop cancer of the stomach. The last-mentioned cause is the more active, if the stomach inclines to be attacked with acute or chronic catarrh, in which case carcinoma originates very readily in the disorganized mucous membrane. Carcinoma of the stomach is most usually a primary disease, with reference to other cancerous disorganizations, but may readily give rise to cancerous formations in other localities.

Inasmuch as an intelligent comprehension of the symptoms of carcinoma of the stomach implies a knowledge of the anatomical structure and locality, we here furnish a short view of its pathological post-mortem degenerations. Carcinoma of the stomach has most generally the form of scirrhus, the fibrous carcinoma, less frequently that of medullary fungus, and still less frequently of any other form; in exceptional cases these two forms may occur in combination. The seat of carcinoma, from where it generally starts, is, in the majority of cases, the pylorus; next to that the cardia; after that, the small curvature, and very seldom the fundus. Carcinoma prefers spreading like a ring, in opposition to the longitudinal axis of the stomach. The disposition to decomposition, and the dissolution in ichor, is greatest in the case of medullary fungus, taking place with more or less rapidity, whereas the parts not destroyed by dissolution are sometimes simultaneously metamorphosed into fungoid growths. The secondary alterations, caused in the stomach by the carcinomatous process, differ according as their locality differs. If the carcinoma is seated near the cardia, we have stricture and shrinking of the parts; if near the pylorus, the stomach becomes dilated. In the former case the œsophagus is apt to become involved in the disorganization, in the latter the duodenum. If the disorganized portion of the stomach does not form any adhesions with adjoining parts, as is often the case, the carcinoma is apt to draw the stomach downwards, out of its normal situation.

It is easily seen that the symptoms of carcinoma of the stomach must vary a great deal. A precursory stage, properly speaking, can hardly be supposed to exist. If the carcinoma develops itself out of other diseases, they cannot well be regarded as an ordinary preliminary stage of the disorganization, but the carcinoma and this disease coincide accidentally, and without obeying any fixed law. As soon, however, as the carcinoma begins to form, the signs of a chronic gastric catarrh at once make their appearance. The patient experiences a pain after every meal, the prevailing character of which is a hard pressure; digestion takes place slowly, a quantity of gas forms, whence distension of the pit of the stomach, eructations, etc.; moreover, heartburn, nausea, waterbrash. These symptoms are not characteristic of carcinoma, and they may continue for a long time, even if the carcinoma should continue to grow all this time; a perfectly certain diagnosis, at this stage of the disease, is impossible. As soon as a reliable diagnosis can be made, we meet with the following symptoms: A spot in the region of the stomach becomes painful, both when pressed upon or without pressure, the pain being worse after every ingestion of food. The pain is at times like a hard pressure, at other times burning, and very often lancing or cutting, which is so often characteristic of cancer.

Food does not cause as intense a pain as in ulcer of the stomach, but the pain lasts longer. Generally the pain is associated with vomiting, at first rather of water and mucus, and afterwards of the ingesta. The vomiting does not occur at regular periods, at the commencement, particularly, the paroxysms may be separated by longer intervals. At a later period, the time when the vomiting sets in, depends upon the seat of the cancerous degeneration. If the cardia is the locality of the disease, the vomiting takes place soon after eating; if seated around the pylorus, a few hours may elapse before the vomiting takes place. Vomiting may likewise occur early in the morning, before any food has been swallowed; this accident, however, apparently does not occur unless blood has become effused into the cavity of the stomach, in consequence of the ichorous dissolution or separation of the diseased mass. It being speedily decomposed by the gastric juice, the blood, when vomited up, looks like coffee dregs, grumous, having a chocolate color, which is pathognomonic of cancer. This metamorphosis of the blood occurs only when it oozes from the capillary vessels, ramified over the lining membrane. If a larger vessel is destroyed by the ichorous process, the blood is vomited up in the shape of a black mass, and in large quantity. This last circumstance does not often occur in carcinoma. When the pain and vomiting set in, the constitution begins to show the disastrous inroad of the disease. The body begins to waste away, and the strength becomes very much impaired. The appetite is entirely gone, or, if there is a little appetite left, the patient dares not gratify it on account of the pain caused by the food. The alvine evacuations are, of course, very scanty, sometimes black, if blood accumulates in the stomach. This fact can often be inferred from the character of the stools, provided the blood is not evacuated by the mouth. At an early period of the disease, the face assumes an expression of suffering, the corners of the mouth become depressed, and the face assumes a dingy yellowish-gray or livid hue. The spirits are always very much depressed, and an irresistible hopelessness adds to the patient's tortures. The emaciation becomes excessive; œdema of the extremities supervenes, less frequently ascites. If the cancer is located in the neighborhood of the cardia, the sufferings of the patient are the most acute. The inability to swallow food, condemns the sufferer to die of starvation; and the certainty of having to meet such a terrible end, frequently drives him to commit suicide. We do not always succeed in verifying the existence of carcinoma by palpation or percussion; sometimes we fail even in the most characteristically marked cases. Scirrhus, in the region of the pylorus, is most easily diagnosed as a solid bunch in the pit of the stomach; or, if the stomach had gravitated downwards, near the umbilicus. The vomiting may sometimes abate, or even be suspended for some time, without any corresponding improvement. If the tumor becomes detached, or melts away into ichor, the patient may experience a corresponding degree of ease, in consequence of the passage through the cardia, or the pylorus, having become temporarily freed.

These phenomena are not always found united, otherwise the diagnosis would be very easy. Sometimes one, and sometimes another symptom is absent, and there are cases where the pains are comparatively very slight. This last-mentioned circumstance is often witnessed in the case of old people, who barely complain of the symptoms of a slight catarrh of the stomach, while they are rapidly wasting away under the cancerous disease.

A few circumstances modify very essentially the course of the disease. The wasting of the strength goes on more rapidly when the cardia or pylorus is attacked, than when the disease is located in the curvatures. Scirrhus grows more slowly than medullary fungus, nor does it encroach as much upon the cavity of the stomach. Hemorrhages, of course, complicate the prognosis; the same takes place, if, side by side with the local carcinomatous affection of the stomach, carcinomatous tumors and excretions are discovered in other organs, as is very frequently the case in the further course of the disease. Unless serious untoward circumstances arise, the disease runs a somewhat protracted course, at least for several months, and sometimes even for years. Of all carcinomatous degenerations, the medullary fungus runs the most rapid course. One of the secondary accidents, which sometimes puts a sudden end to the sufferings and life of the patient, is the perforation of the coats of the stomach consequent upon the decay of the scirrhous tumor, with rapidly following and fatal peritonitis. Death generally takes place amid the most marked signs of general prostration and decay, which is most generally indicated by the appearance of more or less extensive dropsical symptoms.

Without determining whether a remedy for this disease has been properly chosen, the diagnosis of carcinoma of the stomach is of particular importance, in so far as it enables us to decide whether the disease can be acted upon by internal treatment, and whether the reported cures really were carcinoma. The importance of a correct diagnosis is particularly interesting in our relations towards our professional opponents, and, we are sorry to confess, is very much underrated in this respect. The most important points for a correct diagnosis of the disease are: In the first place, the distinctly perceptible swelling somewhere in the region of the stomach, which does not change its location. Afterwards the peculiar color of the vomit; this, however, may likewise occur in slow and scanty hemorrhages of the stomach from other causes, but is especially copious from perforating ulcer of the stomach. The pains likewise may contribute to corroborate the diagnosis. In cancer they are mostly constant, somewhat aggravated by the ingestion of food; whereas, in the case of ulcer, the pains have sometimes complete intermissions, but are excited to a high degree of intensity by eating. The age of the patient and the duration of the disease constitute important diagnostic aids; for, whereas nutrition is not much interfered with by other chronic affections of the stomach, even after they had lasted a long time; in the case of carcinoma, the strength vanishes rapidly and very soon. Moreover, other affections of the stomach have occasional, although very trifling, remissions; carcinoma progresses steadily without any interruption.

Treatment. In the presence of a disease which is considered incurable by every physician, we are bound to ask ourselves, very seriously, what is the extent of our means, and how far we can hold out the hope of curing a patient who is willing to trust himself into our hands. We have no right to promise the cure of carcinoma by homœopathic means, with the same readiness as we promise a cure of cardialgia, or some other chronic affection. That there are homœopathic physicians who make such rash promises without meaning to do wrong, can easily be proven. But if we inquire whether a case of carcinoma of the stomach, that had been diagnosed with undeniable accuracy, has really been cured by homœopathic means, we have to deny the correctness of such a statement. In taking charge of such a patient, we have to confess our inability to promise anything, at the same time that we resolutely and conscientiously undertake to afford him relief. For the circumstance that a reliable cure of carcinoma has not yet been reported, does not show that we may not, at some future time, be able to achieve such a success, and then we may be fortunate enough to discover new and better remedies that may finally conquer the disease. In such desperate cases we have to follow strictly the law of similarity, with so much more boldness, as we are convinced that the patient's distress will never be increased by such a course. A correct selection of the remedial agent affords us an advantage, that no other curative method can boast of; we sometimes succeed in mitigating and even suspending symptoms that are peculiarly tormenting. Such palliative effects have occurred in the practice of every homœopathic physician, and, although they may only occur exceptionally, yet they are an abundant reward for the trouble it cost to find a remedy capable of producing them.

Hartmann introduces the treatment of carcinoma of the stomach with the following remarks of Canstatt: "To check the further development of the threatening destroyer is a much more thankful task than to undertake to remove the fully-developed, incurable degeneration." From this quotation, and from his subsequent remarks, we infer that Hartmann adopts the existence of a precursory stage. This theory is antagonistic to practical observation, and the measures proposed in accordance with it, deserve but little consideration. It seems to us that Canstatt's opinion would be more properly enunciated in this wise: Considering the great difficulty of distinguishing an incipient carcinoma of the stomach from other, even chronic, derangements of this organ, and in view of the perfectly correct supposition that chronic inflammatory affections of the stomach favor the formation of carcinoma, it becomes a sacred obligation for every physician to watch and to treat every affection of the stomach with the greatest care. It is exceedingly doubtful whether the retrograde metamorphosis of an incipient carcinoma is at all possible; but we must admit that, if a cure is possible, it can best be achieved during the incipiency of the cancerous growth. From this stand-point, the treatment of cancer includes all the remedies that have been recommended for chronic catarrh of the stomach, and perforating ulcer, and will afterwards be recommended for cardialgia. Our previously expressed reflections will, moreover, induce us to attend to the diet, in affections of the stomach, with the utmost attention, since every dietetic transgression, every improper habit in our mode of living, may entail the most disastrous consequences. Although this kind of prophylactic treatment may not be sufficient to prevent carcinoma, yet, if such a misfortune should occur in spite of all dietetic care, it is a consoling thought that nothing had been neglected on our part to prevent it. Further particulars concerning diet are not necessary, since they have been fully explained in our article on chronic catarrh of the stomach. Particular care must be had, to spare the patient all depressing or exciting mental emotions, since every symptom becomes aggravated immediately after such an occurrence.

If called upon to treat a fully-developed, undoubted case of carcinoma of the stomach, every homœopath will undoubtedly first think of *Arsenic* as a sheet-anchor. It cannot be denied that the pathogenesis of Arsenic contains very accurately the symptoms characterizing carcinoma of the stomach, for which we refer the reader to our Materia Medica the more urgently, since Arsenic is one of our best stomach remedies. We do not know of any cure of carcinoma by means of Arsenic, but we do know that in a number of cases Arsenic has arrested the progress of the disorganization for weeks, and even months, and has effected a consequent suspension of the patient's sufferings. Among the latter, we notice more particularly the vomiting and sleeplessness; altogether, Arsenic often acts like Opium. On the other hand, we must not expect too much of this drug; the vomiting, for instance, which is caused by stricture of the orifices of the stomach, cannot possibly be arrested by any kind of medicine. We infer from a number of observations that the higher attenuations of Arsenic, in this disease, palliate the pains more certainly and permanently than the lower, and that the dose should not be repeated too often.

Nux vomica is another of those medicines that palliate many of the distresses in carcinoma of the stomach. It has a favorable effect in the excessive acidity of the stomach, the distressing heartburn early in the morning, vomiting of mucus when it does not occur immediately after eating, the painful flatulence, and finally the obstinate constipation. The last-mentioned symptom is relieved by *Nux*, as by magic; likewise if the constipation had been caused by the excessive use of Opium.

Lycopodium bears great resemblance to Nux. In the chapter on catarrh of the stomach we stated that Lycopodium is particularly indicated, if the symptoms lead us to suspect the presence of some malignant disorganization. It is especially suitable if the patients are much distressed by sour stomach and heartburn, accompanied by burning pain in the pit of the stomach; if the vomiting consists of mucus, takes place at night or early in the morning, or if the constipation is very obstinate and the fæces are enveloped in mucus. Lycopodium is likewise specially indicated by the condition of the mind and feelings.

Veratrum album is only useful for the vomiting of the ingesta. It has afforded relief even in cases where Arsenic seemed powerless.

For occasional attacks of vomiting, especially vomiting of mucus, it is of no use.

Mezereum is recommended for carcinoma of the stomach; whether such a recommendation is properly based upon symptomatic similarity is very doubtful. Kallenbach reports two cases where the vomiting was arrested by this medicine. Our objection to such cases is, that the dissolution of the cancerous growth had most likely cleared the passage in or out of the stomach; for in Kallenbach's cases, both patients died soon after the cessation of the vomiting. The symptoms seem to point out Mezereum as a more appropriate remedy for perforating ulcer, and hemorrhage from the stomach, than for carcinoma.

Plumbum does not seem entirely homœopathic to carcinoma of the stomach; the local symptoms do not indicate it. On the other hand, the manner in which the vomiting takes place, the excessive anguish during the vomiting, the nature of the vomit, the obstinate constipation, the emaciation like that of a skeleton, the condition of the mind, are well calculated to recommend this medicine as an excellent palliative. A very striking case, related by Widumann, in the Hygea VII, should invite similar experiments with Plumbum. We have to observe that Widumann employed the Acetate of Lead, not metallic Lead.

Hartmann mentions, beside these remedies, *Carbo vegetabilis* and *animalis*, likewise *Conium*, but a merely superficial perusal of their pathogenesis, shows that not one of them fully corresponds to the pathological series of carcinoma, and they at most cover a few single symptoms, hence cannot be properly assigned a place in the front rank of cancer-remedies.

Creasotum is recommended by some homœopathic physicians, the same as by physicians of the Old School. The pathogenesis of Creosotum is, however, very imperfect, but, inasmuch as any remedy that may possibly be of some use in the treatment of carcinoma of the stomach, ought to be received by us with a hearty welcome, we deem it our duty to give it a place in our list.

For other medicines that might possibly be of some use in carcinoma, we refer the reader to chapters 2 and 4. A precautionary rule, that cannot be too often or too earnestly enjoined upon beginners, is not to change the medicine too often, nor to indulge in too frequent a repetition of the dose. By the former mistake we are led to be deceived regarding the efficacy of our remedies, and to abandon a good remedy because it has not yet had time to display its effect. In this as in other similar affections, where we are constantly obliged to prescribe a remedy without the least hope of doing the patient any good, we often have to resort to a simple powder of sugar of milk in order to appease the sufferer's impatience.

[*Cuprum aceticum* will sometimes relieve the distressing vomiting in carcinoma of the stomach. H.]

6. Hæmatemesis, Hemorrhage from the Stomach.

This is scarcely ever an idiopathic affection, but almost always symptomatic of some other disease. If we devote a special chapter to this accident, it is because vomiting of blood always excites our most serious apprehensions, and, therefore, is of great importance in a therapeutic point of view. For this reason we place this subject immediately after those processes which mostly occasion the disorder.

Hæmatemesis may depend upon a variety of pathological causes, and if it inclines to become profuse and threatening, it is of the utmost importance in practice to investigate with accuracy and care the precise etiological causes in each attack. Bleeding may occur, even if the vessels of the stomach are all left intact, even if a postmortem examination does not reveal the least rupture of any bloodvessel. As a complicating symptom bleeding occurs, more particularly, in diseases characterized by a peculiar alteration of the whole mass of blood, such as typhus, scurvy, yellow fever, etc. The hemorrhage may be very copious, although none of the larger vessels are ruptured. A second cause of the bleeding is a rupture of the walls of vessels. It may be caused by excessive accumulation of blood in the stomach depending upon disturbances, engorgements, etc., of the vena porta, liver, spleen—hence it is not of unfrequent occurrence in the case of individuals afflicted with piles; or the hemorrhage may be caused by menstrual suppressions and stoppages, on which account it occurs more frequently at the climacteric age; it sometimes seems as if the hemorrhage took place as a vicarious substitute for the menstrual discharge. The vomiting during pregnancy is very frequently stained with blood. In the cases we have mentioned the bleeding is very copious, and generally takes place from the ruptured capillaries. Hemorrhages depending upon an impeded circulation of the liver, spleen, etc., mostly arise from varicose distension of the veins of the stomach, and incline to be very copious. The worst kind of bleeding arises from injuries of the vascular walls, consequent upon ulcerations of the mucous membrane. It is met with in chronic catarrh of the stomach, as well as in cases of perforating and carcinomatous ulcers. If there is an idiosyncratic disposition to bleeding, it may be provoked by a blow upon the stomach, a fall, or a violent emotion.

The symptoms of hæmatemesis differ, according as the bleeding is more or less copious, and arises from different causes. If the bleeding is but slight, and the blood is not vomited up, the accident remains sometimes entirely unnoticed. If the vomited substance only contains a few streaks of blood, it has no particular significance at the time, but the patient has to be watched with more care, because we can never be sure whether a more dangerous hemorrhage is not threatening. The blood should likewise be examined, with a view of discovering pathological changes that had remained latent heretofore. The bleeding likewise acquires importance from the circumstance, whether the blood is discharged with violent straining, or is vomited up easily; in the latter case the bleeding is much more significant, on account of its indicating ulceration of the mucous membrane, or some important change, dilatation, etc., of the vessels, whereas a little blood may be discharged in consequence of violent straining, even if the vessels are perfeetly intact.

As soon as a somewhat considerable quantity of blood is vomited, a series of characteristic symptoms are evolved. The morbid symptoms that already happen to be present, become associated with a constantly increasing dull pressure in the pit of the stomach, and a distressing feeling of distention of the stomach, generally attended with nausea. If the bleeding takes place slowly, the preliminary symptoms may be confined to these few; on the contrary, if the blood is expelled with rapidity and force, the patient experiences the usual symptoms of a considerable loss of blood, such as anxiety, paleness, cold sweat, cold skin, vertigo and even fainting. A large quantity of blood is vomited up at once, and with great force. The action of the gastric juice imparts to it a blackish hue, and has the consistence of coagulated sour milk. The quantity discharged at one vomiting often exceeds one quart, so that it seems scarcely possible that the stomach could have contained such a large quantity at once. Immediately after the vomiting the patients feel faint and exhausted, and are tormented by an almost unquenchable thirst; at the same time a visible throbbing occurs in the pit of the stomach, of which the patient himself is conscious. After this paroxysm, a period of rest and comparative ease sets in, until another attack of bleeding occurs. The interval to the next bleeding, lasts from a few hours to several days; in violent cases four or five attacks may occur on the same day; of course in such a case, severe symptoms of anæmia may set in even unto convulsions, and death may be the immediate consequence. If so much blood is expelled from the stomach, the stools are likewise black as coal, and very thin; it may even happen that the blood is not vomited up first, but that the black stools may be the first sign of the bleeding. Regarding a return of the bleeding, we cannot speak with certainty, it depends entirely upon the primarily exciting cause. If there is a frequent return of the bleeding, anæmia and dropsy are unavoidable results. Recovery from a single attack usually takes place slowly, the patients being at the same time tormented by a variety of gastric disorders, such as a burning distress in the region of the stomach, foul taste, sweetish or foul eructations, horrid thirst, and by a long-continued abdominal pulsation. Under all circumstances there is great danger lest the bleeding should return, hence the patient cannot be too careful in not overtaxing the stomach. Bleeding resulting from ulceration may not afford much relief, but in cases of hæmatemesis, of which we are unable to discover the exact cause, or which depend upon the suppression of other hemorrhages, the relief afforded by such bleedings may be quite considerable.

As regards diagnosis, two circumstances may deceive us. In the first place a violent paroxysm of hæmoptysis may be mistaken by patients for vomiting of blood, and the deception may be kept up if the physician does not himself examine the vomit, since patients, often, are so overwhelmed with anxiety that they lose all calmness and presence of mind. In other respects the black color of the vomit, and the absence of the bloody expectoration, which always follows a paroxysm of bloody cough, furnish the surest indications regarding the true character of the attack. It likewise happens that a person may have a violent attack of nose-bleed over night, and that the blood may be swallowed: if the quantity of the swallowed blood becomes excessive, it awakens the person, and the blood is then vomited up, and may look precisely as it does when true hæmatemesis takes place. It is difficult to distinguish one from the other; our diagnosis has to be more particularly determined by the absence of all precursory symptoms and subsequent gastric derangements. The use of whortle-berries and similarly-colored fruit may likewise occasion a momentary deception, more particularly if the patients are very anxious.

As a general rule, the prognosis in all ordinary cases, is favorable, except where the hemorrhage is at once so excessive that death results from the mere loss of blood. The prognosis, however, is always doubtful, in so far as a first bleeding leaves an inclination to a renewed attack, and the bleeding always indicates the presence of dangerous alterations in the stomach. Hence a permanent cure is never absolutely certain.

Treatment. Hartmann (Vol. II. 183) relates a case from his own practice, which we transcribe literally, with so much more pleasure as it suggests many interesting observations.

"My patient was a man of about sixty years, of a plethoric, atrabilious constitution, who, on previous occasions had several attacks, but none equalling the present one in violence. I arrived at the moment when the patient was vomiting up a quantity of dark-colored carbonized blood, after which he sank back on his couch in a fainting condition. Shortly after, another attack took place, after which the weakness became excessive; the blood which had been vomited up in three attacks, filled half a chamber, yet the disease did not yet seem disposed to intermit, for the horrid visibly perceptible throbbing in the pit of the stomach, perceptible even to the patient, the nausea, eructations, and the other precursors of a renewed attack, continued; the patient's skin felt cold; the features were sunken and he moaned and groaned while drawing breath. No remedy seemed better indicated than *China*, of which he took a drop of the 18th attenuation. In three hours, another but milder paroxysm set in, and on the next morning the patient had recovered so far as to be able to exchange a few words with me; he likewise complained less of the feeling of qualmishness in the pit of the stomach, in the place of which he experienced a burning distress; the sighing inspirations had disappeared, but the visible throbbing in the pit of the stomach with anxiety was still present; the least motion aggravated the nausea, which likewise became worse at night, together with all the above-mentioned complaints. The appetite was entirely gone, the bowels constipated, the patient was tormented by great thirst. Although I allowed the China to act for four days, yet upon the whole there was no improvement; on the contrary the attacks returned every day twice, and the patient had likewise several stools a day, which weakened him still more. The burning distress in the region of the stomach, the unquenchable thirst, the increasing pulsations in the pit of the stomach, together with intense attacks of anxiety, etc., were sure indications for the exhibition of *Arsenicum album,* which I administered on the fourth day early in the morning, after which such a steady improvement set in, that on the fifth day after the patient took the Arsenic, he was able to leave his bed. The bloody stools continued for two days after the Arsenic had been taken, after which they gradually changed to fecal evacuations. The throbbing and the burning distress in the pit of the stomach continued unchanged for a fortnight after the Arsenic was taken, so that I was led to suspect the existence of an aneurism in the aorta descendens. *Calcarea carbonica* had a good effect, but *Carbo vegetabilis* removed the whole of these symptoms."

A superficial comparison of this case with the above-mentioned symptoms, shows that it took a course as though no remedy had been given. It would seem as though Hartmann had treated but few cases of melæna, otherwise he would have held different opinions regarding the correctness of his choice of remedies. Hartmann seems to think, for instance, that *Carbo vegetabilis,* in arresting the abdominal pulsations, likewise arrested the whole trouble, because an apparent feeling of comfort succeeded its administration. But we know that this result takes place in the majority of cases, and that the vomiting of blood occurs again for all that. At all events Hartmann ought to have informed us how many years, after this cure was accomplished, the patient's health remained good. This whole report shows us how cautiously we have to proceed in taking it for granted that a certain remedy had effected a cure.

The treatment of hæmatemesis has to proceed from a twofold point of view, first to arrest the hemorrhage and provide against its immediate consequences, and afterwards to prevent the return of the accident. Our best plan will be, not to give the pathogenesis of each remedy separately, but to group the remedies with reference to the above-mentioned indications.

For the hemorrhage itself we know of no better and more efficacious remedy than *Ipecacuanha,* unless very peculiar accessory symptoms should render some other medicine necessary. Hence it is indicated against a first attack, rather than against the subsequent and alarming symptoms of anæmia. The less the hemorrhage is depending upon some anterior pathological disturbance, the more efficacious Ipecacuanha will prove. But it is necessary to give large doses and frequently repeated; triturations of the root are, moreover, preferable to the tincture. *Nux vomica* is more suitable for hemorrhages accompanied by vascular excitement, they are not very copious, and the vomiting is accomplished with difficulty, and attended with severe retching; Nux is more particularly indicated in hemorrhage arising from some acute affection of the stomach. Under such circumstances the dose has to be adapted to the vascular excitement, lest it should be increased by too powerful medicinal action. It is emphatically suitable in cases where the hemorrhage is but trifling, and the blood bright-red. In such cases *Belladonna* will prove serviceable. If we are called to the patient after he has vomited several times; if the above-described symptoms of anæmia are very prominent; the pulse quick or thready, the skin cool and the nausea unceasing, *Veratrum* deserves a preference. *Secale cornutum* competes with this remedy; Secale, however, is decidedly preferable if convulsions have set in, whereas Veratrum is required rather by the fainting sort of weakness, or by actual syncope. On the contrary *Arsenicum album* is preferable if the anguish is very great, the thirst unappeasable, the restlessness extraordinary and the skin is not too cool.

The above-mentioned remedies will prove generally sufficient to arrest the hemorrhage. We will add that *Arnica* is recommended for hemorrhage caused by mechanical injury. We should likewise state that hæmatemesis, and ordinary bleeding from the stomach, frequently occur in the case of new-born infants, for which *Aconite* is the chief remedy [The sphere of Aconite in this disease is much more extensive. It will be found generally adapted to hemorrhage with great vascular excitement, quick and small, but hard and jerking pulse, or else the pulse is full, bounding, and accelerated, the skin is warm and dry, the face flushed, there is vertigo and headache, the extremities are cold, epigastric region bloated and sore, with pulsative throbbing in the same, nausea and sometimes even palpitation of the heart, great thirst. In Hartmann's case, we should have given Aconite, instead of tampering with other medicines. Aconite would have arrested the hemorrhage at once, and would have effected a cure of the case. Arsenicum was not indicated as the leading remedy in this case, because one of the most characteristic indications for Arsenic in hæmatemesis, is trembling of the lower extremities, with violent chilliness, even in front of a big fire. H.]

China is generally indicated for the secondary phenomena succeeding the bleeding. It is only exceptionally, however, that the symptoms will be found to be strikingly similar. *Nux vomica* is undoubtedly more suitable, provided the hemorrhage had not been too profuse, or else *Veratrum* and *Arsenicum*, the former particularly if the black stools occur very frequently. Not till the more threatening symptoms have abated, is China in its place.

Hemorrhages depending upon decomposition and fluidification of the blood, will be mentioned when the various affections to which they are related as effect and cause, are treated of. Such hemorrhages require to be managed from entirely different points of view.

Where the bleeding is caused by suppression of the menses, we have to think first of *Pulsatilla;* not so much for the purpose of arresting the hemorrhage, as for the purpose of restoring the menstrual flow. If congestive symptoms are present, *Belladonna* is preferable; likewise, if the arrest of the menses is incidental to the climacteric period. Under such circumstances, *Lycopodium* may prove useful.

If the primary affection, upon which the vomiting of blood depends, can be correctly diagnosed, it is not so very difficult to operate against it; the treatment is the same as that of chronic catarrh of the stomach, perforating ulcer, carcinoma of the stomach, or such affections of the liver and spleen as may have caused the disturbances of the circulation. If the fundamental trouble cannot be found out, we have to confine ourselves, almost entirely, to rigid dietetic and hygienic instructions, and we should try to remove every little irregularity in the digestive functions as speedily as possible by appropriate remedies. *Nux vomica*, most generally deserves a preference; if the symptoms do not point to any exceptionally characteristic affection of the stomach, it may be well to continue the use of Nux for a long time at distant intervals.

In order not to omit any remedy that may afford relief in such an important accident, where speedy help is sometimes absolutely required, we add the following remedies to our list as worthy of mention: *Hyoscyamus* is said to be particularly useful in arterial hemorrhage; *Phosphorus, Carbo vegetabilis, Mezereum*. Of the last-mentioned remedy, we have never seen the least effect in hæmatemesis. Hartmann likewise mentions *Millefolium*, (because it is said to be useful in any kind of hemorrhage?) *Cantharides, Natrum muriaticum, Zincum, Sulphur, Cicuta virosa*. It is true Cantharides cause vomiting of blood, but most likely, only by their intensely irritating, local action, not by virtue of their constitutional effect. In melæna proper, they are not specifically appropriate.

[Among the remedies that have been introduced into American practice in the last few years, *Erigeron*, or the Canada fleabane;

Eryngium, or the button snake-root; *Hamamelis*, or the witch-hazel, and *Sanguinaria*, or the common blood-root, have been used by American homœopathic physicians with more or less success. Of Hamamelis especially, a number of excellent cures of epistaxis, hæmatemesis, and hemorrhage from the intestines, have been reported. H.]

It can easily be imagined, that in a disease of this kind, the desire to afford help as rapidly as possible, and to quiet the apprehensions of surrounding friends, lest their impatience should prove injurious to the patient, should induce us to resort to external applications in connection with internal treatment. The most usually employed external means are cold applications, and counter-irritants. It is hard to decide whether a bag of ice laid upon the stomach, exerts a truly favorable effect upon the bleeding. What is the object of such a proceeding? Certainly not to effect a direct deviation of the blood from the vessels of the stomach, since the cold repels the blood from the place where the ice is applied. Hence the driving away of the blood from the skin, would only tend to accumulate this fluid in the vessels of the stomach. That the most intense cold does not act upon the stomach directly, admits of no doubt. But even if no favorable effect can be expected from the ice-bladder, let it be laid upon the stomach, were it only to quiet the family. Only let the patient be protected from excess. We cannot speak much more favorably of the different cutaneous irritants. Among them, dry cupping has most in its favor, and least against it. It should not be tried, however, if striking signs of anæmia are already present.

It is of particular importance that the general dietetic and hygienic habits of the patient should be carefully regulated. As soon as hemorrhage sets in, the patient should remain in a state of perfect bodily and mental rest. A strictly horizontal posture is indispensable, and every motion that is not absolutely necessary should be avoided. The horrid thirst of such patients presents some difficulties. To quench it, small pieces of ice should be swallowed, or should be allowed to melt in the mouth; this is much better than to swallow liquids. Ice is certainly very refreshing to the patient, and he may partake of it safely, whenever it can be procured; the dread of cold water, which seems to control some people, is ill-founded. It may be that drinking large quantities of water, prevents the formation of a thrombus in the stomach, but the frequent use of small quantities of this fluid has no such effect. We know that in cases of severe hemorrhages, the organism desires to repair the quantitative loss of vital fluids by absorbing water, hence the agonizing thirst, hence nothing better can be done than to give the patient, very frequently, a small quantity of fresh, cold water. There can be no harm in reasonably gratifying a natural desire that is so pointedly, and so emphatically expressed. Even the most generous wines are given, if the weakness becomes excessive, simply because Nature seems to require this kind of treatment. There are circumstances when wine is, indeed, the only means from which a favorable effect can be expected, as rapidly as the imminent danger seems to require. We can testify from experience that wine, if properly administered, is not by any means hurtful.

As long as there is danger of a return of the bleeding, the patient has to be kept on a low diet, or, if he has no desire for food, he may safely be allowed to do without it. Otherwise, slimy soups are his best nourishment, only they must be eaten when quite cool. As soon as the hemorrhage is arrested, the waste should be repaired as speedily as possible by giving the patient more invigorating nourishment. As long as there is any sign of abdominal pulsation, solid food had better be avoided; not till every trace of pulsation has disappeared, can the ordinary mode of living be resumed

7. Cardialgia, Spasm of the Stomach.

With a view of facilitating the comprehension of the following chapter, we will state that our remarks apply to all the various conditions that have been designated as gastrodynia neuralgica, gastralgia, neuralgia cœliaca.

By these expressions we understand a very painful affection of the stomach, existing without any material changes in the tissues of this organ, and which, on this account, we regard as simply emanating from the nerves of the stomach.

Regarding the nature of this pathological process, we have not as yet arrived at any very definite explanation.

Cardialgia is, at times, a primary, at other times a secondary affection. The causes of idiopathic cardialgia are: A generally increased sensitiveness and irritability of the nerves of the stomach, without any definite dietetic transgressions being discoverable as the primary cause of the disease. Such an abnormal irritability does not continue uninterruptedly, it appears in paroxysms, without any demonstrable cause, so that at certain times the distress is excited by a variety of articles of food, which at other times can be eaten without the least inconvenience. One cause of cardialgia is the disproportion between waste and supply; hence we find this affection prevailing among persons leading a sedentary life, or indulging in excessive living. In many individuals, especially in the summer season, a common cold is very apt to cause cardialgic pains. The chief causes of the primary disease, are medicinal articles of diet, and medicines themselves. We see cardialgia remain after other severe diseases that had been treated with a quantity of violent drugs; this is known to every homœopathic physician. The disease is likewise caused by abuse of spirits and green tea. Coffee, however, is the beverage to which most individuals owe their attacks of cardialgia—we mean badly prepared coffee. According to our experience, strong, filtered coffee, that has not been boiled, and is free from adventitious admixture, scarcely ever causes gastric derangements, provided it is not partaken of in too large a quantity. This, however, is very seldom the case; and, if it does produce gastric derangements, it is not cardialgia, but such disturbances as we have described under the general designation of catarrh of the stomach. For this reason, women are much more frequently attacked with cardialgia than men. Hartmann may be correct when he says that the sedentary mode of life to which women are so frequently condemned, prevents them from neutralizing the deleterious effects of coffee by plenty of exercise; but this is not the only cause, in proof of which we point to the frequent occurrence of cardialgia, among country women of the poorer class. That coffee is the sole cause of cardialgia among them, has become evident to us by abundant experience, for we have cured many cases of this disease, in a very short time, by means of a few powders of sugar of milk, simply recommending strict avoidance of coffee. But if we do not wish to be deceived, we should proceed very cautiously in examining the patient concerning the use of coffee; for women do not mind telling a falsehood if their favorite beverage, coffee, is at stake. More than one woman has confessed to us that she would have resorted to homœopathic treatment, if it had not been for the dread of having to do without her coffee. We would advise the physician to visit his patient unexpectedly, at the time when she is in the habit of sipping her coffee, in order to satisfy himself what horrid brew she calls by that name; and, at the same time, to become convinced that this so-called coffee, with its admixture of chicorea and the like, is sufficient to cause sickness. Another drug, which, however, does not cause cardialgia as certainly as coffee, is tobacco. The pains caused by tobacco are of a peculiar crampy kind, and often continue the whole day, but do not become seated as easily as the pains caused by coffee. Whether cardialgia can be caused by tight dresses alone, without any other injurious influence, is difficult to determine, for the reason that women who wear such dresses are, generally, predisposed to derangements which culminate in cardialgia.

As a secondary affection we meet with cardialgia in various conditions of the organism which produce nervous debility as a leading result, such as anæmia, chlorosis, leucorrhœa, and affections of the sexual organs generally, likewise onanism, spermatorrhœa, and finally during convalescence from very severe diseases, such as typhus. That hysteric women frequently complain of cardialgia, is well known. Affections of the spinal cord are likewise to be suspected, but it is difficult to determine whether the spinal irritation is the cause, or effect, of the cardialgic disorder. The supposition that the suppression of habitual foot-sweats may cause cardialgia, is likewise very hypothetical. The most violent attacks of cardialgia which we have yet seen, in the case of two female patients, were evidently caused by an excess of uric acid, for during the attacks, which came on periodically, a sandy sediment was discharged with the urine, or very copious crystals were deposited in this fluid. The connection between the two orders of phenomena is not very clear.

Regarding age and sex we meet with cardialgia more frequently among women, very seldom before the age of pubescence, most frequently between thirty and fifty years. The mode of living does not seem to exert a prominent influence, except in so far as the substances, to which we have called attention in previous paragraphs, may give rise to the disease.

In view of the changeable character and multiplicity of the symptoms of cardialgia, we are unable to exhibit them in a connected series, and we, therefore, prefer describing them in detail. The pathognomonic symptom, of cardialgia, are pains, the principal seat and starting point of which is the region of the stomach, and which break out at intervals, at least at the commencement of the disease. The chief character of the pain, is a constrictive, crampy, twisting pain; the pain is likewise tearing, boring, burning, cutting, throbbing, gnawing; indeed, it may assume every possible shape. In the lesser forms of cardialgia, the patient does not suffer much, since the pain is nothing more than a dull painful pressure. Generally, however, shortly after a sensation of malaise, eructations, a feeling of goneness or weariness in the pit of the stomach, the pain suddenly increases in intensity to such a degree that the patient is compelled to cry out. It is characteristic of cardialgia that slight pressure should cause pain, whereas hard and continued pressure is not only easily borne, but affords relief, hence we see the patients pressing their stomachs against the edge of the table, or bending double over the back of a chair, in order to obtain relief from their distress. The pain either remains confined to the region of the stomach, or else it radiates towards the back, the chest, or the abdomen. The respiration is frequently interfered with, hence we often hear cardialgia described as a spasm of the chest. The paroxysm is excited by certain kinds of food and certain emotions, or it may occur at regular intervals, or without any apparent cause or periodicity. Some individuals are attacked early in the morning, when they have nothing on the stomach; others late in the evening or at night, or after a meal. At one time the pain is excited by everything that is taken into the stomach; at other times it is ameliorated by eating. These differences in the time of the appearance of the paroxysms, and in the effect of external circumstances, are not only met with among different individuals, but likewise in the same patient.

The morbid phenomena which may manifest themselves during the intervals of the paroxysms, are exceedingly variable. One of the most common is vomiting; there is seldom vomiting of food except when it occurs shortly after a meal, most generally the patient brings up a slimy-watery fluid. The vomiting usually terminates the paroxysm, it is very rare that the pains continue after the vomiting. Beside the vomiting we frequently meet with an excessive development of gas in the stomach, which sometimes takes place all at once; the gas distends the stomach so that the patient is obliged to loosen his clothes, belching up a quantity of wind affords relief and even arrests the distress. Heartburn, nausea and canine hunger, frequently accompany cardialgia, not so much as constituent symptoms of this affection as accidental symptoms of some other affection of the stomach.

Beside these derangements emanating from the stomach exclusively, we have disturbances in other organs. During the attacks we frequently meet with palpitation of the heart, colicky pains, convulsive motions, debility even unto syncope, etc. After the attack the patient complains of great weariness, the urine is secreted in large quantity and clear as water, very seldom saturated, and the region of the stomach remains sensitive for a short time after.

A single paroxysm, when the disease first commences, seldom lasts longer than one hour. If the disorder increases, the attacks may succeed each other so rapidly that the pain seems to be continuous, with only short remissions, and raging for days. In some cases the general organism does not seem to be affected by the cardialgia, between the paroxysms the patients seem quite well; usually, however, nutrition suffers, especially if the spasm is provoked by certain kinds of food, so that the patients are afraid of eating. But even without this inconvenience the digestive powers gradually become weaker, the alvine evacuations are retarded and difficult, the face puts on an expression of suffering and acquires a pale and livid hue. A transition into other complaints does not take place. Where such a transition is supposed to have been witnessed, it was not cardialgia, but some other affection that the patient had to deal with. That any interference with the functions of the stomach may, under certain circumstances, give rise to chronic catarrh of the stomach, is self-evident; we can likewise readily admit that genuine cardialgia may become combined with some other morbid process, and that both may coexist for a certain period.

It is not always possible, either at the commencement or at the very height of the disease, to diagnose cardialgia with absolute certainty. If the disease is comparatively recent, the paroxysm may be mistaken for an acute attack of gastritis; this mistake is very soon discovered by a cessation of the pains. Beside gastritis it is with the round ulcer that cardialgia may be confounded. The absence of a circumscribed, localized painfulness; the circumstance that in cardialgia the ingestion of food either ameliorates the distress or, at any rate, does not excite the attack; the circumstance that cardialgic pains usually develop themselves gradually, that they disappear without any regularity, and that they are diminished by hard pressure, are pretty safe diagnostic indications in almost every case. With carcinoma, cardialgia can only be confounded if the cardialgic distress continues without interruption, however, the fact that cardialgia does not result in emaciating the system, generally removes all uncertainties regarding the distinctive differences between carcinoma and cardialgia.

Treatment. We are justified in asserting that the rapidity and safety with which cardialgia yields to homœopathic treatment, constitute one of the bright points of Homœopathy. We lay so much more stress upon this advantage, as every other method of treatment generally consumes years in combating this disorder without success. Moreover, in the case of a chronic trouble like cardialgia, the result of the treatment is much more indisputable than in acute affections, where all sorts of imaginable objections are made against the method of treatment, in order to evade the logical necessity of having to admit the reality of the cure by medicinal means. Hence the sure cure of one of the most common and most obstinate affections, is better evidence in favor of Homœopathy, than the most evident success in treating an acute disease.

The treatment of cardialgia is one of the least difficult problems for a homœopathic practitioner, since we have only to deal with subjective symptoms, and hence the selection of the proper remedy depends entirely upon a very careful comparison of the symptoms. Detached suggestions derived from practice, are easily made available in a given case, and constitute in this very affection the safest guides; another reason why cardialgia is easily cured, is that physicians are so frequently called upon to treat it. Of the large number of remedies most of which have been tried practically, we give the more important ones with all their leading indications; the balance can only be mentioned very generally.

Nux vomica. We may safely assert that a majority of all the cases of cardialgia are suitable to this remedy and either yield to it entirely or partially. It is characteristic of Nux to cause pains when the stomach is empty, which afterwards are moderated by eating; on the other hand there are pains caused by Nux which are either excited or aggravated by eating. The early morning-hours are generally the time when the pains to which Nux is homœopathic, are either excited or aggravated; although pains which are felt during the day, are likewise adapted to the curative action of Nux. The circumstances under which cardialgia is either excited or aggravated, are exceedingly varied, likewise the time of their occurrence. In addition to such general indications which are, however, very important in selecting a remedy for cardialgia, the more special symptoms furnish a striking picture of cardialgia, especially of that form the diagnosis of which cannot easily be doubted. Hartmann furnishes the following apt description of the disease: "The characteristic pains are: Contracting, pressing, crampy, tearing pains in the stomach, with sensation as if the clothing were too tight in the region of the stomach and caused an oppression, a sensation that is somewhat like the sensation as if flatulence were pressing against the hypochondria; this sensation as well as the cardialgia itself, are generally aggravated after a meal and by drinking coffee; it is associated with a feeling of oppression and constriction of the chest, spreading in many cases as far as between the shoulders and the small of the back, or causing a sensation as if a tight band were encircling the chest. If the pain is already felt early on rising, if the patient is awakened by it, the curative power of Nux may be certainly depended upon. But Nux is likewise indicated when the following phenomena of reflex-action and synergy are associated with the pain in the stomach: Nausea, especially during the attack, waterbrash, rising of a sour-bitter fluid with or without heartburn, vomiting of the ingesta or of mucus, also ineffectual retching, palpitation of the heart with anxiety, sour-putrid taste in the mouth, constipation, flatulent distension of the abdomen, occasionally hemicrania, pressing pain in the forehead. Nux is likewise indicated in the case of women whose menses are profuse, the pain setting in with particular violence about the time of the catamenia.

"The more delicate and more sensitive the individual, the weaker may be the dose; the more robust the individual, the stronger should be the dose. So far I have never been obliged to give below the third attenuation; if I have once become satisfied that Nux is the remedy in a given case, I do not hesitate to repeat it; nor have I seen any ill effects in the few cases where I have given Nux morning and evening, although I mostly give it only in the evening."

We will add to this characteristic picture that Nux is particularly adapted to men and to women of a sanguine and quick temperament, also to individuals who are troubled with symptoms of impeded circulation in the digestive apparatus. Nux vomica is specifically adapted to cardialgia, caused by the use of coffee, spirits, and the abuse of chamomile tea. It is less frequently suitable in cases arising from some violent emotion; again, on the other hand, it is indicated if the attacks set in after severe diseases, or in consequence of self-abuse.

Arsenicum album. In treating of other affections of the stomach, we have had occasion to point out the strikingly specific action of this drug upon the stomach, and we feel likewise bound to place it in the front rank of our remedies for cardialgia. Hartmann has described the cardialgia, to which Arsenic is homœopathic, under the name of neuralgia cœliaca, and we here transcribe the most essential parts of his statements, because they embody the essential characteristics of the pathogenesis of Arsenic in their correspondential relation to this disease.

The real paroxysm is preceded by a certain restlessness for a longer or shorter period; next, the patient experiences, all at once, a pain under the ensiform process, of a burning, tearing, stitching or pressing nature, as from an incandescent coal, or as if the parts were violently torn asunder. The pain is sometimes so intense that robust persons become raving mad, delicate individuals faint away. After the pain has lasted at this circumscribed spot for half an hour, it leaves this part and, like a flame, shoots upwards under the sternum towards the neck, or else it divides in two currents, ascending towards the neck on both sides of the vertebral column, following the tract of the sympathicus, or finally it scatters suddenly in all directions, more particularly towards the hypochondria, in the direction of the plexus lienalis and hepaticus. Towards the end of the paroxysm the patient generally belches up wind, or water accumulates in his mouth. After the attack he experiences a feeling of emptiness in the abdomen, lassitude and a feeling of weary exhaustion in the whole body. The tongue remains quite clean, the appetite normal, the digestion likewise. The majority of cases occur at night or early in the morning, more frequently among men than women. For attacks of this kind the best remedies are *Arsenicum* and *Nux vomica*. Hartmann establishes the following contrast between the two:

"Nux vomica is more frequently suitable for the male, Arsenicum for the female sex; if the male individual is of a delicate and sensitive frame, Arsenicum may likewise be appropriate. Nux, as is well known, is adapted to a lively, sanguine temperament, an irritable disposition; it is indicated, if the attack is in a measure owing to suppressed hemorrhoids, and if the pain is so acute that the patient is driven by it to madness. It is likewise indicated where sedentary habits, mental labor, have favored the outbreak of such a disease. Arsenicum, on the other hand, is especially suitable in the case of melancholy or nervous temperaments, and the pains are so intense that they cause the patient to faint. Nux deserves a preference if the paroxysm occurs in the morning hours; after it stops, the patient sinks into a heavy slumber, disturbed by dreams, from which he wakes more tired than he was the evening before; during the paroxysm the patient feels more relieved in a recumbent posture than when standing up or walking about. Arsenicum is required if the paroxysms set in about midnight, awaken the patient from the soundest sleep and abate somewhat when he walks about. The burning pain corresponds more to Arsenic, the tearing, stitching, pressing pain to Nux, both kinds of pain are attended with anguish which, when excessive, decides in favor of Arsenic."

Cardialgias characterized by such symptoms, are not very frequent, nor is Arsenic the only remedy in such cases. This agent plays an important part in cases where the diagnosis is uncertain. It is the acute burning pain that points to Arsenic, so much more when it is accompanied by great restlessness, nervous excitability, palpitation of the heart, and an unequal temperature of the body, and the attacks set in more particularly at night.

Chamomilla. According to Hartmann's excellent description of the curative sphere of this drug, it is particularly suitable for irritable dispositions that are disposed to flare up, and if the attack is provoked by a fit of anger. The pain is a hard pressure, as from a stone in the pit of the stomach, and painful bloating of that region and of the left hypochondrium; the pain is attended with shortness of breath and anxiety, is worst at night, so that the patient is beside himself with anguish and restless tossing about; a throbbing headache in the vertex sometimes supervenes, obliging the patient to get up. It is only during rest and when the body is doubled up, that some ease is obtained. It is important to know that such an attack is mitigated by drinking coffee, whereas the cardialgia to which Nux is suitable, is aggravated by coffee. On account of this circumstance Chamomilla may be required in cardialgias caused by coffee, more particularly if Nux alone is not sufficient to a cure.

Belladonna is not often suitable to cardialgia, more particularly to cardialgia of a more violent degree of intensity. The symptoms are very much like those of an incipient acute gastritis, the pain is a gnawing pressure or a tensive pain, is relieved by stretching the region of the stomach when reclining backwards, arrests respiration, spreads over the adjoining parts, is excited or aggravated by the ingestion of warm food, and is so peculiarly intense that it causes syncope. This form of cardialgia is usually caused by a severe cold and on this account breaks out quite suddenly. It is generally attended with considerable accumulation of gas. As far as the origin of the disease is concerned, Belladonna is nearly related to *Colocynth*. This remedy is more suitable if the attacks set in in rapid succession, the pains are crampy and caused as by a twisting of the stomach, oblige the patient to bend double, abate by external warmth, are aggravated by the ingestion of any kind of aliment; there is nausea, but scarcely ever any vomiting. Eructations afford much relief. The pain is attended with chilliness and even a cold perspiration. Such cases are scarcely ever met with except in warm months about the time when colicky pains are common. If the cardialgia to which Coloc corresponds, occurs in a more chronic form, *Cocculus* is the best remedy. It is more particularly indicated when the cardialgia is accompanied by the accumulation of gas in the intestines, crampy pains and obstinate constipation.

Ignatia is like Nux vomica, characterized by a painful pressure in the region of the stomach, as from a stone, which is excited by the ingestion of any kind of food, and, as a spontaneous distress, occurs principally at night. It is attended with a feeling of hunger and aversion to food. If grief and care are the cause of the disease, Ignatia is said to be the more indicated. [A characteristic indication is a feeling of goneness in the pit of the stomach, with sensation as if a number of needles were pricking the inside of this region. H.]

Sepia has a pain similar to that of Ignatia; here, too, it is apt to set in after eating, but seems to prevail early in the morning before breakfast, and between breakfast and dinner. The characteristic distinctions of both drugs are particularly seen in the accompanying mental conditions· Ignatia is more especially adapted to delicately-organized, sensitive, hysteric individuals, upon whom depressing emotions exert an overpowering influence; Sepia, on the contrary, to individuals with sanguine, excitable temperaments, and inclined to congestions. Both remedies are more especially suitable for females; Sepia is more particularly depending upon the accompanying symptoms of the sexual range for its homœopathicity to cardialgia.

Argentum nitricum has already been mentioned in our chapter on perforating ulcer. We there stated that Hartmann's enthusiastic recommendation of this remedy cannot well be applied to its relation to simple, uncomplicated cardialgia. Considering the large number of well-proved and practically tried remedies which we possess for cardialgia, it would be ill-advised to place an uncertain agent, like the Nitrate of Silver, with uncertain indications in the rank of our remedies for cardialgia.

It remains for us to mention three remedies, which we class together, because their action coincides in one important particular. They are *Pulsatilla, Ferrum,* and *China.* We have stated above that cardialgia is frequently met with in individuals who are afflicted with chlorosis, or generally with anæmia or hydræmia, and that it likewise does not unfrequently occur in the stage of convalescence from severe acute diseases, such as typhus. We cannot as yet, show how the altered composition of the blood is related to the nervous derangement of the stomach; that such a relation exists, admits of no doubt.

Pulsatilla is particularly adapted to the cardialgia of chlorotic patients, provided it is of recent origin, more particularly if the spasmodic distress breaks out early in the morning, when the stomach is yet empty. It abates for a while by eating, but afterwards reappears with so much more intensity; it is accompanied by nausea and a desire to vomit, but there is scarcely ever vomiting of water. The symptoms of this form of cardialgia vary a good deal, and have a multitude of secondary or accessory ailments, which are embodied with great completeness in the pathogenesis of Pulsatilla, and to which we refer in our Materia Medica.

Ferrum is likewise, though less exclusively, adapted to the cardialgia of chlorotic females. This remedy corresponds more particularly to the higher grades of the disease; its selection is not very difficult, because the symptomatic indications are very uniform and precise. Ferrum corresponds to cardialgia with violent pressure or a crampy pressure, which is excited or aggravated by the ingestion of the least quantity of aliment, and during which the region of the stomach appears decidedly distended. At the same time there is nausea and vomiting of mucus and water, especially early in the morning before breakfast; another characteristic indication is the excessive and insipid eructations after every meal.

China is particularly appropriate, if the cardialgia depends upon a general weakness caused by loss of animal fluids, or by the excessive use of cathartics, after copious artificial or spontaneous losses of blood, after a protracted diarrhœa. The pain always is like a hard pressure or a crampy pain, and is either mitigated or aggravated by eating. Bodily rest relieves the distress. Beside spasmodic eructations, we likewise have an excess of acid in the stomach; vomiting constitutes the exception.

We do not mean to assert that these remedies are the only ones capable of curing cardialgia; they are the leading remedies in this disease. In the cardialgia of chlorotic patients, *Arsenicum* and *Calcarea carbonica* act an important part, Arsenicum particularly, if we suspect the existence of perforating ulcer. Next to China, Nux vomica deserves special consideration.

Phosphorus is likewise recommended for cardialgia, to which, however, it is not homœopathic symptomatically. The successful cures of this disease with Phosphorus, were not, in our estimation at least, cures of genuine cardialgia.

Carbo vegetabilis likewise is no remedy for pure cardialgia, but is better suited to affections of the stomach, attended with material alterations. Its use in the cardialgia of nursing females is undoubtedly problematical; *China* and *Nux vomica* are preferable.

Beside the remedies we have mentioned, the following likewise deserve our attention: *Platina, Secale cornutum, Lycopodium, Plumbum, Coffea cruda, Magisterium Bismuthi, Staphysagria, Stannum.* [*Acidum hydrocyanicum* is likewise an important remedy for cardialgia. In some of the last numbers of the New England Medical Gazette, some highly interesting cures of cardialgia by subcutaneous injections of Morphia are reported by Doctor Gallinger of Concord, N. H. H.]

Diet does not require any special remarks at our hands. The same rules are to be observed here that we have laid down for chronic catarrh of the stomach. The cause of the distress has to be carefully considered. If the disease arises from weakness of the stomach, all strong, substantial nourishment should be avoided. Fat food is hurtful altogether. That coffee should be avoided, may be inferred from what we have said on the subject of coffee in a former paragraph. The dread of an attack of cardialgia induces many patients to prescribe for themselves a series of privations, so that their assimilative system and general constitution suffer more in consequence, than they would have done under the tortures of simple cardialgia, so that the diagnosis becomes exceedingly uncertain. To such patients, simple, substantial, easily assimilated food is indispensable; cardialgia is not benefited, much less cured, by a regular starvation diet. A marvellously favorable effect is often obtained by the methodical application of cold water. Nothing facilitates the cure of cardialgia as much as a daily ablution of the whole body with cold water, or at least of the trunk and head. The favorable effect of this proceeding is most strikingly visible in the female sex, but likewise in men who do not take much exercise, and have to undergo exhausting mental labor.

These categories of diseases of the stomach, are not sufficiently exhaustive to enable us to assign a place to every possible derangement of the stomach in one of them. It is impossible to furnish such a comprehensive exhibition of all such diseases, at any rate less possible than to range the affections of other organs in such a general series. The stomach is exposed to the action of external influences more than any other important organ. If we understand by health, the power inherent in a healthy organ or organism to equalize all external influences without any striking or lasting disturbance, we may well say that a sound stomach is a rare occurrence in the present condition of civilization. We are satisfied with a moderate degree of normal equilibrium in the functions of the stomach, and do not regard an unimportant disturbance of this organ as anything very abnormal, provided the disturbance does not continue too long, or increases by degrees. It is, indeed, as difficult to draw a sharp line of demarcation between the health and disease of this part, as it is impossible to set up a fixed normal line for the process of nutrition. All these transition forms, from health to disease, the different forms in which a disturbance of the process of digestion may appear, cannot possibly be indicated with approximate completeness, with a view of pointing out the correct treatment. In order to hit upon the proper remedy in all such cases, we must either possess a perfect knowledge of the appropriate remedies, or else consult a Repertory, where the correct remedy will be found, the more readily, the more disconnected the symptom to be removed, appears in the series.

Pathology unites all these conditions under the common name of dyspepsia, and by thus classifying the most diversified conditions in one series, shows how little the practical wants of the sick are responded to by a pathological scheme. It is dyspepsia, if the digestion takes place too slowly, but likewise if it is too fast. The same name is applied to a too copious, as well as to a too scanty secretion of the gastric juice, a disposition to excessive development of gas, etc. Now, can such a designation be expected to be of any use therapeutically? We shall find that physicians who regulate their Therapeutics by pathological categories, fare badly when in face of such trifles as are met with every day in practice; and we ought to be grateful to Homœopathy for her safe guidance in such cases, giving us more reliable means of cure than mere dietetic rules. On the other hand we should do wrong were we to lose sight of the necessity of dietetic restrictions, and simply depend upon medicine. A simple suggestion regarding the diet, will sometimes remove an obstinate gastric trouble; we must only take care to be thoroughly acquainted with the patient's mode of living. How many recover their health simply by eating slowly, and masticating their food with care, or by not eating it too hot, or not smoking immediately after a meal. Such habits have to be inquired into with great care; no medicine can afford help, if the vicious habits which cause the disturbance are kept up.

The medicines that may afford aid in all such cases, are those that have been recommended for acute and gastric catarrh of the stomach; in most cases of gastric disturbance, these medicines will be found sufficient; all we have to do is to carefully compare their pathogenesis with the phenomena of the pathological series, and to impress them well upon the memory. This is so much the more advisable, as the gastric difficulties occur in so many different shapes, and so frequently, that it is impossible to consult the Materia Medica in every case where our assistance is sought.

B. DISEASES OF THE INTESTINAL CANAL.

1. Catarrhus Intestinalis, Intestinal Catarrh.

If it is difficult to present the different forms of the diseases of the stomach under a few heads, in such a manner that the series shall present corresponding advantages in a therapeutic point of view, it seems still more difficult to thus range the diseases of the intestinal canal, for the following reasons: In the case of the stomach, the anatomical disturbances can be harmonized, without much difficulty, with the nomenclature that a simple symptomatology had suggested to former schools; whereas, the affections of the intestinal canal present such a chaos of names and definitions, and such an uncertainty regarding the diagnosis of the diseased locality, that we hardly know what road to pursue in order to write intelligibly from the stand-point of the old-fashioned pathology; and, on the other hand, to satisfy the demands of the more modern classifications. Neither one nor the other is a sufficiently safe guide alone. In order to anticipate the hasty censure of critics, we will state that we have adopted our present plan for the purpose of responding fully and satisfactorily to the necessities of the practical physician; not to gratify a dogmatic pathology. By following the latter, we should have to confine ourselves to discussing higher and lower grades of catarrh, so that the essential distinctions which often separate these grades, together with their most common complications, might be overlooked, to the great disadvantage of the therapeutical part, where the practical treatment of these derangements is exhibited. With a view of showing the fundamental process underlying the forms of disease that will be discussed in the subsequent paragraphs, we have deemed it advisable to group the whole under the general denomination of intestinal catarrh, and to designate them as so many subdivisions; whereas in the older treatises on Pathology they constitute so many leading heads. By pursuing this course, the reader will obtain the desired information, in whatever direction he may look for it.

In order to avoid repetitions, it is advisable to separate only the symptomatic indications; the etiology, and the most prominent anatomical conditions, being the same for all.

As regards etiology, we refer the reader to our statements in the chapter on catarrh of the stomach. The deleterious influences which cause catarrh of the stomach, may likewise affect the intestinal canal, either alone or together with the stomach. A few circumstances, however, deserve particular mention. Many substances that are not apt to cause catarrh of the stomach, very readily disturb the intestinal canal. Among them we mention more particularly fruit, wine that has not been thoroughly fermented, and sour beer. Some persons are affected by coffee, which acts upon them as a very mild cathartic. All sorts of purgatives belong in this category; they not only cause transitory catarrhal symptoms, but likewise more acute intestinal catarrhs, that may interfere with the good effects of homœopathic treatment, and may lead astray in making up our diagnosis, which is, in any case, a subject of considerable difficulty. In some individuals, every cold, whether general or local, causes intestinal catarrh; in others, on the contrary, the catarrh is only excited at certain periods, so that the catarrhal irritations assume the form of an epidemic. Such catarrhs have been traced, perhaps with reason, to a peculiar genius epidemicus gastricus. Generally, however, such epidemics depend upon certain definite atmospheric conditions, only we are not able to account for the connection between cause and effect. What is the reason that in a warm spring, catarrhs of the respiratory organs prevail, whereas in the fall we have more particularly catarrhs of the intestinal canal? Why are the violent catarrhs of the summer season characterized by a deficient, and, sometimes, all but suspended secretion of bile? Observation, likewise, seems to have established the fact that in the summer season the catarrhal irritation seems to be located more particularly in the upper part of the bowels, whereas in the fall season it seems to prefer the larger bowels and rectum. Persons are apt to account for the summer and fall catarrhs by reasons suggested by the dietetic habits of the season, more especially the use of fruit. There is no denying that the abuse of fresh fruit may easily cause irritations of the intestinal canal. That there must prevail a special atmospheric tendency in this direction, is shown by the fact, that persons who have not eaten the least particle of fruit are attacked with intestinal catarrh. As a complication, it supervenes during the most varied morbid processes, sometimes as their regular companion, and at others as an exceptional occurrence. It scarcely ever has a critical significance, which has been taken for granted, rather by the force of habit than that of sound reason.

The anatomical changes superinduced by intestinal catarrh, are so insignificant in a majority of cases, that they need not be expatiated upon in this place. The changes which occur in the intestinal canal during the course of other diseases, will be described when these diseases are treated of. It may suffice in this place, to call attention to the fact, that violent diseases of the intestines, especially if they run a protracted course, may easily lead to ulcerations of the mucous lining. This circumstance must not be lost sight of, otherwise convalescent patients might prematurely indulge in the use of quantities of substantial food, and the copious and solid fæces might easily occasion the discharge of an abscess into the abdominal cavity. This circumstance will be more fully dwelt upon in the chapter on typhus.

a. *Simple Intestinal Catarrh.*

The ordinary acute intestinal catarrh, generally commences with a short preliminary stage of a few hours' duration, consisting of a disagreeable uncomfortable feeling, aversion to food, general chilliness, sometimes vertigo, and dulness of the head. If the attacks are more violent, the affection sometimes sets in at once with a copious, diarrhœic evacuation mingled with a quantity of gas. At the same time, the symptoms of constitutional disturbance increase in intensity, among which a sudden disproportionate general debility, holds a prominent rank. Fever is very seldom present at the commencement, but the temperature rises somewhat later. The tongue is, and remains clean, as long as the intestine is the only part affected. The diarrhœic stools come on repeatedly at irregular intervals; three or four stools may occur in the course of a single day, and again in the course of an hour. The more frequent and copious the discharges, the sooner they become watery, and the less fecal matter they contain. At first the color is normal; it is only at a later period that it becomes lighter, mingled with greenish streaks and small somewhat darker fecal lumps. At first they smell like ordinary fæces, after lasting some time the evacuations almost become inodorous. Local pains are almost always present; at times they are crampy, at others cutting, at times a simple pressure, at others they are felt before or after the discharge, and again they continue all the time. The appetite is less, but never entirely suspended.

This form of catarrh seldom lasts longer than a few days, provided the patient does not commit any serious dietetic mistakes. The discharges become less frequent, and the pain abates. The complete cessation of the diarrhœa, is often succeeded for some days by constipation, the health being otherwise perfectly good. Under particularly unfavorable circumstances this acute form may pass into the chronic.

The treatment is not quite as simple as it might seem at first sight, because it is of importance not to omit even the most trifling circumstances in our choice of the right remedies, of which the number and changeable character of the symptoms suggest a goodly supply. In every case of importance it is best to consult the Materia Medica.

Rheum is suitable in the intestinal catarrh of full-grown persons, as well as of children; more particularly, however, in that of children, especially when caused by a cold. The discharges are not quite watery, usually only papescent, having a sour smell in the case of little children; they are frequently mingled with mucus, and have a dark color. Gas is developed in large quantity, the abdomen being perceptibly distended, with pinching pains before and during stool; these cease for some time after the bowels are relieved. The urging to stool is felt very suddenly.

Dulcamara acts very similarly to Rheum; it is particularly suitable to summer-diarrhœa, with colicky pains around the umbilicus, which are only relieved, not arrested, by an evacuation. The discharges have little color, are mixed with green streaks, papescent, and occur mostly in the afternoon or at night. *Dulcamara* is particularly suitable, if the colicky pains and the accumulation of gas have preceded the diarrhœa for a day or more, so that the seat of the derangement is properly traced to the lesser intestines.

Chamomilla is adapted to catarrhs caused by violent emotions, such as anger or chagrin, also to the diarrhœa of children, especially during the period of dentition. The evacuations are papescent, mixed with mucus, green, (in the case of children,) of the consistence of stirred eggs, excoriating the anus, smelling sour or like rotten eggs. The stools do not follow each other in very rapid succession, are accompanied by severe colicky pains; sometimes however they are painless and occur principally at night.

Mercurius solubilis is particularly suitable for children during the period of dentition; in the intestinal catarrh of adults this remedy is less frequently indicated. There are only a few evacuations in the twenty-four hours; they are not very copious, mixed with mucus, portions of them are tinged dark-green, contain fecal matter, excoriate the anus, and have a sour smell. The pains are cutting or pinching, and precede the diarrhœa, attended with chilliness.

Ipecacuanha corresponds more particularly to the intestinal catarrhs of the summer-season, more especially to the most acute forms thereof. The discharges occur frequently, they are thin, have a foul smell, little color, are rather painless, but accompanied by frequent and sudden prostration.

Colocynthis has not very frequent, papescent stools with a marked bilious tinge, attended with much gas, and paroxysms of severe crampy pains. The flatulence escaping with the stool is very fetid. The patient complains of chilliness.

Colchicum is related to Ipecacuanha; the stools are watery, have little color, are not very copious and painless, it is particularly suitable to individuals who are attacked with intestinal catarrh, from every trifling provocation.

Pulsatilla has nightly diarrhœa without much pain, the discharges are slimy, tinged with green, attended with chills, and succeeded by pinching colicky pains which last some time.

For this milder form of intestinal catarrh, the above-mentioned remedies will generally be found sufficient; for more acute forms, the medicines mentioned in the following chapter may have to be resorted to.

b. *Cholera Sporadica seu Nostras, Cholerine.*

This pathological process is a union of a high grade of intestinal catarrh, with a violent catarrhal affection of the stomach.

Cholerine either takes place only in isolated cases, or as a mild epidemic, in which case it always depends upon peculiar atmospheric influences. It seems to be favored, not so much by warm weather, as by an excess of atmospheric electricity, on which account, cholerine may likewise occur in the fall and winter. Single cases may depend upon previously mentioned etiological influences.

Generally the disease has precursory symptoms, such as a general feeling of malaise, weariness, nausea, aversion to food, cephalæa gastrica, pains and rumbling in the bowels, pressure and a tight feeling in the region of the stomach, and diminished secretion of urine. Violent attacks occur suddenly. The disease generally breaks out at night; the patient is awakened by a feeling of oppression in the pit of the stomach, which is soon followed by copious and repeated vomitings, even to such an extent that the patient sometimes imagines the vomiting uninterrupted. At first the food, which had been partaken of last, is thrown up, after which the vomited substance becomes more or less watery and copious, and is so much the less mingled with remnants of food, or tinged with bile, the longer the vomiting continues. Diarrhœa sets in, either at the time the vomiting occurs, or it supervenes soon after. At first the stools have more consistence; soon, however, they become watery and lose their color, so that in very violent attacks, the evacuations by the mouth as well as by the rectum may assume a rice-water appearance, as in Asiatic cholera. Local pains, (even in the most acute attacks,) may be entirely absent at the commencement, or there may be colicky, crampy, or cutting pains in the umbilical region, which are always heightened by the vomiting. Vomiting is excited by the ingestion of the slightest quantity of food into the stomach; moreover, the patient is prevented from eating, by a distressing aversion to food. Sometimes in a few hours the intensity of the pains abates, and the patient gradually becomes quiet. If the disease lasts any length of time, a number of distressing difficulties supervene. In consequence of the constant efforts to vomit, the stomach becomes very painful, as in cardialgia, the abdomen is meteoristically distended, or else is spasmodically drawn in, and the patients are tormented by agonizing anguish and an unquenchable thirst. The skin becomes remarkably cool, is even covered with a cold sweat, the pulse is less perceptible, the respiration is embarrassed, the features are unusually sunken, and the face has a cyanotic hue. In these higher grades of the disease, muscular spasms are not wanting; they first affect the lower extremities like tonic spasms. The weakness finally becomes so great that the patients have not strength enough left to vomit, and the expulsive action of the stomach is limited to a mere hiccoughing. With these phenomena death takes place very rapidly, although the consciousness sometimes remains undisturbed, even to the last moment. In case of recovery, the urging to vomit first ceases, the skin resumes its functions, and the pulse increases in volume. The evacuations resume a normal color at a later period, convalescence is very slow; very frequently the affection changes to another form which we will designate as mucous fever.

In the case of children, the symptoms and course of this disease are somewhat altered; in their case the affection has even been designated as cholera infantum. Cholera infantum never attacks as suddenly as the cholerine of adults, on the other hand the disease is of longer duration and intensity, hence the danger is more threatening. As in the case of adults, so in that of children, the affection usually breaks out at night, excepting, that either the vomiting or diarrhœa is more prominent. If the vomiting is more frequent, the diarrhœa is less so, and *vice versa*. There is always fever. The substances evacuated from the stomach or bowels have almost always more color than in the case of adults; the quantity and number of the evacuations are likewise proportionally smaller. A single paroxysm is not dangerous; the danger consists in the continuance of the exacerbations and remissions of the disease, which are generally more marked at night, the symptoms abating somewhat during the day. The strength departs very strikingly and rapidly, and the bodily weight diminishes greatly in a few days. Recovery is indicated by a gradual abatement of the evacuations, more gradual than in the case of adults. A fatal termination, which is not unfrequent, is announced by excessive prostration, the supervention of convulsions, delirium, sopor, and the fetor of the evacuations, which become foul and decomposed, and are sometimes mixed with blood. The transition into another form of the catarrhal disease is proportionally of rare occurrence. The danger is the more imminent the younger the infant, it is greatest in the case of infants at the breast, whose feeble existence is so easily extinguished, even by a simple attack of catarrh of the stomach.

Treatment. Since this disease runs its course within very definite boundaries, the number of remedial agents which we employ against it is limited, and our practical knowledge of their action is much more certain and comprehensive. Whereas there is very little danger for adults in the treatment of their cholerine by other than homœopathic means, and this danger seems confined to children and very old persons, we may, on the contrary, be sure of a successful termination of the disease under homœopathic treatment, except, perhaps, in the case of old and decrepit individuals, and feeble children disposed to convulsions, to which they succumb, rather than to the cholerine, as in the case of any other very severe disease.

The leading remedies against cholerine are: *Ipecacuanha, Veratrum album,* and *Arsenicum;* it is not a very difficult task to discriminate between the respective symptomatic indications of these drugs. Ipec. corresponds to the less violent attacks, as long as the discharges have a bilious tinge, and the vomiting and retching are very severe. Hence it is one of the leading remedies for cholera infantum, because the stools scarcely ever become colorless, and is likewise suitable for adults if there is little or no diarrhœa. Ipec. is not counter-indicated by a cold skin, cold sweat, anguish, restlessness, or cramps of the extremities. *Veratrum album* is particularly adapted to a case where the evacuations are colorless; these are always the most difficult to manage. This characteristic of the evacuations may be expected with tolerable certainty, if the disease sets in at once with violent, copious and frequent vomiting, and the accompanying diarrhœa is equally violent. Under such circumstances, it is advisable to at once give *Veratrum* instead of Ipecacuanha. The greater the resemblance of this disease to Asiatic cholera, the more urgent the necessity of giving Veratrum. To substantiate this, we refer the reader to the chapter on Asiatic cholera. In the case of children, Veratrum will seldom be found the most suitable specific. *Arsenicum album* is never indicated at the commencement of this pathological process; it is only suitable when, in the further course of the disease, the pains in the stomach and bowels become unusually severe, the vomiting has been replaced by a distressing retching, the diarrhœa is indeed less copious but more frequent, and is more or less tinged with blood. These symptoms of the intestinal tract are always associated with extreme anguish, embarrassed respiration, inextinguishable thirst, collapsed features, and a small or even imperceptible pulse. As a general rule, Arsenicum is more suitable after Ipecacuanha than after Veratrum. In cholera infantum it is one of our main specifics, if the diarrhœa threatens symptoms of decomposition, such as a gray or black color, admixture of blood, and putrid odor. In the case of adults, cholerine scarcely ever has this termination, more especially if it had been treated homœopathically from the start.

Beside these three remedies, others may be required under certain circumstances. *Chamomilla* is often a good remedy at the commencement of cholera infantum, only it is difficult to decide whether the disease is cut short by the medicine. In the case of adults, we must not expect a striking effect from Chamomilla, although it is constantly recommended for this disease, if mortified or vexed feelings were the exciting cause. The last-mentioned cause seldom occasions an attack of cholerine, but may produce simple catarrh of the bowels. *Colocynthis* is suitable in a proportionally rare form of cholerine, where the patient vomits but a few times, and after that experiences a fearful nausea with paroxysms of retching, which at most results in the expulsion of some phlegm; the stools are diarrhœic, but not watery; they have a marked bilious tinge; are not very frequent, on an average, and are always preceded by intolerable colicky pains. The disease is generally caused by a cold, sometimes by chagrin. *Colchicum autumnale* deserves a preference over any other remedy, if, after one or two, or, at all events, scanty vomitings, the diarrhœa increases to a violent degree, the stools assume a watery consistence, are not entirely colorless, and even take place without warning.

If recovery has fairly commenced, if, after the diarrhœa has ceased, the patient still complains of lassitude and want of appetite, *Nux vomica* sometimes has a surprising effect. Against a protracted diarrhœa, *Acidum phosphoricum* is a most efficient remedy, unless severe pains continue to be present; in such an event, *Phosphorus* is more suitable. If chronic intestinal catarrh should result, the remedies proposed for this condition are to be used. A transition into the febrile form of intestinal catarrh requires the medicines indicated in the subsequent chapters.

As regards dose, most physicians agree that the lower attenuations are most efficient; we need not, on this account, go below the second. Considering the rapid course of the disease, the medicine may be repeated as often as every half hour; in moderate cases, the dose may be repeated every two hours without incurring any risk. The root of Ipecacuanha seems to act more positively and decisively than the tincture.

The diet need not cause any serious thought, for the reason that the patients have an aversion to all kinds of nourishment at the onset of the disease. Small quantities of thin, slimy decoctions, alternated with very cold, fresh well-water, likewise in small quantities, are alone admissible. After the attack is over, the stomach has to be exerted very sparingly for some days; solid food should be allowed only in the smallest quantities, nor should aught but the simplest kind of nourishment be partaken of. In cholera infantum the diet is of more importance. This has generally a number of attacks, and inclines to relapses. The slightest dietetic transgressions and irregularities are strictly to be avoided. The children need not starve; they bear very well beef-tea, milk, good bread, and light soups, only the quantity has to be regulated with great care. If the patient is much emaciated and exhausted, small quantities of a generous sweet wine are very appropriate; in teaspoonful doses it may be given even to children of one year old without the least risk; even at this early age, it sometimes effects a sudden and striking revolution in the digestive functions.

[The *Iris versicolor*, or blue-flag, is used by American homœopathic and eclectic physicians, as a very efficient remedy in cholera infantum. Some use the lower attenuations, others the tincture. The discharges are greenish, worse at night, or they occur principally at night; in severe cases they even resemble the rice-water discharges of Asiatic cholera. In our own experience, and that of many of our friends, Iris has not led to the satisfactory results obtained from it by other practitioners. Acute attacks of cholerine, with slight febrile excitement, prostration, and watery discharges without any, or having a fetid smell, have been arrested promptly and permanently, by means of the lower attenuations, or even one or two drops of the tincture of the root of Aconite. H.]

c. *Catarrhus Intestinalis Chronicus*, *Chronic Intestinal Catarrh*, *Chronic Diarrhœa*, *Cholera Infantum*, *Summer Complaint*.

This form of disease is observed as an accompanying complication in a number of other pathological processes, especially in affections of the liver, spleen and stomach, and very prominently in tuberculosis. Chronic intestinal catarrh develops itself as an idiopathic affection, out of acute attacks of the disease, either because they had been neglected, or else frequent relapses had caused obstinate alterations in the intestines. The affection may likewise be a purely primary one of gradual growth, and which had finally acquired a higher degree of significance.

The symptoms and meaning of this affection differ in the adult and child, and, therefore, require to be described separately.

The intestinal catarrh of adults, at times, is attended with obstinate constipation, at others with diarrhœa. In the former case, the fæces consist of hard dark-colored, little lumps, resembling sheep's dung, which are covered with a viscid, glassy mucus, sometimes mingled with a few streaks of blood. The diarrhœa is either continued, or alternates with constipation. The fecal matter is not very thin, or else it consists of a slimy watery fluid, mixed with a few lumps of hard fecal matter; the peculiar glassy or jelly-like mucus, is always found in them. If the diarrhœic stools occur alternaterly with obstruction of the bowels, the former generally have a very fetid smell. If considerable alterations in the structure of the intestines are present, we find an admixture of pus or blood from the ulcerative surfaces. The stools in one day are never as frequent as in cholerine. With these symptoms of disturbed digestion, a variety of other ailments are always more or less observed. The tongue has usually a thick coating, especially at the root, the appetite is either gone or perverted ; in a few cases there is excessive hunger. If the bowels are constipated, there is always an accumulation of gas, if they are loose there is much less of it. The presence of this flatulence often distresses patients in an extraordinary degree. This distress is generally attended with pains at the anus, caused by hemorrhoidal tumors. The temper is always affected by chronic intestinal catarrh ; the patient is gloomy, sometimes even desperate, like an hypochondriac. Symptoms of irregular circulation supervene, such as cerebral congestions, continued headache, palpitation of the heart, abdominal pulsations, and coldness of the lower extremities. If the stomach sympathizes with the disease, as it always does if the disease lasts any length of time, a loathing of food is experienced, and the patient has perverted desires for unnatural substances, with retching, vomiting of water and mucus, and vomiting of food.

In most cases the disease is one of the most obstinate, without being particularly dangerous. Naturally enough, in view of such a persistent derangement of the digestive faculties, the patient gradually loses flesh and strength. In spite of this, the patients may live to an old age. If the diarrhœa prevails, emaciation sets in very rapidly, marasmus results, and towards the end an effusion of serum into the cellular tissue and the abdominal cavity occurs. If the duration of the disease is determined by intestinal ulcers, the patient's prospect is much worse, because the wasting of the vital strength goes on so much more rapidly. Speaking of ulcers, their existence may be suspected in chronic diarrhœa generally, for as chronic ulceration feeds the catarrh, so does the catarrh feed the ulcerative process. Another malignant complication which is not very unfrequent, is the contraction or stenosis of the intestinal tube, which may occur in consequence of cicatrization, as well as through a bend in the gut, or in consequence of hypertrophy of the mucous membrane. This accident is the more important, as a sure diagnosis is only possible exceptionally, and the treatment may consequently be conducted upon a mistaken basis. Obstinate constipation, and the small size of the discharged fæces, justify the inference, that stenosis may exist. This diagnosis becomes the more certain if, by some means or other, the contraction of the intestine becomes so great that an antiperistaltic movement arises, with consequent fecal vomiting, without any signs of intussusception. Moreover, the continued arrest of the fæces at one place in the intestines, may cause an incidental catarrhal irritation, readily resulting in ulceration. As an excess of flatulence may disturb the circulation, and cause cerebral congestions, so it may likewise derange the functions of the liver and spleen; nevertheless, the phenomena on the side of the liver may likewise be accounted for, by the changes in the digestive functions, and the consequent anomalous direction of the bile.

Among the constitutional complications of other affections, diarrhœa, as a representative of intestinal catarrh, is one of the most significant, since nothing consumes the strength of the patient more rapidly than a persistent case. Above all, it is tuberculosis whose fatal termination is threatened by diarrhœa. It may, however, happen that intestinal catarrh, as an accompaniment of acute affections, may run into the chronic form, on which account convalescence is very much retarded. A result of this kind is more particularly met with in typhus, and likewise in various other diseases. It is always a disagreeable sign, because intestinal ulcerations are very apt to occur under such circumstances.

The chronic intestinal catarrh of children has more definite symptoms than that of adults. If there is no invasion of the stomach by the catarrhal irritation, the leading symptom is an obstinate diarrhœa, with hourly or less frequent discharges. The evacuations are at times very copious, and not so frequent; or else they are scanty and more frequent. At first there is considerable admixture of bile, and the color, after a short exposure to the air, is green; afterwards the discharges assume a lighter color, until finally they often resemble clay. As regards consistence, they are not entirely watery, sometimes papescent and semi-liquid, until the fecal matter gradually disappears. The smell is generally sour, and there is always more or less admixture of bile. The other symptoms vary; there is either an entire loss of appetite, or else a ravenous desire for food; such kinds as the little patient used to be very fond of are refused, and others are grasped at with avidity. If the stomach is involved, all the symptoms of stomach catarrh show themselves, and the diarrhœa is mixed with remnants of undigested food, or flakes of milky coagula. The strength vanishes very rapidly. If the diarrhœa continues any length of time, the patients are reduced to mere skeletons, with the skin dangling loosely around, and their hollow eyes sending forth an erring and confused look from among a multitude of wrinkles.

The causes of this very dangerous affection of childhood, are all those circumstances that have been indicated as the causes of stomach catarrh in the case of children, and to which we refer the reader. The more frequent appearance of this disease among children that have just been weaned, is owing to the peculiar nature of the teething process, as well as to the change of diet. Among children over two years of age, the disease is met with only exceptionally.

Lest this disease should be confounded with the intestinal tuberculosis of children, the so-called tabes meseraica, the diagnosis should be made with the greatest care, for the tubercular disease requires a different kind of treatment. If there is no swelling of the mesenteric glands, and no sign of tubercles in the lungs, it will be found very difficult to draw a line of distinction between the two diseases, with reliable certainty. The probabilities are in favor of intestinal catarrh, if the new diet, or a change of diet for the worse, or the cutting of the first teeth, usher in the first signs of the disease.

Under homœopathic treatment, the prognosis, as long as the disease has not reached its highest degree of intensity, is favorable, although this disorder, as managed by the adherents of other schools, is generally considered a very fatal disease. Of course no successful result of the treatment can be expected unless the strictest diet is observed.

In the case of adults as well as children, the first object of the treatment should be the enforcement of strict dietetic rules. The rules for children, and partially for adults, have been laid down in the chapter on catarrh of the stomach. We must always see that the nourishment can easily be assimilated, it must not be of a stimulating kind, or of one that will throw down much fecal matter; the children should be fed with the most perfect regularity and never to excess. In the case of convalescents, the greatest caution has to be observed in eating; quantities of solids have to be avoided, food should be partaken of frequently, but not in copious quantities.

Nux vomica is the chief remedy for the chronic intestinal catarrh of adults, especially if the stomach is involved in the disease, likewise if it is not. The most important symptoms are: constipation, if not too obstinate and long-lasting, with discharge of small, dark-brown, very hard lumps with mucus or blood, likewise constipation alternating with frequent papescent stools; stitches, painful constriction of the rectum, hemorrhoidal tumors of the rectum, urging to stool; a great deal of flatulence, with difficult stool; pains in the liver; congestions of the head. Compare, moreover, the symptoms referring to the stomach, likewise the symptoms of the emotive sphere. Numberless observations have satisfied us that Nux alone is sufficient to permanently cure, in a short space of time, almost every case of moderate intensity.

Lycopodium acts in this disease with scarcely less certainty than Nux, and has been tried with equal success. It is more appropriate to inveterate and more advanced cases. The moral symptoms, and the looks of the patient, constitute a very safe line of demarcation between the action of Lycopodium and Nux. The mind is very much depressed; the patients have lost all hope; they seem a prey to the deepest hypochondria; their complexion is of a jaundiced, yellowish-gray, or dingy-sallow hue. The constipation is obstinate and long-lasting; there is frequent and ineffectual urging; hemorrhoidal tumors, with secretion of blood; the fæces look like sheep's dung, encircled with mucus. There is a great deal of flatulence, the expulsion of which rarely affords relief. The liver, stomach, and even the spleen participate in the affection. The coating on the tongue is not very thick, or the tongue is even quite clean. The effect of these two remedies upon the alvine discharges is sometimes very rapid; we have often relieved a constipation of years' standing with a single dose on the very first day, so that the diet could not possibly have induced the curative change. Lycopodium likewise affords rapid aid against a distressing flatulence, but it is only palliative, since it is impossible to arrest the tendency to an excessive development of gas, with a few doses of this remedy.

Sulphur is a specific in inveterate cases, when affections of the liver are present. The stools are dry, hard as stone, of small size, and a dark color, lined with mucus, accompanied by frequent ineffectual urging, pains in the anus, swelling of the hemorrhoidal tumors. The moral symptoms and the symptoms of the stomach and abdomen are like those of Lycopodium. Sulphur likewise corresponds to constipation alternating with diarrhœa, or to evacuations composed almost exclusively of mucus, as sometimes occur side by side with the most obstinate constipation. There is always a great deal of bile in the secretions. It is only exceptionally that Sulphur will develop its curative effects in a very short time. This agent suits children, if the stools are mixed with a quantity of mucus or even with some pus. Altogether, if there are traces of ulceration in the intestines, we have to think in the first place of Sulphur.

Graphites acts so similarly to Sulphur, that, instead of repeating our remarks on Sulphur, we prefer referring the reader to our Materia Medica. The remedy is often effective in cases where Sulphur seemed suitable, but did not show any effect. *Natrum muriaticum* also acts similarly to Sulphur, only the accessory symptoms have to determine its appropriateness in a given case, since the local symptoms are not sufficiently decisive.

[Regarding the treatment of intestinal constipation as a symptom of intestinal catarrh, Kafka offers the following remarks: "If a diminution of the peristaltic motion is associated with obstinate constipation, and it is evident that the fecal masses have accumulated in the intestinal canal, all that is left for us to do, is to remove this mechanical obstacle by exciting the peristaltic motion, by means of some suitable cathartic, which will cause a secretion of serum in the bowels, by which means their contents will be dislodged. According to the teachings of physiological pharmacodynamics, *Rheum* fulfils these requisites more completely than any other drug. It is not well to administer this remedy in massive doses, for the reason that they cause an excessive secretion of serum without touching the fecal masses.

"When administered in small quantities, at the rate of five grains per dose, giving a dose every two or three hours, it excites the peristaltic motion. This effect is evidenced by the pinching and rumbling in the abdomen, and emission of fetid flatulence. At the same time serum is secreted in the intestinal canal, after which a few liquid, fetid evacuations take place. After the remedy has been taken two or three days, lumps of fecal matter are passed; under the continued use of the drug, these discharges of lumpy fæces have to be kept up, until no lumps can be felt in the bowels.

"If five grains are not sufficient to produce the desired effect, the quantity may be increased to ten grains; in most cases, however, five grains will be found sufficient.

"If the torpor of the intestinal canal is very great, and Rheum has no effect, we recommend Aloes, from two to three grains per dose, a dose every two or three hours. Both remedies may be taken in the form of pills, or enveloped in a wafer. The passage of the stagnant fecal masses can be powerfully aided by means of stimulating injections of soap-water, with a little sweet or castor-oil and common salt; if the fecal mass is lodged in the upper part of the intestinal tract, it may be reached by fastening to a suitable injection-pipe, a long, elastic tube.

"In the first years of our homœopathic practice, we repeatedly tried to overcome an obstinate stasis of the fæces by homœopathic treatment. Several failures on our part drove the patients back into the hands of allopathic physicians, who, although they treat this condition empirically, yet, as a rule, meet with more success in relieving the patient. In a case of constipation of this kind, we do not hesitate to advise the avoidance of all round about attempts at relief with the usual homœopathic means, and the use of such medicines as we are taught by physiological pharmaco-dynamics will most speedily and safely secure the desired end.

"Many of our readers will undoubtedly find it strange that measures should be recommended in a treatise on homœopathic therapeutics, which are indeed derived from the domain of physiological pharmaco-dynamics, but in reality belong to that of the empirical School. But we have stated at the commencement of our work that we occupy a practical stand-point. At the sick-bed it is often impossible to succeed with theories. Whether a certain method of treatment is correct, feasible, and useful to the patient, has to be decided by experience, and the weight of experience should never be underrated. The sick-bed is the touch stone for our theories; these will survive, if they stand the test of a practical trial; their uselessness in practice is their doom.

"Moreover, it is our duty to deliver our patients from their sufferings by the shortest and safest road. We shall adhere to these motives, and are not afraid of *proclaiming the fact, that the infinitesimal doses of Homœopathy are incapable of removing the accumulation of indurated masses of fæces in the intestinal canal.*

"If, upon examination, fecal masses are no longer accumulated in the bowels, we return to the homœopathic treatment, and remove the intestinal catarrh and the continued torpor of the bowels by means of *Nux vomica*, *Natrum muriaticum*, etc.

"If these remedies should not have the desired effect, we send our patients to Karlsbad, Marienbad, Kissingen, or Homburg. The two first-named springs are particularly efficacious." In our own country, the Congress and Rockhill springs of Saratoga have a distinguished reputation for their excellent effect in habitual constipation. H.]

Phosphorus and **Acidum phosphoricum** correspond to intestinal catarrhs, having taken the form of chronic diarrhœa, both in the case of children as well as adults. Whereas the stools to which Phosphorus is adapted always contain fæces and a considerable admixture of bile, with rather copious traces of blood, and are attended with severe colicky pains, the fæces for which Phosphoric acid is suitable are lighter colored, or even colorless; there are no pains in the abdomen, but a good deal of flatulence. Phosphorus is, moreover, the main remedy for ulceration of the intestinal mucous membrane; next to which, *Nitri acidum* deserves a preference. This remedy is likewise adapted to chronic diarrhœa, more particularly if the fæces contain pus and blood.

In chronic diarrhœa, associated with lienteria, *China*, *Ferrum*, and likewise *Phosphorus*, are the main remedies, *Arsenicum* being less frequently indicated. *China*, together with *Nux vomica*, or *Phosphori acidum*, corresponds most nearly to the intestinal catarrh of convalescent patients; China deserves attention in all diarrhœas of long duration, only it is difficult, in view of the extraordinary diversity of the symptoms, to determine the cases to which it is specifically homœopathic.

Sepia is efficacious in the chronic intestinal catarrh of females. Obstinate obstruction is occasionally interrupted by papescent stools without much bile.

Plumbum has such characteristic symptoms that it would seem specifically, and, as it were, exclusively adapted to certain forms of chronic intestinal catarrh. The obstinate constipation caused by lead-poisoning is well known as a pathognomonic symptom, likewise the peculiar colic. We desire to call attention to the fact that Plumbum corresponds very prominently to the symptoms of stenosis of the intestine and of atonic ulceration of the bowels.

In offering a concluding remark concerning the chronic intestinal catarrh of children, we have to call attention to one other remedy beside Sulphur, Phosphorus, Phosphori acidum, China and Acidum nitricum: we mean *Calcarea carbonica*. As yet, the therapeutic lines between the different kinds of Calcarea have not been distinctly drawn by adequate provings; we do not know how far the Carbonate of Lime is distinguished from the Acetate or Phosphate. Nor has the practical experiment shed sufficient light on these differences. Without any special reasons, one prefers this, another that preparation of Calcarea, the Carbonate being most generally employed in practice. It might be difficult to show what symptoms in chronic intestinal catarrh indicate Calcarea. The whole process, including all its various modifications, is adapted to the action of this drug, and any homœopath who does not avail himself of this agent at the very beginning of the treatment, would commit a very great wrong. The very first dose of this remedy is apt to produce a change in the whole vegetative activity of the childlike organism, without it being possible to attribute the amelioration to a mere change of diet. Such a remedy should occupy a prominent place in the memory of every physician; hence, instead of giving the whole pathogenesis of the drug, we indicate only two leading points that argue in favor of Calcarea: we mean excessive acidity of the stomach and a partial or total deficiency of biliary secretion. We have frequently verified the fact in our own practice that Calcarea carbonica acts better in the form of a liquid attenuation than a trituration of the same number. We cannot account for this circumstance, although there is no doubt that our observation is correct.

Arsenicum album is rarely ever indicated at the commencement of the disease; in cases where the continued exhausting evacuations, and the intensity of the disease, have superinduced septic symptoms, this medicine sometimes affords speedy help, even in cases that seem hopeless. Under such circumstances, Arsenicum is likewise suitable in the case of adults; in their case, however, Arsenicum produces curative effects less frequently, for the reason that symptoms of decomposition do not set in until all help is impossible. In the case of children, however, the disease is still curable even after it has reached the climax. The selection is determined much less by the peculiar nature of the evacuations than by the rapid prostration, the œdematous swellings, the constant anguish and restlessness, the fearful thirst and the extreme emaciation. In the presence of such general symptoms, the stools may be light-colored like those of Calcarea, nevertheless Arsenicum may be indicated; of course, if the stools are dark-colored, mixed with blood and purulent mucus, having a pungent, putrid smell, Arsenicum is the only remedy of which a curative effect may be expected.

In the lesser grades of the disease, where there are but four or five diarrhœic stools a day, papescent, of a light-yellow color, with occasional watery discharges, the evacuations being largely mixed with mucus, the stomach being excessively sour, without any great signs of emaciation, *Borax* is decidedly in its place.

Beside these remedies, *Argentum nitricum*, *Zincum*, *Cuprum*, and *Nitrum* deserve attention. We have no prominently characteristic indications for *Arg. nitricum*; it may be tried where Calcarea is suitable. *Zincum* and *Cuprum* are indicated where the symptoms of chronic intestinal catarrh are attended with general convulsions. Beside these remedies, those indicated for cerebral anæmia are likewise appropriate. Nitrum acts very similarly to Borax; if, in this lesser grade of the disease, the discharges are mixed with blood, *Nitrum* deserves the preference. [*Podophyllum*, 6th to 12th, and *Croton tiglium*, 6th to 18th attenuation, have had good effect in chronic diarrhœa. H.]

Inasmuch as it is very important that the strength of the little patients should be raised as soon as possible, and yet it is very difficult, on account of the deficient activity of the stomach, to accomplish this end, we have to try very carefully what kind of food the stomach can best bear. A very common domestic remedy are raw eggs without the white, but there are many children who cannot bear them. On the other hand, finely shaved raw beef is highly to be recommended, because it is very nutritious and easily digested. If it is not readily digested, we recommend the broth that we have indicated in our chapter on gastric catarrh, which suits even the most debilitated stomach. Particular attention is due to ablutions of the skin, especially among the poorer classes, that consider water rather hurtful than useful as a remedial agent. Very cold ablutions, however, should not be resorted to at once, but gradually from a higher to a lower degree.

d. *Febris Gastrica Catarrhalis, Mucosa et Biliosa; Gastric Fever.*

These forms of fever have a large number of synonymes, of which the principal are: febris saburralis, gastrico-venosa, pituitosa, splanchnica; mucous fever, and bilious fever. We comprehend them in one series, because by so doing we avoid a great many repetitions in the therapeutic section.

The following forms of disease belong all to the catarrhal intestinal affections, which generally make their appearance over a large region of country, and hence depend upon peculiar atmospheric conditions, and cannot be demonstrated as the results of dietetic transgressions, which only furnish the first impulse towards the breaking out of the disease. It is undeniable that severe depressing emotions may give rise to such diseases.

A catarrhal gastric fever is distinguished from a simple gastric fever, of which mention has been made in the chapter on diseases of the stomach, by the fact, that the intestinal canal is involved in the pathological process. The disease scarcely ever begins suddenly, but has precursory symptoms. These consist in the symptoms characterizing the lesser grade of acute catarrh of the stomach. Gradually, seldom suddenly, these symptoms become associated with fever, the patients frequently complaining of chilliness followed by heat. Little by little the fever increases until it becomes continuous, generally with unimportant evening exacerbations. The headache, which at first is dull, now becomes more violent, the thirst very severe, the pulse hurried; the nausea increases unto vomiting; water and mucus, which is at times sour and at other times tasteless, being thrown up. The patients feel so languid and exhausted, that with the best will they are unable to remain out of bed, more particularly in the morning and evening. The evening exacerbation continues till far in the night, so that the sleep, if it is not entirely wanting, is very much disturbed. Morning is the best time for the patient, although even then the fever is not entirely absent. Upon the whole, it slowly increases during the first week. The appetite is entirely lost, the tongue has a thick, white coating, the taste is insipid, pappy, slimy; the region of the stomach and afterwards the whole abdomen, becomes sensitive to the touch; at the commencement of the disease the bowels are somewhat constipated. The symptoms increase in number and intensity, sometimes to the fifth and even to the ninth day. In violent attacks the tongue becomes dry, also brownish, the abdomen is distended, so that the idea of typhus suggests itself, the more as a mild delirium is not unfrequent; the skin is very dry and the urine saturated to excess. If the febrile symptoms abate after the fifth day, more particularly if up to this period they have continued in all their intensity, the evacuations become softer, and finally diarrhœic; however, they do not occur in rapid succession. For all that, convalescence does not date from the period when the fever abates. The patients, overcome with an intense feeling of illness, have to keep their beds, and now only begin to realize their weakness. The tongue remains coated and the appetite is entirely gone. The former exacerbations and remissions of the fever still continue, in the shape of evening-aggravations of the symptoms. It is mostly only at the end of the second week that convalescence fairly commences; however, it may not begin till the fifth week and even later, if the natural course of recovery is interrupted by wrong management. Increased action of the skin and a copious sediment in the urine are the surest signs of the real beginning of recovery; the appetite may not return until some time after; not as in typhus, where with the first signs of recovery the patient is sometimes devoured by an unappeasable hunger. If, on recovering from this fever, the patient should experience a strong appetite, he runs great risk of having a relapse which may prove more dangerous, and last much longer than the original disease; for every error in diet, were it even trifling, is apt to cause an aggravation of the disease, which is sometimes so violent that it is scarcely possible to distinguish it from typhus. The diarrhœa sometimes continues for a longer period, it may even change to chronic intestinal catarrh. If the disease terminates favorably, the organism gradually resumes its normal state. It is characteristic of this fever that it takes a long time, sometimes even months, before the patients recover their strength.

Bilious gastric fever is generally nothing more than a higher grade of the pathological process we have just now described, the phenomena of a disturbance of the biliary functions being particularly prominent. Like the former, the affection sets in with the symptoms of gastric derangement; sometimes even before the fever sets in, the symptoms of disturbed functions of the liver supervene, the patient feeling exceedingly languid, depressed in spirits, the appetite, especially for meat, being lost, and the patient, with a bitter taste in his mouth, craving particularly sour food. The invasion of the disease is generally announced with a chill, followed immediately by great heat; like the gastric fever this form of fever generally sets in in the evening, except that the febrile symptoms are much more intense, and the morning and day-remissions are much less distinct. If the skin had not yet assumed an icteric hue, it now shows itself in the eyes and face. The patients are tormented by a violent boring headache that almost drives them to madness. The pulse is accelerated, the temperature perceptibly heightened. The tongue exhibits a yellowish-white coating, is hot and dry; thirst very great, the patient craves sour drinks. The region of the stomach and liver is sensitive. The nausea and loathing increase to bilious vomiting, which occurs more frequently than in gastric fever, and alternates with retching, accompanied by a feeling of intense anguish. The vomiting consists of green masses, having a bitter and rancid or sour taste. The bowels are constipated; the scanty fæces are tinged deep-brown. The urine shows a bilious pigment. The patient is tormented by an unceasing restlessness, and is very irritable and low-spirited. In this disease likewise, the appearance of diarrhœic stools denotes the beginning of an improvement. The evacuations are sometimes so deeply charged with bile that it seems as though nothing but bile came from the bowels. They are almost painless, are attended with an abatement of the fever, and an increase of cutaneous action; thus convalescence runs its course, as in the former fever, unless interfered with by improper management or dietetic transgressions. In case the disturbance of the hepatic functions is deep-seated, the diarrhœa may not only continue for a longer period, with a corresponding increase of the general languor and weariness, but we likewise perceive the presence of an excess of bile in the blood. The skin remains inactive, the icteric hue becomes more prominent, the patient feels very languid, drowsy, and the pulse becomes sluggish. This condition of things naturally retards convalescence beyond the usual period.

This bilious-gastric fever sometimes bears a closer resemblance to typhus than the catarrhal fever, and there is the more danger of a severe attack of illness, as bilious fever, together with typhus and intermittent fever, generally sets in under the influence of some miasm. It frequently happens that bilious fever runs into intermittent fever, and *vice versa;* as we have had occasion to observe quite recently in a region of country where the flood of last summer had given rise to a prevalence of these two fevers. The same, however, may be said of gastric fever, so that the affection of the liver does not seem the cause of a transition into intermittent fever. It is more difficult to show a transition into typhus, for the reason that both these fevers commence with nearly the same initial symptoms; there is no reason, however, to suppose that such a transition is impossible, since both diseases originate under the same influences, except that one is more local, the other more general. Under the continued action of the causative miasm, the lighter disease may easily assume the more aggravated and more general form.

Of these three forms of fever, the gastric mucous fever, febris gastrica mucosa, is the most dangerous and most inveterate, and the more to be dreaded, as it attacks more particularly old or enfeebled individuals. A characteristic feature of this fever is the accumulation of quantities of mucus upon the mucous membranes of the digestive tract.

Like the other two forms, the mucous fever likewise usually develops itself out of a simple gastric derangement; the transition, however, is less marked, for the reason that the febrile phenomena do not set in all at once. There is a more gradual increase of the symptoms. The appetite soon vanishes; an irresistible aversion to all kinds of food is present; the languor and prostration increase from day to day; the tongue shows a thick coating of mucus. Sooner or later these symptoms become associated with fever, which, however, never reaches the high degree of intensity as in the other forms. At first the chilliness prevails, after which the heat becomes continuous but moderate. The pulse is never much accelerated; in cases where the heat is wanting, it is even slower than the normal pulse. Very rarely the fever has distinct periods of exacerbation, especially at the commencement; whereas, in the later course of the disease, a tertian type becomes more or less prominent. With the fever, all the symptoms increase; the coating of the tongue becomes thicker, and incommodes the patient still more, because the mouth and pharynx are likewise lined with mucus; the taste is flat, pappy, offensive. The region of the stomach is seldom sensitive; as soon, however, as a little food is partaken of, it becomes distended, the patient experiences a feeling of anguish and restlessness, and with much retching the patient vomits up the ingesta, with a quantity of mucus. Even without eating, the patient in the morning may be troubled with retching and vomiting of mucus. The bowels are very torpid; only in the subsequent course of the disease the evacuations are occasionally soft, and mixed with large quantities of mucus; the stools may likewise consist of pure mucus. The urine is diminished in quantity, has a loam color, and is thickly clouded with mucus. In more acute cases, the respiratory organs participate in the secretion of mucus. What imparts to this disease a very peculiar character, is the constitutional condition of the patients; they lie in a state of sopor and apathy; it seems as if the organs of sense had less power to perform their respective functions;

they do not seem to notice the surroundings; yet they are seldom delirious, and the consciousness remains undisturbed; it seems as though the patients had sunk into a state of utter discouragement. At an early period, the strength is reduced entirely; the patient does not complain of pain, properly speaking; his head feels dull, and there is buzzing in the ears. In this way the disease continues unchanged for weeks, sometimes abating a little, and at others increasing. Among older persons the tongue is apt to become brown and dry; with younger ones, the tip and edges become red and dry, or smooth and red. In the end, the vomiting becomes less frequent; the skin remains almost uniformly dry. As the whole course of the disease is so remarkably protracted, recovery takes place but slowly, imperceptibly as it were, interrupted by the least error in diet, by the least unusual physical or mental effort. Not until the production of mucus diminishes very sensibly, can we hope for recovery. Convalescence is generally slow; it sometimes takes months before the patients recover their former condition. The cause of this, next to the extraordinary prostration, is, that the appetite returns only very gradually, and the patient cannot bear any considerable quantity of food. It is only exceptionally that the occurrence of diarrhœic stools denotes a change for the better; as a general rule, diarrhœa aggravates the disease by consuming the strength. Only where a general improvement occurs, after a copious discharge of mucus by the anus, can such an evacuation be looked upon as a favorable crisis.

The danger to life in mucous fever is not so great as the complexity of the symptoms would seem to indicate. It is considerable in cases of old or debilitated individuals, and if continual relapses take place.

No disease is more frequently and more easily confounded with typhus than mucous fever. In this fever the shortness of its course is not, as in the other two forms, decisive of its true character. The difference between febris nervosa lenta and febris mucosa will be shown more fully in the chapter on typhus; we here content ourselves with stating, that the mucous fever is scarcely ever epidemic, hence, less depending upon atmospheric conditions, whereas it arises more readily in consequence of depressing mental emotions, grief, care, and excessive mental labor. Usually the persons who are attacked by this disease have been suffering for a long time with digestive derangements, catarrh of the stomach, constipation, etc., in consequence of which, their constitutions have become debilitated and impoverished. Robust individuals are scarcely ever attacked with mucous fever.

Treatment. Since we have to deal with processes whose course is by no means regular, but exhibits a variety of modifications and transitions, our best plan is to describe the various remedies each by itself, instead of indicating the possible course of the treatment in a continuous series. A general view of the remedies appertaining to this group is the more necessary, as it affords us the means of meeting more easily the relapses and incidental complications occurring in this disease.

Among these different remedies, *Belladonna* is almost the only one suited to the breaking out of the first and second class of these fevers, if, after a severe chill, violent heat is felt in the evening, which increases as night approaches. Its effect is particularly striking on women and children, yet it has an equally good effect on men. This remedy usually moderates the fever and arrests the vomiting and retching. As soon as the heat and redness of the face and the restlessness have abated, other remedies had better be employed. We cannot well recommend *Aconite* at the commencement of gastric fevers; we doubt whether Aconite has ever produced a good effect under these circumstances. In mucous fever, which has scarcely any fever from beginning to end, neither one nor the other remedy is appropriate. If Aconite can be used at all, it will be more particularly at the commencement of bilious fever, if it sets in suddenly without any precursory symptoms.

Mercurius vivus generally is applicable in bilious fever during the best part of the disease. Characteristic symptoms of Mercurius are, the intense fever-heat which sets in in the evening, and is most violent at midnight; the raging, mostly boring headache, which does not permit the patient to lie down; the sensitiveness of the region of the liver and stomach; the yellow tinge of the eyes and skin; the bitter taste and loathing; bitter eructations, vomiting of bile, an intense desire for sour drinks, an excessive restlessness and anguish. If in the subsequent course of the disease, the evacuations contain a large quantity of bile and some mucus, this would be an additional indication for *Mercurius*. Hartmann recommends Mercurius for mucous fever in the following words. His remarks, however, apply more to bilious fever than to what we have described as mucous fever. "It corresponds to the precursory symptoms, as well as to the more fully developed disease; the appetite decreases more and more; the tongue is lined with a whitish mucus; the throat and pharynx are distressingly dry during deglutition; foul taste and smell; loathing and nausea, with tearing, burning pains in the temples; pressure and tension in the pit of the stomach, region of the stomach and liver; rising of an acrid fluid into the mouth; turbid, slimy, sedimentous urine; irregular stools, with frequent urging; pale, sallow, yellowish complexion; debility, apathetic mood. Characteristic indications are more particularly a thick, dirty, slimy coating on the tongue; flat, pasty, soapy taste; great desire for piquant articles of diet; dryness in the mouth and throat; torpor or entire suspension of the alvine evacuations, or else slimy, diarrhœic, fetid stools; considerable mental and physical prostration of strength." Of course the patient must not have taken large doses of Mercury just previously, or even some time before his sickness.

Bryonia resembles Mercurius in many respects, but has a much larger sphere of action in these fevers. It is not only suitable in bilious and catarrhal, but likewise, although less frequently, in mucous fever. The origin of the fever in a cold, or in an error of diet, a fit of chagrin, and during the heat of the summer, points to Bryonia. We cannot enumerate the whole series of the symptomatic indications, which can better be studied in the Materia Medica. The distinctive differences between Bryonia and Mercurius are: The Bryonia-fever generally commences in the afternoon, has slight remissions, but is, at the same time, less intense. The headache is a painful pressure, or a tearing pain, and is considerably relieved by lying down quietly. Patients do not exclusively crave sour or piquant things. The tongue is thinly lined with mucus and the taste is rather flat and pasty, than intensely bitter. The bowels are constipated, or else the alvine evacuations consist of not very frequent diarrhœic discharges, of a deep brown color, and mixed with a good deal of mucus. The cases of mucous fever where Bryonia is to be used, have distinctly marked febrile motions; it will be found particularly suitable during the first eight days of the disease.

Pulsatilla is suitable in the first and second class of these fevers, principally in the second. There must be an increased secretion of bile, if Puls. is to be depended upon. It does not so much correspond to cases with violent fever, as to those that run a slow course, It is more suitable for children and women than for men. The most noteworthy symptoms are: bitter taste and bitter eructations; vomiting of mucus and bile; irresistible aversion to animal food; absence of thirst, or else a desire for sour and piquant beverages; sensitiveness of the region of the stomach and liver; bilious diarrhœa, mixed with mucus; severe evening-exacerbations of the fever, with chilliness prevailing during the day; whining mood, restlessness, with lowness of spirits.

Antimonium crudum is the chief remedy in the genuine mucous fever, especially if the fever is very slight, or has passed off in a measure. It is indicated when a good deal of mucus is secreted on all the mucous membranes. Among the symptoms we have: A great deal of mucus in the mouth, and especially in the fauces; vomiting of mucus; stools consisting of pure, tenacious mucus; copious slimy sediment in the urine; cough, with expectoration of tenacious mucus. In addition, we have: lying in a state of apathy; chilliness, thick coating on the tongue; feeling of hunger, without any appetite; distension of the abdomen after every meal; desire to vomit; obstinate constipation, or else alternate mucous diarrhœa and constipation; excessive debility, prostration. Such a complete image of mucous fever is not to be found in the pathogenesis of any drug; moreover, the curative power of this agent has been verified by a number of practical observations. Only the medicine should not be given up too soon; the long duration of mucous fever renders a sudden cure impossible. *Tartarus stibiatus* acts, in many respects similarly to *Antimonium crudum*, but it is not a very suitable remedy for mucous fever, for the reason that *Tartar emetic* does not prostrate; on the contrary, it elevates the reactive powers of the organism. The catarrhal affection is characterized rather by the production of balls of mucus, which is not viscid, and is first seen in the respiratory organs, and afterwards, but much less intensely, in the digestive organs. All local affections to which Tartar Emetic is homœopathic, have an inflammatory character; whereas those to which *Antim. crudum* is adapted, are distinguished by the character of torpor.

Veratrum album manifests curative virtues more particularly in cases where copious vomiting and diarrhœa are chief symptoms. It is not only an excellent remedy for these symptoms, but is likewise suitable where Ant. crudum seems indicated. Like this remedy, so has Veratrum album the secretion of excessive quantities of mucus upon every mucous expanse, the rest of the symptoms likewise correspond. The more specially distinctive characteristics may be studied in the Materia Medica Pura. We content ourselves with stating, in this case, that the Veratrum album disease is much more acute and searching, whereas the action of Antimony is slow, and imperceptibly increasing in intensity. Veratrum is generally preferable, if the respiratory organs participate in the pathological process.

Phosphori acidum is very seldom indicated in genuine febris mucosa, because it lacks, in some degree, the chief symptom, the characteristic secretion of mucus. However, it is indicated above all other remedies, if the disease resembles lentescent typhus, and consists principally in a soporous condition of the patient, who is lying down overwhelmed with a general debility, without any marked local symptoms. If these symptoms become associated with other alarming symptoms portending a fatal termination, such as complete inactivity of the skin and of the secreting organs, a very small and feeble pulse, complete prostration, real sopor, *Carbo vegetabilis* may be tried. We have already stated that such symptoms only occur among old and decrepit or much enfeebled individuals; otherwise, the diagnosis must have been erroneous, and the typhoid character first manifests itself at a late period.

Digitalis purpurea is likewise an appropriate remedy in mucous fever, but of great significance in this disease, much greater than the present limited use of this medicine would seem to imply. Independently of the other symptoms belonging to this group, all of which are embodied in the pathogenesis of Digitalis, it is, more particularly, the condition of the pulse that points to Digitalis. It is not so much the very slow pulse that furnishes the most important indication, but the alternate acceleration and slowness of the pulse, with weakness of the impulse, that constitute the chief indications for Digitalis. If the patients, while lying in their beds, show from 40 to 45 pulsations, and, on raising themselves, the pulse at once rises to one hundred and more beats; if the pulse is at the same time intermittent and irregular, Digitalis is eminently in its place. Even without any marked change in the pulse, the remedy is adapted to cases for which Acidum phosphoricum has been recommended, if there is obstinate constipation. It is one of the most remarkable peculiarities of the action of Digitalis, that, without any increase of the secretions and excretions of the body, the weight of the body and the strength, decrease with extraordinary rapidity. There is another remedy which, in this respect, bears great resemblance to Digitalis, it is

Cuprum. Since the effects of this poison vary so very greatly, according as it acts with more or less rapidity, and since the natural groups of symptoms can only be learned imperfectly from our Materia Medica, we here subjoin a number of cases of poisoning by copper, which furnish a picture of the Cuprum-disease as it was observed by Frerichs in the well-known case in Mengershausen, near Gœttingen, where a whole village was poisoned by soup that had been boiled in copper kettles. The first effect of the poison was a gradually increasing lassitude and prostration in the whole frame, attended with a feeling of weight in the head, and afterwards vertigo. In addition to this cephalæa gastrica, there was complete loss of appetite, constipation, and now and then fugitive, drawing pains in the abdomen. Very soon the features became collapsed, and the patients tumbled about like shadows. The subsequent symptoms were: Excessive dulness of the head, vertigo which did not even permit them to sit up in bed; headache; restless sleep, disturbed by dreams, also with bland delirium, or else continued sleeping almost like coma, in the case of some, complete sleeplessness; great pallor of the face with an expression of excessive prostration, and stupidity; the eyes had lost their lustre and were deeply sunken in their sockets. Excessive languor and weariness, a fainting fit, whenever they tried to move about; the tongue looked pale, not much coated, was moist, but in the case of some red, dry, and rough; thirst considerable, aversion to all kinds of food. Abdomen soft and painless; occasionally a slight colicky drawing pain; the pulse was somewhat accelerated and small, the urine turbid and cloudy. This condition lasted at least six days and only disappeared gradually, the weariness and languor passing off last. Frerichs himself compares this Cuprum-disease to a light typhus, except that the characteristic diarrhœa, which is seldom wanting in typhus, was not present, so that the symptoms resembled more nearly an attack of mucous fever. We shall revert to this point afterwards when speaking of typhus.

China is an important remedy for both bilious and mucous fever. In either disease it will berarely found indicated at the commencement; in bilious fever if, in spite of bilious stools, no improvement takes place; on the contrary, the disorder seems to increase, and shows more or less distinctly an intermittent type; in mucous fever, if the disease approximates convalescence, without any decided critical change seeming really to make its appearance.

Nux vomica is one of the few remedies that are equally appropriate in the three forms of fever. In the simple gastric fever, the best period for its employment is the time when an improvement seems to set in, and the pains decrease very slowly, with poor appetite, the diarrhœa having either ceased or occurring only at times; the greater the disposition to relapses, the more we may expect of the curative action of Nux. In bilious fever this remedy occupies a high rank as a curative agent, in consequence of its relation to the biliary functions. In view of the multitude of symptoms it is almost impossible to furnish only an approximative list of the symptoms that belong to this group; all we can do in this place, is, to indicate the difference between this remedy and Bryonia. In the Bryonia-fever, the patient lies quietly, the mental and sensorial functions are inactive, whereas Nux vomica has an excessive irritability of the mind as well as of the senses, together with a strikingly rapid decrease of strength. Bryonia has a pale complexion, Nux vomica a bright-red complexion, with a yellowish tinge. The symptoms of buccal catarrh are much more significant under Nux vomica, the tongue is somewhat dry, or coated white, with bright-red edges. The taste, besides being bitter, is sour or putrid, whereas Bryonia has more especially a flat, pasty taste. Nux vomica has aversion to certain kinds of food, Bryonia to all kinds. Bryonia has a marked disposition to perspire, Nux vomica a dry and hot skin. These are a few salient points; for more detailed contrasts the Materia Medica will have to be consulted. In mucous fever, Nux vomica is indicated under similar circumstances as China; it frequently removes very rapidly the peculiar remaining atony of the digestive organs, and regulates the action of the bowels, not unfrequently by first superinducing a few diarrhœic stools. It is well, in selecting a remedy, not to lose sight of the more general conditions of the system. Nux vomica is suggested by an irritable, sanguine, excitable temperament, hemorrhoidal symptoms, derangements of the digestive organs of some standing, origin of the disease in a fit of anger or chagrin. Nux is likewise required in the bilious fever of drunkards, persons living luxuriously, and of individuals exhausted by mental labor or leading a sedentary mode of life. It is generally more suitable for men than women.

Ammonium muriaticum according to Hartmann, corresponds perfectly to the symptoms of a status pituitosus. The tongue is lined with a white mucus; there is constant hawking, on account of a quantity of tenacious mucus in the throat; disagreeable, pappy taste, with accumulation of water in the mouth, aversion to food, empty eructations, gulping up of a bitter-sour fluid, feeling of emptiness and hunger in the stomach, malaise and warmth in the stomach, discharge of a glassy, tenacious mucus by the rectum; these are some of the leading indications for this drug. For all that, striking cures by it are not recorded in our publications.

With these remedies, all ordinary cases of bilious-gastric fever can be cured. Hartmann gives a number of other remedies without any precise indications, which we here transcribe, because the symptomatic differences of these three forms of fever may require a more extensive list, from among which the right remedy can be selected. The catarrhal form may require *Colchicum, Capsicum, Cocculus* and *Staphysagria;* bilious fever, *Chamomilla, Ignatia, Ipecacuanha,* also *Cocculus;* mucous fever, *Dulcamara, Rheum, Sepia, Rhus toxicodendron, Spigelia, Mezereum, Baryta, Arsenicum, Senega.*

As a general rule, a larger dose of the medicine may safely be given in these fevers than in other acute diseases. For the catarrhal and bilious fever, stronger doses of the remedy are necessary, because there is a well founded prospect that larger doses will produce a crisis in a shorter space of time. However, if, as in mucous fever, the disease runs a slow course, it is not well to give large doses, or to repeat them too frequently. This rule is the more urgent the longer the disease has lasted.

During the fever it is not very difficult to regulate the diet, the patients not showing any desire for any kind of food. Piquant and sharp articles of diet have to be forbidden, although patients may evince an extraordinary craving for such things; after eating them, the condition of the patients is always worse. The best beverage is pure, fresh water; a little milk and water is good nourishment. Where it can be had, sweet beer is not only a refreshing and beneficent beverage, but likewise an excellent means of promoting the appetite. Neither diarrhœa nor vomiting need prevent its use; only, if the beer contains a great deal of carbonic acid, it is well to add a little sugar and to first allow the gas to escape. In mucous fever, especially, this beer is excellent, and patients generally crave it. Fruit, especially when stewed, agrees with the patients, and is very refreshing. During the period of convalescence, small quantities of wine often do more good in stimulating the activity of the stomach than medicine. Inasmuch as every error in diet is apt to cause a relapse, it is of the utmost importance to make a proper selection of the food, and to increase the allowance very gradually. On the other hand, the patient, for fear of a relapse, should not be kept too long on lean soups; this would retard convalescence unnecessarily.

2. Enteritis, Inflammation of the Bowels.

We apply this designation principally to an inflammation of the smaller intestines, and more particularly to the most frequently occurring form of this inflammation, ileo-colitis, or inflammation of the ileum and colon. It is difficult to sharply separate the inflammations of the various parts of the bowels, because the different parts are almost always inflamed together, nor would this separation be of much practical value. Duodenitis scarcely ever occurs alone, but almost always as the companion of gastritis. Moreover, it is almost impossible to diagnose this disease, and hence we omit it entirely.

The causes of enteritis are mostly the same as those of intestinal catarrh, dietetic transgressions; the use of irritating, readily decomposed, sour substances; overloading the stomach; abuse of spirits; a cold. In addition, we have poisonous substances; mechanical irritation by fecal matter, the progression of which in the bowels is arrested, in consequence of which the vessels become compressed, or finally, though rarely, the inflammation may be caused by entozoa. Besides these causes, enteritis occurs as a continuation of other inflammatory processes, gastritis, peritonitis, and as a form of reaction against ulcerations of the intestinal mucous membrane.

The anatomical changes differ in accordance with the degree, extent and duration of the affection, and likewise with the constitution of the diseased organism. The inflammation is, at times, very diffuse, or affecting only scattered portions of the intestinal canal; or the whole thickness of the bowel may be invaded by the inflammatory process, or only the mucous membrane. The affected parts are injected and more or less red, or mixed with dark-red extravasations. The mucous membrane is puffed up, interstitially distended; in the later stages of the disease it may become infiltrated with pus, and sometimes falls to pieces in shreds. Ulcerations may likewise occur, but really only under the influence of some constitutional disease, in which case they may spread over a larger surface, whereas, in individuals free from any constitutional taint, the ulceration is confined to single follicles. In very acute cases, a thin, croupous exudation is sometimes seen on the free surface of the mucous lining. If the serous membrane is involved, a thin layer of exudation is likewise observed on its free surface. The appearances in the colon are the same as those in the ileum, except that follicular ulceration is met with more frequently and is more numerous.

If the inflammation is not spread over a large surface, and confined to the lining membrane, the symptoms are not very grave. There are few local pains, little fever, loss of appetite, constipation, feeling of fulness in the umbilical region; nausea occurs very seldom; there is never any vomiting. In this manner the affection may exist for a short time and disappear again almost imperceptibly, or it may increase and continue to spread; very rarely the disorder breaks out at once in all its violence. The pains now become intense, burning or tearing, or cutting like colic, until they sometimes grow intolerable; they spread over the whole abdomen; are generally most violent in the umbilical region, where the least pressure causes an intense aggravation of the pain, which is increased even by the act of breathing; coughing causes extreme pain, which is likewise intensely aggravated every time the patient attempts to turn the upper part of his body, on which account he remains lying motionless on his back. At all times the pain has more or less prolonged exacerbations like colic, evidently caused by the progressive descension of the contents of the bowels. At the same time the abdomen is distended, but not to excess, as if tympanitic. Where the ileum is alone affected, there is obstinate constipation; where the colon is involved in the inflammation, we have sometimes, not always, diarrhœic, colored, frequently bloody stools, not unfrequently attended with tenesmus, or alternate constipation and diarrhœa, or, finally, obstinate constipation. In such cases the colicky pains are more frequent and extensive, the distension of the abdomen more considerable. In violent attacks of this disease the constitutional symptoms are always very marked. A general chill only precedes a very sudden invasion of the disease. The patient feels the heat more perceptibly than others; he is constantly complaining of an intolerable thirst; the pulse is accelerated, even to one hundred and twenty beats, small and contracted, not seldom unequal and intermittent; the skin of the body is hot and dry; the extremities are frequently cool; the forehead is covered with a perspiration as from anguish; the appetite is entirely gone; the tongue has at times a light coating, at times it is clean and very soon becomes dry. If the affection increases in violence, the first symptom generally is nausea, which soon becomes associated with retching and vomiting. At first, bile and mucus are vomited up with the food; but if the inflammation is extensive, even fecal matter may be thrown up; the vomited matter very soon acquires a smell like that of fæces, The signs of collapse now become more apparent;

the face has a cadaverous appearance, expressive of deep suffering, with elongated features and sunken eyes. Under such circumstances, the patient often wanders, the skin becomes cool, and is covered with a cool perspiration. Convulsions and fainting fits occasionally complicate these symptoms, and death may ensue under such circumstances. In enteritis this is rarely the case in the first days of the disease, as in peritonitis; the disease does not so often terminate fatally, by virtue of its own inherent intensity, as by the morbid derangements which it causes in other respects, and, according to their nature, more or less rapidly; a supervening peritonitis leads the more rapidly to a fatal termination, ulcerations of the intestines more slowly. A rapid and complete recovery only takes place exceptionally.

The prognosis is always uncertain, because the disease is apt to pass into insidious chronic complaints, even after recovery seemed to be fairly under way; at all events, enteritis always constitutes one of the more important diseases.

The diagnosis of enteritis, although somewhat difficult, yet, with proper care, can be made in the majority of cases with positive certainty. The disorder is most easily confounded with incarcerations, simple cholerine, colic. The last two can become dangerous, if the trouble is esteemed too lightly, and, as is often the case, is treated with deleterious domestic remedies, among which we class the use of strong alcoholic beverages, and wine. Since it is not always possible to make a sure diagnosis until the disease has run along for a time, the employment of irritating domestic remedies cannot be sufficiently guarded against in cases of colic and cholerine.

Treatment. Hartmann begins this section with the following remarks: " Concerning the treatment of enteritis, I flatter myself that I have been one of the first homœopathic physicians who proposed to continue the use of *Aconite* in enteritis, until every trace of inflammation had disappeared; of course, the dose is not to be repeated until the former dose has exhausted its effect. This period cannot be indicated with positive certainty, since it does not even remain the same in the same individual, lasting at times four, at other times twenty-four hours. The more acute the inflammation, the sooner the medicine exhausts its action; on the contrary, the more the inflammation decreases, the longer the medicine acts, so that at first it may be necessary to administer the medicine three or four times in the course of twenty-four hours, whereas afterwards one dose may be sufficient in the twenty-four hours. I have never repeated the medicine more than six or seven times in a case of enteritis, nor do I believe that it need be given more frequently at any time. We may observe that the constipation attending the enteritis does not counter-indicate Aconite, nor does it require another remedy, since it disappears of itself, as soon as the inflammatory symptoms begin to abate. Under this treatment the disease generally passes off without danger, and within a much shorter period of time. There is no remedy that corresponds to enteritis as perfectly as Aconite, in all the finest shades of the disease."

It would seem to have been hazarding a great deal, if Hartmann had undertaken to recommend an uncertain remedy with so much positiveness; a number of cures have more or less demonstrated the correctness of his statements, and our Materia Medica shows that the law of similarity justifies the selection of Aconite in this disease. Nevertheless, not all forms of enteritis correspond with Aconite, and Hartmann should have restricted his recommendation of Aconite within narrow limits. His advice, not to repeat the dose until the previous one has exhausted its action, is mere theory, for at the commencement of the disease the symptoms but too often increase in intensity up to a certain point, and yet Aconite will at last produce a most satisfactory change in the disease. How are we to wait, under these circumstances, for the completion of drug-action? Aconite corresponds perfectly to the form of enteritis described by Hartmann, but he has only described one form of the more acute disease, namely: where constipation is a prevalent symptom. If, as is not unfrequently the case, the inflammation is attended with profuse diarrhœa, *Belladonna* is much more appropriate; however, this remedy will be rarely found sufficient, which is likewise the case in regard to Aconite. It is particularly two remedies that are most frequently required after either Aconite or Belladonna, namely: *Bryonia* and *Colocynthis*. The former is generally suitable after Aconite, much less frequently after Belladonna; it is obstinate constipation that most frequently points to Bryonia. Colocynthis, on the contrary, is preferable if the diarrhœa is less frequent, the colicky pains continue intense, and the bowels are very much distended with gas, so that their convolutions can be felt through the integuments. Bryonia is, moreover, adapted to the scarcely apparent inflammations, setting in without violent pains or marked fever, and likewise to enteritis involving the peritoneum, so that a layer of exuded fluid is distinctly perceptible.

These four remedies will be found sufficient in all cases of enteritis that run a somewhat regular course, and have no dangerous complications, and were treated homœopathically from the commencement. Instead of Belladonna, *Mercurius* may sometimes be more appropriate; *Nux vomica* is likewise deserving attention in the later stages of the disease. If the disease reaches its climax, *Arsenicum* is the only remedy of which help can be expected, provided help is still possible.

Intestinal inflammations, occurring as a consequence of other diseases, present peculiar difficulties. As a general rule it is advisable, under such circumstances, to regard enteritis as the most important disease, and to direct our treatment against it in the first place.

If the disease assumes the form of a lentescent fever, which is very seldom the case under homœopathic treatment, *Phosphorus* and *Sulphur* will prove the most efficient remedies to secure a favorable turn. Phosphorus will be found necessary if there are unmistakable traces of ulceration of the bowels.

We have to revert once more to the constipation, which is such a common accompaniment of this disease. It is an object of terror to lay-people, and even to many, or rather a majority of physicians. Nevertheless, it is of no essential importance, and is much less dangerous than the means which are generally used to remove it. If these means had no other effect than to cause an increase of the peristaltic movement of the bowels, their employment might be pardonable. In this respect simple injections of water are commendable. But if medicines are used, we not only hasten the action of the bowels, but have to apprehend other hurtful effects, for the reason that we are dealing with a diseased organism. Moreover, we do not always succeed in opening the bowels by cathartic drugs. Homœopathic physicians know better than any others how unnecessary all such violent means of treatment are, for as soon as the inflammatory symptoms have subsided under homœopathic treatment, the constipation ceases of itself. Embrocations of tepid water, applied to the abdomen, and not changed too often, are an excellent palliative. Dry warmth does not act well in enteritis.

In enteritis, as in all other intense diseases of the bowels, the diet has to be regulated with the greatest care. In the first days of the disease, the patients do not eat anything; if they begin to feel hungry, a weak broth is better than lean watery soups. The patient's own desire to partake of a little broth, is the best indication for giving it. Solid food must only be given in gradually increasing quantities.

3. Typhlitis, Perityphlitis, Inflammation of the Cæcum.

This inflammation is one of those that occur most usually as an uncomplicated and idiopathic disease. Sometimes the intestine alone is involved, sometimes only the parts surrounding the intestine, and sometimes both.

The etiology is uncertain; what is certain is, that the peculiar anatomical relations of the cæcum have a great share in the disposition of this intestine to become inflamed. The retarded or impeded passage of the fæces is most frequently accused of having caused the inflammation, whence the disease has been named typhlitis stercoralis. It remains, however, a question, which was the cause and which the effect. Ulcerations of the vermiform process, which are easily caused by foreign bodies that had remained lodged in it, incline to spread to the cæcum. Typhlitis not unfrequently occurs as a complication in inflammations of the female sexual organs, more especially if these arise from puerperal causes. It is difficult to show how far a cold, or the use of sour or easily spoiled food, may be instrumental in producing this disorder. Idiopathic perityphlitis seems to be easily caused by a cold attended with violent exertions, and is principally observed in young persons; whereas typhlitis stercoralis only occurs in advanced age. Nor is typhlitis of rare occurrence in a high grade of tuberculosis, and, in that case, is probably the result of intestinal ulcerations.

The most important anatomical changes caused by typhlitis, are. More or less considerable interstitial puffing of the mucous lining, with infiltration, or in the further course of the disease, with liquefaction and ulceration of the same; the vermiform process is full of pus; ulcerated perforations, with adhesions to the adjoining parts, or having caused peritonitis by opening into the peritoneal cavity, or fistulous openings through the integuments; inflammatory infiltration in the cellular tissue; inflammatory affection of the serous coat and peritoneum. In wide-spread perityphlitis we discover depositions of pus in the parts adjoining the intestine, with descension of the matter towards the thigh.

According to the degree of intensity, locality and extent of the inflammation, the symptoms of typhlitis vary considerably; this circumstance renders a separate description of the disease indispensable.

The most violent acute attacks of the disease begin at once, without any precursory symptoms, with violent, cutting, colicky pains in the right iliac region, which are considerably aggravated by contact. From the commencement of the disease the alvine evacuations are entirely arrested. The whole abdomen gradually becomes much distended, and is more or less painful. The appetite is entirely gone; there are frequent and painful eructations, soon followed by retching and vomiting which, in violent cases, may even contain fecal matter. The fever is high, the skin hot, the pulse accelerated and small; the tongue, although generally clean, soon becomes dry, not unfrequently the extremities are cool, and the face is covered with cool perspiration. The anxiety is very great, prostration complete. The urine is sometimes voided with great pain, or the urinary secretion is entirely suppressed for a long time. The patient is unable to extend the right thigh fully. Very soon a swelling in the cæcal region becomes distinctly perceptible, giving a faint sound on percussion, of various dimensions, and increasing with more or less rapidity in size. When the exudation has reached its climax, the gut is distinctly felt in the right side, like a hard, firm sausage. When the exudation is completed, the pains decrease considerably, sometimes disappear entirely, without, however, the constitutional condition of the patient improving in the least. The intense fever is now replaced by an extraordinary prostration and languor; the expression of the countenance is that of great suffering, the pulse is not retarded. Death may take place with all the signs of an increasing loss of strength; or else the symptoms of perforation of the bowels and diffuse peritonitis may suddenly supervene, and cause a speedy dissolution. In favorable cases recovery may take place very speedily, the exudation being rapidly absorbed. More frequently, however, reabsorption only takes place slowly. In such a case recovery is a slow process, the strength only returns very gradually, digestion is carried on irregularly. Even after the patient's health is apparently restored, the exuded mass remains perceptible for a long time.

If, instead of being reabsorbed, the exudation of the cellular tissue is transformed into pus, the constitutional symptoms, of course, remain in full force, and the symptoms of a higher grade of purulent metamorphosis supervene besides. The swelling becomes more and more fluctuating; the skin grows red, and sooner or later the pus is discharged through the integuments. If the intestine remains intact, only a fistulous opening forms; if the intestine breaks, fecal matter is discharged through the fistula. Or else the pus finds an outlet into the gut, and quantities of pus and blood are discharged by the rectum. Or, finally, the pus may burrow downwards towards the thigh, in which case the abscess discharges in the groin. All these terminations are comparatively favorable, because the formation of pus results in adhesions which prevent the discharge of the pus into the abdominal cavity. Under all circumstances, however, the healing of such abscesses proceeds very slowly, and leaves one or the other derangements of the gastric functions.

This very violent form of typhlitis is not the most frequent. The disease generally arises more gradually, with symptoms that do not allow it to be recognized with any certainty. This generally happens with typhlitis stercoralis. The arrest of the fæces in the cæcum leads to inflammatory phenomena which, with the exception of a most trifling sensitiveness, are scarcely recognizable by the senses. The evacuations are irregular, too scanty, there is a quantity of gas in the bowels, the patient does not feel well, although he is not altogether sick. Remissions take place, during which the parts seem to be restored to their normal condition. Sooner or later another aggravation sets in, which exceeds the former attack in gravity; there is more fever, more languor. Soon after, the exudation in the intestine and the surrounding parts is distinctly felt. The constipation becomes more complete and persistent. Unless the patient recovers at this stage of the disease, the symptoms of the above-described acute attack, set in sooner or later.

Extensive inflammatory processes in the cæcum cannot take place without causing prominent disturbances of the constitutional equilibrium; this applies more particularly to ulcerative inflammation of the vermiform process. Many fatal cases of peritonitis that have arisen most unexpectedly, and have run a rapid course, are, after death, found to be the result of a perforation of the vermiform process.

The terminations of typhlitis have already been enumerated in a previous chapter. If we include all kinds of possibilities, these terminations are very numerous. Beside the above-mentioned terminations, the following are particularly important: adhesions of the intestine; ulceration and chronic inflammation; chronic exhausting suppuration; inflammation of the adjoining bones.

The disease seldom runs its course under two weeks; owing to the peculiar modifications of the exuded matter, the affection may continue for many months, before a complete cure takes place. The most favorable sign of recovery is a frequently occurring, fetid, fecal discharge, with decrease of the frequency of the pulse. Frequent evacuations, at the height of the disease, have no particular significance. Such evacuations generally consist only of mucus, or of mucus and blood, and evince the participation of the colon in the morbid process. Unless the discharges have been examined by the physician, the report of the patient alone may deceive him.

The diagnosis is only difficult if the disease runs an almost latent course; if it is fully developed and exudation has set in, a mistake is impossible.

An absolutely certain diagnosis can hardly be imagined, in view of the many possibilities that may occur during the course of the disease; as long as there are traces of the exudation still existing, as long as the bowels do not yet act with perfect regularity, and the bodily strength seems slow to return, we cannot be perfectly sure that the disease has been removed.

There are comparatively few cases of typhlitis reported in our publications, although the disease is not by any means of rare occurrence. Some years ago *Mercurius* and *Hepar sulphuris* were recommended for perityphlitis, in one of our periodicals. Since then we have treated several cases of this disease, and have always derived the best results from the exhibition of Mercurius. According to our physiological provings, this remedy is only approximatively homœopathic to the disease, but the practical results justify its employment. As regards the use of Mercurius, we have to observe that it is only suitable as long as the exudative process continues, or as long as there is danger of ulterior disorganization, or where suppuration has actually set in. The intensity of the incipient symptoms need not prevent the use of this drug. As far as Hepar is concerned, we have never seen it do the least good. Where the absorption of the exuded fluid is retarded, and the disease assumes the character of a lentescent fever, *Bryonia* is always the best remedy. When treating of peritonitis, this point will be eliminated more fully. Bryonia is likewise appropriate at the commencement of typhlitis stercoralis, and is much relied on to restore the regularity of the alvine evacuations.

In the fortieth volume of the Allgem. Hom. Zeit. we have three cases of perityphlitis reported by Gauwerky, which he cured with high potencies of *Rhus toxicodendron*. On considering these cases more carefully, we find that the action of the drug on these occasions is highly questionable. Complete recovery, that is to say the complete disappearance of the exudation, required seven, eight and ten weeks. Under such circumstances we cannot suppose that the medicine accelerated the absorption, the more as the patients were young persons. Although the disease had assumed a lentescent type, yet it could not possibly have run such a long course, if the medicine had anything to do with abbreviating it.

Of much more significance is Black's cure of two cases of typhlitis, by means of *Lachesis* (see British Journal, 1847). Here, too, we have to ask ourselves whether the previously-given Mercurius was not the true curative agent in these cases. This hypothesis is not weakened by the fact, that the disease continued to increase for a short time after Mercurius had been given, for we cannot suppose that it is within the power of any medicine to at once arrest an incipient exudation. The favorable action of a drug has to be measured by the whole course of the disease. If, as is generally the case, we do not witness any pus after the exhibition of Mercurius, or no excessive exudation, and finally a rapid absorption, all this is proof enough of the curative agency of the drug. Lachesis might lay claim to the cure of these cases, if it had been given alone, from the very commencement. For these reasons it is highly essential to sound observation, that, in morbid processes whose course is definite and demonstrable from beginning to end, the remedy should not be changed, unless such a change is rendered necessary by the supervention of extraordinary occurrences or changes; this method is more especially to be recommended in the use of Mercurius in typhlitis. We have laid down a similar rule when speaking of *Aconite* in enteritis, and we shall have other opportunities to allude to this circumstance. In evidently recognized typhlitis, *Aconite* is no remedy, because it only corresponds to the fever of the first few days, not to the local process. *Belladonna* is much more suitable, because it has a number of symptoms pointing to typhlitis. It is particularly adapted to inflammation confined to the intestinal mucous membrane, or where the serous coat of the intestine, not the cellular tissue, is involved. *Veratrum* should not be lost sight of in typhlitis, if the acute febrile phenomena are very soon replaced by threatening symptoms of paralysis of the intestine, if the pulse is exceedingly rapid and filiform, the skin of the extremities and the face is cool, or covered with a cold perspiration attended with anguish and prostration. Inasmuch as such symptoms scarcely ever occur at the very beginning of the disease, Veratrum will seldom be found indicated; for the subsequently appearing and very similar symptoms require more particularly *Arsenicum* and *Lachesis*. In typhlitis, *Sulphur* holds the same rank as Bryonia. Whereas Bryonia has its use when the disease assumes the form of a lentescent fever, Sulphur is required after the characteristic fever has subsided and the exudation does not seem disposed to yield. It not unfrequently happens that the disease comes under homœopathic treatment at this period, after other means had been tried in vain for some time. Sulphur will scarcely ever fail to afford aid in such cases.

If the disease should assume an abnormal course by the supervention of diffuse peritonitis, we have to employ the remedies of which we shall make mention when speaking of this disease. If pus has become deposited in large quantities, medicinal action will prove fruitless until the pus has been discharged either internally or externally. Not till then, *Silicea*, *Graphites*, or *Sulphur* may be tried, in order to prevent the formation of incurable fistulous canals and osseous disorganizations. If possible, the opening of the abscess should not be left to nature, for the reason that the thickness of the soft parts through which the pus has to pass, is too great, and a further descension of the purulent matter is to be apprehended. Such results of a case of typhlitis that has been treated homœopathically from the start, are unquestionably very rare, and generally come to us from the hands of Old-School physicians. If distinct traces of ulceration of the mucous lining are perceived, as is so often the case in the typhlitis of tuberculous individuals, the prognosis is extremely unfavorable, although we sometimes succeed in deferring the fatal result by the use of *Phosphorus*, *Iodium*, *Arsenicum*. Iodium, especially, has a surprising effect.

Typhlitis stercoralis proper, always requires a long after-treatment and a careful supervision of the patients, since relapses are apt to set in unless the bowels are kept well regulated. *Nux vomica*, *Lycopodium*, *Sepia*, are appropriate remedies; but they have to be continued for some time.

The diet is the same as that recommended for enteritis, except that, in a case of typhlitis, the use of solid food has to be avoided for a much longer period of time; it is of great importance that not too much fecal matter should pass over the diseased surface. Applications of tepid water to the bowels have an excellent, although only palliative, effect.

4. Catarrhal Inflammation of the Rectum, Proctitis.

[According to Kafka, this inflammation is either acute or chronic. Acute proctitis has no other anatomico-pathological phenomena than those which characterize inflammations of the mucous membranes generally. Its passage into ulceration or inflammation of the cellular tissue surrounding the rectum (peri-proctitis) is a very rare occurrence.

Primarily acute proctitis is caused by a cold, by the action of external cold upon the rectum, as when sitting on cold stones, on fresh grass, lying on the cold floor, or by the use of cold injections, cold sitz-baths, etc It may likewise be occasioned by the action of external irritants upon the mucous membrane of the rectum, such as the too frequent use of irritating injections of soap-suds, vinegar, salt, etc., or by the introduction of plugs into the rectum for the purpose of facilitating a passage from the bowels; or by the action of worms, ascarides, foreign bodies, such as sharp-cornered plumpits, the accumulation of indurated fecal masses, or by abuses of the rectum for vile purposes.

Secondarily proctitis may accompany the ulcerous processes of the mucous membrane, such as tuberculosis, carcinoma, dysentery, typhus, syphilis, etc.; or inflammations of adjoining organs, cystitis, metritis, oophoritis, prostatitis.

Catarrhal proctitis is recognized in the majority of cases by a violent tearing, stitching, throbbing or burning pain in the rectum, which is always accompanied by tenesmus. The patients experience a sensation as if a foreign body were lodged in the rectum, which they endeavor to expel by hard pressing. While making this effort, the rectum either protrudes from the anus like a raw lump of flesh, that seems to be held tightly by the surrounding anus, or else the anal orifice is spasmodically contracted and at the same time drawn up, without any prolapsus of the rectum taking place.

The pains spread from the region of the coccyx to the perinæum, to the sexual organs or the abdomen, and are often intolerable. They reach the acme of intensity during an alvine evacuation, more especially if the fæces are hard and dry, in which case these generally appear tinged with blood. In case of diarrhœa, the stools cause a burning sensation and, when passing through the anus, an excruciating pain; they are likewise mixed with blood, and frequently excoriate the anus.

On examination, the mucous membrane of the rectum looks dark-red, interstitially distended, hot and dry, the veins of the rectum are swollen.

If the inflammation reaches a high degree of intensity, it is generally attended with disturbances in the urinary secretions, especially with stranguria, dysuria, or even ischuria. Febrile symptoms only occur if the inflammation is intense; in the lower grades of the inflammation, they are entirely absent. If the pain spreads to the abdomen, it is usually accompanied by vomiting and sometimes even by collapse.

The disease commonly runs its course in two, three, or five days, amid a gradual abatement of the symptoms, and most generally terminates in recovery without passing into the chronic form. If symptoms of peritonitis are present, the disease may run a longer course; it may likewise become dangerous if the walls of the rectum should become perforated.

Secondary proctitis terminates together with the disease occasioning it; if this should be dysentery or syphilis, the healing of the ulcers may result in stricture of the rectum.

In general, the prognosis is favorable; it is only when complicated with peritonitis that the perforation, caused by the dissolution of the exudation, may endanger life.

In treating an acute, primary proctitis, the existing causes have first to be discovered.

If fever is present in catarrhal proctitis, occasioned by a cold, we first give *Aconitum* 3; this remedy usually causes a copious perspiration, after which all the symptoms diminish in intensity.

If the fever is not very intense, the pain, however, very acute, the patient hardly able to bear it, and complains of a distressing tenesmus; if the protruding rectum is hot and constricted, if a throbbing is felt in it, if the anus is spasmodically contracted without any prolapsus of the rectum, and if strangury is present, we give Belladonna 3, in solution, every hour. If no improvement takes place in eight to twelve hours, we resort to *Sulphate of Atropine* 3, in the same form and dose.

These remedies can be depended upon; they not only diminish the capillary hyperæmia, but likewise the excessive sensibility of the rectum, and very soon initiate a dispersion of the inflammation.

In case of diarrhœa, with violent pains before and during stool, discharges of mucus and blood which excoriate the anus, we give *Merc. sol.*, 3d trit., every two or three hours.

If the stools are hard, the evacuation is attended with great pain, and very often causes prolapsus of the rectum, or is accompanied by swelling of the veins of the rectum, we have derived benefit from the exhibition of *Nux* 3, or *Sulphur* 6.

If tenesmus prevails, with spasmodic closing of the bladder (Ischuria), we recommend *Hycscyamus* 3.

Secondary phenomena of the rectum, in the course of ulcerous processes, require, according as the symptoms may indicate, *Arsenicum* 3 to 6, *Hepar sulphuris* 3, *Phosphorus* 3, or *Silicca* 6.

Proctitis, setting in in the course of adjoining inflammations, constitutes a painful complication, and generally yields to *Belladonna* or *Atropine*; these remedies at the same time act favorably upon metritis, cystitis, or oophoritis.

Among external applications, we recommend the application of moist and tepid cloths, or moist and tepid poultices of flaxseed, to the anus; the distressing tenesmus is relieved by injections into the rectum of warm almond or olive oil, by means of a small syringe, or greasing the anus with Atropia ointment, in the proportion of one grain of Atropine to two or three drachms of fresh, unsalt butter. Warm sitz or vapor-baths relieve the pains in the rectum and the tenesmus. Excoriations of the anus are benefited by the application of linen rags soaked with oil, or greased with fresh, unsalt butter, or with sweet cream. A prolapsed rectum has to be replaced by manual interference; if the anus is too much constricted to admit of the operation, the Atropine ointment will have to be applied round the anus, after which the reposition of the rectum will very soon become feasible.

If the stools are hard, and cannot be passed without much pain, we give *Bryonia* or *Nux vomica*, and resort to injections of oil, and a few glasses of loosening mineral-water, (Congress or Rockhill.)

While the inflammation lasts, the diet must be restricted, and the patient must not be permitted to leave his bed.

Chronic proctitis is characterized by interstitial puffing, and thickening of the lining membrane; livid color of this membrane; the presence of a mucous exudation on the surface of the lining membrane; thickening of the sub-mucous cellular tissue; polypous excrescences occasioned by the long continuance of the catarrh, and considerable secretion of mucus; erosions, and ulcerations of the mucous membrane; engorgement of the veins of the rectum, giving rise to frequent bleedings. Under certain circumstances the thickened cellular tissue surrounding the rectum, may become inflamed, (periproctitis.)

Chronic proctitis is either a remnant of the acute form, especially if repeated relapses have taken place, or else it arises in consequence of chronic obstructions of the portal system, that occur in diseases of the heart, lungs, pleura, liver, or of the vena porta itself, etc.

Secondarily, chronic proctitis accompanies the various ulcerous processes of the rectum, more particularly carcinoma and tuberculosis.

Chronic proctitis occurs more frequently than the acute form.

The most constant symptom is the secretion of mucus from the rectum; if the mucus is secreted in small quantity, the fecal masses are generally lined with mucus; if the secretion of mucus is more copious, a muco-purulent substance is either expelled from the rectum, after much urging, or else it continually passes away through the anus, which it keeps moist. The pains are inconsiderable, and are generally felt only during an evacuation.

The patients complain of a sensation of pressure or tension, burning or tickling in the rectum. If the mucous membrane is thickened, the passage of the fæces is rendered difficult. The hemorrhoidal veins are almost always engorged, and, in case of ulceration taking place, bleed frequently. In chronic cases, accompanied by constipation and copious secretion of mucus, prolapsus ani is of frequent occurrence.

This disease runs a slow course, sometimes for weeks or months, and sometimes, if the causes giving rise to the disease cannot be removed, continues until death. Cases remaining after frequent attacks of acute proctitis, or after improper treatment of such attacks, admit more easily of a cure. Chronic proctitis of long duration, frequently gives rise to ulcers of the rectum, with undermined edges. Sometimes the cellular tissue around the rectum becomes perforated and inflamed, in consequence of which, fistulæ of the rectum may take place. The great relaxation of the rectum, consequent upon the copious secretion of mucus, or attended with habitual constipation and the passage of indurated fæces, may lead to permanent prolapsus of the rectum.

In cases of chronic proctitis, remaining after frequent relapses, the prognosis is rather favorable. Proctitis occasioned by obstructions of the vena porta, or of a secondary character, is difficult to cure and sometimes incurable.

In treating chronic proctitis, we have to direct our attention to the quality and quantity of the mucus discharged from the anus, to the quality of the evacuations, to the sensations accompanying them, to the condition of the veins of the rectum, and to the prolapsus, and ulcerations of the rectum, if such should be present. Nor should we lose sight of the possibility of periproctitis setting in.

Special inquiry should be instituted, whether polypi are present in the rectum; they may be both the sole cause, and likewise the consequence, of proctitis. On this account, we examine every patient, without regard to sex. Polypi of some size protrude at the anus, in the shape of dark-red or bluish, smooth, or fringed bodies. Some bleed more or less at every evacuation; physicians who neglect to institute a proper examination, are misled (by such an occurrence) into a belief that the bleeding is owing to hemorrhoids. Some do not bleed, but cause intense pain at every evacuation. On examining the anus, sometimes no polypi are seen; but on requesting the patient to bear down, the polypi are observed, as described above. By introducing the finger into the rectum, we easily discover if the polypi are seated on pedicles, or whether they have a broad base. The polypi are either ligated, or they are twisted off, or removed by means of the recently introduced galvano-caustic methods. After the removal of the polypi, a perfect cure is generally obtained.

In former years, we used to treat polypi with the high and low attenuations of Calc. carb., Phosph., Silic., and Thuya, but without the least result.

If no polypi are present in the rectum, and copious quantities of mucus are secreted, we give *Borax* 3 to 6, two doses a day; at the same time we inject the rectum with this drug, in the proportion of ten grains to one ounce of distilled water. This remedy acts most favorably in cases of chronic proctitis remaining after frequent acute attacks.

In secondary proctitis with venous hyperæmia, we use *Carbo vegetabilis* 6, *Pulsatilla* 3 to 6, *Sulphur* 6, [also *Hamamelis* from the tincture up. H.]

If the mucus is purulent and has a fetid odor, as when ulcers are present in the rectum, we give *Hepar sulph.* 3, or *Sulphur* 6, two to three doses a day. In such cases the symptoms may likewise indicate *Thuya* 6, especially if the mucus is sanguinolent; or *Arsenicum* 6, or *Carbo veg.* 6, if the mucous discharge is attended with burning pains at the rectum; or *Phosphorus* 6, when there is tickling at the anus, or *Nitri ac.* 6, or *Calcarea carb.* 6, when there are pressing pains in the rectum.

For fungoid growths and thickening of the mucous membrane, we recommend *Phosphorus* 6, and *Natrum mur.* 6; the last-named remedy especially if the stools are hard, and passed with difficulty.

If the veins of the rectum are engorged and painful, we give *Pulsatilla* 6, *Carbo veg.* 6, or *Sulphur* 6, [also *Hamamelis*. H.]

For hemorrhage from the veins of the rectum, we prescribe *Phosphorus* 6, *China* 3, or *Sulphur* 6. [See also the remedies recommended for hemorrhoids. H.]

Prolapsus of the rectum is strikingly relieved by *Nux vom.* 3, and *Sulphur* 6, [also by *Mercurius* 2d or 3d trit., and *Ignatia* 6. H.]; if caused by relaxation of the mucous lining, we prescribe *Calcarea carb.* 6, or *Lycopodium* 6, and after replacing the rectum, we support it by a compress, which should be held in place by a T-bandage.

It is important that the bowels should be moved easily. This object is accomplished, in most cases, by using the above-mentioned remedies, by drinking a good deal of water, eating fruit, etc.

The diet to be observed during the treatment of chronic proctitis, should be nourishing without being heavy. Light meats and a great deal of water are most suitable. Heating food and beverages have to be carefully avoided.

Chronic blennorrhœas of the rectum, of long standing, are often benefited by cold sitz-baths, cold douches on the sacrum, the use of such mineral springs as Karlsbad, Marienbad, Kissingen, Homburg, sea-bathing and cold-water treatment.

For anæmia we give *Ferrum metallicum* 1, two or three doses daily, we likewise prescribe country-air, a strengthening diet, and chalybeate baths.

5. Cellulitis,

Inflammation of the Cellular Tissue of the Intestinal Canal.

It occurs most frequently at the rectum, (periproctitis,) and at the cæcum (perityphlitis.)

Periproctitis represents an inflammation of the cellular tissue surrounding the rectum. Primarily it is caused by traumatic agencies, or by a cold, by continued sitting, or by some unknown causes. Secondarily it may be a sequal of chronic catarrhal proctitis, ulcerous processes in the rectum, or in adjoining organs, such as the prostate, bladder, uterus, etc.

The patients experience pressing, or stitching pains, in the region of the rectum; sitting inconveniences them very much; even walking aggravates the pains, which sometimes reach a high degree of intensity. Gradually a swelling is seen in the neighborhood of the rectum, either near the perinæum or coccyx; or else no swelling is visible on the outside, but amid a gradual increase of the pains, a throbbing is felt in the rectum, accompanied by chills, which denote the formation of an abscess near the rectum. The abscess sometimes remains undiscovered, even after the most careful examination. Its locality might be ascertained by means of a digital exploration of the rectum, but this operation is so painful that the patients obstinately refuse to submit to it. The abscess encroaches upon the capacity of the rectum, and causes an obstinate constipation, which is not unfrequently accompanied by dysuria. Sensitive patients have more or less fever, and are generally deprived of sleep.

This inflammation runs a course of from eight days to a fortnight, if the abscess is visible externally; it gradually fills, becomes softer, and discharges outwardly. If the abscess can neither be seen nor felt, it frequently discharges internally by perforating the rectum; fecal matter penetrates through this opening, accumulates outside of it, causes a new inflammation, and another opening in the neighborhood of the anus, giving rise to fistulæ of the rectum.

Abscesses, finding an outlet externally, generally heal perfectly; abscesses perforating the rectum often lead to extensive suppuration or ichorous disorganizations, which, for the most part, cause death by exhaustion, or with all the symptoms of pyæmia.

Traumatic periproctitis is treated with *Arnica* 3, and cold applications to the anus.

Periproctitis caused by a cold, with pressing pains, requires *Bellad.* 3, *Ignat.* 3, *Nux v.* 3.

For stitching pains we give *Bryonia* 3, and *Phosph.* 3. In either case we resort to cold or warm applications to the anus, according to the sensitiveness of the patient.

If the inflammation is not too acute, we often succeed with these remedies in dispersing it, and preventing the formation of an abscess. Absorption of the remaining exudation is effected by *Mercurius* 3, and *Bryonia* 3.

As soon as a swelling becomes visible on the perinæum, or in the region of the coccyx, we cause warm flaxseed poultices to be applied, in order to accelerate the suppurating process.

At every visit the resistance of the swelling should be inquired into. If the abscess is sufficiently matured, a free incision should be made with a lancet, and a quantity of badly-smelling pus will be discharged, to the great relief of the patient. The abscess should be kept discharging, by inserting a plug of lint or a strip of linen into the opening, until all the pus is let out. A premature closing of the abscess may lead to a new attack of periproctitis and fistula of the rectum.

If no swelling is visible, and the symptoms denote the existence of a deep-seated abscess close to the rectum, the physician has to examine the parts around the anus with great care, at every visit. As soon as he discovers a spot in the periphery of the anus, which is softer and more yielding than the other parts, a deep incision should be made, without loss of time, parallel to the longitudinal axis of the rectum. Perforation can only be prevented by thus securing a free outlet to the foul-smelling pus, which will be found mixed with blood. The subsequent treatment is the same as described above.

Perityphlitis is an inflammation of the cellular and connective tissue, which attache the cæcum and the ascending colon to the iliac fascia. It is either caused primarily, by a cold, or by traumatic agencies; or is a consequence of typhlitis; or it occurs secondarily in the course of typhus, puerperal fever, pyæmia, etc.

The most constant symptoms of traumatic or catarrhal perityphlitis, are: pain in the ileo-cæcal region, increased by pressure, motion, deep breathing; or swelling in this region, occasioned by the rapid exudation; it is generally sharply defined, and very sensitive to pressure. If there is considerable meteorism, and the abdomen is very painful, it is sometimes difficult to find the swelling. Its pressure upon the cæcum sometimes causes inveterate constipation; in bad cases symptoms of ileus may be occasioned; the pressure of the swelling upon adjoining nerves may give rise to severe pain, a sensation of formication, and even complete suspension of sensibility in the lower extremities; pressure upon the veins may cause œdema, or symptoms denoting phlebitis; pressure upon the psoas or iliac muscle renders the motion of the right lower extremity painful.

If this condition is accompanied by bilious vomiting, it generally denotes a co-existing peritonitis. If the bowel is entirely closed, fecal vomiting may take place.

According as the inflammation is more or less intense, the fever is likewise more or less violent, the features are sunken, extremities cold; the formation of abscess sets in with chills. The supervention of peritonitis is attended with meteorism, singultus, ischuria, a small, filiform pulse, etc.

The diarrhœa, which is present in some cases, may be attributed to a coexisting catarrh of the large intestines.

Perityphlitis arising from typhlitis, has almost the same phenomena. In every case of typhlitis and inflammation of the vermiform process, there is danger of perityphlitis, especially if obstinate constipation is present. In such cases the swelling is more deep-seated, and is not unfrequently covered by the cæcum, which contains air, on which account the percussion-sound over the swelling is not unfrequently quite resonant.

Secondary perityphlitis generally sets in with chills.

Its course is so much more rapid, the more violent the inflammation, and the more extensive the coexisting peritonitis. In favorable cases the exudation is reabsorbed, and the inflammation is dispersed; this takes place more particularly in catarrhal and traumatic perityphlitis. As the inflammation decreases, the swelling diminishes in size, the pains become less, and the patients recover their health and strength very rapidly. If the inflammation is not dispersed, the swelling gradually increases in size, a fluctuating abscess forms on the abdomen, or in the inguinal region, which, if it discharges outwardly, and the strength of the patient is good, may heal and terminate in recovery. If the patient's constitution is weak, and the suppuration profuse, or the pus changes to ichor, the patient may die of exhaustion

If perforation takes place into the ascending colon, or into the rectum, vagina, or uterus, the pus or ichor is evacuated by the rectum or vagina, and the result may be favorable. If the pus is discharged into the peritoneal cavity, fatal peritonitis sets in very speedily.

If in favorable cases the pus is either absorbed or evacuated, as stated before, adhesions or partial occlusions of the intestine may remain, occasioning obstinate constipation. Chronic suppurations or discharges of ichor always endanger life.

The prognosis in perityphlitis is always dubious. Primary inflammations are always less dangerous than secondary. An important circumstance is the coexisting peritonitis. Puerperal and pyæmic perityphlitis are almost surely fatal.

To moderate the inflammatory pain in primary perityphlitis, we give *Belladonna* 3_v every quarter of an hour, half hour, or hour, without any regard to the presence or absence of fever or collapse.

If Belladonna does not relieve, we give *Atropine*, and if signs of anti-peristaltic motion manifest themselves, we give *Opium* 1, or *Morphia* 1; after which the pains generally abate, and the signs of ileus disappear.

If the swelling shows signs of decrease, we favor the process of absorption by giving *Bryon.* 3, or *Merc. sol.* 3 ; applying at the same time warm poultices to the swelling, or resorting to tepid baths, which means should not be omitted even during the period of inflammation.

If the swelling increases in size, the abdominal integuments become tense and red, and the swelling shows a tendency to discharge on the outside, we apply poultices day and night, in order to facilitate the suppurative process. As soon as the abscess is sufficiently matured, we make a free incision to prevent the pus from gravitating downwards.

During this period we order a strengthening diet, and, if the discharge of pus is very profuse, we give *China* 1, internally, every two hours. If the patient is anæmic, we give *Ferrum* 1, two or three doses a day. Peritonitis, caused by the discharge of pus into the peritoneal cavity, is fatal. H.]

6. Dysenteria, Dysentery.

If we comprise under this general name the inflammatory processes of the colon and rectum, it is simply because we are anxious to do justice to the practical tendency of this work, even if we should have to pursue this course at the risk of doing violence to pathological systems. We comprehend in this class all those conditions that have the pathognomonic sign of dysentery, tenesmus, with deficient or very much diminished evacuation of fecal matter; hence the symptoms of colitis and proctitis will be found more or less completely in the following descriptions of diseases. If we had rigidly adhered to a principle of classification, it would have been necessary to treat of simple catarrhal dysentery in this place, and of epidemic dysentery in a subsequent part of this work, simultaneously with typhus, cholera, etc. This would have compelled us to resort to many repetitions in the therapeutic section of the work, and would have rendered it difficult to contrast many points of diagnosis and treatment.

a. *Catarrhal Dysentery.*

This form represents the simple catarrhal inflammation of the colon and rectum. The etiology scarcely differs in any respect from the previously described affections of the bowels. It is worthy of note that dysentery inclines to supervene during other important local and general diseases ; and, although it is not, strictly speaking, a pernicious complication, and, as a general rule, is much less dangerous than an inflammation of the ileum, when occurring under similar circumstances, yet it deserves more particular attention on account of the pain it causes, and the weakness which the constant disturbance of the patient's rest entails.

The anatomical changes in this disease are only found completely developed in the rectum and at the lower extremity of the colon, more particularly in the region of the sigmoid flexure, and not at all, or only very slightly, towards the cæcum; whereas the reverse is the case in ileo-colitis.

The mucous membrane is red, interstitially distended, more or less infiltrated; the follicles are slightly ulcerated, and ulcerated patches are found in the mucous membrane. A characteristic sign is, the disposition to plastic exudations upon the free surface of the mucous membrane, which often results in the formation of extensive pseudo-membranes.

Symptoms. The disease sets in without any definite precursory symptoms, or suddenly with violent pinching, cutting, or cutting-pinching pains, radiating from the umbilical region downwards, and which are speedily succeeded by a violent urging to stool, with discharge of fecal, soft or watery masses. After the evacuation, the pains abate for a shorter or longer period, after which they return with renewed violence, and more particularly with increased urging, attended with tenesmus and severe pressing pain, during which a small quantity of white, and subsequently blood-stained, mucus is discharged, without any admixture of fecal matter in most cases. At the same time the patients experience an acute burning pain in the anus, and with every new discharge the tenesmus increases. In slighter cases the disease sometimes runs its course without any fever; the more acute cases may be attended with violent fever; the stomach is at times involved in the affection, at times not at all; there is loss of appetite, retching, nausea, vomiting; the tongue is usually quite clean. The duration of the disease usually depends upon its extent, which is pretty accurately measured by the extent of the pain. The slighter cases sometimes do not last more than a day, the severer cases last weeks, and then are disposed to pass into the chronic form. In the case of children the non-admixture of fecal matter in the stools is an exception to the rule; blood, pus, and scrapings of intestinal membrane, shreds of mucous membrane, and false membrane, are met with the more frequently, of a green, not homogeneous, color. The dysentery of children assumes more easily a chronic form than in the case of adults, and almost always leaves a peculiar disposition to relapses. The so-called teething-dysentery is just such a catarrhal affection, and arises less frequently in consequence of the process of dentition than of other influences acting upon the little patient, especially an erroneous system of preparing and administering nourishment. In the case of children, even if there is no sign of fever, convulsive symptoms are apt to supervene, imparting a higher degree of importance to the otherwise not very important disease.

A fatal termination of catarrhal dysentery, in a person of an otherwise good constitution, is a rare occurrence. Even where the disease sets in as a complication of other diseases, the danger incident to its course is only of mediate importance.

The treatment will be shown when we come to speak of dysentery proper.

b. *Dysenteria Epidemica, Dysentery Proper.*

However trifling catarrhal dysentery may seem, dysentery proper is an important and dangerous disease, and so much more interesting to the homœopathic practitioner, as the homœopathic treatment of dysentery is infinitely superior to any other method of treatment. Nothing is better calculated to expose to view the advantages of a method of cure than the prevalence of some epidemic malady.

The etiology of dysentery, although in a measure founded upon positive data, rests likewise upon hypotheses which it might be difficult to demonstrate. The importance of this subject must be our excuse if we dwell upon this point more at length.

Dysentery usually breaks out in an epidemic form; the few cases of sporadic dysentery that come to us for treatment, are either not dysentery, properly speaking, or else they are very rare occurrences. Dysentery is more particularly a disease of young persons and those of middle age, and very seldom attacks either the very young or very old. Epidemic dysentery almost always breaks out late in the summer, or in the beginning of fall, in very hot and dry seasons; it seldom lasts until winter is somewhat advanced; it seems to occur more frequently among the lower than the higher classes; its spread is promoted by the living in crowded rooms; nothing shows this clearer than the devastations which dysentery causes in the ranks of armies. Neither city nor country people are spared; it even seems as though the latter were more fearfully visited by this plague. If a disposition to dysentery prevails, errors in diet and catarrhal exposures excite the attack; the statement, however, that the use of fruit favors the breaking out of dysentery, is not yet proven. This assertion, at most, only applies to unripe fruit, or to such kinds as are apt to cause cholerine, diarrhœa, etc., such as the early cherries, plums, etc. There are, undoubtedly, individuals whose bowels are irritated by the use of any kind of fruit, and in whom it may cause an attack of dysentery.

These detached and well established etiological data, cannot well be harmonized in one series, except by the supposition that there exists a peculiar virus, which has a special relation to the colon and rectum; for it is only in these parts that the phenomena of dysentery become localized. In this respect, dysentery is very near to Asiatic cholera, and likewise to other infectious epidemics. What the quality of the dysenteric virus is, has not yet been decided with any degree of certainty. That the virus is of a vegetable nature might be accepted as true, where dysentery spreads over extensive districts; but this theory does not apply where dysentery attacks whole armies. A discussion of this point is not as useless as it might seem, since its proper solution is intimately connected with the prophylactic treatment of dysentery. This question may perhaps be better elucidated by subsequent epidemics. It is certain that the virus is engendered in the patient, and is transmitted by him like the poison of cholera. Contagion does not take place by contact, but the infection is propagated by water-closets, close-stools, etc. This theory, which is now received as explanatory of the spread of cholera, explains the fact, why the disease decreases and disappears with the appearance of frost; the cold destroys the poison. This may be the reason also why dysentery sometimes continues as long as mid-winter, provided the warm weather lasts, and there is no frost. The circumstance that during an epidemic all the inhabitants of one house, but not all the houses in the neighborhood, are attacked, and that epidemics spread more extensively, and more frequently in the country where the exhalations from excrementitious matter are more freely diffused through the air, speaks likewise in favor of the theory, that infection is communicated in the manner above described. Among armies in the field, the epidemic is propagated in a like manner, whereas the soldiers lying in barracks are protected much more efficaciously, and the cases of dysentery occurring among them are less numerous. Even if the views which we have here expressed, are not absolutely accepted as true, yet no reasonable physician will neglect to arrest the spread of the disease, by effecting the removal of the various circumstances, which we have pointed out as exciting causes of the epidemic. Another important question regarding the etiology of dysentery is, whether an alteration in the functions of the liver does not constitute the chief exciting cause of the disease. The origin of the epidemic, at a time when the action of the liver is known to be altered, and the affections of the liver which so often prevail, during and after epidemic dysentery, seem to confirm this opinion. Hence individuals in whom abnormal changes in the functions of the liver, have developed a disposition to be attacked with dysentery, are most likely to be assailed by this plague; this circumstance again shows why middle-aged persons should be most liable.

The anatomical changes caused by dysentery, bear the greatest resemblance to the pathological process taking place in diphtheritis. An exudation forms upon the surface and within the tissue of the lining membrane, which shows an extraordinary disposition to purulent or gangrenous disorganization, and upon which all other phenomena depend. The resemblance of this process to that of diphtheritis is the more striking, if we take into consideration the etiology of the disease. The changes occur more particularly in the rectum, and sigmoid flexure, and become the more insignificant as they approximate the ileum, which is but exceptionally involved in the pathological process. In the lighter grades of dysentery, the mucous membrane exhibits here and there, narrow streaks of redness, the streaks extending transversely across the axis of the intestine, and mostly running parallel to one of the semilunar folds. The mucous membrane here is infiltrated, likewise the subjacent cellular tissue, and the red places are lined with a soft, reddish-gray secretion, covered with bran-shaped pieces of epithelium, or else the epithelium is raised in the shape of a small vesicle. In the higher grades of the disease, the affected parts of the lining membrane are of larger size, more numerous, and more widely scattered. The mucous membrane is covered with gray or dingy-red membranous masses of exudation, of a gelatinous consistence; they can only be pulled off together with the mucous membrane. The cellular tissue is considerably infiltrated, and usually so unequal, that the mucous membrane is raised like warts, in consequence. The intestine is dilated and filled with a blood-tinged fluid, containing no fecal matter but a good many epithelial and exudative shreds. The farther the wart-shaped elevations are extended, the more generally we meet with a purulent infiltration of the cellular tissue, by which the detaching of the infiltrated mucous membrane is facilitated. Ulcers now form, which are the more widely extended the more intense the attack had been, with shaggy, thickened, considerably undermined edges, and having a base of dingy-gray or blackish-colored cellular tissue; sometimes the infiltrated muscular coat forms the base of the ulcer. In the severest cases, the mucous membrane looks greenish-black, or as if carbonized; the purulent or ichorous infiltration is wide-spread; the cellular tissue is necrosed; the muscular coat is softened; the bowel is much dilated, and filled with a blackish, or brown-red purulent ichor. In the higher grades of the disease, the serous coat of the bowels, the peritoneum, and the omentum, are involved in the inflammatory process. We find an exuded fluid in the peritoneal cavity, which inclines to be transformed into pus. The most frequent phenomenon in other organs are hepatic abscesses.

Where the ulcers are not too extensive, they heal without much cicatrization. If the loss of mucous lining is considerable, contracting cicatrices are the result, so that the bowel looks as if twisted around by cords, or presenting valve-shaped contractions. It is upon the duration of this process that the length of the period of convalescence depends.

Symptoms. The breaking out of the disease is almost always preceded by precursory symptoms. The patient feels languid, prostrate, and out of humor; the appetite is, more or less, wanting; there is oppression of the stomach, deranged digestion, and an increased accumulation of flatulence. These symptoms soon increase to nausea and desire to vomit, with coated tongue and foul taste; sleep is disturbed; there is drawing in the extremities, sensitiveness to external cold, shiverings, and an accelerated pulse. These symptoms show that the disease has invaded the organism. Above all, it is the diarrhœa which denotes the local sphere of the disease. Even if all the other precursory symptoms are wanting, diarrhœa generally precedes the attack, in company with slight colicky pains, and without any further characteristic peculiarities. As these pains increase, the diarrhœic discharges occur more frequently, but are, at the same time, more scanty; in the same proportion the tenesmus, which precedes every discharge, begins to distress the patient. At times, after a few fecal evacuations, and at others after a somewhat longer duration of the simple diarrhœa, fecal matter ceases to be excreted; this is the commencement of the real disease. The colicky pains, which are seldom wanting, increase in intensity, become more continuous, and are attended with a painful urging to stool; a sensation as if the bowels would press out of the abdomen, or as though a heavy weight were suspended from the anus, or as if the sphincter ani would tear. When these pains reach their acme, there occurs a scanty discharge, attended with an intense burning at the anus. At first a remission of the distress takes place after this discharge, but the more frequently it occurs, the more the tenesmus increases in violence, and the less it intermits after the evacuation has taken place. The evacuated substance, which, for some time, continues to show a little tinge, soon becomes a mere mucus, with a grayish admixture, or a more or less copious admixture of blood, (dysenteria rubra et alba, red and white dysentery,) and of a peculiar insipid odor. In more violent cases, pure blood is evacuated. According as the disease is more or less intense, the discharges occur every hour, sometimes every few minutes, so that the patient scarcely dares leave the chamber, however difficult it may be for him, owing to the continued violent and colicky pains, to sit up. The pains now become more tearing, cutting, radiating from the umbilicus downwards. The constitutional equilibrium is not much disturbed at the outset. In mild cases the fever is scarcely perceptible, but there are frequent chilly creepings. The pulse is but little accelerated, the temperature of the skin is not much increased. In proportion as the discharges increase in frequency, the pulse becomes correspondingly accelerated, hard and small, the skin hot and dry, the thirst distressing; the desire to vomit increases to real vomiting, although not regularly; the appetite is entirely gone. The patient soon loses his strength, and feels unable to sit up. The affection may continue at this stage for a week, after which it may gradually terminate in recovery. If the local lesions are more considerable, the disease increases in intensity. The pulse grows frequent, small, and feeble, the thirst becomes agonizing, the temperature unequal, the extremities feel cool to the touch, the tongue can hardly be kept moist, the face has a cadaverous expression, and the prostration is complete. Usually the abdomen is meteoristically distended and sensitive. The discharges follow each other more rapidly, and the tenesmus continues uninterruptedly. The discharges, together with the blood, contain shreds of mucous membrane, and a number of membranous fragments. When the disease reaches this height, delirium is not an unusual occurrence. If the disease approaches a fatal termination, the discharges either become fetid, or else they cease entirely, or take place involuntarily, as a sign that the bowel is paralyzed. It is always a bad symptom, if the discharges diminish in frequency without any corresponding improvement. Death supervenes amid symptoms of general prostration, meteorism, delirium, coma. The termination in recovery may be considered certain, if a general improvement is accompanied by a decreasing frequency of the stools, and the colic abates, although the tenesmus still continues. As soon as the discharges evidence fæces, and the fecal odor is restored, recovery may be considered under full headway. The pulse generally continues somewhat more rapid, yet becomes fuller and stronger, and the febrile symptoms disappear. After a severe attack of dysentery, recovery scarcely ever takes place very rapidly; which, as we said above, is owing to the slowness with which the ulcerated surfaces heal; it may also be owing to the fact, that the condition of the digestive organs does not admit of a rapid reparation of the waste, by a copious supply of food.

In armies, especially, the transition of acute into chronic dysentery is not a rare occurrence. The symptoms of chronic dysentery correspond with those of ulceration of the bowels, which indeed constitutes the basis of the chronic form. In such a case the fever disappears entirely, but the diarrhœa continues, consisting at one time of fecal masses, lined with pus and blood, and at other times of a sanguineo-purulent mucus, or changing about with obstinate constipation. At the same time the appetite does not return, and the patients continue to lose flesh. Death is apt to terminate such sufferings, though frequently not until they have lasted a long time.

The severest forms of dysentery, the septic, putrid or typhoid form, are of very rare occurrence in our latitude; they are more frequently met with in hot climates. Such forms arise either because the milder form assumes a malignant type, with all the signs of gangrenous destruction of the bowel, or else they break out at once with an extraordinary degree of intensity, characterized by the signs of a most acute typhus, and rapidly terminating in death.

Strictly speaking, there is no transition into other affections; the hepatic abscesses which do not occur unfrequently, even among us, after a violent attack of dysentery, are most probably due to the absorption of pus into the vessels; or possibly to a disease of the liver, running its course simultaneously with dysentery.

The prognosis, in the dysenteries of our own climate, is emphatically favorable under homœopathic treatment. In the epidemic dysentery of 1846, where old-school physicians lost from ten to twenty per centum of their patients, Dr. Elwert, of Hanover, did not lose one among nearly three hundred. This difference is too striking to be accounted for on any other ground than the inherent superiority of the homœopathic treatment. We do not mean to assert, however, that every case of dysentery can recover under homœopathic treatment.

Treatment. According to our remarks on the etiological causes of dysentery, it is evident that there must be a prophylactic treatment of dysentery, and that it must result in great good. From what we have said on the subject, the single points of this prophylactic treatment can easily be inferred. In this place we desire to call attention to the absolute necessity of keeping the evacuations of dysenteric patients separate. It is, moreover, of the utmost importance to treat every diarrhœa that may occur during epidemic dysentery, with great care, and to arrest it as soon as possible, since it is an established fact that a diarrhœa produces an increased sensitiveness to the dysenteric virus.

Among the remedies for dysentery, *Mercurius* occupies the first rank, and among the mercurial preparations it is the *Corrosive Sublimate*. This remedy corresponds to the symptoms of ordinary dysentery so perfectly, that it may safely be regarded as a specific remedy for the whole process. The leading phenomenon of dysentery, the sanguineo-mucous evacuations without any fecal matter, attended with the most violent tenesmus and cutting colic, is a characteristic and constant symptom of poisoning with Corrosive Sublimate. As evidence that these effects of the Sublimate are not the result of a local action of the poison, we offer the following case of poisoning, from the Dublin Journal, February, 1856: A woman of twenty-five years, of lax constitution, was ordered injections of the Bichloride of Mercury, for ulcers of the vagina. About noon, she injected, by mistake, one third of a drachm in an ounce of water. Immediately after, she experienced violent, labor-like pains, followed by a copious secretion of thin mucus from the vagina. Shortly after, continual vomiting, a burning heat in the stomach, dry and hot tongue, with red edges, dryness in the fauces; afterwards frequent evacuations of a bloody mucus, with violent tenesmus before and after; coldness of the extremities, spasmodic symptoms in the fingers and toes. Pulse frequent and small. The tenesmus continued three days. At the end of this period, symptoms of stomatitis made their appearance. This case is significant, since we rarely meet with a more specifically marked case of poisoning.

These few features of the case contain the whole picture of dysentery, even the preliminary symptoms. The fifty-one symptoms of Corrosive Sublimate, which Hahnemann mentions in his Materia Medica, likewise contain all the essential phenomena of dysentery, among them one, which we did not mention in our previous description of the disease, and yet, is of tolerably frequent occurrence; we mean ischuria accompanying the tenesmus. Here we evidently are in possession of a specific simillimum, and if anywhere, the homœopathic law must find its verification in the application of this remedy. Indeed our literature offers abundant evidence of this fact; we can point to a number of cases, where Corrosive Sublimate alone effected a cure in a very short period of time. The side-remarks with which various observers accompany their recommendation of this drug, are generally of very little consequence. Griesselich informs us, that it is particularly applicable where the local symptoms are very definite, with little fever, and an absence of the acute distress, except the tenesmus; these statements contradict the action of the Sublimate in many respects. It is precisely the violently-cutting pains, proceeding from the umbilicus downwards, that indicate Sublimate; the fever, although generally not very violent in dysentery, is sufficiently well marked. All physicians, however, agree, that the lower attenuations of this remedy are preferable, and that it should not be given higher than the sixth; they likewise agree, that the dose should be frequently repeated. The best plan is to give a dose of the remedy after every discharge: as the discharges diminish in frequency, the medicine will likewise have to be repeated less frequently. The effect of the remedy is perceived very soon, in most cases within thirty-six hours. Of course we cannot expect to perceive a striking improvement in twenty-four hours; nor would it be advisable to follow Griesselich's plan, and select another medicine, if no improvement takes place in that space of time.

It is difficult to draw the line between Mercurius corrosivus and solubilis, as therapeutic agents in dysentery. The Sublimate almost always deserves a preference in epidemic dysentery; Mercurius sol. is preferable in the so-called white dysentery. In epidemic dysentery, the so-called white dysentery is of rare occurrence, and then only a very transitory phenomenon. On the contrary, catarrhal dysentery, is, in every respect, adapted to Mercurius sol., and it is only in exceptional cases that this remedy will prove unavailing. As long as the evacuations contain fæces, although in small quantity, it is well to give the solubilis the preference, no matter whether blood is discharged with the stools or not. On this account, this remedy is especially appropriate in the dysentery of children, especially during the period of dentition. The triturations of solubilis are preferable, whereas the Sublimate acts better in solution. [The *Mercurius vivus* is preferred in this disease by many physicians. H.]

To give *Aconite* at the commencement of dysentery, as Hartmann recommends, is not even justified by the violence of the fever; this kind of treatment only leads to a rather important loss of time. [This slur on Aconite will undoubtedly be objected to by thousands of our physicians. Although not a panacea, yet it deserves honorable mention in this disease, especially when there is considerable loss of blood, and a burning distress in the anus, fever, thirst, foul tongue, headache, dizziness. The lower attenuations, from the first to the sixth, are to be preferred. H.]

Next to Mercurius *Belladonna* is without doubt the most important remedy in dysentery, both the catarrhal and epidemic. As far as local symptoms are concerned, *Belladonna* is indicated by the violent urging to stool, with or without scanty discharge; violent pains in the distended abdomen, they are aggravated by pressure or else evidently of an inflammatory character; liability of the rectum to protrude. Other prominent indications for Belladonna are: considerable urinary difficulties, even retention of urine; violent fever, also with delirium, severe gastric derangement, nausea, vomiturition, vomiting. Belladonna is most frequently suitable for children; less so for adults.

Colchicum is the main remedy in dysenteria alba proper, that is, the weaker forms of epidemic dysentery. The discharges are less frequent, but the tenesmus continues unabated; the colic is not severe, and restricted to the lower portion of the colon, it is a colicky pain; catarrhal irritation of the stomach; tendency to bilious vomiting; not much fever, but great chilliness; urine saturated, dysuria.

The catarrhal form of dysentery being exceedingly varied, a number of other remedies might be recommended for this disease. *Chamomilla*, for instance, is a main remedy in the dysentery of teething children, if the local symptoms are accompanied by acute fever, restlessness, sleeplessness, constant cries, vomiting of bile, nightly exacerbations of the symptoms, or the symptoms only show themselves during night-time. Another remedy is *Ipecacuanha*, when the tenesmus only sets in after the discharge, and there is frequent and distressing vomiting of bile, while the fever is not very considerable; *Dulcamara* and *Pulsatilla*, when the discharges consist of mere mucus; they mostly take place at night. *Baryta*, for the dysentery of children, when it threatens to become chronic, provided there are no striking symptoms of ulceration of the intestines. *Calcarea carbonica*, is adapted to the same form of dysentery as Baryta, likewise applicable to ulceration of the bowel, here it is even a chief remedy for children.

We have already stated, that the above-mentioned remedies are sufficient in epidemic dysentery, unless it should pursue an entirely exceptional, abnormal course, or be complicated with various accessory symptoms. This statement likewise, only applies to cases that have been treated homœopathically, from the commencement. But we are also called upon to treat dysentery in its more advanced stages, or after the system has been saturated with powerful medicines. For such abnormal forms of dysentery, the above-mentioned remedies are not sufficient, and one or more of the following list will have to be selected.

Arsenicum album is never indicated at the commencement of dysentery, only when evident signs of putrid decomposition become apparent, together with paralysis of the bowels and anus, in a slight degree. The evacuations have no longer a peculiarly insipid smell, but are fetid, of a blackish-brown color, mixed with numerous shreds of mucous membrane. The pains are uniformly severe, the fever is intense, attended with signs of rapid prostration.

Of **Rhus toxicodendron,** Hartmann says: " It is particularly applicable in protracted cases, where the violence of the symptoms has been diminished by the previous treatment, but where all the symptoms that characterized the attack from the commencement, are still present; it is prominently indicated by excessive prostration, the blood is greatly deficient in plasticity, the organic activity threatens to become extinct; typhoid symptoms supervene." In other words, Rhus is suitable in typhoid dysentery, if septic phenomena threaten. Hence, Rhus is related to Arsenicum. A noteworthy symptom, is the circumstance that the evacuations appear at night; there are also involuntary discharges.

Colocynthis is scarcely to be regarded as a remedy for dysentery proper, although it may be suitable to some extent, in the catarrhal form. It is variously recommended, but the reasons are not sufficient. The symptoms of Colocynth, bear no very striking resemblance to dysentery. Nor is *Nux vomica*, a medicine that deserves more particular attention than other remedies. On the other hand, it is of importance in lentescent conditions, such as sometimes remain after dysentery. *Aloes* is not yet sufficiently proved, either theoretically or practically, to justify its use, in preference to so many other well tried remedies in this disease.

Concerning **Plumbum,** Hartmann, uses the following language: "The dysenteries to which Plumbum is homœopathic, are very severe, they constitute the so-called red dysentery, where nothing but blood is discharged; they are characterized by violent fever, severe, cutting pains in the stomach, and bowels, burning at the anus during the passage of the blood, and subsequent tenesmus." These statements do not correspond with the physiological action of lead. In the first place, violent fever-symptoms, are an exception in poisoning with lead; and then poisoning with lead acts slowly, like a lentescent fever. Nevertheless, Plumbum is an important remedy in this disease; nor is the constipation caused by lead, a counter-indication to its use. Constipation is an essential symptom of dysentery, for the discharges do not contain any fæces. One case of poisoning, contains the following important symptoms: pain in the right hypochondrium, pressure at the stomach, empty eructations, nausea, aversion to food and drink, a sweetish-pappy taste; dry tongue with a thin whitish coating; frequent, dysenteric discharges resembling rice-water, these are often mixed with blood, with violent tenesmus; cool skin; general prostration. Occasional paroxysms of colicky pains. Afterwards the abdominal walls are drawn in, hard, the stools become involuntary, but the patient is conscious of them. This last symptom is of particular importance, since it points out the period when Plumbum should be preferred to any other remedy, namely: when the rectum and sphincter are paralyzed. Septic, putrid phenomena, are unsuited to Lead; hence, it could not be administered in cases where the violence of the attack had caused gangrenous destruction of the parts, together with paralysis. In such a case, beside *Arsenicum*, *Secale cornutum* would deserve our attention.

According to Hartmann, *Sulphur* is indicated after the intensity of the characteristic symptoms of dysentery has been diminished by appropriate treatment up to a certain point, after which the improvement ceases, and the patient seems to grow worse again. *Acidum sulphuricum* may meet this new condition, unless the present symptoms should point to *Sulphur*. It is most efficacious in dysenteries with nocturnal exacerbations, with discharges of blood, mucus, and pus, fever, loss of appetite, colic, the patient wants to lie down; the colic often sets in with so much vehemence that it causes nausea, and such profuse perspiration, that the patient seems drenched with it. The fever seems to consist of flashes of dry heat, without much thirst. Next to Sulphur, we have *Hepar sulphuris*. This picture corresponds to chronic dysentery with ulceration of the intestines, at the period when colliquative phenomena set in.

We have a few other important remedies adapted to this stage. namely: *Acidum nitricum*, *China*, *Phosphorus*, also *Calcarea carbonica*, The great diversity of symptoms characterizing ulceration of the bowels does not allow of a detailed description of the symptomatic indications for each of these drugs. Moreover, such a condition affords sufficient time to compare the proper remedies with great care.

Regarding diet, the views are very much divided. It is questionable whether the deprivation-diet proposed by Hartmann, and most physicians, is necessary or advantageous to the patient. Slimy decoctions are undoubtedly the best as a regular article of diet, but why the patient should have to drink boiled water, does not seem very clear. Small quantities of fresh water certainly cannot hurt any one, were he ever so sick; at any rate, this requires to be proven. Considering the arrest of digestive activity, it is, of course, absolutely necessary to avoid substances which, when digested, leave a considerable residue of fecal matter. As soon, however, as the patient can make up his mind to taste of it, let him partake of a little pure broth, or rather beef-tea; for we should not forget that the dysenteric discharges carry off a good deal of albumen, and that it is principally this loss which promotes the rapid sinking of strength and the disposition to œdematous swellings. Even when convalescent, the patient should be very cautious in his diet, so that, in case ulcers should exist which cannot be recognized by any perceptible symptoms, the danger incident to such ulcerations should not be increased by avoidable aggravations.

7. Enteralgia, Colic.

Colic is a morbid condition that does not admit of any precise definition. Nevertheless, modern pathologists have felt compelled to allow it a place in their pathological systems, although it does not rest upon any perceptible anatomical changes. We understand by the term colic, peculiar pains in the abdomen, occurring in paroxysms, and attended with a feeling of illness, although not connected with any other ostensible disease of the intestinal canal.

In spite of the scanty rays of light which have as yet been shed upon the true nature of this pathological process, a knowledge of its etiological causes is of great importance, and has considerable influence upon the choice of the homœopathic agent. In one respect, colic may be viewed as a purely neuralgic process, seated in the mesenteric plexus; as such, it is a thing of rare occurrence, and is seldom diagnosed with perfect certainty. In the next place, colic may be caused by the action of certain poisons, more particularly lead and copper, among whose effects upon the organism colic is a standing symptom. Finally, colic is almost always present in every disease of the bowels; of this kind of colic we only range in this category such colicky pains as do not hold a relation of effect and cause to any other special disease. This kind of colic is caused either by the contents of the bowels or the condition of the intestinal walls. With regard to the former, we have a colica flatulenta, stercoracea, verminosa, occasioned by an excessive development of gas, or an impeded motion of the gas through the intestinal canal, by an accumulation of fæces, worms, especially tænia. As regards the latter cause, we only have rheumatic colic, arising from a cold and affecting the muscular coat of the intestines in the same manner as rheumatism affects the muscles of other parts of the body. The colic described as bilious does not belong here, since it evidently depends upon other morbid processes. A genuine hemorrhoidal colic is hypothetical rather than practical; what might be denominated as such, does not belong in this group. Regarding the causes of flatulent colic, we have to name the various deleterious agencies that produce acute and chronic catarrh of the stomach and bowels; rheumatic colic originates in suppression of the cutaneous secretions.

Our best plan is to describe each kind of colic separately, and to add the particular treatment to each description.

Flatulent colic arises from the accumulation of large quantities of gas in the intestines, or from the incarceration of smaller quantities within a definite locality. The former condition is brought about by the use of flatulent food, or of such things as are easily decomposed and occasion the formation of gas; it may likewise be caused by violent emotions, in the case of sensitive persons, especially hypochondriac and hysteric individuals. Among children who are principally fed on milk, and such as are brought up by hand, colic is of almost daily occurrence. An impeded movement of the gases may give rise to colic in such persons as are afflicted with habitual constipation; this kind of colic has the same etiology as constipation. As regards symptoms, we transcribe Hartmann's own statement:

"The pain is as if the bowels were stretched apart, stitching, drawing, cutting, and is alleviated by compressing the abdomen. It is frequently shifting, with rumbling in the direction of the bowels, especially the colon, in which case the pain, moving all round the abdomen as it were, frequently involves the stomach, sometimes even the chest, where the impeded motion of the diaphragm causes dyspnœa. The abdomen is unequally distended in some parts, without hardness or great sensitiveness; sometimes a tense, elastic, painful swelling is felt somewhere, giving a tympanitic sound on percussion, and at one extremity of which, the hard, incarcerating fecal masses can be distinctly felt. In persons of spare habit, and if the bowel is unusually distended, it can be distinctly felt through the abdominal integuments, likewise its peristaltic motion. An emission of flatulence, upwards as well as downwards, affords more or less relief, which is likewise obtained by friction and pressing on the abdomen; if the attacks are very severe, this constitutes an excellent symptom, by which flatulent colic can be distinguished from enteritis. Sometimes the flatulence only reaches as far as the region of the left hip, where it causes an agonizing pain, after which it soon returns again with a noise. If the colic is very acute, it is sometimes accompanied by ischuria, painful erections, coldness of the extremities; in such a case, the pulse is small, even intermittent.

"One such attack does not last very long, but the attacks are apt to come on in a successive series until they sometimes become habitual."

Treatment. To select the proper remedy, it is important to ascertain the origin of the colic. We, therefore, divide our remedies into two categories, those for excessive accumulation, and those for incarceration of gas.

Belladonna. The bowels are only partially distended by gas, and their convolutions are distinctly felt through the abdominal integuments. The pain is pinching or pulling, a clutching as if with nails; is aggravated by an erect posture; ameliorated by bending double, by external pressure, and by lying down. There is retching, anguish, congestions of the head. It deserves special consideration in the case of children, if the bowels are more or less regular.

Chamomilla is suitable in cases to which Belladonna is adapted, likewise principally in the case of children. The flatulence fills the abdominal cavity, moves about violently, and frequently gives rise to a sensation of ineffectual urging to stool. This kind of colic frequently precedes, for days, an attack of intestinal catarrh; the stools sometimes are passed more frequently from the commencement of the attack, without showing any marked changes of any kind.

Cocculus, for constrictive, crampy and tearing pains, principally in the lower part of the abdomen, with partial distension, not relieved by emission of flatulence, with violent pressing downwards, especially on the bladder; very frequently the stomach is full of gas, with frequent eructations. The attacks are easily excited by eating, or they set in during the night. Cocculus is likewise suitable, when there is great disposition to relapses.

Nux vomica is, according to circumstances, appropriate in either of these two varieties of flatulent colic. Hartmann recommends Nux, if the pains are deep-seated in the hypogastric region, and are accompanied by a sensation as if a cutting or sticking instrument were working on the bladder, the neck of the bladder, the commencement of the urethra, the perinæum, rectum and anus, as if cutting flatulence would press out at all these places; the pains are intolerable at every step, so that the patient has to bend double, whereas in rest, when sitting or lying, the pains disappear very rapidly. Where Nux vomica is indicated, the abdomen is never distended, is rather hard and drawn in, the pain is not keen, it is a distressing pressure; the bowels are constipated. Such attacks are not only met with singly as exceptional events, but likewise habitually, after a dietetic transgression, and without any apparent cause, more particularly among persons who, being of plethoric habit, lead a sedentary life.

Lycopodium is a leading remedy where the bowels are obstinately constipated, and where the colic is caused by the stagnant fecal masses, and the attack has been of frequent occurrence. The patients are afflicted to a great degree with habitual flatulence, which increases only at times to colicky paroxysms, more especially at the conclusion of the process of digestion, towards night, or early in the morning.

Carbo vegetabilis should be mentioned in this place as a remedy for colic, where gas is engendered to excess, the emission of flatulence is difficult, and the stomach is involved in the whole morbid process. The distress is felt soon after eating, continues for some time, and only moderates if, after digestion is ended, the gas which is emitted in large quantities, can no more be replaced.

For the colic of hysteric women, Hartmann recommends *Ignatia amara*, and *Asafœtida*. *Veratrum* is frequently an appropriate remedy in such cases, likewise *Cocculus*. The attacks are always very obstinate and, owing to their capricious behaviour, it is a very difficult thing to obtain positive information concerning the effect a medicine has produced.

For the colic of hypochondriacs we give, besides *Nux vomica* and *Lycopodium*, more especially *Natrum muriaticum*.

Beside the remedies we have named, almost any capable of removing constipation, may be administered for the colic of hypochondriacs, which is almost always an habitual condition of the system. [*Dioscorea villosa*, or the wild yam; a few drops of the tincture, every five or ten minutes, is an admirable remedy for this form of colic, likewise for bilious, neuralgic, and rheumatic colic. H.]

Rheumatic colic is next to the form of colic, of which we have treated in the previous section, the most frequently occurring form of this disease. It is always the result of cold, occurs most frequently in the hot season, and in the transition-period from summer to fall. During this period it occurs so frequently, that it seems to act like an epidemic on a limited scale, even side by side with cholerine, and catarrhal dysentery. It is of very rare occurrence in winter.

This kind of colic generally breaks out all at once. In the morning, the patient is roused from sleep by a slight pinching pain in the umbilical region, with urging to stool, yet without diarrhœa; the pinching soon changes to real colic. This colic is seated round the umbilicus, whence it moves downwards, mostly to the left side. It sets in paroxysmally, every hour, half hour or more frequently; is a violent crampy, constrictive pain, attended with rumbling in the bowels, in the region where the pain is felt; this part is somewhat sensitive to contact during the attack, whereas hard pressure affords relief. The violence of the pain often causes a cold perspiration to break out, and even syncope, may occur in consequence, or else the patients moan and hardly know how to keep quiet; the pain is somewhat relieved when the patients bend double, external warmth and an uniformly quiet recumbent posture, with warm covering, afford the most relief. The intermissions are almost entirely, or even quite free from pain. The alvine evacuations are either normal or retarded, or there are three to four papescent stools a day, which, however, afford no relief. The flatulence is not increased, but its passage through the bowels is exceedingly painful. The tongue is clean, the taste normal, the patient has some appetite, though not a great deal; yet the pain is excited whenever he eats a little more than usual. If the pain is severe, the patient may experience some nausea, but he does not vomit. There is no fever, but great chilliness. The attack is frequently accompanied by urinary difficulties.

If left to itself, the affection runs a slow course; while the frequency of the attacks is gradually diminishing, the disorder drags along from two to three weeks, and every slight cold makes it worse again. The strength is not impaired, since the appetite continues, and the patient's sleep, although somewhat restless, is not materially disturbed. It is only when the pain is very severe that a general feeling of weakness takes possession of the frame. In a few cases, the affection is connected with a more deeply penetrating intestinal catarrh, in which the colic continues after the catarrh has come to an end.

The *treatment* of such a colic is very satisfactory. We possess a remedy against it which is almost always effective, whereas every other method of treatment seems without any avail. We mean *Colocynthis*. It acts like a real specific in this disease. All the above-mentioned symptoms are contained in the pathogenesis of this drug, and we have here a fine illustration of the prompt and thorough manner in which a true specific *simile* cures. After giving this remedy the pains seldom continue longer than twenty-four hours, and at the end of this period are, at any rate, very much diminished. Without treatment the colic, if moderately violent, never abates or disappears, under four to six days. It is, however, necessary to give the medicine in a low attenuation, say the second, and to repeat the dose quite frequently, otherwise the certainty of a curative result is very much diminished.

Except Colocynthis, we are not acquainted with a single remedy that acts as promptly and successfully as this one. The disease has such positive indications, without any side issues, that it seems useless to multiply remedies. The only remedy that might possibly be of use, is *Bryonia*, but a mere glance at its pathogenesis shows that the symptoms of rheumatic colic are only very sparingly to be found in it. This disease is only rarely associated with acute intestinal catarrh; the colic, however, will always require our first care, on account of the severity of the pain. We first remove it by means of Colocynth, and afterwards proceed against the intestinal catarrh.

Inasmuch as the colicky pains are very much increased by frequent and copious eating, especially by the ingestion of solid and flatulent food, it becomes a matter of course, that the patients should confine themselves to soups and slimy beverages. In severe cases they should lie down, in milder attacks they may enjoy a little open air. Embrocations of tepid water are not advisable; external warmth, if applied at all, should be applied dry.

Neuralgic colic, which is the real colic, is, as we said above, a rare occurrence. If it does occur more frequently, it is then mistaken for some other disease. How far endemic colic belongs to this category, has not yet been established, *à priori*, however, it does not seem that this colic is a purely neuralgic affection. The following case from our own practice may serve to illustrate the disease.

The son of one of our merchants, eleven years of age, had been afflicted with a very painful abdominal affection, from his sixth year. The painfulness of the disease had been speedily relieved by homœopathic treatment; a subsequent attack of paralysis had been cured by some other homœopathic practitioner. For three years the boy enjoyed good health, until three months previous to our first examination of him, when the old affection, according to the statement of the parents, had set in again. This time the family physician was unable to relieve the child; on the contrary, the distress increased continually. We found the following condition of things: The child had a slender frame, without being strikingly thin. He looked pale, with an expression of suffering in his face, and dark margins around the eyes. He complained of an exceedingly violent colic; it came in irregular paroxysms, independently of the time of day, meals, or other circumstances. It was located in the parts close to the umbilicus, sometimes radiating upwards, or downwards, in which latter case it was accompanied by an increased urging to urinate, with tenesmus of the bladder; it was a crampy, pinching pain, as though the bowels were clutched and twisted with nails. At first these paroxysms of pain had occurred at long intervals, latterly, however, the intermissions had been of short duration; the paroxysms lasted so long a time, that the pain seemed to be continuous. During the paroxysm the patient looked pale as a corpse, the skin was cold, with cold sweat on the forehead. He was very restless, moaned all the time, with his abdomen firmly compressed, nausea, occasional eructations, but no vomiting. The abdomen was contracted, hard, tense. The appetite only began to fail when the paroxysms became more frequent, the child being afraid of eating, lest the pains should grow worse; the bowels acted normally. A careful examination revealed no abnormal condition in the abdomen.

From November 24th to December 28th, the patient took successively: *Cuprum* 6th trituration, *Cocculus* 3, *Plumbum* 6th trituration, *Colocynthis* 2, without any marked signs of improvement being perceived. On the 29th of December he was given *Plumbum* 30, two pellets every third day. From this day the improvement continued rapidly. After taking four doses the patient recovered, nor has any relapse taken place so far. It is now four years ago.

This case corresponds perfectly with Romberg's description of neuralgia, and the treatment suggests a good many reflections. This is one of those cases where the same remedy had no effect in a low preparation, and when given in a high potency, effected a rapid cure. Was this owing to the neuralgic nature of the disease, or to other circumstances? This is difficult to decide, but the case shows that a remedy which is, in all respects, the true simile, should not be given up until it has been tried in its various potencies. *Plumbum* and *Cuprum*, and in some violent cases, *Arsenicum*, are the only remedies from which we can expect curative results in this form of neuralgia.

Saturnine colic is the most constant symptom of lead-poisoning. It is most frequently met with among individuals whose daily business requires them to handle substances containing lead—we mean painters, miners, potters, tin-founders, type-founders, compositors; or it may be caused by water running through leaden pipes, or by snuff packed away in lead, or by hair-dyes containing lead. How carefully we have to investigate, in cases resembling lead-colic, whether the disease is or is not caused by poisoning, is shown by Herapath, in the London Med. Gazette, 1850, where a whole village were attacked with lead-colic, by using water from a brook that flowed at some distance from lead works, and in eight hundred thousand parts of water contained one part of carbonate of lead.

Beside the pains, the characteristic symptoms of lead-colic are: violent contraction of the abdominal muscles, retraction of the abdomen, slow pulse, obstinate constipation. We transcribe Hartmann's description of the disease.

"The colicky pains are at first dull, intermittent; as the disease increases in violence, the pains become twisting, constrictive, boring; they concentrate in the pit of the stomach and umbilical region, whence they spread towards the chest, back, hips, into the upper and lower extremities. Finally, the paroxysms run into each other, the pain becomes continuous, and is often so agonizing, that the patients endeavor to moderate it by tossing about, writhing and twisting, crying and moaning; compressing the abdomen sometimes seems to moderate the pain. The abdominal muscles are sometimes contracted so rigidly that the abdomen is quite tense and hard, drawn in towards the spine, which can be felt through the abdominal integuments. The bowels are obstinately constipated; sometimes an evacuation is obtained, only with incredible effort, in a week or a fortnight, consisting of hard little balls resembling sheep- or goat-dung."

Other symptoms are: loss of appetite, nausea, retching, vomiting of a verdigris-like, or dark bitter substance; strangury or ischuria; retraction and contraction of the sphincter ani; the testes are spasmodically drawn up towards the abdominal ring; the breathing is anxious, oppressed, and even asthmatic, especially during the attacks of colic; the voice is hollow and without resonance, occasional singultus.

Other symptoms of lead-disease, which are frequently observed in the course of lead-colic, are: tearing pains in the limbs, sometimes alternating with the colic, especially at night; if these pains last any length of time, they result in weakness, trembling and paralysis; lead-paralysis has this peculiarity, that the extensor muscles are paralyzed, and the flexor-muscles gain the ascendency, so that, where this phenomenon is particularly striking, the hands are drawn inwards, towards the forearm; very often the pain in the limbs continues at the same time. Other nervous paroxysms are: epileptic spasms, amaurosis, delirium. The patients emaciate very rapidly, the skin becomes dry, brittle, yellowish.

Lead-colic lasts, at an average from a week to a fortnight. Under homœopathic treatment the colic is very speedily cured, yet even under this treatment relapses are unavoidable, unless the cause of the disease is completely removed. After every relapse the lead-poisoning leaves permanent traces behind; the constipation becomes habitual; the patient retains a pale-yellow complexion, remains emaciated, feeble, becomes paralytic, dropsical. A termination in enteritis, or ileus, is of rare occurrence.

Treatment. If there is a disease that can be regarded fixed, remaining always the same, and always reappearing under the same form, this disease is undoubtedly lead-colic. The above-described picture of the disease embodies two forms, acute and chronic. The latter is a sort of slow poisoning by lead that cannot be removed as speedily as an acute attack, for the reason that, when the disease is chronic, the poison indeed penetrates the organism more slowly, but at the same time more thoroughly, affecting every single organ, whereas in the acute form, the abdomen alone is invaded.

In this disease **Opium** is undoubtedly a most valuable specific, acknowledged as such even by allopathic physicians, who prescribe it in connection with oil, in order to prevent the constipating effect of Opium. Homœopathic physicians explain the curative action of Opium in this disease, in a very different manner, for, it is upon its constipating action that the curative power of this drug in lead-colic depends. Hahnemann says: "Opium cures lead-colic homœopathically because the constipation produced by lead, yields to the Opium constipation." According to a vast number of observations, Opium is one of the most efficient remedies againt lead-colic; in prescribing Opium, there is no need of administering at the same time, Alum, purgatives, Hyoscyamus, etc., in which allopathic physicians indulge. In comparing the effects of Opium upon the healthy human body, with the poisonous effects of Lead, we discover a great similarity between these two orders of phenomena; and the curative action of Opium in lead-colic is easily accounted for. The cures reported by Opium are not numerous, but sufficient to show, that a small dose of Opium is capable of curing the colic caused by lead.

Platina is recommended in accordance with the observations of Franz, as even more efficient than Opium. So far, however, this recommendation has not been confirmed by practical experiments. Frank communicates a case, where a few doses of Platina effected, some improvement, after which *Nux vomica* completed the cure. This remedy is variously recommended for lead-colic. For the subsequent paralytic conditions Hartmann praises *Stramonium*, for amaurosis, and deafness, *Belladonna* and *Hyoscyamus*, also, slight electric shocks. According to this author, *Alumina* likewise renders essential service in the after-treatment of lead-colic.

Regarding copper-colic, colica æruginalis, we are as yet without any therapeutic observations; it may suffice if we transcribe Hartmann's views concerning this matter.

"This disease is comparatively of rare occurrence among workers in copper, for the cases of poisoning, which, because they were attended with colic, have been interpreted as cases of copper-colic, have not by any means, been satisfactorily demonstrated as such. The disease commences with a decrease of strength and gradual emaciation, attended with depression of spirits and despondency. Next the bowels act irregularly, we have alternate diarrhœa, and constipation; after these symptoms have lasted for a time, the colic sets in quite suddenly. It is more distressing than lead-colic, the whole abdomen is involved in it. The pains intermit only during short periods, and resemble a severe enteritis; the abdomen is very sensitive to contact, and somewhat distended. At the same time the whole body participates in the affection. The face is pale, sunken, of a greenish-yellow color; the lips are livid, the gums have a slate-color. Paralytic symptoms in the extremities and in the tongue, are seldom wanting. An attack of this kind, which may not recur again until a year has elapsed, may last from four to eight weeks. The difference between lead and copper-colic depends principally upon the distension and painfulness, and the simultaneous involvement of the whole body, and also upon the alternate diarrhœa, and constipation, the former generally prevailing, and being associated with tenesmus."

The treatment must first aim to moderate the phenomena bordering on inflammation. For this purpose *Belladonna* is the best remedy, and if the sensitiveness is not excessive, *Mercurius*. Beside these remedies, we have next in order: *Hepar sulphuris*, *Nux vomica*, and *Veratrum*. Hartmann does not make mention of *Arsenicum*, which, to judge by the symptoms, is certainly very suitable.

The other species of colic, either are no affections of the intestinal canal, and derive their names from the peculiar character of the pain, like menstrual or uterine colic, hemorrhoidal colic, bilious colic, or else they belong in other sections of the work; for instance worm-colic, which will be treated of in the chapter on helminthiasis. [In these different forms of colic, Bæhr omits the mention of *Aconite*. In fla'ulent and rheumatic colic, we have used this remedy with remarkable success. In neuralgic colic it has likewise rendered good service. We use the German tincture, five or six drops, in half a tumbler of water, a dessertspoonful every half hour until an improvement is obtained. We remind the reader of our previous remark on Dioscorea in colic. H.]

8. Stenosis of the Bowels, Occlusion, Obstruction of the Bowels.

There are many causes which either contract the intestine, or render it impermeable to fecal matter. With a view of remedying this defect by therapeutic means, with a prospect of success, it is important that we should be well acquainted with the changes that take place in the bowel.

Simple stenosis of the intestine is sometimes congenital, and, as such, incurable by internal therapeutic means. Acquired stenosis proceeds from the intestinal wall, which may be infiltrated with exuded matter; or it may be caused by the contracting cicatrices of healed ulcers; by the contraction of the intestinal walls in consequence of a continued emptiness of the bowels; and finally by fecal matter, or a foreign body remaining lodged in a certain locality of the intestinal canal.

A second form of stenosis depends upon causes outside of the intestine; among these we number, a twisting of the intestine around its own axis, in consequence of being pulled on by the omentum, or by the inherent weight of the bowel; a sharp bend in the intestine, resulting from adhesions; and finally a contortion of the bowel, in consequence of recent adhesions with the peritoneum, with other organs, or with some other portion of bowel; these adhesions being remnants of more or less extensive inflammatory processes.

One of the most important forms of occlusion, is that caused by incarceration of the intestine. It is either internal, caused by recently formed cords, or openings in the omentum, into which the intestine has forced itself, or else external, if a protruded portion of intestine has become detached from the rest of the bowels by strangulation.

Finally, the bowels may become closed by the process of invagination, or volvulus. In this process, a piece of bowel slips into the bowel situated below it, in such a manner that the latter surrounds the former like a sheath. Since during this process the bowel is at the same time pulled upon by the omentum, the diminution of the diameter of the intestine becomes so much more considerable.

Of the various forms of stricture of the bowels, that caused by an inflammatory infiltration of the intestinal wall, or by incarceration or invagination, may possibly become a subject for therapeutic experiments; hence it is important to obtain an exact knowledge of the kind of occlusion we have to deal with, in order not to injure the patient, and one's self, by futile efforts to effect a cure.

In all the essential points, the symptoms of these different forms of stricture are pretty much the same; they only differ in degree.

The occlusion caused by an infiltration of the intestinal wall, is only partial, so that the passage of the fæces is only impeded, not entirely prevented. That this difficulty is of great importance to the physician, is evident from the circumstance, that an obstinate and long-lasting constipation, is often caused by a stricture of the intestine, whether depending upon a bend, twist, or infiltration of the intestine. Hence, the want of success in attempting to combat such constipations by internal treatment; whereas if the constipation sets in after an inflammatory affection of the bowels, there is some prospect of relieving it, by succeeding in removing the existing exudation. The only characteristic sign of stenosis, is the size of the fæces, which is always very small if the stenosis is situated close above the rectum. If this is not the case, the diagnosis can only be based upon probabilities. Leading diagnostic points are: a partial distension of the abdomen at one place, which does not change; perhaps the possibility of discovering the fecal mass at this place by the touch; the peculiar form of the excreted fecal matter; the symptoms of intestinal catarrh, attended with constipation; and sometimes eructations, having the odor of fæces.

The remedies that have to be tried for this disease, are of the class of those, that either stimulate the activity of the intestines, or exert a decided influence upon the resorption of exudations. In this last respect *Sulphur* is our choice, and if the accident is quite recent, *Bryonia;* in respect to the former, we prefer *Nux vomica*, and *Lycopodium*. If none of these remedies effect even a trace of improvement, it is certain that no cure is possible; and in such a case it is much better to check the disorder by a suitable diet, rather than by means of ineffectual medicines. The patients should use such food as will nourish them as much as possible, without giving rise to much fecal residue. Acute inflammations arising from the local irritation of incarcerated fecal matter, have to be watched and treated with special care.

The symptoms of genuine stricture of the bowels by intussusception or incarceration, are the same at the beginning of the accident. Sometimes several days before more serious phenomena set in, the patients experience a slight, constantly increasing distension of the abdomen, complain of constipation and slight colicky pains. Sooner or later eructations, nausea, and finally vomiting supervene, and it is at this period that a physician is generally sent for. Sometimes these symptoms of stricture set in soon after incarceration has taken place, in which case the patients know at once and without the least doubt, where the somewhat sensitive spot is situated; very seldom, however, the pain is very considerable at the outset. If the above symptoms are associated with hernia, an error in diagnosis is not well possible; a mistake could only occur if the patient should deny the existence of hernia, which is often done by women. Hence a careful examination should be made, if our suspicion of the existence of hernia should be excited in the least. In a case of invagination, an examination will reveal the affected part, where the intestine feels harder or not entirely hard, and is somewhat sensitive to pressure. The whole picture of the disease becomes more distinctly marked, if the invagination is, at an early period, associated with a limited peritonitis; in consequence of which the pain becomes somewhat more acute. After the first vomiting, the symptoms rapidly increase in intensity, so much more so if, either with or without the physician's consent, the patient takes a cathartic. After a cathartic the pains increase in intensity, and the vomiting becomes much more frequent. At first remnants of food, mucus, and bile, are thrown up, very soon, however, the evacuations acquire the odor of fæces. They are often preceded by violent, crampy, or colicky pains, which continually increase as the disease lasts longer. The abdomen becomes more and more distended. At an early period the face assumes the expression of great suffering, with pendulous features and a cadaverous complexion; the extremities are cool, the pulse small and frequent. At times the patient is unable to partake of any nourishment, or only of liquid diet, any other kind of food is very soon thrown up, and with so much distress, that the patient declines partaking of anything in the shape of food. If the abdomen is very much distended, the protruding and distended intestines are seen or felt. While the strength is constantly sinking, a condition of this kind may drag along for a fortnight, of which we had an instance some time ago, in the case of a man seventy-nine years old. With full consciousness death generally takes place amid infinite torture. The exhaustion is, of course, chiefly caused by the inability to partake of food, and, moreover, the excessive painfulness of the spasmodic attacks, which continually increases in proportion as the bowels become more distended.

The symptoms change somewhat, if the invagination does not result in a complete incarceration of fecal matter. Some fæces may pass through and be evacuated, so that we may be mistaken regarding the magnitude of the danger. This, however, is the case, only at the commencement of the trouble, since the opening is soon rendered impassable, either in consequence of the intestine being pulled on by the omentum, or a more advanced penetration of the intestine through the opening. Generally the gases alone have power to overcome the incarceration, so that the distension does not increase so rapidly, and all the phenomena develop themselves more slowly.

On the contrary, the course of the disease is much more rapid, if a more or less extended peritonitis supervenes during the incarceration. Under such circumstances, death generally takes place in a short space of time. We shall revert to this point hereafter.

The terminations of occlusion of the intestines are not numerous; the most common of them is death. If inflammatory symptoms are wanting, the more complete is the incarceration, the sooner death takes place, though seldom before the eighth day. Invagination may heal by sloughing of the intussuscepted portion, and adhesion of the ends of the intestine; generally, however, a more or less considerable degree of intestinal contraction remains behind. Incarceration may likewise terminate favorably, either by sloughing of the intestine, and the consequent formation of an artificial anus, or by establishing a communication with some other portion of intestine.

The prognosis is very unfavorable from the start, if no operative aid can be rendered as a *dernier resort*. It is the more unfavorable, the longer the occlusion has continued, in which case, the probability of exudative adhesions having formed, is the greater. This likewise, applies to incarcerated hernia. Here, however, we have to add, that the strangulation of the vessels very soon causes gangrene, which would render an operation useless. Where the strangulation had existed for several days, all aid by internal treatment will prove ineffectual, and we regard all opposite assertions as resting upon a doubtful diagnosis.

Treatment. We are just as certain that every non-homœopath will smile at the proposition that hernia or invagination can be cured by internal treatment, as we are certain, that in a multitude of cases, the favorable action of internally administered remedies cannot be doubted. On this account, in every case of occlusion of the bowels, we are bound by the sacred obligations of our calling, to associate with appropriate surgical and mechanical means, the use of our own internal remedies, more particularly if the stricture is internal, and cannot be reached by external means. We shall not attempt to reply to the question, how, in such cases, internal treatment can be of any use, and refer, in the place of an answer, to the many practical cases, that abundantly testify to the successful employment of our remedial agents. Moreover, the process of the incarceration itself is a very obscure one. At the same time we should observe, that it is only at the beginning of an occlusion of the intestine, that internal remedies can be employed with success.

The remedies which have been employed, or rather recommended for incarceration or intussusception, are: *Nux vomica, Opium, Veratrum, Cocculus, Cuprum, Aconitum, Belladonna, Bryonia.* Among these medicines Nux vomica holds the first rank, not only as to the number of cases treated successfully by this drug, but in regard to the positive certainty of success. In every case of occlusion, of whatever nature, this remedy should first be used, unless there are evident signs of inflammation. These require either *Belladonna* or *Aconite*. The former deserves consideration, if the distension of the bowels progresses very rapidly; the latter if signs of general peritonitis are apparent. As far as we know, there are no cures with Opium published; its recommendation is based upon general principles; Hartmann likewise admits that he has no observations to offer with this agent. Nor have we any practical observations to advance with Cocculus. The characteristic symptoms of Plumbum emphatically contradict the symptoms of incarceration. It is the constipation that seems to have singled out Lead as a remedy for ileus; whereas Lead causes a severe contraction of the abdomen, which becomes hard as a board: in incarceration, on the contrary, it is always very much distended. *Veratrum* and *Arsenicum* are indicated if a high degree of prostration, or rather inanition sets in. *Veratrum* is preferable if paralysis threatens to set in at an early period of the disease, attended with fainting fits, and cold perspiration; *Arsenicum*, if signs of gangrenous disorganization begin to show themselves. Both *Cuprum* and *Bryonia* are recommended for ileus.

For fecal vomiting (ileus, miserere) without any signs of invagination, we have often given *Colocynthis* with the best result; violent colicky pains were always the precursory symptoms of the act of vomiting.

We would warn the reader against believing, that a cure by any of the above-mentioned remedies is reliable; on the contrary, it is very uncertain and of rare occurrence. But it is on this very account, that, in an affection which is so inaccessible to internal treatment, those remedies should be tried, the more as the patient cannot possibly be injured by them, for no conscientious physician, at the same time that he uses internal treatment, will omit using all proper surgical appliances. In this respect we will add, that the taxis is often considerably facilitated, by placing the patient on his back, with his head low, and the pelvis raised very high; many ruptures which are otherwise hard to replace, sometimes re-enter the peritoneal cavity of themselves, by resorting to this posture; this rule likewise applies to incarcerated hernia. Applications of cold water or ice cannot be recommended, either in hernia or volvulus; in the case of the former, they will neither prevent nor diminish the gangrenous sloughing caused by strangulation of the vessels; nor can they prevent or arrest peritonitis in a case of intussusception. Copious cold injections, on the contrary, are said to have frequently produced excellent results; but they must be cold as ice, and given in rapid succession.

We need scarcely add that in any form of occlusion of the bowels the use of food that may leave a considerable residue of fecal matter, has to be avoided.

[In number 13, vol. IX, of the United States Medical and Surgical Journal, a case of reduction of strangulated hernia by Doctor Bourillon is reported, where the operation that had been decided upon, was rendered unnecessary by the following preparation of Coffee:

Take one hundred grammes of burnt and freshly ground coffee, and five cups of boiling water; make an infusion and strain; half a cupful every hour, taken cold, and a swallow at a time, not to provoke vomiting; such was the prescription. The next morning this hard and unyielding hernia had suddenly relaxed, after the sixth dose, and had returned to its place, with a gurgling sound. A truss was applied at once, and the hernia has not returned to this time.

The following case has all the characteristics of volvulus, except that the stercoraceous vomiting had not yet made its appearance.

It occurred in the practice of Doctor Jacob Reed, Jr., Grand Rapids, Michigan: "Called July 12th to see H. C., ten years of age—a well developed boy, who had passed nine days without having had a movement of the bowels. Found the little fellow suffering from the effects of a large dose of castor oil, which, with other purgatives, had been administered by the mother; no fever; tongue moderately coated; no nausea; tormina, tenesmus, frequent but ineffectual calls to stool; no tenderness over the abdomen, which was somewhat distended and dull upon percussion, except over the course of the colon, which was normally resonant.

"Ordered rest, abstinence from all medicines; a large stimulating injection, which being immediately returned, was replaced by a soap suppository.

"July 13th, eleventh day of retention; tormina and tenusmus increased, and extremely painful towitness; countenance troubled and fretful; fever, vomiting; abdomen tender upon pressure; tongue heavily coated.

"Ordered warm fomentations to abdomen, with a full dose of opium per rectum; this administered at noon, gave the child two or three hours, quiet sleep, after which several copious liquid evacuations relieved the little fellow from his suffering.

"No further treatment was called for."

In a case of volvulus reported in the August number of the New England Medical Gazette, 1867, a cure was effected by giving Nux vomica, Opium and Arnica. We think the Arnica might have been omitted. H.]

9. Hemorrhoids, Piles.

Hemorrhoids undoubtedly belong in the class of the most frequent and most obstinate ailments, and these two circumstances have imparted to them, from time immemorial, a peculiar importance in the eyes of both physicians and lay-persons. Physicians of former schools, guided in their views of peculiar notions, have traced the fact of hemorrhoids to a peculiar disease, the hemorrhoidal disease, a morbific entity, about as fabulous as Hahnemann's psora, from which every possible disease has been, and still is derived by lay-persons. We admit that we do not believe in the existence of such a disease, nor do we require to believe in it, in order to obtain a rational understanding of its supposed phenomena. We look upon hemorrhoids as varicose enlargements of the veins of the rectum, depending upon a variety of causes, and symptomatic of some internal, frequently undefinable pathological process, which, as a consideration of its etiology will soon show us, may assume diversified manifestations. We deem it important to give more emphatic expression to this circumstance, because the hypothesis of an idiopathic disease must necessarily have an injurious effect upon the treatment to be pursued.

Etiology. Hemorrhoids are, almost without an exception, a disease of middle-aged persons; we meet them seldom or never before the age of pubescence; and, if they should exist at this early period, they gradually disappear again in a more advanced age. They occur most frequently among males, in the first place, because the reasons for their existence are more abundant and more deep-seated among men; and, in the second place, because an accumulation of blood in the veins of the rectum is, in a measure, prevented by the menstrual function. Spare individuals, without much adipose tissue, are more frequently attacked than well-fed persons; the temperament does not seem to have any influence in the matter. There is, doubtless, an hereditary disposition to hemorrhoids, but its influence must not be extended too far, for as bodily ailments are transmitted by birth, so, also, are bad habits of the vital process; this latter circumstance accounts for the so-called hereditary hemorrhoids, just as readily and intelligibly as the gloomy mystery of an hereditary constitution.

The varicose distension of the veins of the rectum takes place in the same manner as that of the veins of the thigh, or the less frequent distension of the veins of the arms or neck, in consequence of the impeded reflux of the blood. Whatever is capable of stopping this reflux, must be capable of giving rise to hemorrhoids. From this point of view, the liver and vena porta are some of the primary localities giving origin to hemorrhoids. If the circulation of the liver is disturbed, if the blood received by the vena porta is not carried onward with a corresponding rapidity, the veins lying back of this system become dilated. In a similar manner, but less immediately, disturbances in the pulmonary circulation give rise to hemorrhoids. Thus we find hemorrhoids coexisting with a high grade of emphysema and heart disease; they impede the circulation in the lungs. In a more mechanical manner, varices of the rectum are caused by accumulations of fæces, the pressure of the gravid uterus, swellings in the pelvis. In some few cases none of these more general causes can be traced; the patients are robust individuals, of a healthy appearance, taking a great deal of exercise. In their case, it is not improbable that the disease may arise from a real abdominal plethora, since more nutriment, and consequently more blood, is carried to the vena porta than it can well control. The peculiar appearance of hemorrhoids in persons recovering from a severe disease, may be owing to various circumstances, all of which it is impossible to enumerate in this place.

All those influences which give rise to the above-mentioned impediments in the circulation, may cause hemorrhoids. Among these we number a sedentary mode of living, accompanied by persevering mental labor; a luxurious diet, and the use of quantities of farinaceous substances; the habit of retaining the stool, to which females are particularly addicted from social reasons; the abuse of wine, beer, spirits, strong coffee, sharp condiments; the frequent use of violent drastics; abuse of fat, or starch-containing substances, or such aliments as tend to produce an excess of gas in the bowels. In general, most of these deleterious influences that give rise to chronic catarrh of the stomach and bowels, belong in this category. Hemorrhoids are very frequent among persons who ride a great deal on horseback. It is not very clear why such an otherwise healthy exercise should cause such stagnations in the circulation, whether by arresting the reflux, or promoting the afflux of the blood.

Symptoms. We have to distinguish with becoming care the hemorrhoidal symptoms proper, and those of the ailments that occasion the disorder. The appearance of the varices is almost always preceded, for a longer or shorter period, by a particular feeling of discomfort, or a constitutional condition responding to the ailments which occasion the hemorrhoids. In addition, we have the local symptoms in the rectum, such as tension, pressure, burning, especially itching, also tenesmus. Persons who have not yet been troubled with varicose tumors, complain, moreover, of pains in the small of the back, which are sometimes very severe. The general health is almost always affected in a very specific manner; the patients are easily exhausted by work, are entirely out of humor, irritable, and disposed to feel vexed; not inclined to attend to any kind of work, complain of tightness and dulness of the head, diminished appetite, eructations, restless sleep, also urinary difficulties. The constitutional condition is not improved with the appearance of the hemorrhoidal tumors; on the other hand, an extraordinary improvement is sometimes suddenly effected by a voluntary discharge of blood from the varicose vessels. This bleeding may take place in the very first days of the disease, and sometimes not till weeks have elapsed; it may be very slight, or else it may resemble a perfect hemorrhage, and cause all the phenomena attending a profuse loss of blood. Where no blood is discharged, a copious secretion of mucus sometimes has the same good effect, only the improvement proceeds more slowly. The worst is, when no discharge of any kind takes place, in which case the disorder lasts so much longer. The degree of pain does not always correspond with the size of the swelling; small tumors sometimes are exceedingly painful, large tumors not at all. It is usually when sitting that the patient feels this pain most. After the blood is discharged, the tumor either disappears, or shrinks in size, and remains for some time in this diminished form, or else it continues unaltered. This is generally the case, if the affection has been of long standing.

An attack of this kind lasts from a few days to several weeks. Its return is indefinite; in some it seems to be typical, every month, three or six months; even years may elapse from one paroxysm to the next, until the disease is again provoked by some gross error in diet, or the resumption of some former mode of living in contravention of all natural laws. The influence of the seasons is sometimes undeniable, since most attacks occur in the spring or fall of the year. The whole duration of the disease, from its inchoation to its final termination, extends over a long period; its spontaneous cure scarcely ever occurs before the fiftieth or sixtieth year, and even later. It is only under certain circumstances that the disease runs a shorter course. The hemorrhoids of convalescent patients are not usually very obstinate, and often disappear in a few months. If varices set in during pregnancy, they disappear again a few weeks after the birth of the child.

According to the explanation we have given of hemorrhoids, a recession of these tumors, or a metastasis to other organs, cannot, of course, be thought of. The phenomena that are supposed to have been observed in this respect, can easily be accounted for by the local affections occasioned by the hemorrhoids.

Our remarks on the etiology of hemorrhoids show that the treatment should be conducted, in the first place, with a view of meeting the present attack, and in the second place, with the object of eradicating the whole disease. We cannot possibly expatiate here upon all the details of such a radical cure; these particulars will be found contained in the various sections on affections of the liver, chronic intestinal catarrh, etc. However, we must not flatter ourselves that the hemorrhoids disappear in every case, together with their cause. We find it just as difficult to cure old hemorrhoids as we do to remove varicose veins on the legs; whereas, as we stated before, the varices of pregnant women are easily cured after the birth of the infant. The prospect of a radical cure, in a great measure, depends upon the time the affection has lasted. Where the disease cannot be traced to any particular cause, it is, at any rate, advisable to regulate the patient's mode of life; regularity in going to stool, and moderate eating and drinking, should be insisted upon, in order to deprive the plethora, that may possibly exist, of all sustenance.

The remedies that are at our disposal against this affection cannot well be separated into remedies for the present attack and those for the whole disease, hence we mention them indiscriminately in one series.

Nux vomica is often capable of removing the whole disease, whether the hemorrhoids are fluent or blind. It is indicated, if the hemorrhoids had been excited by the use of strong, heating beverages— wine, brandy, heating beer, and coffee; or by mental labor, deep studies, with a sedentary mode of life, continued compression of the abdomen; or by hard fæces, worms, especially ascarides, (in which case *Valeriana*, *Mercurius*, *Ignatia*, *Marum verum*, may sometimes be indicated; and finally, by the pressure of an impregnated uterus, swelling of the abdominal organs, organic defects of the rectum, or of adjoining parts. If the patients complain of large-sized hemorrhoidal tumors, with burning, stinging pains; if they experience a sensation as if the rectum were constricted, and the passage for the transmission of fæces were too narrow, accompanied by jerking, dull stitches in the small of the back and the ischiatic bones; if the least movement of the body causes a pain in the small of the back, as from a bruise, which causes the patients to exclaim, to walk and stand bent over; if after or between the evacuations pure blood is discharged, attended with urging to stool: *Nux vomica* is the remedy. (Hartmann.) To these statements we will add that what we have said regarding Nux when treating of intestinal catarrh, shows very satisfactorily where this remedy is capable of effecting a radical cure. It is equally adapted to hemorrhoids depending upon a general abdominal plethora, especially if the hemorrhoids cannot be made to bleed, and pain as if they were inflamed.

Lycopodium is equally applicable to isolated attacks, as to the general disease; it is particularly indicated for hemorrhoidal tumors of long standing and large size. The pains are not so very severe, as the influence upon the general health is unfavorable. The leading indications for this remedy are: a yellow-gray complexion, depression of spirits, lassitude and restlessness, which deprives the sufferer of sleep; obstinate constipation and excessive flatulence; considerable distension of the abdomen; discharge of a great deal of mucus with the fæces, liability of the rectum to protrude. Confirmatory indications are: congestive symptoms in the thoracic organs; participation of the bladder in the hemorrhoidal disease, which is revealed by frequent urging to urinate, with discharge of urine rendered turbid by an admixture of mucus, or with streaks of dark blood floating in the liquid. This drug scarcely ever effects a radical cure, but palliates the pains.

Belladonna affords powerful aid against single attacks, if the following symptoms prevail: symptoms of general plethora, congestions of the head, violent pains in the back, febrile restlessness; and with reference to the locality of the pains: violent stitching and darting pains in the anus, sensitiveness of the tumors to contact; colicky pains previous to every evacuation; copious discharge of blood without any special relief. Retention of urine, and spasms of the rectum, afford additional indications for this drug. Belladonna is likewise used externally by physicians of other Schools, and with excellent success. *Aconite* is recommended for the same symptoms as Belladonna, but the favorable results obtained with it, are not quite as numerous as those yielded by Belladonna.

Arsenicum album is only appropriate as a means of cure, in single attacks; its good effects, at such times, are extraordinary, if the whole organism is deeply affected by the extreme violence of the attack. The pains in the anus are intensely burning or stinging, worse at night and during motion; the tumors or bunches are hot, dark-red, and painfully sensitive. The stools are accompanied by tenesmus and great increase of the pains, even to such an extent, that they cause the patients to faint; at the same time they lose their flesh and strength very rapidly. The pains in the rectum, are often associated with urinary difficulties, and violent burning pains in the back, and small of the back. There is much bleeding which, however, does not afford any relief. The blood is of a dark color.

Carbo vegetabilis acts very similarly to Arsenic; the difference is mostly determined by the general phenomena. Hartmann recommends this remedy if there is violent rush of blood to the head, nose bleed, and a continual secretion of mucus from the anus, which stains the linen. For the last-mentioned symptom, *Antimonium crudum* may be compared.

Sulphur is, with Nux vomica, the most distinguished remedy for the hemorrhoidal disease; it corresponds to all the phenomena of the attack, and to many of the general ailments that cause the disease, more particularly to chronic catarrh of the intestines, and to affections of the liver. It is equally adapted to blind, fluent, and mucous hemorrhoids; it is indicated by a constant urging to stool, with either diarrhœic discharges, or hard stool; violent pains in the protruding anus, as if inflamed; considerable pains in the back, and small of the back; painful urination with frequent urging; colicky pains in the bowels; hypochondriac depression of spirits; tendency to copious and exhausting perspiration; congestive distress in the head, and chest. In such cases, if not occasioned, and kept up by local disorder of a malignant character, *Sulphur*, sometimes aided by *Nux vomica*, will often effect a radical cure.

Space is wanting to furnish a detailed enumeration of the symptomatic indications of the other remedies; we mention them, in connection with their more general spheres of therapeutic action.

For copious bleeding, like hemorrhage, the chief remedy is *Arsenicum;* next to it, we have *Creosotum, Sabina, Acidum muriaticum, Millefolium*.

If the varices are inflamed and pus begins to form, we give *Mercurius;* compare, moreover, *Phosphorus* and *Hepar sulphuris*.

If women are afflicted with hemorrhoids, we may have to give, beside the remedies mentioned at the commencement of the chapter: *Ignatia amara, Sepia*, and *Pulsatilla*.

If the bladder is involved, we give, next to *Belladonna, Arsenicum, Sulphur, Lycopodium: Cantharides, Hepar sulphuris, Graphites*.

The general symptoms may likewise point to *Calcarea carbonica, Chamomilla, Acidum nitricum, Capsicum, Phosphori acidum*.

In view of the diversity of symptoms which characterize the hemorrhoidal disease, we could not well help recommending a large number of remedies for it; this multiplicity cannot possibly create the least confusion and uncertainty in the selection of a remedy, unless we lose sight of the circumstance, that the selection of the appropriate specific remedy in the case, is generally determined by the general phenomena, the local symptoms of most remedies resembling each other almost to a hair.

The urgent wish of the patient to be relieved, as soon as possible, of his sufferings, in connection with the conviction, that internal treatment cannot possibly effect a radical cure in a short space of time, will, of course, make it incumbent upon us not to ignore certain external applications that may have power to palliate the patient's distress. Local depletions have scarcely ever had a favorable effect, and should be avoided, if for no other reasons, than that leech-bites are very apt to become inflamed. Moist applications, on the contrary, have an excellent effect. It is impossible to determine *a priori*, whether cold or warm applications are preferable; this should be settled by a practical trial. It may, however, be taken for granted, that when the rectum is dry, cold applications act better, and when a great deal of mucus is secreted, tepid, moist applications deserve the preference. Sitzbaths do not act as favorably, for the reason that their effect is more general, instead of being restricted to the affected locality. Ground flax-seed is the best material for warm moist poultices. If the stools are hard, difficult and painful, tepid-water injections are very appropriate, and better than cold-water, only they must not be used too frequently in accordance with a mechanical routine. Ice-bladders alleviate the pain, but are apt to exert a bad effect generally, on which account they should be used carefully, and not too long at a time.

[For fluent hemorrhoids, when the attack is characterized by profuse bleeding, with a burning distress at the anus, and general weakness, *Aconite*, first and second attenuation of the tincture of the root, will prove an admirable palliative.

Among the new remedies lately introduced into homœopathic practice by Dr. E. M. Hale, several have done good service in the treatment of piles. We call attention to the horse-chestnut, *Æsculus Hippocastanum;* the stone-root or Collinsonia Canadensis; the witch-hazel or Hamamelis Virginica; the golden seal or Hydrastis Canadensis. For particular indications, and clinical observations, we refer the reader to Hale's New Remedies, second edition; published by E. A. Lodge, Detroit, Mich. H.]

10. Helminthiasis, Worms.

The number of intestinal worms that are found more or less frequently in the human bowels, is pretty large. A detailed enumeration of the different kinds of worms is, however, unimportant, and we, therefore, confine ourselves to naming only the oxyuris vermicularis, the ascaris lumbricoides and the tænia solium.

The oxyuris vermicularis, or pin-worm, is the smallest of the three, is one-third or one-half of an inch long, of the thickness of an ordinary thread, and a distinctly perceptible swelling in the place of a head. Usually it is only found in the rectum, seldom through the whole colon, and sometimes even in the vagina, into which it crawls from the anus. At times, only a few are seen together; sometimes, however, they occur crowded together in large masses, most generally among children. The etiology will be discussed afterwards.

The phenomena occasioned by this worm, vary a great deal. One of the most common, is a violent, distressing itching of the anus, especially in the evening and at night, and disturbing sleep a great deal. Some children are driven almost frantic by this itching, and are tormented by an almost unaccountable nervousness in consequence of it. Among adults, this itching is scarcely ever so painful and severe. The irritation caused by the worms, sometimes occasions a catarrhal affection of the mucous membrane of the rectum, or a spasmodic contraction of the sphincter, with a constant urging to stool, which is not less distressing than the itching. If a large number of them penetrate into the vagina, they cause severe itching, fluor albus, and the constant rubbing is apt to give rise to self-abuse. Beside these less important results, we sometimes meet without any otherwise assignable cause, with more important disturbances, principally of the central nervous system, sometimes resulting in indefinite spasmodic movements, and at other times in eclampsia, epilepsy, chorea, etc. We cannot prove that these affections are caused by worms, but this seems the more probable, as a removal of the worms is sometimes succeeded by an entire disappearance of the nervous disease. The treatment will be described in a subsequent chapter.

Ascaris lumbricoides, the intestinal long worm, is the most common of all. It is from six to twelve inches long, has a cylindrical body, tapering at both ends, of the size of a goose-quill. Its common abode is the ileum and colon, the latter, however, less frequently; exceptionally the worm sometimes wanders into the stomach, the duodenum, the biliary duct; it has even been found in the larynx, and the peritoneal cavity. Very seldom only one worm is present in the intestine, generally there are several together, sometimes as many as twenty or thirty, and even many more; in the case of a young man of twenty years, we have seen upwards of one hundred and seventy worms expelled in one week.

The symptoms caused by the presence of these worms, vary greatly. In the majority of cases there are no very prominent symptoms present; it is only by accident that the presence of worms is generally discovered; the only symptom is perhaps an increased longing for rye-bread, and potatoes; and perhaps a less fresh and healthy complexion. More deep-seated and more general derangements, may be caused by a number of worms together, (in the above-mentioned case of the young man, the symptoms were of no account whatever,) or by the agglomeration of the worms into large balls, or by their entrance into some other organ; or else the bowels may be exceedingly irritable, in consequence of which a small number of worms may cause intestinal catarrh or enteritis, together with their consequences. Among these latter, we number the nervous phenomena caused by worms, which have already been mentioned in the paragraph on pin-worms.

The ailments caused by lumbrici, often resemble greatly other more or less important processes, such as gastric fevers, typhus, dysentery, and likewise the above-mentioned nervous derangements; it is of no small importance to ascertain their origin at an early period. These nervous derangements manifest themselves by various phenomena, of more or less constant occurrence. The appetite becomes fitful, or the patient has a more or less exclusive or at any rate, decided hankering for farinaceous food; the nose and anus itch violently; the pupils are considerably dilated; the eyes are surrounded with dark margins; the patients are of a changeable and irritable mood; the fever is irregular and of variable degrees of intensity; bowels act irregularly, at times constipated, at other times alternately constipated and loose, with frequent changes of this character. It sometimes happens, that the helminthic irritation occasions a real gastric fever, which does not always disappear immediately after the removal of the worms; large balls of these worms, may even cause the same functional or structural changes as hard masses of fecal matter. Properly speaking, it is only in children, that lumbrici cause nervous derangements, and it is well, when these derangements manifest themselves, that the physician should direct his attention to the presence of worms.

The tænia solium or tape-worm, is found in the northwestern parts of Europe, in the place of the tænia lata to be met with in other regions of country. It is twenty and more yards long, is smooth the best part of its length, and about a quarter to a third of an inch wide; towards the extremity representing the head, its shape is more rounded and thin, and the head itself is thin as a thread. The color is of a faintish white, with a yellowish tint. The worm consists of the very small head, which is sucked fast in the intestinal mucous membrane, and to which a neck of the thinness of a thread, and half an inch in length is attached, from which neck, the single links of the worm afterwards proceed. At first these links are narrow, but rather short than broad, so that the worm exhibits a series of closely-crowded transverse lines; the further removed from the head, the more the length of these links increases in proportion to their breadth, until the last links acquire a length of one inch and more. A more detailed description of the structure of these worms does not seem required in this place. The worm grows in length from the head outward, until the last full-grown links, become sooner or later detached, and are expelled with the stool. The tænia has its principal abode in the ileum, and is only exceptionally met with in the colon. Generally there is only one tænia found in the same individual, although we are acquainted with one case where twenty-one worms were discharged by the same person. Such cases are, of course, very rare.

As in the case of other worms, so are the disturbances caused by the tænia exceedingly various, both in kind and degree of intensity. It may be safely asserted, that in the majority of cases the tænia causes very little trouble, and that the patients do not become aware of its existence until a few links have been expelled with the stools, when a variety of ailments and distresses are forthwith traced to the tænia, which, in reality, are the work of the imagination, rather than of the tænia. The mildest disturbances which the tænia occasions, are winding, twisting, colicky pains around and in the navel, not very intense, setting in paroxysmally, more particularly after eating certain kinds of food, and in the morning when the stomach is yet empty. Generally these pains are associated with a little nausea, or even with a sensation of canine hunger, but these symptoms are so trifling that they are only complained of when the patient has become perfectly certain that a tænia is growing in his bowels. Under circumstances, which it is difficult to analyze, more intense disturbances may show themselves, a disconnected enumeration of which we here subjoin: violent colicky pains in the bowels, or a creeping or crawling sensation as from a worm, around the umbilicus, with increased secretion of saliva, nausea, even vomiting, especially after eating fermented food, herring, sharp condiments, sour fruit. Increased appetite, canine hunger, in spite of which the patient emaciates; itching of the nose and anus; sickly complexion; hypochondriac and irritable mood; irregular stool, alternately normal and diarrhœic; headache; disturbed sleep, vivid dreams;

palpitation of the heart; changes in the sound of the voice. Finally, the above-mentioned more striking affections of the general nervous system, which can be traced with more certainty to the presence of tænia. The author of this work had an attack of epilepsy at the age of eighteen, occasioned by the presence of tænia; after the expulsion of the worm the attack never returned. Nevertheless, not every case of epilepsy complicated with tænia, must be regarded as a consequence of the tænia, and the physician should be guarded in hastily establishing a prognosis in accordance with this hypothesis; it is only in very recent cases of epilepsy, when the disease is not yet deeply rooted in the organism, that there is a fair probability of the epileptic paroxysms originating in the irritating action of the tænia.

The presence of tænia can only be diagnosed with perfect certainty, if the patient has actually passed links of the worm. Many lay-persons are too anxious to attribute their ailments, gastric derangements, such as heartburn, water-brash, etc., to the presence of tænia; especially if they experience a sensation as if a worm were crawling about in the stomach, or up the œsophagus; if, in such a case, no links are passed within a few weeks, it is pretty certain that there is no tænia. Most links are passed spontaneously at the time of the new moon. We know this from personal experience, for at such a time we have often passed dozens of links in one day; whereas, at other periods no links were seen for days. The discharge generally takes place a few hours previous to the desire for stool, and stops for a few hours after the evacuation.

Etiology. We have preferred discussing the etiology of helminthiasis, after describing the symptoms of the different forms of worm-disease, because the former is very nearly connected with the therapeutical management.

We cannot afford space or time to combat the views formerly entertained, regarding the formation of worms, and content ourselves with repeating what the most careful investigations have established as the truth in this respect; to which we propose to add a refutation of Hahnemann's own views.

Regarding the formation of oxyuris vermicularis, commonly termed ascarides, no definite results have yet been arrived at. In the intestine, female worms are principally found, very seldom male ones, nor are eggs, or embryonic worm-formations met with; this seems to show that the larva of the worm must have been introduced, as such, into the intestine. It is certain, that this worm is principally met with among children, and adults, who partake of a great deal of farinaceous diet. It makes no difference, whether the individual is of a robust or weakly frame. The fact that in many families every member of the household is afflicted with worms, is accounted for by the circumstance that all use the same kind of diet.

The origin of lumbrici is likewise enveloped in a mysterious obscurity. Although of a very general occurrence, they are principally found in children who eat a great deal of bread and farinaceous food, which imparts to them the peculiar habit of body to which the term scrofulous is generally applied. By this means the causal connection becomes, at all events, more intelligible and amenable to a philosophical analysis, than if the worms are regarded as the cause of such a condition. Female lumbrici likewise exist in larger number in the intestine than male, although the number of male lumbrici exceeds that of the female oxyuris; every specimen seems to have progressed in its development; there is no embryonic stage, no deposition of eggs; here too, we seem compelled to adopt the theory, that the worm must have been introduced as such into the bowels.

The adoption of an hypothesis of this kind becomes the more a necessity as we are perfectly acquainted with the manner in which the tape-worm is introduced and originated, and are somewhat justified in reasoning from analogy, concerning the formation of other worms. Tænia arises from the cysticercus cellulosæ, an animal parasite, which changes to a bladder of a larger size, to which a head, seated upon a neck, is attached. This head is provided with a crown of retractile hooks, and with four suckers. If the cysticercus reaches the interior of the intestine, it hooks on to the intestinal wall, throws off the tail-shaped bladder, and from the neck grow out the above-described articulations. This proceeding has been demonstrated, by Küchenmeister's investigations, as an undeniable fact. The cysticercus is most frequently met with in the hog, and less frequently in cattle; it is killed by roasting, boiling, and thorough smoking; hence can only be introduced into the human economy as an animated parasite, by the use of raw or badly smoked meat. This circumstance accounts for its rare occurrence in districts where little pork is eaten, or among the Jews; and the frequency of its occurrence in middle-aged individuals. Since the fashion has recently been introduced, of feeding children on raw meat, we have met with several instances of tape-worm, even among children scarcely fifteen months old.

After what we have said, and according to all well-established facts bearing upon this point, it seems to be undeniable, that not one of the various kinds of worms owes its existence to a peculiar pre-established disposition in the intestinal canal, but that they may develop themselves in every individual living under like external circumstances; hence that helminthiasis is not a disease *sui generis*. At the same time, we must not omit to state that worms may cause derangements that may still continue after the removal of the parasites, for the reason that their peculiar character, or their intensity, have made them independent diseases.

Treatment. The question now is, how far these recently established facts, concerning the formation of worms, affect the treatment of this abnormal condition. Hahnemann asserts that the cure of helminthiasis consists in removing the morbid disposition in the intestine, which engenders and sustains the worms. This view corresponded perfectly with Hahnemann's time, and we must not deem it an original idea of his, if he considered the removal of the worms as perfectly indifferent, and depended, for a complete cure of helminthiasis, upon the action of infinitesimal doses of the homœopathic remedy. It is inconceivable, that there are homœopathic physicians at the present time who still advocate Hahnemann's doctrines on this subject. Even if we admit that many morbid conditions, caused by worms, can be moderated, and even entirely removed, without the expulsion of the worms, this, certainly, does not mean that the helminthiasis is cured by such a result. It is not by any means true that an intestine which is morbidly affected by worms, must have been previously diseased, otherwise, the worms could have had no influence over it. Nor can it be alleged, in favor of Hahnemann's views, that morbid conditions of a very obstinate character sometimes remain after the removal of the entozoa; if an enteritis, caused by worms, has resulted in ulceration of the intestines, it takes, of course, time to heal the ulcers.

We need not extend these remarks farther, as homœopathic practitioners generally no longer share Hahnemann's views on this point. If we mean to act as true physicians, we have to proceed in the treatment of helminthiasis as in that of any other pathological process; and have first to remove the cause, provided we are certain of having a correct knowledge of what it is, and where located. After having accomplished this object, we proceed to the further treatment of the remaining ailments. Hence, in the present case, our first aim should be to remove the definitely known cause, or in other words to exterminate the entozoa. If, after having allowed the organism sufficient time to resume its normal condition, any derangements of the normal functions still remain, they will easily and permanently yield to the influence of suitable homœopathic specifics. Of course the diet will have to be regulated in accordance with what we have stated in the etiological chapter; otherwise, the same deleterious causes might reproduce the same morbid results.

Of all three kinds of worms, the expulsion of the oxyuris vermicularis, is, by all odds, the most difficult, because the least certain. This may be owing in a measure to the fact, that after the worms have once been expelled, a continuance of the former faulty mode of living soon causes a reproduction of the parasites. The mode of proceeding being very simple and harmless, it can, and may be easily repeated quite frequently. Internal remedies are inadequate, for the reason that the worm is lodged in the rectum, and does not easily come in contact with the poison. Remedies used internally may, moreover, cause hurtful accessory symptoms, which had better be avoided. Hence the proper method is to employ remedies exter nally, since they come immediately in contact with the entozoa. For this purpose we resort to injections, for which a variety of substances may be used, from simple cold water to solutions of Corrosive Sublimate, *Sabadilla, Cina, Hepar sulphuris,* etc. All these remedies have been employed with success; some, however, are too dangerous agents to be employed, without further thought, against such trifling inconveniences as worms. We have generally been able to proceed to our perfect satisfaction with simple garlic, or *Allium sativum.* A few drachms of fresh garlic are cut fine, boiling water is poured over it, and this infusion is used as an injection, as soon as it has sufficiently cooled. The worms which this injection reaches, are certainly killed by it; hence it is well to use a large injection, in order to secure its ascension high up in the bowels. If worms should again show themselves, the injection must be repeated without loss of time. After the expulsion of the oxyuris, morbid symptoms will seldom remain visible; at any rate, they will soon disappear, such as the discharge of mucus from the anus. The remedies which homœopaths use against the ailments caused by oxyuris, either have reference to single ailments, or to the removal of such changes in the intestinal canal as have hitherto been regarded as the causes of worms. These remedies are: *Aconite, Cina, Ferrum, Mercurius, Cuprum;* a second series are: *Calcarea carbonica, Sulphur, Ferrum.* After what has been said, we do not deem it necessary to enter into any further details concerning the use of these agents. The same diet has to be pursued as indicated in the subsequent paragraphs, where the management of lumbrici is treated of. [Weak injections of *Fowler's solution,* from fifteen to twenty drops to an ounce of water, or *Carbolic acid* in the same proportion, or stronger, will often destroy the worms; the injection must not be thrown up high in the rectum. H.]

The lumbricus, being lodged in the ileum, is not immediately accessible to external remedies; hence can only be reached by internal treatment. *Cina* seems to act as a true specific against this parasite, and, with proper management, no other medicine need be used. As regards the administration of the *Semina cinæ,* we find it particularly inconvenient in the case of little children; accessory medicinal symptoms are likewise frequently caused by their use. They occur only feebly, and not very often after the use of *Santonine,* which is now almost universally used. Children mostly prefer it in the form of *Troches Santonini,* which generally contains one grain of the drug. From two to four troches, according to the age of the child, are given at night before bed-time, on two successive evenings. Care must be taken not to feed the children too much on farinaceous diet, on the day previous. The period between full and new moon is generally looked upon as the best time for the administration of the drug. Adequate experiments in an opposite direction have not yet been made; the method proposed commends itself from the circumstance, that at this time the worms are most frequently discharged spontaneously. Cathartics are entirely unnecessary. If the troches are not to be had, the Santonine can just as easily be given with sugar of milk. Frequent doses should be administered, if the worms are numerous.

The homœopathic remedies against ailments caused by lumbrici, are the following: *Cina, Nux vomica, Spigelia, Belladonna, Mercurius, Calcarea, Pulsatilla, Antimonium crudum,* and a few others less frequently used. It is difficult to say where each of these remedies should be given. According to Hartmann, *Nux vomica* is indicated in worm difficulties, if the abdomen is distended and sensitive, with a feeling of heat in the bowels; the stool is hard, there is a disposition to vomit, nervous irritability and aggravation of the symptoms early in the morning. For such symptoms, Nux should be given, whether worms are present or no.—Likewise *China:* nightly aggravation of the pains; after every meal the patient complains of a painful colicky pressure under the umbilicus, with repletion of the abdomen, heartburn with accumulation of water in the mouth, oppression at the stomach and retching; extreme nervous sensitiveness, with spasmodic muscular twitchings and tremulous weakness. Worms are certainly not required to indicate China for such a group of symptoms. *Cina* is an important remedy if the worm-symptoms are complicated with symptoms of cerebral derangement; it is here that the symptoms might easily lead us to the adoption of some other remedy. Where Cina or Santonine has already been employed in large quantities, neither will be found adequate when given in small doses; nevertheless, if the worms are not to be expelled immediately, a small dose may be found sufficient to remove the following more or less threatening symptoms: evening-chilliness, with small, rather hard, frequent pulse; not much sleep; tossing about in bed, crying out and starting during sleep; ill-humor, imbecile appearance, passing attacks of delirium, heaviness of the extremities; the face is at times pale and cold, at other times red and hot; dilatation of the pupils; constant rubbing at the tip of the nose; obstruction of the nose; slimy coating on the tongue; offensive eructations; vomiting; heat and distension of the abdomen; colicky pains in the bowels; constipation, involuntary emission of urine.—Beside the above-mentioned remedies, *Zincum* and *Valeriana* deserve especial attention if spasmodic symptoms are present. As a general rule worm-ailments should be treated as if no worms were present; hence it is unnecessary to single out any other remedies.

In the case of lumbrici, as well as ascarides, the diet should strive to attain a twofold object; in the first place to prevent the production of new parasites, and in the second to protect the already enfeebled or diseased intestinal canal. Respecting the first point, farinaceous food has to be partaken of as little as possible, and, if used, good sweet flour should be employed. Respecting the second point, the same precaution will have to be used, that has been recommended regarding the chronic intestinal catarrh of children. If Hartmann cautions against the use of milk, we cannot conceive of any possible reason for such advice. Milk is the best nourishment for the human organism, at any rate it never does any real injury. Much sugar or pastry should of course be avoided, were it only for the reason that even the best digestive powers are weakened by such abuse.

In order to remove the ailments caused by the tænia solium, the worm will in the first place have to be extirpated. The remedies that have been recommended for this purpose, not to mention the horse-cures that were formerly in vogue, are: *Punica granatum, Polypodium filix mas, Kousso,* and *Rottlera tinctoria,* (Kameela.) Every one of these four remedies is reported to have effected radical cures; which of them is the best, has not yet been decided with certainty. If the superiority of any of them is measured by the trifling nature of the drug-symptoms it produces, Kousso undoubtedly carries off the palm. The powder of Kousso is best administered in the following manner: From two and a half to three drachms are placed at night in a common tumbler, and cold water is poured upon it; care must be had to prevent any of the powder floating on the liquid. Early next morning this mass, after having been well stirred previously, is swallowed in two portions, leaving an interval of half an hour between. A preparatory treatment is not exactly required, except that no farinaceous food should be used for a day or two previous to the cure. To prevent nausea, a small cup of black coffee may be drank before taking the medicine, and if a disposition to vomit should be experienced nevertheless, a little lemon-juice may be swallowed. One and a half to four hours after taking the medicine, the worm is expelled without the use of cathartics. We have found this proceeding efficacious in a number of cases treated by ourselves, only one case acted differently. The patient was a robust young woman. She had taken the medicine as directed, but twenty-four hours elapsed without any worm being passed. Without my advice she took several mild cathartics, but no worm came away with the diarrhœic stools. Not till full eight days had elapsed, the worm was expelled in the shape of a hard ball wrapt in mucus and fæces. The bark of the Punica granatum is given in infusion, or in the shape of an extract; Filix mas is given in infusion or as an extract, also in tincture-form. If we do not at once expect the most complete success, namely the expulsion of the whole worm, head and all, Kousso is the best remedy. If the tænia should grow again, the cure can easily be repeated; for the expulsion of the worm does not leave the least medicinal symptoms. So far we are only acquainted with one case where the tænia grew again, after having been expelled by Kousso.

A refutation of the rules laid down by Hahnemann, Hartmann, Hering and others, concerning the treatment of tænia, is deemed by us superfluous. At the time when these rules were published, the conditions which give origin to tænia, were absolutely unknown. If any ailments remain after the worm is expelled, we treat them without the least reference to the previous presence of the worm. Those who do not wish to be again molested by this parasite, have to abstain from the use of smoked or raw meat.

C. DISEASES OF THE PERITONEUM.

There are, strictly speaking, three kinds of idiopathic diseases of the peritoneum, namely: inflammation, puerperal peritonitis, and ascites. But inasmuch as, for many reasons, the second kind had better be treated of among the diseases of the female organs of generation, and ascites in the chapter on dropsy generally, all that remains for us to do here, is to treat of the first kind.

Peritonitis, Inflammation of the Peritoneum.

In Hartmann's Manual a description of true peritonitis is entirely omitted, although the acute or phlegmonous enteritis corresponds tolerably well to peritonitis. An omission of this kind can only be accounted for upon the ground, that Hartmann supposed the peritoneum is always inflamed if the intestines are. As little, however, as pleurisy and pneumonia can be regarded as one, as little can enteritis and peritonitis be considered identical. Peritonitis acquires importance for the reason that the peritoneum is a serous membrane and, moreover, a serous membrane that is the most extensive of its kind in the whole body.

If we include the circumscribed forms of peritonitis, this inflammation is one of the most frequent we know of; as peritonitis diffusa it is, of course, of less frequent occurrence. If affects more particularly, middle-aged persons, and is very seldom met with among children, or among old people. The disease, for reasons which will be stated bye and bye, is more frequently met with among women than men. It is infinitely less frequent as an idiopathic affection than as a secondary disease, probably because the peritoneum is well guarded by the thick abdominal integuments, against the action of external deleterious influences.

In the main, the origin of the disease is traceable to the following causes.

After all injuries which bring the peritoneal cavity in contact with atmospheric air, peritonitis may be expected in the majority of cases. Although the inflammation very often remains confined to the injured locality, yet it will almost certainly spread over a larger portion of the peritoneum, if blood, pus, or a certain quantity of atmospheric air enters the peritoneal cavity. This point deserves the utmost consideration in operations upon the abdominal cavity. The danger of inflammation is likewise greater, if the abdomen is very much distended before the operation, and collapses after it; hence, peritonitis is very apt to occur after the Cæsarean operation, after tapping for ascites, and after operations during confinement.

An intense cold will sometimes cause peritonitis among persons, who are otherwise perfectly healthy. Among women, a cold may be a matter of great importance. There is no question, that confinement and the menses are very apt to cause peritonitis; especially if a cold supervenes at such times. This observation is so common, even among lay-people, that women have become accustomed to be very careful at such times. The disappearance of the menses, or of the lochia, at the commencement of the inflammation has given rise to the theory, that it is this suppression which causes the inflammation; it seems to us more simple, and more natural, to reverse this relation of cause and effect. During confinement, the collapse of the distended abdomen exerts a powerful influence; hence, peritonitis is more apt to occur in the case of women, who have borne several children, than among primiparæ.

One of the most frequent causes of peritonitis are the inflammatory conditions of the organs, situated close to and within the peritoneal sac; the inflammation being communicated, either in consequence of its proximity to the serous covering, or else in consequence of the pus gradually penetrating to the peritonæum. Thus the disease is met with as an accompaniment of gastritis, of affections of the bowels, ushered in with hyperæmia, or inflammation; more particularly, in consequence of conditions which occasion an occlusion of the bowels, or in consequence of affections of the liver and spleen, metritis, inflammation of the psoas-muscle, abscesses on portions of the abdominal walls. All these causes, at times result in circumscribed, at others in diffuse inflammation.

By far the most violent forms of peritonitis, and which run the most rapid course, occur if an organ becomes perforated, and its contents, or even the smallest portion thereof, escape into the peritoneal cavity. This occurs most frequently in the case of perforating ulcer, ulcerations of the intestines, perforation of the vermiform process, and gangrenous destruction consequent upon stricture of the intestine.

Symptoms and course. These of course not only differ in degree, according as the inflammation is confined to small portions of the peritoneum, or, as diffuse peritonitis, invades the whole of the peritoneal expanse; even the diffuse form differs, according as it develops itself suddenly, or by degrees.

Acute, diffuse peritonitis, either if caused by perforation, or when setting in as an idiopathic affection, almost always commences with a severe chill, attended with pain in the abdomen. This pain, which is the most characteristic symptom of the disease, is most intense from the very moment it is first felt. The pain is, as though a pointed knife were plunged through the abdomen, from above downwards, without the patient being always able to indicate the precise starting-point of it. Immediately after, a feeling of illness overtakes the patient, he feels unable to remain up, and he is satisfied that a severe sickness is upon him. If peritonitis sets in, in consequence of the gradual spread of some other affection of the bowels, its own development is gradual; the existing local pains increase in intensity, and gradually spread over the whole abdomen, at times rapidly and at others more slowly. In violent cases the invasion of the pain is not at once followed by violent fever; on the contrary, the patients die in a state bordering on syncope, with cold faces and cool extremities, and it is only the extremely hurried pulse that indicates the approach of a violent fever, which is scarcely ever more than twenty-four hours in coming. From its first beginning, the pain never abates one moment, except, that it sometimes seems more like a colicky pain; as the pain spreads the abdominal walls become so sensitive, that the patients cannot bear the least pressure, so that it is even a relief to them, if the blankets or sheets do not touch the abdomen. The least motion increases the intensity of the pains to such an extent, that the patients have to lie on their backs motionless, and dare not draw a deep breath, because the pain is aggravated by the pressure of the descending diaphragm; they even have to speak in a low whisper. The pains are at times tearing, at others stinging, lancinating, but most of the time fiercely burning, and with a soreness as from an open wound. Sometimes the disease sets in with violent vomiting, and diarrhœa, almost like cholerine; in such a case, the act of vomiting causes intense suffering. The general symptoms betray at first sight the existence of an intense disorder. At the first onset of the disease the face looks pale, with a peculiar expression of distress and anxiety, and with pendulous features; afterwards the face looks flushed, or else the paleness remains throughout the whole disease, in spite of the fever. The eyes are dull and unsteady. The breathing is hurried, is carried on with the ribs only, the speech is short, a mere whisper. The tongue is usually quite clean; there is a craving for cold water, yet only a small quantity can be drank at one time. Retching and vomiting, unless present at the first, are very apt to supervene; otherwise these phenomena and the diarrhœa disappear as the disease increases in intensity; as a general rule, the peritonitis is attended with complete retention of stool the first eight days of its existence. The urine is always less; voiding it is often painful, or there is a constant urging, yet no urine is voided. The pulse is hurried, from one hundred and twenty to one hundred and sixty beats, and soon becomes small, hard and tense. The skin is dry and constricted, although profuse and exhausting sweats sometimes break out; the temperature varies from a burning heat to a disagreeable coolness. An examination of the abdomen is difficult on account of the pain, which is aggravated by the least attempt at percussion. Soon after the pains are felt, the abdomen becomes more and more distended, so that the distended bowels can be felt through the abdominal walls. The percussion-sound, which at first continues tympanitic, soon changes to a dull sound at the pendulous portions of the abdomen; but it is only in exceptional cases that the sound becomes perfectly empty, for the reason that the exudation is never sufficiently copious; in one very violent case, however, the dulness extended over the abdomen from one side to the other, as high up as the umbilicus. In the subsequent stages of the disease, the boundaries of the exudation, if it acquires sufficient consistence, can be distinctly felt through the abdominal walls. At the commencement of the disease, the brain and the sensorium seem unassailed, except that the patient sometimes complains of violent headache. The sleep is very much disturbed; if the patients sink momentarily into a sort of slumber, they at once become delirious. All such patients habitually lie on their backs, with the lower extremities slightly drawn up toward the abdomen.

In the further course of the disease, the symptoms generally undergo the following changes: The distension of the abdomen increases more and more, although its painfulness to contact generally decreases in proportion as the exudation becomes more copious; it even happens that the sensitiveness disappears entirely. This however, is a bad symptom, if at the same time the whole condition of the patient seems to change for the worse. The difficulty of breathing corresponds to the degree of meteoristic distension. The anguish increases, the lips become bluish. The pulse is a little slower than at the commencement of the fever, but its quality remains the same; it does not indicate any remission of the fever, whose intensity continues unabated. If the disease terminates fatally, the general sensorium is overwhelmingly brought under its influence, the patients grow apathetic, do not feel any pain; the pulse becomes imperceptible, the face has a sunken, cadaverous appearance. Death may take place in thirty-six hours, and seems to be principally caused by paralysis of the bowels; the disease, however, seldom terminates in such a short period of time; it generally continues until the seventh day.

If death does not take place at this first onset of the disease, its further course depends upon the quantity of the exudation, and the changes it undergoes. In order to more clearly comprehend these processes, we will first give a description of the anatomical changes that take place in this disease.

At the commencement of the attack the peritoneum appears slightly red, sometimes even ecchymosed. The redness is seldom general, on the contrary, it occurs in isolated spots, of greater or less extent. At the same time the surface soon acquires a faintish velvety appearance, without lustre, and soon becomes covered with a thin layer of exuded, mucus-like fluid. At this period we already begin to discover traces of exudation in the peritoneal cavity. The thin layers of exudation, which likewise loosely line the intestines, may remain the sole product of the inflammation; in such a case, adhesions easily take place between the bowels and the peritoneum, or between the bowels themselves, which either remain, or by the dragging action of the bowels are changed to ribbon or thread-shaped bridges, between the peritoneum and the abdominal viscera. The thicker these layers of exudation, the more copious the fluid exuded in the peritoneal cavity. This fluid contains a great deal of fibrin, is more or less turbid, mixed with flocks, even with fibrinous coagula, and generally contains pus-corpuscles in varied quantities. Sometimes an excess of serum is poured out, in which case the fibrin is, of course, much less, and a copious admixture of albumen generally occurs; in such a case the color is always darker, with a reddish or brown tint.

The changes in the exuded fluid generally vary greatly. In favorable cases the fluid is first reabsorbed, and the solid parts remain for some time behind, before their gradual removal is effected; generally, however, isolated thickenings of the serous coat, or more or less considerable adhesions, remain as traces of the previous inflammation. Or a larger quantity of pus may form, in consequence of which a great deal more of the serum is reabsorbed, and more copious adhesions take place, spreading like sacculated foci over a large extent. Here, too, reabsorption is possible, leaving, however, considerable thickenings behind. Or an abscess may form which, when situated near the surface, and without too much resistance on the part of the abdominal walls, will break outwardly; whereas in the opposite case it finds an outlet into the interior of the intestine, or burrows downwards, following the course of the psoas-muscle, and causing further alterations in the lower extremity. The copious serous exudation, unless absorbed at a very early period, may lead to phenomena resembling those of ascites, and may obstinately persist for some time. If the peritoneum is only partially inflamed, the exudation in the peritoneal cavity is usually quite unimportant, and the super-imposed layers of exudation have the greatest disposition to form adhesions which, however, do not preclude the local formation of pus. A malignant change is the metamorphosis of the exudation into tubercular masses, which may easily occur in individuals of a tuberculous habit.

In accordance with these anatomical changes, the disease assumes a different form as it progresses. If a most favorable metamorphosis should occur, and the effused fluid should be reabsorbed without any further difficulty, the abdomen gradually becomes softer, the bowels are less distended, and begin to move, which is always looked upon as a very favorable symptom, and, above everything else, the respiration becomes less embarrassed. At the same time the pulse may remain accelerated for a long time, at any rate it is only exceptionally that it falls below 120 before convalescence is complete. The expression of the countenance likewise is a sure sign that a favorable change has taken place. Sometimes the improvement sets in with a copious increase of the urinary secretion. Percussion and palpation soon reveal a considerable decrease of dulness, showing that the absorption of the fluid is going on, while the solidified exudation is, at the same time, more distinctly perceptible to the touch, and feels like a row of callous, unequal, bunchy indurations. Under certain circumstances the disease may remain stationary at this point for weeks; the pulse remains hurried, the strength will not return, the appetite continues indifferent, and the exudation does not diminish. The patient is, moreover, tormented by frequent colicky pains. Not.unfrequently sudden aggravations set in at this time, giving rise to the most serious apprehensions, and greatly prolonging the disease. From fear, the causes of such aggravation are sometimes kept concealed from the physician, especially if dietetic transgressions had been committed, or the patient had been very much excited by untoward occurrences. In a case of diffuse metro-peritonitis, which occurred in our own practice, a dangerous aggravation was caused four times in succession, in consequence of which the disease was protracted for a period of sixteen weeks, which delay we were unable to account for, until the patient herself, having fully recovered from her disease, explained the cause. All sorts of mortifying communications concerning her husband and sister had been whispered into her ear by a relative. This shows how delicately and carefully such patients should be treated, as long as the exudation is not entirely absorbed. It is remarkable how rapidly the absorption of apparently solidified masses is carried on in women whose constitutions are otherwise sound, at least up to the point when the exuded substance becomes imperceptible to the touch. A single week is sometimes sufficient for this purpose. From this time the patient begins to feel decidedly better; the appetite improves, the pulse almost becomes normal, the cutaneous functions are restored to their natural condition; only the colicky pains still continue to be experienced in the diseased locality, although the evacuations have resumed their natural course. For some time a considerable tendency to unimportant aggravations remains.

On the contrary, if the exudation becomes purulent, the fever likewise abates at first, the pains become less, the meteorism and the consequent oppression of breathing and retention of stool decrease, the dulness on percussion is less extensive, and the solidified exudation is felt more and more distinctly. But there is no increase of strength, on the contrary, the patients become evidently weaker, and look much worse. After a previous violent chill, the fever gradually returns, in paroxysms, to the original degree of intensity, the skin remaining mostly dry. It is only in the later stages of the disease that the fever assumes the full type of a hectic fever, and is accompanied by colliquative sweats. The exuded fluid forms distinct sacs, imparting a striking irregularity to the abdominal walls; they are less hard, and have a doughy feel. In this way the patient may linger along for many weeks; even if we succeed, which is seldom possible, in effecting absorption, it proceeds slowly, and is scarcely ever complete. Death may simply take place from exhaustion, without the pus having been liberated. If an abscess should form, or the pus should penetrate into other organs, the question always will be what course the organism will pursue in trying to counterbalance this abnormal process. The relief succeeding the discharge of the pus is either permanent and followed by an increase of strength, or else it is only momentary; and colliquative phenomena set in rapidly, and with redoubled violence. Finally, the purulent discharge may give rise to another inflammation and consequent death.

Peritonitis, with prevalent tendency to decomposition, has its prototype in puerperal peritonitis, when treating of which, full information will be communicated on this point.

The transition to tubercles is marked by similar symptoms as the purulent metamorphosis, except that the fever is less violent. The disease runs its course with all the symptoms of phthisis, concerning the details of which the chapter on tuberculosis may be consulted.

According to what we have stated, it is not always possible to determine the duration of the whole disease with anything like certainty at the commencement of the outbreak. If in a violent case, with extensive inflammation, the first week is happily passed without any unfavorable changes, the prospect of a good recovery is well founded. But if the reabsorption of the effused fluid is delayed beyond the fourth week, the danger is great; nor is it diminished by the longer duration of the disease. Under the form of a so-called chronic peritonitis, the disease may drag along for many months, and its consequences may remain visible throughout the patient's lifetime.

The terminations of peritonitis differ according as the disease has been treated homœopathically or allopathically. We feel at liberty to give a more favorable prognosis in this disease, which is generally regarded as very fatal, than any other method of treatment is authorized to do. Our remedies not only prevent the exuded fluid from changing to pus, but they likewise promote absorption. The most unfavorable forms of peritonitis are those caused by perforations, and likewise those that set in at once with typhoid symptoms. For the same reason we meet under our treatment much less frequently with such consequences of inflammation as are caused by adhesions, breaks or bends of the bowels, dragging or strictures of the intestine, or as otherwise depend upon considerable, callous thickenings of the peritoneum. The best criterion for a reliable prognosis is, after all, the pulse; as long as it is not nearly restored to its normal condition, the danger is not passed, although the other indications may seem favorable.

Treatment. Before we pass to the homœopathic treatment of this disease, we will cast a glance at the manner in which it is treated by physicians of other Schools, in order to show the great superiority of the homœopathic treatment over any other. Without an exception the diagnosis of peritonitis is so certain, that it can hardly be said that the reported cure of a case of peritonitis was mistaken for that of some other disease. Peritonitis is one of those diseases which neither a so-called rational nor physiological physician fancies can be treated without blood-letting, and where the omission of bleeding is looked upon by a lay-person as downright murder. It behooves us the more to fight against such a method with all our means, for venesection exerts undoubtedly a bad effect upon this disease. When speaking of apoplexy we took occasion to condemn the practice of blood-letting, but owing to the inability of establishing a reliable diagnosis, we had to build our argument upon an uncertain basis. The case is different with peritonitis, which is far more accessible to a rational comprehension. It is an inflammation which results in a very short time in copious exudation, more copious than takes place in any other inflammation in the same space of time. Most probably this is mostly owing to the slight resistance of the bowels, and to the great extensibility of the abdominal walls; whereas the pleural cavity, although in other respects constructed very similarly to the peritoneal cavity, consists externally of the firm thoracic wall, and internally of the much less yielding pulmonary parenchyma. The copiousness of the peritoneal exudation accounts for many phenomena that are not otherwise peculiar to inflammations; we mean, for instance, that in many cases a tolerably high degree of anæmia sets in, which gives rise to the cold skin, the cadaverous paleness, the peculiar headache, the contracted smallness of the pulse, and the almost cyanotic appearance of the patient. It is moreover certain that the abundance of serous exudation at the commencement of the disease is exceedingly threatening to life, or perhaps presents the only real danger at this stage, since it is the pressure exerted by this exudation that causes all the threatening symptoms. What can local or general depletions accomplish against this chief danger? Is the serous exudation arrested by bleeding? Certainly not; for the bleeding deprives the blood of its plastic ingredients, hence it is the more disposed to form serous exudations. Moreover, the integrity of the whole volume of blood is rapidly restored by the absorption of serum from every part of the organism, except from the morbidly altered parts of the peritoneum, and the really dangerous symptoms of general anæmia are rendered still more intense. Again, is the plastic exudation diminished or arrested? Supposing this is so, yet in view of the present danger and the final termination, there is no advantage in bleeding. For the fluid that had been exuded in the first stage of the disease, before bleeding was resorted to, remains where it is, only it is not increased; but the conditions under which the process of absorption can be carried on, are much more unfavorable, and the chances of a purulent metamorphosis are greatly increased. Finally, we may ask the question, whether the influence of bleeding upon the general organism is such as to justify this process in spite of its disadvantages in other respects. What can here be said in favor of this proceeding in the presence of a disease which destroys life so rapidly by a premature exhaustion of the vital energies? Even if we were willing to admit the propriety of bleeding in a case of circumscribed peritonitis, yet in a case of this kind bleeding is unnecessary, since this form of peritonitis is very seldom suddenly dangerous.

From these *a priori* reasons we deem every sanguineous depletion in peritonitis unjustifiable. In addition to this we have absolute evidence that peritonitis treated with bleeding, becomes more readily fatal at the onset, or that in the opposite case the convalescence is very much retarded, and that the complete reabsorption of the exudation is a rare event; whereas the transformation into pus occurs quite frequently. Who, in the presence of such arguments to the contrary, can talk of rational proofs in favor of blood-letting? If we were disposed to invoke personalities, we could easily show that rational and physiological physicians do not insist much upon a rational demonstration in favor of bleeding, and that they simply take refuge, if need be, behind the old adage that it is so, and cannot be otherwise. Dire necessity is a very soft cushion to rest one's head upon. Other external applications will be discussed by and by, they do not constitute the most essential part of the treatment. To the internal remedies, on the contrary, we have to devote a few words. At present only two remedies are really in use, Opium and Calomel. The former is to restrict at the onset the activity of the intestines, and if no diarrhœa is present; the last-mentioned remedy, Calomel, is to excite stool. How absurd, however, in a disease where the intestine is exquisitely paralyzed from the commencement of the attack, to give a medicine that diminishes the functional activity of the bowels still more! Moreover, are not extensive and firm adhesions the more certain, the less they are disturbed and loosened by the movements of the bowels? We are amazed at the assertion of a well-known pathologist and professor of clinical medicine, that in peritonitis Opium does not constipate the bowels, and that, on the contrary, it rather has a tendency to gently loosen them. Every homœopath knows how to account for this; why does not the pathologist likewise try to account for this phenomenon, which is certainly sufficiently striking? The use of Calomel for the purpose of causing stool, is just as absurd as the use of Opium, the more as generally no stool follows. We shall afterwards find that the use of Mercury in this disease is justifiable, but not by any means as a symptomatic remedy. Calomel and Opium, sanguineous depletions, cold or warm applications and injections, constitute the whole therapeutic apparatus, with which modern Medicine combats one of the most dangerous diseases; hence nobody can wonder that peritonitis should have a mortality of seventy to seventy-five per cent., while the remaining twenty-five per cent. remain diseased the balance of their days, or at any rate retain the seeds of a variety of other ailments. Would it not be just as well, with just such a prospect before them, that Old-School physicians should pursue a strictly expectant treatment?

As we said above, Homœopathy can boldly dispute the palm with any other method of cure, for the reason that it cures more cases of peritonitis, that its cures are throughout more complete, and that it effects a convalescence in a much shorter period of time. These results are obtained with the following remedies:

Aconitum. When treating of enteritis, we gave it as our opinion, that Hartmann's recommendation of Aconite was not intended for enteritis, but for peritonitis, which is entirely omitted in his work, because he regards it as synonymous with enteritis; a view that it is difficult to comprehend, if we look at the extreme difference of the tissues composing the intestine and the peritoneum. For many forms of peritonitis, Aconite is undoubtedly the most suitable and surest remedy, but not to the extent that Hartmann imagines. There is a vast difference between the two kinds of exudation, which we recognize very speedily. Aconite is the specific remedy, if the inflammation either spreads further from a circumscribed spot, or in cases where it sets in with more local symptoms, without the accompaniment of the general disturbances, which are sometimes truly fearful, except perhaps the presence of an intense fever. It is in this manner, that inflammations with an excess of plastic exudation generally announce themselves; here meteorism never reaches the high degree it does in other forms of inflammation, and percussion usually yields a dull sound very indistinctly. We do not understand Hartmann's advice, to continue the Aconite until all the inflammatory symptoms have disappeared; for this would mean until the disease is cured; he meant probably febrile instead of inflammatory, but this likewise does not happen as he fancies. Observation has shown, that in inflammations Aconite is only useful until the exudation is completed. At this stage the pulse, in inflammations, for which Aconite is indicated, becomes somewhat slower and stronger, and the pain abates in a marked manner, which is seldom the case before the fifth day of the disease. All physicians agree, that one of the lower attenuations should be given in repeated doses.

Belladonna is suitable only at the commencement of peritonitis. It competes with Aconite, if the local symptoms are accompanied by severe congestions of the head and chest, with anguish, dyspnœa, restlessness, dark-red and bloated face; and continual and distressing vomiting of bile, which changes about with retching. The exudation is profuse, and the intestines are distended at an early stage of the disease, so that the single convolutions can be distinctly felt through the abdominal integuments. Intestinal catarrh, which may be present during the first days of the disease, is an additional recommendation for this drug, so is the development of this inflammation from enteritis. Belladonna is likewise an excellent remedy for the vomiting, which is apt to set in, in the subsequent stages of the disease; in this respect it is only surpassed by *Arsenic* in a few cases. The abatement of meteorism designates exactly the period when Belladonna is indicated.

Veratrum album is related to Belladonna in some respects. If the disease sets in in the form of cholerine; more particularly, if the vomiting is copious and frequent, at the same time the patients look pale and sunken, and feel cool to the hand; the pulse is small at the onset, and the anguish, restlessness and thirst are exceedingly distressing, Veratrum is the appropriate remedy. As a general rule, the disease assumes this form in the first three days;

afterwards other remedies have to be employed; although, if we judge of the homœopathicity of a remedy by mere symptoms, Veratrum should correspond to the disease throughout its whole course.

Mercurius is less adapted to peritonitis than to enteritis. It seems to us a mistake to give Mercurius from the beginning; except in the entirely local inflammations. The tendency to suppuration is the best indication for this remedy. Hence, it is in the second and third week, that Mercurius must be given; and the more special indications are the above-mentioned phenomena, characterizing the process of purulent metamorphosis. It is the frequently exacerbating fever, with creeping chills, and copious perspiration after the heat, which points to Mercury. In partial peritonitis, on the contrary; as soon as the inflammation is localized, Mercurius may be given at the onset. It is likewise appropriate if the purulent exudation seeks to penetrate to the outside and form an abscess.

These four remedies are the only ones that need be given in the first stage of the disease. In the further course of the disease we may have to administer:

Bryonia alba. Hartmann's assertion that peritonitis cannot be cured without Aconite, seems to us more applicable to Bryonia. It comes into play at the most decisive period in the development of the disease, namely: when we desire to remove the effused fluid as soon as possible. In saying this, we may be accused of generalizing too liberally, but we appeal to what we have said in the introduction, namely: that these general statements are only intended as a guide to the Materia Medica, not as a means of superseding its use. In comparing the second stage of peritonitis with the pathogenesis of Bryonia, we shall find, that in the majority of cases this remedy is indicated by its physiological effects upon the healthy; it is almost certain, that under the influence of Bryonia the exuded fluid is reabsorbed without causing any further derangements; hence, that no suppuration will take place. But the medicine should be used consistently; we cannot expect to obtain results in a day, that can only be obtained in from ten days to a fortnight. As a general rule, Bryonia is not indicated, if a copious diarrhœa is present; this, however, is a rare occurrence in the second stage, and, if it does occur, it is a bad omen.

Sulphur is a second remedy we make use of in order to promote, or indeed, to excite the absorption of the exuded fluid. In cases where Bryonia leaves us in the lurch, or effects the absorption of the exudation only to a certain point, *Sulphur* is entirely appropriate. It acts even when the remaining portion of the exuded fluid had been left for months without any alteration. However, no hectic or colliquative symptoms must be present; the exuded substance should be lying in the abdominal cavity like a dead mass, and except the great weakness and the deficient reaction, no other abnormal phenomena must be present. If symptoms of ulceration have appeared, Sulphur can only cause a loss of time. An appeal to the Materia Medica is less feasible in the case of Sulphur, than in that of any of the above-mentioned remedies; such remnants of intense inflammations often furnish but a small number of morbid phenomena, which are entirely insufficient for a correct selection of the drug in accordance with mere symptoms.

Arsenicum album is very closely related to Veratrum album symptomatically.; in a present case, it is difficult to decide between the two remedies, especially at the commencement of the attack. In the further course of the disease, it is particularly the continued, violent, colicky pains, that point to Arsenicum; which is, likewise, sometimes indicated by the gradual development of the inflammation out of gastritis, the perforating ulcer, or ulceration of the bowels. Arsenic exerts, moreover, a striking influence, when the exuded fluid is copious and obstinately persistent, the abdomen, when percussed, simulating the phenomena of ascites. For all that we must not allow ourselves, by the peculiarities of the picture of the disease, more particularly by the extraordinary restlessness and anxiety, to be too readily induced to use Arsenic, as is so easily the case at the commencement of the disease. If Arsenic acts as a homœopathic specific, the reaction must not be prostrated, on the contrary it must be vehement; hence the fever must be violent and continued. For the rest we refer the reader to our remarks on puerperal peritonitis, which will be found in the chapter of diseases of the female organs, and where the use of Arsenic will be discussed more fully. In the same chapter, more detailed statements will be found concerning the use of *Rhus toxicodendron*, of which, we here simply remark, that it is an excellent remedy in this disease, if it sets in all at once with all the fierceness and characteristics of typhus.

It remains for us to mention several drugs, to which attention must be directed under certain circumstances. *Opium* is sometimes useful against the paralytic weakness of the intestinal canal, which often remains after the disappearance of the exudation; the intestine is unusually distended and the constipation is complete. *Nux vomica* is still more preferable under such circumstances, only the meteorism must not be too great. In general it is an excellent remedy in equalizing the remaining trifling irregularities in the digestive functions, especially the torpor of the bowels. *China* will only be found applicable in the subsequent course of peritonitis; it is the more suitable, the more the copious exudation, or other previously existing conditions, have impressed upon the organism the appearances of anæmia. *Phosphorus* corresponds to conditions for which *Mercurius*, *Arsenicum*, or *Rhus*, had been given previously, and is to be exhibited when suppuration has set in, together with evident symptoms of colliquation, exhausting diarrhœa and hectic fever. Finally we recommend *Colocynthis*, which we gave in a case of diffuse peritonitis, with a mass of solidified exudation and uninterrupted colicky pain, with such success, that the disease took a favorable turn so suddenly, that in view of the length of time this pathological process had been going on, there could be no possible doubt that the medicine had produced the favorable change.

The medicines we have indicated are most probably sufficient in every case of peritonitis without any unusual complications. Single striking complications, such as may occur during convalescence, especially in the region of the liver, bladder or uterus, cannot be dwelt upon in extenso, since the diversity of their forms would not admit of a full description of their symptomatology. Complications of this kind always increase the difficulties of the treatment; this cannot be taught in a manual of Therapeutics, but the Materia Medica will have to be referred to for further information.

Although we have every reason to depend upon the efficacy of our means of treatment, yet the disease is so dangerous, its first invasion fills the patient with so much anxiety, and it is so excessively painful, that we are anxious to find out and apply such remedial agents, as will afford a momentary relief from the pains; and will perhaps exert a curative influence upon the morbid process generally. We should resort to such palliative means with the more willingness, as thereby the attention of surrounding relatives is diverted from the patient. The chief palliatives are injections and fomentations. It is impossible to decide *a priori* whether cold, or moist, or dry and warm applications deserve a preference. At first, when the pains are very violent, the patient usually prefers cold applications, ice-cloths, or even a bladder filled with ice. There are, however, exceptions to this rule, more particularly the circumstance that patients cannot bear the least weight on their bowels, on account of the extraordinary sensitiveness of these parts. Warm and moist fomentations are generally best applied on the fifth day, in some cases the patients prefer them at the very beginning of the disease; they are more especially useful, if the patients transpire very copiously. They should never be applied too hot, for too high a temperature is prejudicial. What had best be applied in a given case, will have to be decided by an actual trial, but such an experiment should be instituted with great care, lest obstinacy in waiting for a result should prove injurious. As a general rule, the fomentations that do not afford relief to the patient within a few hours, or are otherwise than pleasant to his feelings, are not adapted to his condition. As regards the wet sheet, which is praised by many, we have no experience of our own to offer. At first these wet clothes should be applied to the abdomen alone. In view of the great sensitiveness of the abdominal walls, it is doubtful whether such an application can be frequently repeated. Simple injections of water, whether cold or tepid, never have such a penetrating action, that their use should be insisted upon, in spite of the pain which they may inflict upon the patient. If used at the commencement of the disease, they will prove insufficient to remove the paralysis of the intestinal canal. During convalescence, on the contrary, injections of water often render excellent service.

In scarcely any other disease, the diet deserves more careful attention than in peritonitis. There is no necessity of enjoining special rest, since the pain which the patient suffers renders movement almost impossible. The case which we have related in a previous paragraph, shows, however, how important it is to keep all mental or emotional excitement away from the patient, since it will undoubtedly exert an injurious influence. Moreover, the room should be kept at a uniform temperature of about fifty degrees F., the air should be kept fresh, and the patient should only be lightly covered. Feather beds should never be used as a covering. Very frequently all kinds of covering should be kept from the abdomen by some suitable contrivance, such as barrel-hoops. At the commencement of the disease, the patients are tormented by an agonizing thirst which can only be quenched by fresh water. Small lumps of ice in the mouth, likewise, render good service, and are particularly suitable, if there is much retching and vomiting. Afterwards, if the appetite commences to return, such food should be used as will leave the smallest possible residue of fecal matter; the administration of beef-broth should not be delayed too long, as exhaustion might prove fatal to the patient. Solid food should only be given gradually, and with the greatest care; the patients should be kept on a lean diet for some time, even though they should seem convalescent. If exhaustion should set in suddenly, and at an early period, the use of small quantities of good wine will be attended with beneficial results.

FIFTH SECTION.

Diseases of the Liver, Spleen and Pancreas.

A. DISEASES OF THE LIVER.

In no other division of Pathology have such great revolutionary changes been effected by recent investigations, than in the doctrine of diseases of the liver; but these changes do not date further back than some twenty or thirty years. Until then, the views concerning the functions and morbid changes of the liver were so confused and untenable, that the Pathology which had prevailed up to that time was really of no use; at least, no reliable system of Therapeutics could be built upon it. This circumstance is the more interesting, as the subject presents even now many obscure and uncertain points; and the material out of which we might build up a therapeutic edifice, based upon experience, is exceedingly scanty. It is in accordance with these views that the following chapters should be judged; it is not probable that all will be pleased with them. If, in making their reports, homœopathic physicians would take the small trouble of presenting a diagnosis corresponding with the demands of pathology, the chapter of affections of the liver would become one of the most promising in the Therapeutics of our School, for the reason that we have a right to be proud of the brilliant results we have achieved in this direction.

In order to avoid continual repetitions, it is best to introduce the subject of affections of the liver, with a statement of the manner in which their physical examination has to be conducted, which will yield most important information in many cases.

An objective examination is conducted by means of inspection, palpation and percussion.

Inspection yields a distinct result only in cases of unusual enlargement of the liver. In these cases the last ribs bulge more prominently, or the sharp edge of the right lobe of the liver becomes distinctly visible below them; else the left lobe is felt in the pit of the stomach as a swelling. These symptoms are most prominently marked in persons of a slender frame, the more so as the abdominal walls are drawn towards the vertebral column.

Palpation likewise yields marked results only under certain circumstances. If the liver has its normal size, the thoracic walls interfere very much with an examination by the hand; all that can be accomplished, is to satisfy one's self of the sensitiveness of the liver to external pressure. If the liver is enlarged, the lower sharp edge can often be distinctly felt; the left lobe can likewise be traced all around. We sometimes succeed in feeling biliary calculi through the abdominal walls, or swellings proceeding from the liver. Sometimes we are misled in our diagnosis by swellings in the abdominal cavity, hard excrements in the intestines, hypertrophy of the pancreas, and an irritated stomach. To institute a proper examination, the patient has to lie down, with the head somewhat raised, but not too high, and the lower extremities drawn up; at the same time the respiration should be carried on quietly and uniformly; nor should the inspirations be too deep. Palpation is most successfully carried on during the act of expiration.

Percussion is the best diagnostic aid, for the reason that it almost always yields some positive result. In its largest extent, the liver yields a perfectly dull sound, except that the upper edge is somewhat higher, on account of the organ encroaching, in a degree, upon the thoracic cavity; and the lower sharp edge and the boundary of the left lobe, do not yield much dulness, on account of the subjacent intestines. The upper margin of the liver extends from the lower extremity of the sternum along the lower border of the sixth rib as far as the side, where it reaches downwards below the eighth rib; whereas, close to the vertebral column it is bounded by the eleventh rib. Expiration and inspiration may drag it an inch higher up or lower down. The lower margin of the liver is pretty exactly described, anteriorly and laterally, by the lower edge of the last rib, beyond which it usually descends to a certain distance, without, however, a dull sound being yielded by the overreaching portion. Posteriorly the twelfth rib overreaches the liver. In the middle region, the left lobe of the liver overreaches somewhat the curve of the ribs, and generally extends as far as the mesian line of the abdomen. By these boundaries we are enabled to judge whether the liver is enlarged or not, and to what extent—a circumstance of great weight in affections of this organ. Various circumstances may render an exact delineation of the boundaries of the liver impossible. Among these circumstances we number all diseases that cause such changes as will give rise to a dull percussion-sound along the boundaries of the liver: infiltration of the right lung, exudation in the right pleural cavity; in the middle region of the liver it is the accumulation of serum in the pericardium, especially if attended with a change in the position of the heart; along the lower edge, it is swellings in the abdominal cavity. Considerable exudations in the thoracic cavity may also push the liver downwards. During an examination by percussion, the respiration should be calm and uniform, and not too deep; and the patient should be in a horizontal posture, with easy extension of the body, so that the abdominal integuments are neither too much relaxed, nor too tightly stretched.

For an analysis of the secretions, which is sometimes important, with a view of determining the presence and amount of bile, we refer to Chemical Manuals. Information of this kind is of little value, unless it is complete.

1. Hyperæmia of the Liver.

The structure of the liver, more particularly the arrangement of the vessels which conduct the blood to and from the liver, suggests *a priori* the probability that a sanguineous engorgement of this organ can not only easily take place, but is, indeed, of frequent occurrence. However, we are not able to diagnose, with perfect certainty, an hyperæmia of the liver, unless it is so considerable that the volume of the liver is greatly increased. We can only conclude with some certainty, from the symptoms and other circumstances, that certain conditions, which will be discussed presently, must depend upon an increased quantity of blood, to be found at that time in the liver; and hence, that these conditions are the consequence of active sanguineous congestion. To give a minute account of the causes that occasion an accumulation of blood in the liver, by impeding the flow of blood from this organ, is not within the province of this book. We will simply state that hyperæmia of the liver is more particularly occasioned by diseases of the heart, which interfere with the reception of the venous blood, and by pulmonary affections, with a considerably impaired faculty to respire freely. We will merely call to mind the circumstance, that tuberculous patients are frequently afflicted by liver complaint.

The etiology of active hyperæmia depends in the main upon the following circumstances: The various deleterious influences that give rise to obstinate constipation or hemorrhoids; inordinate eating, with disproportionate scantiness of waste, cause hyperæmia of the liver. Hence it is frequently met with among individuals who consume a great deal of nourishing food, and at the same time lead a very sedentary life, or who work too little in proportion to the quantity of food they eat, and in this way bring about a real plethora of the abdominal organs. Congestion of the liver is, moreover, frequently met with among women whose catamenia are not sufficiently copious, or even entirely suppressed, especially during the critical age. It is likewise undeniable that a disposition to this disease may be hereditary; we are acquainted with families in whom every adult member seems to have inherited liver complaint from the mother. Certain poisonous substances, which cause congestion of the liver in a majority of cases, are of great importance in this respect. In a subsequent part of this work, where we treat of intermittent fever, we shall likewise dwell upon the influence of malaria, and upon the action of China on the liver. Beside these influences, it is principally alcohol and Mercury that cause such congestive symptoms in the liver as are so frequently met with in practice. Nor can the influence of atmospheric and climatic conditions be denied. In the torrid zone, diseases of the liver are much more frequent than in the temperate zones. Northerners who have resided a long while in hot countries, are very apt to contract a striking disposition to derangements of the liver. Even with us affections of the liver are much more frequent in the hot summer and fall. They more particularly attack persons who use improper food, such as quantities of fat meat and the like, which cause derangements of the liver, not only in hot countries, but likewise among us during the heat of summer. Finally, it is certain that violent emotions increase the afflux of blood to the liver. If an attack of congestion of the liver has once existed, it always leaves a tendency to relapses, which sometimes become so seated in certain individuals, that the attacks return at almost definite intervals, more particularly in the months of May and September until November, without apparently having been excited by any irregularities in the mode of living, or by any deleterious influences whatsoever.

Symptoms. The phenomena of liver-hyperæmia not only differ in intensity, but likewise in extent and distinctness; this difference is best observed among patients who are frequently attacked with this disease, and with unequal degrees of violence. As preliminary symptoms, we may regard the disturbances caused by the above-mentioned deleterious influences in the intestinal canal, or in various other organs; and which differ a great deal on this account. An error in diet may cause catarrh of the stomach and bowels; mental excitement may cause slight headache and loss of appetite; alcohol may occasion gastric derangements, etc. Otherwise the preliminary symptoms are of no importance, because they never point to the disease with absolute certainty. The first real symptom of disease, is a sensation of tension and fulness in the region of the liver, and a not very painful, but disagreeable pressure in that region. This is generally accompanied by a peculiar disturbance of the mental equilibrium; the patients feel languid and weary, they are restless; the thought of not being able to succeed in their business, drives them about from place to place; they look on the dark side of everything, are irritable and out of humor; their sleep is disturbed. According as the hyperæmia is more or less considerable, the local symptoms likewise vary in intensity, but really acute pains are rarely felt, nor is the sensitiveness to pressure very great, yet tight clothing is not agreeable. The appetite is not very much impaired, the bowels may act regularly, but are generally constipated; the urine becomes dark at an early stage of the disorder, and deposits a sediment. Occasionally the patient vomits. The secretion of bile is not always uniformly affected, the stools sometimes containing more, and at other times less bile; the patient looks somewhat jaundiced, but never to a great extent. Febrile symptoms are only present when the attacks are severe. It is only in the more marked forms of this disease that percussion reveals an enlargement of the liver, and then only very prominently in case the attacks return very often; in such a case the eye alone is sufficient to recognize the more marked convexity of the liver.

An attack lasts from a few days to several weeks. It generally terminates in recovery, unless the patient, who never feels sick enough to keep his bed, commits gross mistakes. The trouble either decreases gradually, or else it disappears all at once and is replaced by a perfect feeling of health. If the disorder returns frequently, it never leaves again entirely. In such a case it looks more like a chronic disease with occasional exacerbations. In the course of time the liver becomes enlarged, more particularly during an exacerbation of the symptoms. The constitutional condition of the patient remains permanently disturbed in various ways, he complains of derangements of the stomach, constipation, and want of clearness of the head; he becomes fitful, irritable, and his complexion remains sallow. Off and on he vomits bile, and has at the same time violent attacks of headache. From such apparently trifling symptoms, a more formidable disorganization will sometimes result.

In isolated attacks the prognosis is always favorable, provided the cause which provoked the attack, is not allowed to act permanently. In chronic cases of this kind, the prospect of a cure is more uncertain. All we can do, in many cases, is to effect a general improvement, and a less frequent return of the paroxysms. Women passing through the critical age, often recover spontaneously, in proportion as the organism gets the upper hand of the disturbances caused by the stoppage of the menstrual functions.

The affections of the liver caused by Alcohol and Mercury, will be treated of more fully in subsequent parts of this work. Nor is this the place for such forms of hyperæmia, as are apt to supervene during catarrh of the stomach, or to result in an attack of bilious colic, bilious gastric fever and the like. The affection of the liver being symptomatic in such cases, such complications will be discussed in connection with the main diseases

Treatment. From what we have said it is evident that the treatment should be conducted with reference to the exciting cause, and the special attack, as well as with reference to the chronic form of the whole disease. Our remarks on the ëtiological causes of the disease will suggest the proper mode of meeting the indicatio causalis; in selecting a remedy, homœopathic practitioners may likewise keep this object in view; the diet will likewise have to be regulated accordingly.

For a single attack the most frequently homœopathic remedy is *Nux vomica.* This medicine has, as it were, a more specific relation to the liver than to the stomach. The phenomena caused by Nux in the region of the liver, designate every degree of hyperæmia, even to fully-developed inflammation. Pressure and tension, stitches during motion and contact, sensitiveness of the region of the liver to contact, swelling of the liver, and jaundiced complexion: all these symptoms point to Nux as an important remedy for diseases of the liver. In addition to this we have the phenomena in other organs, especially in the digestive organs, (which need here not be mentioned more in detail, and the peculiarities of the mental and emotive sphere; together with the exciting cause. Nux vomica is particularly suitable if, the symptoms corresponding, the complexion has a bright hue, with a slightly yellowish tint; however, we do not mean to suggest that this alone constitutes a sufficient indication for Nux. This remedy is likewise indicated in chronic hyperæmia, where, however, it is not sufficient and will have to be associated with other remedies.

The liver-symptoms of **Ignatia amara** are almost the same as those of Nux; they differ more particularly in their accessory symptoms. Ignatia is particularly suitable for women, whereas Nux is more adapted to the female organism. The genuine nervous constitution is its proper sphere of action, together with the mental disturbances to which such patients are liable, and the ailments caused more especially by grief, fright or chagrin. If the menses are profuse, irregular, and always attended with violent pains and congestions, Ignatia is indicated so much more specifically. This remedy is likewise adapted to the chronic form.

Chamomilla is one of the best remedies if the attacks have not yet occurred very frequently, and consequently if the liver has still preserved its normal condition, and the attack was brought on by a fit of anger or chagrin. The region of the liver is not exactly painful, but the patient experiences a distressing dull pressure in that region, which is not aggravated by either motion or contact. On the cortrary, the patient complains of colicky pains in the umbilical region and in the stomach, attended with bilious vomiting, dyspnœa, anxiety, and the complexion has an icteric hue. There are always symptoms of catarrhal irritation of the intestine.

Bryonia alba is only appropriate to a few obscure cases where the patient experiences a painful pressure in the region of the liver, with sensitiveness to pressure in that region; but the symptoms are otherwise indistinct, and the affection seems more like an attack of excessive debility.

Belladonna is indicated in cases of hyperæmia bordering very closely on inflammation, from which it is at first distinguished with difficulty, more particularly if the patients are plethoric individuals. The region of the liver is painful and very sensitive to pressure; there is considerable headache with flushed face and feverish pulse; the stomach is likewise affected, and there is frequent vomiting of a watery mucus mixed with bile. The patient complains of intense thirst.

Mercurius is next to Belladonna in similarity of action; it is more adapted to hepatitis than to simple hyperæmia. For further details we refer to the chapter on hepatitis.

Beside Nux and Ignatia, we have to employ several other remedies in the chronic form of the disease, provided a cure is at all possible. *Sulphur* holds the first rank. We shall have to dwell upon its relation to the liver more fully and frequently in subsequent chapters; hence we shall content ourselves with a brief allusion to these points in the present instance. It is suitable in hypertrophy of the liver; the organ is sensitive to contact; there is little icterus, nor is less bile passed with the stool; the circulation in the intestinal canal seems impeded, and symptoms of catarrh of the stomach are not wanting. An occasional attack of distressing itching of the skin, which, without any visible change in this organ, is present in affections of the liver generally, and more especially in hyperæmia, is a characteristic indication for Sulphur. Next to Sulphur, *Sepia* is the most prominent remedy. It is more particularly suitable for women in the critical years; the menses appear irregularly, sometimes remain suspended for months, and are attended with more or less violent uterine difficulties. The local pains in the region of the liver are not considerable, generally amounting to a continued crampy pressure, with occasional fugitive stitches, especially about the catamenial period, without any marked swelling of the liver or icterus, although the complexion is somewhat jaundiced. Sepia, too, corresponds to the cutaneous symptoms of individuals afflicted with liver-complaint, more especially if the local symptoms are very prominent, and are attended with violent itching. Beside the digestive symptoms which always furnish very marked indications for Sepia, we have to call attention to the sudden and violent, but not long continuing congestions to the heart, chest and head, revealed more especially by rapid changes of color in the face.

Few drugs are in such characteristic rapport with the liver as *China*. We know that the continued use of China, as well as Quinine, in intermittent fevers, is usually succeeded by a considerable swelling of the liver, which cannot well be looked upon as anything else than a fully developed hyperæmia. This circumstance alone is sufficient to direct our attention to China in affections of the liver. The local symptoms are not sufficiently characteristic to establish a distinction between the action of China and that of other medicines; they are a sensation of pressure or stitches, with sensitiveness in the region of the liver, to external pressure, attended with bloat in this region. Hence, the selection of China will have principally to be determined by the multitudinous symptoms which it causes in the same organs. The chief symptoms among them are: A pale, grayish-yellow, icteric color of the skin; sickly appearance; aggravations at night or after a meal; sensitiveness to external cold; origin of the disease in consequence of other slow morbid conditions, or after losses of blood, or abuse of Mercury; a general debility out of all proportion to the other symptoms. Beside these three remedies we have to direct particular attention to *Lycopodium* and *Staphysagria*. For other remedies we refer to the chapter on chronic hepatitis.

During a first attack, the diet and mode of life are of not so much consequence, since the patients feel badly enough to eat and drink cautiously, and generally to behave with a great deal of discretion. Knowing, however, how easily patients may relapse and contract chronic hyperæmia and enlargement of the liver, it behooves us to give them full instructions regarding their behavior during the paroxysm. Our remarks on the etiological causes of the disease are sufficient to show what ought to be avoided; we must add that coffee and tea should likewise be avoided, as well as the habit of sleeping or sitting in a stooping posture after a meal. In the spring, and more especially in the fall, patients should be doubly careful, live moderately and with great regularity, and avoid beer. The copious use of fruit in any form, drinking a great deal of water, sour milk, or butter-milk, are much to be commended. The favorite bonny-clabber, however, should be used with a great deal of discretion, since an otherwise perfectly sound stomach is easily spoiled by it. In judging of the effect of bonny-clabber upon the process of nutrition, we should not be guided by the results obtained at spa's or hygienic establishments; the radical changes in the whole mode of living which prevails in these places is much more decisive than the use of clabber. [In chronic hyperæmia hepatis, *Carduus marianus* in infusion will be found an excellent remedy. H.]

2. Hepatitis, Inflammation of the Liver.

In consequence of numerous repetitions, we should have to extend the therapeutic portion of this section too far, if we were to treat the different forms of hepatitis separately. Hence we prefer adopting the general classification into acute and chronic, which comprises all the more important differences. The acute form comprises not only the inflammation of the parenchyma, but likewise, that of the capsules of the liver, and the vena porta.

a. *Hepatitis Acuta, Acute Inflammation of the Liver.*

Inflammation of the parenchyma of the liver is of rare occurrence in our temperate zone, whereas it is frequently met with in some of the tropical countries, and diminishes in frequency in proportion as we approximate to the poles. It cannot be denied that Northerners who emigrate South are taken sick more frequently than natives; this may be owing to an altogether unnatural mode of living. But even there, it is only exceptionally that the disease occurs as a purely primary malady, but it is generally a consequence of septic or ulcerative processes, especially dysentery which, with us, is very seldom succeeded by abscesses of the liver. Moreover an inflammation of the vena porta may extend to the liver. Injuries of the brain constitute a peculiar, hitherto unaccountable, cause of hepatitis. It may likewise be caused by mechanical injuries, contusions, wounds, etc., and by biliary calculi.

The anatomical changes caused by hepatitis in the beginning of the disease, are very difficult to demonstrate, since other derangements may produce similar effects. Parenchymatous hepatitis never affects more than a portion of the liver; generally it has only one focus, seldom several; the right lobe of the liver is, by far, the most frequent locality of the inflammation. A post-mortem examination, generally only reveals the termination of the inflammation in the cadaver; we find an abscess which often creates large caverns, seldom a number of small foci. The seat of the inflammation is more or less close to the surface; in the latter case the abscess may open externally, and either discharge into the abdominal cavity, or break through the integuments. Since, before the abscess breaks, its surface usually forms adhesions with the neighbouring parts, a discharge into a free cavity is of rare occurrence. At the same time the whole organ is more or less swollen, at times, only the diseased lobe of the liver, at times both.

Symptoms. The phenomena of suppurative hepatitis differ in degree, extent, and distinctness. The local symptoms are sometimes so few in number, or so obscure, that a sure diagnosis is scarcely possible, and becomes peculiarly difficult if the inflammation is a complication of other affections, by which it is more or less completely obscured. This may readily happen during the course of malignant dysenteries, where the liver may swell up and become painful, even if no inflammation is present. Hence, in many secondary cases of hepatitis, we only meet with a portion of the symptoms; to be subsequently indicated as the symptoms of a distinctly recognizable, idiopathic hepatitis. Generally, it is very difficult to define the commencement of the inflammation with anything like certainty; it scarcely ever sets in with a chill, which almost always ushers in other important inflammations. The region of the liver becomes painful, sensitive to pressure, and frequently bulges very visibly. The pain is more or less violent, seldom lancing or burning; more frequently it is a dull pressure. The faint dulness of the percussion-sound extends over a larger surface, sometimes the edge of the liver can be plainly felt under the short ribs. Icteric symptoms are seldom marked, sometimes they are entirely absent. The intestinal canal is generally very much involved in the morbid process; the stomach rejects all food, the appetite is gone, and the patient is troubled with loathing, retching and vomiting. The bowels are generally costive; the discharges are light-colored, or of an ash-gray or clay color, corresponding with the degree of icteric color of the skin. The liver being very painful, breathing, coughing and sneezing are of course correspondingly aggravated and painful, even to a high degree of dyspnœa and other phenomena simulating pleuritis. The fever at first is not very violent, and has marked remissions, the pulse is not much hurried. All these symptoms change as soon as the abscess commences to form. Now the fever becomes continuous and is only interrupted by violent chills; soon it assumes a peculiar adynamic character, and finally, changes to a well-marked hectic fever; or else the whole pathological process looks very much like lentescent typhus. At first, the local pains increase in intensity, but after the abscess is fully formed, they abate somewhat; icterus now is almost always present. The stomach is very much affected, the patients are tormented by a distressing retching. The pain in the right shoulder, and the numbness of the right arm are, if not characteristic, at least somewhat pathognomonic signs of the disease. Sometimes the whole of the right side is painful. At this stage, the brain is very much involved, violent circumscribed headache, sopor and delirium setting in. In addition to all these symptoms, the patient now rapidly emaciates, and, after the disease has lasted a short time, death may set in by exhaustion. Usually, however, the disease drags along more slowly, and without the abscess passing beyond the boundaries of the liver, life is destroyed by ulceration of this organ, attended with hectic phenomena. If the abscess discharges, the course of the disease will depend upon the accompanying circumstances. If the abscess discharges outwardly, we notice a prominent, generally a fluctuating spot, which breaks after a while, and permits the pus to escape. Under favorable circumstances, the opening afterwards closes and heals, or else the suppuration continues and hectic fever sets in. A discharge inwardly, whether into the cavity of the chest, the intestine, the peritoneal cavity or elsewhere, is generally fatal; although at first the patients feel somewhat relieved. A capsular insulation of the abscess is a rare occurence in this disease.

The whole duration of the disease varies from a few weeks to several months, the duration of the abscess is, of course, not included in this period. The prognosis depends upon the various circumstances mentioned in the symptomatology of the disease.

In the majority of cases the diagnosis presents a good many difficulties, because the local symptoms are not very characteristic, and may just as well indicate a severe hyperæmia, as other affections of the liver. A rigid diagnosis can only be established if an abscess can be demonstrated, or the disease runs an acute and characteristic course; otherwise a reported cure of hepatitis should be received *cum grano salis*; not because it is difficult to cure this disease, but that it is of rare occurrence, and it is difficult to show that it was a case of hepatitis.

The treatment will be described at the end of this chapter, together with both the other forms.

b. *Perihepatitis, Inflammation of the Capsules of the Liver, Capsular Hepatitis.*

This form of hepatitis admits of a decided division into acute and chronic; the chronic form will be treated of in the next chapter.

Perihepatitis owes its origin, most commonly, to all the circumstances which we have pointed out as causes of hyperæmia; one form of this inflammation, which will be more fully treated of in the chapter on chronic hepatitis, is more particularly due to the habitual abuse of alcohol. That it may be caused by mechanical injury may be regarded as possible, but is not a very frequent occurrence.

Symptoms. Unless a preliminary stage, consisting of the symptoms of hyperæmia, precedes, the disease generally sets in with the sudden chill that is peculiar to the access of every severe disease, and which is at once followed by more or less violent local pains. At times these pains are a simple pressure, a painful sensation of fulness in the region of the liver, with tension across the whole epigastric region, and a slight increase of sensitiveness to external pressure; or else, which is more frequently the case, they are acute, lancinating, burning pains, darting into the abdomen; the region of the liver is sensitive to the least pressure, and the pain is aggravated by the least motion. The liver is more or less swollen, and corresponding icteric symptoms generally appear. The fever is at times slight, at other times intense and continuous. The symptoms in other organs generally correspond to the intensity and extent of the disease; the stomach is always involved, and, as in the former, so may retching and vomiting be present in this form. The breathing is very often greatly impeded on account of the pain, the movements of the diaphragm, in consequence, being very much interfered with.

The course is either that of a circumscribed peritonitis, (in eight days to a fortnight health being gradually restored,) or else the inflammation spreads, acting like a diffuse peritonitis; or finally the disease terminates in the chronic form. It is only if the second result should happen, that there is danger of a fatal termination; otherwise the disease is one of the less threatening kinds, although very painful. The diagnosis meets with a good many difficulties; the distinctive signs between simple hyperæmia and hepatitis may be entirely missing, and in the next place parenchymatous and perihepatitis may seem entirely alike at the beginning. From hyperæmia, perihepatitis is best distinguished by the fever; parenchymatous and perihepatitis are distinguished from each other by the circumstance, that, in the last-mentioned form the swelling is less, the painfulness is spread over a larger surface and is more intense, and the icterus is less marked. The treatment will be indicated in the next chapter.

c. *Pylephlebitis, Inflammation of the Vena Porta.*

We subjoin this form in this place, because the vena porta exerts a deep influence on the condition of the liver, and its inflammation is very commonly the cause of a suppurative inflammation of this viscus.

The causes of the inflammation of the vena porta are either deleterious influences that affect it directly, or inflammations of adjoining parts; or inflammation of the rectum and colon. The first kind, which is the really primary form of the disease, is by far the least frequent. A progression of acute forms of hepatitis, especially of perihepatitis, is a common occurrence. Among the inflammatory processes it is more particularly dysentery which leads to pylephlebitis, in consequence of the gangrenous destruction of the mucous lining.

Symptoms. Since a post-mortem examination frequently reveals evident signs of pylephlebitis in the obliterations of single ramifications of the main trunk, without any corresponding morbid symptoms having been observed during the lifetime of the patient, we must suppose, that such inflammatory processes can run their course without any prominent symptoms. If the inflammation is more violent and more diffuse, we first notice a violent, generally burning pain in the region of the liver, which is very soon succeeded by a considerable swelling of this organ, with widespread sensitiveness. At the onset, the fever is not as intense as during hepatitis; however, the functions of the stomach and intestinal canal are very much disturbed. The inflammation usually advances rapidly towards suppuration, subsequent to which a change takes place in the character of the fever, which is now frequently interrupted by chilly creepings. Generally the inflammatory process now invades the parenchyma of the liver, where it commonly excites an intense suppurative hepatitis. Pylephlebitis has, moreover, a few, more or less, pathognomonic symptoms. At the head of the list we have the icterus, which is scarcely ever as much marked in any abnormal condition of the liver, as in this inflammation. Next, we almost always have a considerable swelling of the spleen, and the vessels of the abdomen reveal the symptoms of a high degree of plethora, that may easily lead to hemorrhage from the bowels, and serous exudations in the peritoneal cavity

The terminations of pylephlebitis are either in recovery, which is, however, seldom complete, or in adhesions or suppuration. Adhesions are only of importance, if they involve a large number of ramifications or the main trunk of the vein. In such a case we notice all the signs of an impeded portal circulation: hemorrhoids, swelling of the spleen, hemorrhages from the stomach and bowels, violent intestinal catarrhs, dropsical symptoms, which in the long run attain to an extraordinary development, and the icterus which remains unchanged. In suppuration the signs of an abscess in the liver become most prominent, although a metastatic pneumonia may arise, having a fatal termination. Death seldom takes place after a short period of time, generally not till a few weeks have elapsed; with symptoms of a high degree of exhaustion, and complete emaciation. Where pylephlebitis constitutes a mere complication of some other acute inflammation, it is almost always sure to end fatally.

Treatment. If we comprise these three forms in one series, it is because in practice we are very apt to content ourselves with the general diagnosis of an inflammatory condition; and we do not take the trouble to distinguish the different kinds, which are, however, of great importance, so far as the first and second forms are concerned, since they respectively require different remedies. It is likewise of importance to know whether hepatitis emanates from a phlebitis or not; for phlebitis certainly requires to be treated with other medicines, and may possibly be removed before a complication with hepatitis renders it a fatal disease. In order to give the reader an opportunity of making himself acquainted with the remedies that are adapted to the various cases, which may leave us in doubt as to which form of inflammation they belong, we here give the leading symptomatic indication for each remedy separately.

Aconitum is recommended by Hartmann very earnestly at the commencement of hepatitis. But we have already stated that the parenchymatous form seldom sets in with intense fever and other phenomena of acute inflammation; in this form Aconite will not often be found appropriate. It is different with perihepatitis, for which Aconite is probably the best remedy, at least at the onset. Be this as it may, Aconite is not selected in such cases in accordance with the fever-symptoms, a form of homœopathicity which is very much objected to at the present time, but strictly in accordance with its physiological symptoms; among which the characteristic symptoms of hepatitis, even the two first forms, are to be found. As a characteristic symptom we have the short and painful cough, which is more particularly apt to set in when the upper surface of the liver is inflamed.

Belladonna has been found better adapted to this disease than Aconite; this at least is the opinion of most of our physicians. Perihepatitis is more particularly its proper sphere of action, if the following symptoms prevail: stitching pains, rather superficial, like pleurisy-pains, aggravated by pressure, inspiration, coughing or lying on the affected side; they spread as far as the neck and shoulder. At the same time we have dry cough, oppression of breathing, hiccough, congestions of the head, with obscuration of sight, and sensation of fainting; fulness and tension across the pit of the stomach; violent thirst, sleepless tossing about, sometimes with inability to collect one's senses; nausea, retching, distressing vomitting, and continued fever, attended with a high increase of temperature. When the local pains abate, which they generally do as soon as the exudation terminates, we must no longer expect any particular good effects from Belladonna.

Bryonia alba is generally appropriate as a sequel to Belladonna, even in parenchymatous hepatitis, provided it does not set in with too much violence, but, as is generally the case, resembles a light typhus. The icteric symptoms are not very prominent with Bryonia; the fever is continuous, although not very violent, the pain is burning, although not very intense.

Mercurius solubilis is the most important remedy in the worst form of parenchymatous hepatitis. The region of the liver is very sensitive to contact, and is especially painful when the patient draws breath, coughs, etc.; the pain in the liver is a painful pressure or a burning, stinging pain; the liver is enlarged; there is considerable icterus. These local symptoms, however, are much less to be depended upon than the general ones. Mercury should be given when suppuration is about to set in. This period is more definitely indicated by a burning fever, changing about with violent chills. It is, moreover, indicated by striking nocturnal exacerbations, great restlessness, an agonizing thirst, with desire for very cold drinks, and marked jaundice.

Phosphorus is, without doubt, one of the more important remedies in inflammatory affections of the liver, with well-marked icteric symptoms, which it excites very rapidly in connection with inflammatory symptoms. If we consider these effects side by side with its general action upon the organism, we infer that Phosphorus is more especially indicated in those violent forms of hepatitis accompanied by deeply pervading typhoid symptoms, and rapid prostration of strength. It is the only remedy which we can employ in pylephlebitis with any prospect of success; phlebitis is an appropriate sphere of action for Phosphorus; likewise pyæmic phenomena in ulcerations of the intestinal canal, with metastasis to the lungs.

The remedies which we have named so far, are only beneficially applicable during the acute form of the disease; but we know that convalescence, or even a fatal termination, is sometimes slow; in such a case the disease takes upon itself changes that have to be met by a different class of remedies.

Nux vomica will be found of especial benefit after the fever is removed, the liver continues painful and bloated, the skin is still jaundiced, the strength is still down and the digestive functions very much disturbed. The acute stage seldom exhibits symptoms that point to Nux as a true simile. *China* is very similar in its action to Nux vomica; this remedy has already been referred to in speaking of hyperæmia of the liver, and will be mentioned more fully in the next chapter. The acute form of the inflammation is not the proper sphere of action for China; it is more appropriate in combating the residuary consequences of the disease, such as enlargement of the liver, and the accompanying digestive derangements. *Sulphur*, one of the most efficient remedies in diseases of the liver, is essentially adapted to chronic inflammatory conditions, and may likewise be required in a case of abscess whose dispersion Mercury was unable to accomplish, or which had discharged on the outside, forming a fistulous opening. If, in such a case, the general symptoms point to *China*, Sulphur nevertheless is required for the local symptoms. *Phosphorus* likewise is important in the phthisis hepatica proper; *Arsenic* also deserves honorable mention. Owing to the incurable nature of such a condition of the parts, we can hardly expect to obtain curative results from any of these remedies. *Lycopodium*, *Sepia*, *Silicea* likewise come into play; for more special indications we refer to the next chapter.

It is difficult to regulate the diet in these forms of liver-disease. If the patients are very sick, if they are troubled with a disposition to vomit, there is no difficulty in controlling their desire to eat, for they cannot eat anything. But if the stomach is not much affected, or if the appetite begins to return, the greatest precaution is necessary. The aversion to meat and fat which these patients experience, is an important sign of Nature, that this kind of food should either be avoided, or else should be given very cautiously. This circumstance is very unfavorable to convalescence; and the desire to do away with the emaciation and obviate the great prostration of strength, may lead one to hurt the patient in the vain hope of benefiting him. Wine never does any good in the whole course of the inflammation. If the patient desires anything refreshing for his burning thirst, water and mild vegetable acids, either in the shape of syrups or jellies, are most suitable for this purpose.

3. Hepatitis Chronica, Chronic Inflammatory Affections of the Liver.

Under this heading we comprehend divers conditions of the liver which can all be traced more or less directly to inflammation, among which we class the yellow atrophy of the liver, since it does not seem desirable to devote a special chapter to such an obscure disease. In the succeeding paragraphs we therefore group the following diseases side by side: fatty liver, hypertrophy of the liver, waxy or amyloid liver, granular liver, cirrhosis of the liver, nutmeg-liver, and acute yellow atrophy of the liver. If fault should be found for bringing so many different conditions together in one chapter, we will meet the objection by referring the reader to the therapeutic chapter.

The etiology of chronic hepatitis is, in many respects, the same as that of hyperæmia, where particulars may be found. The main causes of these abnormal conditions are: sedentary mode of life, especially when associated with a large supply of food; a disproportionate amount of nourishing, fat-making food, hot climate, excessive heat even in our own temperate zone; abuse of Cinchona, Mercury, Alcohol; miasmatic influences; intermittent fevers, syphilis, excessive emotional excitements, continued deep grief, etc. In this class of exciting causes likewise belong all kinds of diseases which impede the circulation in the liver, especially diseases of the heart and lungs, with greatly diminished capacity of breathing. Such chronic affections of the liver are very apt to supervene in individuals afflicted with so-called dyscrasias. As was said before, acute forms of liver-disease are very apt to change to one of these chronic forms.

It is a very difficult matter to trace the above-mentioned forms of disease to special causes referring exclusively to one particular form, since the same deleterious influences may cause any one of these abnormal conditions; nevertheless, certain influences are almost always succeeded by the same forms. Cirrhosis, for instance, is principally met with in persons addicted to the use of alcohol, whereas the peculiar nodular form of the liver, (syphiloma,) is chiefly met with among syphilitic subjects. Fatty liver is not only found in those who eat much fat, or are disposed to excessive formation of fat, but likewise, (and this has hitherto remained unaccounted for,) in persons who are afflicted with rapidly wasting diseases, especially tuberculosis. Waxy liver is only met with among individuals who are afflicted with constitutional diseases, such as rickets, scrofulosis, syphilis, and hydrargyrosis.

As regards age, children remain entirely free from chronic liver-disease, except syphilitic affections; old people likewise are rarely attacked with liver-disease. It is particularly middle-aged persons who are afflicted with such disorders. Some forms of it attack principally men, cirrhosis, for instance, which is easily accounted for; but as a general rule, women are, under similar circumstances, more liable to the disease than men. As we stated when treating of hyperæmia, some forms of liver-disease are hereditary, although, even in such cases, the disease does not appear until the age of pubescence, whereas not a trace of the disease had been visible before.

The various morbid conditions of the liver differ so greatly, with reference to their anatomical changes and symptomatic manifestations, that we shall have to consider each of them separately.

The so-called *hypertrophy of the liver*, by which we understand an increase of substance of this organ without any apparent exudation, results most probably from repeated attacks of hyperæmia. The shape of the liver is not particularly altered, but upon the whole is larger than the normal size, and the parenchyma is generally much firmer, darker, and contains more blood. Or the liver, with an unequal increase of substance, exhibits unequal patches upon the cut surface, the veins of the liver having become enlarged, and looking like isolated spots in the rest of the organ (nutmeg-liver.) In consequence of the pressure of the blood, this form may afterwards result in a shrinking of the liver-cells, and formation of areolar tissue, so that the tissue of the liver may assume an appearance like that of cirrhosis.

In simple hypertrophy of the liver the symptoms are generally unimportant, and not persistent, but occurring in paroxysms. The commencement of the disease almost always escapes observation, until our attention is excited by local pains, pressure in the region of the liver, enlargement of this viscus, with a slight transient attack of icterus. These symptoms are attended with derangements of the digestive system. The appetite may remain good, but the food does not seem to digest well; after a meal the patients feel lazy, are troubled with eructations or heartburn, and pressure at the stomach. The bowels are costive, the patients are tormented with piles; often fitful and desponding, or irritable. When taken at the onset, the disease is always curable, although only after a long lapse of time; but a cure is no longer possible, if a nutmeg-liver has become atrophied.

Cirrhosis of the liver (granular liver) consists in an excessive formation of adventitious areolar tissue, in consequence of which the substance of the liver becomes atrophied. At first the size of the liver remains unchanged, very rarely it is slightly enlarged; in the subsequent course of the disease it is more or less diminished in size. The shape of the liver changes in consequence of the greater or less shrinking of the margins of the liver, until they finally acquire a membranous consistence of great firmness and density, without any parenchyma; the right lobe becomes more and more globular, and the left is almost entirely atrophied. The capsular covering is thickened, firm, and seems drawn in here and there, which gives a knobby, unequal, granular appearance to the surface. The tissue has a firmer consistence, sometimes as firm as cartilage. When cut, the parenchyma is lighter colored, and of a coriaceous firmness. Here, too, the granulations appear, first of a yellow color, and afterwards showing a grayish tint, embedded in a tenacious, whitish fibrous tissue, which sometimes takes the place of large portions of the parenchyma.

The symptoms of incipient cirrhosis are identical with those of perihepatitis, but are not often very intense, and resemble rather the symptoms of simple hyperæmia. Hence, it is very seldom that they become an object of medical treatment, because the disease mostly affects drunkards, who will not consult a physician for trifling ailments. When the affection is at its height, most of the phenomena are easily accounted for by the compression and obliteration of the ramifications of the portal vein, in consequence of which the circulation through the hepatic vessels is very much impeded. Local symptoms, properly speaking, only exist at the commencement of the disease, whereas, as the disease progresses, all painfulness disappears. The dull sound over the left lobe diminishes more and more, and very soon disappears entirely. The icteric symptoms are never entirely absent, but on the other hand never exist to a high degree, and are limited to a dirty-gray color of the skin and face, a light-yellow color of the sclerotica, and frequently a more or less yellow color of the urine. The phenomena of obstructed circulation in the digestive organs are quite marked. The gastro-intestinal catarrh exists to a high degree; however, there is no increased excretion of fæces, but the bowels are constipated, and a copious quantity of tenacious mucus is discharged. The fæces are either of a light-yellow, or more commonly of a clay, grayish-white color. Hemorrhoids are scarcely ever absent, and the engorgement of the veins of the intestines or rectum, in the long run almost always lead to hemorrhage from these vessels. The appetite being almost entirely gone, nutrition is rapidly and thoroughly prostrated. The urine is always secreted in smaller quantity, and is generally charged with uric-acid sediments. In addition to this, the equally impeded flow of the splenetic blood almost always causes an increased enlargement of the spleen. These symptoms are associated with a more or less rapidly progressing exudation of serum into the peritoneal cavity. The ascites, unless arrested by death, always increases to a high degree, nor does its increase depend upon an increased or decreased secretion of urine. This is characteristic of this form of ascites. The duration of the disease is always protracted. If death takes place prematurely in a few months, it is generally caused by secondary complications; otherwise, the disease may last for years before the patients succumb, with all the signs of a fully developed marasmus.

When the disease has reached its acme, the prognosis is decidedly unfavorable, since it is impossible to remove the newly-formed connective tissue, and to secure a corresponding restoration of the liver-cells. It is even questionable whether the disease can be arrested in its incipiency.

It is only for the sake of completeness, that we mention the syphilitic form of hepatitis. In its essential features it greatly resembles cirrhosis. In syphiloma, likewise, we have the formation of an excess of connective tissue, which causes the hepatic parenchyma to shrivel, except that, in this disease, it forms deeper furrows, which impart to the liver a lobular appearance, and not, as in cirrhosis, fine granulations. This disease is only a partial manifestation of constitutional syphilis, nor is it characterized by striking symptoms, and its treatment is, in all respects, identical with that of general syphilis.

Fatty liver is one of the most common abnormal conditions of the liver; its advent sometimes is so insidious, that the boundary between a sound and abnormal condition of the liver can scarcely be defined; a copious infiltration of fat may even be associated with a feeling of health. Fatty liver may likewise arise in consequence of a peculiar metamorphosis of inflammatory exudations into fat; in such a case, the shape and general condition of the liver depend upon the primary disease.

Hepatitis Chronica.

In a tolerably high grade of fatty liver this organ is always enlarged; it is flattened out, less bulging, its edges are changed, their normal sharpness being superseded by a more or less striking roundness. The enlargement may be considerable. The color is lighter, a yellowish-red or entirely yellow, with irregular red patches. The consistence is much less, sometimes like dough, so that the pressure of the finger remains. On cutting through the liver, the knife is seen lined with a coating of fat.

The symptoms corresponding to this form of the disease, vary greatly, at least in intensity. How far a copious accumulation of fat agrees with every appearance of health, is shown by the fattening of animals, which likewise teaches the important lesson, that the conditions under which the process of fattening is carried on, may develop diseases of the most malignant kind. With men the case is not different. If individuals, having little mental and physical exercise, with a large supply of nutritious food, grow large and acquire very fat livers, they may feel perfectly well, with the exception of a little awkwardness and heaviness; but if they should be attacked with some acute disease, they run infinitely more risk. In other persons, enlargement of the liver causes a pressure in the right side, dyspnœa, but no pain. Peculiar symptoms often arise if the left lobe is enlarged and presses upon the stomach. This may easily give rise to the idea of some malignant disease, for the reason that a distressing vomiting almost always occurs, attended even with violent pains. With fatty liver, the skin is said to contain a great deal more fat than usual, and to consequently acquire a glistening appearance. Icterus is never present. Percussion, and sometimes palpation, are the surest diagnostic means, for this form of enlargement may possibly exist without any pain, and at the same time be attended with a perfect feeling of health.

Fatty liver, such as is often met with in the colliquative stage of tuberculosis, is a bad omen. Probably, in consequence of secondary hyperæmia, it is associated with increased painfulness, so that the pains in the liver become a chief source of distress to patients thus afflicted.

Waxy or *amyloid* liver greatly resembles the former variety in its physical symptoms. The liver is considerably enlarged, its edges are rounded and thickened, and its consistence is firmer instead of being softer, as in fatty liver. The substance of the liver is infiltrated at times with a dense, lardaceous mass throughout its whole extent, while at other times only in parts; this mass causes the parenchyma of the liver to shrivel up. The color is grayish; on the cut surface it glistens like lard, and is uniformly mottled red.

The symptoms of this disorder are less certain, for the reason that amyloid liver is always a partial manifestation of some constitutional disease. Icterus is generally absent, nor do the patients experience much pain. An almost unavoidable consequence is the exudation of serum into the peritoneal cavity. Altogether, its resemblance to cirrhosis is not trifling, except that the symptoms of a considerably impeded hepatic circulation are either wanting, or only present in a slight degree. The disorder is of long duration, since it only progresses very slowly. The diagnosis of fatty liver is somewhat facilitated by the circumstance, that the disease attacks individuals afflicted with some dycrasia, and likewise by an analysis of the secondary phenomena arising from the primary disorganization; from cirrhosis it is most easily distinguished by the great enlargement of the organ.

Acute yellow atrophy is a morbid condition of the liver that has not yet been satisfactorily explained and accounted for; in many respects it resembles softening of the brain. The morbid process consists in decomposition of the substance of the liver, and considerable diminution of its volume. This may have shrivelled up to one half the normal size of the liver. At the same time the organ is flattened out, flabby and unelastic, and its surface wrinkled. The color is a bright-yellow, almost without any admixture of red.

At times the disease sets in suddenly and acutely, at others very gradually. In the latter case various digestive disturbances are observed, such as are characteristic of catarrhal affections of the stomach and bowels, accompanied by slight icteric symptoms. These, however, scarcely ever continue very long. The actual disease sets in with pains in the region of the liver, which is likewise very sensitive to pressure, and with a rapidly increasing and finally very intense jaundice. Very soon percussion reveals a diminution of the natural dulness of sound until in some cases it disappears entirely. Corresponding to the diminution of the size of the liver, the spleen generally increases in size. At an early period, the local symptoms become associated with those of sympathetic cerebral irritation, such as violent headache, restlessness, irritable mood, which are soon followed by delirium and muscular twitches. The fever is very fierce, the temperature very high, pulse frequent, sometimes slow, always small and soft. The appetite is entirely gone; at first there is both retention of stool and urine. These phenomena of severe irritation are very soon followed by total collapse. The patients become comatose, and the pulse grows smaller and more frequent. Stool and urine are discharged involuntarily, the tongue becomes dry and cracked, colliquative sweats break out, petechiæ appear, hemorrhages from the intestinal canal set in, and death soon after supervenes. From the first appearance of the cerebral symptoms a fatal termination is reached very rapidly, mostly in a week.

The diagnosis of this disease is not uncertain, except if an examination of the region of the liver is neglected; in such a case it may be confounded with typhus the more easily, the longer the preliminary stage contiuues. If the normal du'ness of sound disappears, the diagnosis becomes pretty well assured; for in no other disease does this disappearance of the normal dulness take place as rapidly.

Some regard this disease as absolutely fatal, others only conditionally so. Both parties are right to a certain extent. The former diagnose acute yellow atrophy only if the last stage, which runs a very rapid course, has already set in; the other party refer to the disease as recognized in its first beginnings. At all events, no method of treatment can boast of having performed many cures of this disease. It should be observed that no icterus, though scarcely perceptible at first and apparently harmless, should be neglected, because we cannot know what mischief may be hidden behind it. By this means many an acute attack may be avoided, although we may not be able to show how this is accomplished.

Treatment. From what we have said when describing each single form of the disease, it is evident what result we may expect to accomplish by treatment. Whereas, simple hypertrophy, fatty and amyloid liver, may admit of a more or less complete cure, a cure of acute yellow atrophy is of questionable possibility, and fully-developed cirrhosis defies every attempt at a cure. This knowledge is important because it will induce us to search for remedies in all curable forms of liver-disease, and to confine ourselves to palliative treatment in incurable cases. We are thereby induced to heed such affections of the liver as arise very gradually, even the most trifling irregularities of the hepatic functions, since even cirrhosis, if taken at the onset, may be arrested and the incipient disorganization removed by a process of retrograde metamorphosis.

The medicines which will be recommended for these different forms of liver-disease, can only be presented more or less hypothetically, since in the cases of liver-disease reported in our publications, the diagnosis is anything but certain. Nor do our physiological provings present the necessary clearness in their relations to diseases of the liver, so that secondary or accessory circumstances will have to guide us in the selection of our remedies.

Nux vomica, of which mention has been made when treating of acute affections of the liver, is likewise indispensable in chronic liver-disease. Slight derangements, or such as are not attended with material changes, are easily removed by Nux; in more deep-seated diseases it can only act as a palliative, the completion of the cure being left to other medicines. This medicine is best suited to individuals affected with abdominal plethora, using a deal of fat and wine, taking very little physical or mental exercise, or working too hard mentally and being of a sanguine temperament. To genuine inveterate drunkards, Nux vomica is of comparatively little use. Simple hypertrophy and fatty liver are more particularly favorably acted upon by Nux; in the former it is more especially suitable if it arose from repeated attacks of hyperæmia, and the liver is subject to paroxysms of painful sensitiveness. It is appropriate in fatty liver, if this disorder exists without any simultaneous excess of general obesity. It is more especially in the enlargements caused by abuse of Cinchona, that Nux is endowed with a specific power to control. Among the special indications, the phenomena of the stomach and intestinal canal are particularly noteworthy. The distress is excited or aggravated by eating, the bowels are disposed to be constipated; but the constipation is not obstinate, nor are the fæces colorless. Nux is seldom sufficient to effect a cure; in inveterate cases, never. In the more malignant forms of the liver-disease, Nux may at most have a good effect in the beginning, when they do not differ much from the non-malignant forms; afterwards, when the obstructions of the portal circulation become more prominent, even a palliative effect can no longer be expected.

Of all the medicines at our command, *Sulphur* is most frequently applicable in chronic affections of the liver; for the reason that, even when regarded from the most diverse points of view, it is still adapted to the most diversified forms. In non-malignant diseases, where Nux is a suitable but insufficient remedy, it is Sulphur which completes the action of Nux vomica, and effects a cure. In liver-complaint caused by abuse of Cinchona or Mercury, especially the latter, Sulphur is indispensable, as likewise for the residuary consequences of acute inflammatory affections, especially for hypertrophy of the liver. Until now nothing definite can be said respecting the action of Sulphur in cirrhosis. However, since we know that this disorganization is caused by an exudation into the parenchyma of the liver, and that, reasoning from analogy, Sulphur must exert an influence upon it, this alone may be sufficient to induce a trial of this remedy. In amyloid liver this remedy promises better success, in the first place for the above-mentioned reason, and in the second place on account of its action upon inveterate dyscrasic processes of every kind, especially rickets and hydrargyrosis. We must be spared the trouble of enumerating single symptoms; the effects of Sulphur are too numerous; but we have to point out two circumstances that contra-indicate the exhibition of Sulphur. The stools must not be colorless, as is so often the case in the higher grades of this disease, nor must there be much jaundice, two circumstances that are generally closely connected. Much cannot be expected from Sulphur if ascites or intestinal hemorrhage is present, or if the strength of the patient is entirely consumed; for, in order to have its effect, Sulphur must be assisted in its action by the strength required for the reactive endeavors of the organism. The violent itching in diseases of the liver, and the exanthemata which are so often present during these diseases, are good indications for Sulphur.

China has been alluded to very fully when treating of hyperæmia of the liver, where the reader will find more detailed information. A few additional remarks are needed here. Among the symptoms of China there are many indications of icterus, but the bile-pigment is not absent in the excretions. Where China is to act homœopathically, the secretion of bile must not have been entirely suspended. When treating waxy liver we may often be reminded of China, because this kind of liver is only met with in cachectic subjects; a radical cure must not, however, be expected of this drug. In rarer cases, where the affection of the liver is attended with exhausting diarrhœa, or when there is profuse bleeding from the stomach or bowels, or the spleen is much enlarged, China will do efficient service. From the well-known effects of large doses of Cinchona, it is apparent that this drug must have a specific curative action in enlargement of the liver arising from the influence of malaria and being often of considerable size. Sometimes it relieves the liver-pains experienced by tuberculous patients; in such cases the stomach always is deeply involved in the distress caused by the condition of the liver.

Sepia. We have repeatedly stated in former paragraphs that this remedy is specially adapted to females with a bright complexion, disposed to sudden changes of color and having dark-brown margins around the eyes. Such individuals are always very sensitive, irritable, disposed to congestions, having a fine, transparent skin, and being frequently troubled with hepatic spots, they are undoubtedly inclined to diseases of the liver. It is more particularly non-malignant tumors of the liver that come within the curative range of Sepia, if they are accompanied by icterus, and the passage of bile into the intestinal canal is very much diminished, the region of the liver is occasionally painful. A feeling of languor much greater than the looks would lead one to suppose, aversion to meat, distress at the stomach, irregular menses: these symptoms point to Sepia. Among the symptoms of Sepia we have likewise the peculiar itching of individuals suffering with liver-complaint, and also the congestions in various parts of the body. The mental and moral symptoms of Sepia are likewise somewhat characteristic: hypochondriac mood, loss of spirits, looking on the dark side of things, occasional paroxysms of irritability, disposition to feel vexed and to show an irascible temper.

Lycopodium occupies a high rank among the remedies for diseases of the liver, not only by virtue of its physiological symptoms, but likewise on account of the practical results that we expect to accomplish by it. If our literature contains but few cases of cure of diseases of the liver with Lycopodium, it is because Lycopodium is only suited to the most severe among them and is scarcely ever alone sufficient to effect a cure. Lycopodium is particularly adapted to the treatment of cirrhosis, and to such affections generally as are characterized by considerable obstruction of the portal circulation. In speaking of the prognosis of this disease we have shown that our hopes of curing such a disorder are very slim, hence we must not expect too much of Lycopodium. Among the single symptoms those referring to the feelings, and the symptoms of chronic gastro-intestinal catarrh are particularly prominent; of course a variety of pains are experienced in the region of the liver, but they are very imperfectly defined in the pathogenesis. Lycopodium has no icteric symptoms properly speaking; indeed they are mostly absent in this disease, but it has in their place a peculiar sallowness of the complexion. Besides well-marked hemorrhoidal ailments, Lycopodium has likewise vomiting of blood, exudation of serum into the peritoneal cavity, and rapid emaciation.

Hepatitis Chronica.

Digitalis purpurea has been variously tried in liver-complaint; it is not only suitable in slight attacks of icterus, which generally pass off again spontaneously in a very short time, but it is likewise specially adapted to some of the worst forms of liver-disease. In all such cases, however, icteric symptoms have to be strikingly present. We desire to direct special attention to the many points of correspondential relation between acute yellow atrophy and the effects of Digitalis. The marked cerebral symptoms consisting of severe irritation, which is speedily followed by complete depression; the peculiar character of the pulse, varying between extreme frequency and remarkable slowness; the retention of urine; the painfulness of the region of the liver attended with rapidly increasing icterus; the agonizing anguish of the patient, and, finally, the preliminary symptoms while the disease is slowly and gradually preparing for an outbreak, are all to be found in the pathogenesis of Digitalis; and there is scarcely a drug that has such a rapid prostration of strength without any corresponding colliquative phenomena as Digitalis. Among the remedies that could possibly be used, Digitalis is undoubtedly the nearest.

[Some years ago we were called to see an old man of seventy-two years, who was employed in one of the machine shops of this city; an exceedingly sober person who never used a drop of liquor of any kind. This man had up to this time enjoyed a fair share of good health, and had never given much employment to physicians; nor had he taken much medicine of any kind. After having felt more or less indisposed for a few days, he took to his bed, and we were sent for. We found him slightly delirious, jaundiced, tongue not much coated, skin dry and constricted, pulse about hundred. The old man failed from hour to hour, and died in a few days. A post-mortem revealed nutmeg-liver. The parenchyma of the liver was exceedingly rotten throughout its whole extent. The year following, his son, who was a man of about forty years, and had always enjoyed good health, except that he was unable to undergo much fatigue, was taken down with the following symptoms: Saffron-color of the skin from the top of the head to the soles of the feet; even the tongue and fauces had this appearance; the urine had a blackish-yellow appearance and deposited a similarly-colored sediment. Bowels loose, the discharges having the same dark-yellow color. Pulse exceedingly intermittent and irregular, feeble and slow. It was a case of what the people in our part of the country designate as black jaundice. Remembering the condition of his father's liver, we had a right to infer that in this case the liver must be badly diseased; yet there was no tenderness in the region of the liver, nor could we discover any change either in the size or shape of the liver by percussion or palpation. We gave this man *Digitalis*, small doses at first, which had no effect whatever, and afterwards large doses of ten to fifteen drops in half a tumbler of water in the course of the day. No other medicine was given, and the patient was able to attend to business after having been confined to his room three weeks. There was no trace of jaundice left.

The year following this man was taken sick again; he was slightly icteric, but there was no intermission of the pulse; no sensitiveness in the region of the liver, except the left lobe, which was somewhat swollen and painful. The bowels where tumefied; stools very scanty and light-colored; urine dark, depositing a great deal of bilious sediment, and having a foul smell. The patient's spirits were very much depressed; tongue looked foul; he complained of headache and excessive prostration; he soon became very much emaciated. We treated him with Arsenic and Nux. Fowler's solution was often used, in the proportion of ten drops to a tumbler of water, in the course of a day. The man was confined to his room about five weeks. He made a perfect recovery, grew fat and strong and has worked hard ever since. H.]

Phosphorus has a remarkable similarity to Digitalis in relation to acute yellow atrophy. When speaking of hepatitis, we have directed attention to the constant action of Phosphorus upon the liver, which is uncommonly intense even in the first days, and is attended with acute pains in the region of the liver. We are in possession of abundant material showing the anatomical changes which Phosphorus occasions in the liver. According to these results it is not any of the ordinary acute inflammations which Phosphorus causes. The most common changes are a copious infiltration of fat, which may, however, have existed anteriorly to the poisoning; at any rate this point is by no means removed beyond the sphere of doubt. In two cases where death took place after the seventh day, a large portion of the liver showed great resemblance to the liver in a state of acute yellow atrophy, especially so far as the liver-cells are concerned, and where the gall-bladder, instead of bile, contained a pale-yellow, slimy, ropy fluid. According to these changes, with which the general symptoms correspond, Phosphorus may be fairly tried in acute yellow atrophy. The frequent occurrence of fatty liver would likewise seem to suggest the employment of Phosphorus in this disease. Here the accumulation of fat cannot be accounted for in the same manner as in tuberculosis; however, although it takes place very rapidly, yet a condition of this kind furnishes an additional important indication for the use of Phosphorus in this disease.

There are but few symptoms in the pathogenesis of **Iodium**, that point clearly and unmistakably to affections of the liver; at all events they are insufficient to warrant a recommendation of Iodium in diseases of the liver. The praises that have been bestowed upon Iodium in hypertrophy of the liver, amyloid liver, mercurial affections of the liver, are entirely based upon the well-known general indications. There may be a great deal of truth in them, but they are more or less vague and hypothetical, and the use of the remedy is purely empirical. Hartmann has the following more particular indications: " In jaundice, not in simple icterus as the following symptoms show, Iodium is indicated if the skin is of a dirty-yellow color, there is a high degree of emaciation, irritable and desponding mood, yellow or almost brown, dark complexion, thick coating on the tongue, a good deal of thirst, nausea, clay-colored stools changing about with constipation, dark, yellowish-green, smarting urine, etc.; it is suitable after Mercury has been used to excess. This agent has a large sphere of action, for it comprehends even jaundice with structural changes in the liver, dyscratic conditions, hectic fever, etc." This last recommendation is undoubtedly intended for the last-mentioned pathological process.

[The July number, 1868, of the American Journal of the Medical Sciences, contains an interesting article by John Homans, M. D., of Boston, Mass., on acute atrophy of the liver, with remarks upon the similarity between this disease and the effects of poisoning by Phosphorus. His remarks are illustrated by a number of cases. In concluding his article the writer offers the following observations: " Much has been written on the physiological action of Phosphorus during the last six or seven years. All writers, so far as I have examined their statements, agree that Phosphorus, taken internally, produces a fatty degeneration of the secreting portion of the kidney and liver; in many instances the heart and lungs were in a state of fatty degeneration and even the brain also. Lewin (see Sydenham Soc. Year-book, 1863) made experiments on rabbits and frogs, and found fatty liver in six out of eight rabbits which had lived eight days after the administration of Phosphorus.

" Numerous papers on poisoning by Phosphorus are to be found in the foreign, and especially in the German Journals for the past year, which fully confirm the modern views of the similarity of the symptoms with those of acute atrophy of the liver, and of the rapidity with which fatty degeneration of almost all parts of the body occurs in these cases," (Sydenham Soc. Year-book, 1863.)

"This subject is considered and accounts of cases may be found in the Union Médicale, in the Archives Générales, in Virchow's Archives, in Canstatt, in Schmidt's Jahrbuch, in Wagner's Archives, in the Medico-Chirurgical Transactions for 1867, in the Vienna Medical Journals, and other Periodicals. From what I can learn, it seems to me that the action of Phosphorus on the liver is secondary to a change in the constitution of the blood, and that fatty degeneration of the liver is not necessarily the cause of death, because sometimes a fatal result follows poisoning by Phosphorus, and the liver is found to be neither atrophied nor fatty."

After giving the symptoms in eight cases of poisoning by Phosphorus in the human subject, the Doctor remarks: " The similarity in the symptoms of the two affections, (acute atrophy of the liver and poisoning by Phosphorus,) is, I should judge, rather more marked than in the post-mortem appearances. In both there may be vomiting, either of an hemorrhagic character or not; there may be pain at the epigastrium, restlessness and irritability, rigors, jaundice, tympanitis, retention of urine, delirium, somnolence, convulsions, and coma. After death there may be found, in both, extravasations of blood in various tissues and organs, blood liquid and dark-colored, bloody fluid in alimentary canal, fatty degeneration of the liver and kidneys, and ascites, (generally slight.) But, so far as my observations or reading of descriptions have extended, the gross appearances of the liver are very unlike. It is not so limp, and shrunken, and atrophied, nor has it the peculiar rhubarb-like color, (in many parts,) in cases of poisoning by Phosphorus, that it has in acute atrophy." H.]

Conium maculatum. Rentsch has communicated an interesting cure by this drug in the "Allg. Hom. Zeitung." It is not very certain which of the above-described affections of the liver was cured by Rentsch, but the liver was very much enlarged and the constitutional disturbance was very great; as it is only met with in severe diseases of this viscus. There are but few cases of liver-complaint reported in our Journals, that have been cured with Conium. This medicine is evidently not used a great deal, nevertheless, but few medicines can show more distinct and striking liver-symptoms than Conium.

Calcarea carbonica is, like Conium, scarcely ever recommended for affections of the liver without being associated with some other medicine. Considering, however, what an influence this medicine exerts upon the most deep-seated gastric derangements, especially when the secretion of bile is either diminished or entirely suspended, Calcarea must certainly appear one of the most important remedies in liver-complaint. It is particularly adapted to such complaints in the case of women and children. The local symptoms are numerous, but not very distinct; the constitutional symptoms are very significant. Calcarea likewise exerts an influence upon liver-complaint in the case of tuberculous and chlorotic patients. Waxy liver seems to come more particularly within the range of Calcarea, the more as this disorder only occurs among cachectic individuals.

Silicea is closely related to Calcarea carb., it is particularly suitable in the case of cachectic persons, especially if the affection of the liver is associated with diseases of the bones. The attending intestinal catarrh should not be accompanied by an increase of fecal evacuations. Neither our practical observations nor the physiological provings inform us very precisely in what particular class of liver-disease this remedy will prove most serviceable; at all events, in the liver-complaint of tuberculous individuals Silicea will prove very useful. In addition to these statements we will mention a symptom that seems to be met with exclusively in diseases of the liver, although it does not exactly state how the liver is diseased; we allude to a peculiar, almost sudden change in the finger-nails. they lose their transparency, assume a yellowish hue, crack longitudinally, increase considerably in thickness, and, in a few months, become quite ill-shapen. This change is a sure evidence of some existing liver-disease, and points to a small number of remedies, all of which exert a powerful influence upon the liver: *Silicea, Sulphur, Antimonium crudum*, and *Graphites*, [also *Mercurius vivus*. H.] In many cases this one symptom contributes a great deal towards establishing the diagnosis upon a firm basis; it may be further remarked that this symptom is only observed in diseases of the liver that are not of a malignant character.

Nitri acidum is another medicine having a decided action upon the liver, although we are as yet unable to state in what special form of liver-disease it is indicated. The well marked icterus, the urine full of bile, the colorless stools, and the painful sensitiveness of the region of the liver, show conclusively in what manner the liver is affected. Existing hemorrhoids and chronic intestinal catarrh define still more clearly the specific adaptation of Nitri acidum to the existing case, for they show that no bile enters the bowels from the gall-bladder, and that the ramifications of the portal vein are compressed or even obliterated. Hence it is in cirrhosis, syphiloma and atrophied nutmeg liver, that Nitri acidum may prove useful. The antidotal power of this remedy against the mercurial disease is well known, and we need scarcely state that the diseases of the liver caused by Mercury find their remedy in Nitric acid.

Carbo vegetabilis is not only to be considered in its special relation to the liver, but likewise in its general relation to the organism. The reactive energies of the organism are entirely prostrate. Viewed from this point, *Carbo vegetabilis* will not be suitable in the less important diseases of the liver, nor generally at the commencement of the more important ones, but not until the circulation begins to be very much impeded, the patient shows signs of emaciation, and the serous exudation into the peritoneal cavity has commenced. In addition to these symptoms we always have a high degree of gastro-intestinal catarrh, the hemorrhoidal vessels are very much engorged, vomiting of blood sets in. Hence, cirrhosis seems to constitute the proper sphere of action for Carbo veg., especially if the disease occurs among drunkards. Moreover, Carbo is frequently indicated in the chronic affections evidently resulting from continued losses of animal fluids, such as metrorrhagia and excessive lactation.

Arsenicum album acts pretty much in the same way as the former remedy; the symptoms resemble each other greatly, in most respects, except that Arsenicum is not appropriate when the reactive powers of the system are entirely prostrate. Waxy liver evidently depending upon dyscrasia, is favorably acted upon by Arsenicum. We have already shown that in certain stages of liver-disease only a palliative result can be obtained; this is more particularly the case when remedies like Arsenic and Carbo veg. are required. A great deal is done if the urinary secretion is increased, and the general dropsical symptoms are diminished, which will likewise lessen the patient's anxiety.

We should commit a sin of omission should we here close the list of our remedies for liver-complaint. There are other medicines, the special indications for which it is beyond the sphere of this work to state, that may likewise be required by certain specific symptoms; they are *Graphites, Hepar sulphuris calcareum, Antimonium crudum, Kali carbonicum, Lachesis, Chelidonium majus, Mercurius, Natrum muriaticum, Ferrum, Magnesia muriatica.* Regarding these drugs we are greatly in need of more extensive practical observations; their local symptoms are only obscurely hinted at in our provings, and the utmost care will be required, in order to establish their homœopathicity upon an accurate knowledge of the symptoms.

Although a frequent change of medicines is not advisable in diseases of the liver, yet we should not, on this account, overlook intercurrent morbid conditions, since a good share of success frequently depends upon their speedy removal, especially if the abdominal viscera are concerned in this exceptional treatment. The frequent congestions of the liver deserve particular consideration.

This is not the place to dwell upon the effect of certain mineral waters, since we are not as yet in possession of provings, instituted with reference to their homœopathicity to certain diseases. However, we know that certain desperate cases of disease of the liver have either been cured, or materially improved by the Karlsbad, Marienbad, etc., and this should induce us, in doubtful cases, not to postpone the use of such remedial agents beyond a certain limit of time. It not unfrequently happens that an affection of the liver, which seems beyond the reach of our remedies, is improved by the Karlsbad, or some other mineral water, and that then our medicines act with much better effect.

In every form of chronic hepatitis the diet is a subject of the utmost importance. If the disease is curable, a sound diet will promote the cure; if it is incurable, it will help to preserve the organism as long as possible. The above-mentioned etiological influences sufficiently show what and where certain restrictions are required. Dietetic rules cannot be laid down too rigidly; a single error in diet may entail pernicious consequences. Fat food, especially boiled or fried fat, is to be forbidden, likewise coffee, tea, spirits, and sharp condiments. On the contrary, the use of any kind of fruit should be encouraged; carbonated water may be used as a beverage. Wine and beer have to be used cautiously and moderately, except if the patient is very weak. The condition of the digestive tract will have to be considered with so much more care, as it is opposed to every undue attempt to preserve the vital strength. Where sedentary habits or a luxurious mode of living has caused the disease, vigorous and continued exercise is indispensable, so far at least as the existing strength will permit.

In conclusion, we will mention a palliative means that is often resorted to too soon—we mean tapping. It is difficult to lay down a rule in this respect; nevertheless, it is always well to delay the operation as long as the fluid is confined to the peritoneal cavity It generally accumulates again with great rapidity, and the patient is thus deprived of his last remnant of strength; on this account alone, if on no other, such extreme means ought only to be resorted to very sparingly. In general dropsy, tapping acts much more favorably, and the effect is much more lasting. After tapping it is proper to compress the abdomen, for the purpose of preventing the extension of the abdominal walls; such a compression is best effected by suitably arranged corsets, not by means of a bandage, which is easily pushed out of its proper position.

4. Icterus, Aurigo, Jaundice.

We apply this name to the deposition of bile-pigment in the skin and eye; in some of the preceding chapters we have had frequent opportunities to call attention to this characteristic phenomenon. The essential process in jaundice is a retention of bile in the liver and gall-bladder, and consequent transition into the blood. Hence, this affection is not an independent disease, but one that occurs in connection with other morbid changes, and we should not here devote a special chapter to it, if it were not in most cases beyond our power to recognize the causal or primary disease, so that the morbid process generally seems to us purely idiopathic.

In part, the causes of jaundice have been stated in the preceding chapter on the various diseases of the liver. We have shown that all the morbid processes implying a compression of the biliary ducts, result in icterus. In these cases jaundice is simply a symptom of some other disease. More directly, and apparently more idiopathically, the disease may likewise be caused by deleterious influences acting directly upon the gall-bladder and excretory ducts of the bile. In this respect, the disease may be caused by biliary calculi remaining for a longer or shorter period in the excretory duct, an occurrence that is undoubtedly much more frequent than is generally supposed, since it may be perfectly painless, and only in the smaller number of cases causes such distress as is generally attributed to the passage of biliary calculi. The excretory ducts of the bile may be compressed by adventitious formations, cicatrices, or abscesses, without being themselves diseased; or else their diameter is lessened, in consequence of a morbid affection of their mucous membrane. This last-mentioned circumstance causes catarrhal icterus, very rarely as an idiopathic disease, but in consequence of the catarrhal process spreading from the duodenum to the gall-bladder.

Whether icterus can be the consequence of spasm of the excretory ducts, is questionable. Without any demonstrable changes in the liver, jaundice may occur during the course of various severe diseases, such as pneumonia, typhus, intermittent fever, affections of the spleen. Jaundice occurring after violent emotions, and sometimes very rapidly, is a very curious occurrence, defying every physiological explanation.

Next to these more directly acting causes, which it is sometimes very difficult to explain, we have to consider other more indirectly acting ones, which are of importance so far as the selection of proper remedies is concerned. Under this head we have to enumerate all the etiological influences mentioned previously in connection with acute catarrh of the stomach and bowels, likewise the various causes of diseases of the liver, to which chapter we refer the reader. We may observe that various circumstances, which usually or very readily cause intestinal catarrh, may likewise directly lead to icterus; among these causes we note, more particularly, immoderate eating and pregnancy.

A special disposition to jaundice seems to be more frequent than it really is; it is often not only difficult but impossible to make out specific changes in the liver; and thus it is that an affection of this viscus which is the real cause of the jaundice, seems to have nothing to do with it. As regards age and sex, neither seems to show any particular predisposition for jaundice. Infancy manifests a tendency to icterus, which seems even to constitute a part of the normal physiological life of new-born infants, and it is sometimes very difficult to decide whether the icteric process remains within the boundaries of this normal development. Most new-born children have a jaundiced appearance in the second or third week; however, this is not real jaundice, for the yellow tint of the eyes is absent. Hence icterus neonatorum can only be talked of, if the eye shows the characteristic yellow tint; the yellow color of the skin arises from the copious quantity of the blood accumulated in the dermis of new-born infants, on which account the bright redness which usually succeeds the yellow color, soon changes to the normal white color.

These remarks show that, as a rule, icterus is symptomatic of some other disease, and that it is only in rare instances that icterus is an idiopathic process.

Symptoms. It is very seldom that the disease sets in without precursory symptoms; but they are trifling and the patient is only reminded of them after the yellow color has made its appearance. In the attacks of primary as well as secondary jaundice the patients feel faint, sick, out of humor, their appetite is less and they complain of bitter taste and pains in the limbs. In the secondary forms of jaundice all these symptoms or only single ones of them are added to those already existing. The characteristic color of the skin may set in suddenly or only gradually. Generally the bile-pigment is first seen in the urine, the fæces lose their color more and more, after which the conjunctiva and finally the skin become icteric. There are cases where the skin remains free from the yellow tint, although the conjunctiva and urine show a marked yellow color. The color changes between a bright yellow and a dark-brown, sometimes assumes a reddish, and more frequently a greenish tint; the urine especially inclines to assume this color. The skin is generally tinged unequally. In intense cases the mucous membrane of the mouth is likewise distinctly tinged. As the disease continues the color becomes more intense, although it may remain unchanged for weeks. The color of the urine does not always keep even pace with the color of the skin; the urine sometimes exhibiting an intensely yellow tinge whereas the skin remains colorless; or showing only a slightly yellow appearance, while the skin looks bronze-colored. The presence of bile-pigment is shown by Nitric Acid containing a small quantity of nitrous oxide. Fill a glass tube full of urine and allow the acid to trickle down the side of the tube; very soon layers of different colors, green, bluish, violet and red, will be seen in the fluid, after which the yellow color of the urine reappears. The perspiration likewise sometimes contains so much bile-pigment that it stains the linen yellow. The more the bile is prevented from mixing up with the fæces, the less color they will exhibit, until they finally look like common loam, and, in the highest degree of the disease, like clay. The nature of the stools is an important aid in determining how far the bile is retained out of the bowels and what are the patient's prospects of being cured. The color of the stools is indeed the only safe criterion of an improvement, since even days after the bile has resumed its flow, the skin and conjunctiva may retain their yellow color. The excrements are always remarkably devoid of cohesion and dry; diarrhœa is a rare occurrence.

These characteristic symptoms of jaundice are attended with various derangements of the general organism, of course independently of the causal disease. It is only in rare cases that, after the breaking out of the icterus, the general organism does not suffer; the patients feel well, have a good appetite, and are at most a little less vigorous and enduring than before, their sleep is likewise more restless; in such a case, although the color of the skin may be intensely yellow, the secretion of bile is not entirely suspended, and the stool is still somewhat tinged, though less than usual. The digestion is apt to suffer from the beginning. The tongue is thickly coated, the taste disgustingly bitter, the appetite is gone, at least there is no desire for animal food, the nausea seldom increases to actual vomiting. The stool is very fetid and of the above-mentioned character, attended with copious flatulence which distends the abdomen. The pulse acts very strangely, it is generally less frequent than the normal pulse, seldom more so. This decrease in the frequency of the pulse must be an effect of the bile, for it likewise sets in if the jaundice is a complication of febrile diseases; frequency of the pulse, under such circumstances, is always ominous of unfavorable results. The loss of strength is usually proportionate to the intensity of the icterus and there generally supervenes an exceedingly irritable, desponding state of mind which looks on the dark side of everything and which the patients cannot possibly get rid of. Sleep is generally restless, disturbed by dreams; the skin is very dry. The distressing itching, to which allusion has been made in former paragraphs, is seldom absent. That this itching is not caused by a contact of the reabsorbed bile with the cutaneous nerves, is proven by the fact that it is met with in affections of the liver without any jaundice. The duration of such light attacks varies; if we calculate the duration by the period when the bile commences to reappear in the alvine evacuations, it may be only a few days; but more commonly it extends to several weeks. The yellow color of the skin sometimes does not disappear until weeks after the patients have recovered their natural feeling of health.

But it is not always that jaundice runs such a mild course; sometimes it breaks out as a malignant disease, or assumes a malignant character while running its course. The pulse, in such a case, becomes more hurried, and the temperature rises with occasional attacks of intercurrent chills; the nervous system likewise suffers, as is seen by the violent headache which attacks the patient at the commencement of the disease and by the subsequent delirium. The patient loses his strength very soon, and emaciates very rapidly. There is a striking disposition to petechial effusions. Such a malignant change may take place very suddenly, but may likewise set in very gradually under the form of a lentescent or hectic fever. When at its acme this malignant form may only last a few hours, but it may likewise drag along for months. It is one of the most fatal diseases.

The icterus neonatorum is not essentially distinct from that of full-grown persons. We have said that the mildest forms of this disorder do not seem to be a deviation from the normal condition of the organism, and that the icteric nature of the disease itself is problematical. As in the case of adults, so in that of infants do the real retentions of bile either present the symptoms of a malignant disease, or else are without any noticeable symptomatic manifestations. Malignant symptoms, however, are more readily noticed in infants, because they are always more easily affected by hurtful influences and assimilation is so suddenly and radically interfered with. This last-mentioned result generally depends upon the diarrhœa, which is always present during the icterus of children in its worst form. In addition to this we have the symptoms of a deeply-pervading gastro-intestinal catarrh, tendency to convulsions, and, in the highest grades of the disease, symptoms of putrid decomposition.

Ordinary simple forms of jaundice mostly terminate favorably; the malignant forms are decidedly rare. New-born infants, of course, run the greatest danger. In adults, the appearance of a rapid pulse and diarrhœa, is a bad sign and renders the prognosis exceedingly doubtful. Whether jaundice can terminate fatally, unless it is symptomatic of some other severe disease, is questionable.

Treatment. From what we have said, it is evidently important to the successful treatment of jaundice that we should be acquainted with the internal changes upon which it depends. While we have no means of removing the pressure caused by abscesses, adventitious formations, cicatrices, etc, from the biliary ducts; or of removing the obstacles occasioned by the presence of a biliary calculus; and while our aid, in malignant diseases of the liver, seems of questionable utility, we are in possession of a number of excellent remedies against the benign forms of jaundice. Only we must not stop to judge of the result of our remedial agents by the color of the skin and conjunctiva, for this might deceive us; but we should be guided by the color of the stools, where a favorable change in the secretion of bile is first made manifest, and, after that, by the urine, which shows more definitely than any other secretion, whether, and how much, bile is still reabsorbed. If, in giving the indications for the different remedies, we seem to indulge in too many generalities, the reader will please remember that for the primary causal affections of jaundice, he is referred to the chapters where these are treated of.

According to Hartmann, the following medicines contain in their pathogeneses the symptoms of jaundice: *Aconitum, Arsenicum, Bryonia, Calcarea carbonica, Cantharides, Carbo vegetabilis, China, Conium, Cuprum, Digitalis, Iodium, Mercurius, Acidum nitricum, Nux vomica, Plumbum, Pulsatilla, Ranunculus, Rhus toxicodendron, Secale cornutum, Sulphur, Acidum sulphuricum.* We might transcribe the whole passage if it contained more characteristic indications for each special remedy, but will endeavor to give the more essential parts. For all that, Hartmann has left out some important remedies, such as *Phosphorus;* and so far as the practical necessities of the physician are concerned, the list is too large, for some of the medicines are only of use in the more severe affections of the liver, not in simple jaundice.

When treating of the etiology of jaundice, we showed that this disease is often caused in consequence of a catarrhal irritation of the mucous membrane of the stomach and duodenum, spreading to the mucous lining of the excretory ducts of the bile. Since this need not necessarily be an acute catarrh, but may result just as well from a chronic form of this disease, many of the remedies that have been recommended for chronic gastro-intestinal catarrh, will likewise come into play in the treatment of jaundice. The first among these is

Mercurius. It is not only appropriate in jaundice with fever, but equally so in jaundice without. It is, however, more particularly adapted to the former. The secretion of bile should not be entirely suspended, or else the stools should be liquid. The stomach shows the symptoms of acute catarrh: loss of appetite, perverse desires, eructations, loathing, vomiting, increase of the gastric symptoms after every meal, and thickly coated tongue; in addition we have painfulness of the region of the liver. The skin has a moderate yellow tinge, not very deeply marked. In the icterus neonatorum and of children generally, the remedy is particularly useful. Among the chronic forms, Mercurius is eminently suitable in jaundice caused by abuse of Cinchona.

Nux vomica has a still more extensive sphere of action than the former drug. It is likewise principally adapted to the treatment of catarrhal jaundice with fever. The liver has all the symptoms characteristic of hyperæmia, moreover, spasmodic symptoms, as occur in colic from the presence of biliary calculi. The secretion of bile is almost entirely suspended. The bowels are torpid, the patient is troubled with swellings of the hemorrhoidal vessels. The stomach symptoms are similar to those of Mercurius, but they may likewise occur when the stomach is empty. The disease is chiefly caused by a sedentary mode of life, a large supply of food, abuse of fat, wine, coffee, spirits. The chronic forms of jaundice to which Nux corresponds, can easily be inferred from our remarks on the subject of gastro-intestinal catarrh; we may add, that no remedy has effected better and more numerous curative results than Nux.

Bryonia alba is particularly appropriate in jaundice with fever, where its choice is more particularly determined by the peculiar symptoms of the gastric range: thick whitish coating of the tongue; nausea, retching and vomiting, which is excited both by eating and drinking; obstinate constipation. The complexion is pale and sickly, whereas Nux has a bright color of the face, together with the yellowish tint. The secretion of bile is not entirely suspended, the evacuations remain slightly colored. Bryonia is specifically indicated by extreme languor, or rather by a general feeling of illness.

Aconitum has been recommended and used in jaundice, but it seems to us very improperly in what we call simple jaundice. It is undoubtedly adapted to jaundice depending upon an hyperæmic enlargement of the liver, or upon capsular hepatitis, but not in painless or catarrhal jaundice. According to our provings Aconite has no colorless stools, hence is not appropriate in jaundice of the highest grade.

Belladonna has among its symptoms the two most essential characteristics of jaundice, yellow color of the conjunctiva and completely colorless stools. We have shown before, its intimate relation to the liver. In our Periodicals, we indeed find some cases of chronic jaundice reported cured with Belladonna; we imagine, however, that it will prove much more efficient in the acute forms with fever, both if the jaundice is caused by an acute catarrh, and likewise in the more malignant forms of the disease. The peculiar pulse, first slow and afterwards very rapid, and the intense headache, which easily becomes associated with violent delirium, are two circumstances that we do not find in any other remedy, with more marked and definite distinctness, than in Belladonna; these render this remedy one of great importance in malignant jaundice.

We here subjoin the remedies that compete with Belladonna in the more malignant forms of this disease:

Digitalis purpurea is superior to Belladonna, on account of its remarkable action upon the pulse. What distinguishes Belladonna from Digitalis is, that with the former the face is injected and flushed, whereas Digitalis is indicated by paleness of the countenance. For the rest we refer the reader to our remarks on Digitalis, in the article on chronic hepatitis. The objection that Digitalis manifests its action upon the liver subsequently to that upon the heart, whereas in jaundice the liver is primarily affected, is easily met by the suggestion that it is not by any means shown what causes the slow pulse in jaundice, and hence which organ is first acted upon by Digitalis. A good deal in this respect depends upon the individuality of the patient, and for the present we shall have to content ourselves with the peculiar and exceedingly characteristic totality and connection of the symptoms.

Phosphorus has likewise been alluded to in the article on chronic hepatitis. It is strange that Hartmann should have omitted this remedy among those that cause symptoms of jaundice; and that even Sorge, in his treatise on Phosphorus, does not seem to think much of the relations of this drug to the liver. We are guided by several cases of poisoning, which evidently have not come under Sorge's knowledge, and which have induced us to speak favorably of Phosphorus in acute atrophy of the liver.* We cannot dwell upon this subject more fully in this place, on account of its special character, only it seems to us that Sorge restricts the sphere of Phosphorus in diseases of the liver too much, when he says: "In chronic catarrh of the stomach this case authorizes the employment of Phosphorus as a homœopathic remedy, if bile-pigment is at the same time found in the urine in consequence of a sympathetic affection of the biliary ducts;" and when he afterwards points to Phosphorus in fatty liver in connection with uræmic and slight icteric phenomena. It is our opinion that at the present time we are not as yet acquainted with a better homœopathic remedy for the tolerably obscure connection between pneumonia and jaundice than Phosphorus; likewise for the connection of jaundice with symptoms of a highly developed affection of the brain. At all events the curative sphere of Phosphorus, in this respect, has to be verified by clinical observations, and all we can do is to point out the great similarity between the disease and the action of the drug.

---

* See remarks in brackets, page 549. H.

Sepia has been repeatedly found useful in the case of patients, especially females, who look as if they were afflicted with liver-complaint, or who are inclined to affections of the liver; their complexion is of a bright rather than pale color, with brown-yellow color of the eyelids. Besides other symptoms showing the homœopathicity of this drug to jaundice, we find among its pathogenesis the leading symptom, namely, the absence of color in the alvine evacuations. The general character of Sepia shows that it is not so well adapted to the acute as to the chronic form of jaundice, with frequently recurring paroxysms.

Sulphur, the importance of which has been already pointed out, is likewise suitable only in chronic cases, and then only if material changes exist in the structure of the liver.

Chamomilla is recommended more frequently than it deserves. It is particularly indicated in the icterus neonatorum, which, however, may likewise pass off without any treatment, generally in a short time, and favorably.

China, one of our chief remedies in hepatic diseases, is likewise suitable in the chronic, but not in the febrile form of icterus. China is particularly indicated by the condition of the stomach. Aversion to food, especially meat; perverse appetite; nausea, with canine hunger; distention of the abdomen after every meal; oppression of the stomach; eructations; bitter or bitter-sour taste; vomiting of mucus; a sallow and sickly complexion; dryness and roughness of the skin; languor and weariness; constipation, alternating with diarrhœa; clay or loam-colored fæces, constitute the main indications. China renders good service if the liver-complaint was caused by Mercury or malaria, and likewise in the threatening form of icterus, caused by excessive loss of animal fluids, blood, etc. Females passing through the critical period, are frequently attacked with symptoms of icterus, without any great changes in the liver having taken place.

There is no necessity of dwelling any further upon the special indications of other remedies in jaundice. This is the more unnecessary, as chronic jaundice is simply a symptom of the various forms of liver-complaint that have been described in previous chapters. We here subjoin some of the more important medicines that have not been mentioned before. In febrile jaundice: *Pulsatilla, Rhus toxicodendron, Veratrum album,* also *Conium* and *Cuprum,* the last-mentioned agent under the same circumstances as *Belladonna, Digitalis purpurea, Phosphorus,* if the blood is poisoned by the bile.

Icterus, Aurigo, Jaundice.

In chronic jaundice: *Arsenicum, Aurum, Acidum nitricum*, or *sulphuricum, Carbo Vegetabilis, Calcarea, Iodium*,—Acidum nitricum and Iodium are of particular use in jaundice caused by Mercury. According to Hartmann, Iodium is more especially indicated in the deeply-penetrating icterus of dyscrasic individuals.

We deem it advisable to transcribe Hartmann's arrangement of the remedies for icterus, in accordance with the exciting causes of the disease; he says, Part I, page 466: If the jaundice is caused by vexation, anger, mortified feelings, we use: *Aconitum, Bryonia, Chamomilla, China, Ignatia, Nux vomica, Natrum muriaticum, Sulphur.* If caused by a cold, sudden change of temperature: *Dulcamara, Nux vomica, Chamomilla;* if caused by overloading the stomach and indulging in improper diet: *Pulsatilla, Antimonium, Bryonia, Carbo vegetabilis, Chamomilla, Natrum, Nux vomica;* if caused by abuse of chamomile: *Ignatia, Nux vomica, Pulsatilla, China,* by abuse of Mercury: *China, Hepar sulphuris, Sulphur, Acidum nitricum, Asafœtida, Iodium, Arsenicum*; by abuse of Cinchona: *Pulsatilla, Arsenicum, Mercurius, Ipecacuanha.* The jaundice caused by the pressure of the impregnated uterus upon the liver, is probably most promptly relieved and removed by *Nux vomica, Ipecac,* and *Natrum muriaticum.* The dyspeptic phenomena which sometimes remain after an attack of jaundice, such as loss of appetite, aversion to food, nausea, oppression at the stomach after eating, obstinate constipation and the like, most commonly yield to *Bryonia.*

The diet of icteric patients should be regulated with the same care as if some important disease of the liver had to be removed, the more as in jaundice running a long course, we cannot be sure whether some important defect in the condition of the liver ought not to be suspected. Marked symptoms of gastro-intestinal catarrh should not be overlooked. Avoiding fat food, spirits and fermented articles of diet, is of great importance; the use of ripe fruit, in any shape and mode of preparation, is much to be recommended.

[To the list of remedies indicated in the preceding paragraphs we will add the following: *Gelseminum* or the yellow jessamine; it causes creamy, papescent stools, and seems to exert a depressing influence upon the secretion of bile. *Hydrastis* or the golden seal, has cured several inveterate cases of jaundice; it was given in large doses of the mother-tincture. We refer the reader to Hale's New Remedies, second edition, page 576. *Podophyllum peltatum*, or mandrake, has cured jaundice; it may be given in the second or third trituration, or even higher. We have found it excellent in moderate attacks of jaundice without fever. *Sanguinaria* or the common blood-root, is likewise frequently used in jaundice by eclectic physicians. In homœpathic practice our experience with this remedy is not yet very extensive. H.]

5. Cholelithiasis, Biliari Calculi.

The tendency inherent in the bile to form firm concretions, is quite considerable; hence biliari calculi are a common occurrence. The causes of such concretions are very obscure; they occur in individuals of the most varied constitutions, and pursuing the most diversified occupations, diet and habits of life. Their formation seems to be most promoted by a copious supply of animal food, and by the use of lime-water. As a rule, such calculi are not met with until after the thirtieth year; they occur more frequently among females, and their formation is promoted by every circumstance that causes an arrest of the flow of bile.

Biliary calculi are chiefly found in the gall-bladder; here they are met with in large numbers, seldom as solitary concretions. In the latter case their form is oval or rounded; where several concretions are present they assume an angular form with more or less curved surfaces, in consequence of the sides being rubbed off, and of the pressure and counter-pressure they exert upon each other.

They mostly consist of a nucleus, round which a lighter-colored layer of lime has been deposited, which is again surrounded by an envelope composed principally of cholesterine and bile-pigment. Their color is at times light, at others white, yellow, dark-brown, dark-gray or black. They are not very firm; in their recent state they are friable and can easily be crushed.

Bilious concretions may be without any danger to the individual affected with them; they may be expelled without any pain; on the other hand they may acquire importance from the pains which they cause and from the lesions to which they give rise. In this respect, the size of the concretions is of much less importance than their shape and the internal condition of the gall-bladder; biliary calculi of the largest size sometimes cause the least distress.

Hence the symptoms caused by these concretions vary a great deal according to their shape and intensity of pain. In slight cases a short-lasting spasmodic pain corresponding to the region of the gall-bladder, accompanies the expulsion of the calculi into the bowels. In other cases the pain is continuous but not violent sometimes it is paroxysmal. It is only in the smallest number of cases that the calculi cause regular attacks of colic. This colic commonly sets in all at once, the patient feeling otherwise perfectly well; it is attended with a more or less violent pain in the region of the gall-bladder. Generally this pain increases very rapidly in intensity; it is an intolerably burning, boring pain, and, while increasing in intensity, radiates over the chest and abdomen to varying distances. At the same time the region of the liver becomes exceedingly painful to pressure, it is apt to bloat, and, in consequence of the contraction of the abdominal muscles, the abdomen becomes hard as a board. The pain is generally so distressing and acute, and the patients find it so difficult to breathe, that they toss about in the greatest agony. The general constitutional condition is likewise affected by the pain according to the sensitiveness of the patient and the duration of the pain. Although there is no fever, yet the pulse soon becomes small, filiform, almost uncountable, disappears even entirely, although the heart is in tumultuous motion; the skin becomes correspondingly cool and is covered with a cold perspiration, the complexion is cadaverous. The pain is most commonly associated with distressing vomiting and retching which terminates in a painful hiccuping. The nervous system participates in the violent racking of the frame; the patient is attacked by violent chills or local cramps, especially of the gastrocnemii muscles, or else by violent convulsions at times tonic, at others clonic, which are apt to terminate in syncope. Such paroxysms sometimes last a few hours, at others a day and longer. The pains usually all cease as soon as the calculus enters the intestine; sometimes they disappear gradually or have complete remissions according to the condition of the excretory ducts of the gall-bladder, or to the peculiar shape of the calculus which at times adheres and at others moves on again. After the pain ceases, all the incidental ailments generally disappear very rapidly, and nothing remains but languor and weariness. About this time icterus makes its appearance in different degrees of intensity. The appearance of icterus depends upon the length of time that the excretory ducts of the bile remain obstructed. If the obstruction only continues a short time, the icterus may not break out at all; on the contrary, if the obstruction lasts long, the jaundice may already set in during the pains. As regards frequency the attacks vary, but the same individual is scarcely ever attacked once only; because, as we stated before, solitary concretions cause pain only exceptionally, whereas a multitude of smaller concretions that have become sharply angular by rubbing against each other, penetrate more easily into the excretory duct and cause a more acute irritation.

The terminations of colic from the presence of biliari calculi, or rather the consequences of cholelithiasis, vary a great deal. Death scarcely ever takes place in consequence of an attack of such colic. If the calculus remains incarcerated for a long time, and fills at the same time the whole space of the excretory duct, we obtain a picture of a fully developed icterus with the various symptoms previously described. If the incarceration is not removed, suppurative hepatitis, inflammation of the gall-bladder and its excretory ducts may be the consequence. In the last-mentioned case the patients succumb to peritonitis arising from perforation of the gall-bladder, or, if the gall-bladder should have become adherent to the surrounding parts, the patients fall away gradually until death ends their sufferings.

The diagnosis of biliari calculi is generally very easy and sure. The seat of the pain, the sudden beginning and the equally sudden cessation of the pain, and above all the discharge of bilious concretions with the fæces, establish the diagnosis. If the concretions are soft, they may not appear in the fæces, for the former may break up and scatter during their passage through the intestines. If the colic is not violent, it is difficult to recognize its true character, especially if the symptoms of the stomach are not very prominent and the attack runs a slow course. The swelling and painfulness of the region of the liver may remind one of hepatitis, or else the symptoms may be those of acute hyperæmia of the liver. The spasmodic symptoms do not generally follow immediately after the commencement of an attack, so that it is scarcely possible to confound it with eclampsia, epilepsy, etc.

The treatment involves an abbreviation and mitigation of the attacks of colic, and a prevention of all further mischief from it; at the same time we must try to prevent the return or reproduction of new concretions by proper treatment.

In treating this form of colic, every independent observer must deem it highly improbable that medicine can act upon these biliary concretions, the examples of cure with which all such objections are met, do not remove the suspicion whether the biliary calculi might not have passed through the duct with equal rapidity without any medicine being administered for that purpose. But if the interests and feelings of the patient and his relatives impose upon us the duty of trying the effect of proper medicines, on the other hand we should not be in too great a hurry to attribute our success to the action of the medicine and, in accordance with former favorable observations, to establish a prognosis that might fail us to our detriment. With these restrictions and reservations we here transcribe Hartmann's remarks concerning this form of colic, observing at the same time that, in our own practice at least, we have never yet obtained any degree of evident success by adopting the treatment he proposes.

"One of the leading remedies in this disease is *Chamomilla*, in frequently repeated, not too powerful, doses. It is appropriate, for the consequences of suppressed mortification of the feelings during a meal, in persons of a choleric temperament, but will prove ineffectual if the exciting cause continues to act afresh all the time. Chamomilla is indicated by the following symptoms: painful pressure in the pit of the stomach, in the stomach and hypochondria, especially after eating, with regurgitation of the ingesta, followed by bitter or bilious vomiting, with restless, desperate tossing about and violent headache as if the head would burst."

"Under similar circumstances, only with greater intensity of the symptoms, after suffering an internal, gnawing humiliation or some unworthy treatment, *Colocynthis* ranks above Chamomilla in colic from biliary calculi. These causes will always invite the physician's attention to this drug, more especially if bilious vomiting and a painful pressure in the region of the stomach are present.

"Both these remedies failed us in several cases where I fancied I had chosen the right remedy, until the yellow color of the skin led me to *Digitalis*. It acted with remarkable promptness when the aching and heavy pain in the stomach was accompanied by excessive and violent green vomiting, a rapid and sudden prostration of strength and frequent attacks of syncope. The stools generally had a whitish color, had to be brought away by injections, and the urine had a dark color. In this fearful disease I have likewise employed *Laurocerasus*, *China*, *Veratrum*, *Cuprum* with more or less success in accordance with the most prominent symptoms. It is a difficult matter in this terrible agony, where the patient is unable to give the least explanation of his sufferings, and the physician has to be guided altogether by his own surmises, to hit every time upon the right remedy. *Nux vomica* and *Nux moschata* have likewise done some good, the former if the spasm was centred in the stomach, and had been preceded for some days by retching and eructations. Injections of oil always afforded some relief, even if no fecal matter came away; the intermissions, at least, seemed to last longer after such injections; likewise after frictions with warm oil in the hypochondria.

"No remedy, however, has seemed to act with more lasting benefit than *Arsenic*, even in the most violent cases, when the patients lay without consciousness, with the pallor of death in their countenances and covered with the sweat of anguish, in a state of perfect apathy; when the syncope never ceased, and was only interrupted by occasional fruitless efforts to vomit. After a single dose the vital reaction seemed to be restored in five minutes, and went on until the disease was entirely subdued. At a later period, whenever the disease set in with unceasing cardialgia and colicky pains of the most violent kind, with horrid burning in the affected parts, frequent vomiting, excessive weakness, constipation and a visible reflection of the distress in the countenance, I gave Arsenic from first to last."

Let every reader pass his own criticism on the preceding statements and draw his own conclusions relative to the errors they contain. If we take symptomatic similarities for our guide, Arsenic is undoubtedly the best remedy, the more as it generally exerts a wonderfully soothing influence upon the irritated nervous system; it seems to us as though no other medicine could dispute the rank with Arsenic. Beside this remedy, *Veratrum* and *Cocculus* are excellent in this disease; likewise *Belladonna* although less frequently. Of more decisive value than Hartmann's injections of oil, are the moist and warm fomentations in the region of the liver, which will likewise attract the attention of the horrified and impatient relatives. They may be applied as warm as possible. Where the parts are not too painful, gentle kneading with the fist has a decidedly soothing effect.

Against a tendency to the formation of biliary calculi, a careful diet is the most effective remedy, and *Nux vomica* and *Sulphur* are admirable supports. If the biliary calculi are numerous, which can be inferred with tolerable certainty from the angular shape of those that are passed, the truly sovereign remedy is the water of Carlsbad, the waters of Marienbad and Kissingen being less efficient. We cannot accede to Hartmann's opinion, who advises us to use the artificially prepared water, if the natural waters cannot be had. Whether a fruit-cure, especially the grape-cure, will prove efficient, has not yet been clearly ascertained; at all events vegetable acids are the best means to properly regulate the functions of the liver. Whether *Turpentine* alone is sufficient, has not yet been satisfactorily shown. It is a chief ingredient of Durand's celebrated remedy for this trouble, and probably the only efficient one. Generally the same diet should be adopted that has been recommended in affections of the liver; it cannot be regulated with sufficient care.

6. Carcinoma Hepatis, Cancer of the Liver.

The deposition of carcinomatous growths in the liver is one of the most common accompaniments of what is generally designated as the carcinomatous diathesis. Where the carcinoma is restricted to the liver, the causes of the disease are quite obscure, and it is so much more difficult to trace them to their first beginning as their development is gradual and had commenced long before the time when the patient first complained of his trouble and the physician was able to establish a certain diagnosis. Carcinoma of the liver is most commonly a consequence of surgical operations on carcinomatous degenerations in other parts of the body, in consequence of which the cancerous virus was excited into action throughout the body. For these reasons carcinoma of the liver constitutes one of the most frequent forms of the carcinomatous disease.

The most common kind of cancer of the liver is the fungus medullaris, which generally has several foci, and seldom appears as a solitary fungus, but, as an infiltrating substance, may likewise permeate a large portion of the liver. The single tubercles vary from the size of a pin's head to that of a fist, and beyond; they generally exhibit a whitish tint, and, only when very soft, their color is red or even black in consequence of hemorrhagic effusions. They are most commonly located near the surface, beyond which they grow in the form of semi-globular elevations, which generally present an umbilical depression. They may be changed to ichor, or degenerate into fat or form capsular cysts.

The symptoms caused by carcinoma of the liver, differ in intensity according to the size and locality of the degeneration, so that the disease sometimes remains without any symptoms. Usually the disease commences with the vague symptoms of hyperæmia or of fatty liver, with pressure and a feeling of fulness in the right hypochondrium. As the cancerous tubercles near the surface, partial peritonitis usually sets in, with occasionally more or less considerable painfulness, which is, of course, less than in acute hepatitis, but as a rule exceeds that of any other affection of the liver and, on that account, is an important diagnostic sign. If the carcinoma is deep-seated, the pain may be entirely absent. An important item in the diagnosis of carcinoma of the liver is the rapid enlargement of this organ even to an enormous size, and the consequent bulging of the margin of the ribs. The carcinomatous protuberances upon the surface of the liver can generally be felt. The immediate consequences of carcinoma are, a suspension of the biliary secretion and obstructions in the portal circulation. Icterus may be entirely absent; but if biliary ducts are compressed by carcinomatous tubercles, a more or less marked icterus develops itself, the stool retaining its color; it is only when the excretory ducts of the bile are compressed, that the icteric tint becomes excessive, in which case the icterus constitutes a valuable diagnostic sign. If the carcinoma is seated on the portal vein and compresses it, serum very soon accumulates in the peritoneal cavity, the quantity of which is proportionate to the degree of the compression and the size of the compressed branches, even as we stated in a former chapter when treating of the pathological processes accompanying chronic hepatitis. The constitutional symptoms vary a great deal. Sometimes the stomach and intestinal canal are much disturbed by the affection of the liver, and sometimes they remain perfectly free from all traces of trouble. This circumstance cannot always be accounted for by the influence of the carcinoma upon the secretion of bile. On the other hand the nature of the affection shows itself at an early stage, by the changes it produces in the general condition of the patient, who becomes a prey to the peculiar depression of spirits engendered by the carcinomatous cachexia, emaciates and falls away without any apparent cause for these changes; for the appetite may remain normal, nor are the excretions increased. Indirect consequences are: the spread of the carcinoma to neighboring organs, carcinomatous degenerations in the peritoneal cavity, diffuse acute or chronic peritonitis, ichorous dissolution and discharge outwardly.

As a rule, Carcinoma of the liver is an incurable affection which must prove fatal sooner or later. The duration varies from a few months to a number of years, and depends upon the rapidity with which the cancer grows. Carcinomata that break out after operations, are generally more speedily fatal, than such as are restricted to the liver.

A treatment pursued with a view of curing the disease, has very small chances of success. Reported cures should be received with a great deal of distrust. Our duty, therefore, seems to be to pursue a palliative course by endeavoring to remove single prominent symptoms, without troubling ourselves about the general disease. No remarkable success can even be expected by this treatment. It is not possible to point out the medicines that may have to be used for such a purpose. If we desire to act upon the liver, the medicines that will answer our purpose in this direction, together with the necessary therapeutic instructions, may be found mentioned in chapters 3d and 4th. For other disturbances we refer the reader to the respective chapters where they are treated of. It is strange that no mention is made of this not unfrequent disease in Hartmann's work, as though he considered all treatment futile. We have already stated that our Periodicals do not contain a single reliable cure of carcinoma of the liver. The water of Karlsbad is said to have effected a few cures. The use of this remedy should not be delayed too long, nor the chances of a cure be lessened by an obstinate adherence to other remedial agents.

We have dwelt upon carcinoma of the liver somewhat extensively, because the diagnosis and prognosis of the disease are of great importance. The following points are essential to a correct diagnosis. Extraordinary enlargement of the liver with bulging of the margin of the ribs; unequal, knobby feeling of the surface of the liver; paroxysms of great painfulness; a high grade of icterus with swelling of the liver; marasmus which cannot be accounted for from any other causes, and is accompanied by derangements of the liver; carcinomatous symptoms in other organs; carcinomatous degenerations that had been operated on previously. [Some years ago we treated a lady for headache; for years past she had been subject to the most agonizing attacks of a stupefying headache; during the attack her generally sallow complexion changed to a dark-brown hue. For the last few years the attacks of the headache had been fiercer and more frequent. Nothing relieved her but a dose of Aloes, which opened her bowels which were habitually costive. A post-mortem examination revealed extensive cancerous degenerations in the liver and spleen, that had remained utterly unknown and unsuspected for years. During the last six weeks of her life the carcinomatous degeneration invaded the mammæ and the inguinal glands. There was no enlargement or painfulness of the liver or spleen. H.]

We have made no mention of the echinococcus, another affection of the liver; this parasite is of very rare occurrence in our climate, nor are we acquainted with any remedy by means of which this disease could be cured, hence a treatise on the diagnosis of this disease would be valueless in a therapeutic point of view.

B. DISEASES OF THE SPLEEN.

THE pathological conditions of the spleen belong to the most obscure and least known points of Pathology. This is mostly owing to the circumstance that it is only during the last twenty years that more careful investigations concerning the functions of this organ have been instituted, which, on account of inherent difficulties and a liability to deception, have not yet yielded any very brilliant results, and have more especially shed very little light on the functional disturbances to which the spleen is liable. We know most undoubtedly that in leucæmia the spleen is generally very much diseased; but whether the disease is the cause or consequence of the leucæmia, is not yet decided; for the circumstance that the spleen is one of the great organs of sanguification, does not justify the hypothesis that leucæmia originates in the spleen as an abnormal physiological process; we have not as yet got that far in our knowledge. However, although we are not yet able to draw many conclusions from the still mysterious functions of the spleen, the anatomical structure of this organ suggests an explanation for many of its morbid conditions. The tissue of the spleen is softer than that of any other glandular body, and contains a number of cavities that seem to be formed by the veins. This circumstance alone enables it to receive a quantity of blood into its interior. In addition to this, however, the capsule of the spleen is very flabby, and only capable of slight resistance to the pressure of the blood from within. The tissue of the spleen, moreover, possesses only a slight degree of elasticity, so that, if engorged with blood, it returns to its former condition only with great difficulty. After receiving the larger veins of the stomach and other less important ones, the veins of the spleen pour their contents into the vena portarum. The spleen is only held loosely in its place by folds of the peritoneum.

These anatomical data account for the frequent participation of the spleen in diseases of the abdominal viscera, for the influence of affections of the spleen upon the stomach, and the proportionate scarcity of a separate disease of the spleen. Hence we see diseases of the liver that impede the flow of blood from the vena portarum, or, in general, all diseases that interfere with the reflux of the blood from the abdominal cavity, such as emphysema of the lungs and diseases of the right heart, accompanied by considerable enlargement of the spleen. The loose attachments of the spleen explain to us how this enlarged viscus may sometimes leave its normal position by gravitating downwards. Again the connection of the veins of the stomach with the vena lienalis explains how obstructions in the circulation of the blood in the spleen can easily result in vomiting of blood.

The changes which the spleen undergoes in acute infectious diseases, are so far, however, inexplicable. Enlargement of the spleen is principally seen in typhus and intermittent fever; in the former it is said to determine the character of the disease, which is not so. Leaving out intermittent fever, where a well defined anomalous change in the blood cannot well be proven, splenetic tumors are principally caused by such morbid conditions as result in a striking alteration of the composition of the blood.

Beside these morbid changes in the spleen where the enlargement of this viscus appears like an isolated symptom, without having the character of an idiopathic disease, we meet with splenetic tumors that do not seem to originate in any specific or known cause, but probably because the patients do not know how to account for them. These tumors are exactly like hypertrophy that had arisen from continued sanguineous engorgement, and which, after the removal of the primary disturbance, remained behind as an idiopathic disease. For instance, in malarious districts they are often met with in individuals who never had fever and ague.

From these statements it is evident that there is no special therapeutics for hypertrophied conditions of the spleen, any more than it is possible to present them as some special form of disease. If, however, we should be called upon to treat an hypertrophy of the last-named kind, the chief remedies would be: *China*, *Arsenicum*, and *Natrum muriaticum*, less frequently *Lycopodium*.

Splenitis, Inflammation of the Spleen.

A fully developed splenitis is a very rare disease, the lower grades of this disease are undoubtedly more frequent, although not easily recognized with positive certainty on account of the vagueness of the symptoms.

The causes of this disease are very indefinite. Injuries, running, excessive bodily exertions, a cold, suppression of normal or habitual losses of blood, spread of the inflammation of adjoining organs, are mentioned as such causes, but with very doubtful propriety.

The inflammation is either seated in the capsule or substance of the spleen; the former is the more frequent of the two, in which case the splenitis is a sort of circumscribed peritonitis which does not affect the organ itself. An inflammation of the substance of the spleen almost always affects only a part of the organ, and very commonly terminates in the formation of an abscess. We transcribe Hartmann's statement of the symptoms, with this remark, however, that his definition of a splenitis will seldom be found applicable to the fully developed disease.

"Violent, stitching, boring, tensive, throbbing pains in the left hypochondrium, region of the spleen, spreading to the shoulder, clavicle, nipple, or else to the stomach, back, and downwards to the kidneys; they interfere with the act of respiration, constrict the epigastrium, are aggravated by pressure on the left hypochondrium, by motion and deep breathing, coughing, sneezing, etc., and make it either difficult or impossible for the patient to lie on the left side. This painfulness continues unabated; sometimes the temperature in the region of the spleen is sensibly higher, and, if the lower and anterior portion of the spleen is affected, it is felt anteriorly in the region of the ninth and tenth rib like a hard, round, not very movable body which is exceedingly painful to pressure. The following accompanying symptoms are frequently present: Oppression of breathing, anxiety, cough, dyspeptic symptoms, vomiting, burning in the region of the stomach, frequently a bitter or sour taste with burning eructations, retching, vomiting which affords no relief, hiccough. Most every attack of splenitis is attended with vomiting of blood, almost at the beginning of it; at first the blood is usually mixed with bile and mucus; it looks like serum, except that it has the blackish color of venous blood. Afterwards the blood that is vomited, is thicker, blacker and thrown up in larger quantity. Obscuration of sight, vertigo, disposition to faint, are frequently present, especially in the erect position. The fever is a synocha, the thirst distressing, pulse changing, at the left radius it is often suspended, intermittent; the urine is burning-hot, dark-brown, less frequently of a dirty, saffron-color. The fever is of the remittent type, sometimes even quartan or tertian."

The disease runs its course in from a week to a fortnight, after which sweat, critical urine, phlyctænæ around the mouth, and occasional attacks of moderate epistaxis set in, and the inflammation and swelling are dispersed. Induration and permanent enlargement of the spleen may remain as consequences of the inflammation. Death rarely ensues; it is brought about by softening or suppuration of the parenchyma.

A slight degree of inflammation of the capsule is not a very rare occurrence. The violent stitches which are suddenly felt in the region of the spleen after a violent effort, such as running immediately after a copious meal, and which stop one's breath and are distinguished from ordinary splenetic stitches by continuing unabated for one or more weeks, are undoubtedly manifestations of this capsular inflammation. The general health is not much disturbed, and there are no symptoms present that might lead one to infer the existence of functional disturbances of the spleen. Such a condition can scarcely be regarded as a simple hyperæmia.

In order to obtain a correct diagnosis of organic alterations of the spleen, it is important that the situation of the organ should be carefully determined, and that the direction which the enlargement generally takes should be exactly known. The normal spleen yields a dull sound on percussion, from the free border of the eleventh rib upwards and backwards, within a space of two inches to two inches and a half. As a rule the spleen enlarges first anteriorly, hence the dulness is more sensibly perceived towards the margin of the false ribs, beyond which it is scarcely ever felt to a great extent. It is only when the enlargement is considerable that the dulness is felt beyond the eleventh rib; and in such a case the spleen can be distinctly felt. In particular cases the dulness is felt along the whole of the left half of the abdomen, down to the iliac bone.

The homœopathic treatment of splenitis has not yet been firmly established by practical experience; Hartmann's statements in this respect are speculative and require to be verified by clinical observations. We here transcribe his remarks concerning the treatment of splenitis, because they contain the names of all the leading remedies in this disease.

"In idiopathic splenitis the fever is generally more acute than in splenitis complicated with other diseases; a few doses of *Aconite* will always improve the case. If this remedy only moderates the fever without removing any of the main symptoms, it would be foolish to persist in the use of the drug with a view of obtaining a result of this kind by sheer force as it were. Under such circumstances a remedy in homœopathic rapport with the symptoms should be given. We have such a remedy in *Nux vomica*, more particularly if the sensation of an internal swelling; the stitching pain which is aggravated by contact and motion; the spasmodic pain in the left hypochondrium, with qualmishness, especially in the pit of the stomach; the aversion to food and the fainting fits; the vomiting of blood or the mere gulping up of a dark blood from the stomach are attended with other gastric derangements, dyspeptic conditions, constipation, etc., and previous derangements, the constitution and temperament of the patient likewise point to Nux.

"*Arnica* is an excellent remedy in this inflammation, if the blood, which is vomited up, is coagulated, the color is between bright- and dark-red, and the respiration is interfered with by a continued aching, stitching pain in the left hypochondrium.

"Next to this remedy we have *Cantharides*, not, however, unless the kidney of the same side is inflamed and there is a continual retching with discharge of a small quantity of blood, a stitching pressure and feeling of fulness in the left hypochondrium as far as the dorsal vertebræ, with tossing about as if in a desperate agony.

"*Belladonna* is undoubtedly an efficient remedy in splenitis, sanguineous congestions constitute the proper sphere of action for Belladonna, and congestion of the spleen is the forerunner of inflammation of this organ. Although the symptoms of splenitis are very obscure, yet even if the inflammatory symptoms, as we see them, should lead us to suspect an inflammation of some of the adjoining organs, Belladonna would still be indicated by its homœopathicity to the latter. *Chamomilla*, likewise, deserves being mentioned, for a tensive and burning pain in the left hypochondrium is characteristic of this drug, likewise a pressure in the pit of the stomach, frequent hiccuping.

"Although *China* is of very little use in really inflammatory diseases, yet I am satisfied that, after the fever has been moderated by a few doses of Aconite, it will prove of eminent service, if the vital strength has become depressed by the frequent vomiting of blood, and the pinching pressure, which is experienced at the commencement of the disease, is changed to sharp, cutting stitches, with swelling and hardness of the spleen. Nor is it out of place, if frequent diarrhœic stools set in, with discharge of a dark, coagulated blood, although *Arsenic* may deserve the preference under such circumstances, especially if the patient complains of a violent burning pain in the spleen with swelling of this organ, in connection with an uninterrupted anxiety and throbbing in the pit of the stomach which is distinctly felt by the finger; likewise if the spleen is swollen and painful and the patient is prevented by the tearing stitches from lying on that side. The accompanying fever is characterized by a dry, burning heat, with great thirst, restlessness, præcordial anguish, sallow complexion, dry and cracked lips, white coating of the tongue, bitter taste in the mouth, nausea, aversion to food, etc."

"*Bryonia* is homœopathic in the absence of diarrhœa and vomiting of blood; the stitching pains in the region of the spleen are attended with constipation. In my opinion, *Bryonia* and *Pulsatilla* are most frequently indicated in inflammation of the capsule of the spleen, if the stitching and aching pain is very much aggravated by every motion, and a swelling is distinctly perceptible in the painful region."

"Homœopathic physicians, myself included, have found the curative power of the above-mentioned medicines in splenitis confirmed by experience; however, they are not the only remedies in this disease, but, to judge by the symptoms, the following may likewise prove efficacious: *Laurocerasus*, *Mezereum*, *Drosera*, *Stannum*, *Plumbum*, *Spigelia*, *Lycopodium*, *Carbo vegetabilis*, and others."

To these statements we take the liberty of adding a few remarks. Hartmann's predilection for Aconite has undoubtedly induced him to assign to this agent a high place among the remedies for splenitis, although he admits that the homœopathicity of Aconite to this disease is not very striking. *Belladonna* seems the more appropriate even at the onset, especially if the stomach is very much affected, which is almost always the case. Among Hartmann's last series, *Mezereum* is the only remedy that may prove useful, the balance are not at all appropriate in such an acute disease, at any rate they have no very strikingly characteristic symptom. On the other hand *Stannum*, *Plumbum*, *Carbo veg.*, and more particularly *Lycopodium*, may be tried, if the inflammation persists and finally passes into the chronic form in the shape of a splenetic tumor. Beside the above-mentioned remedies we have: *Berberis*, *Bromum*, *Agnus castus*, and *Mercurius;* the last-mentioned remedy more, from general reasons based upon analogy, than by virtue of physiologico-homœopathic similarities. In the chronic form, *Iodium* and *Sulphur* are likewise indicated. It is desirable, on account of the scanty material, that every case of splenitis, treated homœopathically, should be published. This is the only method of obtaining satisfactory evidence regarding the reliability of the above-mentioned drugs as homœopathic remedies for this disease.

C. DISEASES OF THE PANCREAS.

In our opinion the pancreas is much less accessible than the spleen, and the knowledge we possess of its morbid alterations is as yet so imperfect and uncertain that it is impossible to infer the nature of these alterations from the phenomena on the living; we can at most decide that the pancreas is diseased. We have communicated a case in the Zeit. für Hom. Klinik, 1857, which, as far as we know, is the only clinical case of this disease that has as yet been recorded in our Journals, and corresponds to the picture of what our modern pathologists have designated as sub-acute inflammation of the pancreas. We here subjoin a brief recapitulation of the symptoms.

Appetite slight, but occasionally a sensation of hunger; tongue thinly coated, taste bad but not particularly definable; directly under the stomach, above the navel, extending from the mesian line to the left, and at a corresponding spot of the back, insufferable pains that cannot be described, exacerbating in the evening or during the early part of the night. The painful region is somewhat sensitive to hard pressure, but no swelling can be discovered. Five or six hours after eating solid food, vomiting sets in, which is sometimes sudden and violent, never preceded by nausea, and mitigating the local pain; a slimy fluid resembling serum is vomited up, containing food if any had been partaken of shortly before, not otherwise. In addition: headache, languor, anxiety and desponding mood, restless sleep, scarcely any fever, expression of suffering; marked emaciation with occasional diarrhœa. There was, however, no icterus which is always present to some extent in pancreatitis.

Nux vomica, Cuprum, Iodium, Veratrum album, Arsenicum were given in vain. *Mercurius* and *Sulphur* might perhaps have been tried. After the *Sulphate of Atropine* a most decided improvement set in. *Belladonna* might perhaps have acted just as well; at any rate we should try it in a similar case. The above-mentioned symptoms might likewise suggest *Digitalis purpurea* which is their homœopathic simile. *Phosphorus* has the chief symptom, the vomiting.

It is of importance to fix the diagnosis in this affection. It has peculiar difficulties, especially if the vomiting is not sufficiently characteristic. The disease is readily confounded with an affection of the stomach, especially with chronic catarrh of this organ. But if we keep an eye on the fact that actual stomach-symptoms are absent; that the vomiting, in case it should occur in an attack of catarrh of the stomach in such a manner and at such a time, must always depend upon considerable changes of the pylorus having no symptomatic manifestations; that the pain is felt in a different locality from what it is in catarrh of the stomach; that the course of the disease is subacute, not chronic; that finally the stool is characterized by peculiarities that are not present either in catarrh of the stomach or bowels; it would seem as though the diagnosis could not be very difficult.

Pancreatic affections attended with a decrease of the secretion of saliva, are beyond the reach of our present means of diagnosis. It has frequently happened that an emaciation that could not be accounted for by any morbid action taking place in other organs, has been traced to structural alterations of the pancreas. Considering what a powerful influence the saliva has upon the digestion, we can easily understand that a defective quality or a deficient secretion of the pancreatic juice must give rise in a superior degree to the symptoms which are caused by a deficiency of saliva.

SIXTH SECTION.

Diseases of the Uropoiëtic System.

A. DISEASES OF THE KIDNEYS.

It is not very long since the diseases of the kidneys have become a special subject of the attention of physicians. Whatever important part the renal secretions have played in the practice of medicine from its earliest beginning, the changes in the urine were attributed more to general than to local causes. It is only since the beginning of the present century that the united efforts of chemistry and pathological anatomy have effected an essential progress in the diagnosis of the morbid conditions of the kidneys, to which Bright's discovery has furnished the most important incentive. These improvements dating only as far back as the last twenty years, it becomes self-evident that Hahnemann, in spite of his excellent knowledge of chemistry, knew but little of the urine and its changes. Hence the great deficiency, in our Materia Medica, of useful objective symptoms of the urinary organs, which subsequent provers have in vain or but imperfectly tried to remedy. That the importance of objective symptoms, especially in the domain of renal affections, should not be undervalued, must be clear to any one who, in view of our modern means of diagnosis, undertakes to treat such morbid conditions in accordance with our homœopathic provings; for in no disease are we more easily misled by the general symptoms than in affections of the kidneys. It is probably on this account that such affections occupy but a small space in the literature of our school, and we wish to have it understood that the therapeutic portion of this section contains a great deal that is hypothetical and unproven.

In order to render further repetitions unnecessary, we will here discuss more fully certain points referring to the diagnosis of renal diseases.

The situation of the kidneys on both sides, and close to the vertebral column, where they are surrounded by a thick layer of fat and loose cellular tissue, and covered externally by a heavy layer of muscular tissue, renders it impossible and always uncertain in most cases, to obtain a knowledge of their condition by palpation and percussion, the more so as percussion must necessarily lead to deceptive results on account of the peculiar situation of the intestine, and palpation cannot be conducted with certainty on account of the movable position of the kidneys. For an appreciation of local sensations of pain it is sufficient to know that the kidneys are situated on both sides of and near the upper lumbar vertebræ, from the lower edge of the eleventh or the upper edge of the twelfth rib as far as near the upper rim of the os ilium.

An analysis of the urine remains the only sure means of diagnosis. It cannot be expected that we should furnish here a detailed statement of the different points referring to this subject; this would take up a very considerable space. In his Vierteljahrsschrift, Clotar Müller has collated the most important items of urinary analysis; for special data we refer the reader to this article and content ourselves in this place with communicating the most necessary facts.

The chemical composition of the urine is of little or no significance in diseases of the kidneys; the deviations from the normal quantity of uric acid, salts, etc., scarcely ever points to a primary, idiopathic affection of the kidneys, and is of importance only with a view of arriving at a correct diagnostic appreciation of various other morbid conditions, but more particularly of constitutional diseases. We infer the existence of renal diseases from an abnormal quantity of the urine, from deviations from the specific weight of the urine, and from the substances mixed up with this fluid.

The quantity of normal urine cannot well be defined. It depends upon the supply of food, upon the quantity of the liquids drank, upon muscular and mental action, upon the activity of the skin, upon the condition of the atmosphere, and upon individual and not further demonstrable peculiarities. How difficult it is to determine these different influences correctly, is only clear to those who have persistently measured the quantity of their urine. In spite of large quantities of liquids having been drank, the urinary secretion may be comparatively small, if the cutaneous exhalations are very copious, or a good deal of salt food has been used. Beer, especially hop-beer causes a profuse flow of urine in most persons; in exceptional cases, the quantity of urine is lessened. Coffee and tea retard the secretion of urine, yet the quantity voided, is increased; wine, on the contrary, diminishes the secretion of urine in almost every one. That more urine is voided in winter than in summer, is easily accounted for by the increase of perspiration in the summer season; but the weather being apparently unchanged, perceptible changes may take place in the quantity of urine, depending upon differences in atmospheric pressure, and the amount of electric tension. Continued bodily exertion diminishes, continued mental exertion increases the urinary secretion; after great commotions of the mind or feelings we likewise often have a large increase of urine. We mention these points in order to show how important it is to investigate and observe all these circumstances before jumping at the conclusion that the urine is morbidly increased. In addition to these normal variations in the quantity of the urinary fluid we have others belonging more or less in the domain of disease, and being of great importance to the physician. We have shown how the normal cutaneous activity affects the urine; this influence is still more strikingly observed in many disturbances of the cutaneous functions. In extensive burns the renal function is much interfered with; likewise in consequence of sudden colds, inflammations of the skin and the epispastic action of vesicatories, not so much in consequence of their specific stimulating effect. Finally the urine is much less in all febrile conditions, and likewise in some affections without fever, especially heart-disease; here the quantity of urine is always more or less sensibly diminished.

The question now is when the quantity of the urine justifies the conclusion that we have an affection of the kidneys to deal with. The normal quantity of urine, when a moderate quantity of liquid is taken, varies from 24 to 40 ounces per day, or from 800 to 1,200 cubic centimeters. This quantity is about equal to the volume of one and a half ordinary wine-bottles. A continued increase or decrease of this quantity justifies the suspicion that the kidneys are diseased, unless some very acute febrile affection should be present, in which case an extremely small quantity of urine is sometimes secreted. For ordinary purposes, and with a view of securing an approximate determination of the quantity of urine, a bottle and a half full of water may be poured into the chamber, and the quantity of urine voided in twenty-four hours, may be measured accordingly; if we desire a more exact measurement, a glass-cylinder provided with a centimeter-scale is absolutely required.

The specific gravity of the urine is subject to the same variations as the quantity. In the normal condition it is so much higher in proportion as the quantity of urine voided in the course of a day is less; this is inferred from the circumstance that the excretion of solid substances in the course of twenty-four hours remains about the same; the specific gravity being determined by the quantity of the solids, it becomes self-evident that this gravity is increased or diminished according as there is more or less water in the urine. The normal specific gravity is between 1,010 and 1,032, also 1,034, the latter figure being very questionable. The less the specific gravity when the quantity of urine is very much diminished; or the higher when the quantity is very much increased, the more we are justified in suspecting the existence of renal disease; in doubtful cases the use of the areometer becomes indispensable. Even if the results obtained by means of this instrument are not extremely accurate, yet they are sufficiently so for all practical purposes, and the facility with which the instrument can be used, commends it to our favorable consideration.

The urine is mixed up with a great many substances. Independently of those that are rarely found in it, it sometimes contains blood, coloring matter, pus, mucus, gravel, coagula, albumen and sugar.

The admixture of blood is generally recognized by the red, or even brown-red, blackish color, sometimes with a bluish tint. If there is but little blood, it cannot well be confounded with bile-pigment. The presence of blood-corpuscles as revealed by the microscope, places the presence of blood beyond all doubt. Sometimes these are absent, although the urine may be intensely colored like blood; this occurs only in diseases with a typhoid composition of the blood. If bloody coagula are present, an error of diagnosis cannot possibly be committed. From which of the urinary organs the blood is derived, will be shown when we come to treat of renal hemorrhage.

The diagnostic value of the coloring matter of the urine is not yet firmly settled. We have already alluded to the hæmatine in the urine; the presence of albumen and sugar in the urine is likewise often revealed by a peculiar color of this fluid, the presence of albumen by a feeble bluish-green tint, and that of sugar by a yellowish-green. This, however, is of trifling value, for even without this peculiar color, the symptoms will demand a careful examination of the urine.

Pus and mucus form almost the same appearances; they can only be distinguished by the microscope. Such a microscopic examination is important because pus points rather to a disease of the kidneys, mucus to some abnormal condition of the bladder. We must not overlook the fact that even in the normal condition of the system mucus is often secreted with the urine. In the clear urine mucus floats as a transparent cloud at some distance from the bottom of the vessel.

Gravel is scarcely ever found in the urine, except when the kidneys are diseased. We do not mean to say that the structural changes of the kidneys must be considerable, for the formation of gravel generally results from defective nutrition. However, it is also met with in individuals who lead a very uniform and simple life; under such circumstances it is most probably the result of some abnormal change in the kidneys. Of the larger concretions, such as renal calculi, we shall speak hereafter.

Coagula, either in the shape of granular conglomerations, or as cylindrical formations, constitute one of the most important admixtures of the urine. Their presence can only be determined by the microscope. We shall recur to these foreign elements in the urine when we come to treat of Bright's disease.

Albumen is not only found in the urine in Bright's disease, but likewise in smaller quantity in physiologically normal conditions, such as pregnancy. Its presence is of importance only when there is an excessive quantity of it, small quantities being of no moment. A large quantity of albumen in the urine always indicates an intense disease of the kidneys. Albumen can be tested for in two different ways. After having first satisfied ourselves that the urine has an acid reaction, we fill a test-tube half full of this fluid. If there is no acid reaction, we first add a little acetic acid, until a feeble degree of acid reaction is obtained. After heating the urine over the flame of a spirit-lamp, the fluid, as soon as the boiling point is nearly reached, shows a cloud at its surface, which gradually spreads towards the bottom of the vessel, and is caused by the coagulation of the albumen. Its density increases in proportion as the urine contains more albumen. If there is but a small quantity of albumen, the cloud becomes visible only after the urine has been allowed to settle and cool, and the coagulated particles have collected at the bottom of the tube. If there is much albumen, the coagulation generally takes place in larger flocks. Inasmuch as the Phosphates, by boiling, yield a precipitate resembling albumen, the urine has either to be further tested with nitric acid, or a little dilute muriatic acid should be added to the boiled liquid, in which case albumen will remain undissolved, whereas the cloudiness caused by the presence of Phosphates is soon dispersed. The second test consists in dropping into a like quantity of urine, as before stated, drops of nitric acid. A precipitate of coagulated albumen will likewise be thrown down. It is always advisable to resort to both these tests.

Sugar in the urine is not a symptom of some specific, idiopathic disease of the kidneys, but of an intensely penetrating constitutional affection. Since we have classed diabetes among the diseases of the kidneys, it is proper that the means by which sugar can be detected in the urine, should be explained in this place. If, independent of general morbid phenomena, the urine is excreted in excessive quantities, having a somewhat dim or cloudy appearance, with a very slight, greenish-yellow tint, and a specific gravity, which never falls below the highest figure above mentioned, or even exceeds it, we may almost certainly conclude that the urine contains sugar. The chemical methods of testing for sugar are too complicated for the practical physician, and can only be employed with great loss of time. Since all he cares to know is, whether sugar is present in the urine, whose increase or decrease is indicated with more or less positiveness by the rise and fall of the specific gravity, we propose the following methods of testing for sugar as the most practicable. We will indicate several methods, in order to enable the physician to verify the results of his experiments by applying a variety of tests, for not one of them singly can be depended upon with absolute certainty. This is easily accounted for by the differences in the composition of the urine.

1. Dissolve in the urine to be examined, a small quantity of extract of ox-gall, add gradually concentrated sulphuric acid, and stir carefully with a little glass rod. If a purple-red color ensues, the liquid contains sugar.

2. Equal parts of urine and lime-water are made to boil in a test-tube; if no color is seen, there is no sugar; on the contrary, if the mixture shows more or less color, it contains sugar.

3. In a test-tube, mix equal parts of urine and a solution of the Carbonate of Soda (consisting of one part of crystallized Carbonate of Soda and three parts of distilled water;) add to this mixture a pinch of the Nitrate of Bismuth, and heat the whole until it begins to boil. If, after boiling, the snow-white salt of Bismuth shows

the least blackness or gray color, the presence of sugar is indicated with positive certainty; no other constituent of the urine is capable of changing the salt of Bismuth to a sub-oxide, or even to metallic Bismuth. Pure rock sugar does not induce a reaction of this kind, but glucose does.

4. Dissolve a drachm of the Bichromate of Potash in two ounces of distilled water, add two drachms of concentrated sulphuric acid; let the mixture settle, and pour the clear fluid cautiously off the sediment. Heat equal parts of this liquid and diabetic urine, until they boil; if sugar is present, even one half per cent. of it will yield a characteristic blue-green color, whereas a whitish precipitate indicates the presence of albumen. Reaction sets in even without the urine being heated, except that it takes more time, whereas boiling excites the reaction at once. The blue-green color becomes more or less striking, according as there is more or less sugar, so that, with a little practice, the increase or decrease of sugar can be determined by this method. If there is no sugar in the urine, a dirty brownish-red color ensues, at most with a very feeble greenish tint, which, however, does not indicate the presence of sugar. The presence of albumen, bile-pigment, or bile-acids does not prevent the reaction.

With these four tests, all of which are simple, and can be applied without any outlay for instruments or reagents, the presence of sugar can be detected in every case, which is the main point in practice.

We deem it unnecessary to dwell here more fully upon general pathological or therapeutical data concerning the kidneys, the more as we shall refer to this subject as far as may be necessary, in the following chapters.

1. Nephritis, Inflammation of the Kidneys.

In opposition to other inflammatory affections of the kidneys of which mention will be made hereafter, we apply the name of nephritis, or nephritis vera, or insterstitial inflammation of the kidneys, to an inflammation of the tissue connecting the tubuli uriniferi.

The etiology is in many respects very obscure. The disease occurs chiefly among middle-aged persons, and befalls men more frequently than women. Proximate causes of the disease are: Contusions of the region of the kidneys, sharp or adhering renal calculi, violent colds, employment of various drugs, such as oil of turpentine, cantharides, nitre, also savin, whether used internally or externally; sometimes violent, extensive burns. Secondarily the disease is often caused by suppurative inflammations in other organs, affections of the brain and spinal marrow, heart-disease, etc.

Insterstitial nephritis usually sets in, like other acute inflammatory diseases, with a violent chill, which is almost immediately succeeded by the local pains. After they have reached the acme of their intensity, they extend over the whole region of the kidneys, on both sides; they are continuous, of different degrees of acuteness, cannot easily be described according to their nature, they are considerably aggravated by pressure upon the renal region, likewise by violent contractions of the diaphragm, or by motion generally, also by lying on the affected side and by the warmth of the bed. They are scarcely ever restricted to the kidneys; on the contrary, following the course of the ureters they radiate into the bladder, testicles, and, in the case of females into the round ligaments and thighs. Sometimes the testicles are found drawn up spasmodically towards the abdominal ring. With the appearance of these pains the urinary secretion diminishes in proportion as the inflammation involves a larger portion of the kidneys, so that the secretion of urine may be entirely suspended. At first the urine is only saturated, sometimes tinged like blood; but it may likewise preserve its normal color, if one kidney is sound and the other does not secrete any urine at all. The general constitutional equilibrium is very much disturbed. The fever is very violent, the pulse hurried and soon becomes small and contracted, the skin is hot and dry, the thirst agonizing. The patients feel sick to the core. Vomiting is a frequent occurrence without the stomach appearing much deranged, for the tongue may be quite clean. At first the bowels are quite constipated, the appetite is gone. The further course of the disease varies in accordance with the peculiar anatomical changes in the kidneys, on which account we here subjoin a description of them.

The inflammation very seldom invades the whole extent of the kidney, generally only a part of it; sometimes it is confined to single foci. At the beginning of this morbid process the kidney is enlarged, intensely red, its parenchyma is permeated by a thickish, bloody fluid, through which the internal structure of the kidney is but indistinctly perceived. Very soon the infiltration becomes discolored, somewhat yellowish, then grayish or of a brownish-gray color, after which isolated yellow points are seen in it which denote the commencement of suppuration. These points increase in size, either forming detached foci of suppuration, of different sizes and usually of a cuneiform shape, or else they run together into one

Diseases of the Kidneys.

large cavernous abscess which may even fill the whole of the kidney. Side by side with the purulent deposits a number of small, or else a few detached more considerable hemorrhagic effusions, may often be seen. The suppuration may heal by forming cicatrized tissue; or else the pus may become encysted, and, its solid constituents being absorbed, may become inspissated; or it may find an outlet into the pelvis of the kidney, or into adjoining organs. In less frequent cases the inflammatory infiltration acts as in cirrhosis of the liver, giving rise to an excess of interstitial cicatrized tissue which results in atrophy of the kidney. The atrophied kidney shows many depressions on the surface, which is covered with granulations and has a pale appearance. A larger abscess may likewise result in atrophy of the renal parenchyma, although less extensive than when the suppuration of the cortical substance is more diffuse.

The further course of nephritis corresponds with the changes that have been indicated. Recovery may take place after the first onset of the disease, without any suppuration having taken place, or by arresting it, the completeness of the recovery being shown most conclusively by the urine resuming its normal quality. On the contrary, if suppuration sets in, the local pain decreases, becomes duller and more like a painful pressure; the fever, however, increases, frequent chills or shiverings are experienced by the patient, the tongue becomes coated, the stomach is still more disturbed, pus is found in the urine at an early stage of the disease and there is frequently an admixture of blood. The patient becomes anxious, restless, the pulse is more frequent and smaller. The subsequent phenomena depend upon how far the urinary secretion is suspended. If only one kidney is diseased, or only a small portion of both, there is no material diminution of the quantity of urine secreted ; an abscess forms, with the usual phenomena characterizing the suppurative process, the abscess either discharging and recovery taking place, or else renal phthisis setting in, with all the symptoms of marasmus gradually supervening. This last mentioned result may drag along for months, the urine containing pus all the time. Characteristic features of renal phthisis are, a great tendency to malignant affections of the skin, dermatitis, decubitus. If the urinary secretion is considerably impeded by an infiltration of the kidneys, symptoms make their appearance which denote the supervention of uræmia. They set in most suddenly when the excretion of urine had been completely suspended from the beginning, and the patients die in a few days, with all the symptoms of an intense cerebral typhus. They may likewise set in gradually, so that the disease, by slow degrees, assumes a typhoid character. The patients sink into a state of sopor, are attacked with a more or less violent delirium, convulsions, and finally die comatose. This uræmic intoxication may likewise supervene, if the disease runs a very chronic course, so that it is almost impossible to recognize it as such, because the morbid renal symptoms are not very important, at any rate very indistinct.

The diagnosis of nephritis cannot always be made with perfect certainty, because the symptoms are sometimes very trifling, and, moreover, very little characteristic. The difference between nephritis and Bright's disease will be pointed out in a subsequent chapter. The distinction between typhus and nephritis is often difficult, unless the attack has been watched from the commencement. It is, to some extent, pathognomonic of a high degree of nephritis, that the urine is excreted in an extremely small quantity, and always contains pus-corpuscles. In nephritis the bowels are almost always obstinately constipated; if the disease terminates in phthisis, the constipation changes to diarrhœa.

The prognosis is unfavorable only if the symptoms of uræmia become more and more manifest, until they reach the highest degree of intensity. In other respects the disease becomes the more threatening, the more protracted a course it runs, until it finally terminates in phthisis. If the pus has an outlet through the ureters, the renal abscess is of not so much importance; but from the moment it seeks another outlet, there is great, although no immediate danger.

We here subjoin a few remarks on the inflammation of the pelvis—pyelitis—the treatment of which is in many respects like that of nephritis.

Pyelitis easily arises from the same causes as nephritis, more particularly from the presence of urinary concretions; or it may result from the spread of other inflammatory processes, accompanied by violent general catarrhal inflammatory phenomena.

The symptoms likewise resemble each other very closely, except that the disease does not set in so suddenly and with as much intensity; the symptoms of gastric derangement are less regularly present, and the painfulness is not so great, especially at the commencement of the attack. The urine becomes turbid and purulent at an early stage of the disease, and is usually tinged with blood.

The excretion of urine takes place very frequently and is very painful. Uræmia occurs rarely as the disease progresses, which becomes immediately threatening only if an existing concretion cannot be removed and speedy ulceration is the consequence. On the other hand the affection is exceedingly disposed to become chronic, and, in that case, becomes dangerous by the constant loss of pus. While voiding the urine it is uniformly turbid, of a greenish, bright-yellow or whitish color; after settling, the super-natant liquid is clear, and a loose, white sediment is formed, being sharply separated from the liquid and consisting of pus and mucus. Since these substances likewise coagulate, their nature cannot be inferred exclusively from applying the tests for albumen, but they have to be examined microscopically. Chronic pyelitis is a very obstinate, and, when highly developed, a very dangerous affection, although years may sometimes elapse until a fatal termination is reached.

We omit mentioning an inflammation of the capsule of the kidney because, if existing separately and alone, it is difficult to diagnose, even if abscesses have formed that discharge their contents into the adjoining organs, for their origin cannot be traced to the kidney with any positive certainty.

Treatment. Among the remedies for nephritis we have to select those whose external as well as internal use results in this disease; they are principally: *Cantharides, Terebinthina, Sabina, Nitrum,* whose specific action upon the kidneys has been satisfactorily and abundantly revealed to us by the ignorance of lay-people as well as by the shortsightedness and boldness of physicians. They are mostly appropriate only as long as the disease retains its acute character, not in its chronic form.

Cantharides. From Schroff's experiments with this drug we transcribe the following poisoning with *Cantharidin* because it contains a full and striking image of nephritis. For particulars we refer to the "Zeitschrift der Gesellschaft der Ærzte in Wien," 1855, No. VII. and VIII.

At half-past four in the afternoon 0.01 gramme of Cantharidin was swallowed, without any admixture. Soon after, an increased feeling of warmth on the tongue, where a number of hyperæmic spots became visible; increased secretion of saliva. Next, a burning in the stomach, eructations, nausea and oppression on the chest; tongue and lips extremely sensitive; deglutition, even of liquids, is impossible. The pulse falls from 62 to 56. In the evening, copious, papescent stool; the urine is voided without any difficulty. After the lapse of eight hours marked blisters break out on the tongue and gums. Between midnight and four o'clock in the morning the chill gradually gives way to an increase of warmth, the pulse increasing to 90. At the same time involuntary, but painless discharges of urine, which become more and more frequent, and finally painful, until they take place every two or three minutes, attended with such a violent spasm, that stool becomes impossible. The urine now is mixed with blood. At four in the morning, stool with tenesmus. From this time a drawing, stitching pain in the region of the kidneys, aggravated by external pressure. Violent vomiting in the morning, after tasting a little water, again in three hours, with expulsion, first of greenish, afterwards reddish, and finally chocolate-colored substances. The stool likewise contains blood. At one o'clock at noon, twenty-one hours after taking the drug, flushed face, hot skin, pulse 80; in the mouth the effects of the local action of the drug are visible; violent pains in the stomach, bowels, and kidneys; constant urging to urinate, burning of the urine in the urethra, the mouth of which is red and swollen. The urine is voided in tolerable quantity, but averages less than usual, deposits a copious, loose, slimy sediment, and shows here and there a reddish tinge. Under the microscope degenerated blood-corpuscles and normal pus-globules are seen, a quantity of epithelium and fibrinous cylinders. The reaction is feebly alkaline. Upon the addition of concentrated nitric acid, a dense cloud is thrown down. The pains in the kidneys lasted until the fifth day, whereas a fortnight after some traces of poisoning still remained visible.

To this picture of nephritis, which can scarcely be drawn with more completeness and accuracy, we will add a few data from other detached observations. In Schroff's case, the evident action of Cantharidin did not become visible until after some time. Usually it sets in after six or twelve hours. In a case related by Jaffe, it began three hours after the poison had been administered, with the most marked intensity. According to Bouillaud, vesicatories, if applied to scarified surfaces, act with a high degree of intensity; albuminuria is always present in such cases. After Cantharidin a post-mortem shows inflammation of the kidneys more or less fully developed and extended, but it is never stated in what parts of the kidneys the inflammatory process is principally located. The rapid appearance of pus-globules in the urine seems to imply the existence of pyelitis. In the next chapter we shall revert to this subject more fully. The symptoms of a moderate degree of uræmic intoxication are noticed in some cases of poisoning with Cantharidin.

These statements show that, if anywhere, it is in the treatment of nephritis with Cantharides that the law of similarity must prove true. Hartmann considers Cantharides as one of the chief remedies for nephritis, and gives the following indications for its use : "Stitching, lancinating, and tearing pains in the renal and lumbar region, aggravated by the least motion, even until they seem intolerable, and sometimes arresting the breathing by the suddenness of their appearance; painful urination, which is sometimes even impossible, or discharge of the urine drop by drop; it is mixed with blood, and the emission is attended with the most agonizing, burning pains, in which case it is very likely that both kidneys are inflamed. The accompanying fever is usually very acute, the pulse frequent, full and rather hard, thirst great, cheeks hot and flushed; loss of appetite, constipation; the sleep is disturbed by the violent pains and the urging to urinate, which is generally more frequently experienced during the night; or the patient sleeps only by snatches, and feels much worse in the morning."

These symptoms embody not only an inflammation of the kidneys, but likewise of the other urinary organs. The inflammation superinduced by Cantharidin always runs a rapid course, is not inclined to become chronic, nor is there a trace of suppuration. Hence, the remedy is especially applicable in the first stage of nephritis.

Regarding **Terebinthina** we refer the reader to our remarks on the subject of Bright's disease.

Sabina, if we may judge from its pathogenesis, is not particularly appropriate in nephritis; at any rate, the pathogenetic effects of this drug in the urinary sphere, are not sufficiently precise. My attention was directed to Sabina by a tolerably violent nephritis, which it excited in a female who had swallowed a large dose of it for the purpose of producing a miscarriage, which attempt, however, did not succeed. The nephritis caused by this drug is not a consequence, but independent of the abortus.

Nitrum causes a nephritis that generally assumes a chronic form, with evident signs of pus in the urine. This effect, if caused by poisonous doses, is at first covered up by the extreme depression of the whole organism, and does not become manifest until at a later period. At that time the urine looks pale and turbid, or has a bloody tinge, depositing a thick, sharply delineated, white sediment which, when shaken, floats upwards in the shape of large flocks. The renal region is very painful, the emission of the urine more or less impeded.

Copaiva, Cubebs and **Mezereum** likewise cause inflammatory symptoms in the urinary organs. We have no adequate provings of either of these drugs. Nevertheless, they deserve our most attentive consideration.

We now have reached the better known and more frequently used drugs, namely:

Aconitum, which corresponds to nephritis, not only on account of the fever, but likewise in its special action upon the urinary organs. The secretion of urine is much less, takes place more frequently and with more difficulty, and is painful; in a case of poisoning the kidneys are found strongly engorged with blood. These local symptoms, in connection with the more general ones of a case of Aconite-poisoning, justify the selection of Aconite, especially in the first stage of the disease.

Next to Cantharides, **Belladonna** is undoubtedly the main remedy in nephritis. Hartmann recommends it if the pains in the kidneys are stinging-burning, extend towards the bladder, come in paroxysms, like colicky pains; at the same time cardialgia, a fiery urine which is passed in small quantities, anxiety, restlessness, constipation. Pus is likewise found in the urine. The local inflammatory symptoms, in connection with those of the brain, show that Belladonna corresponds fully with incipient uræmia, or even when attended with violent delirium, the more as complete retention of urine is one of the effects of Belladonna; hence, it is in a very acute attack of nephritis where symptoms of uræmia appear already in the first few days of the disease, that Belladonna is indicated.

Mercurius does not yield to Belladonna in importance as a remedy for nephritis. If we recommend Mercurius as adapted to the incipient stage of suppuration, we do not base our recommendation upon a few isolated inflammatory symptoms in the pathogenesis of Mercury, but upon the special symptomatic homœopathicity of this drug to the disease. This homœopathicity is proven by the pathogenesis of the drug. We have diminished secretion of urine, with increased urging; urine saturated, dark-brown, mixed with blood, cloudy, with a white sediment that looks like flour, or a white sediment which, when stirred, looks like clouds of flocks and shreds. These phenomena alone are sufficient to justify the selection of Mercury the more since the ailments that generally co-exist with Mercury, can be found in the pathogenesis of this drug, more especially the peculiar fever and the gastric derangements. Mercurius likewise corresponds to the course of uræmia; it has power to cause a condition simulating typhus, with powerful convulsions. The distinction between Belladonna and Mercurius, beside the special data, rests in the circumstance that the Belladonna-convulsions break out speedily, when the poison first begins to act; the Mercurius-convulsions, on the contrary, not till the poison has acted for some time, which shows that Mercurius is more appropriate where, after the inflammation has lasted for some time, symptoms of suppuration and subsequently those of uræmia gradually become manifest. If the question is asked: What mercurial preparation is most homœopathic to nephritis? we answer *Mercurius corrosivus.* A severe poisoning with Calomel or metallic Mercury sometimes is without any symptoms of nephritis; in a poisoning with sublimate, they are almost as characteristic as dysentery. Among my pharmacodynamic records there are three cases of poisoning with Corrosive Sublimate, with the following post-mortem symptoms: The kidneys are enlarged, dark-red on the cut surface, the pyramids and the cortical substance can scarcely be distinguished one from the other. (The urinary secretion had been almost entirely suppressed.) Three days after the poison had been swallowed, no more urine was secreted. The left kidney was of looser texture than normally; it contained a small abscess filled with pus; the bladder completely empty, and exceedingly contracted. Here we have the anatomical picture of nephritis from the first bloody exudation to the formation of an abscess. At the time when the kidney containing this abscess was dissected, (the report of the case is to be found in the Edinburgh Med. and Surg. Journal, 1811, vol. VII., page 150,) the anatomy of the kidney was still imperfectly known, and hence a detailed description of the post-mortem symptoms is wanting.

But the data are sufficient to show that Corrosive Sublimate occupies the first rank among the Mercurial preparations as a remedy for nephritis.

Hepar sulphuris is likewise a remedy for nephritis, although Hartmann is wrong in placing it side by side with Belladonna. Hepar has no retention of urine, nor any symptoms of incipient nephritis, but it seems appropriate in nephritis threatening to become chronic. The renal region is painful, the paroxysms of stitching pains radiate to the bladder and thigh, they are not violent; the urine is pale, turbid, even when being voided, depositing a white, flocculent sediment. The blood, if there is any, is discharged with the last drops of urine; it most likely indicates a disease of the bladder, not of the kidney. The fever denotes suppuration, a violent chill alternating with burning heat. These symptoms likewise show that Hepar is not indicated at the beginning of suppuration, but after the suppurative process is completed.

Nux vomica seems to us little suitable in nephritis; however, we will transcribe Hartmann's statements on the subject: "If a suppression of habitual hemorrhages or abuse of spirits is the cause of the nephritis, which, in such a case, results from abdominal congestion, Nux will be found the best remedy, if distention of the abdomen, pressure, heat, burning in the region of the kidneys and loins are present. Experience has shown, moreover, that Nux is likewise adapted to other nephritic difficulties, whose symptoms are strikingly similar to the primary effects of Nux, even to kidney-diseases caused by renal calculi or by suppressed hemorrhoids."

Colocynthis is likewise mentioned by Hartmann as a renal remedy, but whether correctly or not, is still an open question. The characteristic symptom: "Foul-smelling urine, which, after settling, soon becomes thick like jelly or coagulated albumen;" is so isolated that too much importance should not be attached to it. Colocynthis might, perhaps, be appropriate in inflammatory renal affections caused by calculi, and, according to the above-mentioned symptom, in violent catarrh of the bladder.

Phosphorus is undoubtedly of much more importance in affections of the kidneys, than in the use that has thus far been made of it, and Sorge's treatise would lead one to suppose. Phosphorus being more homœopathic to Bright's disease than to any other affection of the kidneys, we shall postpone our remarks on Phosphorus until the next chapter.

Cannabis is recommended by Hartmann in the following words: "Too little attention has been paid to Cannabis generally, and to nephritis in particular. Cannabis will always prove useful for a drawing, ulcerative pain from the region of the kidneys down to the groin, accompanied by an anxious sensation and nausea." Among a large number of cases of poisoning by Cannabis, the records of which are in our possession, there is no action on the kidneys denoting inflammation of this viscus, perceptible. The retention of urine is evidently a consequence of the narcotic action of the drug. The Indian hemp, hashish, may perhaps differ from our own native Cannabis in this, that it acts more intensely upon the urinary organs, for we find the following symptoms recorded in our Materia Medica: Ulcerative pain in the region of the kidneys, with or without contact; this pain spreads down into the thighs;

frequent urination, but diminished quantity of urine; retention of urine; urine bloody, turbid, as if mixed with pus and whitish shreds. According to these symptoms, Cannabis should not be overlooked in nephritis.

Pulsatilla is said to be excellent if nephritis is caused by suppression of the menses. It seems, however, as if Pulsatilla acted less specifically upon the kidneys than upon the bladder, and did not cause inflammation, but simply a catarrh of the bladder. In practice it cannot be placed in the front rank of renal remedies.

Beside the above-mentioned remedies we have for acute nephritis: *Cocculus*, *Veratrum*, *Clematis*, and *Rhus toxicodendron*. For the chronic form of nephritis, a more detailed list of remedies will be found in the next chapter. The reader will there also find a few other remedies of particular importance in uræmia, Rhus tox. being one of the most efficient.

In nephritis the diet is a subject of considerable interest. Above all things we must take care to avoid articles of diet that might impart too many solid constituents to the urine. Although most patients would feel a natural disinclination to solid food, yet it is well that the physician should emphatically protest against its use. In few diseases is a strict deprivation cure more necessary than in nephritis. At the same time our object is attained in a different way, by ordering the patient to drink much fresh water, even carbonated water; the use of stewed fruit is both refreshing and advantageous to the patient. Under certain circumstances, tepid drinks may agree better with the patient, at any rate, they need not be objected to; a mixture of water and acidulated juice of some fruit, especially apples, is more particularly to be commended.

2. Morbus Brightii, Bright's Disease of the Kidneys.

Under this heading we class the different conditions described as nephritis parenchymatosa, crouposa, desquamativa, and as cirrhosis of the kidneys, in so far as they all have the characteristic signs of Bright's disease: inflammatory exudation into the tubuli uriniferi with their various terminations and sequelæ.

The etiology of this disease cannot be traced with any positive certainty. Although, as a rule, it sets in as a secondary affection, yet the question may fairly be asked whether it does not sometimes break out as a primary disease.

Bright's disease chiefly befalls persons of middle age, less frequently children, and still less old people. Males seem more disposed to contract this disease, probably because they use such noxious substances as predispose to it, more frequently than women. Feeble individuals are more frequently attacked than vigorous persons. Damp and cold weather is considered one of the most frequent causes of this disease, which is supposed to account for its frequent occurrence in the countries of the Northwest of Europe, especially England, Holland, and the coast of the North Sea. Even if we admit, however, that colds, which are so common in these countries, may give rise to renal diseases, in consequence of a suppression of the cutaneous exhalations, on the other hand we must not forget that the abuse of alcoholic beverages, which is such a prevalent vice in these countries, likewise is a main cause of the nephritis, which is so frequently met with among their inhabitants. But it is not only alcohol, but likewise the above-mentioned drugs and poisons that cause both nephritis and Bright's disease. Among general febrile diseases, it is particularly after cholera and scarlatina that parenchymatous nephritis occurs, although it may likewise develop itself after other acute affections, but rather exceptionally. Among chronic diseases, it is dyscrasias, such as rachitis, arthritis, and scrofulosis, which are often accompanied by this disease. We are no more able to account for the connection between these dyscrasias and Bright's disease, than we are for the frequent occurrence of Bright's disease during extensive suppurations of bones, although we may know that the quality of the urine, during such conditions of the system, undergoes considerable changes.

Symptoms and course. Since a knowledge of the anatomical changes are of great importance to an accurate comprehension of the symptoms of the disease, we first furnish a short description of these changes. They may naturally be classified in three stages. In the first stage the kidney is enlarged to double its size and weight, its surface is smooth but injected, and unequally reddened ; the albuginea can easily be detached; it is opaque, and beneath it small extravasations are frequently observed. On section the cortical substance is chiefly found altered. It is considerably thicker, of a dark-red or brown-red color, with isolated bright-red points, sometimes completely mottled, friable, and soaked with a turbid and viscid fluid, which can be squeezed out, and under the microscope reveals cylindrical casts of the size of the tubuli uriniferi, partially covered with epithelium and blood-cells. The other parts of the kidney are likewise more or less vividly injected. In the second stage the volume of the kidney is still larger, the surface mostly continues smooth, or is covered with single granulations, no longer injected red, but the color passing more and more into a gray or yellowish tint; it is unequal, and sometimes looks as if sprinkled. The albuginea can still easily be detached. On section the cortical substance looks still larger than during the first stage; its color is no longer dark, but of a reddish-gray, and finally of a yellowish-gray or clear yellow. The cut surface has a greasy lustre. Under the microscope the tubuli uriniferi of the cortical substance appear considerably enlarged, filled with exudation, which already shows partial traces of fatty degeneration, and with copious epithelium; the granulations on the surface are found to be dilated tubuli uriniferi. The third stage includes the retrograde metamorphosis of the exudation. In consequence of this process, the volume and weight of the kidney decrease again more and more, until they finally shrink, sometimes quite considerably below the normal figure. The surface appears uneven, knobby, covered with detached granulations, and traversed by depressions or furrows; the albuginea adheres very firmly. On cutting through the kidney, the tissue is found to be denser and more tenacious, and the cut surface is strikingly dry. The cortical substance now is seen to be the real focus of the disease. It gradually shrinks away, sometimes to such an extent that it seems like a narrow border round the cut surface. Its color is a mixture of gray, red and yellow, sometimes striated. The rest of the kidney is but little altered in appearance and size, or some parts may still appear injected. These changes are seldom witnessed in both kidneys; it is even a rare occurrence that the whole of only one kidney is invaded by this morbid process; very commonly the symptoms of two stages are found side by side in the same kidney.

A division of Bright's disease into acute and chronic, is a very difficult task. What can at most be asserted is, that the disease only passes through the first stage, or goes on its course further into the other stages. It is only the characteristic nephritis during scarlatina, very seldom during the course of other exanthematic fevers, to which the name of Bright's disease can properly be applied, for the reason that in most cases it passes only through the first stage. The cause of it, in our opinion at least, is not so much a difference in the etiological influences, as the age of the patients. Nephritis after scarlatina is scarcely ever met with, except in children or young persons, in whom the reactive efforts of the organism differ greatly, especially in regard to the kidneys, from those of middle-aged persons. This difference is likewise clearly manifested by the symptoms, as the following description sufficiently shows.

The acute form of Bright's disease, after scarlatina, generally sets in with distinct febrile phenomena, sometimes with pain in the renal region, and almost always associated with vomiting at an early period, a circumstance that deserves to be considered with great care in convalescents from scarlet fever. Only in rare cases the disease develops itself without the above-mentioned symptoms, in a more insidious manner, or is covered up by the other morbid phenomena accompanying the exanthem. From the onset, the quantity of the urine is considerably lessened, but a day seldom passes that some urine is not voided. The urine has a very dark color, red or brown like beer, makes a very consistent foam, and, after settling, deposits a dark sediment, in which the microscope discovers numerous blood-cells, a quantity of epithelium and fibrinous casts. The previously mentioned tests for albumen yield copious coagula. The excretion of the urine is interrupted; there is a good deal of urging, with scanty discharge. These symptoms of disturbance of the renal functions are very soon succeeded by an œdematous swelling over the whole body, which is first strikingly seen in the face, and attains a high degree of intensity. During this stage, the fever is generally not very violent, the patients may even feel tolerably well, and have some appetite. The thirst is always great, they desire cold drinks; the skin is entirely inactive, cool, feels dry, and has a pale, sickly color. The bowels are generally confined; the presence of diarrhœa is not a favorable symptom. If the disease has a favorable termination, which may take several weeks, the urine is again secreted in larger quantity, the morbid products in the urine decrease, the skin resumes its functional activity, and without any special signs of disordered functions, the disease soon yields to perfect recovery. Not unfrequently, however, such patients succumb to inflammations of other organs, or, which is less frequently the case, the second and third stage of the disease may appear. The supervention of uræmia is of rare occurrence, and, if a prominent œdema after scarlatina is accompanied by cerebral symptoms, meningitis may be suspected. If the disease runs a rapid and favorable course, there is no great loss of strength, and the patients generally recover very rapidly.

Where Bright's disease is not a sequela of acute diseases, it has an entirely different beginning. Under such circumstances, the first stage may indeed pass away very rapidly with the more or less marked symptoms of typhus, which, however, is generally associated with convulsions, and where the accompanying œdema of the face generally shows the true character of the disease. If both kidneys are affected, and the urinary excretion is entirely suspended, an acute dropsy may suddenly cause death. But almost always the disease commences without any preliminary symptoms, without chilliness or heat, and without local pains, at any rate these pains are not very prominent. Thus it happens that the patients are unable to indicate the beginning of their trouble. Insensibly they begin to complain, their strength diminishes, they feel that some illness is about to overtake them, the appetite is less, symptoms of stomach-catarrh become manifest, the intestines may likewise be similarly affected. The urine is voided as usual, seldom less, rather more, and should the disease set in with much severity, the urine shows the above-mentioned darker color, and diminishes in quantity. Usually it is feebly turbid, even while being voided, of a pale color, of a bluish-green tint, foams very strongly, and the foam lasts a great while. Only at the commencement of the disease, blood is found mixed up with it. The test for albumen shows decisive results. The microscope reveals numerous fibrinous casts, at first accompanied by blood-cells and epithelium, afterwards covered with fat globules and granules. The specific gravity is always much less, even down to 1005; this is owing to the great decrease of urea, and of the urates and other salts. Under these circumstances, an anæmic appearance and other signs of impoverished blood soon set in, which point to the existence of some important constitutional malady, without its locality being indicated with positive certainty, and the ominous significance of which can only be determined by a careful investigation of the urine. Much less rapidly than with the acute form, sometimes even at a remarkably late period, but rarely before the termination of a few weeks, a symptom makes its appearance, together with the dropsical phenomena, which renders any error in diagnosis almost impossible. Here, too, one of the first symptoms is œdema of the skin, which has the peculiarity to be more prominent in one place or the other, and at times to disappear entirely. It is always most marked in the face and on the lower extremities. While the œdema of the skin is constantly increasing, water finally accumulates in the cavities, and the patient succumbs to the injury which the increasing pressure of the water inflicts upon the most important organs.

This, however, is not the only manner in which the disease can terminate. It is a peculiarity of Bright's disease to easily develop malignant affections in other organs, such as inflammations of the thoracic viscera and of the peritonæum, the dangerous nature of which is increased by the renal affection, and which generally terminate fatally. It seems as if the increase of danger resulted from the altered relations of waste and supply, or, perhaps, from the extreme anæmia. The very frequent pulmonary and intestinal catarrhs are likewise threatening prognostics; they are principally characterized by the secretion of chiefly serous substances that seem to act as a substitute for the disturbed renal and cutaneous functions, but take down the patient's strength at a rapid rate. The most obscure diseases, although their presence has been demonstrated in a number of cases, are the diseases of the heart which are so frequently met with in albuminuria. Beside the products of former pericarditis or endocarditis, we mostly meet with hypertrophy of the left ventricle. The connection of these diseases cannot always be definitely shown, for the reason that we have not always an opportunity of watching the patients from the commencement of the disease. Although the heart affection seems, in most cases, to be of a secondary character, yet in many cases it must evidently have been the primary disease and the first cause of the renal disorder. Nor is the action of nephritis upon the eyes cleared up; all we know is, that the renal disease is very frequently associated with a more or less complete amaurosis, which the most careful examination of the eyes is not always able to trace definitely to sanguineous extravasations or disorganizations of the retina. Uræmia does not usually supervene during this disease, or, at any rate, not to a very great extent; this may, however, be owing to the premature supervention of death by dropsy, or in consequence of some malignant inflammation.

In the more acute cases the disease hastens, with uniform rapidity, onward towards a fatal termination. If the disease runs a more chronic course, its intensity varies; remissions that almost seem intermissions, and of various duration, are observed, during which the strength of the patient not only increases, but the albumen disappears from the urine down to a scarcely perceptible trace. Accordingly, the disease at times lasts months, and at others years; there are no positive landmarks by which the duration of the disease can be determined *a priori* even approximatively. The prognosis is always very doubtful; in cases of long standing it is absolutely unfavorable. A complete cure is most easily effected in recent cases that do not run a too rapid course. An actually existing cirrhosis of the kidneys cannot be removed; at any rate, such a thing is improbable. The danger is essentially increased, if there is a tendency to inflammation of other viscera, or by the presence of heart-disease. If the disease had been caused by external circumstances, a damp climate or dwelling, or frequent colds, the removal of these causes may be of great importance.

Treatment. Our literature has very few cures, or even mere reports of cases of Bright's disease. Some of them have even to be regarded as doubtful. Nor are there any more cases of albuminuria to be met with in our periodicals. The cause of this is undoubtedly that in Hahnemann's time albuminuria was not yet thought of. After Hahnemann something has been accomplished in the domain of the diseases of urinary organs and their treatment; but not enough to enable us to oppose an exact pathogenesis to the pathological group. When treating of other affections, we have often taken the opportunity of calling attention to this inconvenience, which is scarcely ever more acutely felt than in renal diseases, for the reason that the characteristic symptoms have to be left unnoticed, and the other symptoms are either so unimportant, or have so little reference to the real focus of the disease, that they are absolutely insufficient to guide us in selecting the true remedy. These remarks are particularly applicable to the last stage of Bright's disease, which is at the same time the worst, because it holds out so little hope of recovery. On this account we cannot help admitting that the therapeutic chapter of this disease is not yet based upon experience, and this has induced us to indicate a more than usual number of remedies that may be found suitable for it.

Terebinthina. In the All. Hom. Zeit., vol. LI., we read the following concise but interesting case of poisoning: "A healthy man who had never been suffering with any special disease of the kidneys, took for tænia one and a half ounces of spirits of turpentine, with an equal quantity of castor oil; soon after he was attacked with dulness of the head, vomiting, and diarrhœa. In eight hours he experienced frequent urging to urinate, with scanty discharge of a burning urine containing bloody coagula. During the night he urinated fourteen to fifteen times, and the whole of the following day the urging continued, but with less pain. The urine, which was copiously mixed with blood and albumen, showed under the microscope cylindrical casts, inflammation-cells, crystals of the oxalate of lime, but no epithelium. At the end of seventeen days, the blood and albumen gradually disappeared, and the urine resumed its normal quality. This case is instructive. It plainly shows a tolerably acute attack of Bright's disease, except that no epithelial debris were found in the urine, although, with such symptoms, it is difficult to understand why renal epithelium should not necessarily have been detached. It seems as though, in this particular, the examination of the urine must have been defective. Corresponding with the above-mentioned symptoms, we find in the Materia Medica: violent pains in the kidneys, extending downwards along the course of the ureters; painful, greatly diminished excretion of a bloody urine, which afterwards becomes more copious, turbid and slimy, and of a whitish color. In addition to these symptoms we have anasarca and general prostration. These symptoms fully justify the use of Turpentine in Bright's disease, but only in the first, and perhaps in the second stage, not in the third. The peculiarity of this medicine, in causing an erythema similar to the scarlet eruption, affords an important indication for the use of this drug in post-scarlatinal nephritis. As yet our reports of cures with Turpentine are very scanty.

Cantharides. To what we have said in the preceding chapter, to which we refer the reader, we add a few items belonging in the same group. We have given, in a previous chapter, the pathological evidences upon which the diagnosis of an acute attack of Bright's disease can be predicated with positive certainty. Clemens has likewise seen a long-lasting, violent albuminuria result from Cantharides. Although this remedy seems, properly speaking, only suitable in the first stage of the disease, yet the previously-quoted observation will undoubtedly induce us to try Cantharides, even if no trace of inflammatory symptoms are present. At this stage, however, all similarity between the natural and the drug disease will most likely have disappeared.

Phosphorus. Sorge, in his well-known essay on Phosphorus, dispatches this drug in its relation to the kidney, with a very few words. He gives this abstract: "The urine contained several times a number of epithelial scales, pus, and mucus-corpuscles, albumen in six cases, in two cases exudation-casts, and in one case blood-corpuscles. Hence Phosphorus may prove a remedy against Bright's disease, although there is as yet no cure of this disease recorded in our works." He then mentions a cure which, however, is only that of a post-scarlatinal croupous nephritis. We have to extend these notes still further, and begin with furnishing a few detached toxicological data. Nitsche (Wiener Wochenblatt, 1857) found in a man who had always enjoyed good health, and who had perished four days after having swallowed the Phosphorus: kidneys disorganized as in Bright's disease, the cortical substance not very granular, the corpora and rete Malpighii considerably injected, the tubuli uriniferi filled with exudation-casts. In addition an incipient pneumonia. While the patient was still alive, the urine had shown albumen and exudation-casts, but a higher specific gravity, an increase of the Sulphates and Phosphates, and a diminution of the Chlorides. In several rapidly fatal cases, a somewhat advanced pneumonia was found associated with considerable hyperæmia of the kidneys. After poisoning with Phosphorus, the skin is almost always pale and anæmic; mention is often made of a waxy color of the skin, or of its having a yellowish tint. By contrasting with these toxical symptoms, which were obtained by means of large, rapidly destroying doses of the poison, the pathogenetic symptoms of Phosphorus, as contained in the Materia Medica, we shall find that Phosphorus is not only homœopathic to the first stage of Bright's disease, but likewise to post-scarlatinal nephritis, and to the whole course of the disease. It is to Phosphorus that we more particularly resort, in cases of Bright's disease depending upon suppurations of bones, or associated with pneumonia or malignant pulmonary catarrh. Phosphorus is likewise adapted to Bright's disease, complicated with amaurosis. A copious, watery diarrhœa is one of the most constant effects of Phosphorus.

Arsenicum album is frequently recommended as a remedy for Bright's disease, but whether correctly so, should be carefully ascertained. Among a number of acute and chronic cases of poisoning with Arsenic, we have only met with one case that had hyperæmia of the kidneys, but no other sign of degeneration. This is no accident. If Arsenic had a specific effect upon the kidneys, symptoms of the arsenical disease, both of a subjective and objective character, would be met with in every case of slow poisoning by Arsenic, which is, however, not the case. The kidney-symptoms contained in the Materia Medica, are indeed calculated, upon a first cursory review, to excite our attention; but, when examined more closely, they appear much more like manifestations of the general effect of Arsenic than of the local action. In the same manner marked urinary difficulties are witnessed in severe constitutional diseases, without the kidneys being affected. No more than in the first stage, is Arsenic adapted to the second stage of Bright's disease. We have stated above that this disease causes a slow sinking of the vital energies, without any striking local symptoms, but with the well-defined character of anæmia. But we are unable to conceive what great similarity exists between this stage of Bright's disease, and the effects of Arsenic. Hence, we think that we should commit a mistake, were we to prescribe Arsenic for the dropsy which supervenes during Bright's disease. This remedy will be found the more useful if the heart is involved in the disease, for instance in carditis.

Digitalis purpurea is undoubtedly an important remedy in Bright's disease, although there is, as yet, no case of poisoning on record where albumen has been found in the urine. Digitalis does not cause a renal affection like parenchymatous nephritis; on the contrary, the similarity between the third stage and the effects of Digitalis is very great, more particularly as regards the general constitutional symptoms. It would carry us too far were we to go into particulars regarding this point, on which account we refer to our essay on Digitalis, and call attention to the fact, that Christison has given Digitalin in two cases of Bright's disease, in doses of one seventy-fifth of a grain, two or three times a day, with the most decided advantage. But even if we would admit that the uncomplicated form of Bright's disease does not belong to the therapeutic domain of Digitalis, yet this remedy is undoubtedly of the utmost importance, if the renal affection is combined with heart-disease. A peculiar indication for Digitalis are the apparently rheumatic pains which are not unfrequently met with in nephritis; and, moreover, the characteristic pulmonary catarrh, with profuse serous expectoration.

Colchicum autumnale exerts a very constant and decided action upon the kidneys. Unfortunately the post-mortem examinations, made in the cases of poisoning with which we have become acquainted, on account of their rapidly fatal end, showed no other significant changes of tissue, than a marked hyperæmia of the kidneys. The urinary secretions and excretions, on the contrary, show a number of characteristic changes, among which the extraordinary inaction of the skin is very prominent. This last-mentioned circumstance leads us to propose Colchicum as a remedy for the post-scarlatinal Bright's disease. This remedy is not appropriate in the chronic form of the disease.

Colocynthis acts very similarly to Colchicum, as far as the local symptoms are concerned, and deserves a place among the remedies for post-scarlatinal Bright's disease. The pathogenetic differences between the two remedies are restricted to the general symptoms.

Nitri acidum has no very definite symptoms pointing to Bright's disease, but deserves careful attention. Its selection depends upon a few general points of importance, such as albuminuria resulting from suppurations of bones, abuse of Mercury, and dyscrasias. It is curious how greatly this drug is praised by other physicians in this disease.

Secale cornutum is recommended by Trinks for scarlatinal dropsy. He relates several undeniable cures. Corresponding symptoms are: Diminished urine · turbid, bloody urine, depositing a copious sediment, or else watery, colorless urine, which is turbid even while being voided. Accordingly, Secale cornutum corresponds to the last stage of Bright's disease, the more as the rest of the symptoms will likewise be found to correspond, more particularly the œdematous swellings.

Helleborus niger is recommended as a remedy for scarlatinal dropsy, although no special cases are reported. [Not long ago we cured a case of scarlatinal dropsy with this remedy. The patient was a consumptive boy of seven years. There was a highly developed general anasarca, and the sexual organs were fearfully swollen. We put the boy on five drops of the tincture in half a tumbler of water, for about a fortnight; the patient recovered without any further untoward symptoms. H.] Symptomatically, however, this remedy does not correspond to Bright's disease, and will most likely prove of small value in this malady.

Lycopodium is sufficiently known as one of the most efficient renal remedies, but we are not yet acquainted with the exact nature of its action. No attempt has, as yet, been made to clear up this point. Among the urinary symptoms we have: Increased secretion of a whitish-turbid, foaming urine, which is easily decomposed. These are important symptoms. In addition we have: great weakness, an anæmic appearance, symptoms of heart-disease, excessive tendency to pulmonary catarrhs, great depression of spirits, etc. These symptoms might justify the use of Lycopodium in the third stage of Bright's disease.

Sulphur. We have already stated that it is difficult to pick out the characteristic, or rather the constant symptoms of Sulphur in the pathogenesis of this drug. This remark likewise applies to its urinary symptoms. All we know is, that Sulphur causes important changes in the urinary range, and that many of the symptoms point to Bright's disease, more particularly the cloudiness of the colorless urine while being voided, with rapid decomposition. Other considerations, in the absence of definite symptoms, direct our attention to Sulphur. Parenchymatous nephritis results in copious exudation, upon the speedy removal of which everything depends. In most inflammations Sulphur is unquestionably an excellent remedy to promote absorption, even if the symptoms do not indicate it. How much more good may we expect from it, if its physiological effects seem to correspond with the case before us. Moreover, in most dyscrasic affections, Sulphur is indispensable, and we know that dyscrasic individuals are easily attacked by Bright's disease.

To **Calcarea carbonica** the same remarks apply as to Sulphur. The local symptoms are very distinct, more so than with most other remedies, and the other symptoms frequently correspond. Its relation to scrofulosis and to suppurations of bones, is very specific. In general, Calcarea carb. is suitable for impoverished individuals whose constitutions have been impaired by perverse modes of living.

To the above-mentioned remedies we add the following more or less important ones, in order to enlarge the means of treating a disease which, therapeutically speaking, has as yet been very poorly provided for: *Pulsatilla, Bryonia, Thuja, Mezereum, Sabadilla, Creasotum, Ferrum, Conium maculatum, China.*

Beside these medicinal agents we have to mention another one which, under certain circumstances, is more powerful than either of the foregoing—it is water. In any form of Bright's disease, the skin is very inactive; we know, moreover, that an interruption of the cutaneous functions is very apt to result in nephritis. Hence, the self-evident conclusion, that a restoration of the normal activity of the skin must favor, or perhaps of itself cause, a restoration of the normal functions of the kidneys. Water is, at all events, the safest and mildest means to accomplish this purpose, provided a correct use is made of it. Its use is most evident in scarlatinal dropsy. If, as soon as the first symptoms of nephritis, or even of anasarca show themselves, the patient is wrapped in a wet sheet, the danger of these morbid processes is much lessened; at any rate, our own experience has shown us that the skin, and hence the kidneys, recover their activity in from six to eight days at the latest. To accomplish this purpose the patients were wrapped up for about five hours every day, and after that rubbed dry. A hurtful influence was never perceived after such a pack. Many may perhaps be frightened away from this use of cold water by the antiquated dread of using this liquid in acute exanthemata. Let such persons inquire of hydropaths what results they obtain by employing cold water even from the beginning. Cold water has not only curative, but likewise prophylactic virtues. We, at least, have become satisfied of the great probability that patients who are washed all over when the period of desquamation is setting in, and after the washing are well rubbed down, are not attacked with dropsy. Regarding the use of water in chronic parenchymatous nephritis proper, opinions are very much divided. Tepid baths are generally recommended. But their usefulness is very questionable, because they do not incite an independent activity of the skin. Under such circumstances the vapor bath would be preferable, although we place the cold wet pack ahead of the latter. The result may never be as favorable as in scarlet-fever, probably for the reason that the cold water is not immediately resorted to as soon as the scarlatina breaks out; but even at a later stage a successful palliation may be hoped for with certainty. Drinking quantities of cold water may be of more questionable utility. Many persons are benefited by this proceeding as much as others are injured by it. This has to be determined by careful experiments.

In this disease the diet is an object of much importance. That spirits, condiments, all articles of diet that have a powerful action upon the kidneys, or coffee and tea, celery, parsley, onions, etc., have to be rigorously avoided, is a matter of course. It is equally clear that etiological influences, as far as they can be ascertained, have to be adequately met. Positive means have likewise to be employed. The anæmic appearance of the patients shows of itself that they require an abundant quantity of invigorating, animal food, were it only to replace the loss of albumen. Too much cannot be done in this respect, provided the stomach of the patient is not made sick by excessive quantities. The cautious use of good wine, and still more of good beer, containing but a small quantity of hops, can only be useful, more particularly in the case of persons who have been addicted to the use of spirits. Of course this can only apply to chronic nephritis, not to the really inflammatory stage. Milk is an important article of diet. It is only in exceptional cases that it does not agree with patients' stomachs; as a rule it will prove the best, it being the mildest and most perfect nourishment, and its use cannot be insisted upon with sufficient force. Good fruit in any shape, more especially such as contains a good deal of sugar, like grapes, may likewise be used by the patient without fear.

This is not the place to dwell upon the effect of various mineral waters. They are scarcely ever ordered at the beginning, when they might, perhaps, afford help. In the last stage it is not likely that they will do more good than any other method of treatment.

If the disease has to be treated during its acute course, the diet is of course the same as that of acute nephritis. [Grauvogl professes to have cured acute attacks of Bright's disease with teaspoonful doses of *Cochineal*. We call the reader's attention to an interesting article on Bright's disease, in the 13th volume of the British Journal of Homœopathy, by Doctor Joseph Kidd. Helonin is efficacious in this disease. H.]

3. Hemorrhage in the Kidneys.

The blood may be discharged into the tissue of the kidneys, as well as into the tubuli uriniferi, or into the pelvis of the kidney. In the former case ecchymoses or small extravasations or real apoplectic foci arise, the beginning of which it is, however, difficult to diagnose, and hence cannot become a subject for therapeutic measures. It is only when the blood finds an outlet outwardly, that we can, to some extent, infer from what organ the hemorrhage comes.

The blood-mixed urine may proceed from any part of the urinary organs. We shall presently show what means are at our command to determine the origin of the hemorrhage.

The causes of the affection are, principally renal concretions, which wound the mucous membranes with their sharp corners; moreover, contusions of the renal region, excessive muscular exertions, prominent hyperæmia of the kidneys, medicines that have an irritating effect upon the kidneys, likewise various articles of diet, such as asparagus, celery, garlic, and suppression of physiological or habitual hemorrhages; these are known as the causes of hyperæmia of the kidneys. Hemorrhage of the kidneys is, moreover, an accompanying symptom of inflammatory affections of the kidneys, and of diseases that terminate in, or are characterized by dissolution of the blood, such as typhus, scurvy, and malignant growths in the kidneys.

The symptoms which accompany the renal hemorrhage, depend, in all cases where the hemorrhage is symptomatic of some other disease, upon the symptoms of this disease; it is only where the hemorrhage is very considerable that it may become the cause of morbid phenomena peculiar to it. But even if the hemorrhage exists as an apparently or really idiopathic disease, the accompanying ailments may be very unimportant. This depends mostly upon the circumstance, whether the blood coagulates in the kidney or in the ureter. If this is the case, the impediment to the excretion of the urine causes pains in the renal region, being at times a dull pressure or a tearing distress, and at others increasing to violent colicky paroxysms, without their enabling us to determine the amount of resistance which the coagulated blood opposes to the urine. On this account subjective symptoms of this kind have but little value, and serve at most to render the diagnosis in such cases more secure, whereas the objective symptoms alone would leave us in the dark. The accumulation of a quantity of bloody coagula in the bladder sometimes causes so much distress in the interior of this organ, that we feel tempted to locate the seat of the trouble in this region. The retention of the urine is really the important fact in the case. Sometimes it has a pale-red color, at times a brown and even a black color; after settling, a scanty dark-brown, amorphous sediment, or a bloody clot, is deposited at the bottom of the vessel. In renal hemorrhage the blood is always more or less decomposed and discolored; this circumstance can be made available with some certainty, as a distinctive sign that the blood does not come from the bladder. The coagula coming away with the urine have a vermiform shape, so fashioned by the ureter. A microscopic examination is of special importance. If the blood had been discharged into the uriniferous tubules, we see cylindrical casts, covered with blood-cells; this phenomenon alone is sufficient to diagnose renal hemorrhage. If the hemorrhage proceeds from the pelvis of the kidney, the cylinders are of course absent, and only the blood-cells are principally altered. Chemical analysis results in a scanty yield of albumen from the blood, but may likewise show, in dubious cases, whether the color of the urine arises from the presence of blood or from some other admixture, and is of particular importance if no blood-corpuscles are excreted with the urine. Heller's test for hæmatin is simple, and can be conducted without loss of time. To the heated urine we add a mixture of caustic potash, and then heat it again. A sediment is thrown down which, when the light shines *upon* it, has a dingy, reddish-yellow color; but, when the light shines *through* it, has a bright, blood-red appearance.

The course of renal hemorrhage depends, in the first place, upon the primary causative affection, and secondly upon circumstances which it is not in our power to determine *a priori*. Sometimes the disorder is confined to a few discharges of blood, and sometimes it lasts for weeks without an interruption. Even if the hemorrhage is considerable, there is particular danger only in exceptional cases; except the consequences of a loss of blood, which are never very marked, the accident leaves no serious disturbance behind. This applies, however, only to idiopathic hemorrhage, whereas symptomatic hemorrhages may, of course, cause a great deal of exhaustion.

Treatment. We should not hesitate to transcribe Hartmann's whole passage concerning the treatment of renal hemorrhage, if he did not generalize too much, whereas it certainly is not the same thing whether the blood comes from the kidney or bladder. Moreover, since a distinction between these two kinds of hemorrhage cannot always be made, we refer the reader to the chapter on hemorrhage from the bladder, where the remedies that are not mentioned here, will be found indicated.

In every hemorrhage from the urinary organs, we have to examine with great care whether there is an inflammatory or some other prominent morbid condition present. If the hemorrhage is the main symptom, the following remedies will have to be resorted to:

Terebinthina. It is only exceptionally that this drug has a discharge of pure blood with the urine; the blood is most usually intimately mixed with the urine, which has a dirty brown-red or even blackish color. If this symptom of itself denotes hemorrhage from the kidneys, this fact derives additional confirmation from the circumstance, that Terebinthina generally acts upon the kidneys rather than upon the bladder. Hartmann recommends it more particularly, if the bloody urine is accompanied by violent burning and drawing pains in the kidneys, spasmodic urging and pressing in the region of the bladder, which, when in a sitting posture, moves upward towards both kidneys, and disappears on motion; moreover, previous to urination, during rest, the patient complains of tenesmus and cutting in the bladder, alternating with a similar sensation in the umbilical region. Terebinthina is likewise an excellent remedy if the hemorrhage is the result of a peculiar composition of the blood, which sometimes exists without any considerable constitutional symptoms in scurvy; for instance, among mariners who return home after a long voyage, or among people who live in damp and close dwellings.

Arnica is recommended by many physicians, and likewise by Hartmann, for renal hemorrhage caused by mechanical injuries, such as concussion, etc., but such recommendations are not based so much upon the physiological action of the drug, as upon the well-known general indication, that Arnica is a remedy for mechanical injuries.

Nux vomica is likewise a remedy for renal hemorrhage, not simply a means, as Hartmann teaches, for subduing vascular irritation. The bloody urine of Nux evidently depends upon other causes than a simple bleeding.

Cantharides. We transcribe all the essential parts of Hartmann's own statements: "This remedy is one of the chief remedies for renal hemorrhage, especially if no evident cause can be assigned to it; among its primary effects we have not only the bloody urine, but likewise the pains accompanying its discharge. The most common pain which a bloody urine occasions along the course of the urethra, and which this remedy relieves with perfect certainty, is a burning pain, which is the more keenly felt the less blood is passed at one discharge, either with or without urine; hence, the pain is felt most acutely when the blood is discharged drop by drop. Sometimes this difficulty of urinating depends upon an obstruction of the orifice of the urethra in the bladder by coagulated blood, sometimes upon a spasmodic contraction of the sphincters; in the former case bloody shreds or blackish clots of coagulated blood are passed with every drop of urine, as long as any coagulated blood remains in the bladder, after which pure, clear blood is discharged. In the latter case relief is afforded by vapors of hot milk or water ascending to the region of the bladder and sexual organs. In either case, when there are violent cutting, pressing, and spasmodic pains in the region of the bladder extending along the ureters to the kidneys, Cantharides will be employed with advantage, and afford the desired relief. Cantharides are not only indicated if the blood in the urine proceeds from the bladder, but likewise if it originates in an affection of the kidneys or ureters, and is attended with burning, stinging, drawing, keen pains in the lumbar and renal region." That which in the preceding paragraph refers to hemorrhage from the bladder, has been left by us purposely united to other parts referring to the kidneys, otherwise the meaning of this passage would have been obscured. With reference to renal hemorrhage, however, we will add a few remarks. Cantharides never cause a copious discharge of blood from the kidneys; this discharge is always associated with marked symptoms of severe hyperæmia, or even incipient inflammation. This distinguishes Cantharides, most prominently, from Terebinthina. If the blood from the kidneys is filled with exudation-casts, as above described, Cantharides are indicated above any other remedy, likewise if the hemorrhage is caused by renal calculi. At all events they are more efficient in hemorrhage from the bladder than from the kidneys. If the hemorrhage is caused by the abuse of Cantharides, the best antidote is *Camphora*, together with the copious use of tepid water.

Ipecacuanha is an important remedy, if the hemorrhage is very copious, and phenomena of anæmia make their appearance, such as paleness, faint feeling, cold skin, nausea; such cases are rare.

Millefolium. The pathogenesis of this drug is not sufficiently accurate to enable us to use it in accordance with homœopathic indications. Used empirically, it has shown great excellence as a specific remedy in hæmaturia, with painfulness of the kidneys, from which the blood evidently proceeded.

The same may be said of **Uva ursi.** Hartmann says of this drug: "In a case where no other remedy seemed disposed to do any good, and where the discharge of blood was attended with loss of mucus, painful urging previous to urination and constipation, I have employed this remedy with remarkable success." It was given in the form of a decoction.

Secale cornutum has not been known or used much as a remedy for urinary affections, and can only be recommended for bloody urine if the blood-disks are entirely, or nearly absent in the urine, which may be regarded as a sign of a peculiar dissolution of the blood. For this reason Secale cornutum may prove useful in certain very severe febrile conditions, if the bloody urine occurs as a complicating symptom.

Phosphorus is indicated under the same circumstances as the previous remedy, but is likewise adapted to chronic hæmaturia, if the discharge of urine is very painful and the urinary excretion much less. If the trouble is caused by sexual excesses, onanism, Phosphorus is, next to Nux vomica and China, a leading remedy.

Arsenicum album is an efficient remedy, both in the acute and chronic form of renal hemorrhage. The local symptoms will scarcely ever be sufficient to determine the selection of Arsenic; the general symptoms should indicate and sanction its employment. It is chiefly indicated by the following symptoms: The emission of urine is very painful, the urine is much less in quantity, there is strangury, wide-spread burning pains in the urinary organs, paralytic phenomena in the bladder, rapid decomposition of the urine in the vessel, deficiency of bloody coagula, the urine being, however, of a very dark color.

Lycopodium will have to be selected in accordance with the general symptoms, rather than the local, the latter being but vaguely defined. It is only adapted to the chronic form when existing in decrepit individuals, in connection with chronic catarrhal affections of the lining membrane of the urinary organs.

Colchicum autumnale deserves especial consideration, if the disease is caused by a cold or by getting wet, with scalding urine.

Cannabis, Capsicum, Pulsatilla, Squilla, Zincum, are mentioned here for the sake of completeness; we shall recur to these remedies when we come to speak of hemorrhage from the bladder. [*Aconite* should not be forgotten as a remedy for renal hemorrhage; we have effected cures of this disease with Aconite, without calling in the aid of any other drug. It is indicated by swelling and soreness of the renal region, heat, throbbing. H.]

Regarding the diet, we refer the reader to what we have said on this subject in the chapter on nephritis. Excessive care may, perhaps, not always be necessary; but in hæmaturia it is better to do a little too much than not enough. The abuse of liquids should be forbidden; they can only be allowed if bloody coagula prevent the urinary excretion; liquids exert an increasing pressure upon them. That external means, such as cold, dry, or moist warmth, foot or sitz-baths, act favorably, cannot well be proven, nor should they be recommended.

4. Renal Calculi, Gravel.

The formation of urinary concretions in the kidneys is a common occurrence, but frequently remains unnoticed, because no abnormal symptoms are caused by them. In most cases, the causes of this affection are obscure, or very indefinite. Although the concretions of uric acid are generally met with in plethoric individuals who mostly live on animal food, yet they likewise occur in weakly persons, who use a very spare diet. Without doubt, the mode of living is the cause of the concretions; although a peculiar disposition must likewise exist, which is as yet unknown to us.

The urinary concretions in the kidneys generally consist of Urates, less frequently of Phosphates, or the salts of lime. Their size varies; at times they form a fine sandy deposit, gravel; at other times larger bodies, whose shapes vary according to their locality and their place of origin; they may even be large enough to fill the pelvis of the kidney. Their surface is, at times smooth, at others rough; the number of calculi contained in one kidney is very indefinite; sometimes their sides, where they had been in contact with other calculi, form regular facets.

The symptoms caused by renal calculi, are very important to the physician, because they frequently attain a great height, and have the appearance of great danger, as though life itself were imperilled by them. Gravel may exist without any morbid symptoms; in other cases, the passage, and perhaps the formation of gravel are attended with marked derangements of the functions of the stomach, the main feature of which, generally, is an excess of acidity. We have pointed out this connection when speaking of chronic catarrh of the stomach. Even larger calculi may exist and be passed without any pain. This depends upon the size of the calculus, its smoothness, roughness, or the angularity of its form, upon the width of the ureters, upon the sensitiveness of the urinary passages to the foreign body, whether and what severe disturbances the passage of the calculus occasions. These symptoms together, are generally designated by the name of renal colic. It should be observed, however, that other obstacles to the excretion of urine, such as the presence of bloody coagula in renal hemorrhage, may cause renal colic, except that such colic is usually less persistent, violent, and distressing; for the reason that the obstruction is not fixed, and does not irritate or wound the mucous membrane.

Renal colic generally breaks out suddenly, after a severe effort or concussion; its gradual development from indefinite pains in the renal region, whence they spread to adjoining parts, is of less frequent occurrence; the former generally takes place if the pains announce the entrance of a renal calculus into the ureter; the latter, if the pain is occasioned by a gradual irritation of the renal pelvis, or by a change in the position of the concretion. The pains generally are very violent, are felt in the region of the affected kidney, whence they spread to the bladder and the thigh, and, when excessive, generally affect the whole side. The patients suffer a great deal, are tortured by an agonizing anxiety, and have no rest in any position or place. Their face is at times pale as death, at others bright-red; the body is cool, the pulse small and frequent. If the parts are very sensitive, convulsive symptoms are apt to set in. The passage of urine is impeded and painful, sometimes the strangury is complete. The pains sometimes continue gradually to increase, until the abdomen shrinks from the least touch, or else they remain unchanged, or they remit at intervals until they finally cease entirely, and the patient again enjoys perfect health. In such cases the concretions usually pass off, soon after, with the urine. Very often hæmaturia takes place after the passage of the calculus. If the calculus has not passed, the pain may continue and nephritis result in consequence. The passage through the ureter, which, after the intense pain has somewhat abated, the patient is able to watch and point out as the calculus progresses, lasts from a few hours to several days.

The diagnosis of renal colic is not always very easy; at the commencement the affection is often confounded with peritonitis, cardialgia, enteralgia; a misapprehension that is amply justified by the apparently threatening symptoms. The most common characteristic indications of the disease are: the fixed starting-point of the pain, together with the urinary difficulties. The prognosis is unfavorable only, if the concretions remain in the kidney and cause a dangerous irritation in this viscus. An arrest of the calculus in the ureter is a rare exception.

Treatment. The main object of the treatment must be to prevent the renewal of the concretion, which is most essentially accomplished by attending to the diet. How to prevent the renewal of the calculi, composed of the salts of lime or of Phosphates, seems to remain a mystery for the present; whereas a good deal can be accomplished so far as the urates are concerned. If the individual is affected with catarrh of the stomach or excessive acidity, this should be corrected; the patients must content themselves with a moderate and lean diet, partake sparingly of animal food, and entirely avoid all fat; on the other hand they may eat vegetables and a great deal of fruit, drink quantities of water, and discard the use of spirits entirely. By such means we have it, at any rate, in our power to acquire an influence over the disease. An attack of renal colic itself is most likely beyond the reach of strictly medical treatment, whatever may be asserted to the contrary by many practitioners. The calculus has to pass through the ureter, and no medicine can hasten this passage. Moreover it is impossible to judge of the effect of any medicine, because we cannot decide *a priori* how soon a calculus will pass if no medicines are employed. A young woman, one of our own patients, passed two small calculi in about sixteen hours, and a third, an inch in length, in four days, in spite of the remedies that were employed to facilitate the passage.

Nux vomica and *Colocynthis*, perhaps also, *Cantharides*, are most likely to exert an influence. Of more importance are external applications, more especially a tepid or warm bath, perhaps also, the cold sitz or foot-bath, and drinking copious quantities of water, in order to increase the pressure of the urine upon the calculus. Renal colic is one of those diseases, where even the strictest homœopath will sometimes feel called upon to prescribe a large dose of Morphine; but the dose should be large enough to exert its narcotic action, in spite of the intense pain. Narcotizing inhalations of Chloroform are perhaps preferable to Morphine, although neither always secure relief from this great distress.

[Doctor Becher of Muehlhausen, employs with great success, for renal calculus and gravel, the *Citrated Borate of Magnesia*, which has a slightly acid taste, and with sugar resembles lemonade powder, and which can very easily be taken. Two cases are reported in the 24th volume of the British Journal of Homœopathy. Dose: As much as will stand on the point of a knife, every two hours, or less frequently, if the case will permit. Very soon after the commencement of the administration of the drug, the pain diminishes, and the calculi are passed without pain. The Borate can be obtained from the apothecary, Doctor Kayser, at Muehlhausen. H.]

5. Diabetes Mellitus, Melituria, Glycosuria.

If we locate this morbid process among the diseases of the kidneys, we do not mean to be understood as though we regarded diabetes as a renal disease. In so far, however, as the main symptom of this affection proceeds from the kidneys; in so far as the urine is the most important diagnostic sign in this disease, we have deemed it proper, because of the opportunity of explaining the necessary examination of the urine, to offer our remarks on this disease in this chapter, instead of giving it its proper place among the constitutional diseases. The problematical character of the whole process, its comparatively rare occurrence, and our comparative ignorance of a suitable treatment of this disease, will be accepted as our excuse, if we content ourselves with briefly mentioning the main data. If a case should occur in a physician's practice, he will have an abundance of time to consult special works on the subject.

The etiology of diabetes is enveloped in complete obscurity; all data referring to it are purely hypothetical, and rest upon the patient's endeavor to trace his disease to some cause, in order to meet the questions addressed to him by the physician. The true cause is the more inaccessible to observation as the disorder commonly sets in gradually, and is not communicated to the physician until, by its long continuance, it has become an inveterate malady. It is important for us to know that sugar is said to have been discovered in the urine, after poisoning by lead or copper. Nor does age shed light on the subject; although most cases of this disease occur between the ages of twenty-five and fifty years, yet children and old people are likewise known to have been attacked with it. It is an established fact, that the disease prevails chiefly among males, and that it occurs much less frequently in the torrid than in the temperate zone.

In diabetes, pathological anatomy leaves us completely in the lurch: not one structural change has either been discovered in the kidneys or liver as a constant phenomenon; a very general post-mortem appearance in this disease, is a rather high grade of pulmonary tuberculosis.

The symptoms of this disease cannot well be ranged together in a coherent series, but have to be considered one by one.

The main symptom is the excretion of sugar by the urine, saliva, and perspiration. In the introduction to this section, we have mentioned the methods how sugar can be detected in the urine. Although this fluid looks very pale, yet it has a high specific gravity, which varies between 1020 and 1050, and may even rise to a higher figure; this is the more remarkable, as an extraordinary quantity of urine is usually discharged. A specific gravity of 1037 to 1039 indicates, almost certainly, the presence of sugar in the urine, for we are as yet unacquainted with any disease where the specific gravity of the urine rises so high. The color of the urine generally is of a dim straw-color, with a greenish tint; the dimness is considerable only in case other renal affections are present. On voiding the urine, it makes a foam, which generally lasts for some time. The percentage of sugar in the urine varies at different times of the day and at different periods, between two and twelve per cent. and above. For some hours after a meal, the quantity of sugar in the urine is larger; hence, if we desire to obtain results of reliable and undisputed validity, the urine will have to be tested for sugar for a period of at least twenty-four hours. It is a known fact that sugar is derived from the starch contained in the food, although this is not the only source of sugar, for it does not entirely disappear, even if we restrict the diet to animal food exclusively. This observation is of particular importance in regulating the diet of diabetic patients.

The second main symptom is, an unusual increase of the urinary secretion, which is almost always present, and, when the disease is at its height, is never absent. In the course of a day, the patient voids ten times and upwards the normal quantity of urine, corresponding to the quantity of liquid that had been drank in the same space of time. The assertion that the quantity of urine voided in twenty-four hours exceeds the quantity of liquid drank in this space of time, has been shown by recent investigations to be, most likely, fallacious. The quantity of urine is not always in definite proportion to the quantity of sugar in the urine. This may increase, whereas the urine decreases in quantity, and vice versa. At all events, the largest quantity of urine is voided after a meal.

The third and never-failing main symptom is the ravenous hunger, which it is impossible to account for. Many patients consume incredible quantities of food without experiencing any derangements of the stomach. We have known a diabetic patient who consumed every day from seven to ten pounds of meat, without, however, eating anything else.

From these three main phenomena proceed a series of others, with more or less regularity and distinctness.

The skin is almost always extremely dry and inactive, so that the patients do not perspire, even in the greatest summer heat. Since this condition of things will naturally occasion a suppression of habitual perspiration, of the feet for instance, this suppression has often been regarded as the cause of diabetes, whereas the reverse is the fact. The great dryness of the skin renders it very sensitive to cold, and creates a remarkable tendency to catarrhal irritations.

The thirst is proportionate to the quantity of urine, hence is sometimes perfectly agonizing. It is particularly intense after a meal, and in the night. It is scarcely credible what immense quantities of water a diabetic patient is capable of swallowing in the course of a day; the thirst is quenched only for a short time, even if the patient drinks ever so much water.

The buccal cavity is very seldom remarkably dry; the tongue is mostly clean, the taste sweetish, the breath has a nauseous odor; the teeth readily turn black, and become carious, and the gums look ulcerated and spongy, as in scurvy. The stomach is seldom affected; acid eructations are very frequent; the patient has a particular longing for farinaceous food; the alvine discharges are always very dry; the bowels are costive. Almost always, a decrease or complete loss of sexual power takes place at an early period of the disease; the lens very frequently becomes dim, and the hair falls out. If the disease lasts any time, the cerebral energy decreases even unto complete imbecility, a tendency to furuncles and decubitus becomes manifest, and pulmonary tuberculosis very often closes the scene. A striking symptom is the extraordinary emaciation, which continues to increase, in spite of eating, and is particularly striking in the face, whose bony framework is distinctly seen, even if the patients still seem very vigorous.

With such symptoms the disease runs a slow course, unless the patient's constitution was previously tainted with disease. This disease scarcely ever terminates fatally under a year, unless other inflammatory or gangrenous affections, to which the patients incline, suddenly cause a fatal termination. With careful nursing and proper diet the patients may last for years, and even be capable of doing some work; hence it is, that in the lower walks of life diabetes terminates fatally much more rapidly than in the higher. Generally the disease has longer or shorter remissions, or even intermissions of some length, which are frequently regarded as a cure without being so.

Diabetes generally terminates fatally, either with the symptoms of hectic fever, or in consequence of intervening complications of a malignant character. Only a few permanent and complete cures are recorded. Reports of diabetic cases are incomplete and unreliable, for the reason that, owing to the peculiar course of the disease the same physician scarcely ever attends the same patient from the commencement to the end of his trouble.

Treatment. What we have said in previous paragraphs shows that the treatment of diabetes is almost hopeless; indeed, we must confess that even under homœopathic treatment patients have not been materially benefited. Before giving a list of the remedies usually employed in this disease, it may be proper to cast a glance at the usual method of treating it.

It is literally true, that there is scarcely a medicine that has not been used and recommended in diabetes. The remissions, which are very apt to take place in this disease, have most probably been regarded as an effect of the medicine. It is an admitted fact, however, that so far we are not acquainted with any medicine or group of medicines that have evinced reliable curative powers in diabetes. Most prominent are the Carbonates of Potash, Creasotum, and Quinine; a cure by the last-mentioned drug is reported in the "Deutsche Klinik" of last year, the Quinine being used in very large and continued doses of the drug. The most frequent and most reliable curative effects have so far been obtained from the waters of Karlsbad and Vichy; both have effected radical cures, which have been reported in the journals.

Great stress has recently been laid on the diet. It is a fact that the exclusive use of animal diet diminishes the quantity of sugar in the urine to an extraordinary degree, but yet some sugar remains. Such a diet, however, cannot be carried out, even with the most iron will, not even if small quantities of farinaceous food are permitted. Moreover, the result of such a severe regimen does not compensate for the great sacrifice; a cure is never obtained by such means, even the apparent improvement loses its importance, for the reason that the diminished quantity of sugar in the urine is owing to the circumstance that fewer substances are introduced into the organism capable of being eliminated as sugar. We do not mean to be understood as though a rigorous diet were entirely useless, for it is undeniable that under a strict animal diet the patients last longer; what we contend for is, that the diet need not be so severe. Many physicians bear testimony that their diabetic patients did very well with a moderate farinaceous and a copious invigorating meat diet; whereas other physicians will admit that but few of their patients were able to live through such a rigorous meat diet, and preferred abandoning it, together with their physician. Those delude themselves who fancy that they have obtained great results by causing a diminution of the sugar by artificial means. An improvement only exists if, with the same quantity of food, the amount of sugar grows less, and hence the tendency of the organism to this abnormal elimination of sugar has been diminished. We subjoin a few rules for a proper diet. We have already stated that any kind of animal food may be permitted, hence the question is: What kind of vegetable diet may be allowed? This should be regulated by positive instructions, so as to prevent the patient from giving himself up to his ravenous appetite. He may be allowed a certain quantity of bread, that need not be too scanty; he may likewise indulge now and then in the moderate use of potatoes or a certain quantity of rice. These three articles of diet are sufficient, and everything else should be forbidden. Vegetables containing the least quantity of sugar are best adapted to our purpose, such as cabbage, asparagus, spinage, beans, salad of different kinds. Fruit may be allowed, if the stomach can bear it; strawberries and peaches are the best kinds. The excessive thirst of the patients likewise requires to be attended to with great care. Bouchardat has set up the proposition, that the metamorphosis of starch into sugar requires a considerable quantity of water, hence that the degree of thirst is proportionate to the quantity of sugar produced. It would seem, therefore, that the intense thirst is a natural desire of the organism, and that there can be no danger in appeasing it. But, inasmuch as the patients may be tempted to drink too much, it is well to regulate the quantity of the liquids they drink, as nearly as possible, by fixed rules. The best beverage is fresh water, although the patients like to have their usual allowance of coffee and tea. In view of their copious meat diet, the moderate use of good claret with their food is likewise to be commended.

Coming to the treatment of diabetes by strictly homœopathic remedies, we confess that we are as yet unacquainted with any specifics against this disease. So far we are not aware that the provings of any of our drugs have yielded sugar in the urine. It is from the presence of sugar in the urine that most of the other symptoms of the disease arise; hence, this symptom is the most important and of indispensable necessity to establish a relation of similarity. It is evident that the absence of this symptom renders the reliable selection of a drug impossible, and that of any drug exceedingly difficult. We cannot, therefore, wonder that our literature should not have a single cure of diabetes to boast of.

Having no corresponding remedy to oppose to the main symptom, we have to be guided in the selection of a drug by the accessory symptoms, although but few of them are contained in the pathogenesis of our drugs. The remedies that have so far been recommended for diabetes, are: *Argentum metallicum, Arsenicum, Plumbum, Sulphur, Cuprum.*

Argentum is recommended even by Hahnemann as a suitable remedy for diabetes, and Rueckert reports in his "Klinischen Erfahrungen," a cure of diabetes by means of Argentum, where, however, the main business, an analysis of the urine, had been neglected. We do not see in what way Argentum is homœopathic to diabetes, since the characteristic symptoms are wanting. In many respects *Arsenicum* may be regarded as a simile; it has the sudden, extensive emaciation, the sinking of strength, the disposition to gangrenous inflammations of the skin, an increase of the urinary secretion together with an agonizing thirst. But the excessive hunger and the unquenchable thirst are wanting; for the Arsenic-thirst only admits of small quantities of liquids being drank very frequently. Hence, these symptoms do not point to Arsenic as a strictly homœopathic remedy; indeed, we do not possess any reports of cures effected with this drug. [Granvogl, in his Homœopathy, Vol. II, page 175, relates a cure of diabetes mellitus with Arsenic. The patient was reduced to a skeleton, his mouth excessively dry, thirst agonizing; he fancied that somebody standing by performed every occupation for him, ate, washed, in short did everything for him; he was forty-eight years old, and very dissipated; he was cured in three months. H.]

Cuprum has more homœopathic similarity than Arsenic. Cuprum is more especially indicated by the following symptoms: Slowly-progressing, extreme emaciation, symptoms of tubercular suppuration in the lungs, violent cerebral depression, increased hunger, sweetish taste in the mouth, increased secretion of urine, especially at night, dry and scanty stool, decrease of sexual excitement.

Plumbum has all these symptoms in a more marked degree, and, what is more important, much more constantly. We know that the emaciation caused by Plumbum gradually reaches an extraordinary degree, that the symptoms of suppuration in the lungs are very common, that a genuine hectic fever sets in, and that impotence is a very common result of lead-poisoning. The constipation is very obstinate; the urine, although generally less, is sometimes very much increased; the hunger is very great, the taste almost always sweetish, alternating with sour. The disposition to catarrhal ulceration of the mouth, and to malignant inflammations of the skin, is likewise present, and we admit with Kurtz, that our Materia Medica does not contain a single drug whose symptoms are so strikingly similar to diabetes as Plumbum. Practical results, however, are altogether wanting. *Sulphur,* too, has some of the more prominent symptoms of diabetes among its symptoms, such as; the great emaciation, the sweetish taste, the constipation, the increased flow of urine, etc. In our practice we have made a persistent use of the drug in two cases without witnessing the least result from its employment. We must add, however, that we gave the thirtieth potency; of course, lower potencies, as may easily be imagined, had a better effect.

To these remedies we must add, *China, Creasotum,* and *Lachesis.* In a previous paragraph, we have alluded to a cure of diabetes with large doses of Quinine, but large or small doses, Quinine achieved the cure. The similarity of the effects of Cinchona to the symptoms of diabetes is not very striking; it does not affect the special symptoms, but is rather of a general nature. A cure by Creasotum is related in the Prussian Vereinszeitung, of 1855. The sugar at once diminished in quantity quite considerably, but the general condition of the patient grew worse, (probably in consequence of taking too large doses,) after which an improvement was effected by *China*, subsequently to which, a return to the Creasotum was followed by a complete disappearance of the sugar, and at the same time by a general amelioration of the constitutional symptoms. In comparing the symptoms of Creasotum, more especially the urinary symptoms, to those of Diabetes, we shall find that this cure can be accounted for by the law of Homœopathic similarity. The urine is excreted in larger quantity, is colorless, turbid, has an offensive odor; the bowels are constipated and the fæces very dry; impotence. *Lachesis* has many symptoms that seem to refer to this disease, but it is well known that the value of these symptoms is very unsteady and uncertain. According to P. Frank, the bite of the dipsas causes diabetes, and the connection of serpent-poisons with affections resembling diabetes has frequently been noticed. One of our colleagues was acquainted with a man, sixty years of age, in whom the excessive use of salt developed every symptom of diabetes, which disappeared as soon as he stopped this pernicious habit. About four years ago, a French physician made the discovery that daily doses of 1.5 centigrammes of the *Muriate of Uranium* caused sugar to appear in the urine. If we had had a fair opportunity for instituting provings, we should have done so at once, but we found it inconvenient to carry out such a purpose. However, we had a chance to experiment with the drug on two diabetic patients, a boy of thirteen years and a farmer aged forty years. Unfortunately, on account of the distance at which these patients resided from our office, and their own want of perseverance, we were unable to make many or perfect observations. Both pursued their accustomed mode of living; nevertheless in the case of the boy, the specific gravity fell from 1042 to 1030, and in the case of the man, from 1039 to 1031; the thirst, hunger, and the quantity of the urine likewise diminished very greatly. Doctor Weber made two similar observations on two patients, both of whom died of typhoid, probably uræmic symptoms. After taking *Uranium*, second trituration, the specific gravity always decreased.

These results would be trifling, if they did not concern a disease against which our means of treatment have so far proved inefficient; the drug, undoubtedly, deserves to be subjected to further trials.

In conclusion, we repeat, that the use of the waters of Karlsbad and Vichy has constantly shown such favorable results in diabetes, that it is a physician's duty to send every patient, whose circumstances will admit of it, to those springs. These spa's being only visited during the fine season, time enough remains during the winter, to try other remedial agents in such cases.

B. DISEASES OF THE BLADDER.

1. Cystitis, Inflammation of the Bladder.

CYSTITIS, in most cases, involves the mucous lining of the bladder, and as such is designated cystitis catarrhalis; or it is accompanied by diphtheritic exudation, cystitis crouposa, or else it may be located in the connective tissue enveloping the bladder, in which case the name of peri-cystitis is applied to it. The two last-mentioned forms being very rare, and the necessity of diagnosing them being of rare occurrence, we here only speak of cystitis catarrhalis, both acute and chronic.

The most frequent causes of cystitis are irritations affecting the mucous lining of the bladder directly; they are either mechanical: catheterism, injections into the bladder, stone, or medicinal: acrid diuretics, Cantharides, Copaiva, Cubebs, or even the decomposing urine itself. In other cases the disease may occur as a complication; inflammatory disturbances of adjoining organs may spread to the bladder, or the cystitis may simply be symptomatic of some acute general affection. In rare cases only a cold alone will be sufficient to cause an inflammation of the bladder.

The symptoms of acute cystitis vary. The local symptoms may amount to no more than a slight feeling of pressure in the region of the bladder, and are scarcely ever as intense as Hartmann describes them. Amid more or less febrile motions, the patient always experiences at first a pain when urinating. When the attack first sets in, a larger quantity of urine is voided with a painful urging; soon, however, the urine is voided only in drops, and amid the most agonizing pains, as though burning embers were passing through the urethra. This symptom is most strikingly witnessed in the most acute form of cystitis after the use of new beer; it is characteristic of this inflammation. Very soon the difficulty of urinating becomes associated with a constant pain in the region of the bladder; it is a cutting or stitching pain, and is aggravated by motion, urging to stool, coughing, sneezing, pressure from without; it spreads upwards and downwards to the penis, perinæum, and thigh. At the outset of the disease the urine is clear; after a while it becomes slightly tinged with blood, and, in the further course of the disease, mixed with flocks of mucus and pus-corpuscles, turbid, inclined to decomposition. The general health is not always disturbed correspondingly to the abnormal sensations proceeding from the bladder; at the commencement of the disease the general health is not much impaired, and it is only at a later period that restlessness, chills, loss of appetite, and even vomiting set in.

The disease very frequently runs such a rapid course, that an improvement and even complete recovery may take place in a few days. If the disease increases in intensity, the tenesmus of the bladder may increase to complete retention, the bladder becomes extremely distended, and threatening symptoms of prostration set in, which may end in death. Usually, however, the disease, unless recovery takes place, assumes a lentescent character, and becomes chronic.

In the chronic form the pains decrease considerably, only the constant urging remains. The mucus is secreted in considerable quantity, and along with it pus, so that the urine has a marked white-yellow appearance, sometimes like milk, and deposits a very tenacious mucous sediment. The tendency to decomposition is very great, the reaction decidedly alkaline, less frequently neutral. However, the urine is decomposed only, if it remains for a long time in the bladder. Unless peculiar circumstances hasten the loss of strength, it generally takes place very slowly, and the disease may continue for years before death takes place from exhaustion. Complete recovery is a rare event. Among the sequelæ, we distinguish ulceration of the mucous membrane, hypertrophy of the walls of the bladder, paralysis of the detrusor muscle; it is particularly the two first-named sequelæ that hasten the fatal termination of the disorder, by causing hectic fever and a real phthisis of the bladder.

What we have said shows that the prognosis is quite uncertain. Even if we usually succeed in overcoming an acute catarrh of the bladder, yet ailments sometimes remain for a long time after the slightest attacks, to which the careless or improper conduct of the patient may impart a high degree of gravity. Chronic catarrh of the bladder is always a dangerous disorder, whenever a great deal of mucus and pus is secreted.

Cystitis.

Treatment. The most important remedy against the acute form are *Cantharides*. In a previous paragraph we have called attention to the constant and characteristic effect of Cantharides upon the kidneys, and we will here observe that the relation of this medicine to the bladder is much more definite and profound. In order to avoid unnecessary repetitions, we refer the reader to what we have said on the subject of Cantharides when treating of nephritis; here we simply describe the symptoms that specially refer to cystitis, and which characterize every case of poisoning by Cantharides, whereas the symptoms of nephritis are of less frequent occurrence. Spasmodic, distressing pains in the perinæum and along the urethra, spreading into the testicles, that seem to be drawn up, as if by force; burning, almost insufferable pains in the bladder, spasmodic pains in the thighs; cutting pain through the abdomen; burning pains in the glans; the excretion of urine is more or less obstructed, dribbling of the urine drop by drop, during which it seems like molten lead, the pains are very much increased, and the tenesmus is frightful. The urine is at first clear, afterwards saturated, turbid, tinged with blood, and sometimes drops of pure blood are passed. Great tendency to painful erections; excessive restlessness, with marked fever. These symptoms embody a perfect image of acute cystitis, and we may include the profuse secretion of mucus taking place in a case of chronic poisoning, likewise an image of the further course of cystitis. It cannot be denied that this effect of Cantharides seldom lasts beyond the fifth day, and hence, in long lasting cases of cystitis, we had better look about for other medicines. This remedy deserves especial consideration if the cystitis arises from nephritis, or else caused this latter disease, and likewise in cystitis caused by gonorrhœa. In the chronic form *Cantharides* are scarcely ever appropriate. There is good reason why the medicine should not be given in too large a dose; we have frequently seen instantaneous aggravations take place after the third trituration.

Aconitum is scarcely ever indicated in cystitis; the intense fever only accompanies very violent inflammations, to which the symptoms of Aconite do not by any means correspond. [We think that Baehr undervalues altogether the usefulness of Aconite in this disease. In *rheumatic cystitis* Aconite is not only invaluable, but the true specific remedy, superior to Cantharides. H.]

Cannabis. The bladder symptoms of this drug so nearly resemble those of Cantharides, that it is very difficult to distinguish them from each other. At most the action of Cannabis is less intense. If the particular remedy is not clearly indicated by the accessory phenomena, it may be well, as Kreussler advises, to give Cannabis, if Cantharides have afforded no relief within twenty-four hours.

Colocynthis. The characteristic differences between this drug and Cantharides are more marked. We have tenesmus of the bladder, but less intense, and the pains at urinating are felt over the whole abdomen. The main difference resides in the quality of the urine, which is quite dim, even while being voided, and deposits a tenacious, ropy sediment. Hence, Colocynthis is not adapted to cystitis at the commencement of the disease, but during the period when the pains begin to abate, and mucus begins to be discharged, which scarcely ever takes place before the fifth day. In the chronic form Colocynthis is likewise indicated, provided the disease had not been of too long standing, and no important anatomical changes had taken place.

Mercurius solubilis is very nearly related to the former drug; it has likewise a profuse secretion of mucus at urinating, together with the other diagnostic symptoms. The difference between this and other remedies, will easily be determined from a comparison between their accessory symptoms; violent fever with chilly creepings, and great sensitiveness in the region of the bladder, are characteristic indications for Mercurius; gonorrhœal cystitis likewise requires Mercurius. If the urine contains pus, Mercurius is preferable to Colocynthis under all circumstances.

The remedies that have been named so far, will be found sufficient in all cases of acute cystitis. In addition the following may be considered: *Hepar sulphuris, Nux vomica, Pulsatilla, Belladonna, Mezereum.* In chronic catarrh of the bladder, the following remedies may have to be used:

Acidum phosphoricum for the so-called milky urine, or in other words urine with excessive secretion of mucus, so that the mucus coagulates even in the bladder; the urine is rapidly decomposed, even before being voided. *Arsenicum album* may have to be used in cystitis running a rapid course with threatening symptoms, more particularly, however, in chronic cystitis, when the extraordinary ischuria gives rise to violent distention of the bladder, and threatens to paralyze this organ, and symptoms of ulceration are evidently present. The strength of the patient sinks rapidly, amid febrile motions: the urine is dim, mixed with pus rather than mucus, decomposing very rapidly, and occasionally, but not always, mixed with blood. *Lycopodium* may be required in old cases; the patients' constitutions are worn out, blood is discharged occasionally, as in the so-called hemorrhoids of the bladder. The pains are trifling, but there is a constant distressing urging, although but little urine in the bladder. Causticum; the detrusor urinæ is paralyzed, in consequence of the long-lasting retention of urine, so that in spite of the large quantity of urine in the bladder, very little urine is emitted, or only by fits and starts. *Carbo vegetabilis* is likewise adapted to vesical catarrh attended with paralytic symptoms.

Beside these medicines, the following deserve attention: *Graphites*, *Sulphur*, *Alumina*, *Conium maculatum*, *Sepia*, *Aurum*, *Senega*, *Capsicum*, *Sarsaparilla*. [In chronic catarrh of the bladder, originating in gonorrhœa, *Copaivæ balsamum* may be the best remedy. Some time ago we cured a case of this kind with Copaiva and Cinchona, giving fifteen drops of the Copaiva three times a day. The patient was a middle-aged man, and had consulted some of the first physicians in New York. He had been afflicted with the disease for several years, which had been caused by improper treatment of gonorrhœa with injections. The discharge had been suppressed, and left him with chronic catarrh of the bladder. This came on in paroxysms, with distressing urging every few minutes; at each urination he only passed a few drops of urine and a quantity of purulent mucus. The patient improved very rapidly, indeed immediately after taking the Copaiva, and has remained free from all trouble for the last few years. H.]

The diet has to be regulated with great care. In acute as well as chronic cases, such a diet should be observed as will keep the urine as free from solids as possible, although this is not an easy task to accomplish, because the patients have to use substantial nourishment in order to sustain their strength. In acute cases the patient should eat as little animal food as possible, and should avoid all kinds of spices, coffee, tea, wine, spirits; the use of copious quantities of water should, however, be insisted on. Carbonated water has an unmistakably beneficial effect.

2. Hematuria. Bloody Urine.

Bloody urine not depending upon the above-described renal hemorrhage, but proceeding from the bladder, originates most commonly in injuries of the mucous membrane of the bladder by foreign bodies, or by concretions. Moreover, hematuria and malignant growths in the bladder may arise from cystitis and its consequences, ulcerations and dilatation of the vessels. It is seldom the case that hemorrhage from the bladder occurs without any evidently material cause. As in the kidneys, so in the bladder, certain poisons may cause hemorrhage, though in the latter less frequently than in the former.

Excepting the symptoms of the causal affection, the symptoms of hematuria are generally trifling, determined, for the most part, by the coagula that form very readily and interfere with the easy flow of urine. Hence, we have urging, tenesmus, spasm of the bladder, burning or cutting pains, and very frequently a perfect absence of pain. The symptoms are always restricted to the bladder, and do not involve the kidneys in any way. As a rule the blood is not intimately mixed with the urine, is not decomposed, and, if the hemorrhage is at all considerable, the blood coagulates in such quantity that the catheter is often required in order to effect a passage for the urine. The flow of blood from the bladder very easily exceeds the quantity flowing from the kidneys, and hence superinduces more readily the phenomena entailed by loss of blood. On the other hand, an hemorrhage from the bladder usually has a shorter duration than hemorrhage from the kidneys, and scarcely ever lasts uninterruptedly for weeks. Of itself it is scarcely ever an accident of any great importance.

Treatment. The remedies recommended for renal hemorrhage are likewise appropriate in hematuria; we, therefore, refer to the former, and add the following particulars in this place.

Cantharides may only be found suitable in hematuria accompanied by violent symptoms of irritation; they are not adapted to hemorrhage without much pain. Particulars may be found in the chapter on renal hemorrhage; likewise regarding *Terebinthina*, which we are seldom called upon to use in this affection. *Arnica* is the best remedy if the bleeding is occasioned by the catheter, by an operation or by concretions. *Ipecacuanha* is indicated in copious hemorrhage, with coldness of the skin, nausea, vomiting, fainting, retention of urine on account of the bloody coagula, dark color of the lost blood. *Cannabis* in the same cases as Cantharides, and likewise if the blood is lost from the urethra. For the so-called hemorrhoids of the bladder, which usually occur in consequence of, or attended with chronic catarrh of the bladder, and where the loss of blood occurs periodically, but sometimes in large quantity, the chief remedies are: *Lycopodium, Arsenicum, Sulphur.* If pure blood is discharged, especially immediately after urinating, *Meze-*

reum is required. If the hemorrhage is caused by irritating drugs, especially by Cantharides, *Camphora* is the remedy. There are many other remedies that have bloody urine among their symptoms, but we have not deemed it necessary to enumerate them in this place. [We have often cured hematuria with Aconite root, first attenuation, especially in the case of bilious individuals, with sallow complexion, a wiry frame, and bilious-nervous temperament. We can recommend the Canada flea-bane, or the Erigeron canadense, and Hamamelis virginiana, or witch-hazel, as far superior to many of the above-mentioned remedies. Small doses, however, will not answer. *Trillium pendulum*, or the beth-root, is highly recommended by some physicians; we have no experience of our own to offer. H.]

3. Enuresis Nocturna, Wetting the Bed.

This inconvenience would be of little consequence, except for the crying abuses to which the endeavor to remove it has led. Physicians as well as parents have supposed that this weakness could be done away with by purely educational means, which were, moreover suggested by the most insane views regarding its causes. Latterly, physicians have improved their methods of meeting this accident; lay-persons, however, are still true to their absurd prejudices in this respect.

Wetting the bed is an accident to which children are liable; it seldom lasts beyond the age of pubescence, still less beyond the age of twenty years. Healthy individuals scarcely ever wet their beds more than once. This trouble generally dates from the earliest infancy, and rarely makes its appearance at a later period. Various causes have been assigned for it, and corresponding methods of treatment devised for its cure, however with varied results. Laziness may give rise to it in many cases, but more frequently it is the fear of getting up in the dark. A common cause of the trouble is, that children sleep too soundly to be roused from their sleep by the irritating action of the urine upon the bladder. Yet the bladder need not be weak or paralyzed; if so, the accident may take place even during a light sleep. The children generally say that they dreamed of wetting the bed, showing that the irritation was not sufficiently powerful to wake them. The quality of the urine may cause a passing attack of enuresis: we see this in children who are liable to catarrhal attacks, and, under such circumstances, immediately void a saturated urine. The irritation caused by pin-worms may likewise induce enuresis.

Corporal punishment should never be resorted to as a means of curing this weakness, which is rather made worse by it than otherwise; older children are made so nervous by this treatment, that they sometimes remain wide awake half the night. On the contrary, their sense of honor and will should be appealed to. It is of no use to keep the ordinary beverage from them in the evening; this may cover up the weakness for a time, which returns again as soon as a little more liquid is again partaken of. Nor is it of any more use to frequently rouse children from their sleep at night. If no abnormal conditions forbid, the best plan is to gradually accustom the bladder to hold larger quantities of liquid. Children should be accustomed during the day to retain the urine as long as may seem proper, and not to yield to the least desire to urinate, as is their usual custom. This system, if carried out consistently and vigorously, is often alone sufficient, in otherwise normal cases, to effect a cure, of course not in a few days. By measuring the quantity of urine at every discharge, we can determine *a priori* the time when the enuresis will cease. The more the quantity increases the nearer we are to a cure. This method has the advantage of being readily adopted by the children, provided they are promised a speedy delivery from their trouble.

The reader may infer from what we have said, that we do not entertain a very high opinion of the efficacy of internal remedies in this disease, except when enuresis is a purely secondary affection, in which case we resort to the remedies for catarrh of the bladder, helminthiasis, etc. But inasmuch as no torturing effects need be apprehended from the remedies proposed by homœopathic practice for this disease, like those inflicted by one of the leaders of the Physiological School, whose means of cure recommended for it are truly startling and even frightful, we here name the remedies that may be given with more or less good effect: *Belladonna*, *Pulsatilla*, *Cina*, *Causticum*, *Sepia*, *Sulphur*. One of our oldest practitioners recommends the last-named medicine in the thirtieth potency, and at long intervals; but we confess that we have never derived the least benefit from it, unless the above-proposed precautionary measures were at the same time adopted. [The *Nitrate* or *Muriate of Uranium* may have a very good effect. H.]

4. Cystospasmus, Spasm of the Bladder.

This spasm is a symptom in many affections of the urinary organs, and, as such, is not referred to in this place. There is no doubt that it may likewise represent a pure neurosis of the bladder, although its occurrence as such is comparatively rare.

The disease may break out at any age, but is most frequent in middle-aged individuals of the male sex. All persons with weak and irritable nerves are predisposed to this affection, hence it is most frequently met with among hypochondriac and hysteric individuals. Hence, a sudden emotion, an outburst of passion, great depression of strength, violent exertions during sexual intercourse, onanism, may be proximate causes of the disease. Whether a simple spasm of the bladder may be caused by a cold, is questionable.

A spasm of the bladder commonly sets in quite suddenly, the patient being otherwise in the enjoyment of good health, as a violent, constrictive pain, proceeding from the neck of the bladder, and extending along the dorsum of the penis towards the glans, attended with partial or complete erection, sometimes radiating to the groin, testes, thighs, and very often, at the same time, along the perinæum towards the anus, accompanied by a pain resembling tenesmus. If the spasm affects the detrusor muscle alone, the least accumulation of urine excites a violent desire to void it, so that the patients are sometimes unable to prevent the flow of urine; if the sphincter is affected, the urine is either voided drop by drop or cannot be voided at all; if the detrusor and sphincter are affected at the same time, we have the most violent urging to urinate, attended with a more or less complete inability to void the urine; this last-mentioned case is most apt to cause nervous phenomena of a different kind, such as anguish, restlessness, trembling, convulsions, violent tenesmus. An attack of spasm may last from one or more minutes to half an hour. After the pains begin to abate, the urine sometimes passes off in a full stream, clearer and paler than usual. The return of the paroxysm is not governed by any rule, since the spasm sometimes only takes place once, sometimes a number of times, even on the same day.

Treatment. Hartmann's therapeutic recommendations not only refer to the mere spasm, but likewise to a spasm symptomatic of other morbid complications. Our previous remarks concerning *Cantharides, Cannabis, Terebinthina*, etc., show that these remedies may cure the latter kind of spasm. We want to know the remedies that will cure spasm of the bladder when occurring as a pure neurosis. We have very few practical indications to guide us in the selection of a remedy, most probably because cystospasmus is a very rare affection. We may take it for granted, however, that such remedies will prove most effectual as are capable of exciting genuine spasms in other organs and systems. *Nux vomica* ranks first among such remedies. It not only meets all the bladder-symptoms, but likewise the consequences of sexual excesses, onanism, etc.; likewise hypochondria and other conditions that have been referred to among the etiological causes. A second important remedy is *Hyoscyamus*, well known to veterinary surgeons as a good remedy for the spasmodic urinary difficulties of horses; clinical observations of this kind on the human species are as yet very scanty. *Belladonna* and *Cocculus* likewise deserve mention. Although we place these remedies in the front rank, yet we are willing to admit that the other remedies, which we have indicated for acute catarrh of the bladder, may likewise prove useful, more especially *Colocynthis*, and likewise *Colchicum*, *Pulsatilla*, *Sarsaparilla*. Hartmann recommends the last-mentioned remedy as particularly efficacious for spasms of the bladder caused by stone in the bladder. [Spasm of the bladder, caused by a cold, yields speedily and permanently to Aconite, first attenuation of the tincture of the root, or to a few drops of the German tincture in half a tumbler of water. H.]

The peculiar character of this disease suggests the propriety of trying to relieve the patient by external applications. Water is most adapted to this purpose. As a rule, warm sitz-baths or warm fomentations to the region of the bladder afford the most relief; it is only now and then that very cold water, or a cold-water injection may be preferable. The patient may likewise be advised, as soon as the spasm commences, to drink large quantities of water, either cold or warm. In thirty minutes the water will have entered the bladder. The use of water is especially desirable, if the attack was caused by acrid medicines or beer.

5. Cystoplegia, Paralysis of the Bladder.

Although this form of paralysis has been alluded to in the first section of this work, yet we deem a few additional remarks on the subject indispensable, for the reason that paralysis of the bladder sometimes occurs as an idiopathic disease, independent of affections of the spine or brain, and becomes a source of great distress to those who are afflicted with it.

The causes of this affection, beside those that originate in the central organs of the nervous system, are of three kinds, namely: advanced age or premature marasmus, excessive distention of the bladder, and sexual excesses, particularly onanism. The symptoms vary, according as the sphincter or the detrusor muscle is paralyzed. In the former case, and if the paralysis is complete, the urine flows off involuntarily, as soon as the bladder is somewhat distended, whereas, if the paralysis is incomplete, in a case of so-called paralytic weakness, the patients are indeed able to retain the urine for a short, but never for any great length of time. This last-named condition is met with quite frequently, and many persons are afflicted with this weakness without consulting a physician on the subject. If the detrusor is paralyzed, the bladder acquires an undue distention before it overcomes the normal resistance of the sphincter, and only a portion of the contents is voided, always with the co-operation of the abdominal muscles. If both muscles of the bladder are paralyzed at the same time, it becomes excessively and permanently distended, and only the smallest portion of the urine is voided voluntarily.

We shall here speak only of the two forms of paralysis that originate in excessive distention of the bladder and in sexual excesses, onanism, etc.; for paralysis of the bladder, which befalls old people, is not amenable to systematic treatment. In the former cases, the patients are generally younger persons. The first form of paralysis from excessive distention, is caused by an undue retention of urine, which young girls are particularly apt to indulge in, a paralysis similar to that which may attack the rectum from an analogous cause. In such a case, the physician may interfere, not only with prophylactic, but likewise with curative means. The prophylactic treatment consists in advising mothers to warn their children against indulging in such unreasonable prudery, and to explain to them the consequences of such foolish conduct. The curative treatment consists in prescribing *Ignatia*, *Rhus tox.*, *Ruta graveolens*, or *Baryta carbonica*, the precise indications for which we omit, for the reason, that each case will have to be treated in accordance with its own special symptoms. Paralysis of the bladder, arising from abuse of the sexual organs, is generally only a semi-paralysis, a more or less marked weakness. Of course, a successful treatment implies a mode of life in accordance with sound hygiene and morality. The remedies are: *Nux vomica*, *Ignatia*, *Phosphorus*, *China*, *Causticum*. In both these forms of paralysis, cold water is an important means of cure; it may be used as a cold sitz-bath, or wet sheet, or as an injection. Paralysis of the bladder, consequent upon severe labor, has to be treated in the same manner; it generally disappears of itself, but may likewise remain as a permanent weakness.

VOLUME II.

THE SCIENCE
of
HOMOEOPATHIC
THERAPEUTICS

BERNHARD BAEHR, M.D.

TRANSLATED AND ENRICHED WITH NUMEROUS ADDITIONS

from

KAFKA AND OTHER SOURCES

by

CHARLES J. HEMPEL, M.D.

VOLUME II

B. JAIN PUBLISHERS (P) LTD.
NEW DELHI

> **Note from the Publishers**
>
> Any information given in this book is not intended to be taken as a replacement for medical advice. Any person with a condition requiring medical attention should consult a qualified practitioner or therapeutist.

THE SCIENCE OF THERAPEUTICS

Reprint Edition: 1996, 2004

No part of this book may be reproduced, stored in a retrieval system or transmitted, in any form or by any means, mechanical, photocopying, recording or otherwise, without any prior written permission of the publisher.

© All rights are reserved with the publisher

Price: Rs. 300.00

Published by Kuldeep Jain for
B. Jain Publishers (P) Ltd.
1921, Street No. 10, Chuna Mandi,
Paharganj, New Delhi 110 055 (INDIA)
Phones: 2358 0800, 2358 1100, 2358 1300, 2358 3100, 5169 8991
Fax: 011-2358 0471, 5169 8993; *Email:* bjain@vsnl.com
Website: www.bjainbooks.com

Printed in India by
J.J. Offset Printers
522, FIE, Patpar Ganj, Delhi - 110 092
Phones: 2216 9633, 2215 6128

ISBN: 81-8056-426-2
BOOKCODE: BB-2272

CONTENTS OF THE SECOND VOLUME.

SEVENTH SECTION.

	Page
Diseases of the Sexual Organs	1
A. *Diseases of the Male Sexual Organs*	1
1. Urethritis. Gonorrhœa, Catarrh of the Urethra, Blennorrhœa of the Urethral Lining Membrane	1
2. Orchitis, Inflammation of the Testes	13
3. Spermatorrhœa	16
B. *Diseases of the Female Sexual Organs*	20
1. Vaginitis, Catarrh of the Sexual Mucous Lining. Fluor Albus, Leucorrhœa, Whites	20
2. Metritis, Inflammation of the Womb	27
3. Metritis puerperalis. Puerperal Fever, Inflammation of the Uterus during Confinement	34
4. Oophoritis, Ovaritis. Inflammation of the Ovaries	45
5. Menstrual Anomalies	47
a. Derangements attendant upon the appearance of the Menses	53
b. Amenorrhœa, Suppression or Delay of the Menses	55
c. Menstruatio Nimia, Profuse Menses	57
d. Dysmenorrhœa, Scanty Menses	60
e. Difficult Menstruation, Ailments accompanying the Menses	61
6. Metrorrhagia. Uterine Hemorrhage	66
7. Carcinoma Uteri. Cancer of the Womb	81
8. Various Morbid Conditions in the Sexual System of the Female	87
9. Vaginodynia, Neuralgia of the Vagina	92
10. Mastitis, Inflammation of the Breasts	95
11. Mastodynia	99
12. Carcinoma Mammæ. Cancer of the Breasts	100

EIGHTH SECTION.

Diseases of the Respiratory Organs	107
A. *Diseases of the Larynx and Trachea*	107
1. Laryngotracheitis Catarrhalis acuta. Acûte Laryngotracheal Catarrh	107
2. Laryngotracheitis Crouposa. Croup, Membranous Croup	112
3. Laryngotracheitis Chronica. Chronic Laryngotracheal Catarrh	129

Contents of the Second Volume.

		Page
4.	Œdema Glottidis, Laryngitis Submucosa, Œdema of the Glottis	137
5.	Spasmus Glottidis, Spasm of the Glottis	140
6.	Ulcers of the Larynx, Helcosis seu ulcera laryngis	145

B. Diseases of the Lungs 149
    1. Hyperæmia of the Lungs. Congestion, Plethora of the Lungs 150
    2. Pneumorrhagia, Pulmonary Hemorrhage 154
    3. Bronchitis Acuta, Acute Bronchitis 164
    4. Influenza, Grippe 182
    5. Tussis Convulsiva, Pertussis, Whooping-Cough 193
    6. Bronchitis Chronica, Chronic Bronchitis, Chronic Pulmonary or Bronchial Catarrh 210
    7. Bronchiectasia, Dilatation of the Bronchia 234
    8. Emphysema Pulmonum, Emphysema of the Lungs 235
    9. Pneumonia, Inflammation of the Lungs 243
    10. Gangræna Pulmonum, Gangrene of the Lungs 303
    11. Œdema Pulmonum, Hydrops Pulmonum, Œdema of the Lungs, Dropsy of the Lungs 307
    12. Asthma 311

C. Diseases of the Diaphragm 321
    1. Diaphragmitis, Inflammation of the Diaphragm 322
    2. Singultus, Hiccup 323
    3. Hernia of the Diaphragm 324

D. Diseases of the Pleura 325
    1. Pleuritis, Pleurisy, Inflammation of the Pleura 325
    2. Hydrothorax, Dropsy of the Chest 342
    3. Pneumothorax 343

NINTH SECTION.

Diseases of the Organs of Circulation 345
  A. Diseases of the Heart 345
    1. Carditis, Pericarditis, Endocarditis, Myocarditis. Inflammation of the Heart, Pericardium, Endocardium, Substance of the Heart 347
    2. Hypertrophia Cordis, Hypertrophy of the Heart 372
    3. Dilatatio Cordis, Dilatation of the Heart 381
    4. Adipositas Cordis, Fatty Degeneration of the Heart 382
    5. Anomalies, Abnormal Conditions of the Orifices of the Heart, Valvular Diseases 388
        a. Insufficiency of the Mitral Valve 388
        b. Stenosis of the left Auriculo-ventricular Orifice 389
        c. Insufficiency of the Aortic Valves 394
        d. Stenosis of the Aortic Orifice 396
        e. Defects of the Orifices and Valves of the Right Heart 399
    6. Palpitation of the Heart 399
    7. Stenocardia, Angina Pectoris 405

Contents of the Second Volume. VII

TENTH SECTION.

Page
Derangements of Single Systems 410
   A. Diseases of the Bones, Muscles, Articulations 410
      1. Ostitis, Periostitis, Pott's Disease. Inflammation of the Bones and Periosteum 410
      2. Rhachitis, Rickets 416
      3. Enchondroma, Pædarthrocace, Spina Ventosa 420
      4. Psoitis, Inflammation of the Psoas-muscle 421
      5. Lumbago 422
      6. Progressive Muscular Paralysis 424
      7. Inflammation of Joints 426
         a. Coxalgia, Coxarthrocace, Inflammation of the Hip-joint 427
         b. Gonarthrocace, Tumor Albus Genu, Gonitis, Inflammation of the Knee-joint 430
         c. Inflammation of the Tarsus 433
   B. Diseases of the Arteries, Veins, Lymphatics and Lymphatic Glands 435
      1. Diseases of the Arteries 435
      2. Diseases of the Veins 436
         a. Phlebitis, Inflammation of the Veins 436
         b. Phlebectasia, Varices, Dilatation of the Veins 438
      3. Diseases of the Lymphatic Vessels and Glands 442
         a. Lymphangioitis and Lymphadenitis Acuta 442
         b. Lymphadenitis Chronica, Chronic Inflammation of Lymphatic Glands 445
   C. Diseases of the Nerves 447
      1. Ischias 447
      2. Neuralgia Intercostalis. Intercostal Neuralgia 450
   D. Diseases of the Skin 452
      1. Erythema 453
      2. Erysipelas 455
      3. Roseola, Rubeolæ 465
      4. Urticaria, Nettlerash 466
      5. Miliaria, Rash 469
      6. Pityriasis, Dandruff, Dandriff 470
      7. Psoriasis, Scaly Tetter 472
      8. Ichthyosis, Fish-skin, Porcupine Disease 473
      9. Lichen, Strophulus, Tooth-Rash 474
      10. Prurigo 476
      11. Acne, Stone-pock 478
      12. Sycosis, Mentagra 480
      13. Acne Rosacea, Gutta Rosacea, Copper-nose, Bottle-nose ... 482
      14. Lupus, Wolf, Jacob's Ulcer 483
      15. Herpes, Tetter 486
         a. Herpes Facialis 487
         b. Herpes Præputialis 487
         c. Herpes Zoster, Zona, Shingles 488
         d. Herpes Iris and Circinnatus 490

		Page
16.	Eczema	490
17.	Impetigo	497
18.	Ecthyma, Rupia	499
19.	Pemphygus	501
20.	Furuncle, Carbuncle, Anthrax	503
21.	Seborrhœa	505
22.	Favus, Honey-comb Tetter, Scald-head	506
23.	Scabies, Itch	507

ELEVENTH SECTION.

Constitutional Diseases 513

A. *Acute and Chronic Contagious Diseases* 513

1. Morbilli, Measles 513
2. Scarlatina, Scarlet-fever 522
3. Variola, Small-pox 532
4. Syphilis 542
   a. Primary Chancre 543
   b. Secondary Syphilis 548
   c. Tertiary Syphilis 551

B. *Epidemic and Endemic Infectious Diseases* 563

1. Intermittent Fever, Fever and Ague 563
2. Typhus 576
3. Febris Icterodes, Yellow Fever 602
4. Cholera Asiatica 613

C. *Constitutional Diseases without Definite Infection* 624

1. Chlorosis, Green-sickness 624
2. Rheumatism 630
   a. Acute Articular Rheumatism 630
   b. Acute Muscular Rheumatism 632
   c. Chronic Articular Rheumatism 633
3. Arthritis, Gout 640
4. Dropsy 645
5. Scorbutus, Scurvy 649
6. Scrofulosis 652
7. Tuberculosis 658
8. Constitutional Plethora, Polyæmia, Hyperæmia 681
9. Anæmia, Oligæmia. Deficiency or rather Paleness of the Blood 687
10. Congenital Anæmia 701
11. Consecutive Anæmia 709
12. Secondary Anæmia 711
13. Marasmus, Tabes 711
14. Obesitas, Adiposis, Polysarcia, Obesity 714
15. Uræmia 720
16. Pyæmia. Purulent Decomposition of the Blood 728
17. Septicæmia. Putrid Decomposition of the Blood 732
18. Gastromalacia, Softening of the Stomach 737
19. Goitre, Bronchocele, Derbyshire Neck 743

SEVENTH SECTION.

Diseases of the Sexual Organs.

A. DISEASES OF THE MALE SEXUAL ORGANS.

1. Urethritis.

Gonorrhœa, Catarrh of the Urethra, Blennorrhœa of the Urethral Mucous Lining.

IF we have not made a distinction between virulent and non-virulent gonorrhœa, it is because the last-named disease is so vague and indefinite and, moreover, of such rare occurrence, that a bare allusion to the same will suffice for all practical purposes.

Etiology. The non-virulent blennorrhœa is caused by the irritation produced by foreign bodies in the urethra (calculi, etc.); or it may be caused by excessive sexual intercourse, intercourse during the menstrual flow, irritating drugs, etc., although not frequently by the latter; it may likewise have a catarrhal origin and, finally, may constitute a symptom of other inflammations, more especially of the bladder and prostate gland. In a case of blennorrhœa we should never be too hasty in not attributing it to the contact with an infectious virus. Gonorrhœa proper or an infectious blennorrhœa of the urethra, is always occasioned by infectious contact; and, although we cannot deny the possibility that gonorrhœa may result without sexual intercourse, yet in the majority of cases it may be boldly asserted that an impure coition is the cause of the disease. Of course, the patients make every possible effort to conceal the origin of their trouble. What conditions and influences have to co-operate in order to produce an infection, is difficult to determine: all we know is, that the same woman will infect one person without infecting the other. The degree of sexual excitement may possibly constitute an additional cause of infection; at all events it is remarkable that novices are almost always caught.

Regarding the nature of the gonorrhœal contagium, opinions still differ. Some deny the specific nature of the contagium, placing it in the same category as the secretion of epidemic blepharophthalmitis; they assert that gonorrhœa is caused by contact with the secretion caused by an intense catarrhal inflammation of the vagina. This view is not entirely unfounded, and is more particularly supported by the circumstance that gonorrhœa does not superinduce constitutional diseases. Others attribute to the gonorrhœal virus a specific character, and the power of producing constitutional maladies, concerning whose essential actuality and nature, we shall offer some further remarks in the following paragraphs. The gonorrhœal virus has even been supposed to be identical with the chancre-poison; this opinion has, however, been abandoned. We cannot afford time or space to enter upon a more extensive discussion of these points, to which we shall, however, refer somewhat more fully in the next paragraph. [Jahr's recent work on Venereal Diseases, translated and edited with numerous notes and additions by Chs. J. Hempel, M. D., and published by W. Radde, No. 550 Pearl St., New York, is the best work on this important subject now extant, in the literature of our School; no physician who desires to have a full and accurate knowledge of the various opinions now prevalent regarding the nature of the gonorrhœal virus and the syphilitic contagium, or of the manifold disorders which they are capable of producing, from the simplest blennorrhœa to the most terrible disorganization, or of their homœopathic treatment as conducted in accordance with strictly and unimpeachably scientific principles, can do without this work. H.]

Symptoms and Course. The time between the first communication of the gonorrhœal disease and its actual manifestation is from three to eight days, very seldom either less or more, although the patients are very apt to indicate a longer period. Usually, however, this is an intentional deception, but may likewise be an error, for the reason that the disease sometimes sets in so mildly that it may have existed for some days without having been noticed. The duration of the stage of incubation may likewise differ, in consequence of differences inherent in the degree of infectiousness of the secretion, as has already been noticed when speaking of blennorrhœa of the eyes. The affection commences with a titillating, painless, sometimes even voluptuous sensation in the urethra, from which a small quantity of a transparent, slimy secretion is discharged by which the orifice is glued together in the morning. At this stage the visible portion of the urethral mucous membrane is already redder and swollen. The peculiar titillation is followed by an increased desire to urinate and increased erections, sometimes also by nocturnal emissions. In a few days the titillation changes to a pain, the urging to urinate becomes more frequent, the pain at urinating becomes intolerable, and the urine of which only a few drops are emitted, becomes scalding hot, so that it seems like fire. If the urine is emitted in larger quantity, the pains during the emission are less severe, but so much more violent immediately after. The concentrated urine, moreover, causes an increased pain, on which account the first discharge of urine early in the morning is the most distressing. The orifice of the urethra now begins to swell quite perceptibly, the lips look very red. The secretion still remains scanty, looks yellow or greenish-yellow, is thick, stiffens the linen with yellow or greenish-yellow stains, and, in the morning is easily squeezed out in an increased quantity. The sensitiveness of the urethra to pressure now extends to the fossa navicularis. The erections, especially at night, become more frequent and continuous, causing the patient great pain in consequence of the stretching of the exceedingly sensitive urethra; emissions now occur very rarely. Shortly after this, the purulent secretion increases in quantity, but preserves its greenish-yellow color. The parts stained by the discharge, the glans and prepuce, swell; the smegma is secreted more abundantly, excoriations and small superficial ulcers show themselves. The inflammatory irritation of the prepuce easily results in phimosis or paraphimosis. The further extension of the disease is evident from the fact that the urethra now is sensitive in its whole length. It is only in a few cases that the gonorrhœa remains confined to the anterior portion of the urethra. This so-called inflammatory stage seldom lasts less than eight days, generally a fortnight. General febrile symptoms are seldom present; what might be considered as such, is owing to the mental excitement of the patient and to the intensity of the pain. Towards the end of this first stage the discharge generally becomes very copious, but its color changes more and more to that of a whitish mucus, and assumes a more fluid consistence. At the same time the pains at urinating abate almost entirely, leaving at most only a disagreeable feeling, the erections become less frequent and painful; on the other hand, the nocturnal emissions are apt to be more frequent and to be followed by slight exacerbations. The white secretion leaves gray and stiff stains on the linen, with a yellowish point in the centre. In favorable cases the whole disease is terminated in five to seven weeks amid a gradual abatement of all the symptoms.

Such a simple and favorable course does not by any means constitute the rule; generally we meet with one or more complications.

In the first stage, we not unfrequently meet with a considerable inflammation, on which account a gonorrhœa of this kind has been termed erythematous, with distinct febrile motions. The inflammatory stage may be protracted beyond the above-named period. In the next place we sometimes observe inflamed spots in the neighborhood of the urethra, elongated or rounded infiltrations which sometimes terminate in abscesses, but are not always of great importance. The extension of the inflammation along the whole course of the urethra is apt to superinduce a simple congestive or even inflammatory affection of the prostate gland, rarely of the bladder. An inflammation of the prostate gland involves danger, because it may result in a more or less complete retention of urine, or terminate in suppuration. Orchitis will be spoken of more fully by and by. Inflammatory swellings of the inguinal glands, so-called gonorrhœal buboes, are very common. They are of no special importance, and disappear of themselves as soon as the inflammatory stage has run its course.

Isolated deviations from this picture of gonorrhœa, exert little or no influence upon its general course. The so-called dry gonorrhœa consists in a short-lasting suspension of the purulent secretion, which is most commonly accompanied by an exacerbation of the inflammatory symptoms. It not unfrequently happens that at the commencement of the disease streaks of blood are mixed up with the pus, which does not influence the further course of the disease. The so-called torpid gonorrhœa which has the peculiar characteristic of being totally or partially without any inflammatory symptoms, is of rare occurrence and mostly attacks individuals who have had the disease more than once. It cannot be denied that repeated attacks of gonorrhœa and the cauterizing action of the injections used during the treatment of such attacks, diminish the disposition to contract an inflammatory gonorrhœa.

One of the most painful complications is chordée by which is understood the curving of the penis downwards during an erection. It arises when the corpora cavernosa have become involved in the inflammation and the consequent infiltration of these bodies does not permit the interstitial swelling of these parts during an erection. This trouble is so much more serious as this condition of the corpora cavernosa may remain a permanent disorganization.

One of the most ordinary consequences of gonorrhœa, which is so common, that it may almost be considered the rule, is gleet, a chronic urethritis or secondary gonorrhœa. It arises gradually from the acute form, the discharge becoming more and more scanty, clearer and thinner, and continuing all the time, sometimes for years, unless arrested by medical interference. It often defies all treatment. A discharge of this kind would be of comparatively trifling importance if we knew to a certainty whether it is infectious or not, the latter supposition having undoubtedly the larger amount of probability in its favor. The treacherous stains on the linen are, of course, a source of great anxiety to the sufferers, and it is not to be wondered if they desire to be freed from their distress. Finally, exacerbations will occur during gleet, which, if they do not result in an attack of acute gonorrhœa, cause some pain at urinating and an increased, whitish discharge. Such exacerbations sometimes set in after slight colds, after drinking beer or wine, or even after coition. Gleet is no guarantee against a fresh infection, but this may absorb it instead of rendering it more inveterate.

Among the sequelæ which may involve the bladder, prostate gland, etc., we note more especially strictures of the urethra. One cause of stricture may be a contracting cicatrix in the urethra, in which case the bougie is alone capable of affording help. Or the stricture may depend upon infiltration and subsequent callous hypertrophy of the tissue surrounding the urethra, in which case it is sometimes felt externally like a hard, elongated swelling.

We shall devote a few lines to the so-called gonorrhœal disease and gonorrhœal metastases. Hahnemann speaks of two kinds of gonorrhœa, a benign kind which may be regarded as a local disease of the urethra, and another kind depending upon the sycosic contagium. Hartmann observes, that the two kinds cannot well be distinguished in a given case. It can scarcely be supposed that condylomata constitute a distinct phenomenon in gonorrhœa, which may run its course as completely and rapidly with, as without them. If blennorhœic condylomata constituted a specific product, ophthalmic blennorhœa ought to be a result of the sycosic miasm, since condylomatous growths likewise occur in the former disease. Be this as it may, it is of very little consequence whether there are two kinds of gonorrhœa, for in practice we cannot make this distinction even if we would. It is an established fact, that the gonorrhœal bears no resemblance to the syphilitic contagium, by which is meant that the former does not develop, as a more or less regular consequence, a constitutional malady, and that it acts like the contagium of the ophthalmic blennorhœa and similarly to the contagium of small-pox, scarlatina, etc. Or shall we consider these contagia as syphilitic because their respective diseases sometimes leave severe constitutional derangements behind them? In our opinion, a gonorrhœal epidemic disease neither exists, nor is it at all possible. At all events, if an intense gonorrhœal infection, including, of course, the absurd manner in which it is often treated, gives rise to a constitutional disease, it is wrong to hold the gonorrhœa responsible for it, any more than that it may have acted as the exciting cause or the spark that may have ignited the accumulated combustible material. This view is supported by a number of analogies, whereas the other view requires for its proof a mass of speculative hypotheses. Let the partisans of this doctrine be invited to point to a case of gonorrhœal constitutional disease. If such a thing did at all exist, it certainly cannot be difficult to pick out a dozen cases among the tens of thousands that have been treated for gonorrhœa. And then it would be incumbent upon them to show that in those cases the gonorrhœa was a simple blennorrhœa and not caused by a syphilitic ulcer. Hartmann has not made this distinction, nor is it probable that Hahnemann did so.

Gonorrhœal metastasis, is likewise a theory of very questionable authenticity. Orchitis is certainly not to be regarded as such a metastasis and, as regards gonorrhœal rheumatism, which is admitted even by the most obstinate sceptics, we are not quite sure whether the medicines which the patient took, have not more to do with it than the gonorrhœa. Under homœopathic treatment we have never yet met with a single case of pretended metastasis.

Treatment. Hartmann's views in respect to the treatment of gonorrhœa differ from our own in many respects.

According to Hartmann, Hahnemann gives the following instructions for the treatment of gonorrhœa: "Sycosic gonorrhœa is cured most certainly and radically by the internal use of *Thuya*, which is homœopathic to this disease, giving one dose of a few pellets of the 30th potency, which, if no improvement has taken place in twenty, thirty or forty days, is to be followed by an equally small dose of the 12th potency of *Nitric acid* which must be permitted to act for an equally long period. The miasm of the other benign kinds of gonorrhœa does not seem to infect the general organism, and to remain localized in the urinary organs. This kind of gonorrhœa yields to a single drop of the fresh juice of parsley (succus Petroselini), provided the frequent urging to urinate indicates this drug, or to a drop of an alcoholic solution of Copaiva, unless the intense inflammation and the debilitating treatment have roused the latent psora which hitherto had been slumbering in the organism of the patient, in which case it often happens that a lingering gonorrhœa is excited into action which will only yield to an antipsoric treatment." Hartmann replies to these statements in the following words: "The simple gonorrhœa yields only in a few cases to the tincture of parsley or to the alcoholic solution of Copaiva: nor have I been able to cure sycosic gonorrhœa with nothing but Thuya; in general this kind of gonorrhœa cannot well be separated from the benign form, unless condylomata are present, or the patient knows positively that the woman who infected him, had sycosis. The same remark applies to figwarts. Quite recently I treated a case of sycosic condylomata which would not yield to Thuya, but got well in ten days after a single dose of Nitric acid 1; in another case I effected a cure with two doses of *Cinnabaris;* in other cases other mercurial preparations were required." At a later period he adds: "In many cases of gonorrhœa all three remedies proposed by Hahnemann, and even many others, have to be used for a cure."—"I know now that gonorrhœa which sets in with great violence at first, is much more easily managed, if Thuya is used at once at the commencement. Nevertheless, I admit that I am as yet unable to distinguish sycosic gonorrhœa from any other form unless condylomata are present. Gonorrhœa attended with condylomata is in most cases a secondary affection, as may be inferred from the fact that it disappears simultaneously with the sycosic disease against which the treatment has to be directed."

The idea of a so-called gonorrhœal disease is very plainly enunciated in the preceding paragraph. It is evident that the doctrine of a sycosic miasm owes its origin to the difficulty of explaining the frequently peculiar and chronic course of gonorrhœa; but it is wrong to undertake to explain that which requires to be explained by resorting to an explanation which is itself unintelligible. If any one should consider a statement of this kind as disrespectful to Hahnemann, let him consider that it is much better to admit defects than to wilfully close one's eyes to them. How many cures has any homœopathic physician made in accordance with Hahnemann's precepts? A normal gonorrhœa runs a course of five to seven weeks. How can we talk about cures if we are to let remedies act for forty or eighty days? If a gonorrhæa disappears under Hahnemann's treatment, what has Thuya or Nitric acid to do with the cure?

We boldly assert that most homœopathic physicians employ other means and methods in order to secure the cure of gonorrhœa. If the gonorrhœa disappears in the fourth week, we are entitled to consider this a cure. It will scarcely ever yield in a shorter period of time. Hartmann admits that this disease cannot be cured by means of a strict comparison of the symptoms, and that we cannot get along without resorting to a certain empiricism. We fully agree with him in this opinion; hence the reader must not expect to find the use of each of the following remedies accounted for by an enumeration of the symptoms.

For the first stage of an uncomplicated gonorrhœa there is no better simile and no more efficient remedy than *Mercurius solubilis*. This drug has the whole group of symptoms; tickling in the urethra when touching it at urinating, the tickling is of a voluptuous sort, attended with violently excited sexual desire; greenish-yellow purulent secretion from the urethra, with traces of blood; inflammation of the prepuce and glans with balanorrhœa; breaking out of little sores; urging to urinate, with frequent and painful emissions, etc. The choice of Mercurius is therefore in strict accord with homœopathic principles, but does not depend, as Hartmann fancies, upon the resemblance of the gonorrhœal to the chancre-virus, for it does not exist. If Hartmann states that he has cured but few cases of gonorrhœa with Mercurius, we do not find this strange; Mercurius is not sufficient to a cure, and even if it were, it would not cure the disease at once, for it cannot be cut short by internal treatment. Let it suffice to state that most homœopathic physicians prefer Mercurius as long as the inflammatory symptoms continue. Some of the above-mentioned complications likewise require Mercurius. We allude more particularly to inflammatory infiltrations of the prostate and to the parts adjoining the urethra. It is surprising that such infiltrations scarcely ever occur if the gonorrhœa is treated with Mercurius from the beginning. If chordée sets in, Mercurius is indicated by the cause producing the chordée. Gonorrhœal buboes likewise require Mercurius. The doses should not be too small; we have always had more success with the second trituration than with the higher attenuations; one or two grains every morning or even every other morning are quite sufficient; it may not be advisable to continue the use of this drug longer than ten days or a fortnight.

Urethritis.

Hepar sulphuris is the best remedy to give after Mercurius. The symptoms referring to the disease are not very characteristic, but the success obtained in very many cases, is remarkably striking. This medicine is given as soon as the discharge assumes a whitish color and the pains abate quite considerably. This usually takes place about the ninth or tenth day. Under the persevering use of this remedy, the discharge will either cease entirely in the fourth week, or else become so trifling, that the pain will almost cease; nor will a secondary discharge remain, except in a very few cases. Mercurius and Hepar sulphuris are tolerably sure remedies for an uncomplicated gonorrhœa of moderate intensity. The various deviations from the average course of the disease will require a few additional remedies.

For the excessive sexual excitement during the inflammatory period of gonorrhœa, with almost unceasing painful erections, especially at night, violent urging to urinate, with inability to void more than a few drops, discharge of blood, or if there is no discharge as in dry gonorrhœa, *Cantharides* will be found excellent. This remedy should not be given too strong; even the third trituration may still cause an homœopathic aggravation.

If the gonorrhœa sets in without any marked inflammatory symptoms; if the discharge is copious, rather white than yellow, and causing a superficial inflammation of the glans and prepuce, *Cannabis* is preferable to Mercurius at the outset. Marked sexual excitement argues against, rather than in favor of the remedy. In the subsequent course of the disease where Hepar has been advised, Cannabis sometimes has a very good curative effect. This medicine should be given in the lowest attenuations.

The true torpid gonorrhœa which is more particularly met with in individuals that have been infected several times, requires for its cure *Thuya*, *Acidum nitr.*, *Sulphur* and likewise *Hepar sulphuris*, and in general, the remedies recommended for secondary gonorrhœa.

As we said before, gonorrhœal buboes are best treated with Mercurius; but after they have passed into a chronic-inflammatory condition, *Clematis erecta* or *Kali iodatum* should be employed.

Chordée does not require any special treatment: it is best acted upon by Mercurius. If the erections are frequent and continuous, Cantharides may relieve them. An admixture of blood in the discharge is not an alarming symptom, and is met by most of the previously-named remedies.

If the bladder becomes involved in the inflammation, the medicines indicated for cystitis, will have to be used.

Secondary gonorrhœa constitutes, so to speak, a separate affection; it is one of the most obstinate plagues both to the physician and patient, and its removal is so much more difficult as it presents a great uniformity of symptoms which greatly interferes with the selection of the suitable homœopathic agent. The published cases shed very little light regarding the preference that should be given to one or the other remedy; it is, indeed, very difficult to distinguish between a cure effected by the action of Nature and that of the remedy.

According to the experience of most physicians *Thuya occidentalis* is the best remedy. It should not be given as long as inflammatory symptoms are present; nevertheless, it is recommended by many, and even by Hahnemann, at the outset of gonorrhœa. In the acute stage Hartmann only derived benefit from Thuya if condylomata were present; on the contrary, in secondary gonorrhœa, he found it very efficacious, which many other practitioners confirm by their own experience. Although the presence of condylomata is a good indication, yet Thuya likewise acts well if no condylomata are present.

Nitri acidum competes with Thuya, but will scarcely ever prove useful, except in the secondary form of gonorrhœa. As a rule it seems to act best in cases where Thuya had proved useless.

Petroleum has been recommended in former times, but is now very generally abandoned on account of its inefficiency in this disease. It has likewise been recommended in the acute form, more particularly if the neck of the bladder is very much involved. *Capsicum* may likewise prove useful under such circumstances.

Sulphur sometimes has a good effect if all the other remedies have proved fruitless; nevertheless it cannot be depended upon for certain. In strictures occasioned by chronic-inflammatory infiltrations it is an important remedy. *Clematis erecta* and *Nitri ac.* should, however, be tried first for this trouble. Strictures depending upon the presence of cicatrices in the urethra, are beyond the reach of internal treatment and have to be managed by surgical means, the bougie, etc.

The following remedies have likewise either been used or recommended. In acute gonorrhœa: *Balsam. copaivœ, Tussilago petasites, Petroselinum;* the last-named remedy deserves the most attention, although it is not used much by practitioners generally. In gleet: *Cubebæ, Agnus castus, Mezereum, Iodium, Phosphori acidum.*

[In several inveterate cases of gonorrhœa, where injections had been used for several months without the least benefit, a cure was effected by Kafka by means of the internal use of *Matico* 1, a Peruvian plant known in Peru as the Yerba del soldado, (the soldier's weed or herb.) H.]

It cannot be denied that Homœopathy cannot boast of any very brilliant results in the treatment of gonorrhœa. It is only exceptionally that a real gonorrhœa yields in a few days to internal homœopathic treatment; it generally takes weeks to cure the disease, and even then the gradual transformation of the disease into a gleetish discharge cannot be avoided. Have we not yet discovered the right remedies? Or do we not make a proper use of the remedies we have? In this condition of things it certainly behooves us to ascertain how gonorrhœa is treated by physicians of other Schools. The most common method now in vogue is a vigorous cauterization of the urethra with Nitrate of silver, zinc, etc. Not even the most inveterate doubter can deny that a gonorrhœa is sometimes cut short by such a proceeding; on the other hand, it is certain that a cure does not always take place in this way, that this treatment is attended with severe pain, and that it is not without danger as regards the supervention of strictures. This last circumstance is of course flatly denied by the partisans of this checking or aborting method. Astringent injections after the inflammatory stage is passed, frequently lead to good results, nor are their secondary effects attended with the danger involved in the former method; nevertheless they are not absolutely reliable, and it often happens that the gonorrhœa breaks out again after a suppression of several days. Large quantities of Copaiva and Cubebs sometimes suppress the discharge for a few days, but it frequently returns again with a renewed fierceness and changes to a most obstinate gleet. In addition to these disappointments the gastro-intestinal canal is sometimes very much weakened by these drugs. Moreover it is our conviction that these two drugs are the most frequent cause of gonorrhœal orchitis and of the peculiar gonorrhœal rheumatism, neither of which conditions has ever occurred to us under a strict homœopathic treatment.

Upon the whole, we are willing to admit that these severe methods of treatment are now and then crowned with brilliant success; but on the other hand we believe that they do not counterbalance the dangers incident to this treatment; we believe that a gonorrhœa treated in this manner, without being cured, becomes exceedingly inveterate. Hence we prefer, under all circumstances, the slower but safer homœopathic treatment, were it for no better reason than that it never does any positive harm. It might be worth while to ascertain how often a strict homœopathic treatment of gonorrhœa has resulted in orchitis, strictures, cystitis, etc. Such cases will be few indeed. Another advantage of the homœopathic treatment of gonorrhœa, which is readily perceived and appreciated by the patients, is the circumstance that they need not impose upon themselves distressing inconveniences. It is well, however, that the attention of the patient should be directed at the very commencement of the treatment to the difference between the allopathic and the homœopathic methods.

The patient's mode of living constitutes an important part in the treatment of gonorrhœa. The views of physicians differ greatly in this respect. Some doctors torment their patients half to death by their pedantic dogmatism in regulating the diet and general mode of living. Abundant experience has satisfied us that so much pedantic care is uncalled-for. The patient may take exercise, but should avoid all severe exertions and remain as much as possible in a recumbent posture. Every patient should wear from the start a good suspensory which we do not, however, regard as a preventive against orchitis. The usual diet may be pursued with the following exceptions: The patient must abstain from fat food, eat meat moderately, avoid spices, spirits, wine and beer, and likewise coffee during the first period of the treatment; during the subsequent treatment coffee may be drank without hesitation. In order to avoid the nocturnal erections, the supper should be very light and eaten in good season; after supper all beverages should be abstained from. Balanitis and phimosis are best prevented by frequently washing the penis with tepid water; if the glans is covered by the prepuce, the water should be injected under the prepuce. Physicians should never omit to direct their patients' attention to the danger of gonorrhœal virus getting into their eyes. By systematically drinking cold water, the urine becomes much less concentrated. My patients drink a glassful every hour. The night-urine is especially irritating; on this account the patients should drink two or three glasses of water on rising in the morning, and should then wait forty or fifty minutes before urinating; during this period the larger portion of the water will have passed into the bladder. By pursuing this course we have always got along tolerably well, and our patients enjoy the advantage of being able to attend to their usual avocations. That even severe exercise may not always have an injurious effect upon gonorrhœa, has become evident to us by the example of dozens of soldiers who, in order not to be sent to the hospital by their regimental physician, were treated by us secretly and who attended to their military duties all the time, even those who served in the artillery. We have never seen any injurious consequences result from this management. As a matter of course, the presence of important complications during the course of gonorrhœa will require corresponding modifications in all these arrangements. In recent cases of secondary gonorrhœa, the use of cold water, as above recommended, should likewise be resorted to; in cases of long standing it has no effect. The injections which Hahnemann likewise concedes as proper, have sometimes, but not always, a favorable effect. Excellent injections are prepared of *claret* diluted with water, to which small quantities of *Tannin* may be added. We have never obtained equally favorable results with weak solutions of Nitrate of Silver, Muriate of Gold, Sublimate, Thuya; nor have we done any better with lime-water, or solutions of Zinc, Copper, or Lead.

2. Orchitis.
Inflammation of the Testes.

Now and then this affection is met with as the result of mechanical injuries, but most frequently originates in gonorrhœa. It not only supervenes during the course of acute urethritis, but it may likewise set in suddenly during gleet, generally without any apparent exciting cause. Severe exertion or the discontinuance of the use of suspensories are said to sometimes cause the disease, but this is not an established fact. The excessive use of beer or wine is a much more active cause of the disease, probably because the inflammation is very much increased by such stimulants. Both Cubebs and Copaiva hold the same relation to gonorrhœa. They have a specific effect upon the urethra, and it is easily conceivable that, instead of effecting a cure when given in large quantities, they aggravate the inflammatory symptoms and, owing to the specific action which they likewise exert upon the testicles, communicate the inflammation to these organs. This point has not yet been substantiated by provings on the healthy. At any rate it is strange that the exhibition of these two drugs should be so frequently and speedily followed by orchitis which is scarcely ever observed under strictly homœopathic treatment unless the patient should commit some gross indiscretion. It might be well to inquire into this circumstance; the result might suggest additional reasons for preferring the homœopathic treatment of gonorrhœa. That orchitis takes place in consequence of the spread of the urethral inflammation through the seminal vesicles to the vas deferens and the epididymis, is distinctly shown by the painfulness of the former organs. A gonorrhœal metastasis is out of the question, because the gonorrhœal discharge either continues side by side with the orchitis, or only disappears after the orchitis is fully developed, not before, in the same manner as a nasal catarrh disappears during the supervention of a more serious disease of the respiratory organs.

Symptoms. Orchitis seldom sets in suddenly. Ordinarily it commences with slight drawing pains in the spermatic cord which is sensitive to contact. At the same time the patient experiences violent tearing pains in the thigh of the affected side. The weight of the testicles at first is troublesome, then becomes painful and finally intolerable. In one or two days the epididymis becomes painful to pressure, swells with more or less rapidity, and shortly after is succeeded by an inflammatory effusion into the tunica propria, in consequence of which the testicle very soon enlarges to the size of a fist. The pains now become agonizing; the patient has to confine himself to a horizontal posture with the testicle properly supported. The pain is a burning-tearing pain, most frequently with remissions after the fashion of rheumatic pains. The general condition of the patient does not suffer much, only in violent cases there is fever or even vomiting. The discharge usually disappears after the orchitis is fully developed, and does not re-appear until the inflammation has run its course; only in a few cases it does not re-appear after the subsidence of orchitis.

The inflammation in its acute form does not often last beyond the tenth day, sometimes the improvement commences on the fourth day. This, however, is not very rapid, since it sometimes takes weeks before the testicle resumes its former size; very frequently an obstinate swelling of the testicles remains.

Treatment. Most physicians prescribe in the first place *Mercurius sol.* or *vivus*, especially if the orchitis had its origin in a recent attack of gonorrhœa. We give the first trituration and continue it until the inflammation begins to abate. For orchitis arising from chronic urethritis, *Clematis erecta* is preferable. This medicine does good service after Mercurius, even better than Pulsatilla which, however, has more decided symptoms referring to such a case. It is very difficult, in a case of this kind, to select a remedy in accordance with the symptoms, for the reason that the symptoms of the different drugs are so very much alike. Beside the above-mentioned drugs, we likewise recommend *Acidum nitr.*, especially if the patient is tainted with syphilis and has taken a good deal of Mercury. The subsequent enlargement of the testicle, if of recent origin, requires in the first place *Clematis*, likewise *Iodium;* Hartmann also proposes *Staphysagria*, and, if the enlargement had lasted sometime, *Aurum met.* and *Sulphur*. *Colocynthis* has helped us out very promptly in two cases of violent rheumatic pains in the thighs which emanated from the testicle and had remained behind after an orchitis.

If the orchitis does not originate in gonorrhœa, a few other medicines deserve attention. If caused by a contusion of the testicles, *Arnica* has to be given, afterwards *Conium* or *Pulsatilla*, to which Hartmann adds *Calendula officinalis*. If it is caused by a cold or a metastasis of parotitis, *Rhus tox.*, *Belladonna*, *Bryonia* have to be given together with the above-named drugs. [We have subdued the most intense phlegmonous inflammation of the testes consequent upon sudden suppression of gonorrhœa by means of the 18th attenuation of *Aconite;* the first tablespoonful of a solution of a few globules in half a tumbler of water, produced an almost instantaneous relief from the most agonizing distress. In rheumatic orchitis the lower attenuations of Aconite act more specifically, or in other words are more specifically adapted to the pathological process.

In a case of terrible orchitis caused by suppression of the gonorrhœal discharge, with swelling and inflammation of the spermatic cord of the affected side, high fever, flushed cheeks, glistening eyes, intolerable restlessness, *Belladonna* given internally and applied externally, in the proportion of fifteen to twenty drops of the fluid extract to half a cupful of water, controlled the inflammation and swelling, after other remedies had been tried in vain. H.]

These remedies are likewise to be used in chronic primary swellings of the testes. Some of these swellings are, indeed, past all cure, especially those having a tubercular origin; in some cases, however, even of long standing, the result of our treatment is, indeed very striking.

External applications generally are of very little use in orchitis. Neither warm nor cold fomentations are easily born, nor have they any good effect, not even palliative. Of course the testicle should be supported so that the spermatic cord is not pulled upon. A suspensory should be worn even some time after the disease is cured. Strapping the testicle with strips of adhesive plaster so as to exert a slight compression, frequently exerts a strikingly beneficial influence. Those who have recovered from the disease, will have to behave with great discretion in order to avoid relapses which are apt to take place.

3. Spermatorrhœa.

By this heading we, strictly speaking, comprehend a flow of semen without any sexual excitement. However, in order to avoid the necessity of resorting to a number of sub-divisions, we have classed together in this chapter abnormal nocturnal emissions as well as various other morbid derangements of the male sexual organs; an additional motive for this arrangement is the circumstance that the treatment of most of these conditions is the same.

The functions of the male sexual organs vary in accordance with temperament, mode of life, constitution, etc., to such an extent that it is often difficult to decide whether these differences are of a morbid nature or belong to the normal standard. This can only be determined by the manner in which the male sexual sphere is generally affected by the local phenomena; whether the organs are not abnormally disturbed, or whether the procreative powers are impaired or even suspended.

The etiology of these various abnormal conditions of the sexual sphere is pretty much the same. Debilitating constitutional diseases, or acute diseases during the period of convalescence are apt to cause a so-called irritable weakness in the sexual sphere, which, in the former case is permanent and in the latter case only temporary. This fact is most strikingly witnessed in diabetes and tuberculosis. In the last-named condition the excessive irritability of the sexual organs contributes to hasten the general decay. A second cause are cardiac and nervous diseases, which may, however, likewise result from the sexual weakness. Hypochondria is a frequent cause, and still a more frequent consequence of sexual weakness. The most common cause of sexual weakness is the vice of onanism, which is too much overlooked by physicians. Yet it is certain that thousands might, by a timely warning, be saved from unspeakable mental and physical disease.

Excessive nocturnal emissions generally take place between the years of 20 and 25, and exceptionally at an ealier age, even 16.

They are of a morbid nature if they occur almost regularly without rousing one from sleep, and if they do not occur often, yet leave for days a sensation of languor and debility, and of mental depression. They are likewise abnormal if they occur several times in one night or week. Moreover every emission that takes place in the waking state, with or without any special cause, at stool for instance, is to be regarded as abnormal. The consequences of such abnormal losses very soon show themselves: Paleness of the face with dark margins around the eyes; insufficient sleep; drowsiness with inability to sleep; dulness of the head; aching, pressing pain in the head; vertigo; irritable, sensitive temper; aversion to society, to work, and, after a while, a deranged appetite and digestion, deficient assimilation.

Spermatorrhœa, properly speaking, consists in a loss of semen at every emission of urine, at stool, without any cause or after the most trifling erections. The pernicious consequences of this sort of spermatorrhœa manifest themselves much more speedily than after nocturnal emissions, most probably because spermatorrhœa never occurs in organisms whose physiological functions had been carried on in a normal manner.

Irritable weakness of the sexual organs is sometimes the cause, but more frequently the consequence of both the previously-mentioned anomalies. The sexual excitement occurs too easily and too vehemently, without possessing sufficient energy and consistence for the act of coition. The ejaculation of the semen takes place too soon, or even not at all, or the introduction of the penis into the vagina is prevented, by a premature cessation of the erection. The sexual weakness may be characterized by all sorts of abnormal manifestations in the sexual sphere. The mental disposition exerts a powerful influence in this direction. Hypochondriacs are particularly disposed to irritable weakness which, under abnormal mental influences, sometimes attains to such a degree of intensity that it seems to amount to complete impotence.

Complete impotence, by which is meant an entire suspension of the ability to perform the sexual act, is upon the whole a very rare and frequently only temporary disorder, except when depending upon debilitating incurable constitutional diseases, such as diabetes or tuberculosis, or when depending upon the loss of one testicle.

An excess of sexual excitement (satyriasis) besides taking place at the commencement of gonorrhœa, as we have already stated, may likewise occur in consequence of debilitating conditions, first as a passing increase and subsequently to be succeeded by a decrease of excitability. It is frequently met with in the case of persons who have been addicted to the vice of onanism, or among worn-out roués; very rarely without such a cause, and then mostly as a symptom of some deep-seated disease of the brain.

In treating most of these forms of sexual weakness, the diet, mode of life and psychical agencies exert an important influence; hence we place them in the front rank.

We cannot lay it down as a rule that these morbid conditions require either a lean or a strengthening diet. Some are afflicted with weakness of the sexual organs, more especially with excessive pollutions, because they live too well; it is a mistake to suppose that this waste is repaired by a nourishing diet, since it is well known that some persons are living in circumstances which preclude the possibility of indulging in good living. Hence it becomes a matter of interest to inquire whether a lean or a rich diet is the more suitable. All such patients must be cautioned against going to sleep with a full bladder or a full stomach, either in the daytime or at night. Certain beverages, such as spirits and hop-beer, must be strictly avoided. Beer-drinkers are very apt to deny the debilitating influence of hop-beer on the genital organs; that this influence exists, must be evident to all who are acquainted with the effects of Lupulin. It is well known that drunkenness, either partial or total, causes an irritable weakness of the sexual organs. Coffee, and in some even tobacco, have to be interdicted; among the secondary effects of coffee we notice a depressing excitability and irritability of the nervous system. In general all strongly-spiced and stimulating food is hurtful. As regards bodily exercise, it is certain that bodily fatigue diminishes sexual excitement and brings it back again to a normal standard; muscular exercise has also the advantage of preventing the mind from dwelling upon erotic subjects. Viewed from this point, walking is not the best kind of exercise, for the reason that it leaves the mind free to revel in all kinds of fancies; onanists are very apt to be fond of walking. Severe mental labor is sometimes preferable to bodily exercise, especially in the case of hypochondriacs and onanists. This leads us to a consideration of psychical influences as a means of cure. Every physician knows that the evil consequences of nocturnal emissions, and even to some extent, of self-abuse, are more imaginary than real. Numbers are made hypochondriacs by reading books that fill them with fear and trembling at the excesses they may have been guilty of in former days. Encouraging advice does them more good than medicine. Self-abuse is prevented much more certainly by comforting encouragement than by picturing the consequences of such a crime in the most frightful colors. In dealing with sexual weakness, it is in the first place necessary to depress the fancy, and in the second place to strengthen the will. On this account, reading novels is so hurtful, and cold-water treatment has such an excellent effect.

We deem a special enumeration of the medicines, referring to this subject, inappropriate; the multiplicity of the phenomena would leave too many gaps. The symptoms being all confined to one set of organs, they can easily be compared with the symptoms in the Materia Medica. It is only because the chapter entitled "Male genital organs" is so replete with symptoms and remedies that we furnish in the next paragraph a list of the remedies whose practical value has been verified by experience, and we classify them in accordance with the different divisions adopted for the symptoms of the disease.

For excessive emissions, with increased irritability: *Cantharides, Nux vomica, Camphora, Phosphorus;* with diminished irritability; *Conium maculatum, Phosphori acidum, Clematis erecta, Digitalis purpurea, China.*

For spermatorrhœa: *Phosphori acidum, Calcarea carbonica, Conium, Cantharides.* Among all these remedies Digitalis, and more particularly *Digitalin*, has the best effect. A few doses of the third trituration of this medicine are generally sufficient to effect a complete cure or at least a marked improvement. The medicine should be given in the morning; in the evening it is very apt to disturb the night's sleep. [*Gelsemin*, given for a period of time, has cured spermatorrhœa. *Stillingin* is likewise an excellent remedy for both nocturnal emissions and spermatorrhœa. H. 7.]

Irritable weakness requires besides the remedies mentioned for spermatorrhœa and nocturnal emissions, the following medicines: *Caladium seguinum, Selenium, Nitri acidum, Agaricus muscarius,* and, if the weakness borders on impotence, *Agnus castus, Cannabis, Baryta, Capsicum annuum, Lycopodium, Natrum muriaticum.*

Satyriasis requires particularly *Cantharides* and *Phosphorus*, the latter more particularly, if the affection is caused by disturbances of the central nervous system.

The consequences of self-abuse are so varied that we cannot in this place indicate all the remedies that may have to be employed against them. Moreover we have made it a point to allude to this vice in treating of the various functional derangements of the different organs. As far as the sexual organs and their functions are involved, we may have to resort to *Phosphori acidum, Nux vomica, China, Calcarea carbonica.*

Among the external agents that may prove useful in the treatment of these affections, cold water occupies the first rank. In some forms of irritable weakness cold ablutions of the sexual organs or sitz-baths are sufficient; but where the whole nervous system is involved, a rigorous and systematic water-cure treatment is preferable; it not only helps to invigorate the constitution, but likewise to give exercise and tone to the mental energy, which is impaired by nothing more than by abuse of the sexual organs.

B. DISEASES OF THE FEMALE SEXUAL ORGANS.

1. Vaginitis, Catarrh of the Sexual Mucous Lining.
Fluor Albus, Leucorrhœa, Whites.

CATARRH of the female sexual organs may be distinguished as simple and virulent catarrh.

The virulent catarrh or gonorrhœa of the female is caused, like gonorrhœa of the male, by contact with gonorrhœal matter, and never develops itself from an intensified simple catarrh. Simple catarrh is one of the most common derangements of the female sex. It originates in a variety of causes. In the first place we have to mention as exciting causes such as act directly upon the sexual organs: excessive coition, self-abuse, miscarriage, and to some extent confinements which, if occurring in too rapid succession, almost always cause leucorrhœa. Ascarides likewise cause catarrhal discharges from the vagina, by crawling from the anus into the last-named organ; pessaries should likewise be mentioned. The main causes, however, are not local, but have a constitutional origin: menstrual disturbances, a sedentary mode of life, abuse of coffee, chlorosis, scrofulosis, tuberculosis, and the various defects inherent in our modern systems of education, which have already been alluded to in the chapter on hysteria. A vaginal catarrh is scarcely ever owing to a mere cold, except perhaps at the time of the menses, at which period the tendency to this derangement is most marked. With reference to age, the trouble occurs most frequently between the first commencement and the cessation of the menstrual period; it is likewise met with among children, and very often among women who have ceased to menstruate, the less frequently, however, the longer the menses had ceased to make their appearance. Tumors in the uterine cavity are accompanied by a tolerably profuse catarrh as a symptomatic appearance.

We transcribe from Kafka the following concise description of acute vaginal catarrh. The mucous lining of the vagina is attacked by an acute catarrhal inflammation, in which sometimes the labia majora and minora and the entrance to the vagina, and at other times the whole length of the vagina, are involved. In bad cases the inflammation may communicate itself to the cervix uteri, to the internal cavity of the uterus or to the urethra.

The mucous membrane is dark-red, swollen and interstitially distended; the papillæ are swollen and form numerous prominences imparting to the mucous lining a granular appearance. The granulations are at times scattered, at other times confluent, at times occupying isolated portions of the vagina, at other times the vagina in its whole extent. The hyperæmia induces a sub-mucous œdema which narrows the vaginal space. The secretion of mucus is very scanty at first, or even entirely suppressed; afterwards it becomes more copious, of a yellow or yellowish-green color and opaque. Not unfrequently we find in the course of the inflammation superficial numerous erosions on the external and internal labia and at the entrance of the vagina.

A benign acute catarrh of the vagina is most generally occasioned by local injuries affecting directly the mucous lining of the vagina, such as: excessive sexual intercourse, self-abuse, sudden exposure to the action of cold, foreign bodies in the vagina, such as badly-fitting pessaries, or corrosive injections, or else the inflammatory process in the vagina may simply be a continuation of a similar process in the uterus.

The symptoms of acute vaginal catarrh are an itching in the vagina with which a burning sensation afterwards becomes associated. Walking, the introduction of the finger, of a speculum, and sexual intercourse, are exceedingly painful. If the urethra is involved in the inflammation, the patients experience a violent desire to urinate; in such a case urination causes a burning distress in the urethra. The yellow secretion stains the linen yellow; if acrid, it inflames and excoriates the parts adjoining the vulva, and often spreads a pungent and offensive odor.

An examination with the speculum would show whether the secretion proceeds from the uterine cavity or the vagina; but the introduction of the speculum is not only very painful, but often causes hemorrhage.

An acute vaginal catarrh lasts from eight days to a fortnight, or else passes into the chronic form. The prognosis is generally favorable.

We recently treated an acute vaginal catarrh in a girl of nine years. It was caused by sitting on a cold stone. The vagina and vulva were much inflamed, and the purulent and yellow-greenish discharge exceedingly profuse. The disease was radically cured in about a week with the German tincture of Aconite and a few doses of Iodine. H.]

A simple acute catarrh is, upon the whole, a very rare disorder. Inasmuch as, with the exception of slight differences, it is identical, as far as intensity is concerned, with the virulent form of catarrh, we confine our description of the disease to the latter.

Female gonorrhœa commences with a feeling of heat and dryness in the vagina, attended with a peculiar titillation and sensitiveness to contact. Soon after, the mucous membrane is seen injected, urination becomes painful (which is never the case in simple catarrh), the external pudendum becomes swollen and inflamed, in consequence of which walking is impeded, and a muco-purulent discharge makes its appearance the same as in gonorrhœa of the male, only more copious and generally of a bad odor. Some individuals, according as the disease is more or less intense, experience febrile motions, lassitude, depression of strength, drawing pains in the lumbar and sacral regions, dull pains in the pelvis, sensitiveness to contact, difficulty of urinating. Upon the mucous membrane, as well as in the neighborhood of the vagina, we often notice erosions and small flat ulcers. This inflammatory stage lasts, as in the case of the male, from eight days to a fortnight. As the pains abate, the discharge becomes thinner, more milky, and, in favorable cases, abates little by little until it ceases entirely in a few weeks. More commonly, however, the discharge continues for months, and in case the uterus is considerably involved, the gonorrhœa becomes chronic and exceedingly obstinate. The infectiousness of the discharge does not become extinct until it has lasted a long time.

Chronic catarrh very generally arises from the acute form, but in most cases takes place without any preliminary acute stage. A scanty slimy secretion from the vagina occurs in most females, either as a constant discharge, or before or after menstruation, and even a profuse discharge after several confinements still constitutes a normal secretion; at any rate the women themselves do not look upon it as anything unnatural. It is only when the discharge is excessive, or when it occurs in children, that we are justified in regarding it as a morbid phenomenon. Under the operation of one of the above-named exciting causes the discharge continues to increase in quantity and to gradually disturb the constitutional equilibrium. The discharge is at times of a glassy transparency, at times milky, and less frequently purulent; it may become so profuse that the patients may not be able to leave their room; the stains on the linen are generally stiff and grayish, less frequently yellowish; it often excoriates the external parts and the thighs; this is not owing to the quantity of the secretion, but to its quality and perhaps to the sensitiveness of the skin. The discharge is scarcely ever uniformly the same; sometimes it has remissions and even intermissions, is generally most copious before or after the menses, and frequently even takes their place entirely. If the uterine secretion is very tenacious, mucous plugs are easily deposited in the cervical canal, and an increased accumulation of mucus takes place in the uterus which causes labor-like pains that cease all at once as soon as the mucus has been expelled. The anatomical changes accompanying this condition of things, consist in an interstitial puffing and swelling of the mucous lining which may result even in polypous formations; the follicles, known as the ovula Nabothi, are likewise altered, their orifices becoming closed by the continued secretion; they are particularly seen at the cervix in the shape of small, prominent, transparent vesicles. The ulcers are either flat, catarrhal erosions, or else the suppurating follicles are transformed into more deep-seated rounded ulcers. The erosions not unfrequently give rise to the granular ulcers of the cervix, the ulcerated surface becoming uneven and very much disposed to bleed. More recently a degree of importance has been attached to this ulcerative process of which it is not possessed in reality. In every chronic catarrh, simular ulcerations take place without the catarrh being on that account derived from the ulcers, or the constitutional symptoms from the ulcerative process generally. Why should this be done in a case of uterine catarrh? It cannot be denied that the last-named ulcers give rise to pain, especially during coition, and that they may even cause slight hemorrhages; but it is questionable whether such accidents impair the general health as much as is supposed. It is much more natural to regard the general irritability and the nervous phenomena as simple consequences of the catarrhal disease, and to derive the ulcers from the irritation produced by the act of coition in individuals with a peculiar predisposition for such derangements. On hearing of so many physicians who make female diseases a speciality and trot around with their specula, promising the afflicted a speedy cure, we cannot forbear suspecting such vagabonds of impure designs. These ulcers of the cervix fare no better than many other modern discoveries in medicine; at first everything is explained by means of them, until repeated disappointments satisfy us, that the discovery was no great thing after all.

The consequences of catarrh to the general organism vary both in extent and in intensity. Many women who have been afflicted for years with profuse leucorrhœa preserve an appearance of perfect health; others, on the contrary, are very much affected even by an inconsiderable discharge. One of the most common consequences, and, on the other hand, one of the most common causes, are menstrual irregularities, generally scanty menses. Moreover, an unusual nervous irritability, backache, aching pains in the small of the back, hemicrania, hysteric spasms set in. The patient looks sick, with a grayish, dingy complexion and dark margins around the eyes. If the discharge is very profuse, symptoms of anæmia make their appearance. The faculty of conception is not very much influenced by uterine catarrh, otherwise women afflicted with it, would not conceive so readily. If the mucous lining is considerably puffed up, and the uterine canal closed by plugs of mucus, it is a matter of course that conception must be very much interfered with. The worst thing that can happen to the patient is the shock to the nervous system caused by a co-existing titillation of the genital organs and a violent excitement of the sexual instinct.

Treatment. Whether an acute vaginal catarrh is virulent or not, can be inferred from the symptoms with tolerable certainty. The non-virulent catarrh scarely ever affects the parts with much intensity, but usually makes an inroad upon the constitutional well-being, and leaves the urethra unirritated; at least no pus can be squeezed out of its orifice.

As in the male, so in the female gonorrhœa, *Mercurius solubilis* or *vivus* is the first and most important remedy. The employment of aconite in this disease, as recommended by Hartmann, simply involves a loss of time. Mercurius has all the symptoms of the inflammatory stage: Itching, smarting and burning in the sexual organs; increased sexual desire; inflammatory swelling of the vagina and external pudendum, with sensitiveness to contact; whitish, thick, purulent and greenish discharge, of an offensive odor, causing erosions and ulcerations in the surrounding parts, with painful emission of urine; tenesmus of the bladder and rectum. These phenomena constitute a complete image of the gonorrhœa of females, for which Mercurius will be found as efficient a remedy as it is for gonorrhœa of the male.

The symptoms which remain after the inflammation is removed, may require a variety of remedies. It is advisable to first find a suitable remedy among those that have been recommended for gonorrhœa of the male. *Hepar sulphuris* may be required, or else *Nitri acidum* or *Thuya*. *Nitri acidum* is particularly suitable if the discharge looks bad, is mixed with blood and has a bad odor; *Thuya* is more suitable if condylomata are present. For marked urinary difficulties *Cannabis* and *Cantharides* may be resorted to.

If we are sure that an acute attack of vaginal catarrh is of the non-virulent kind, *Aconite*, whatever Hartmann may say in favor of this drug, is scarcely ever required, at any rate much less frequently than *Belladonna*. As a rule Belladonna is preferable to Aconite in all diseases of the mucous membrane; in this instance it is likewise more specifically indicated by the symptoms.

Regarding *Arnica*, Hartmann has the following: "A condition characterized by an increased sensation of warmth, fulness and tension in the internal pudendum, constant titillation, sometimes even a burning sensation at urinating, slight fever, is sometimes met with in the case of newly married people. It would be wrong to attribute these symptoms to infection; they are caused by too great a narrowness of the vagina and by the contusion caused by intercourse, as is likewise made evident by the swelling and redness of the external labia, attended with an intense burning pain at urinating, and even retention of urine, owing to the inflammation and swelling of the urethra and of the internal organs. *Arnica* meets this condition. [*Belladonna* and even *Aconite* are often required to control the swelling and inflammation of the labia. H.]

If the patient complains of a burning in the vagina and labia, with discharge of a thin but acrid mucus from the genital organs, constant chilliness, disposition to lie down, sadness, depression of spirits, etc., *Pulsatilla* answers this condition better than any other remedy.

Other remedies which are likewise adapted to the acute form of catarrh, will be indicated in the subsequent paragraph; altogether the transition from the acute to the chronic form of leucorrhœa is scarcely noticeable.

Chronic leucorrhœa is one of the most inveterate derangements, and is much more difficult to cure than an obstinate gleet, although the use of local remedies is much more practicable in the former than in the latter. We merely mention the names of the remedies, since it is impracticable to enumerate the symptoms of each which, in order to effect a cure, will have to be compared with the utmost care with the pathological phenomena; the large number of drugs bearing upon this affection, renders the use of a good Repertory indispensable. The most important and most frequently required remedies are: *Calcarea carbonica, Ferrum, Graphites, Lycopodium, Natrum muriaticum, China, Sepia, Kali carbonicum, Mezereum, Phosphorus, Platina, Sabina, Iodium, Conium, Alumina*. We will endeavor to classify these drugs in accordance with some of the most important indications, referring the reader for more minute symptomatic particulars to the Materia Medica.

The most important item to be considered is the appearance of leucorrhœa at the beginning or during the course of the menses; this point alone may furnish us a clue to the whole character of the discharge. For leucorrhœa previous to the menses the following remedies are suitable: *Calcarea carbonica, Sepia, Phosphorus, Graphites, Alumina, Natrum muriaticum;* for leucorrhœa setting in in the place of the menses: *Pulsatilla, Sabina, Zincum, China, Natrum muriaticum;* and subsequently to the menses: *Bovista, Iodium, Ruta, Calc. carb., Sepia, Graphites, Lycopodium.*

In the case of chlorotic individuals, if fluor albus is the consequence, not the cause of the anæmia, we resort to: *Ferrum, Puls., Calc. carb.*, and *Arsenicum;* if the anæmia is caused by the loss of fluids involved in the leucorrhœal discharge, *China, Ferrum, Lycopodium, Natrum muriaticum, Stannum* are required.

The nervous phenomena attendant on the discharge, are most generally found under *Ignatia* and *Platina;* and if self-abuse is one of the causes, *Zincum, Nux vomica* and *Ignatia* may be exhibited. In the case of patients of a somewhat advanced age, the following remedies may be preferable: *Kali carb., Natrum mur., Mezereum, Lycopodium, Sepia.*

In dietetic respects all that is needful to do is to avoid everything that has a tendency to excite or keep up the discharge; this is easily neglected if the patient's whole mode of living is chargeable with the disorder. In such a case marvellous cures are related from a visit to these or those springs, whereas a little common sense might teach that the same results can be obtained with much less trouble and expense by pursuing a regular course of proper diet and general hygiene at home. It is not our object to single out and recommend in this place certain springs that are really of use in this affection; all we have to say is, that salt-water bathing is sometimes a sovereign remedy for the most obstinate uterine catarrh, agreeable to the indications furnished by the physiological experiments instituted with common salt.

Injections of water by means of a good vaginal syringe keep the parts clean and free from soreness and ulcerations; otherwise they have no curative effect. But we should not pedantically insist upon cold water being used under all circumstances and by everybody; tepid water sometimes has a much more certain palliative effect.

2. Metritis.
Inflammation of the Womb.

This inflammation may involve the internal lining as well as the substance and the external serous coat of the uterus. If the mucous lining alone is invaded, we have the picture of an acute uterine catarrh which, however, almost always accompanies both the other forms, parenchymatous and peri-metritis.

The common causes of metritis are, like those of acute catarrh, deleterious influences acting directly upon the uterus, more especially excessive coition, obstetrical operations or foreign bodies in the cavity of the uterus; or the causes may be more general, such as a cold, or violent emotions; these influences affect the uterus so much more readily at a period when the organ is in a state of congestion, for instance at the time of the menses. If the menses suddenly cease at the commencement of inflammation, we have no right to conclude that this suppression is the cause instead of the consequence of the inflammation. Chronic metritis generally arises from the acute form, or is occasioned by causes similar to those in which a chronic catarrh of the sexual mucous membrane originates.

Symptoms and Course. The disease usually commences with a chill which is at once followed by pains in the diseased organ. If the parenchyma is alone affected, the pains are not very violent, aching, boring, throbbing, stitching or lancing, they are seated deep in the pelvis, are accompanied by a most painful pressing downwards resembling feeble labor-pains; they are increased by pressing upon the abdomen, by very active respiratory movements, urging at stool, and erect posture, and they radiate to the small of the back and thighs. If the serous covering is likewise involved the pains become more acute, the sensitiveness to contact is greater and extends over a larger surface. The volume of the uterus not being sufficiently increased, it cannot be felt through the abdominal integuments; on exploration the uterus is found to be more sensitive, and the cervical portion is softer, more swollen and shorter than in the normal condition. The constitutional symptoms are of different degrees of intensity. Fever is never entirely absent, but is not generally very violent; the pulse is generally small and rather hard. The stomach sympathizes most readily in this disease; loss of appetite, coated tongue, nausea, retching and vomiting are very common. The bowels are constipated, the passage of the fæces is attended with tenesmus, urination is impeded and sometimes quite impossible. If the disease breaks out during the menses, they cease immediately and in their place a discharge sets in as in acute catarrh of the uterus. If the menstrual period happens within the course of the disease, the menses either remain suspended, or else the flow of blood is more copious, sometimes even amounting to an actual hemorrhage. In the further course of the disease the discharge from the uterus is apt to become purulent, and if, which is a rare occurrence, abscesses form within the substance of the uterus, clear pus is discharged. The disease runs an acute course of about a fortnight, when, if no particular complications exist, convalescence takes place; which, however, is frequently incomplete, inasmuch as either leucorrhœa or swelling of the uterus is apt to remain behind.

Among the most important complications we number an inflammation of the peritonæum which is apt to occur and by which the course of the disease is very much protracted and the metritis itself is very much aggravated. In such a case the inflammation assumes the form of diffuse peritonitis, with a very dubious prognosis. In a case of this kind, the patient being a robust young woman, not pregnant and the attack having occurred between the menstrual periods, a copious discharge of thin pus from the vagina took place about the tenth day, so that it was scarcely possible to keep a sufficient supply of clean cloths under her. This was of course followed by extreme weakness owing to which her recovery was very much delayed. Previous to this discharge nothing of any sort had passed her.

Metritis of pregnant females can scarcely ever be recognized with perfect certainty unless the enveloping membrane of the uterus and the peritonæum generally become involved. It may be supposed to exist if febrile motions, vomiting or retching, meteorism, painfulness of the gravid uterus whether touched or not, set in. During the first months the inflammation extends over the whole organ; afterwards it becomes localized, and the painful sensitiveness is likewise more circumscribed and confined to a definite locality. It is only exceptionally, that the course of pregnancy is affected unfavorably by the inflammation, and if the latter is very intense. If metritis occurs during the period of parturition, labor becomes unusually painful; and, if abscesses should form, rupture of the uterus may easily take place. After confinement metritis generally takes the form of puerperal metritis, of which we shall treat in the next chapter.

Chronic metritis is upon the whole a somewhat obscure condition. It generally remains as a consequence of acute metritis, but may likewise develop itself spontaneously under the operation of the various causes that may give rise to chronic catarrh of the uterus. We discover a more or less considerable general or total swelling of the uterus; enlargement, interstitial distention, hardness and ulceration of the vaginal portion, obstinate leucorrhœa. The pains ordinarily are trifling, consisting of a sensation of pressure and heaviness in the pelvis. During and previous to menstruation the pains increase to such a degree of intensity that they seem like genuine uterine colic. In higher grades of the disease the menses become entirely suppressed, except that about the period for their appearance violent pains set in, as if the flow would really take place. The constitutional equilibrium is more or less disturbed, and so-called hysteric nervous affections almost always make their appearance. If the swelling is considerable, the passage of the fæces and urine is very much interfered with, likewise the circulation of the left or right lower extremity. The faculty to conceive is very much impaired by both the acute and chronic form of metritis, although the possibility of conception cannot altogether be denied.

Treatment. We transcribe a few passages from Hartmann's work: " Having had many opportunities of treating this kind of inflammation I recommend as a chief and frequently applicable remedy *Nux vomica,* which I found useful in the district where I happened to be located, for the additional reason that the women in my district were in the habit of indulging in the excessive use of coffee. Other homœopathic physicians have tested the efficacy of Nux in these inflammations. The selection of a drug, however, neither depends upon the seat of the inflammation, nor upon the fact whether the uterus is impregnated or not, or whether the inflammation occurs during pregnancy or confinement. If the medicine was otherwise homœopathic to the symptoms, I have cured inflammation of the fundus, cervix, anterior or posterior surface of the uterus, with a single dose of Nux. In some cases where the fever was accompanied by a severe chill, followed by intense heat, frequent and tense pulse and violent thirst, I found it necessary to begin the treatment with a few doses of *Aconite*. Nux vomica is indicated by the following characteristic symptoms: acute pressing pains above the pubic bones, increased by external pressure and an exploration of the internal parts; violent pains in the loins and small of the back; constipation or hard stools attended with burning-stinging pains; painful urination or retention of urine; stitching and bruising pain of the abdomen during motion or when coughing and sneezing; increased temperature and swelling of the os tincæ, with simultaneous painfulness of the vagina; exacerbations in the morning-hours." We doubt the correctness of these statements. The symptoms of Aconite do not point to metritis as an homœopathic remedy for this inflammation; not even the accompanying fever is sufficiently intense to justify the use of Aconite. Nor do we believe that metritis can be cured with a single dose of Nux; at any rate we should not expect, nor do we deem it possible to cut a metritis short.

"An equally indispensable remedy in these inflammations is *Belladonna*, more particularly, if the sensation of heaviness and dragging in the abdomen, which frequently increases to a painful bearing-down, becomes very troublesome and is attended with a stinging-burning pain above the pubic bones, pains in the small of the back as if it would break, stinging pains in the hip-joints which cannot bear either motion or contact, (under certain circumstances *China* may here be indicated after Aconite.) If the inflammation sets in after confinement, the lochial secretion is arrested, the placenta adheres, or is discharged in the shape of an ichorous, fetid liquid, with violent burning and a sensation of fulness in the vagina, the employment of Belladonna is called for so much more pressingly." We refrain from commenting upon the last passage, for we hold that if such phenomena occur while the placenta remains adhering to the uterus, we have a strictly puerperal disease before us, which does not belong in this chapter. Without doubt *Belladonna* is eminently suitable in cases of violent metritis, and is even preferable to Nux, more especially if the menses were arrested during the course of the inflammation. Nor have we a better remedy for metrorrhagia setting in at the time of the menses.

"A similar affection occasioned by a violent fit of chagrin, especially after confinement, yields most speedily and surely to a single dose of *Chamomilla*. In such a case the lochial secretion is generally more profuse, and, if it was already white, it again changes to a discharge of quantities of blackish, coagulated blood. Not unfrequently we see metritis set in after the inordinate use of Chamomile-tea, which unreasonable midwives will allow their patients in confinement in spite of all the warnings of physicians. In such cases *Nux, Ignatia, Pulsatilla,* each according to the symptoms of the disease, will be found to be the best antidotes. We here refer to what we have said above concerning the one dose of Nux; moreover we doubt the value of Chamomilla as a remedy in metritis.

Mercurius deserves the same encomiums in this disease as in uterine catarrh. It is indicated by violent febrile heat interrupted by chills; inclination to abundant perspiration; violent thirst; purulent discharge from the vagina; diarrhœic discharge with tenesmus. These are symptoms denoting the formation of pus. Knowing as we do that this is apt to set in in the impregnated uterus, Mercurius had better be prescribed first, when the uterus is partially inflamed.

Sabina may be given if the menses set in in the form of hemorrhage during the course of the inflammation, attended with labor-like pains that spread to the thighs. This remedy will likewise be found applicable in other forms of metritis; we are led to this conclusion because Sabina which is so often employed as a means of producing abortion, is apt to cause inflammatory conditions of the uterus.

Other suitable remedies will be found in the next chapter on puerperal fever; or for the remaining traces of metritis we refer the reader to the remedies recommended for catarrh of the genital mucous lining; or finally, in case the peritoneum should be intensely affected, the remedies for peritonitis may be consulted. It is always well to watch convalescent patients for a time lest chronic metritis should remain behind.

For this disease we do not possess any Similia in the rigorous sense of the term; our provings have not as yet disclosed such pathogenetic virtues in our drugs as can be considered homœopathic to the pathological symptoms. Hence we shall have to select our remedies in accordance with accessory symptoms. A most important symptom is the discharge from the vagina, and next to this the character of the menstrual functions. The most noteworthy remedies in this direction have already been mentioned in the previous chapter. They are: *Sepia*, *Platina*, *Lycopodium*, *Graphites*, *Conium maculatum*, *Arsenicum album*, *Natrum muriaticum*, and finally *Sulphur*. Sulphur is especially appropriate if the chronic disease had remained after an acute attack, in which case it is superior to any other remedy.

[In bad cases of endometritis Kafka proposes *Kreosotum* and *Secale cornutum*. He writes: "If the lochia have a dirty-brown color and a fetid odor, and ulcers have broken out on the external pudendum, the question is to check the further spread of the diphtheritic process as soon as possible. At the commencement of this disease we resort to Kreosotum 1. in solution every two hours; at the same time we order injections into the vagina and uterus, using for this purpose lukewarm water to which from 10 to 15 drops of Kreosote are added. The injections have to be repeated every three or four hours. The diphtheritic exudation soon becomes detached and the lochia and ulcers of the vagina assume a healthier appearance.

In very bad cases of this kind, if the diphtheritic process in the uterus has spread over a large surface, the lochia have a cadaverous smell, and the injections bring away whole quantities of disorganized, gangrened cellular tissue; if at the same time the patients are very much prostrated and become anæmic, and the ulcers on the pudendum assume a gangrened appearance, we prescribe *Secale cornutum* 1, in order to induce more powerful contractions and to bring about the detachment and expulsion of the necrosed cellular tissue. We will relate a striking case of this kind from our former practice. In a case of septic metritis setting in in consequence of a very tedious labor that lasted over 72 hours, the above-described phenomena were all present; the patient grew weaker from hour to hour, she ceased to answer questions and was pale as death; yet she had her senses; the extremities were cool, and the hydræmia which had already set in, had given rise to oedema round the ankle; a gangrenous ulcer in the vagina had already destroyed a considerable portion of the nymphæ. Without being acquainted with the physiological effects of Secale, we proposed the external and internal use of this drug. We gave five grains of the powder every two hours, and ordered injections into the uterus every two hours, of a decoction of the same substance of the strength of one drachm of the powder to one pound of water. After the sixth powder and the sixth injection violent labor-like pains set in which brought away a black, excessively fetid coagulum that had filled the cavity of the uterus and consisted of decaying detritus. The patient who in the mean while had fainted as if dead, was washed with wine and, after her consciousness had been restored by the inhalation of some diffusible stimulant, she partook of small quantities of Malaga. The patient was saved. A good diet gradually restored her strength, and her recovery was soon obtained.

Since we have become acquainted with the effects of small doses, we prescribe in the higher grades of endometritis, if the above described phenomena are present, *Secale cornutum* 1, in solution every hour or two hours, and, by this means, accomplish the same purpose, with this difference, that no such tumultuous reaction takes place in the uterus, that the contractions take place slowly without any pain worth mentioning, and that the exudation is not detached all at once, but gradually. *Ergotin* 1, has given us the same favorable results.

In desperate cases *Sabina* 1, may be given internally and externally. If during the course of septic endometritis the symptoms of puerperal fever supervene (for a description see next chapter), we give *Camphora* 1, one or two drops on sugar of milk every two hours, at the same time ordering injections of Camphor into the uterus in the proportion of one drachm of the spirits of Camphor to one pound of water, for the purpose of rousing the sinking vitality of the uterine capillaries and of the general organism, by quickening the movements of the stagnant blood-corpuscles, increasing the chances of a favorable reaction. This result, however, is a very rare one. However, if we succeed, we then discontinue the Camphor, and resort to *Kreosote* in order to keep up the incipient improvement.

In order to neutralize the bad effects of the fetid odor of the lochia we resort to the use of disinfectants, such as the Chloride of Lime, fumigations with vinegar, etc.

Parenchymatous metritis and metrophlebitis set in with frequently-recurring chills. These chills are more especially ominous if symptoms of puerperal fever are at the same time present. In such cases, which are generally of the worst kind, we at once give *Chinin.* 1, every two hours. The intention is to prevent the rapid failing of strength, and at the same time to exert a favorable influence upon the fluids.

If this remedy does not cause a satisfactory improvement, we resort to *Chininum arsenicosum* 1, for the same purpose, more particularly if the chills are attended with rapid sinking of strength and the integuments at the same time show a remarkable degree of pallor. H.]

3. Metritis puerperalis.

Puerperal Fever, Inflammation of the Uterus during Confinement.

Our excuse for bringing together in this chapter several morbid conditions that ought to have been separated according to the exigencies of a rigorous pathological classification, is a desire to simplify our remarks on the subject of treatment. Consequently we shall discuss in this chapter not only the simple puerperal inflammation of the tissues of the uterus, but likewise puerperal fever properly speaking, and shall, as far as possible, explain the differences between these two diseases in the paragraph on the etiological causes.

Simple puerperal metritis involves, it is true, most frequently the internal lining of the uterus (endometritis), but usually likewise extends to the parenchyma, the veins and lymphatic vessels, and very frequently to the peritonæum, although no specific etiological cause can be assigned for each of these different localizations.

The disease originates more especially in the circumstances under which the act of parturition takes place. The inner lining of the uterus is very easily injured by the process of labor; the place where the placenta adheres, is like an open sore; the uterine involution, even in perfectly normal conditions, is attended with signs of local inflammatory action and a general febrile excitement. Hence, even if the process of parturition takes place ever so normally, we have to carefully weigh every circumstance which the most trifling cause might kindle into an inflammatory affection. If, in addition to this, we have the effects of a tedious labor, perhaps an operation, detachment of the placenta, turning, etc., the uterus is so much more disposed to become inflamed, and the access of atmospheric air which cannot be kept out, increases this disposition by favoring the decomposition of the uterine secretion. This accounts for the

Metritis Puerperalis.

ease with which trifling causes sometimes exert the most unfavorable influence upon women in confinement. Among these we place in the front rank emotions whether joyful or depressing; excessive warmth of the sick-room and bed-covering, with which a want of cleanliness almost always goes hand in hand; stimulating beverages such as chamomile-tea and coffee; and finally a cold, which, however, occurs much less frequently than is generally supposed, to the detriment of lying-in women who are not only deprived of fresh air, but, being kept too warm, are made to perspire, and thus become sensitive to the least exposure.

True puerperal fever, under circumstances of which mention will be made by and by, develops itself from the uterine inflammation, or else it originates without any such special cause. Various hypotheses have been resorted to in order to explain this pernicious malady, but all these hypotheses are still unproven. What is certain is that the composition of the blood is altered, that exudations take place with a most decided tendency to suppuration, and that a general dissolution of the blood, as in typhus, is apt to occur. It seems as though this decomposition of the blood were not depending upon the puerperal condition, but may have existed already previous to confinement, which is inferred from the circumstance that fever and various local symptoms are already perceived during the last few days or even weeks of pregnancy. That the composition of the blood is altered, is moreover evidenced by the circumstance that only such women are attacked as are constitutionally sickly or are exposed to want and oppressed with care and anxiety. If, as Scanzoni asserts, pulmonary tuberculosis is a protection against puerperal fever, the doctrine of dyscrasias would seem to be confirmed by such a fact.

Puerperal fever sets in under the operation of the same causes that have been indicated for simple metritis; two weighty circumstances, however, have yet to be added. One is the epidemic appearance of the disease, which shows that general atmospheric or telluric influences are at work in producing the disease, and it would seem as though stormy and damp cold weather exerted the greatest influence as an exciting cause; and the other circumstance is the communication of the disease by infection. In this respect opinions, although not by any means agreed, incline to the theory that the disease is not communicated by a contagium, but, like cholera, by miasmatic agencies. We do not deem it expedient to discuss this matter more fully in this place. A number of cases in lying-in hospitals undoubtedly originate in this source, although there are exceptions.

Symptoms and Course. In order to intelligently appreciate the phenomena characterizing the morbid process of which we are speaking, it is well to familiarize one's mind with the anatomical changes that this morbid process develops. The disease always commences in the first days after confinement, at a period when the uterus has not yet completed the process of involution. This return to a normal condition is checked by the inflammation, on which account the uterus remains larger than in its normal condition, its walls are soft and flabby. The interstices of the internal lining are sometimes puffed up only in part, and covered with a purulent secretion; and at other times they are covered with a croupous, membranous exudation, more especially round the portion where the placenta was attached. All such exudations incline very strongly to gangrenous disorganization, in which case the mucous membrane is transformed into a fetid, dark-colored pulp. The uterine parenchyma scarcely ever remains uninvaded; sometimes, however, its inner layer only is interstitially distended and infiltrated. If the inflammatory process spreads, exudation takes place here and there in the muscular layer, with abscesses or ichorous deposits, the veins become involved in the inflammation, and likewise the lymphatic vessels, after which a more or less considerable peritoneal exudation is scarcely ever absent. In consequence of a further spread of the inflammation of the veins and lymphatic vessels, the femoral vessels not unfrequently become inflamed and closed up, giving rise to the so-called phlegmasia alba dolens; or else metastatic abscesses originate in consequence of the inflammation communicating itself to remote parts.

Simple puerperal metritis rarely commences before the second, and equally rarely after the eighth day of confinement, almost always with a severe chill followed by burning heat. At the same time or very soon after, the uterus becomes painful, with or without pressure, and very soon shows a decrease of resisting power. Generally the lochial discharge ceases as soon as the inflammation sets in. One of the most common symptoms at the very outset is a violent, painful vomiting and retching, and more or less frequent diarrhœic discharges with tenesmus. The fever is very intense; the pulse, if vomiting is present, is at first empty, but seldom less than one hundred, and afterwards full and hard. The patients are tormented by a desire for cold water, their features are collapsed from the commencement of the attack, and, if the vomiting is severe, an expression of despair is depicted in their countenances. Two or three days after the breaking out of the disease, flat ulcers are usually seen on the external pudendum, which are covered with pus or a croupous exudation. If the disease runs a favorable course, and if no complications develop themselves, it may gradually terminate in recovery in one or two weeks, with a return of the lochia, a decrease of the local pains, and a resumption, on the part of the skin, of its normal functions. The last-mentioned change is frequently attended with the breaking out of a rash and profuse perspiration.

But if decomposition of the inflammatory products in the uterus takes place, we are led to suspect the occurrence of such a change by the supervention of severe rigors followed by heat, the pulse becomes more frequent and smaller, and collapse sometimes takes place with extraordinary rapidity. The vagina now discharges a fetid, dark, ichorous fluid, mixed with exudation-shreds, and the ulcers on the pudendum assume a suspicious look and become gangrened. At the same time the local pain may disappear entirely, at least it scarcely ever increases in intensity; a profuse, colliquative diarrhœa now breaks out, nor are complications in other organs wanting, such as a copious exudation in the peritoneal cavity. With this series of phenomena simple metritis, under the operation of the causes described in the paragraph on etiology, passes into true puerperal fever, that is, a general decomposition of the blood takes place very speedily. The pulse now becomes very small and frequent, all pain disappears, the features collapse, assume a cadaverous appearance, the skin is burning hot and very dry, the tongue looks as in the most violent form of typhus. The diarrhœa becomes foul, bloody or dysenteric, and the vomiting sometimes reappears. Very bad symptoms are a vomiting of the color of verdigris, and an intense meteorism. The secretion from the vagina is either entirely arrested, or else exceedingly ichorous and decomposed. Gangrenous erysipelas of the integuments is a very common attendant on this dreadful disease.

In cases where this putrescence of the uterus sets in as a primary affection, not as the result of a process of decomposition in the course of simple metritis, the signs of an intense constitutional disease are generally manifest already previous to the period of confinement, although the indications may be so vague that it is not always easy to interpret them correctly. The patients have a sickly, cachectic appearance, complain of a feeling of languor, frequent shiverings, without much heat. Labor is tedious, the pains are distressing and feeble, the child is often still-born, the exhaustion after labor out of all proportion, the uterus is sensitive to pressure. If after such preliminary symptoms a violent chill and other symptoms of metritis set in suddenly two or three days after confinement, a malignant puerperal fever may be confidently expected, which most commonly terminates in death after a very short period of time.

Phlegmasia alba dolens is one of the most striking and most frequent metastatic inflammations occurring during the course of metritis. It is occasioned by the inflammation of one or more of the larger femoral veins. Amid severe pain, sometimes high up in the limb, sometimes in the knee or leg, the limb swells very rapidly from above downwards, frequently to an enormous size. The swelling is white, shining, painful, elastic in the lower grades of the disease, and at a later stage retaining, like œdema, the imprint of the finger. The motion of the limb is either rendered difficult or impossible. If the superficial veins are inflamed, they appear down the limb like bright-red, painful streaks of great hardness. The termination is either in recovery by a return of the circulation, or in suppuration of the surrounding cellular tissue and other soft parts, whereby life is greatly endangered.

In severe attacks of puerperal metritis, the prognosis is always rather unfavorable. Although simple endometritis is of itself a less threatening disease, yet accidental unavoidable circumstances may transform it at any time into a putrid inflammation, or may cause a fatal termination by an invasion of the peritoneum. True puerperal fever is undoubtedly one of the most fatal diseases with which we are acquainted.

Treatment.

Aconitum is indicated at the commencement of metritis not so much by the local as by the general constitutional symptoms.

"**Belladonna** 30 is indicated by the following symptoms: Disappearance of the milk from the breasts, or suspension of the milky secretion with cord-like indurations; redness radiating towards one focus, with stitching and tearing pains in the breasts. Short, oppressed breathing; anxiety with oppression; distressing drawing, lancing, labor-like pains deep in the abdomen, with painful pressing towards the sexual organs and the anus, and constant urging to stool which cannot be gratified on account of a contracting spasm in the rectum (for which Belladonna is almost a specific); discharge of a coagulated, fetid, black blood, or suppression of the lochial discharge; meteorism of the abdomen, without eructations or emission of flatulence, attended with stinging-digging pains in the abdomen, aggravated by contact and accompanied by a continual invitation to hack; burning heat of the whole body, especially on the forehead and in the palms of the hands, with perspiration on other parts of the body, and violent, sometimes only moderate thirst, and occasional difficulty in swallowing; violent pressing headache, especially in the forehead; turgescence of the veins of the head and conjunctiva, with contraction or dilatation of the pupils, which imparts to the eyes a glassy appearance; not unfrequently optical illusions are present, such as sparks, luminous vibrations; photopsia, even amaurosis; headache rendered intolerable by motion and noise and also by moving the eyes, the patient sometimes loses his senses and becomes furiously delirious; sleep is generally restless, not refreshing. If constipation is present it will disappear, after the use of Belladonna, together with the pains in the abdomen. Generally speaking, Belladonna deserves particular attention if a puerperal fever assumes the character of typhus, if symptoms of meningitis or encephalitis become apparent, and the affection originates in a violent paroxysm of emotional excitement." This complex of symptoms does not clearly inform us in what particular case Belladonna is really indicated. We make this remark in order to show how impracticable such a vast enumeration of all the symptoms of a drug is in the treatment of a disease whose symptomatic manifestations are so exceedingly varied. Hartmann has omitted the important symptom of spasmodic vomiting with which an attack of metritis is so apt to set in. In our opinion Belladonna should be given if puerperal metritis sets in with great violence and an intense fever; for symptomatic particulars we refer the reader to our Materia Medica. An important indication for Belladonna is the meteorism which may set in even if no marked symptoms of peritonitis are observed. If peritonitis is present, our chief attention should be directed towards it. As soon as symptoms of suppuration in the uterus, or of decomposition of the exudation become manifest, other remedies will have to be resorted to.

As regards Chamomilla and Pulsatilla, we do not, as Hartmann does, regard them as remedies for puerperal metritis; if either of these remedies is supposed to have cured metritis, all we have to say is that no metritis was present.

"**Nux vomica** will frequently be found curative, for the additional reason that coffee which is made use of by women in confinement in such large quantities and so strong, often occasions the disease. (Nux is likewise suitable, if the disease is caused by abuse of Chamomile-tea, provided, however, that the symptoms indicate this remedy.) The prejudice which is even entertained by people of cultivation, that coffee facilitates the secretion of milk, or even makes milk, cannot be removed by anything physicians may say to the contrary. If some of the following symptoms are present, the selection is no longer doubtful: Acute pains in the small of the back or loins; stinging and bruising pain of the abdomen during motion or contact, or when coughing or sneezing; bitter taste and eructations; nausea, even vomiting; dryness of the lips and tongue, slimy or dirty-yellow coating on the tongue; sensation of weight and burning heat in the sexual organs; suppression of the lochia; constipation or hard stool, with burning-stinging pains in the rectum; painful urination or retention of urine; dry, parchment-like, burning-hot skin, with thirst, desire for cold drinks, full and hard pulse, anxiety and oppression reflected in the countenance, constant restlessness; the secretion of milk is very seldom suspended, rather increased, causing a turgescence of the breasts, with pressure and tension in the same." We will add that Nux has afforded aid in the less violent and uncomplicated forms of endometritis, but never in the more intense forms of this disease. A characteristic symptom for Nux is the violent inflammatory pain of the swollen veins of the rectum, with exquisite sensitiveness to contact.

"**Colocynthis** is an important remedy in these fevers when caused by a fit of indignation or mortification on account of unworthy treatment, beginning and progressing with fainting-fits, attended with a febrile heat, hot and dry skin, hard, full and quick pulse, sopor alternating with delirium, during which the eyes are kept open; disposition to escape, heat about the head, stinging in the eyes and forehead, dark-red face, yellowish coating on the tongue, bitter taste in the mouth and of everything the patient eats, colic and diarrhœa after partaking of the least nourishment, and pain in the pit of the stomach when touching this part." These symptoms are not the most characteristic indications for Colocynthis. If the peritoneum is more especially attacked; if the coat of the uterus is invaded by the inflammation, or if, during the paroxysms of violent pain, the complexion shows the pallor of death, the features become distorted, the skin is in part cool, and in part burning-hot,

Metritis Puerperalis.

the pulse is quick and there is distressing vomiting with diarrhœa: Colocynth would be much more appropriate. We request the reader to compare what we have said when treating of peritonitis.

Veratrum album deserves a preference at the outset of the attack, if the disease sets in suddenly and with great violence; there is fierce vomiting and frequent diarrhœic stools, the trunk is hot, while the extremities are icy-cold, the face is pale as death and covered with cold sweat, a particular indication is the presence of delirium from the commencement, attended with an unspeakable anguish. In this respect Veratrum is very similar to Colocynth, and is particularly adapted to attacks that set in with the most intense vehemence.

These remedies, to which we will add *Coffea cruda*, *Arnica* and *Hyoscyamus* for the sake of completeness, are particularly suited in the lighter grades of metritis, and at the commencement of the severer forms of the disease. We now proceed to point out the remedies that have to be resorted to in the further course of this inflammation and for ensuing complications.

Mercurius vivus and **solubilis**. Simple endometritis is altogether the same process as acute catarrh of the uterus, modified by puerperal influences. These modifications, however, being no less adapted to the action of Mercurius than simple catarrh, the similarity of this remedy is not interfered with. The period for its employment is the appearance of ulcers on the pudendum, hence on the second day of the disease. Without describing the general symptoms which manifest themselves as accompaniments of this stage, we will direct the reader's attention to one general indication. As long as the exudation in the uterus or peritoneal cavity does not show any disposition to putrid decomposition, and as long as a simple suppurative process prevails, Mercurius is the appropriate remedy. The condition of the ulcers is the best criterium by which the propriety of using Mercurius can be determined: as long as these ulcers preserve their healthy color, and do not become ichorous or gangrenous, Mercurius may be given, no matter whether the fever is high or only slight.

Bryonia alba, according to Hartmann, is indicated by a feeling of emptiness in the breasts, a copious secretion of urine, no suppression of the lochia, (on the contrary, a re-appearance of a bloody lochial discharge,) no pain in the rectum at stool, sensitiveness of the uterus, violent fever, with great restlessness and depression of spirits, painfulness of the thigh when moving it. In our opinion these indications are exceedingly uncertain and insufficient. We consider Bryonia indicated, if the fever is not very violent, the peritoneum is involved in the inflammation, if no decomposition threatens and no ulcers have formed; disposition to sweat, breaking out here and there, but lasting only for a few moments; general languor and inclination to lie quiet; the digestive organs are very much involved in the attack, but there is no vomiting or diarrhœa; meteorism. Compare peritonitis.

Rhus toxicodendron is, in some respects, similar to Bryonia. It is particularly appropriate if simple metritis assumes a typhoid form without any symptoms of decomposition being present. The typhoid character may be manifest from the very commencement, but as a rule it does not set in until the disease has fairly entered upon its course. The fever is continuous, with a burning heat and dryness of the skin, quick and excited pulse; the sentient sphere is very much irritated; the patients complain of violent headache, feel dizzy and as if overwhelmed with sleep, or they are more or less delirious; the face is intensely red, but the color seems unnatural; the tongue is dry and the thirst excessive. These symptoms may cause us to suspect the approach of puerperal fever. Rhus is likewise suitable if this fever sets in at the outset, or supervenes gradually in the course of puerperal metritis. In such a case Rhus is more especially indicated by two circumstances: first by the appearance of metastatic inflammations of the veins, lymphatic vessels or skin, where a malignant erysipelas or petechiæ are apt to break out; and secondly, diarrhœa is very apt to suggest Rhus. If the decomposition is very far advanced, the ulcers are gangrenous, the discharge from the vagina has a fetid odor, the following remedies will be found more suitable. When giving Rhus, we have to see that the reaction is not prostrated and the fever is not completely adynamic.

Secale cornutum. No remedy in our whole Materia Medica shows such a powerful tendency to decomposition of the blood as this drug; nor is any drug possessed of a more intimate and more characteristic relation to the uterus. Hence it is the true puerperal fever, the putrescence of the uterus which invites the exhibition of this drug; it is indicated by the following symptoms: The abdomen is distended and not very painful; the discharge from the vagina brownish and fetid, the ulcers on the pudendum have a bad color and spread rapidly; the fever consists in a violent burning heat mingled with almost convulsive shiverings, and with a small, almost intermittent pulse; at the same time we notice great anxiety, pain in the pit of the stomach, vomiting of a bad-looking substance, fetid and decomposed diarrhœic stools, almost complete suppression of urine. The skin has a bad appearance, is covered with petechiæ or miliaria, or badly-colored local inflammations become manifest which very speedily terminate in gangrenous disorganization of the integuments. At times the patients lie in a state of quiet, with bland delirium, and then again the delirium may be of the furious kind, attended with marked anxiety and a desire to leave the bed.

Arsenicum album. Hartmann has the following remarks on this drug: "The disease may break out in any form whatever, yet it may exhibit symptoms that may require Arsenic. Such symptoms are: Burning or burning-corrosive pains in the interior of the affected part, with inability to lie on the affected part, and decrease of the pains during motion. Again: excessive anguish attended with a general, rapid prostration of strength, excessive debility, sunken eyes, extinct look, sallow, livid complexion, sleeplessness at night, restless tossing about, and a sensation as if a burning-hot water were flowing through the veins; or the sleep is disturbed by frightful and anxious dreams. The Arsenic-fever is always of a violent kind; dry and burning heat, intense thirst which is quenched by frequently drinking small quantities of water; dry and cracked lips, phlyctæna around the mouth; nausea, loathing of food, and sometimes bilious vomiting, with violent pressing-burning pains in the abdominal viscera, meteorism; oppressive pains in the chest, dizziness and headache, restlessness, delirium, a small, feeble, intermittent pulse, etc." This picture does not reflect every characteristic feature of the Arsenic-group in puerperal fever. The position of Arsenic in this disease is best learned by comparing this remedy with Secale. Both show undoubted symptoms of decomposition of the blood; but in the case of Arsenic the reaction is violent, painful, still active, whereas in the case of Secale it is almost extinct. Hence, if both remedies are indicated by the symptoms, we may say that the prevalence of severe pain would point to Arsenic. This diagnostic distinction is particularly applicable to existing ulcers and erysipelatous inflammations to which Arsenic is homœopathic if they are painful, and Secale if they are painless and atonic. For further points of comparison we refer to the Materia Medica.

Phosphorus deserves honorable mention in this place. Even a cursory perusal of its pathogenesis shows its intimate relation to the female sexual organs. Its curative influence in puerperal metritis cannot be determined a priori without further inquiry. This influence does not depend upon the local symptoms, but is defined by the general phenomena according to which Phosphorus holds an intermediate rank between Rhus and Arsenicum, to either of which it bears a good deal of resemblance, and from either of which it likewise differs a great deal. This can only be decided in every case by a careful comparison of the symptoms. In one form of puerperal fever Phosphorus is preferable to any other remedy, we mean the pyæmic form, more particularly if metastatic inflammations take place in the pleural cavity, the lungs, the pericardium, the femoral veins. The violent fever is mingled with frequent rigors, the conjunctiva and skin have a jaundiced appearance, and soon after we observe the signs of pyæmic inflammation in the metastatically-invaded organ. For this reason Phosphorus is likewise the best remedy in metritis if the disease has assumed the character of metro-phlebitis, which it is not always possible to decide with positive certainty. The symptoms indicating such a change are: Slight signs of endometritis, or disappearance of the symptoms of this disease without any corresponding abatement of the fever, increased painfulness of the uterus with inflammation of the femoral veins, and particularly the above-described febrile symptoms, burning heat alternating with frequent feverish shiverings or rigors.

The following remedies may likewise be useful, although the indications for their use are not very frequent: *Carbo vegetabilis, Zincum, Platina, Stramonium.* [See Kafka's remarks on puerperal metritis, page 32 of this work. H.]

Many remedies have been recommended for phlegmasia alba dolens, although we do not see upon what such a recommendation is founded. We propose: *Mercurius vivus, Phosphorus, Bryonia, Rhus toxicodendron,* and *Arsenicum.* Mercurius corresponds to the white swelling of the thigh caused by an inflammation of the lymphatic vessels, the other remedies are indicated in this form of phlegmasia as well as in that caused by an inflammation of the veins. These few remedies will, in our opinion, prove sufficient to effect a cure. [Bæhr has omitted three important remedies which are indispensable, if we wish to treat phlegmasia arising from phlebitis, as promptly and successfully as such an inflammation can be cured; they are: Belladonna, Aconite and Hamamelis. H.]

4. Oophoritis, ovaritis.
Inflammation of the Ovaries.

This inflammation only occurs during the period when this organ is active, between the age of pubescence and the critical change of life; or likewise previous to the 24th year, very seldom at any other time. The exciting causes are, upon the whole, obscure: it is certain, however, that an inflammation of the uterus during the first week after confinement is very apt to communicate itself to the ovaries. As an idiopathic disease oophoritis is met with among women on the other side of thirty, and among prostitutes who have intercourse with men during the menstrual flow, or it may be caused by a cold; it is likewise said to occur after medicines that are taken for the purpose of producing abortion. Only one ovary is inflamed at a time.

Symptoms and Course. We have to distinguish the acute and chronic form. Acute oophoritis sets in with sudden pains in the region of the ovaries; most commonly they are dull and indefinite, stinging and burning, and aggravated by hard pressure. A swelling at this place cannot be felt, and we only succeed now and then in discovering a swelling by an exploration per rectum. The pain sometimes spreads to the adjoining parts, radiates even to the thigh which feels numb, and is more especially increased by sudden motions, not however so as to enable the patients to aggravate the pain ad libitum. Very generally the uterine mucous lining becomes involved in the inflammation which manifests itself with the symptoms of uterine catarrh. There is no fever, or it is trifling; on the other hand various nervous derangements set in similar to those of hysteria; even nymphomania and vomiting may occur.

Only in very rare cases oophoritis terminates in suppuration; if no dispersion takes place, the inflammation becomes chronic. In the chronic form the swelling is larger and can even be felt externally; the pains remain, but are inconsiderable and only incline to exacerbate during the menses, during pregnancy and confinement. The menses most generally become irregular, scanty; leucorrhœa is very commonly present; in the chronic more than in the acute form symptoms of hysteria become manifest, more especially an irritable, capricious mood. The prospect of a complete cure is more favorable in the acute than in the chronic form; in the latter the exciting cause generally never ceases to be present and keep up the morbid process.

Diseases of the Female Sexual Organs.

Treatment. The scarcity of this disease explains why so few cases are reported in our publications that can be reliably regarded as cases of oophoritis. The affection being almost without an exception without any very great importance, we shall confine ourselves to very general indications regarding the use of the proper remedies.

Belladonna is in many respects the most important remedy in this disease. As a rule, this medicine is specially adapted to diseases of glandular organs, more particularly when located in the interior of the body. Moreover our provings as well as practice have shown that this medicine bears intimate relations to the female sexual organs. Oophoritis is pointed at by the symptoms, as may easily be seen by reference to the abdominal group. Hence, Belladonna is particularly adapted to acute oophoritis attended with severe pain. Experience has likewise satisfied us that Belladonna is useful in the chronic form, provided we do not expect any immediate result.

Colocynthis is recommended for inflammatory ovarian affections; the symptoms, however, do not justify this choice; nor do the pains indicating colocynth emanate from the ovary.

Conium maculatum. Jahr relates a cure of chronic oophoritis effected with this drug; the ovary was very much swollen and had been indurated for a long time. This result and our physiological provings may suffice to recommend this drug.

If in addition to these remedies, we mention *Bryonia*, *Sabina* and *Cantharis*, we have named all the remedies that are of use in acute, and, to some extent, in chronic oophoritis. We must not, however, forget *Apis mellifica* which contains in its pathogenesis a number of symptoms pointing to affections of the ovaries. It is very likely that too much has been expected of this remedy, but we are prepared to assert its efficacy in acute oophoritis from abundant experience in our own practice. [In acute oophoritis we should not forget to associate Aconite 3 with Apis; the former remedy may be exhibited first, and after the inflammatory symptoms are somewhat subdued, Apis may be resorted to, or both may be continued more or less at alternate intervals. H.]

For chronic oophoritis we recommend: *Mercurius*, *China*, *Platina*, *Sepia*, likewise *Ignatia*, *Sulphur* and *Staphysagria*. The selection of the right remedy is often very much interfered with by the existing hysteric difficulties. From Hartmann we take the following indications: If the affection was caused by disappointments in love and consequent dwelling of the fancy upon sexual things, *Ignatia*,

Staphysagria and *Acidum phosphoricum* may be exhibited. *China* may be added to the two last-mentioned drugs if onanism is one of the exciting causes. *Platina* for a continual titillation in the internal sexual organs, compelling the patient to rub the parts and attended with complete nymphomania; by pressing on the parts, the inflammatory pain changes to a pain as if the parts had been contused or bruised, with anxiety and oppression, palpitation of the heart, stitches in the front part of the head, sadness alternating with excessive mirth. According to Hartmann, Platina in connection with Belladonna is particularly suitable in the case of prostitutes. With *Aurum metallicum* and *muriaticum*, *Clematis* and *Iodium*, we close the list of ovarian remedies; other morbid conditions of these organs, in so far as they are curable, will yield to the above-mentioned remedies.

[In the Allgem. hom. Zeit., May 17th, 1862, we have the report of a cure of ovarian cyst by Dr. Hirsch of Prague, of which a republication will be found in the 20th number of the British Journal of Homœopathy. The cyst was the result of an inflammation of the left ovary, which had been treated allœopathically. The disorder was completely cured chiefly by the use of the Iodine water of Hall, of which the patient took three tablespoonfuls every morning fasting, containing the 48th part of a grain of Iodine. Hall is situated near Linz in Austria; the leading constituents of this mineral water are Chlorides of Sodium, Potassium, Ammonium, Calcium, Magnesium; Iodides of Sodium and Magnesium; Bromide of Magnesium; Phosphate of Lime; Carbonate of Lime, Magnesia, and Iron; Silicic Acid. H.]

5. Menstrual Anomalies.

With a view of securing a true definition of menstrual anomalies, we deem it necessary to premise certain observations concerning the normal condition of the menstrual functions.

By menstruation we understand a flow of blood from the female sexual organs recurring at regular intervals. It is a sign that the female organism has attained the faculty of conceiving, and depends upon the following processes: The gradual maturing of an ovulum in the ovaries determines an increased afflux of blood to those organs. If this congestion has reached its acme, the other organs of the sexual system participate in this hyperæmia to such an extent that the blood-vessels become ruptured and a more or less considerable discharge of blood takes place accompanied by a sometimes more extensive and at other times more local detachment of the epithelial lining of the sexual organs. While the discharge of blood lasts, the matured ovulum enters the Fallopian tubes, which renders its fecondation possible. A discharge of blood need not necessarily accompany the passage of the ovule into the tubes; otherwise how could a woman who is nursing her baby and does not see the least sign of a menstrual show, conceive again at such a time? That this happens, is a fact established beyond the possibility of a doubt.

According to circumstances the menses appear at times sooner, and at other times later. They are influenced by climate; the nearer to the equator, the sooner the menstrual period appears; they are likewise influenced by the mode of living: in cities the menses appear sooner than among country-girls; by the mental capacities: the more advanced the mental development, the earlier the menstrual functions make their appearance. The constitution exerts no particular influence; very robust girls sometimes menstruate very late, whereas feeble ones often menstruate prematurely. According to these circumstances the menses may set in between the ages of 10 and 20 years; in our climate they appear in cities between the ages of 14 and 16, and in the country between the ages of 16 and 20 years.

The quantity of the menstrual blood is likewise variable and cannot be determined a priori; stout women sometimes lose a small quantity of blood, whereas feeble and spare-built women lose a great deal. The quantity is from two to eight ounces.

Nor is the duration of the menstrual flow the same in all cases. It generally averages five days, but, without being considered abnormal, may last only two, or may be extended to eight or nine days. Sometimes the bleeding stops for a short time and then reappears again.

The periodicity of the bleeding likewise varies. By far in the majority of cases it returns again every 28th day. In many cases there is an interval of four weeks between the periods; in a few cases we notice an interval of 21 to 30 days. Four weeks may be considered the normal length of the interval between each two successive turns.

The influence of the menses upon the general health is sometimes considerable and at other times none at all. We notice hyperæmia of the vagina and of the external pudendum, sometimes with increased secretion of mucus; tumefaction of the breasts with painful, knotty swelling of single galactiferous ducts. During the menstrual flow the nervous system is much more sensitive and excitable, whence the following phenomena: chilliness alternating with flashes of heat; headache, hemicrania, vertigo, languor, drowsiness without any ability to sleep; irritated, whining mood; loss of appetite, palpitation of the heart. In addition to these derangements we often see a sickly, gray complexion, efflorescences in the face, margins around the eyes; vomiting or nausea; altered voice. These phenomena usually occur only during the first twenty-four hours of the flow, after which they cease either suddenly or gradually.

The total cessation of the menses takes place indefinitely, some women menstruating regularly until the age of 55, whereas others cease to menstruate when they are 40 years old. These differences do not depend upon the time of the first appearance of the menses, or upon the vigor of the individual, upon the number of times a woman has conceived, nor even upon other morbid conditions. The final cessation is not bound by any rule, and may take place quite normally between the ages of 40 and 50 years. It may occur suddenly and completely, or in paroxysms; some periods, even to the number of ten or twelve, being skipped, after which the menses may occur again regularly for months, or a sort of hemorrhage may set in which is again followed by a stoppage of the menses. As a rule the quantity of the menstrual flow is larger as the period of a final cesssation draws near, than in the preceding years.

In the previous paragraphs we have only briefly alluded to the most important points. But they show satisfactorily the importance of the menstrual function to the female organism. Hence it is that menstrual irregularities have at all times excited a lively interest among physicians as well as lay-persons, to such an extent that they have been classified under special heads, although, in reality, they constitute a symptomatic' manifestation of one and the same general or local disease. The question now is, when, in a general sense, menstruation may be said to be abnormal. The menses are abnormal in the first place if they do not harmonize with one of the previously-indicated periods; they are likewise abnormal if, for some cause or other, the usual duration of the menstrual flow in a given case is either shortened or lengthened. A woman who menstruates every 21st day, is not considered sick; but we consider a return of the menses every 21st day abnormal, if heretofore they had occured every 28th day. Finally, whether the menstrual flow is to be considered abnormal, may depend upon the influence which it exerts upon the general organism. A suspension of the menses in the case of a young girl who, after being relieved from the prejudicial influences of school and city-home, goes into the country and there regains her blooming health, cannot be regarded as a morbid condition.

We now transcribe, with a few additions and variations, the following details from Hartmann, whose treatment of this subject seems to us excellent. We will first notice his general dietetic rules.

"Every attention should be given to the mind and feelings of the young woman; her excited fancy should be controlled, and her nervous sensitiveness and excitable temperament which are so apt to cause disease, should be quieted. For this reason a woman should be treated with kindness and attention, especially during pregnancy and the menstrual period. Every depressing emotion, chagrin, fright, anger, acts prejudicially upon persons in health, much more upon those who are diseased." We refer the reader to our chapter on hysteria and to our subsequent chapter on chlorosis, where we shall show that a premature development of the mental faculties, and more particularly of the fancy, exerts a pernicious influence upon the constitution of the growing woman generally, and upon the normal functions of the sexual system in particular.

"Woman's material mode of living deserves a closer attention. A wrong system has, in this respect, become a second nature to such an extent that a physician is expected to allow his patients to indulge in. their accustomed violations of a proper diet, on which account we invite him to pay particular attention to the following points in the treatment of female diseases.

1) "Women who lead a sedentary life, should be induced to take more exercise than usual, and to rouse themselves from their phlegmatic torpor. This is one of the first requisites of health: frequent exercise in the open air, cleanliness, frequent bathing and washing, and frequent changes of linen. During the menses, every heating exercise and every exposure to a cold should be avoided; likewise heavy farinaceous food, freshly-baked bread; violent emotions, sexual intercourse, emetics, purgatives, baths. This caution need not be carried so far as to compel healthy and robust women to lie down the first two days and even to give up their accustomed walk. Even the drinking of mineral water should be discontinued by patients who are on a visit to springs for their health, unless the discontinuance of the water should entail greater damage than the use of it

might occasion by its interference with the menses, in which case it is proper to put up with the lesser evil of the two.

2) "The physician should see to it that his patient drinks more liquid than heretofore. Many ladies drink nothing the whole day, except three cups of coffee at breakfast and dinner; if this quantity is diminished, as it necessarily has to be under homœopathic treatment, some other beverage will have to be substituted, such as cocoa, milk, unspiced chocolate, weak black tea, or roasted rye or barley. We know, however, from experience that these warm beverages relax the stomach and bowels, hence the patient will have to drink every day a few glasses of fresh water or very light beer. Any other spirituous or spiced, heating beverages, such as wine, punch, and the various liquors, have to be strictly prohibited." We cannot forbear offering a few objections to Hartmann's views regarding the use of coffee. As generally prepared and drank by most women, coffee is undoubtedly hurtful, but this does not apply to properly-prepared coffee that is not too weak and whose aroma is properly preserved. In this shape coffee is a beverage whose partisans are so numerous because it is the best medicine against many of the morbid tendencies engendered by civilization, and which has a particularly beneficial influence on females. Only let them use good coffee of which they cannot drink large quantities, and the use of which should always be associated with fresh water. The so-called substitutes for coffee prove in the end more hurtful than even weak and badly-prepared coffee, except perhaps beer which, however, cannot well be drank early in the morning.

3) "A bad habit that is indulged in by many ladies, is eating at any hour of the day. This practice is decidedly injurious to the success of homœopathic treatment, and should be abolished. Order is useful in all things and likewise in our meals, and patients should be given to understand that they must partake every day of a warm dinner at a fixed hour; breakfast and supper may consist of cold articles of food.

4) "Too much sleep, and sleeping too often within twenty-four hours, can only be approved of, if the patients are very weak and anæmic; during sleep the body has to be kept perfectly unrestrained and easy, without the least inconvenience from the pressure of the ordinary clothing; otherwise sleep will not exert the quickening influence that is expected from it. Females especially have the bad habit of lying down with a mass of clothes on. This practice not only prevents the body from getting warm, but interferes with the

free circulation of the blood and thus gives rise to other troubles in addition to those already existing. Tight lacing is another censurable practice which is often the sole cause of menstrual irregularities. In such cases we do not advise to abandon the use of corsets entirely, but simply not to lace too tightly. If the patient is able to sit up and were to dispense with her corsets altogether, she would soon complain of weakness of the back and weakness all over, and would be more inconvenienced by the use of the many strings with which ladies have to fasten their garments, than by wearing loose and easy corsets." In this respect we cannot agree with Hartmann. Corsets, even if laced very loosely, have the disadvantage of supporting the back and occasioning muscular weakness of the back, unless they are worn without interruption. By going without corsets for a time the woman will soon learn to keep her back straight without any such artificial support. If corsets are worn too tightly, they compel the wearer to breathe with the upper portion of the thorax, the lower ribs being not allowed freely to expand on account of the compression exerted upon them. This gives rise to an incomplete respiration, an imperfect introduction of oxygen and a diminution of the elasticity of the pulmonary vesicles. Thus it is that corsets become a co-operating cause of many of the blood-diseases of females. When speaking of chlorosis and tuberculosis, we shall revert to this subject.

5) " The physician will have to inquire whether his patient, as is so often the case in the higher walks of life, uses cosmetics for the purpose of giving more color to her face, or making it look paler by such substances as vinegar, tea, decoctions, lime, chalk, roast oyster-shells, etc. The same objection can be raised against most kinds of pomatum and perfumes for the hair which, if it requires more fat, had better be greased with beef-marrow. This is a subject of great importance, if we consider that Lead and Arsenic are usually employed in the composition of cosmetics.

6) " Regarding the functions of the bowels, it is of importance that our female patients should never suppress an urging to stool, and that they should at least have one evacuation from the bowels every day. Women are much more afflicted with constipation than men; in most cases they are the authors of this exceedingly prejudicial state of the bowels, sometimes on account of neglect, at other times from sheer laziness, again on account of sedentary habits, and finally because they are ashamed of satisfying the calls of Nature.

7) "Women should make it a rule to wash their parts, especially if affected with leucorrhœa or other diseases, several times a day with cold water, and during the menstrual flow with tepid water. More recently the Sitz-baths and the vaginal syringe are now in almost general use. These are not only excellent means of relief in many morbid conditions, but likewise excellent means of prevention, and should be found in every lady's bed-chamber. Cold water is indeed the most reliable nervine at our disposal."

a. *Derangements Attendant on the Appearance of the Menses.*

"It must be self-evident that the awakening of the sexual life, which is the greatest revolution which the female organism can undergo, is accompanied by phenomena that very often partake of the nature of a morbid process. The normal conditions under which the menses should first appear, have been explained in a previous paragraph. A premature appearance of the menses always implies a feeble constitution and powerful sexual instinct. Hence it is of the utmost importance not to accelerate this period because all the ailments which sometimes befall young girls at this age, are supposed to originate in the tardy appearance of the catamenial discharge. Of course, where the delay is evidently of a morbid character, Nature should be assisted by such remedial means as will promote the menstrual flow.

Such morbid phenomena are the more striking, the more sensitive and delicate the young woman who had been reared in the bosom of luxury and ease. Although these ailments may not be very considerable yet their removal often requires the interference of art. Sometimes a judicious diet is sufficient for this purpose, but in many cases medicinal agents have to be used. Conditions requiring the assistance of a physician, are characterized by the following symptoms: Congestion of blood to the head, as indicated by heaviness of the head; rush of blood to the chest, with palpitation of the heart, and sometimes attended with oppression of breathing; sensation of warmth and repletion in the abdomen; feeling of indolence through the whole body; occasional flashes of heat and red flushes in the face; languid feeling in the legs and feet; pain in the small of the back and pelvic region; drawing in the thighs, frequent urging to urinate. These symptoms may be regarded as menstrual distresses which are very speedily succeeded by an actual appearance of the menses and disappear with them. If these simptoms continue for a longer time without any menstrual show taking place, the patient will have to take a good deal of exercise in the open air, use more vegetable than animal diet, more liquids than usual, and spend her time as much as possible in cheerful company.

"If the above-mentioned symptoms become more severe and continuous; if the rush of blood is more violent, causing anxiety, palpitation of the heart, constant heat, a restless sleep full of dreams and interrupted by sudden starts; if the face looks bright-red, and the pathognomonic signs of cerebral hyperæmia and congestion of the thoracic organs become manifest: we resort to the remedies that have been indicated for such conditions in their respective chapters. One of the leading remedies is undoubtedly *Pulsatilla*, especially if the congestive symptoms of the head and chest are accompanied by signs of abdominal and uterine congestion, as if a stone were oppressing the uterus, and the patient complains of chilliness, stretching of the extremities, yawning and other febrile symptoms. *Chamomilla* and *Veratrum* may likewise be indicated by a certain train of symptoms. The above-mentioned dietetic rules shold not be neglected while these medicines are used. *Belladonna* may be added to this group of remedies as one of its most prominent members. Whereas Chamomilla is very seldom indicated, Veratrum and Belladonna will often be required, the former if the functional activity of the heart is very much impaired, as indicated by paleness of the countenance, great chilliness or constant alternation of chilliness and heat, anxious feelings; the latter if symptoms of cerebral congestion prevail, with bright redness of the face, altogether in individuals of full habit.

"The so-called anti-psorics here come undoubtedly into play, since this physiological act is transformed into a pathological disturbance only if a constitutional disease prevails whose symptoms are still very obscure and undeveloped. If such a disease evidently exists, it will have to be met by its appropriate remedies, otherwise we may resort to *Sepia*, *Conium*, *Magnesia* and *Lycopodium*.

"If the young woman has reached the age of pubescence and feels otherwise quite well, although the menses do not show the least sign of making their appearance: the physician would commit a great wrong if he were to drench the organism with medicines; his duty will be to leave Nature alone in determining the period for the appearance of the menses, more particularly if the organism shows signs of being backward in its development. It is only if the organism is sufficiently developed and the young woman's age justifies the expectation that the menses ought to appear, that it is proper to hasten this process by the employment of suitable remedies, more particularly of the anti-psorics. Nevertheless, we do not commence the treatment with this class of remedies, but give in the first place *Pulsatilla* and, if the indications are satisfactory, repeat the dose rather frequently, more particularly in cases where the non-appearance of the menses causes, without any other bodily ailments, an excessive nervous irritability, whining, peevish, timorous disposition, paleness of the face and great flabbiness of the muscular tissue. *Nux vomica*, on the contrary, will be found appropriate in persons of an opposite temperament, an irascible, choleric disposition, a full habit, without any decided congestions, redness of the cheeks and turgescence of the body. If these remedies, to which we shall add a few more by and by, prove fruitless, we recommend as the best remedies: *Causticum* and *Graphites*, more particularly if the appearance of the menses only seems delayed in consequence of the insufficient efforts of Nature, and the discharge finally takes place in small quantity and then again ceases; *Natrum muriaticum* and *Kali carbonicum*, if the menses do not appear at all, and *Calcarea carbonica*, if there is no show, but the whole appearance of the menses indicates a plethoric habit of body. *Sulphur* is under such circumstances one of the chief remedies, a few doses of which ought to be given before any other medicine is resorted to, more especially if a chlorotic state of the blood is indicated by the patient's complexion.

"Among the remedies corresponding to the morbid phenomena which sometimes trouble young girls before the menses first appear, we recommend *Sepia* and *Calcarea* for the violent hemicrania which sometimes attack such persons even at regular periods; *Calcarea* and *Phosphorus* for the violent pains in the back which sometimes resemble spinal irritation; for the convulsive symptoms we give *Cocculus* and *Ignatia*; *Cuprum* is less frequently indicated; for symptoms of anæmia we recommend *Ferrum* and sometimes *Arsenicum* will be found appropriate."

b. *Suppression or Delay of the Menses, Amenorrhœa.*

"This suppression either takes place during the flow, or in consequence of causes acting previous to the actual appearance. In the former case a cold may have operated; or cold washing may be the cause; or the feet may have got chilled; or the patient may not have been sufficiently protected by her clothes; mental or moral emotions, vexations, chagrin, anger, fright, or dancing, sexual intercourse, dietetic transgressions may have led to the suppression. Most of these causes, if operating shortly before the time when the menses were to come on, may cause their retention. A gradual suppression of the catamenia may take place in consequence of deficient nutrition as well as of the abuse of warm beverages and the continued influence of depressing emotions. We have already shown that a change in the mode of living may superinduce a suspension of the menses in the case of young women, without leading to derangements of the general health.

"The more sudden the suppression of the menses, the more violent the changes arising from such an occurrence. Some of the most prominent symptoms are: violent hemicrania, great anxiety and oppression of breathing, nose-bleed, spitting of blood, congestions of the head, heart and lungs, and the like. In some cases a suppression of this kind gives rise to acute uterine catarrh, metritis, peritonitis. If a physician is called in time, he will of course inquire what gave rise to the trouble, and will seek to remove the consequences of fright, mortification, anger, etc., by appropriately-specific remedies. If the physician is not called until some time after the morbid symptoms have existed, the aforesaid remedies will no longer be applicable and the constitutional condition generally will have to be acted upon by corresponding remedies. The remedies mentioned in the preceding chapter under "a" will often be found indicated.

"If at the time of the menses they do not appear, and violent abdominal spasms occur, we commend *Cocculus* as the most suitable remedy, especially if the spasms are accompanied by anxiety and oppression of the chest, moaning and groaning, a paralytic sort of weakness, so that the patient is unable to utter a loud word, and her extremities have lost all power or are convulsively agitated, and the pulse is scarcely perceptible. *Cuprum aceticum,* or still better *metallicum,* acts very similarly to Cocculus. It is particularly applicable in typical paroxysms of the most violent kind, consisting of unbearable abdominal spasms affecting even the chest, causing a loathing, gagging, and even vomiting, affecting at the same time the extremities with epileptiform spasms during which the patient utters a piercing cry.

"The following remedies likewise deserve commendation: *Valeriana, Platina, Ignatia, Belladonna, Magnes arcticus, Mezereum, Digitalis.*

"If these remedies do not restore the menses, the physician will then have to resort to the so-called antipsoric remedies, more particularly *Magnesia carbonica* and *muriatica, Sulphur, Sepia, Zincum, Silicea, Lycopodium, Graphites, Acidum nitricum,* which may even be employed if the menstrual suppression causes no further trouble." We do not share Hartmann's opinion in this respect. Medicines should never be given except where actual morbid manifestations seem to indicate their use; the non-appearance of the menses sometimes is a means, on the part of Nature, to increase, or at least to economize the strength of the organism.

"In the treatment of delaying menses we have to follow the same rules and maxims that have been laid down for menstrual suppression. A suppression or delay of the menses often causes abdominal spasms and other difficulties for which *Pulsatilla* is an excellent remedy. We likewise recommend *Cicuta, Terebinthina, Zincum* (especially when menstrual suppression is attended with a painful swelling of the breasts); *Calcarea carbonica* (likewise for menstrual suppression, attended with marked symptoms of plethora); *Graphites* (when the menses delay too long, and the patient complains of hoarseness, headache, bloating of the feet, chilliness, bearing-down pains in the small of the back); *Natrum muriaticum* (if the menses delay too long and are very scanty); *Strontiana* (if the menses delay too long, and afterwards, when appearing, look like flesh-water and pass off in the shape of coagula); *Sarsaparilla* (when the menses delay, are too scanty and acrid), etc."

These few indications may show that a good Repertory is the best means of securing the selection of the proper remedy. As regards external applications, we do not approve of them; their usefulness is questionable, and in many respects they are decidedly prejudicial. Hot foot-baths are more particularly hurtful; they often exert a very injurious effect upon the brain and heart, not to mention the increased susceptibility of the feet to get chilled which they invariably occasion. If the flow of blood towards the lower extremities is to be promoted, the most efficient and never hurtful means to accomplish this result, is continued and fatiguing walking. Dry cupping on the inside of the thighs is the only palliative means that can safely be permitted.

c. *Menstruatio Nimia, Profuse Menses.*

An excess of loss of menstrual blood, a true menorrhagia, does not occur as often as it may seem to those who complain of it. To constitute menorrhagia, several circumstances have to occur that require to be carefully discriminated. The quantity of the discharged blood has to exceed the ordinary loss quite considerably, and then again we have to inquire whether the scantiness of the ordinary menstrual flow is not an abnormal diminution in the present case. The menstrual flow is likewise considered too copious, if it continues beyond the ordinary period, although this need not necessarily imply that the menses are profuse. The morbid character of the menses is finally and more especially determined by the accessory symptoms, for a copious flow of the menses cannot be considered abnormal as long as the constitutional harmony is in no respect disturbed by it.

All circumstances that cause either permanently or temporarily an increased flow of blood towards the sexual organs, may be regarded as causes of menorrhagia. A temporary excess of the menstrual flow may be caused by the influences that have been pointed out as the causes of metritis; a permanent excess is occasioned by onanism, novel-reading, a constant dwelling of the fancy upon sexual things, and the habitual use of heating beverages. A few other important points have to be added. Under certain circumstances a profuse flow of the menstrual blood becomes a real physiological necessity to the body; for instance, if a larger supply of nourishment than the body requires for its normal support, causes a real plethora. This can scarcely be regarded as a morbid condition. A profuse flow is sometimes occasioned by changes in the uterus, such as acute or chronic metritis, and adventitious growths in the uterine cavity. Nursing exerts a very particular influence. As a rule, nursing women do not menstruate; yet it may happen, even in the case of quite healthy mothers, that the menses reappear again prematurely, in which case the flow is often very profuse. This is not a normal condition, although it does not inconvenience all women. Of a threatening character and exceedingly prejudicial are menorrhagias that set in when the process of nursing is continued too long. Accidents of this kind occur quite often in the country, where the women nurse their children for several years for the purpose of preventing conception, not thinking that by doing so they inflict permanent injury upon their health. We must not forget to record the fact that diseases of other organs, or of the general constitution, exert an influence upon the menses. Without considering the influence of diseases which alter the quality of the blood, such as typhus or scurvy, etc., the influence of heart-disease, of tuberculous infiltration of the lungs, emphysema, accumulations of fluid in the pleural cavity cannot be denied; it is more especially heart-disease that causes menorrhagia, so that the heart had better be carefully examined in every case of menorrhagia. Finally the cessation of the menses at the critical age is almost always ushered in by profuse losses of blood. Particulars on this subject may be found under the heading: metrorrhagia.

The symptoms of profuse menstruation generally may be quite inconsiderable, being no more than feeble indications of anæmia. In most cases, however, profuse menstruation is allied with the symptoms of difficult menstruation of which we shall speak hereafter.

In treating this anomaly we have in the first place to direct our attention to the causal indications as far as such a thing is possible. These indications are so numerous that we cannot well specify them more particularly in this place. They constitute the cases for which Hartmann recommends the antipsorics. Where menorrhagia occurs without being dependent upon some more deep-seated disorder, *Nux vomica* will be found an efficient remedy, more particularly if the nervous system had become very much excited by disturbing mental influences, the patient gets angry at the least remark, shows an irascible and obstinate temper, starts at the least noise, loses her balance on the most trifling occurrence, wants to lie down all the time, and shows an aversion to open air. *Chamomilla* is particularly indicated, if the blood looks dark, almost black and coagulated, with drawing, griping pains from the small of the back to the pubic bones, sometimes accompanied by fainting fits, coldness of the extremities and great thirst. It cannot be denied that the use of Chamomile-tea often has an influence over the quantity of the menstrual discharge. Unfortunately this beverage is generally first resorted to for such ailments as precede menorrhagia which is undoubtedly made worse by the use of this tea. Besides *Nux vomica Ignatia* and *China* are indicated by such symptoms. The indications for *Calcarea carbonica* have been furnished by Hahnemann himself in the following brief but exhaustive remarks: "If the menses appear several days previous to the regular monthly term and to excess, Calcarea is often indispensable, more especially if the menstrual flow is excessive. But if the menses occur at the regular period, or later, Calcarea will do no good even if they are not scanty." We add that Calcarea will afford much relief in cases where anæmic phenomena prevail, with disposition to congestions of the head or chest. *Belladonna* apparently acts similarly to the former drug, except that the congestive phenomena for which Belladonna is indicated, arise from real plethora; the menses are too profuse, not excessively dark-colored and their appearance is accompanied by a pressing downwards, a painful drawing and tearing from the uterus to the thighs. *Phosphorus* is indicated if the menses delay a tolerably long time beyond the natural term, set in profusely and occasion great debility, weariness and languor, paleness of the countenance, a sickly appearance, back-ache. It is more particularly applicable to the menorrhagia of nursing women. *Platina* for a painful and too frequent return of the menses, a copious and dark discharge with labor-like pains, more particularly in the case of sanguine, lively individuals. *Sepia* has similar characteristic symptoms. *Digitalis* is indicated if the menorrhagia depends upon a stasis of the blood caused by heart-disease, if the symptoms of passive venous congestion prevail, the face is pale or livid, the skin is cold.

For further particulars we refer to the chapter on metrorrhagia where more medicines will be found mentioned.

d. *Dysmenorrhœa, Scanty Menstruation.*

It is just as difficult to define what is understood by scanty, as we have found it difficult to define what is to be understood by profuse menstruation. As a change in the mode of living may induce a suppression of the menses, so it may likewise, by exerting a modifying influence upon the internal development of the organism, occasion a diminished flow of the catamenia. This may occur among women of a more advanced age as well as among younger persons, and it would be highly improper to disturb such a change by medicinal interference.

In by far the least frequent cases scanty menstruation is of itself a morbid symptom; generally it is dependent upon some local affection, profuse leucorrhœa, chronic metritis, uterine displacements, or it may be owing to constitutional disturbances such as chlorosis, hydræmia, marasmus, excessive formation of fat, tuberculosis, etc.

These different forms of scanty menstruation do not, in reality, require a separate treatment; it is identical with the treatment of the constitutional disorder, or else no treatment at all is required because the suppression of the menstrual flow may simply bear evidence to the fact that the organism has no blood to spare for such a function. For this reason we deem it unnecessary to indicate remedies for such a condition of things, and refer the reader to the chapter on chlorosis and, for various particular points, to the next chapter on difficult menstruation.

Menstrual Anomalies. 61

e. *Ailments accompanying the Menses, Difficult Menstruation.*

Ailments of various kinds, sometimes preceding and sometimes accompanying the menses, are so common, especially among the higher classes, that, unless they become too troublesome, they are not complained of to a physician; on the other hand, their diversified forms may make them a source of great trouble, or they may cease for a short time in order to reappear with so much more obstinacy some time thereafter.

These ailments may very naturally be classified in three categories. Either they arise from material changes in the sexual organs, a bent in the uterus, retroversion, anteversion, chronic metritis, etc., or else they are occasioned by an excess of menstrual congestion, or finally they may be of a purely nervous kind. Although the first category does not properly belong here, yet we call attention to it in order that their presence or absence be satisfactorily established. The congestive ailments are almost exclusively confined to the pelvic organs, and consist in a variety of pains, sometimes attended with palpitation of the heart, congestive headache, febrile symptoms. The nervous ailments are not restricted to the sexual sphere and very generally involve the whole nervous system. Whereas the congestive ailments abate with the appearance of the menses, and disappear entirely on the second day, the nervous symptoms on the contrary are apt to continue during the whole period.

In most cases the causes of these ailments are very obscure. Although they most generally accompany scanty menses, yet they are not unfrequently attendant on profuse menstruation; moreover, although they more commonly affect sensitive, feeble, irritable, delicate and effeminate individuals, yet they are likewise met with among women of a robust constitution and who menstruate regularly.

These remarks may show that it would be a futile undertaking to indicate the whole series of symptoms which characterize such ailments. Hence we prefer recording a few of the more important difficulties together with their corresponding remedies. We must, however, caution the reader against supposing that the particulars contained in the subsequent paragraphs are intended to render all further reference to the Materia Medica superfluous.

It is proper to ascertain whether the ailments occur before, during or after the menstrual flow.

For ailments previous to the menses, if the patients menstruate too profusely, we recommend: *Belladonna, Chamomilla, Calcarea,*

Lycopodium, Platina, Nux vomica, and if the menses are too scanty: *Pulsatilla, Cocculus, Sepia, Alumina, Baryta.*

Ailments during the menses, if too copious: *Nux vomica, Arsenicum, Phosphorus* (the last-named deserving particular consideration), *Calcarea carbonica;* if too scanty: *Alumina, Pulsatilla, Conium maculatum, Graphites, Sepia, Carbo vegetabilis.*

Ailments after the menses, which, however, are not often noticed unless we mean the prejudicial effect of a considerable loss of blood: *Platina, Ferrum, Graphites, Borax.*

For the colicky pains the seat of which cannot always be traced with perfect certainty, whether it is the intestinal canal or the uterus, with scanty menses: *Cocculus, Conium, Sepia, Pulsatilla,* and with a copious flow: *Belladonna, Platina, Nux vomica.*

For the congestive symptoms in the pelvic organs, if preceding the appearance of the menses: *Belladonna, Bryonia alba, Sabina;* if accompanying the menses: *Phosphorus, Veratrum album, Nux vomica;* if remaining after the menses: *China, Platina.*

For distress at the stomach, if very marked, such as eructations, nausea, vomiting, perverted taste, loss of appetite: *Pulsatilla, Ipecacuanha, Veratrum, Iodium.*

For the toothache which so often accompanies and precedes the menses, and constitutes one of the most troublesome torments of women, if setting in previous to the menses: *Aconitum, Chamomilla, Belladonna, Pulsatilla,* and more particularly *Arsenicum;* if during the menses: *Calc. Carb., Sepia, Phosphorus.*

For hemicrania which generally is present during a scanty, scarcely ever during a profuse menstrual flow: *Sepia, Nux vomica, Pulsatilla.*

Convulsive symptoms may of course vary, sometimes being purely local, at times general, then again tonic and at other times clonic; they may even appear like epileptiform spasms so that they seem much more threatening than they really are. We may consider it as an established fact that the epileptiform spasms which occur at the time of the menses, never partake of the dangerous nature of epilepsy. The most important remedies are: *Ignatia amara, Cocculus, Cuprum, Platina, Secale cornutum* and *Causticum.*

The mental disturbances belonging in this category, mostly partake of the character of exaltation, for which remedies like *Platina, Veratrum album, Hyoscyamus, Belladonna, Stramonium,* are indicated; states of depression which occur much less frequently, require *Lycopodium* or *Natrum muriaticum.*

We will conclude this chapter by giving a general hint bearing upon the selection of a remedy for menstrual difficulties: our chief attention should be directed to the conduct of the discharge, whether it appears at the right season or not, whether it is too scanty or too profuse, or whether it occurs normally. These points are essentially characteristic; if the remedy does not meet them, the correspondence with the other phenomena may be ever so perfect, the remedy will not suit the requirements of the case.

[Recently a number of drugs have been introduced into the Materia Medica of our School, some of which are being used with great success in various diseases, and more particularly in abnormal menstruation.

Aletris farinosa, or the star-grass, is recommended for the preliminary symptoms of miscarriage, such as dizziness, nausea, headache, fulness in the region of the womb, colicky pains.

Caulophyllum thalictroides, or the blue cohosh, has been extensively used by homœopathic physicians for painful menstruation, with a scanty flow of blood, or when the appearance of the menses is preceded by severe spasmodic pains, for which *Cocculus* is generally recommended. We give the Cohosh as soon as the pains commence, and resume the medicine a few days before the next period. This course of treatment has a tendency to effect a radical cure.

Cimicifuga racemosa, or the black cohosh, is eminently useful in the various forms of menstrual disorder, menostasia, amenorrhœa, dysmenorrhœa, also tendency to miscarriage, menorrhagia. The resinoid Cimicifugin, first or second trituration, is very commonly used. In the menostasia of young girls it is generally indicated by headache, hysteric nervousness, pale complexion, debility, loss of appetite, colicky bearing-down pains in the lower abdomen. In amenorrhœa or suppression of the menses from some accidental cause, a cold, etc., the characteristic indications are: congestive or neuralgic headache, febrile motions, chilly creepings, rheumatic pains in the limbs, backach, uterine spasms. In dysmenorrhœa it seems principally indicated by the prevalence of neuralgic pains, spasmodic pains in the uterine region, disposition to faint, nausea, headache. In menorrhagia it is useful when the flow is of a passive character, the blood is dark-colored, coagulated, the patient complains of neuralgic pains in the small of the back, dizziness, headache, obscured vision, great weakness. It will be found admirably adapted to the hemorrhages occurring at the critical age. The doses should not be given too small. If given in sufficiently large doses, this medicine will often prevent miscarriage. It is chiefly indicated by the sudden appearance of violent bearing-down pains, together with such accessory symptoms as headache, nausea, fainting feeling, etc. Cimicifuga is used by eclectic physicians for leucorrhœa with much success. It greatly facilitates labor, not only by accelerating the process itself, but likewise by preventing the harassing and exhausting pains which so often accompany a tedious labor. Dr. E. M. Hale suggests the use of Cimicifuga as a preventive of difficult labor. In the second edition of his "New Remedies" he relates the following case: A lady, the mother of three children, was in the eighth month of pregnancy. Her previous labors had been unusually severe, very tedious, painful and accompanied by fainting fits, cramps, agonizing pain, etc., before the birth, and flooding, syncope, and many unpleasant symptoms after the expulsion of the placenta. She took, for nearly three weeks, about ten drops of Cimicifuga first decimal dilution, four times a day. Labor came on at the proper period, but lasted only six hours; was not painful nor difficult; there was no flooding, no fainting and no cramps. She got up in nine days, and had a better convalescence than ever before.

We know from abundant experience that it is an excellent remedy for the various ailments incident to the critical age of women. The annoying flashes of heat to which such women are so often subject, and for which we have been in the habit of prescribing Sepia, Sanguinaria, etc., yield much better to Cimicifuga. "In the irritable condition of the uterus," writes the London Lancet, "often observed in patients for some time after menstruation has ceased, or irregular when about to cease, and marked by pain more or less periodical in the lumbar region, Cimicifuga affords rapid relief. In neuralgic pains often met with in such patients, in other localities, it is equally beneficial. Females at the period of life we are speaking of, frequently suffer from a distressing pain in the upper part of the head, recurring with greater severity at night. These cases are very satisfactorily met by this remedy. Pains in the mammæ also, whether referable to uterine disturbance or to pregnancy, are relieved by the Cimicifuga very speedily."

Collinsonia canadensis, stone-root. This remedy is recommended by some homœopathic physicians for amenorrhœa, menorrhagia, dysmenorrhœa, miscarriage, and other disorders of the female organs of generation, such as pruritus and prolapsus uteri. It is not supposed to exert a direct specific action upon these organs, but to cure the disorders alluded to by removing the affections upon which the disturbances of the sexual organs are depending. These affections are principally piles and constipation. The curative results of Collinsonia have been mostly obtained by means of comparatively large doses.

Gelseminum sempervireus, yellow jessamine. Dr. Hughes writes, in the British Journal of Homœopathy: "I continue to derive the most brilliant results from this drug in dysmenorrrhœa and after-pains, when these are spasmodic and not inflammatory. Its power over after-pains is so great that the lying-in chamber is well nigh freed from one of its greatest bugbears. But it is antipathic rather than homœopathic to these conditions, and requires to be given in full doses, from three to ten drops of the first decimal dilution." Dr. Hughes would imply that large doses of Gelseminum are antipathic, and small doses are homœopathic to spasmodic pains. If this is the Doctor's meaning, his doctrine is incorrect. We have the testimony of Dr. Douglas of Milwaukie, one of the provers of Gelseminum, that he experienced severe spasmodic pains "a succession of acute, sudden, darting pains, evidently running along single nerve-branches in almost every part of the body and limbs, sometimes so sudden and acute as to make me start. At one time a quick succession of these acute sudden pains coursed down the outside and front of the tibia for over half an hour, leaving a line of considerable tenderness marking its track. These pains, which seemed clearly neuralgic, gave me the palpable indication for its employment in this disease. And it has certainly been successful. But while it has fully cured some distressing cases of neuralgia, in which Aconite had been fully tried without benefit, there have occurred some other cases in which it has failed and Aconite has succeeded. What is the explanation of this? If we suppose that in some cases of this disease there exists a real inflammatory state of the nerve, and in others a mere excess of sensitiveness, the explanation is easy; Aconite cures the first, Gelseminum the last." But then Dr. Douglas writes further: "A majority of all cases of neuralgia will be promptly relieved by Gelseminum, but it sometimes requires to be given *in pretty large doses,* repeated every half hour till the pain is relieved."

Hamamelis virginina has been used with excellent effect in dysmenorrhœa and vicarious menstruation. In Hale's New Remedies a few cases are reported where cures were effected with the middle potencies of the remedy.

Helonias dioica, false Unicorn, of which we prepare the resinoid *Helonin,* which is very frequently used in practice, has been prescribed by homœopathic physicians for prolapsus uteri, a very fine case of which is reported by Dr. Geo. S. Foster of Meadville, Pa., in Hale's New Remedies. It was a case of prolapsus with ulceration of nine years' standing, and was cured perfectly by means of Helonin, after a number of other remedies had been used either without, or with only partial success. Congestive symptoms are prominently present in uterine diseases where Helonias is used, in amenorrhœa, menorrhagia, prolapsus, etc.

Senecio aureus, life-root, is possessed of fine curative powers in painful menstruation when the menses occur prematurely and are very profuse; the patient suffers greatly with violent uterine spasms at the time of the menses. We recommend comparatively large doses during the attack. H.]

6. Metrorrhagia.
Uterine Hemorrhage.

We deem it unnecessary to justify the distinction we have drawn between menorrhagia and metrorrhagia; both differ in their essential characteristics. When speaking of the treatment, we have included among the remedies for ordinary metrorrhagia those that refer more specially to metrorrhagia during confinement as well as during pregnancy.

An hemorrhage from the unimpregnated uterus is mostly due to the same causes as menorrhagia. Every circumstance that has power to determine an excessive flow of blood to the uterus, may become the cause of metrorrhagia. It may likewise occur in consequence of a number of pathological alterations of the uterine substance and of adventitious growths in the uterine cavity. Hemorrhages of this kind are so common that every loss of blood which cannot be attributed to the menses, ought to excite a suspicion that it is owing to the presence of material lesions. Metrorrhagia occurs most frequently at the critical age, when it is difficult to distinguish between menorrhagia and Metrorrhagia.

Metrorrhagia is generally preceded by preliminary symptoms of longer or shorter duration, indicating for the most part a violent determination of blood to the pelvic organs, such as: a painful drawing and pressing in the small of the back towards the sexual organs and thighs, sensation of heaviness and fulness, of increased warmth and throbbing in the pelvis, also colicky pains; frequent desire to void the urine; titillation and burning in the sexual organs, accompanied by chilliness, heat; an accelerated, soft pulse, sometimes with a double

Metrorrhagia.

beat (pulsus dicrotus), palpitation of the heart, swelling and sensitiveness of the breasts, leucorrhœa, etc. These symptoms are particularly prominent during metrorrhagia at the critical age. The hemorrhage itself often sets in with chilliness, paleness of the face, coldness of the extremities, sometimes without any special phenomena; sometimes it is a mere dribbling of blood, at other times large quantities of an usually dark, black blood are poured out periodically, which readily coagulates on account of the fibrin it contains, and forms coagula of considerable size even while yet in the uterus. In addition to this loss of blood we notice the most varied symptoms of constitutional disturbance, such as: excited temperament, anxiety, restlessness, labor-like pains, colic, urinary difficulties, vomiting, convulsions, spasmodic laughter and weeping. If the hemorrhage lasts a sufficient length of time, symptoms of anæmia make their appearance. The importance to the organism of such hemorrhages should not be estimated too lightly; even the most trifling hemorrhage may, by its continuance or by an extraordinary increase of the loss of blood, permanently impair the patient's health and ever threaten her life.

Uterine hemorrhage shortly after the expulsion of the fetus, constitutes one of the most important and dangerous events. Where it is not caused by injuries of the uterine parenchyma, it almost always results from deficiency of the uterine contractions. A deficiency of this kind is not always owing to atony of the uterus such as may result from tedious labor or violent labor-pains, or even from general debility; it may likewise depend upon circumstances that render the necessary contractions even after normal labor-pains impossible. Among such circumstances we number a too rapid labor, partial adhesions of the placenta, and the presence of copious coagula in the uterus. We have only to do here with hemorrhages depending upon atony and deficient contractions of the uterus; these hemorrhages alone are accessible to medicinal influences. Hemorrhages of this kind occur immediately after confinement; they must be expected if the uterus remains large and soft. Sleep, immediately after confinement, may become the cause or at least the promoter of hemorrhage; it should not be indulged in. The symptoms of hemorrhage can only escape detection, if the accident occurs within the womb. The os tincæ and the vagina are so filled with coagula that the blood remains confined within the uterine cavity, which again becomes distended by the accumulated fluid. As in every other copious loss of blood, the symptoms of anæmia become rapidly manifest, such as pallor of the countenance, chilliness, cold sweat, obscuration of sight, fainting, sopor, decrease of the pulse, convulsions; the uterus, moreover, feels flabby, and increases perceptibly in size. This accident is generally unaccompanied by pain.

Hemorrhage occurring at a later period of confinement, is generally less copious; it likewise originates in deficient uterine contractions, or in inflammatory processes, but the prognosis in such cases is unfavorable. Hemorrhages of this kind occur more particularly in the case of women who do not nurse their children; the intense stimulation generally caused by the nursing, now reacts upon the uterus.

Hemorrhages during pregnancy are sometimes of trifling importance, and at other times more threatening. Some women are in the habit of menstruating several times after conception without detriment to the fœtus. It has seemed to us as though children born of such mothers at full term, and having otherwise their full development, were less vigorous and disposed to a variety of ailments. Hemorrhages during the second half of pregancy, if not depending upon placenta prævia, originate in the same causes as those of the first half, of which we shall treat presently; but they usually are of a subordinate significance, because they seldom threaten the life, or interfere with the further development of the fœtus. The most important hemorrhages are those occurring during the first half of pregnancy, for the reason that they mostly precede, cause or accompany a

Miscarriage or **abortus.** Such hemorrhages happen in consequence of the vessels uniting the ovum to the uterus, being torn, either because the natural resistance of the uterus against its contents is too great, or because the resistance of the contents against the walls of the uterus is too feeble. In this way the uterus is excited to premature contractions which may easily superinduce a laceration of the vessels for the reason that in the first three months the ovum is on its whole surface connected with the uterus by means of very delicate blood-vessels. Hence miscarriages take place most easily during the first three months of pregnancy. If the after-birth is already formed, premature contractions likewise lead to the laceration and detachment of the placental vessels. This, however, is of less frequent occurrence, because the contractions affect only a smaller portion of the uterus, and it is moreover well known that the normal seat of the placenta is not the locality usually affected by the contractions, but that they are much more commonly confined to the lower portion of the uterus. It is all-important that the circumstances which cause premature contractions of the uterus should be carefully investigated; a miscarriage can only be prevented by keeping all such exciting causes out of the way. The causes of miscarriage either proceed from the fœtus in consequence of its premature death, or from the mother. The death of the fœtus is superinduced by intensely-debilitating diseases of the mother, especially a far advanced anæmia; next by constitutional syphilis, and finally by violent commotions such as fright. To judge by the changes which are sometimes noticed in the fœtus, it would seem as though certain poisonous substances which will be named by and by, might exert a destructive influence over it. As proceeding from the mother, we have the various circumstances that tend to cause a determination of blood to the uterus, and which have already been named in the chapter on acute uterine catarrh. Plethoric individuals are much more liable to miscarriage than anæmic women, especially if the former are afflicted with profuse menstruation. In their case the hemorrhage is apt to appear at the time of the catamenia. Acute febrile affections and diseases of the heart likewise predispose to miscarriage. Mechanical causes acting upon the sexual organs directly, or transmitting their effect upon the uterus by a general concussion of the system, exert a peculiarly injurious influence; so do depressing mental causes when affecting the uterus unceasingly. It is well known that women who, although again pregnant, continue to nurse their children, become liable to miscarriage on account of the excited condition of the uterus transmitted to this organ from the excited nipple. Lastly we have to mention various poisons which are sometimes resorted to for the criminal purpose of producing miscarriage. These are *Sabina, Crocus, Secale cornutum.* Sabina is so frequently used as a means of producing abortion, that the Juniperus Sabina which grows in the neighborhood of large cities, is usually found pulled to pieces and deprived of its branches. As regards Secale cornutum, we know from the history of epidemic ergotism that the women who were attacked by this disease, generally miscarried. In conclusion we have to observe that a woman who miscarries once, retains a disposition to miscarry a second time, and that this second miscarriage is apt to take place at the same period as the former. Thus it may happen that women miscarry nine or ten times in succession, notwithstanding they had given birth to healthy children heretofore. It almost seems as though the uterus, after the normal function of impregnation has once been interfered with, loses its capacity to again successfully engage in the process of utero-gestation.

Symptoms and Course. We have to examine these points more fully, because upon their correct knowledge and appreciation depends the possibility of preserving the lives of both mother and child.

In the first three months, hemorrhage is generally the first symptom of incipient miscarriage. As a rule, the hemorrhage at once assumes the form of metrorrhagia, even if the woman had been otherwise perfectly healthy, especially if violent external impressions were the cause of the accident. A mere dribbling of blood at this time is of much less frequent occurrence. At first the patient does not complain of any pain; after a short lapse of time, it sets in very gradually as a dull pain, and increases until it finally assumes the character of real labor-pains; this is likewise substantiated by the circumstance that, during the paroxysms of pain, the blood is expelled in larger quantity. These phenomena are mistaken by inexperienced women, if they are otherwise afflicted with difficult and profuse menstruation, for a return of the menses.

In the subsequent stages of pregnancy, metrorrhagia only takes place exceptionally, without a preliminary stage which is determined by the entrance of blood into the uterus whose mouth still remains closed; or by the premature contractions of this organ, or by the death of the fœtus.

In the first of these three cases, the patients complain of a dull pain in the pelvis which extends to the back and is increased by motion, by voiding the urine or by evacuating the bowels. The symptoms are frequently associated with slight febrile motions, diarrhœa with tenesmus, urinary difficulties. All these phenomena rarely precede the hemorrhage longer than five days. It commences with distinct labor-pains.

The premature contractions of the uterus may be allied to the congestive phenomena just described, but they likewise occur as primary symptoms. In such a case the patient experiences a peculiar drawing pain from the uterus across the abdomen, and spreading with peculiar violence to the small of the back, at first intermitting for hours, and finally only for a few minutes. The general organism does not seem to be affected by this pain. Sometimes the pains intermit even for days; nevertheless, they return again. The more continuous and more violent the pains, the more certainly and the sooner the hemorrhage will occur.

If miscarriage is caused by the death of the fœtus, striking precursory symptoms are scarcely ever absent. They sometimes last even for weeks. The patients feel faint and weary, complain of feeling feverish, are remarkably pale, and experience a sensation of coldness in the abdomen and lower extremities. The signs of life that may have been perceived in the fœtus, cease. The patient is very much depressed in spirits, complains of pains in the stomach, increased nausea and distressing vomiting. While these symptoms continue, the pains and contractions foreboding the approaching expulsion of the fœtus set in, and the hemorrhage takes place.

After the blood has begun to flow the course of the trouble is pretty much the same in every case. If the fœtus is separated from the organism of the mother, it has to be expelled. If the hemorrhage is at all copious, the expulsion can no longer be prevented. The course of the difficulty now varies according to the different states of the uterus. During the first months of pregnancy the lower segment is still very rigid, the os tincæ firmly closed; more force or a longer time is required to open the womb, whereas in the subsequent months the vaginal portion becomes more yielding and dilatable. Hence a miscarriage extends over a longer space of time in the commencement than in the subsequent months of pregnancy; moreover, the hemorrhage in the former case is more profuse. As a rule the ovum, up to the third month, is discharged uninjured, sometimes unperceived, whereas, at a subsequent period, the membranes of the ovum are ruptured, and afterwards expelled subsequently to the expulsion of the fœtus. The constitutional symptoms are preëminently those of acute anæmia; even the convulsive phenomena which are not unfrequently present, are only occasioned by the anæmic condition of the patient, very seldom by the amount of pain involved in the hemorrhage. Primiparœ generally suffer most. As soon as the fœtus is expelled, the flow of blood generally ceases very soon. But if the placenta has already been formed, the whole of the fœtus is not always expelled, but fragments of the ovum remain in the uterus and, by preventing the full contraction of this organ, cause the hemorrhage to continue. This is so much more dangerous as it is commonly more copious than at the commencement of miscarriage, the danger being still greater, if we are not able to remove the remnants of the fœtus. In this case the hemorrhage may likewise be internal, if the fœtal remnants close up the os tincæ. Hemorrhages of this kind are always more or less threatening, and sometimes endanger life. What we have said, shows that miscarriage is least apt to occur in the first three months; and that the danger involved in the hemorrhage is greatest, if a placenta has already formed, because remnants of the ovum are easily retained in the uterus.

The whole course of such an accident assumes a peculiar form, if the uterus firmly contracts round the remnants of the ovum. In such a case the flow of blood suddenly stops and complete recovery seems to have taken place, until the hemorrhage returns, sometimes after the lapse of weeks, and these hemorrhages follow each other in such rapid succession that it is impossible to mistake them for the menses. A misapprehension of this kind is, moreover, prevented by the anæmic symptoms accompanying this condition. In such a case a rapid cure can only be effected by the artificial removal of the remnants of ovum whose spontaneous expulsion is sometimes delayed to a remote period. A similar course takes place in the rare cases of miscarriage of twins. After the expulsion of one fœtus the uterus firmly contracts round the other one, and, for a time, the trouble seems at an end, until a second hemorrhage brings away another fœtus.

In a case of miscarriage the prognosis has to consider a variety of circumstances: the possibility to save the life of the fœtus; the danger to which the life of the mother is exposed by the hemorrhage; the further consequences of the accident, and finally its influence upon the faculty of conceiving anew. As far as the preservation of the fœtus is concerned, the prognosis is the more unfavorable, the more copious the hemorrhage and the sooner it takes place, so that, if a profuse hemorrhage sets in during the first three months of pregnancy, the retention of the fœtus can scarcely be hoped for. All morbid processes, especially inflammatory affections, in other organs, and either causing or accompanying the miscarriage, diminish the chances of a successful issue. The indirect consequences of a miscarriage sometimes tell on the whole future life of the patient. One of these consequences is a high grade of anæmia, together with the abnormal conditions of the heart, which it often occasions. Chronic uterine affections are likewise very common; so are leucorrhœa, chronic metritis, displacements and changes in the normal shape of the uterus. A number of nervous derangements sometimes remain after miscarriage. The influence of such an accident upon a subsequent conception is often so trifling that it may be said to amount to nothing; many women conceive and abort by turns; as a rule the second miscarriage takes place about the same time as the former. Other women, having once miscarried, never again go the full term of pregnancy; at a certain period a hemorrhage again sets in. This is a very common occurrence after a miscarriage previous to the fourth month, and is almost a rule in the case of a primipara. The general faculty of conceiving does not seem to become modified by miscarriages.

Before passing to the treatment of uterine hemorrhages generally, we will add a few more remarks concerning miscarriage. Miscarriage, both as regards the prophylactic and curative treatment of such an accident, is a morbid process which sometimes defies the most consistent treatment of the so-called Rational School. On the contrary, the homœopathic treatment of miscarriage is generally crowned with the most brilliant success. For this reason we have deemed it our privilege to lay particular stress upon a morbid process whose importance must be self-evident. In our own practice we can show the records of a number of cases of threatening miscarriage that were successfully prevented by internal treatment, and where the full term of pregnancy was secured even after hemorrhage and severe uterine contractions had already set in in some of them. Quite recently the wife of a most excellent allopathic physician of this city, who had miscarried nine times in succession in spite of her husband's best efforts to prevent such an accident, was successfully carried through her tenth pregnancy by homœopathic treatment. In the presence of so much brilliant success we have a right to say that we possess the means of preventing miscarriage with an almost unerring certainty.

We will now proceed to mention the different remedies that are most commonly resorted to in the treatment of miscarriage, and afterwards review this treatment in a connected series.

Sabina. We have shown on several previous occasions that the action of this drug upon the uterus is specifically characterized by congestion often amounting even to inflammation. This fact should not be lost sight of in cases where Sabina may seem to be indicated. If the metrorrhagia is preceded for some time by a labor-like drawing in the abdomen, sensitiveness to pressure, increase of the sexual passion, a more copious secretion of mucus from the vagina; if the hemorrhage is profuse, painful, and the blood is bright-red and fluid, or is discharged in the shape of firm coagula, Sabina is our best simile that will certainly help in most cases, for a confirmation of which fact we can point to our own experience as well as to our printed records. This remedy suggests itself more particularly in the case of robust persons of a plethoric habit, who have menstruated at an early age and always were inclined to menstruate profusely. We have already stated in a previous paragraph that the specific action of Sabina upon the uterus is known even to lay-persons, and that this knowledge is made available for purposes of criminal abortion even by married women; the evidence of such a crime has been on more than one occasion furnished us in our own practice.

The relation of **Secale cornutum** to the uterus is equally constant and characteristic. This relation is not, as Griesselich fancies, dependent upon the action of this drug upon the spinal cord; it is immediate, but differs greatly from that of Sabina. Secale tends to rapidly destroy the organic activity, without occasioning any very striking signs of reaction which may even be entirely absent. Hence Secale is particularly appropriate in metrorrhagia unattended by symptoms of reaction on the part of the uterus, or the general organism, without any marked pains in the uterus, in the case of individuals of an anæmic or leucophlegmatic habit of body. Secale is therefore indicated in metrorrhagias occurring at the critical age, or in chlorotic individuals whose constitutions are broken down by debilitating diseases; or in post-partum metrorrhagias depending upon atony of the uterus, or which cause or accompany the miscarriages of anæmic subjects, or which are occasioned by the death of the fœtus. The general character of the hemorrhage will prove a better guide in the selection of Secale than mere symptomatic indications, of which we, nevertheless, proceed to point out the most essential: The blood has a dark color and shows very little or no disposition to coagulate; its discharge is either painless, or else the pain is very vague and undefinable; it flows in a rather uninterrupted stream; the hemorrhage is accompanied by great prostration, fainting fits, palpitation of the heart with intermission of the beats, convulsive movements, cold skin. Secale is likewise indicated in the latter stage of hemorrhages that commence with signs of congestions, and likewise in hemorrhages occurring during the latter term of confinement.

Crocus is an important member of this group of remedies, but differing from either of the above. If Crocus is so often recommended for active congestive uterine hemorrhages, we attribute this recommendation to the circumstance that the symptoms of the female sexual organs have alone been considered. They are: Pressure and a feeling of weight, stitches, pressing towards and in the sexual parts, discharge of a dark, tenacious, even black blood, but without any labor-like pains. If, in addition to these symptoms, we consider the general languor and loss of strength, the constant chilliness and a variety of other symptoms, it seems difficult to regard this series of phenomena as an active congestion. A passive congestion, on the contrary, is undoubtedly a reliable indication for Crocus, which is more especially confirmed by the quality of the blood. In general, Crocus is adapted to metrorrhagias at the critical age or which are accompanied by affections of the heart or arise from impediments in the portal circulation, in which case varicose swellings of the veins of the rectum and lower extremities present specific indications for its use. These symptoms likewise point to Crocus in cases of miscarriage and post-partum hemorrhages, although in the former we may seldom meet with the quality of the blood characteristic of Crocus.

We take the liberty of presenting these three remedies as prototypes of the different medicines for metrorrhagia, even if by so doing we should incur the reproach of a generalizing dogmatism. This would, of course, be unjust, since it is the object of this work to lead the reader through general principles to special or individualizing applications, and not to teach the former for the purpose of superseding the latter.

We rank in the Sabina-category the following drugs: *Belladonna, Chamomilla, Platina, Nux vomica, Calcarea carbonica, Hyoscyamus, Ignatia amara, Ferrum,* to which we add these short remarks: Belladonna and Chamomilla are especially applicable in the hemorrhages of lying-in women, with a general excitement of the circulation. Calcarea, Ferrum, and perhaps Pulsatilla, are adapted to the hemorrhages of feeble and anæmic subjects, with excited circulation. Hyoscyamus, if symptoms of convulsion accompany the hemorrhage from the start, more especially shortly after confinement. Ignatia and Platina for hemorrhages with excessive irritability of the nervous system and the general sensorium, especially if the accident was preceded, and probably caused by some violent commotion of feeling or by sexual excitement, Ignatia being more appropriate in the former, and Platina in the latter case.

The Secale-category does not comprehend many remedies; at any rate not one of them shows a complete resemblance to the prototype. *Ipecacuanha, China,* and under certain circumstances *Ferrum, Plumbum* and *Arsenicum* are the few remedies belonging to this category. Ipecacuanha is generally appropriate only for post-partum hemorrhages, or after miscarriage, with cutting, colicky pains around the umbilicus, pressing towards the uterus and anus, great chilliness on the outside and extreme heat within. *China* is mostly required after the hemorrhage had lasted already for some time, especially after confinement if the uterine contractions seem to be utterly exhausted, the patient is cold and blue, and a convulsive shock now and then agitates the frame. The choice of Arsenicum can only be determined by the general symptoms, not by the local sexual phenomena. Regarding Plumbum, we transcribe Griesselich's remarks from Rückert's "Klinischen Erfahrungen": "Among the worst kinds of metrorrhagias we number those that befall females at the critical age and who are afflicted with hypertrophy of the uterus. If the patients have been long weighed down by severe mental distress, the hemorrhage will prove still more unyielding. Other remedies have often proved futile in such cases. The cases where Plumbum afforded help, happened among women of the higher classes who had attained the age of forty; they had had few children in the first years of their marriage; the metrorrhagia had become inveterate, and had assumed a passive character. Generally the patients had lived well, had partaken of quantities of heating beverages, had led a sedentary life and their constitutions had assumed a preëminently venous tendency; hemorrhoidal tumors had made their appearance, constipation, bloating of the bowels after eating, etc. The metrorrhagia had existed for years, with free intervals of four to six weeks and even longer. During these intervals the patients recovered their strength, but another attack brought them down again. The attack was preceded by a sensation of weight and fulness in the abdomen; slight labor-like pains from the small of the back to the front were experienced, amid which dark coagula were expelled mingled with fluid blood and serum, without any unpleasant odor; the discharge was increased by motion; a profuse discharge was attended with syncope, yawning and stretching, twitchings and by such other signs of anæmia as palpitation of the heart, a small, intermittent pulse, etc. The hemorrhage was succeeded by a more or less profuse, inodorous and mild leucorrhœa. On exploration the uterus was found to be uniformly distended. Between the attacks the patients looked sickly, almost chlorotic; the assimilating functions were disturbed, the skin was dry, pale and yellowish, with hepatic spots; the patients complained of languor, shortness of breath on going up-stairs, had a sad and desponding mood. The Acetate of Lead, in doses of one quarter of a grain per day, arrested the hemorrhage in several cases and removed the danger of total destruction which threatened the cachectic body, without, however, correcting the constitutional condition." To these statements we add an important observation: Paul (Archives générales, Mai, 1800) has had an opportunity of watching the effects of Lead upon the female sexual organs in upwards of eighty cases; his observations lead him to infer that this metal favors miscarriages and premature births in a most extraordinary degree, and that it very commonly occasions the death of the fœtus.

The category of Crocus contains a number of remedies some of which are closely related to Secale. The most important are: *Arnica, China, Digitalis purpurea, Lycopodium, Kali carbonicum, Sepia, Kreosotum, Phosphorus, Carbo vegetabilis*. Arnica may likewise be required in active metrorrhagia; it is particularly adapted to post-partum hemorrhages, and is known as an efficient remedy for excessive and painful after-pains. For particulars concerning Digitalis or rather Digitalin, we refer the reader to our Essay on this drug. There is no question that in metrorrhagias occasioned by blood-stasis depending upon heart-disease, Digitalis is one of the first remedies. We are not as yet in possession of more special indications. The cure of a dangerous metrorrhagia which is reported in that Essay, has not yet been interrupted by a similar accident, it is now eight years. Sepia deserves special consideration in cases of miscarriage; it is but seldom indicated in simple metrorrhagia. At all events it is one of our most important remedies as a preventive of miscarriage. Whereas Sabina is especially adapted to active, plethoric and robust constitutions, Sepia responds to nervous irritability associated with a quick circulation; it is such conditions of the system that so often give the first impulse to miscarriage and are associated with obstruction in the abdominal circulation. Reisig recommends Sepia in miscarriage between the fifth and seventh months, if symptoms of abdominal plethora are present; Kallenbach relates several cases where Sepia had a good effect, the following symptoms being present: rush of blood to the head and chest, sensation of weight in the abdomen, swelling of the hemorrhoidal vessels, irritable temper, disposition to syncope. While these symptoms prevail, the movements of the fœtus grow weaker until they finally cease altogether and miscarriage threatens, most probably provoked by apoplexy of the fœtus consequent upon uterine congestion. Experience has demonstrated the curative virtues of Sepia as a preventive of miscarriage in so many cases that it must be owing to indolence if our physicians do not report more cases of cure than they have done, with carefully and distinctly drawn outlines. Lycopodium is likewise recommended as a preventive of miscarriage, but has not the same practical effect as Sepia. Lycopodium is more particularly suitable for feeble, worn-out individuals afflicted with bad digestion, chronic gastro-intestinal catarrh, obstinate fluor albus, symptoms of venous congestion in the extremities and abdomen, varices on the legs and private parts, hemorrhoids, liver-complaint, splenetic engorgements. Such symptoms are not often met with in young persons, on which account Lycopodium is preëminently suitable for middle-aged women. It is of especial value in the metrorrhagias of the critical period, if the above-described symptoms indicate this drug. According to Hartmann, *Kreosotum* is suitable if a quantity of dark blood is discharged, succeeded for a few days by an acrid-swelling, bloody ichor causing a gnawing-itching and smarting of the parts, after which the flow of blood recommences mingled with coagula. At the same time the head feels very much distressed. Such symptoms suggest the presence of malignant disorganizations of the uterus: however, they may likewise occur at the critical age or during confinement without any perceptible organic alterations.

It would lead us too far if we were to particularize the symptomatic indications for more remedies; it may be well, however, to classify the remedies we have named, in accordance with the distinctions which we have pointed out as characteristic features of the various kinds of metrorrhagia.

Hemorrhages of the unimpregnated uterus previous to the critical age, require: *Belladonna, Platina, Nux vomica, Calcarea carbonica, Hyoscyamus, Ignatia, Ferrum;* very rarely *Sabina, Sepia, Phosphorus;* hemorrhages at the critical age require: *Platina, Secale, China, Plumbum, Arsenicum, Digitalis, Lycopodium, Kali carbonicum, Kreosotum, Carbo veg., Crocus.*

For post-partum hemorrhages we recommend: *Sabina, Belladonna, Chamomilla, Bryonia, Hyoscyamus, Secale, Ipecacuanha, China, Arnica.*

Hemorrhages during pregnancy require the remedies that will be presently named for miscarriages.

In treating miscarriages we have to keep two things in view, namely the prevention of the hemorrhage by general means, the arrest of the hemorrhage, and the management of the consequences of hemorrhage in accordance with general principles.

It is undoubtedly possible to prevent miscarriage; the case of the

Doctor's wife to which allusion was made in a previous paragraph, will be accepted as evidence of such a fact. The nature of the prophylactic treatment is more especially determined by the constitutional symptoms of the patient. If the patient is an anæmic, feeble, pale woman, *Pulsatilla, Ferrum, China* have to be prescribed in not too frequently repeated doses; if the anæmia is attended with disposition to congestion, *Calcarea carbonica* is preferable. If the woman had miscarried several times, it is best to give the previously-mentioned remedies about four weeks before the term when the miscarriage is expected to take place, but neither too low nor too frequently; perhaps a few drops every three days, and to continue this treatment until at least four weeks after the term. We avoid strong attenuations lest the medicine should produce primary effects. The remedies proposed for anæmia should not be continued at the time when the miscarriage is expected; at such a period *Calcarea, Sepia* or *Sabina* are preferable each as the patient's personality may indicate. Regarding the necessity of absolute rest in order to prevent a miscarriage, views differ a great deal. It is certainly well for the patient to avoid all physical and mental excitement, but careful and slow exercise in the open air cannot do any hurt, less, at any rate than to constantly be lying down. If this practice is excusable in the case of weakly, nervous individuals, it is certainly inexcusable in the case of plethoric, robust and quick persons. Nor can a scanty, not very nourishing diet be adopted as a rule, for in anæmia we are called upon to improve the composition of the blood by a suitable mode of living; whereas truly robust women are benefitted by a sort of starvation-cure, because they are tormented by a voracious appetite during the first months of their pregnancy. Of greater importance than all these details is the clothing of pregnant females. As a matter of course every tight-fitting garment should be avoided; if it does not directly interfere with the portal circulation, it certainly interferes with the oxygenation of the blood in the lungs. This point, generally speaking, is not sufficiently heeded. Moreover, the strictest abstemiousness is indispensable from the moment that conception has become an established fact. The use of coffee should likewise be forbidden in the strictest manner. It is much more difficult to prevent the vomiting which, on account of the extraordinary strain on the abdominal muscles which the vomiting occasions may easily give rise to obstructions of the circulation. As yet we have no remedy that can be regarded as specific against the vomiting of pregnant females, and it is difficult enough in any given case to select a remedy, for the reason that all cases look so very much alike. All we can do is to experiment, and to give *Belladonna, Iodium, Veratrum, Cuprum, Pulsatilla* and *Sepia*, the choice of any special remedy, being of course determined by the constitution, the accessory symptoms, etc. By employing these prophylactic means we often succeed in carrying the patient through the full term of pregnancy. Of course we cannot promise success in every case.

The treatment of a miscarriage begins with the commencement of the hemorrhage and the uterine contractions. In almost every case where the appearance of the blood is the first morbid symptom, Sabina will prove the right remedy, whether pains are present or not. We have often succeeded in arresting with this remedy an uterine hemorrhage that had already become very copious. We doubt whether any other medicine will act more promptly and satisfactorily at this period. Belladonna ranks next to Sabina. It is indicated, if the hemorrhage commences with violent colicky pains and a sensation in the pelvis as if pressure were made from above downwards, and as if the sexual organs would be pressed out; at the same time there is a good deal of vascular excitement. *Opium* is recommended, if a miscarriage is threatened in consequence of fright.

If the hemorrhage is preceded for some time by distinct labor-pains, Pulsatilla, Belladonna, Secale cornutum may be tried in order to arrest the contractions if possible. If the patients are feeble, with worn-out constitutions, and the blood has begun to flow, *Secale cornutum* is preferable to Sabina. *Crocus* is seldom appropriate at the commencement of the hemorrhage. The cases where the miscarriage is caused by the premature death of the fœtus, may not require any medicinal aid previous to the setting in of the hemorrhage, when Secale will most likely prove the most suitable remedy.

If the above-mentioned remedies do not prevent the miscarriage, and if the os-tincæ dilate more and more, it is advisable not to give too powerful doses, and to calmly await the period when the fœtus will be expelled; for this event can probably only be hastened by manual interference; it is moreover very questionable whether at this period the hemorrhage can be modified by internal treatment.

After the expulsion of the fœtus most of the above-mentioned remedies that have been recommended for simple metrorrhagia, come into play, especially: *Sabina, Belladonna, Crocus, Secale, Ipecacuanha, Chamomilla, China, Hyoscyamus.*

Although we do not believe that a miscarriage can be prevented by keeping the patient all the time in a horizontal posture, yet this posture becomes indispensable as soon as the hemorrhage has commenced. Even after the hemorrhage has been arrested, the patient should be kept quietly on her back for a couple of days. If a miscarriage has taken place, the patients will have to be treated like women in confinement, even with more care, for a return of the hemorrhage, metritis, prolapsus of the uterus are apt to take place. Above all we have to make sure that no fragments of the fœtus have remained in the uterus; the worst consequences of the miscarriage are sometimes caused by such an oversight.

[Besides the medicines recommended by Bæhr for the arrest of uterine hemorrhage and the prevention of a miscarriage, we often make use of the following with perfect success:

Aconitum, if the pulse is full and bounding, the patient experiences a sensation of fulness and heaviness in the uterine region, and drops of blood have already begun to trickle down. We give the lower potencies. In active uterine hemorrhages caused by a sudden concussion, a violent strain, or subsequent to the expulsion of the fœtus, Aconite may likewise help to arrest the hemorrhage. The pulse is full and bounding or else the opposite, the patient complains of headache, the cheeks are flushed, the skin is warm and dry or else cold and covered with a clammy perspiration; the action of the heart is often disturbed, there is a tremulous fluttering of the heart, less frequently tumultuous beating.

Erigeron canadense, an alcoholic solution of the oil, often helps in uterine hemorrhage, if the blood is lumpy and dark-colored.

Trillium pendulum is likewise much used both in the form of an alcoholic tincture and watery infusion. Small doses will not answer.

Hamamelis virg. has been used with much success in passive venous and likewise in the more active form of arterial hemorrhage.

Hemorrhages brought on by mechanical concussions of the uterine region, blows, a fall, etc., require the use of *Arnica*, lower potencies, sometimes in alternation with Aconite. H.]

7. Carcinoma Uteri,
Cancer of the Uterus.

In by far the majority of cases this disease occurs beyond the age of forty, and is very seldom met with in women of a less advanced age. Its origin cannot be accounted for upon well established principles; feeble as well as robust, married as well as unmarried women are attacked by this terrible destroyer. Cancer of the uterus is one of the most frequently occurring forms of carcinoma, and not unfrequently runs its course as a solitary cancer. It is only in rare cases that it breaks out in addition to cancerous degenerations of other organs.

The most ordinary form is medullary cancer, whereas scirrhus and alveolar cancer are very rare; epithelial cancer is a little more frequent. The medullary cancer usually commences at the vaginal portion of the uterus as a very firm, rugged infiltration, whence it spreads to the fundus and to adjoining organs, especially the bladder and rectum. The less firmness it possesses, the sooner it becomes converted into pus or ichor, in consequence of which enormous destructions of tissue may take place. Epithelial cancer always commences with cauliflower-excrescences at the os tincæ so that these excrescences seem to have taken the place of the os, or at any rate coalesce with it. The excrescences seem to grow out of the papillæ of the os; at first they resemble condylomata and afterwards sprout like a fungus, with marked vascular development. As the fungoid growth increases, the elements of epithelial cancer unite with the former and the mass decays and changes to ichor. It is not certain whether these excrescences are really carcinomatous at the outset; at any rate, the fact, that they have been successfully extirpated, throws doubt on the correctness of the cancer-hypothesis.

Hartmann relates a form of disease the carcinomatous nature of which is doubtful, we mean the phagedænic ulcer of the uterus. It likewise emanates from the vaginal portion, but the ulcerative process is not preceded by the deposition of a firm, pseudo-plastic layer or infiltration; the uterine tissue surrounding the ulceration is sound, or else softened, yellow or reddish-brown. The disorganization may gradually spread to the walls of the uterus and vagina, to the rectum, bladder and peritoneum.

Carcinoma of the uterus is frequently mistaken at the commencement for menstrual disorder, leucorrhœa or chronic metritis. The first symptoms usually are menstrual derangements, cessation or a more frequent return of the menses, or in the place of the menses we have irregular hemorrhages and leucorrhœa. The mistake is made the more easily if the patient has not yet reached the critical period, so that these changes may be set down as results of a physiological cessation of the catamenial secretion. If the patient has passed through the critical period, a sudden flow of blood takes place, at first resembling the menstrual flow, but soon increasing to a true hemorrhage. In the beginning the patient often complains only of a feeling of weight, drawing in the pelvis, a pressing towards the sexual organs, or the pains are excited by bodily motion, a concussion, sexual intercourse, touch. An examination shows the vaginal portion harder than in the normal condition, of unequal resistance, swollen, misshapen, rugged and knotty, sensitive to pressure and readily bleeding; the lips of the os tincæ look puffy and notched, the os is patulous. In the course of the disease pains set in, which are at first vague and occur only now and then, but afterwards become more severe and finally, especially at night, exceedingly violent, pressing, stinging, lancinating, burning, not confined to the region of the uterus, but spreading to the small of the back and thighs. Characteristic are the more or less violent burning and stinging-boring pains over the pubic bones and in the small of the back, along the hips and thighs, interfering with walking and even sitting; very often a burning pain is continually felt deep in the pelvis, accompanied by fugitive stitches darting through the uterus. The neighboring lymphatic glands are generally infiltrated and painful. At the beginning of the trouble a serous or slimy secretion flows from the vagina, having but little smell; more usually the discharge is copious, of a brownish-red, suspicious-looking color, having a horrid smell and excoriating the skin. The bleeding becomes more and more frequent and copious, the blood being mixed with detached portions of tissue. These hemorrhages consume the strength of the patient in a very short time. At this stage of the disease the ichorous dissolution of the carcinoma progresses very rapidly. An examination reveals the funnel-shaped ulcer and the soft, readily-bleeding excrescences; the vagina likewise is often very much narrowed by the cancerous infiltration. The patients show the imprint of the carcinomatous cachexia, together with the symptoms of a high grade of anæmia. The disease generally lasts for years, calculating from the first manifestation of distinct symptoms, and without allowing for the influence of special circumstances, such as confinement, which is one of the most pernicious occurrences that can happen to a woman afflicted with cancer of the womb. It is inconceivable how it is possible for the organism to bear up for so long a time under a destructive malady like cancer, without perishing.

Cauliflower-excrescences seldom beget symptoms different from those of carcinoma, and the pains are equally intense. On the other hand, however, life is less rapidly destroyed by the former, because they are not so speedily converted into ichor, and the destruction of tissue does not spread so far. Hemorrhages take place more readily from cauliflower-excrescences than from carcinoma.

Treatment. No more than we reject the possibility of a cure of carcinoma generally, do we believe that carcinoma of the uterus is an incurable disease, although it is difficult to obtain certainty in this respect. A cure is only possible as long as the carcinoma has not spread too far, and has not yet become converted into ichor. In such a case the diagnosis is still uncertain, for sensitiveness and an uneven swelling of the os tincæ do not constitute carcinoma; even a fetid discharge from the vagina does not settle the diagnosis. In the stage of dissolution every attempt at a radical cure is unsuccessful, and all we can do is to mitigate the patient's distress.

A number of remedies have been indicated for carcinoma of the uterus, that have only a partial affinity to this disease, and are, for the most part, suitable only for the various accessory affections accompanying the cancerous destroyer. An enumeration of all these remedies would only lead to confusion; hence we only mention those that can be employed against cancer generally. Our first remedy is:

Kreosotum. Kurtz recommends this remedy when the following symptoms are present: Obstinate leucorrhœa during frequently recurring metrorrhagias, with aching or pressing pains and a gradually appearing fetid discharge of a serous fluid or a bloody ichor. This is attended with burning or lancinating pains in the small of the back and loins. When standing she experiences a sensation as of a weight in the pelvis; coition is painful; all the symptoms are worse at the time of the menses. On examination the vagina is found hot, the interstices of the mucous lining enlarged, the follicles are hypertrophied, the vaginal portion of the uterus is swollen, hard, the os tincæ is garnished with small, wart-shaped or bunchy cauliflower-excrescences. Hartmann describes the following group of symptoms: Electrical stitches in the vagina, as if proceeding from the abdomen, causing the patient to start; voluptuous itching in the vagina, with burning and swelling of the external and internal labia; hard nodosities at the cervix uteri; ulcerative pain during coition; the menses appear from four to ten days too soon, and continue for days, with discharge of a dark, coagulated blood, pains in the small of the back and subsequent discharge of a pungent and bloody ichor; gnawing, itching and smarting in the parts; the menses stop for hours and days, but afterwards return again in a more fluid form and attended with violent colicky pains. The pressing downwards and the abdominal spasms continue after the menses, more especially in the groin and pelvic region; bleeding from the uterus and a continual corrosive leucorrhœa are not wanting. The pains are worse at night. Sensation of fainting on rising, with a peevish and desponding mood, and livid complexion. Kurtz describes cauliflower-excrescences, Hartmann true carcinoma. Of the former several cases of cure are reported in our books, of the latter not any, or at least only palliative results. It is certain that Creosotum has not answered the expectations that Wahle's recommendation had excited in our minds. A weak local application of Creosote often does more good than the internal use of the drug.

Arsenicum album has been given with excellent success in carcinoma uteri not so much on account of the specific action of Arsenic upon the sexual organs, which is rather inconsiderable and hence devoid of any marked significance, as on account of the remarkable correspondence of Arsenic with the general phenomena of a carcinomatous dyscrasia. Arsenic can only be resorted to after the whole organism reflects the picture of a cancerous disease. However, it only palliates the severe pains and the sleeplessness, and perhaps modifies the profuse metrorrhagia, which occurs every now and then in the course of the disease.

Nitri acidum is symptomatically indicated in carcinoma uteri, as it is in many other inveterate dyscrasic conditions of the organism. The most important symptoms are: Irregular menses, they sometimes remain suspended for weeks and then appear again at short intervals; between the menses copious leucorrhœa of a badly-colored, brownish appearance and offensive odor. The patient looks worn, feels nervous and is depressed in spirits. Obstructions in the portal circulation, such as hemorrhoids, indicate this drug. Acidum nitricum can, however, only be used as an intercurrent remedy at the commencement of the disease; if ichorous dissolution has commenced, this drug is no longer of any use.

Graphites. The local symptoms of this drug point to carcinoma uteri not any more than those of Arsenic. Out of respect for Wahle, who recommends this drug, we give the symptoms to which, according to Wahle and Hartmann, this drug corresponds: The vagina is hot and painful; swelling of the lymphatic glands, some of which are as large as small hazel-nuts; the neck of the uterus is hard and swollen, on its left side there are three hard little nodes of various sizes and consisting of several detached tubercles which cause an acute pain and have the appearance as if they might be converted into cauliflower-excrescences; when rising, sensation of a heavy weight deep in the abdomen, with an increase of the pains and great weakness and trembling of the lower extremities; at the time of the menses, which appear every six weeks, the pains are worse, shortly previous to, and during the menses; the blood is black, lumpy and smells very strongly; constant complaint as if a lump of lead were lying in her abdomen, with violent lancinating stitches in the uterus, darting into the thighs like electric currents; the pains are always burning and lancing; frequent lancinating stitches in the uterus, darting into the thighs; not much appetite; constipation from two to four days, followed by stool with much pressing; livid complexion; frequent chilliness, without any subsequent heat or sweat; feels sad, anxious, desponding; pulse frequent and hard.

Conium maculatum is powerfully related to the female organs, but has no specific affinity to carcinoma; the menses are very much diminished, nor has it any hemorrhage from the uterus. We do not see why Conium should be so universally recommended for carcinoma uteri; moreover, there is not a single case on record substantiating the curative virtues of Conium in this disease. It can at most only be used at the beginning, when the diagnosis is still uncertain.

Nor do we see upon what grounds many other remedies have been recommended for carcinoma uteri, *Thuya occidentalis* for instance, which is recommended simply on account of the wart-shaped excrescences, or *Iodium, Carbo animalis, Aurum, Silicea, Sabina*, etc. *Sepia* may perhaps do some good in this disease.

If we expect these medicines will modify the morbid process to some extent, we shall soon find that their influence is uncertain and questionable. For the hemorrhage which is one of the most dangerous incidental symptoms of uterine cancer, we refer to the remedies that have been recommended for menorrhagia and metrorrhagia.

The conduct of the patients, outside of the use of medicines, is of the utmost importance. Their anæmic appearance renders a highly nutritious diet indispensable, perfect cleanliness is likewise needful to their comfort; nor should injections of water into the vagina ever be omitted. [The use of disinfectants in this disease is indispensable; one of the best disinfecting agents is the Permanganate of Potassa to which attention has already been called when speaking of stomatitis and scurvy of the gums. H.]

8. Various Morbid Conditions in the Sexual System of the Female.

Climaxis, Critical Age, Change of Life. The physiological involution of the uterus or the cessation of the faculty of conceiving is attended in almost every woman with more or less marked derangements which, however, cannot be regarded as morbid conditions any more than the ailments announcing or accompanying the appearance of the menses. If the derangements alluded to are disproportionately severe and troublesome, we have of course to regard them as morbid affections requiring medicinal aid. A common complaint at the critical age is the flooding. Before interfering medicinally, it is always best to first inquire whether it is a disease. This question is best determined by the general health of the patient; if this is not impaired by the flooding, medical treatment is not called for. We often see robust women lose a quantity of blood at intervals of six to sixteen weeks and longer, but instead of being made sick by such losses, they get, on the contrary, rid of all sorts of congestive symptoms by which they had been tormented heretofore. Other women, on the contrary, after such flooding exhibit signs of extreme debility and anæmia, which shows that the loss of blood is not a normal physiological phenomenon. The loss of blood may always be said to be abnormal if it occurs more frequently than the menses. The proper remedies are pointed out in the chapters on Menstrual Irregularities and Metrorrhagia.

Other abnormal conditions may arise from the disturbances caused by stasis of the blood. As a matter of course, the organism, after the naturul cessation of the menstrual flow, has gradually to restore the equilibrium of the circulation, and we seldom meet with a woman in whom this restoration takes place without any signs of disturbance. It is most frequently the abdominal organs that suffer, first the liver, next the stomach and kidneys; piles not unfrequently make their appearance. The principal remedies for these derangements are: *Sepia, Belladonna, Lycopodium, Nux vomica* and *Sulphur*. The heart, lungs or head are less frequently affected by these congestions, for which Hartmann recommends *Crocus*. As a rule the remedies for these congestions are the same as those recommended for hyperæmia of the brain, [more especially *Aconite, Veratrum viride* and *Cimicifuga racemosa*. For the sudden flashes of heat to which such patients are liable, we recommend beside the remedies that are usually resorted to, such as Sepia, Sanguinaria, etc., *Veratrum vir.*

and *Cimicifuga*. For congestions of the heart, *Aconite*, *Digitalis* and *Cactus* may be required. H.]

Prolapsus uteri, which is always more or less occasioned by a relaxation of the vaginal mucous lining, can scarcely ever be cured by the exclusive use of internal remedies, and it would be wrong to expect such a result without at the same time resorting to mechanical means. Hartmann recommends as adapted to such conditions: *Arnica*, *Mercurius*, *Nux vomica*, *Sepia*, *Belladonna*, *Aurum* and *Calcarea carbonica;* we confess, however, that we have never seen the least curative effect from any of these remedies. [*Cimicifuga*, *Hamamelis* and *Helonias* are employed with more or less success, most generally in connection with pessaries and supporters. H.]

Sterility depends upon the most diversified conditions of the system. Most commonly it is due to a disharmonious degree of excitability in the man and woman. Generally this want of harmony is owing to the dissolute life which the man may have led before his marriage, and by which he may have reduced his sexual powers below the point of normal action. It may likewise be the woman's fault, if she had indulged in self-abuse. In such cases medicines are of very little use, whereas proper hygienic rules may accomplish a great deal of good. Above all things sexual intercourse should be indulged in very moderately. If the woman is really suffering, her troubles will have to be met by appropriate medicinal treatment. Hartmann has the following brief advice: If the sterility is caused by an excess of sexual passion on the part of the woman, *Platina* and *Phosphorus* are the most promising remedies. If the menses are suppressed, we give *Conium maculatum;* if they are too profuse, *Mercurius*, and at the same time too early: *Natrum muriaticum*, *Calcarea carbonica*, *Acidum sulphuricum*, *Sulphur;* if the menses delay: *Graphites* and *Consticum;* if they are too scanty: *Ammonium carbonicum*. If husband and wife meet normally, and no conception takes place, Hartmann advises them to take frequent doses of *Sabina* or *Cannabis*. So far as we know, no particular results have been obtained by this treatment, and we doubt very much whether the remedies which Hartmann advises can do much good. On the contrary, in our opinion the remedies for menstrual irregularities or for the other morbid conditions of the sexual organs, ought to be resorted to in treating sterility. This defect can only be removed, if both husband and wife endeavor to avoid with scrupulous care every thing that might have a tendency to prevent conception.

Pruritus vulvæ, itching of the pudendum, is symptomatic of many more or less acute diseases of the sexual organs, likewise at the commencement of pregnancy, both among young women as well as among those who are of a more advanced age; very commonly it precedes the appearance of the menses for a few days. Under such circumstances the trouble is not so very distressing, and does not require any special treatment. The real pruritus is generally met with among older females shortly before and after the critical cessation of the menses, more especially if they are unmarried. In their case the itching is horrid, deprives them of sleep and causes a variety of nervous ailments; yet an inspection does not reveal any abnormal symptoms, except perhaps a greater dryness of the vaginal mucous membrane. The trouble often continues unceasingly for months. Most commonly, however, such individuals are affected with hemorrhoidal swellings, and the idea suggests itself that the itching may perhaps be caused by an engorged condition of the veins in the vagina. Among the remedies for this inconvenience *Caladium seguinum* is the most certain and efficacious, as we are able to assert from personal experience. Moreover, we may derive benefit from *Conium maculatum*, *Lycopodium*, *Platina* and *Sepia*. [If the parts are very much swollen and engorged with blood, and the itching and burning are very great, we have have given with perfect relief *Aconite* and *Belladonna* in alternation; sometimes we have derived benefit from the external use of *Hamamelis*. If an inspection through a glass reveals the presence of a fine fungoid herpes on the parts, we use a weak solution of the Sulphite of Soda as an external application. One of Dr. Dewee's favorite local applications was a solution of *Biborate of Soda*. Injections of dilute cider-vinegar are also resorted to. H.]

[*Neuralgia of the Uterus*. Although this affection has been variously alluded to in the different chapters on menstrual irregularities, yet we deem it useful and expedient to transfer the following more compact picture of this disease from Kafka to our pages:

Neuralgia of the uterus consists in a variety of painful sensations in the uterus, previous to, or at the commencement or during the course of the catamenial discharge.

As long as these pains are not excessive, we designate this condition as painful or difficult menstruation. If the pains reach a high degree of intensity, they become colicky, and we describe them as menstrual colic.

If these pains appear between the menstrual periods, they constitute a peculiar form of uterine neuralgia which we shall discuss presently.

Pains in the uterus before or during the menses attack more especially individuals of sensitive or very irritable dispositions, girls as well as women whose uterus had become very irritable partly through psychical and partly through external causes. Amorous fancies, the reading of love-stories, slippery conversation, voluptuous dreams, etc., are just as frequently the causes of painful menstruation as a libidinous rubbing of the parts, amorous dallying, onanism, etc. All these causes keep up a constant irritation in the uterus, the consequences of which are congestion or nervous erethism of this organ.

Uterine neuralgia between the menstrual periods may be caused by catarrhal metritis, especially after confinement with slow or imperfect return of the uterus to its normal condition, chronic infarctions, displacements and flexions of the uterus, protracted lactation, excessive coition as in the case of newly married persons or prostitutes.

Previous to or during the menstrual period the pains set in either in a mild form or with much vehemence. In the former case the pains are at times tearing, at other times cutting, or drawing, pressing, contracting, griping, burning; they are mostly experienced in the region above the symphisis pubis, are either fixed or wandering, and are sometimes felt in the uterus, at other times in the vagina, or at the entrance of the vagina, in the rectum, bladder, and not unfrequently assume the form of labor-pains.

If the pains set in with a great deal of vehemence, they act like colic; they are most generally contracting, tearing, griping or clawing, spread from the umbilical region to the uterus, the vagina, urethra, the anterior surface of the thigh, the small of the back or over the entire hypogastrium, not unfrequently causing a sensation of burning in the parts where the pain is felt. When the pains reach the acme of intensity, females with sensitive temperaments are not unfrequently attacked with nausea or even bilious vomiting; their features look collapsed and the extremities are cold. In other cases, especially if the patients are of a plethoric habit, the cheeks become flushed, the temperature of the body is increased, the pulse is accelerated, the thirst intense, with a longing for acidulated drinks. If vaginal blennorrhœa is present, these phenomena frequently denote a condition like catarrhal metritis which not unfrequently becomes aggravated before or during the menstrual flow.

In case of chronic engorgements or displacements of the uterus pains are not always present, but the neuralgic affection manifests itself in the form of disagreeable sensations such as weakness, languor and pressing towards the small of the back or thighs, patulous condition of the vulva with sensation as if the pelvic viscera would press out. These uncomfortable sensations are sometimes accompanied by frequent but ineffectual urging to stool, frequent desire to urinate with scanty emission of urine.

The pains are sometimes so trifling that they are not even noticed by the patients. The colicky pains are always very penetrating and distressing, and sometimes last for hours and even days.

The pains are often accompanied by other derangements that are of sufficient importance not to be overlooked. At one time it is a pain in the temporal region, on one side of the head, or a pressive pain in the vertex or occiput sometimes increasing to an intolerable degree of intensity; at other times spasmodic muscular contractions are experienced in the œsophagus or larynx, sometimes taking the shape of globus hystericus, laryngismus or aphonia; again, symptoms of dyspnœa with oppression of the chest and increased or unrhythmical palpitations of the heart set in; at other times the patients complain of dyspepsia with accumulation of gas in the bowels, muscular weakness especially of the lower extremities, aggravated by the least exertion; then again we notice symptoms of reflex-action in the sympathic range taking the form of spasmodic weeping or laughing; or the spinal nerves are consensually affected giving rise to convulsions. In many cases the sensorium is disturbed in consequence of reflex-action, resulting in loud and loquacious delirium and even ecstatic conditions. At the same time the menses are either excessively profuse or very much diminished.

The prognosis of uterine neuralgia is generally favorable; if depending upon structural lesions or displacements of the uterus, it is doubtful. In obstinate cases of this kind the age of the patient determines the chances of a successful treatment; if the critical age is near at hand, a speedy cessation of their troubles may be safely promised all such patients; experience has taught us that with the cessation of menstruation the uterine pains disappear.

Beside the remedies that we have recommended for the various forms of menstrual irregularities, more especially for difficult and painful menstruation, we derive particular benefit in these neuralgic affections of the uterus from:

Aconitum, lower and middle potencies;
Gelseminum, generally if given in tolerably large doses;
Cimicifuga racemosa, likewise to be given in reasonably large doses;

Magnesia muriatica, lower and middle attenuations;
Hypericum perfoliatum, lower attenuations.

Aconite is generally indicated by a throbbing or pecking pain in the uterus, sensation of fulness, heat, or a hard aching and seated pain in the uterus, nausea, headache, palpitation of the heart. If Aconite does not relieve,

Cimicifuga may be given, more especially if the symptoms, for which this remedy has been recommended when occurring at the critical age, are present, such as headache at the top of the head, chilliness with flashes of heat, etc.

Gelseminum. We are not aware that this medicine has been much used in uterine neuralgic affections of the womb, except in so far as they are symptomatic of menstrual disorders, dysmenorrhœa, etc., or in so far as they occur in child-birth. The neuralgic pains, to which both Aconite and Gelseminum are homœopathic, are most generally, though not necessarily, attended with signs of vascular engorgement. These two remedies are very often given in alternation with great benefit to the patient.

Magnesia muriatica has shown good curative effects in purely spasmodic affections of the uterus.

Hypericum perfoliatum. Violent tearing in the genital organs, with desire to urinate; tension in the region of the uterus as from a tight bandage; the menses delay in such a case.

If neuralgia of the uterus is a secondary affection, depending upon other primary pathological conditions of the uterus, prolapsus, anteversion, retroversion, lateral displacements, flexures, etc., these causes have to be removed before a cure can be thought of. Chronic engorgements, in connection with neuralgia, may require *Belladonna, Veratrum viride, Aconite, Mercurius sol.,* etc. Subcutaneous injections of Morphia and Atropine have relieved the most obstinate cases of uterine neuralgia. H.]

9. Vaginodynia.
Neuralgia of the Vagina.

We extract from Kafka the following notice of this subject: The mucous membrane of the vagina is neither swollen nor hyperæmic, its secretion is not increased, its appearance unaltered. This disease is either a local affection of the vagina, or else it is complicated with uterine neuralgia. It may be caused by lascivious fancies, masturbation, abuse of sexual intercourse which is only partially gratified; discharge of an acrid, corrosive secretion from the uterus, irritating pessaries, ascarides in the vagina, dust in the uterus, displacements of this organ, etc.

The symptoms are in part local, and in part general. Among the local symptoms we notice a peculiar itching or tickling of the vagina of various degrees of intensity. If not excessive, this titillation of the vagina can be borne; it does not excite the sexual passion, or at least very triflingly; it causes a slight sensation of warmth in the vagina and an irresistible urging to scratch or rub the itching parts of the vulva or vagina, which generally causes a redness of the mucous membrane and an increase of the temperature. In proportion as the warmth of the itching parts increases, they likewise become affected with a striking dryness, which is very troublesome to the patients.

In sensitive and excitable women the sexual passion is first excited by the frequent rubbing of the vulva or vagina; at such a time the eyes glisten, the cheeks look flushed, the head is hot. If the rubbing is continued, a pleasurable sensation is excited, which continues until a seminal vesicle is detached after which the person feels exhausted, the face looks pale and a certain moroseness or sullenness of temper prevails.

An observing physician is not slow to observe these changes in the looks and mood of his patient. They constitute important phenomena in the case of young girls whose sexual passion could not properly be made the subject of professional inquiry.

The titillation in the vagina may become so violent that it may rouse an irresistible desire for sexual intercourse, and may even lead to self-abuse. In one case of this kind, an examination showed that the titillation was excited and kept up by retroversion of the uterus. Excitable, generally sterile women of feeble constitutions, lose their seminal fluid during a paroxysm of titillation, without resorting to friction; others become nymphomaniac and may even go so far as to invite men to sexual converse. Other women experience at the same time violent pains in the uterus, heat in the vagina, an increased secretion of mucus and a high degree of nervous erethism and hysteric irritability of temper, sometimes extending to the sensorium and resulting in delirium or hallucinations.

Sometimes the titillation and the sexual excitement are entirely absent, and the vagina is in a condition of hyperæsthesia. Coition is exceedingly painful; even a digital exploration causes pain, the vagina contracting spasmodically around the finger. Such women generally remain sterile.

These spasmodic contractions may even spread to the urethra and rectum, causing a continual urging to urinate and to evacuate the bowels. Vaginodynia often lasts for years and is very difficult to cure. Cases depending upon displacements of the uterus, are the most obstinate.

Treatment. In order to obtain perfect certainty regarding the true nature of the disease, an ocular and manual examination of the vagina is indispensable.

For simple itching, without any simultaneous excitement of the sexual passion, we give *Sulphur* and *Graphites*, the former if the itching is more of a burning nature, the latter if the itching is attended with a smarting sensation in the vagina.

The troublesome feeling of dryness in the vagina is relieved by frictions with the best kind of olive-oil. If this is not sufficient, and the vagina is cool and pale, we give *Natrum muriaticum* 6 to 30. If there is much heat and redness, we give *Belladonna* 3.

If the titillation in the vagina is attended with lascivious desires, and there is a good deal of nervous erethism, pain in the uterus, meteorism, torpor of the bowels, *Nux vomica* is the remedy. *Cannabis indica* 3 is likewise excellent under such circumstances, likewise if there is a good deal of urging to urinate, burning during urination, and the vaginal lining membrane is hot and dry.

Calcarea carbonica may be given in alternation with, or after Nux vomica.

Zincum met., if the titillation occurs during the menstrual flow; *Mercurius sol.*, if the itching is confined to the labia and the entrance to the vagina.

If symptoms of nymphomania are present, we may give *Nux vomica*, *Platina*, *Zincum met.*, also *Stramonium* and *Hyoscyamus*.

If the titillation in the vagina arises from dust in the vagina, we may resort to tepid Sitz-baths, also to injections of tepid water, castile soap and water, a weak solution of the Sulphite of Soda.

For the itching caused by ascarides, see Helminthiasis.

For painfulness of the vagina during intercourse we give *Ferrum acet.* 3 to 6, also *Ferrum muriat.* 3 to 6.

If the itching is attended with aversion to sexual intercourse, *Phosphorus* is a good remedy.

[Vaginismus must not be confounded with the neuralgic condition of the vagina described in the preceding paragraph. Vaginismus is a spasmodic contraction of the vaginal sphincter which, so far as we know, is beyond the reach of internal treatment. Dr.

Thomas, in his recent work entitled: "A Practical Treatise on the Diseases of Women," informs us that this disease was first described by Burns, who advised an operation which is at present regarded as the only reliable method of cure. This operation has been recently performed by one of our own most brilliant surgeons, William Tod Helmuth, of St. Louis. According to Dr. Thomas the causes of vaginal spasm are: The hysterical diathesis; excoriations or fissures at the vulva; irritable tumor of the meatus; chronic metritis or vaginitis; pustular or vesicular eruptions on the vulva; neuromata. For a full description of the disease and its surgical treatment we refer the reader to Dr. Sims' paper upon "Vaginismus," communicated to the London Obstetrical Society, Nov. 6th, 1861, or to Sims' work on Uterine Surgery. H.]

10. Mastitis.
Inflammation of the Breasts.

The mammæ constituting exclusively a part of the female organism, we prefer treating of inflammation of the mammæ in this place instead of ranging this disease among the diseases of the thoracic organs.

Mastitis proper only occurs during or immediately after lactation. The painful, sometimes rather extensive, indurated swellings of single portions of the mammæ, which sometimes occur among unmarried females or married women who are not nursing, especially about the time of the menses, are evidently transitory states of hyperæmia which never terminates in suppuration. The cause of mastitis is always traceable to the impeded excretion of the milk. By some cause or other, soreness or a bad shape of the nipples, too feeble drawing by the child, one or more lactiferous ducts become closed, the milk in the corresponding mammary lobule becomes stagnant, and an inflammatory process is the result. Another cause of obstruction of the milk-ducts is the improper manner in which some women wear their clothes, owing to which the breasts either hang too loosely or a direct pressure is exerted upon them. The doctrine that mastitis can originate in dietetic transgressions or a cold, is a convenient supposition rather than a scientific fact; but to go so far as to assert with Hartmann that mastitis is one of the multifarious manifestations of psora, is more than can be proved by anybody. What happens with other abscesses, is likewise true in regard to abscesses of the mammæ: in some cases they heal rapidly, in other cases they cause vast destructions of tissue. Mastitis is most apt to occur soon after confinement or shortly after weaning the child; mastitis occurring at the latter period is less apt to lead to the formation of abscesses.

Symptoms. The disease never breaks out all at once. Generally women experience some time previous, a gradually increasing pain both spontaneously or while the child is nursing; and a swelling of one or more mammary lobules, which rapidly increases in extent and induration, develops itself soon after. As a rule the lower or lateral lobes are inflamed, very seldom the upper ones, and still less frequently both mammæ. Sooner or later, sometimes in a few days, and at other times in some weeks, the painful spot becomes red and more sensitive, and the inflammation is intense, the whole organism feels the effect of the inflammatory process and shows its sympathy by febrile phenomena. Soon the infiltrated tissue shows the signs of suppuration, the pus being discharged through a small opening. As soon as the discharge, which is never complete, commences, the pain suddenly ceases and the febrile symptoms abate.

The course of the inflammation depends upon a variety of circumstances. If the inflammation is confined to one lobe, the abscess most commonly discharges close to the nipple, empties itself very rapidly and heals. If several lobes are inflamed, or the inflamed lobe is situated near the base, the suppuration, swelling and pain continue for a long time; months and even years may elapse before the abscess heals, which discharges through several openings near the nipple. This disorder never lasts less than two weeks, and, under corresponding circumstances, may continue for months even in its acute form.

The treatment of mastitis includes above everything else a prophylactic treatment which has to be commenced long before confinement, especially in the case of primiparæ. The preservation and proper management of the nipples and of the mammæ generally should be a constant subject of our attention. After confinement, if women do not intend to nurse their children, they will have to dispense with liquids as much as possible. Nursing women have to keep the following points constantly in view: the breasts must not be kept too warm, must not be enclosed in tight clothing, and must, by some suitable support, be prevented from dragging down; every time after the baby has nursed, the nipple must be washed, but not be kept moist between the acts of nursing; the excessive use of liquids which women fancy favor the secretion of milk, must be avoided; the child should be put to the breast as seldom as possible, for the more hungry it is the more vigorously it will draw and the more completely the breast will be emptied. At the same time the nipples will not be held so long in the child's mouth, and they will not be exposed so much to the risk of being made sore by the constant nursing. By following these instructions, and more particularly by putting the child to the breast every two hours in the early period after confinement, mastitis will generally be prevented. By picturing this disease in its most horrid form, women can generally be induced to comply with the course recommended by their physician; his warning counsels in trying to prevent this disease as well as the gastric catarrh of children, are generally more potent than all the medicines of the drug-shops.

If the breasts have become hard and painful, the best remedy in the case of lying-in women is *Bryonia*, less frequently *Belladonna*, whereas the latter medicine is better adapted to women who are weaning their infants. We sometimes succeed in dispersing the stagnation of the milk by gently rubbing the indurated portion while the child is nursing. The same good effect is sometimes obtained by causing the milk to be drawn by an older, more vigorous child. In no event should the infant be all at once kept from the breast, even if nursing causes pain. It is only if the pain is very acute, and the hardness considerable that the infant should no longer be put to the diseased breast. *Belladonna* will now have to be administered. As soon as redness has set in, the chances of scattering the inflammation are very slim; in some exceptional cases we may sometimes succeed in effecting this result by a few doses of *Mercurius*. Warm poultices should never be omitted; they sometimes favor the dispersion of the abscess as much as in other cases they hasten the process of suppuration. It is best not to apply them until pus has begun to form. *Hepar sulphuris* will sometimes promote the discharge of the pus. A great many authorities teach to open the abscess at an early period in order to prevent the further spread of the inflammation. We doubt whether such a proceeding is justified by corresponding results; after opening the abscess we have often seen the inflammation spread much more rapidly; in the most tedious cases of mastitis, the abscess had been opened in accordance with this suggestion. On the contrary, if the abscess was not opened and the above-mentioned remedies were used, we have never seen mastitis run a tedious course. This cannot have been owing to the mildness of the cases; a coincidence of this kind cannot be supposed probable. Most homœopathic physicians avoid the lancing of such abscesses, and yet can boast of excellent results. This shows that their medicines must have an effect which, in such cases, our opponents are doubly disposed to doubt and to deny. We do not mean to say that the abscess should not be opened if the pus is distinctly seen through the skin; what we oppose is the opening of an abscess where the tissues situated below the epidermis have to be divided. In this respect a mammary abscess is to be treated like any other abscess. If the tissues through which the abscess has to discharge, are of a nature to render every effort towards a spontaneous discharge nugatory, they have to be divided with the knife. A case of this kind occurs very rarely under homœopathic treatment.

After the abscess has commenced to discharge, the course of the difficulty is quite different under homœopathic from what it is under allopathic treatment. In a fortnight at latest the discharge of pus ceases under the use of a few doses of *Mercurius*, and the sore heals. If this is not the case, if the hardness and pain continue and the pus is secreted in small quantity; or if the infiltration keeps spreading, and we are called upon at this juncture to treat the disease, *Hepar sulphuris* is to be given first. After using this remedy, the suppuration generally increases and the pain abates. *Phosphorus* deserves a preference if the inflammation frequently reassumes the acute form after an apparent arrest of the inflammatory process; likewise in the very rare cases of phthisis of the mammæ. If the breast has become callous, and fistulous canals have formed, the healing of the sore will prove a very protracted process. In such cases *Silicea*, *Sulphur*, *Conium* and *Graphites* may prove the best remedies.

[Regarding the use of *Aconite* in mastitis, **Kafka** has the following: If the breast swells in consequence of a cold or of a mechanical injury, and a deep-seated pain is experienced in the mammæ, we at once give *Aconite* 3 in solution every hour; the local hyperæmia will most speedily be scattered under the influence of this remedy, and, if the pain was owing to a cold, a general transpiration will speedily take place, after which the inflammation runs a much milder course and often terminates in dispersion without suppuration.

Our poke or the *Phytolacca decandra* has long been used in domestic practice as a remedy for swelling and inflammation of the breasts. We refer the reader to Dr. H..le's notes on this subject in the second edition of his New Remedies, pages 794 and further.

The medicine should be used internally and applied externally by means of a compress soaked with a mixture of a few drops of the tincture in half a tumbler of water, or with a mild infusion or decoction of the root. H.]

11. Mastodynia.

[Kafka writes: Painful sensations in the breasts, not having any causal connection with pregnancy or with the processes of nursing or weaning, and being most frequently noticed in girls and women as symptoms of development at the age of pubescence or as paroxysms of neuralgia, do not unfrequently become the subject of medical treatment.

At the period of pubescence, either some time before or during or after the first appearance of the menses, some girls experience stitching, drawing or throbbing pains, or a tingling or prickling sensation in the swelling breasts which appear turgid and tense and very often sensitive to contact. If the girls have already commenced to menstruate, the painful sensations most commonly make their appearance before or during the menses. If menstruation has not yet commenced, the pains generally continue until the age of pubescence has been reached. Sometimes the breasts are so sensitive that the least touch, the least friction from the underclothes, or the least pressure, are almost unbearable. This sensitiveness extends either over the whole breast or is confined to the region of the nipples.

The sensitiveness lasts for a longer or shorter period according as the development of the organism is more or less rapid. We are acquainted with cases of hyperæsthesia of the breasts that continued until the patients were married, and spread even to other parts of the body, particularly to the region of the stomach, uterus and pudendum.

The breasts are likewise liable to being attacked with pains that are not connected with the period of pubescence, but depend upon mechanical, traumatic or constitutional causes. They attack periodically full-grown girls or women, are seated in the mammary gland or nipples, come on in paroxysms, are lancing, tearing, drawing or boring; they are generally worse about the time of the menses, are aggravated by pressure, and, if lasting a certain time, result in the formation of small tubercles in the mammary gland, of a rounded shape, smooth and of the size of hazelnuts.

Such paroxysms of pain scarcely ever occur spontaneously, and are generally caused by the continued pressure of tight garments, corsets, whalebones, or they are caused by pinching, pulling, contusions, blows, etc. Sometimes they are the result of chlorosis, tuberculosis, carcinoma or constitutional syphilis. Their duration is determined by the continuance of the exciting causes.

In treating these affections the cause has to be removed before anything can be expected from internal treatment.

For simple hyperæsthesia of the breasts *Belladonna* and *Nux vomica* may be given. If the affection can be traced to a delay in the appearance of the menses, *Pulsatilla, Caulophyllum, Belladonna* may be useful. If the pains are stinging and the patients are at the same time very nervous, we give *Calc. carb.* or *Nux vomica*. If caused by a blow, contusion, etc. *Arnica, Conium* or *Sepia* may be required. For tearing pains we give *Conium* 3 or *Baryta carb.* 6, and if seated in the nipples, we give *Bismuth* 6, or *Calc. caust.* 6. Drawing pains in the mammæ require *Kreosote* 3 to 6, and if seated in the nipples *Zinc. met.* 6. For boring pains in the mammæ we give *Indigo* 3 to 6, and if affecting the nipples *Spigelia* 3 to 6. The sensation of prickling in the nipples is relieved by *Sabina* 3 to 6.

If these pains result from constitutional causes we have to direct our treatment against the latter. If traceable to chlorosis, we give *Iron* persistently, in the case of tuberculous patients *Iodine;* if a carcinomatous diathesis is suspected we resort to *Conium* and *Rana bufo;* if syphilis is the cause, we give *Mercurius jodatus* and *Cinnabaris*. At the same time the breasts have to be covered with soft material, and carefully protected against friction, pressure and cold. H.]

12. Carcinoma Mammæ.
Cancer of the Breasts.

Next to the uterus the mammæ are most frequently attacked by cancer. Cancer of the mammæ is most commonly of a primary nature, hence the beginning of the cancerous disease.

The causes of this disease can scarcely ever be determined with certainty. If a blow or a contusion is generally regarded as the cause of this disease, it is probably because no better cause can be found, not because the disease has ever been known to result immediately from such an injury. The influence of depressing emotions which are so easily and so commonly succeeded by cancerous degenerations, is a much more evident source of the cancerous disease. Cancer of the mammæ most commonly occurs between the ages of 40 and 50, about the period which is generally designated as a change of life. Unmarried women or women who have not had children seem to be more liable to it than married women with children. Before and after this period, it is proportionally a rare occurrence.

The most frequently observed form of carcinoma of the mammæ is scirrhus, next to which we range the encephaloid or medullary fungus, the alveolar or colloid cancer and the epithelial cancer or epithelioma.

[Mr. Maurice H. Collis of Dublin, in his work "The Diagnosis and Treatment of Cancer, and the Tumors analogous to it" 1864, has thrown out epithelioma and colloid growths from the true cancer-group. He regards Colloid as a mere variety of fibroid or recurrent tumors. Virchow says that "its stroma differs in its containing mucus and in its gelatinous nature from the ordinary stroma of cancer," page 526, On Tumors. Mr. Collis says, in rejecting epithelioma from the group of cancerous tumors: "Its superficial origin, its slow progress, its indisposition to infiltrate the deeper structures, or to contaminate the glands, the certainty of cure which follows its timely removal, and the different appearance when occupying similar localities, are of sufficient importance to outweigh the points of resemblance which it undoubtedly bears to cancer in its advanced and secondary stages. In its early stage it is strictly an hypertrophy, and in this condition it may remain for an indefinite period. Its second stage is one of hypertrophy and ulceration combined. This stage also, as far as external or cutaneous epithelioma is concerned, is slow to advance into the third or destructive stage, that of infiltration and secondary deposit," page 226. Speaking of Colloid, Virchow writes: "It remains for a very long time local, so that the nearest lymphatic glands often do not become affected until after the lapse of years, and then again the process is for a long time confined to the disease of the lymphatic glands, so that a general outbreak of the disease in all parts of the body does not take place until late, and only in rare instances." (See his work on Tumors, page 531.) H.]

The commencement of the disease is scarcely ever marked by peculiar morbid phenomena; the patients generally do not notice anything out of the way until a tolerably large tumor is perceived in the breast. It is at first round, smooth, movable, grows with more or less rapidity, and loses its mobility in proportion as it increases in size, and its surface becomes more uneven. At first it is most commonly deep-seated and gradually grows towards the surface, is sometimes entirely painless or becomes painful only at the time of the menses and when receiving some mechanical injury. If the cancer reaches the skin, it coalesces with it, after which the pains are almost constantly felt. At the same time the disorganizing process extends to the deeper tissues, and at an early stage the axillary and other neighboring glands become involved. The patients now commence to feel constantly or at intervals, and particularly at night, lancinating, boring pains in the affected part which very soon become unbearable. The assimilative functions begin to suffer; the patients have a pale yellowish-gray appearance, the spirits are very much depressed. A characteristic sign is the gradual effacement and finally the complete retraction of the nipple which discharges either spontaneously or on pressure a turbid, serous fluid. At the place where the cancerous growth first became interwoven with the skin, the latter by slow degrees loses its healthy color, and finally breaks. An irregularly-shaped ulcer forms showing a disposition to penetrate to the subjacent tissues; the edges of the ulcer are infiltrated, have a sickly color and an uneven base, and secrete at first a thin, serous and afterwards an ichorous, purulent, sanguinolent and most commonly very fetid fluid. If the disease runs a slow course, the incipient ulcer often heals for a time, but again breaks open at a later period; if the disease runs a rapid course, spongy and readily-bleeding excrescences are apt to shoot up from the bottom of the sore. If larger vessels become necrosed, hemorrhages take place which are sometimes very profuse, at other times trifling. The further course of the disease which, having arrived at this stage, always terminates fatally, depends upon the extension of the cancer, upon the invasion, by the carcinomatous process, of internal organs, upon the importance of the hemorrhage and upon the loss of fluids in consequence of the ichorous discharge. Medullary fungus generally terminates fatally more speedily than schirrus; the latter may even continue for years before the skin breaks, whereas medullary fungus terminates in ichorous dissolution in a comparatively short period of time.

The duration of the whole disease varies considerably, ranging from two to twelve and even more years. The younger the patient, the sooner she will succomb to the disease, and the more sudden the cancerous growth, the sooner it will destroy life. The prognosis is very bad with scarcely an exception.

Carcinoma Mammæ.

In many respects the diagnosis is liable to difficulties, because various kinds of benign tumors may occur in the breast. An incipient cancer cannot always be recognized as such, though it may grow rapidly and be painful; these two conditions never occur in the case of benign tumors. At a later period the diagnosis is determined by the retraction of the nipple, the fluid which it discharges, the rugged unevenness and immobility of the swelling, the participation of the neighboring glands in the disease, the failing of the whole organism without any increase of the secretory products. Nevertheless there occur many cases of cancer the true nature of which remains for a long time undetermined and is clearly revealed only after the disease has run a long course.

Carcinoma of the mammæ is generally considered a surgical disease; it is supposed by most authors that internal treatment cannot reach it. The disease, at least in its incipiency, is considered purely local, and an operation the only cure. It is as yet difficult to show what method of treatment is the most successful in this disease, but physicians seem to incline more and more to the belief that the extirpation with the knife simply leads to the transfer of the disease to more vital organs, without affecting its general duration. Homœopathic physicians have, for a long time past, rejected every extirpation of cancer as injurious or at least unproductive of good results.

Unfortunately we are unable to affirm that Homœopathy is acquainted with a safe method of healing cancer; at present we are not acquainted with a single undeniable cure of this disease. We are entitled, however, to claim palliative results for our treatment; it never increases the trouble, and delays a fatal termination were it from no other cause than because it does not rob the patient of her strength.

Hartmann mentions a number of remedies for cancer, with a multitude of indications which we do not repeat here because they have seemed to us irrelevant. The remedies which seem to have exerted some influence over this disease, are: *Belladonna, Arsenicum, Carbo animalis* and *vegetabilis, Clematis erecta, Conium maculatum, Sepia,* perhaps also *Sulphur, Kreosotum, Aurum muriaticum* and *Baryta carbonica*. Belladonna only alleviates the pains if they are lancing or burning pains, attended with sub-inflammatory symptoms, and as long as the carcinoma has not become an open sore. Arsenicum likewise is an excellent palliative against the burning pains of cancerous ulcers, especially when worse at night;

this remedy likewise diminishes or even suspends for a time the suppuration and ichorous decomposition. Conium and Clematis, and likewise Baryta can only be used if the tumor has not yet begun to discharge; the other above-mentioned remedies are principally of use in cases of open cancer.

For further symptomatic particulars we refer to Hahnemann's Materia Medica Pura.

Other medicines have been mentioned which, however, do not seem to refer very particularly to carcinoma, such as: *Nitri acidum, Pulsatilla, Bryonia, Phosphorus; Lycopodium, Silicea, Natrum muriaticum* would seem more appropriate.

Most observers agree that the higher attenuations, if given in not too frequently repeated doses, deserve the preference over the lower. Their palliative effect is much more certain and persistent, whereas the lower attenuations sometimes do not seem to palliate at all. We do not mean to induce any one to accede to our views; we would advise, however, if a lower attenuation has not seemed to have any effect to first try a higher one before the medicine is changed.

The diet should be as invigorating as possible in order to sustain the patient's strength; above all the most scrupulous cleanliness has to be observed.

[The *Hydrastis canadensis* has been used by the American Indians as a remedy for cancer. It has likewise been experimented with by American and English homœopathic practitioners, but the results so far have not been very satisfactory. The medicine may be given internally 3d to 6th attenuation, and applied externally in the shape of an ointment or a solution of the resinoid *Hydrastin*. We have used it in some cases of suppurating cancer, with some success; the destruction was arrested in its course, the pain almost ceased and the patients declared they felt comfortable. One of them was an old lady of nearly 80 years, who is still living.

Bæhr's views regarding the propriety of an operation differ so widely from those of Kafka and leading homœopaths in our own midst that we deem it proper to transcribe them: If the methodical use of appropriate remedies for tumors in the breast remains without any result; if in the meanwhile the tumor gains in size, and becomes less movable, and the axillary glands have not yet become involved in the carcinomatous degeneration, we at once advise to proceed to the extirpation of the tumor. Do not wait until the schirrous swelling has become interwoven with the tissue of the skin, or begins to show signs of a more marked carcinomatous degeneration. As yet the process may be regarded as local and the extirpation succeeds perfectly in a majority of cases. If these changes, however, have already taken place and if the axillary glands already begin to show signs of cancerous degeneration, the operation is very doubtful and fails in almost all such cases.

As soon as the tumor has acquired a stony hardness, the skin over it is no longer movable, and the patients are tormented by severe nocturnal pains in the swelling, a cure by internal homœopathic treatment can no longer be thought of. We at least have never succeeded in performing a cure at this stage of the disease.

Even at this stage the extirpation of the tumor is still feasible, but a successful result is already very doubtful. The axillary or mesenteric glands may not yet be involved; but the operation is succeeded by new disorganizations which very speedily terminate fatally in ichorous dissolution. A successful extirpation at this stage has to be attributed to a fortunate coincidence of favorable circumstances which cannot be arranged according to a definite plan. Hence even under these circumstances we are in favor of extirpation for the reason that it does result in a cure in some cases, whereas without it the cancerous disorganization progresses in its course towards an unavoidable fatal destruction of the tissues.

If the above-described phenomena of cancer of the mammæ have set in and ulceration has perhaps taken place, our treatment must remain purely symptomatic. All we can do is to appease as much as possible the nocturnal tormenting pains, to preserve the patient's appetite and strength, to stop the hemorrhage that may set in, to correct the air impregnated with the pestiferous odor of the foul ichor, to arrest the colliquative diarrhœa, etc.

The treatment is conducted as advised by Bæhr. A few additional remedies are recommended such as *China* 3 for extreme debility, or *China* and *Phosphorus* for the stitching pains, *Arsenic*, *Phosphorus* and the *Arsen. of Quinine* for the colliquative diarrhœa; *Acidum sulphuricum* 1 for hemorrhage at the same time applying ice-water externally, or a solution of the Perchloride of Iron, or even touching the bleeding vessel with the real cautery.

The horrid odor may be neutralized to some extent by covering the bottom of the sore with a thick layer of pulverized charcoal which absorbs the ichor; we cause the ulcers to be cleansed several times a day with tepid water, and we have the sick chamber aired and sprinkled with Chlore or Kreosote-water [or with the Permanganate of Potash.] As regards the use of caustics of any kind, after the cancer is fully developed, we have never seen them do the least good, on the contrary they seem to increase the pain and promote the spread of the ulcer.

If the remedies which we use, do not produce the least favorable result, we give the patient *Morphine* from motives of humanity, as the only efficient palliative at our disposal.

Professor Franklin of the St. Louis College of Homœopathy emphatically recommends a speedy extirpation of the cancerous tumor and claims for the operation an almost uniform success provided every vestige of the cancer is removed, and not a single cancer-cell is left behind. H.]

EIGHTH SECTION.

Diseases of the Respiratory Organs.

A. DISEASES OF THE LARYNX AND TRACHEA.

1. Laryngotracheitis Catarrhalis Acuta.
Acute Laryngotracheal Catarrh.

Next to the catarrh of the Schneiderian membrane, a catarrh of the larynx and trachea is one of the most frequent diseases; yet the liability of these organs to catarrhal affections cannot be accounted for either by their structure or functions.

One of the most common causes of disease is a cold, whether it affects the organs locally or through the skin. This is the reason why such people are most commonly affected as have rendered themselves, and more especially the skin, very susceptible by their effeminate mode of living. We often notice that, by keeping the neck too warm, the larynx becomes easily affected with catarrh, whereas such persons fancied that by enveloping their necks in thick cravats or comforters, they were effectually protected against catarrh. Since we cannot avoid frequent exposures of the neck to the air, the susceptibility of the larynx to catarrh increases in proportion as the skin of the neck is stimulated to action by an excess of warm covering. Why some persons should be affected with laryngeal catarrh from the least cold, whereas others seem to enjoy a perfect immunity in this respect, cannot be accounted for. An excessive use of the organs of voice is one of the causes that begets a particular disposition to laryngeal catarrh; individuals who, not accustomed to talking, have had to make long and fatiguing speeches, or amateur-singers are very apt to contract laryngeal disease. The disposition to such diseases is very much enhanced by the excessive use of spirits, and more particularly of the common beer. We shall afterwards speak of the influence which tubercular infiltrations of the lungs exert over catarrhal affections of the

(107)

trachea; we will here state that the development of laryngeal catarrh from the least exposure very properly excites a suspicion of the presence of pulmonary tuberculosis.

Secondarily laryngotracheal catarrh may result from nasal catarrh working down to the larynx, or from bronchial catarrh working upwards. It may likewise supervene during or in consequence of the presence of measles and variola, and other constitutional diseases.

Symptoms and Course. The phenomena of laryngotracheal catarrh vary a great deal according to the intensity of the disease or the sensitiveness of the individual attacked by it. In mild attacks the disease always commences without fever although usually with a peculiar sensation of languor and heaviness in the extremities. The patients complain of a peculiar tickling, or a soreness and burning in the larynx down to the sternum, which is aggravated by coughing and talking. At the same time the voice is altered, it is hoarse and has a peculiarly deeper and metallic sound; this alteration of the voice increases, according to circumstances, to complete hoarseness or loss of voice. In a few hours already a cough supervenes the particular modifications of which will be described in subsequent paragraphs. At first no phlegm is brought up by the cough, afterwards a clear, tenacious, glassy mucus is raised, which, in a few days, assumes a greenish color, becomes lumpy and has an unpleasant taste until, in a few days more, the expectoration assumes a globular shape, becomes more copious and has a yellowish-white color. At the commencement of the catarrh streaks of blood are frequently seen mixed with the mucus; a copious admixture of blood occurs very rarely.

The higher grades of catarrh which are sometimes described as laryngitis, always commence with fever which is sometimes very violent and continues several days. The pains in the larynx are very acute, stinging and burning, as from a sore; aphonia sets in at once, and every attempt at talking increases the pain to an eminent degree. The cough becomes exceedingly distressing, painful, sometimes convulsive, with a constrictive sensation of the rima glottidis and a real difficulty of performing the act of inspiration. The larynx generally feels sore when pressed upon. In two to five days the fever abates, (it scarcely ever lasts longer,) and an expectoration of mucus with relief of the cough sets in. In this form of catarrh the general constitution is more or less disturbed; the patients may even be compelled to keep their beds for some days.

Laryngotracheitis Catarrhalis Acuta.

The laryngotracheitis of children is of particular importance. The children may have seemed quite well during the day, and often wake about midnight with a hoarse, barking cough which is sometimes associated with constricted inspirations and anxiety, so that, at first sight, the little patients seem to have a violent attack of croup; yet this is evidently contradicted by the fact that on the following day their health seems fully restored. The croupy sound seems to arise from the fact that during their sound sleep in the first part of the night, when the children breathe with their mouths open as they do in laryngeal catarrh, the vocal cords become very dry and are covered with a dried-up mucus; on this account the child's cough in the daytime has no croupy sound, nor if it wakes several times in the night. This affection has been designated as catarrhal croup. If, which is less frequently the case, this affection is associated with a marked inflammatory swelling of the laryngeal mucous membrane, or if, generally, the affection acquires a higher grade of intensity, the croupous sound may be heard for several nights in succession, and may be attended with threatening symptoms of dyspnœa. Some children are remarkably liable to an affection of this kind; this liability is still increased by the excessive quantity of clothing in which the little patients are wrapt by their relatives for fear of croup. It is of such children that physicians hear the report they had had several attacks of croup, and that they have an attack every spring and fall. There are physicians who encourage this kind of belief which is hurtful to both the parents and their children.

We have to add a few words concerning the cough which accompanies this affection. Many individuals whose laryngeal mucous membranes are evidently not very susceptible to catarrhal irritations, have no cough in spite of a most severe attack of catarrh, or they cough only once or twice a day. Others, on the contrary, experience even at the onset such a violent and continual irritation and desire to cough that they cough uninterruptedly, or have violent paroxysms of cough which often last four hours and end with an attack of vomiting, or even become associated with a spasm of the glottis. This kind of violent cough is generally peculiar to the catarrh accompanying measles.

The disease lasts at most nine days, but, if the cough is very violent, it rarely ever disappears entirely at the termination of this period. As a rule, while decreasing gradually, it continues for some time after, or, if the patients are again enabled to go out, it often disappears of itself as soon as a steady and mild weather sets in. More frequently the hoarseness continues for a longer time, were it only just enough to interfere with singing, if not with talking. The transition into chronic catarrh is very frequent, and is favored by the circumstance that patients, not minding the trifling disorder, expose themselves to renewed attacks of acute catarrh which finally assumes the chronic form. Laryngotracheal catarrh does not endanger life unless other diseases should supervene as grave complications.

Treatment. This morbid process is not sufficiently important to require a number of remedies. It may be that a rigid individualization of every case may facilitate the cure, but we cannot indulge in the luxury of furnishing so many details. Whatever Hartmann may say to the contrary, we consider a few practical generalizations more adapted to our purpose and shall therefore confine ourselves to mentioning the remedies which experience has pointed out as the most valuable and reliable in this disease.

Nux vomica is suitable in the milder cases that scarcely ever become the subject of a physician's care; the patients complain of a little hoarseness, a burning tickling in the larynx, frequent cough with tickling, scanty expectoration, and especially troublesome early in the morning, a weary and languid feeling, chilliness, frontal headache. In the more violent cases of catarrh, Nux is only useful if, after the fever has begun to abate, the expectoration continues to remain tenacious and hard to raise, and the patient is tormented by a constant titillating hacking cough.

Aconitum is useful in catarrhs caused by exposure to a sharp and keen dry wind. Upon the whole, this remedy does not seem often indicated in simple catarrhal affections, except perhaps in the case of children in whom the febrile symptoms assume a different shape from what they do in the case of full-grown persons. For catarrhal croup it is undoubtedly the best remedy, which, however, ceases to be indicated, if the physician is not called till the second or third day of the disease.

Belladonna may prove most serviceable in the first few days, if the catarrh is associated with fever. The following symptoms are characteristic: fever with disposition to perspire and sleep; violent stinging pains in the larynx; a dry, barking spasmodic cough coming on in paroxysms, exacerbating more particularly in the evening and before midnight; sensation as if dust had been swallowed; feeling of constriction in the larynx; the catarrh is complicated with tonsillitis; aphonia.

Laryngotracheitis Catarrhalis Acuta.

Mercurius acts similarly to Belladonna in this disease. It is suitable at the commencement of febrile laryngitis, if the following symptoms are present: chilliness and great sensitiveness to cold, mingled with frequent paroxysms of a burning heat; dry, distressing cough occurring more particularly at night and racking the frame; the mucous membrane of the mouth and nose is involved in the catarrh; soreness of the larynx, hoarseness but no loss of voice; disposition to copious perspiration.

Next to Aconite, **Spongia** is the principal remedy in the so-called catarrhal croup, with distinct symptoms of œdema of the mucous lining of the glottis. The cough is barking, hoarse, hollow, comes in paroxysms, especially at night, without expectoration and wheezing inspirations. Spongia is likewise appropriate, if the croupous sound of the cough still continues and lumps of a tenacious, yellow mucus are expectorated.

Hepar sulphuris bears a good deal of resemblance to Spongia. It should be given, if mucus commences to be raised, the barking sound of the cough continues, there is a great deal of hoarseness, symptoms of ulceration of the larynx begin to make their appearance, and a constant rattling of mucus is heard in the larynx. It is an excellent remedy for singers and persons who have to talk a great deal.

Hartmann has moreover the following remedies: *Arsenicum*, when there is glowing fever-heat with constant thirst, yawning, stretching, a prostrate feeling in the whole body, tearing-stitching pains in the head and limbs, oppression of breathing; in the night the pains abate with the appearance of perspiration, and return again early in the morning; constant desire to cough, the cough being dry, accompanied by dryness and burning in the larynx. *Pulsatilla:* titillation with cough, excited by a sensation of scraping and roughness in the throat, spasmodic and setting in more especially in the evening and when lying down, better on sitting up, commencing again on lying down, and sometimes increasing to suffocation; chilliness. *Hyoscyamus*, if the cough only occurs at night. *Euphrasia*, if the cough continues all day, and fluent coryza is present at the same time. He likewise mentions *Rhus, Ignatia, Drosera, Ipecacuanha, Bryonia* and others, which will be more fully dwelt upon in the chapter on chronic catarrh of the larynx.

If patients are very much disposed to relapses, prophylactic measures are of the utmost importance; among these the use of cold water and the abandonment of too much covering around the neck occupy the first rank. If tuberculosis lies at the foundation of the disease, the treatment will have to be conducted in accordance with other considerations that will be expounded in the chapter on tuberculosis.

2. Laryngotracheitis Crouposa.
Croup, Membranous Croup.

Croup is an inflammation of the larynx and trachea resulting in a copious exudation upon the mucous membrane, on which account it is also described as angina membranacea. It is only in the present century that the anatomy, cause and course of this disease have been studied with more particular care. Consequently the literature of croup has become very extensive, owing to the importance of a disease which so often terminates fatally.

Croup is almost exclusively a disease of children between the ages of two and seven years, or between the first and second dentition. It occurs even less frequently before the second than after the seventh year; the cases which are said to have occurred among adults are so rare that it is doubtful whether they were genuine croup. Moreover such cases scarcely ever prove fatal, so that the fact of their being croup cannot be confirmed by post-mortem examinations. According to all statistical tables boys are more frequently attacked than girls; from 60 to 70 per cent. of all cases are boys. As regards the influence of constitution and various other points in croup, opinions differ. Rilliet who can in many respects be regarded as an authority in croup, asserts positively that most children who are attacked with croup, are of a lymphatic habit. In this respect he differs from a number of physicians who maintain that robust, well-fed children are most liable to croup. Upon close examination we find however that these two views only differ in appearance. A lymphatic constitution is often disguised under a full habit, bright complexion, appearance of muscular strength; whereas a marked disposition to eczema, to gastric catarrhs, to angina with copious exudation and subsequent hypertrophied swellings, distinctly betray a bad foundation. Hence it is not perfectly healthy and vigorous children that are predisposed to croup, which is still more evident from the following propositions derived from actual experience. Most of the children attacked with croup belong to scrofulous and tuberculous families where croup has been a prevailing disease for several generations. Moreover croup is much more frequent in the country where the ground is level, than in cities, and here again more frequent in the lower strata of the population. We shall show afterwards, however, how in the country so many circumstances combine for the development of tuberculosis, and how similar circumstances prevail among the lower strata of city-population. In this respect we can account for the frequently observed fact that croup is an hereditary disease or that several members of a family are attacked at once or shortly one after the other, or that the same individual is attacked several times in succession. It cannot be denied that if a child has been once attacked with croup, it retains an increased disposition to inflammatory affections of the larynx.

True croup is secondarily met with, although very rarely, as an accompaniment of measles, typhus, tuberculosis. In a case of measles catarrhal croup is easily confounded with true croup; the measle-catarrh is apt to commence with croupy cough which may continue for several days. The croup which is sometimes observed in a case of scarlatina, is something entirely different from true croup; it is a diphtheritic disease the true characteristics of which have already been described in the first volume.

The exciting causes of croup are not always easy to trace. If croup is a very rare disease in warm climates, nor is very frequent in mountainous districts, provided the locality is at a considerable altitude or otherwise well protected: we still are unable to explain by these facts why so many cases of croup occur in one and so few in another year. A northwest or a north wind, or even a sultry and southwest wind with rain, are very apt to bring a good deal of sickness. A district not far from the city of Hanover and situated in front of a range of mountains extending from northwest to southeast, in consequence of which that district is exposed to the winds blowing in a similar direction, is visited every year from March until June by a good many cases of croup and of severe pneumonia among adults. The flat country from Hanover to the North-Sea is similarly circumstanced. The winds blowing in this region of country, must be possessed of a peculiar nature in order to cause extensive epidemics which sometimes snatch away twenty and more children in one village. According to the investigations of latter years, which indeed are still incomplete, it appears as though the amount of ozone in the air acted an important part as one of the causative influences of croup. This is so much more probable since the amount of ozone contained in the air is liable to the greatest variations during the prevalence of abnormal proportions of electricity such as are apt to be caused by a northwest wind. That croup is caused by a simple cold, is much more easily asserted than proven. The same child has many attacks of violent laryngeal catarrh in the course of the year, but is attacked with croup only during the prevalence of a keen blast from the north. The epidemic character of croup likewise shows that there must be other causes at work in its development beside cold or warm weather. That croup is contagious is only believed by those who regard croup and diphtheria as identical.

Symptoms and Course. For a clearer comprehension of the morbid symptoms we here premise a short description of the postmortem appearances. The mucous membrane shows every possible degree of hyperæmia, from the brightest to the darkest color, but only if death takes place after the disease had run a short course; if it lasts a more considerable length of time, the color of the membrane is sometimes strikingly pale. The sub-mucous tissue is usually infiltrated, the mucous membrane itself less frequently, though the infiltration is not considerable; the muscular tissue of the larynx is likewise found swollen and softened. Upon the free surface of the mucous membrane an exudation of fibrinous plasma takes place, at times only in detached spots, at other times covering a large portion and even the whole surface of the larynx and trachea, and dipping down to the bronchial tubes. In few cases only the exudation has the consistence of cream; usually it becomes tough and firm, in which case these characteristics are more marked on the free surface of the membrane than on the surface adhering to the mucous lining. At times it adheres to this lining loosely, at other times very firmly. The thickness of this membranous exudation sometimes exceeds one line, sometimes it only forms a very thin, transparent layer. The formation of a firm, compact cylinder is of rare occurrence; more commonly the exudation adheres to the mucous lining in the shape of patches of various sizes. Sometimes, side by side with firm membranous patches, a portion of the exudation is seen converted into pus or even ichor, or feeble traces of vascularity are observed on the side adhering to the mucous membrane. Very commonly though not regularly, the pharynx is involved in the morbid process, but always only to a limited extent. Less frequently, but not by any means very rarely, the exudative process spreads to the bronchia and the lungs.

In a majority of cases, croup is preceded by a preliminary stage which is, however, not well defined. T" children are less cheerful

Laryngotracheitis Crouposa.

than usual, they cough with a somewhat unusual sound, are somewhat hoarse, with a little roughness in the throat, have slight febrile motions, etc. These symptoms are so trifling that they are most commonly overlooked, if the children are otherwise strong and vigorous. In very rare, or rather in exceptional cases, croup is preceded by a nasal catarrh which, when present, is a tolerably certain guarantee against the possible occurrence of croup; in general, the transition from an ordinary catarrh of the respiratory organs to croup is not often noticed. The precursory symptoms very seldom precede the outbreak of the real disease longer than a day.

This outbreak generally takes place about midnight. After sleeping quietly for a few hours, the children have a few short turns of cough, or sometimes are roused from their sleep by a severe paroxysm. The cough has a sound that is very difficult to describe; it resembles most nearly the bark of a watch-dog; it is a hoarse cough having a metallic ring and is forced out with great vehemence. These peculiar features are so striking, that the very first turn of cough rouses the family from their sleep by its unusually loud and shrill ring. At the same time the voice becomes husky, loses its resonance, and seems labored; the inspirations are somewhat impeded, although not yet to a very high degree, audible, wheezing, and prolonged. This makes the patient restless and anxious. The fever is scarcely ever very high, but the larynx is very frequently sensitive to contact. Sometimes the child falls asleep again after a short turn of cough, and it is only the wheezing inspirations that betray the presence of the terribly threatening danger. In the morning, the little patient may feel quite well, except perhaps a little weak and languid.

Up to this period, croup resembles an ordinary attack of laryngitis so perfectly that it is often impossible to distinguish one from the other. This uncertainty and vagueness of the symptoms may continue during the second and even third night, although the croupy character of the attack becomes more and more marked as the disease progresses on its course. As a rule, the affection presents all its frightful features on the second day, or even at the very outset of the attack. The cough may not become more frequent or violent, but it is less sonorous, more distressing and wheezing, and fills the children with inexpressible agony. As soon as they become aware of the approach of a paroxysm of cough, they raise themselves in their beds, hold on with spasmodic energy to the person near them, or throw themselves about as if convulsed. The agony is still heightened by the gradually increasing difficulty of drawing breath, which is seldom very marked at the commencement of the attack and is particularly striking during the paroxysms of cough. As the dyspnœa increases, the complexion becomes pallid and finally livid, and the face bloats. The pulse increases in frequency and becomes smaller. The little ones seem to suffer more pain than they really do; the children grasp at their throats and pull at their tongues, not so much because they suffer acute pain as because they are so terribly distressed for breath; at any rate touching the larynx does not seem to cause an increase of suffering. The cough and the agony of breathing do not last all the time; between the paroxysms, the patients lie in a state of sopor and utter exhaustion. True intermissions during which the disease seems on the point of leaving and the patients appear cheerful and in apparent health, occur very rarely. Intermissions or remissions generally take place in the morning; they seldom last all day, and still less frequently a day and a night, but are interrupted by renewed attacks of cough and dyspnœa.

If at this stage of the disease the pathological disease should take a favorable turn, the improvement may announce itself quite suddenly by the expectoration, within a short period of time, of large quantities of membranous patches or even of the whole of the cylindrical tube at once. This last-mentioned change occurs very rarely, and even if it does occur, it is not safe to regard the danger as entirely over until at least two days have elapsed without any trace of a renewed exudation having been perceived. In other cases recovery takes place by the gradual absorption and liquefaction of the membrane, the cough becomes moister, a mucous râle is heard in the larynx and trachea, small pieces of membrane and a yellowish tenacious mucus are coughed up, the signs of congestion in the head and face decrease, the pulse rises and the breathing becomes easier. Several days may pass while these changes are going on, before all danger is past; this point remains more particularly doubtful if the children do not bring up any thing and swallow the detached mucus or membranous patches.

If the disease runs an unfavorable course, every symptom steadily and uniformly increases in intensity, or the increase takes place by fits and starts, with remissions such as we have described. The face now exhibits the pallor of death, the eyes gradually lose their lustre and assume a vague and unmeaning expression. The cough now loses all resonance, the very power to force out a single turn of cough seems to be lost. At times the membranes in the trachea are heard to flutter, and their expulsion is momentarily expected. The dyspnœa now reaches its climax, the children are almost driven to frenzy during the paroxysms of cough or the respiration becomes so restricted and superficial that the dyspnœa apparently does not seem to be as violent as it is in reality. Sometimes the paroxysms become so violent that the child suddenly perishes by suffocation. Between the attacks, the coma becomes more and more profound, and the brain seems to participate in the struggle. This phenomenon, however, like the majority of deaths, has to be attributed to the gradual poisoning of the blood by carbonic acid originating in the deficient access of air to the lungs. This likewise accounts for the slow death. No immediate asphyxia taking place, this suffocative stage sometimes lasts forty-eight hours before death takes place.

There is a form of croup which runs its course without the peculiar croupy cough. Here the gradually-growing danger is overlooked, because the dyspnœa increases more uniformly and slowly. This may be owing to the glottis not being contracted or at least in a lesser degree. Sometimes the diagnosis can only be determined with perfect certainty by the expulsion of membranous patches. This form of croup is scarcely less dangerous than the former, only it usually lasts much longer.

The duration of croup depends upon a variety of circumstances. If the intensity of all the symptoms increases steadily, death may take place in thirty-six hours by asphyxia. In most cases the patients die on the fifth or sixth day, seldom later, and exceptionally only after the ninth day. This period does not include the preliminary stage, but dates from the first outset of the disease itself.

The prognosis is in every case very doubtful. Although homœopathy is justly entitled to claim more favorable results in its treatment of croup than any other method has a right to do, yet even under homœopathic treatment croup is one of the most fatal diseases. Moreover the results of any form of treatment are often very much complicated by another circumstance. Membranous croup, especially if a cure only takes place after the dyspnœa had continued for some time, is very apt to be succeeded by dangerous after-diseases among which lobular pneumonia, bronchitis and acute œdema of the lungs are the most important. These affections are the most common complications of croup, owing to which recovery is often delayed for a long time, or is never complete for the reason that chronic bronchitis, emphysema, etc., remain behind.

Before discussing the diagnosis of croup, we will add a few remarks on diphtheritic laryngitis which differs essentially from croup. Epidemic diphtheria, although more particularly confined to the mucous membrane of the mouth and fauces, is likewise very much inclined to invade the larynx. This occurrence generally shows that the disease is of a most malignant type. The symptoms of diphtheritic croup resemble those of the ordinary form of membranous croup, from which the former differs, however, in some respects. The patients begin to show laryngeal symptoms after the affection of the fauces has existed for some time, and the strength has begun to fail. The dyspnœa is less intense as in membranous croup; the inflammatory swelling is less, and the patients do not die so much on account of the dyspnœa as on account of the general violence of the disease. The characteristic sopor of the last stage of croup does not occur in diphtheria. These distinctions do not occur in every case, but in the majority of cases. They are easily accounted for by the differences in the character of the exudation which in diphtheria involves the tissue of the mucous lining itself, and very speedily results in gangrenous or ichorous dissolution, often attended with considerable loss of substance. If the diphtheritic process invades the larynx, it assumes a very destructive character, sometimes without interfering with the breathing, whereas croupous laryngitis unattended with dyspnœa need not necessarily be a very dangerous disease. In pathological treatises both these forms of croup are generally described as homogeneous, whereas they differ essentially in their natures, which explains the fact that the views concerning croup are so much at variance in the different works on Pathology.

Towards the end of the disease the diagnosis of croup is just as easy as it is sometimes obscure at the commencement. It is most apt to be confounded with laryngitis; indeed, both these forms of disease resemble each other so much that it is very difficult during the first twenty-four hours to diagnose the true character of the attack, in spite of the most careful investigation of all anamnestic circumstances. If we have before us an individual who has had frequent attacks of simple laryngitis; who is otherwise in the enjoyment of bodily vigor and health, and shows symptoms of an incipient or fully developed nasal catarrh: it is almost certain that the idea of croup may be abandoned. The last-mentioned circumstance is of particular importance, for we have never yet seen incipient croup accompanied by a damp nose; and if the nose does begin to discharge during the last stage of croup, the secretion is always of the ichorous character of a diphtheritic discharge. In laryngitis as in croup the dyspnœa may at first be very great, except that in the former disease the dyspnœa decreases in intensity as soon as the children are wide awake and have tasted of a little nourishment; nor does it increase after the first attack, although it may last longer than the first twenty-four hours. If croup prevails as an epidemic, every attack of laryngitis ought to be suspected from the outset; likewise, if in the same family several children had already been attacked with croup. The presence of membranous exudations on the tonsils and in the pharynx, which, however, are not always noticed at the very commencement of the attack, places the diagnosis beyond all doubt. A spasm of the glottis which is but a transitory condition, can only be confounded with croup at the outset, so much more easily if the spasm is complicated with laryngitis. In a few hours already the true character of the enemy is sufficiently apparent.

Treatment. Since Napoleon's famous concourse of 1807 the pathological and pathologico-anatomical changes occurring in croup have been investigated so thoroughly and almost exhaustively by such a number of physicians that it seems almost impossible that the therapeutic management of croup should have been so sadly neglected. Nevertheless this charge is just. The Old School has not a single remedy for croup unless tracheotomy which is the last desperate resort, is considered such. If the numerous therapeutic experiments that have been made during the last fifty-six years on croup-patients, have failed to lead to the desired result, the method according to which the experiments were conducted, must have been erroneous. We place this fact in bold relief in order to show with so much more force the superiority of the homœopathic treatment of croup over any other method. To this effect we first name some of the more renowned remedial agents that are used in croup. At the same time we cannot help expressing our surprise that croup should drive the scepticism of the Physiological or Rational School to such straits; for it is astonishing what remedies even the leaders of this School propose in order to avert the fatal blow. Here the highly praised expectant method is utterly abandoned; on the contrary, the most diametrically opposed agents are brought into requisition one after the other in the most rapid succession, so that, without entertaining the least prejudice, we are naturally led to inquire what has become of the "rationality" of the method.

The most important and most extensively used remedies are emetics, topical and general sanguineous depletions, Calomel internally and the mercurial ointment externally, Antimony, Tartar emetic, Hepar sulphuris, Alum and finally a number of locally applied substances. At the same time cold and warm compresses, watery vapors, wrappings, etc., are not wanting. Emetics which are the most important agents in this list, are indebted for their reputation to the apparent success which they have in simple laryngitis; we call this success apparent because no true laryngitis can be cut short by a simple emetic. No amount of sophistical argumentation is able to show that an emetic can exert the least influence over an incipient croup. Moreover we cannot overlook the fact that the effect of an emetic does not end with the act of vomiting, especially if the Sulphate of Copper is used for this purpose, and that our patients are little children. Children who had an attack of simple laryngitis, often suffer for weeks from the effects of the Sulphate of Copper or of Tartar emetic. The use of an emetic is much more excusable if, after the membrane had begun to be formed, the process of expectoration is to be promoted; there is no difficulty in comprehending that the act of vomiting stimulates the disposition to expectorate. An homœopath will undoubtedly know how to account for the action of Ipecacuanha or Tartar emetic or even of the Sulphate of Copper upon different principles from those in vogue. In the second stage of croup the Sulphate of Copper is now the fashionable emetic; yet this preference is not accounted for upon scientific principles. We know that Copper has a good effect in the spasmodic closing of the glottis, and hence is of advantage in croup. While mentioning this effect of Copper a knowledge of which has been acquired by the most foolhardy empiricism, we at the same time have to remind our readers that not one of our allopathic opponents has been able to account for the good effects of Copper in croup except by the act of vomiting.

As regards the sanguineous depletions, be they local or general, we can dispense with the trouble of dwelling upon them any further. It is inconceivable that they are expected to prevent, arrest or diminish the exudation; what is certain is that bleeding robs the child of the power to develop the necessary reaction against the disease. Even the croup-fever is not sufficiently intense to justify bleeding. As far as Mercury is concerned, the only excuse, we dare not call it indication, for its use is that a quantity of coagulable lymph is effused in croup and that Mercury is a powerful antiplastic agent. But this agent alone has never yet removed a case of croup, but has occasioned such violent attacks of stomatitis that the jaws have united by ulceration. The other remedies will be further dwelt upon by and by, especially the Sulphuret of Lime; this agent which is a true specific in many cases of croup, is only mentioned very cursorily in allopathic works, more like a curiosity than as an useful remedy.

The want of internal remedies naturally led physicians to hunt up external applications. The croup-membrane was to be destroyed, the subjacent mucous lining to be cauterized and the disease was thus to be conquered. Strange fancy, as if we did not know that croup is a special form of inflammation resulting from, or determined by constitutional susceptibilities. A glance at the results of the cauterizing process in diphtheria ought to have discouraged the cauterizers of the croupy membrane. The mucous lining of the larynx has been washed with the Nitrate of Silver, Muriatic acid, Alum, etc., causing the patient the most agonizing distress. The only advantage derived from such a proceeding may be that the irritating action of those agents may cause a violent coughing fit which may promote the process of expectoration. The inhalations to which we shall refer hereafter, are not of very great importance, nor is the application of ice or cold water. If we add to these means of treatment the unavoidable blisters and sinapisms, we have the best part of the medicinal apparatus of the Old School before us. In spite of all these appliances, from 70 to 90 per cent. of all undoubted cases of membranous croup perish. This result is certainly no triumph, nor has tracheotomy increased the chances of recovery.

In opposition to these failures Homœopathy can show a most successful treatment of croup to her opponents without inflicting upon the poor little patients the horrible tortures of Old School practice. We are not sanguine enough to add credence to those who profess to have treated hundreds of cases of croup during a practice of thirty or forty years without losing a single patient; but we do know that by far the larger number of cases are saved under homœopathic treatment; this is an amount of success to be proud of. We do not fall back upon statistical data which may be called in doubt on account of diagnostic inaccuracies or uncertainties; a single fact among many may prove more convincing to the most inveterate sceptic than the most scientific statistical exhibit. At the beginning of this year epidemic croup broke out on a heather about sixteen miles from this city. Several dozens of children had already fallen victims to the above-described treatment. A young gentleman who happened to visit a merchant of the place, advised him to try homœopathic treatment. The results of this treatment were so striking that the house of this merchant was from that day besieged by persons seeking aid. With the aid of a simple domestic manual, this merchant succeeded in saving a number of lives. Is it possible to remain blind to such events? We do not attach implicit faith in the doctrine that vox populi is vox Dei; but in such terrible epidemics even a layman has sense enough to see whether those who are attacked, perish or get well, and what method of treatment is crowned with the latter result.

The remedies which homœopaths use in treating croup, are the following: *Aconitum*, *Hepar sulphuris*, *Spongia maritima*, *Iodium*, *Bromum*, *Phosphorus*, *Cuprum* and several more. We shall consider these drugs in their respective bearing upon each of the different stages of croup, instead of furnishing a detached list of the symptomatic indications of each drug in particular.

If we are called to a case of croup in the night, it is not always possible to at once obtain the conviction that we are dealing with a case of croup; for even the presence of considerable dyspnœa does not always imply that the disease before us is croup. In order to meet this uncertainty the custom has prevailed for a long time already to at once give *Aconite* in alternation with some other remedy. We do not approve of this custom of giving remedies in alternation, but make an exception in favor of croup on account of the uncertainty in our diagnosis. Aconite is excellent in catarrhal, but utterly inefficient in membranous croup. If we suspect a case of membranous croup, we give *Aconite* 2, and *Iodium* 2, in alternation every hour. The Iodine had better be prepared fresh in order that we may be sure of operating with a reliable attenuation. This remedy is not given by all practitioners at the outset of the attack, but Hepar sulphuris or Spongia. We have the following reasons for our proceeding. Iodium exerts a special action on the larynx so constantly, and causes a violent inflammation of the larynx with so much certainty that this effect may be set down as a pathognomonic and highly characteristic symptom of the action of Iodine. That it is capable of healing far advanced cases of croup, is true beyond all doubt. Hence there is no reason why a medicine that embraces in its pathogenetic series all the symptoms of croup and must therefore be adapted to every stage of this disease, should not be given at the very commencement of the attack. We consider this medicine much more appropriate than some other medicine that is only suitable in the incipient stages of the disease. Many other physicians prefer *Hepar sulphuris* at the outset, if the following symptoms prevail: Marked febrile motions, the respiration is almost entirely unembarrassed, but has a peculiar sound; dry, metallic cough with disposition to choke, mingled with a short rattling in the trachea, as if mucus would be raised; or if the cough seems to continue moist, and the croupy sound is present; the larynx is painful; there is hoarseness, but no loss of voice. Spongia is even recommended more strongly than Hepar at the first invasion of the disease. Hahnemann himself regards Spongia as the main remedy in croup and directs to resort now and then to an intermediate dose of Aconite or Hepar; he does not consider Spongia indicated until the respiration has become embarrassed and exudation has commenced. Almost all observers are of the same opinion.

In the first night, it may not matter much which of these remedies is given in alternation with Aconite. It is certain that catarrhal croup will be modified by a few doses of Aconite within twelve hours so fully that whenever this favorable change does not take place within this period of time, we may rest assured, that we are dealing with a case of membranous croup and that the selection of a specific remedy can no longer remain doubtful. This feat is not so easily accomplished if we take the Materia Medica for our guide; moreover, experience has done already a great deal for us in this respect. Experience informs us that Hepar is a suitable remedy on the second day, if mucus begins to accumulate in the windpipe, there is no increase of hoarseness, no dyspnœa or very little of it, and the cough has a uniformly croupy sound; hence Hepar is indicated in the milder cases of croup. Spongia is required if the croup shows its malignant features after the lapse of a few hours, the cough has a hollow sound, less resonance, the hoarseness approximates to aphonia, the dyspnœa is more marked. *Iodium* is to be given if the symptoms steadily increase in intensity, the loss of voice is complete, the dyspnœa has reached the highest degree of intensity, and the cough has lost a good deal of its ringing and shrill sound.

As soon as we have become satisfied of the nature of the disease, Aconite is no longer given in alternation with some other drug, even if violent fever should be present. The question now is whether at this stage of the disease two remedies like *Spongia* and *Hepar*, or *Hepar* or *Spongia* and *Iodium*, had not better be continued in alternation. A good deal may be excused in the presence of such a dangerous malady, and we have not the heart to condemn any one who deems it proper to continue the alternate use of two drugs, more particularly in cases where the life of the patient might be jeopardized if the action of a single drug were allowed to continue for twelve hours and even longer. Alternating drugs does not improve our knowledge of their true action; hence this custom should be abandoned whenever such a thing is possible.

In the vast majority of cases the further progress of croup will be stayed under the operation of one of the above-mentioned three remedies; if this fact is perceived, we have every reason to be satisfied with the treatment, and we must not be anxious to change the medicine until every symptom of the real croup-disease has disappeared. If *Hepar* and *Spongia* seem ineffectual, and the disease steadily continues to grow worse, we give *Iodium* which we continue at least forty-eight hours unless symptoms of asphyxia manifest themselves before this period is passed. In most cases Iodium will undoubtedly have a favorable effect. Only we must not indulge in the expectation of cutting the disease short. A result of this kind only occurs in a very small number of cases. Most commonly the pathological process continues to go on under the action of *Iodine*, after which it retrogrades, as is the case in every other inflammation. What is essential is that it should be kept confined within proper boundaries. Even if the dyspnœa increases at first, this is no reason why the use of Iodine should be discontinued.

Instead of Iodine, many physicians recommend *Bromine*; some successful cures with Bromine are reported, whereas others deny it all power over croup. We are not yet able to express a decided opinion on this subject. The symptoms indicating Bromine are the following: Cough having a croupy sound, hoarse, wheezing, distressing cough which does not give one a chance to speak, attended with sneezing and violent fits of suffocation; spasm of the glottis, whence the symptoms of asphyxia; moist respiratory râle, the breathing is at times wheezing and slow, at other times as if he would suffocate, and then again hurried, superficial, labored, distressed, painful and gasping. This combination of symptoms is furnished by Attomyr, but we would like to ask whether anything in this group points to Bromine? Moreover we confess that we consider a purely symptomatic treatment of croup inadequate, and that, if croup were to be treated according to mere symptoms, we would have to change the medicine as often as the symptoms change, which would be productive of a vast deal of harm. We are acquainted with the effects of the remedies to be employed, but which of them is the best adapted to the exigencies of the case, is best determined by practical experience. We do not mean to reject Bromine, but it is only in mild cases that we would substitute its use for that of Iodine.

If, in spite of all treatment, the symptoms of asphyxia increase more and more; if the dyspnœa continues to increase; if the agony and restlessness of the little patient become more distressing, and the symptoms of cerebral congestion more marked, two remedies remain from which aid may be expected, namely *Phosphorus* and *Tartar emetic*. The former is indicated if the cough has lost all resonance and force, and the mucous râle has ceased; or more especially if the croupous process has invaded the bronchia and the lungs have evidently become hyperæmic. *Tartar emetic* is indicated if the dyspnœa and danger of asphyxia are occasioned by movable patches of membrane, the cough is indeed feeble and without resonance, but a mucous râle is still distinctly heard in the trachea. However it is not advisable to prescribe this remedy in large doses, for the favorable effect of the act of vomiting is very problematical. whereas the great depression caused by the vomiting is sure to follow. Nor is it at all certain whether any emetic at this advanced stage of croup can cause vomiting. Grain doses of the second trituration are sufficiently strong; as regards *Phosphorus* we would not dare give it below the third attenuation.

In this place we will call attention to a few remedies that have no relation to the croupous exudation, but are important in other respects. The danger of suffocation depends in many cases upon a spasmodic closing rather than upon a mechanical disarrangement or an inflammatory infiltration of the rima glottidis. A condition of this kind is pretty certain to exist if the dyspnœa sets in in single, pretty sharply detached paroxysms, the remissions between the paroxysms are quite considerable and no râles are heard in the larynx. If we designate this closing of the glottis as spasmodic, the designation is not entirely correct, because paralysis of the muscular apparatus of the larynx is undoubtedly the chief cause of the asphyxia, whereas a spasm of the larynx could not well be accounted for. If we consider that in the case of children the glottis forms an uniformly narrow chink whose sides incline obliquely towards each other from without inwards, and from below upwards, it is easily conceivable that, in case the sides are somewhat relaxed, they may be forced against each other during the act of inspiration, in consequence of which the glottis will either be very much contracted or even closed. These facts explain how children may die of croup without a membrane being seen after death, and why full-grown persons whose glottis is wider and differently shaped, scarcely ever succomb to an attack of croup. We can meet this paralytic condition by some remedies that are well worthy of our consideration: *Cuprum, Moschus, Nux moschata, Ipecacuanha,* and *Arsenicum.* Of all these remedies, Cuprum is undoubtedly the most important; its effect is in a measure confirmed by the effect of the Sulphate of Copper when administered as an emetic. Arsenicum has shown its favorable effect upon dyspnœa in a most desperate case which terminated in recovery. The other three remedies have been strongly recommended by other physicians; we have no personal experience to offer in their behalf. If these remedies are to be used, they will have to be given in alternation with the true specifics for croup; the best mode of using them is to interpolate a dose every few hours.

If the stage of asphyxia sets in in spite of this treatment,—which will not often be the case,—the question then occurs what will have to be the further object of the treatment. The glottis is paralyzed or its space encroached upon, together with that of the trachea, by membranes; the existing sopor shows that the poisoning by carbonic acid has already made considerable headway; the icy coldness of the skin is evidence that an independent reaction can hardly be expected any longer. The only remaining chance of saving the patient is by promoting the oxygenation of the blood. It would be absurd to prescribe for these apparent symptoms of cerebral congestions remedies like Opium, Belladonna, Hyoscyamus, etc., which will not have the least effect. Nor will the continued use of Phosphorus or Tartar emetic, in the absence of all reaction, produce the least result. Under these circumstances tracheotomy alone can afford help, and it would be just as criminal to leave the operation undone at this stage, as it would have been criminal to perform it at an earlier period. For a description of this operation we refer the reader to works on Surgery. We are decidedly opposed to the operation being performed before the stage of asphyxia has set in; this may be excusable in cases that are not treated homœopathically, for other Schools have no really specific remedies for croup.

If but few patients are saved by this operation, it is not the fault of the operation, but of the period when it is performed. Without the operation all patients die in the stage of asphyxia; where the operation is performed, only some die, though it be the larger number. These results show that the operation is not only justifiable, but eminently necessary and important. However, in order that all possible advantages may be derived from the operation, it should not be delayed too long; otherwise the sopor might progress too far, or recovery might be prevented by an acute emphysema and œdema of the lungs; conditions that may lead to a fatal termination even after the cure of croup is successfully accomplished.

[The reader may peruse with profit an article on tracheotomy in croup, by Doctor Talbot, of Boston, in one of the late numbers of the New England Medical Gazette. H.]

If an improvement sets in, we first notice an abatement of the dyspnœa; it is by changes of this kind that we can measure the probable chances of our final success. Nevertheless, the medicine which induces the favorable turn, had better be continued for some time longer, but at more extended intervals. To continue the use of the medicine is of importance, for the reason that, after a marked remission of the symptoms, the disease sometimes breaks out again with renewed violence. The cough sometimes retains for a long time its hoarse, barking sound; the aphonia likewise often continues for a long time. For the cough we administer Hepar, more especially if it is attended with mucous râle; if the cough is dry, Phosphorus is preferable. This agent is likewise most suitable for the subsequent hoarseness.

The so-called torpid croup does not destroy life as rapidly as the preceding varieties, but is withal a very insidious disease. It is treated with the same remedies as those above mentioned, except that Hepar sulphuris very frequently deserves the preference.

If croup results from a gradual working down of the diphtheritic process from the pharynx to the larynx, it is always more dangerous than the primary form of croup, and, according to the reasons we have advanced when speaking of diphtheritis, requires to be treated with entirely different remedies. In diphtheritic croup Bromine may possibly deserve particular attention. We refer the reader to the chapter on diphtheritis. It is this form of croup that has given rise to the belief in the contagiousness of croup; it does, indeed, seem to be a contagious disease. [Some cures have been made of diphtheritic croup with *Lachesis* highly potentized; and also with *Kali bichromicum*. H.]

External applications in croup are generally without any effect. Whereas some apply hot water to the neck, and cause watery vapors to be inhaled, or order hot arm-baths; others, on the contrary, prefer ice-water or ice itself, and others again resort to the wet pack. This deserves a preference over the other applications, because it most advantageously stimulates the functional activity of the skin. Upon the whole, however, it is our belief that the greatest advantage of these auxiliary means consists in diverting the attention of the family who are generally plunged into extreme agony.

Whether the administration of drugs by means of vaporous inhalations is the most useful method, is still a disputed point. We do not see whether a medicine introduced into the human body through the respiratory organs, should develop its effects more surely or more penetratingly than when administered by the mouth. Moreover, this method is sometimes attended with difficulties, unless we do not mind filling the sick-chamber with vapors. This has the disadvantage that no fresh supply of pure air gets to the lungs and that the medicine ceases to be under our control. The dyspnœa is, moreover, easily increased by inhalation. Apparatuses for inhalation cannot be used, because the little patients are exceedingly restless and tossed about by their agonizing distress. At all events, the inhaling process has to be conducted with great care.

We have no special remarks to offer on the subject of diet in this disease. On account of the dyspnœa, which renders deglutition exceedingly difficult, the greatest trouble is experienced in giving children the least quantity of nourishment; what nourishment is given, should be in a liquid form, and very strengthening. If the strength fails too rapidly, a little good wine proves an excellent stimulant.

There is no real prophylactic treatment against croup, except a regular system of hardening children from the moment they are born, and bringing them up in all respects in accordance with principles of health. If a child with a suspicious habit of body is attacked with a croupy cough whenever it takes cold, and is generally inclined to have an attack of severe laryngitis, let it be kept in-doors during a keen North wind, or let it at least be protected by a sufficient amount of warm clothing. Whether *Calcarea carbonica*, *Hepar* or *Phosphorus* are capable of exerting a protective influence against croup, is not yet decided. After a first attack of croup, a disposition to be again attacked generally remains. It is doubtful whether even such a disposition can be removed; the constitutional diathesis cannot well be remedied.

3. Laryngotracheitis Chronica.
Chronic Laryngotracheal Catarrh.

The chronic form of this catarrh is, like the acute, one of the most frequent diseases both with reference to affections of the respiratory organs specially, and with reference to all other diseases collectively.

This disease befalls children only as an exceptional disturbance; if it does occur in childhood, it is almost always a consequence of a more malignant acute disease, especially of croup and diphtheria. Nor are older people frequently attacked by this disease; hence we say that middle-aged persons between the ages of twenty and fifty years are principally liable to such attacks. Sex has an undoubted influence over the disease; for although women are much less exposed to the unfavorable influences which we shall mention by and by, this does not satisfactorily account for the extraordinary prevalence of the disease among the male sex. Regarding a special disposition, we refer the reader to what we have said in the first chapter of this section.

Chronic laryngotracheal catarrh is seldom a primary, generally a secondary or consecutive affection. Primarily this form of catarrh is caused by the same influences as the acute form, a cold, continued talking, singing, the constant use of spirits, beer, exposure to marked differences of temperature. Secondarily it may represent a slow form of acute catarrh, which is the most frequent cause of the chronic form, especially if the individual had several acute attacks in succession; or else it is a continuation of a catarrhal affection of the nose, fauces, buccal cavity; or it may result from the constant irritation caused by repeated ulcerations or adventitious growths; or finally it may be a manifestation of some constitutional disease. In this respect it sometimes accompanies syphilis or a mercurial dyscrasia; most commonly, however, it is a symptom of pulmonary tuberculosis, so that every catarrh whose persistence cannot be accounted for by any known cause, must necessarily excite the suspicion that the lungs are infiltrated with tubercular matter.

In this affection the anatomical changes are so important for a proper understanding of the symptoms, that we premise a short description of these changes. Usually the mucous membrane is darker than normally, sometimes the dark tinge is quite considerable; the membrane is more or less thickened and puffed up. It is traversed by a multitude of engorged vessels and studded with swollen follicles imparting to it a granular appearance. It is covered with a tenacious, gray, yellowish or transparent secretion. The subjacent tissues, cellular tissues, muscles, ligaments are swollen and softened. If particular circumstances prevail, the mucous membrane ulcerates at an early stage of the disease, but almost always after the disease has lasted some time. Most commonly we observe a simple erosion in the shape of a superficial exfoliation surrounded by a more intensely red border, but without any definite form. These erosions may change to more deeply-penetrating ulcers with blown or puffed edges which eat only in exceptional cases through the whole thickness of the mucous membrane. Another form of ulceration arises from the inflammation of the follicles; in which case small, deep, rounded ulcers form, which very readily penetrate the mucous membrane and propagate the affection to external organs. We observe moreover fungoid growths of single follicles, even polypi; cicatrizations and contracting cicatrices, thickenings and callosities of the mucous membrane. Of special importance are the subsequent changes, especially cicatrices which may lead to dangerous accidents.

The great differences of the anatomical lesions depending upon their nature, locality and extent, render it self-evident that it is impossible to draw a true and striking picture of laryngotracheal catarrh. Hence we shall have to confine ourselves to a delineation of the leading symptoms. The absence of almost every objective aid in establishing our diagnosis, is often seriously felt, nor is it certain whether the laryngoscope has as yet led to striking results, although we are willing to admit that this means of investigation has a bright future before it. The most important symptoms of the disease are: pain, alterations of the voice, cough, embarrassed respiration.

The pain is scarcely ever very considerable, and if it is described as acute, we may be sure that ulcers have formed. It is scarcely ever continuous, but is excited by talking, singing, running, sudden changes of temperature, and most easily by coughing. Sometimes it is a soreness, at other times the pain is stinging, burning, gnawing, and inclines to exacerbate towards morning. An annoying sensation is the feeling as if there were dust or a foreign body in the throat, or the patients complain of a periodically returning tickling in the larynx.

The voice is variously altered. We may lay it down as a rule that every persistent change in the voice points to chronic laryngeal catarrh. The hoarseness runs throughout its whole series of gradations, from simple roughness of voice to complete aphonia. It scarcely ever continues all the time in the same degree of violence; it may even disappear entirely for a while, and then be excited anew by some unusual exertion in using the organs of voice. Sometimes the hoarseness is only perceived during singing. However, it is not by any means a characteristic symptom of chronic laryngotracheal catarrh. A sudden cracking of the voice or an inability to raise the voice beyond a certain pitch, is often met with.

Cough is a very common symptom in this affection. Sometimes it amounts to no more than a hawking occasioned by a titillation in the larynx or oppressed breathing; at other times it torments the patient for days, after which it often intermits for a while; sometimes it breaks out in regular paroxysms which most commonly set in in the morning after rising and abate again after small quantities of mucus have been expectorated. There is nothing characteristic in the sound of the cough, except that a rattling of mucus is most generally heard in the trachea or glottis, and that a dry titillating cough sometimes prevails by way of exception. The expectoration is never very copious except when it is mixed with mucus from the lungs, of a white or grayish color, firmly cohering and globular, sometimes slightly streaked with blood. If it has a purulent appearance, we may almost feel sure that the expectoration does not alone proceed from the larynx and trachea.

The difficulties of breathing, an oppressed, wheezing respiration, and even an asthmatic dyspnœa are occasioned by a swelling and constriction of the glottis, hence do not show the degree of intensity, but the seat of the disease. These difficulties are of importance to a physician for the additional reason that they excite the most fearful apprehensions in the minds of most patients.

This disease generally runs a protracted and even obstinate course. It is mostly determined by the existing anatomical lesions. A simple affection of the mucous membrane is easily cured; what renders the final result doubtful is, when the patients expose themselves to influences that rekindle the disorder as soon as it begins to mend. A simple ulcer is likewise within the reach of remedial influences, whereas the more deeply-penetrating ulcer and the fungoid exerescences of the mucous membrane resist all treatment so much more obstinately as their diagnosis is more uncertain. It is only in very rare cases that laryngotracheal catarrh is dangerous to life, not immediately, but in consequence of some pulmonary affection that may have been superinduced by the difficulties which the air encounters in passing through the larynx. Laryngeal phthisis without tubercles is a very rare occurrence, in which case it most generally depends upon other dyscrasic conditions. The tubercular laryngeal catarrh will be described when we come to speak of tuberculosis; here we will only state that almost all dangerous and obstinate laryngeal catarrhs, especially if attended with emaciation or fever, are caused by tubercular infiltration.

Treatment. We deal with an affection that may occur in the most diversified forms, complications and degrees of intensity, and which on this account alone renders the selection of a large number of remedies expedient. We could not possibly mention every drug that may be required for the treatment of this disease, and have confined ourselves to an enumeration of the more important remedies, referring the reader to a good Repertory as an indispensable auxiliary, if a remedy is to be chosen for a single symptom of characteristic value.

Tartarus stibiatus and **Antimonium crudum.** The former is especially indicated when the acute form passes into the chronic, more particularly in the case of children and old people. There is a frequent desire to cough, attended with an audible rattling of mucus in the air-passages, a thick and white phlegm being brought up after a severe paroxysm of racking cough. Or the cough may set in in detached violent paroxysms accompanied with dyspnœa and ending in gagging and forcing up mucus. Both kinds are principally met with among children and old people. For hoarseness as an isolated symptom, Tartarus stibiatus may not be appropriate; *Antimonium crudum* will be found preferable. The following symptoms indicate this remedy: the hoarseness is made worse by excitement and overheating; disposition of the voice to give out suddenly; sensation of roughness in the larynx, and as if a foreign body had lodged in it.

Hepar sulphuris calcareum is particularly adapted to neglected acute catarrh, and is an indispensable remedy for singers and people who have to talk a good deal, but is likewise suitable in many cases of chronic catarrh. The following symptoms are the most essential: the larynx feels painful as if sore and burning, especially when the patients cough or talk loud; hoarseness sometimes increasing for a short time to aphonia; feeling of dryness in the larynx, although the presence of mucus is distinctly perceived; a hoarse titillating cough with scanty expectoration and rattling of mucus in the trachea; hard, lumpy, yellow or greenish expectoration, very tenacious and sometimes tinged with blood. *Hepar* deserves particular attention in cases of chronic catarrh remaining after croup or measles, or in the case of individuals who had taken much Mercury.

Spongia bears great resemblance to the former drug both symptomatically as well as in its general indications. It too is indicated after croup and measles, in cases of neglected acute catarrh, in the case of singers. It is particularly required for the cough with burning titillation in the larynx, which sets in more particularly at night or after loud talking. The cough has a barking sound, the mucus is hard to bring up, tenacious, yellowish, and the attacks are apt to be accompanied by dyspnœa emanating from the glottis.

Iodium is one of the most important remedies in this affection. Among the general indications for Iodine we distinguish the following: chronic catarrh of scrofulous and mercurialized individuals, or remaining after croup or other acute affections, or complicated with chronic pharyngeal catarrh. The most prominent symptomatic indications are the following: Disposition to take cold, and long duration of the acute stage; the larynx is painful when pressed upon; burning, sore pains in the larynx confined to a definite spot, felt especially during cough; embarrassed respiration, wheezing inspirations causing real attacks of dyspnœa especially at night; a good deal of hawking, with difficulty of bringing up tenacious mucus; a high degree of hoarseness, even aphonia; tickling in the larynx, frequently causing paroxysms of cough without expectoration, or else with scanty expectoration of a tenacious mucus sometimes mixed with streaks of blood. The general organism is very much affected by the disease. The presence of ulcers points more particularly to Iodine, which will again be referred to when we come to speak of tubercular laryngitis.

Manganum is an excellent remedy, although little has been said of it so far. It corresponds more especially to a catarrh accompanying an incipient, not a fully developed tuberculosis, but likewise to forms of catarrh not resulting from a dyscrasic origin, when the following symptoms are present: Slight hoarseness, rather a roughness of the throat, caused by an accumulation of lumps of hard mucus in the glottis, and more particularly marked in the morning, accompanied by oppressed breathing, relieved by expectoration, so that toward noon the voice is perfectly clear; the cough only lasts while the mucus continues to adhere in the glottis; worse in the open air, feels relieved by smoking. This kind of catarrh is very common among persons who use their organs of speech a good deal. We beg the reader to contrast Manganum with *Selenium* which is much praised for these symptoms.

Mezereum is recommended if the disease has a syphilitic origin and the symptoms point to ulceration of the larynx; among these symptoms the livid color of the pharynx and the ulcerated follicles on the posterior wall of this organ are prominent.

Phosphorus has been found reliable in the most desperate cases of laryngotracheal catarrh. A tubercular origin of the affection is indeed a chief indication for Phosphorus, but this remedy likewise cures other forms of catarrh, more especially the chronic hoarseness of preachers or singers. The more important symptoms are: weakness and sensitiveness of the organs of speech, with sensation of dryness, burning, roughness, soreness in the larynx and trachea, more especially after using the voice more than usual; hoarseness, even aphonia, particularly under the operation of exciting emotions; constricted, wheezing inspirations; cough excited by the violent tickling and burning in the larynx, painful, with rattling of mucus, although scanty expectoration; hoarse, dry-sounding cough; sensation, when coughing, as if a lump of flesh would detach itself from the throat; firm, yellowish expectoration, mingled with pus or streaks of blood. If, in addition to these symptoms, we have the general phenomena of a consumptive condition of the system, such as: fever, diarrhœa, emaciation, Phosphorus is indicated so much more decidedly. Experience having confirmed its practical value in chronic laryngeal catarrh, this remedy occupies a deservedly high rank among the remedies for this disease.

Sulphur. The cases suited to the therapeutic range of this medicine, affect principally persons somewhat advanced in age, although they need not be what might be called old people. As a rule, Sulphur is indicated by the following symptoms: Chronic catarrhs of other portions of the mucous expanse, more especially of the intestinal canal, with signs of sanguineous obstructions in the abdomen; enlargement of the liver, hypochondria; catarrh arising from abuse of Mercury; sensitiveness to the open air and dampness in particular. Among the single symptoms a prominent characteristic indication is the cough which sets in in the evening shortly before and after retiring to bed, and is a dry, titillating, distressing cough; or the cough may break out in the morning, and stop during the day, or change to an ordinary moist cough. If tubercles are present, Sulphur has very seldom a good effect, nor does it act favorably in recent cases.

Arsenicum album acts in many respects similarly to the preceding remedy. We shall revert to Arsenic when treating of pulmonary catarrh, to which we refer for the present. Arsenic, too, has great sensitiveness to cold and more particularly to damp air, likewise great nervousness. The hoarseness is not often considerable, and sets in at intervals; it is accompanied by a violent burning soreness of the throat. The cough breaks out in paroxysms with almost completely free intervals, most generally about midnight, resembles a paroxysm of whooping-cough and is accompanied by distressing dyspnœa. There is scarcely any expectoration, except that a morning-paroxysm of cough results in the hawking up of lumps of gray mucus. The constitution feels the influence of the disease. Arsenicum is more especially indicated by the circumstance that the paroxysms of cough are apt to break out when the weather changes.

Next to Phosphorus, *Carbo vegetabilis* is the most important remedy in inveterate catarrh, but acts less favorably than Arsenic in the tubercular form of this disease. Here too, we have extreme sensitiveness to the open air, especially damp air. In consequence of loud talking, the hoarseness may increase to loss of voice; the patient complains of a feeling of great dryness in the throat, with soreness and a stinging pain, together with a copious secretion of a tenacious mucus occasioning constant and sometimes very painful hawking. The cough is wearing, rough, with mucous râles, but only a scanty, greenish or yellowish, lumpy, tenacious expectoration, it sets in more particularly in the morning and is attended with dyspnœa.

We will now mention a few more remedies in the following cursory series:

For the simple protracted chronic catarrh representing an acute attack: *Tartarus stibiatus, Hepar sulphuris calc., Spongia, Pulsatilla;* and for the more acute intercurrent exacerbations principally *Mercurius* and *Belladonna*. The latter is sometimes eminently adapted to a spasmodic nocturnal cough, without expectoration.

For catarrh complicated with ulceration, if not too old: *Iodium,*

Hepar sulph., *Manganum, Silicea, Calcarea carbonica;* for neglected catarrh: *Phosphorus, Sulphur, Carbo veg., Arsenicum album.*

For inveterate simple catarrh: *Sulphur, Carbo veg., Silicea, Arsenicum album.*

For polypous growths: *Phosphorus, Calcarea carb., Silicea.*

For continued hoarseness and chronic catarrhs of singers, preachers, etc.: *Manganum, Phosphorus, Carbo veg., Selenium, Argentum* in older cases; in recent cases: *Hepar sulph., Spongia.*

For catarrh caused by Mercury: *Hepar sulph., Iodium,* and if a syphilitic complication exists: *Mezereum.*

For complete loss of voice, attended with catarrh: *Antimonium crudum, Phosphorus, Carbo veg., Iodium;* if depending upon disturbed innervation: *Cuprum, Opium, Causticum, Phosphorus, Ignatia, Sepia.*

The cure is often promoted and hastened by various dietetic and external means. Individuals, for instance, who have been in the habit of keeping their necks warm, and now take cold from every little exposure, may resort every evening to frictions with lard on the neck with the best results; these will diminish the disposition to take cold. The well known domestic remedy to wear around the neck a rough woollen bandage, is likewise to be commended. The most decided and reliable advantage, however, is obtained from the use of cold water, either by simply washing the neck with it, or by means of wet bandages around the throat. As a matter of course, too warm clothing has to be avoided. There is no better palliative for the distressing titillating cough, which is especially tormenting at night, than inhaling the vapors of warm water. We know from experience that thoroughly practised singers are seldom attacked with permanent hoarseness or pulmonary diseases. A methodical, cautious, uniform use of the voice in singing, especially if confined to the middle notes, is sometimes a better remedy for chronic hoarseness than any other means of treatment; if the vocal chords are morbidly relaxed, this use of the laryngeal muscles would be dictated by the principles of the movement-cure. Only in a case of tubercular hoarseness an experiment of this kind might prove hazardous. Talking in the midst of a noisy company, in a carriage, in rail-cars, etc., should be carefully avoided.

4. Œdema Glottidis, Laryngitis Sub-mucosa.
Œdema of the Glottis.

By this name we understand a sudden infiltration of the submucous tissue of the epiglottis, and of the mucous lining of the larynx extending from the epiglottis to the rima glottidis.

Œdema glottidis is more especially a disease of adults, and in most cases a secondary affection. Primarily it may result from severe burns, by hot food or corrosive substances, but scarcely ever, like common laryngitis, in consequence of a cold. Secondarily we do not often notice it in company with dropsical affections, but most commonly in company with affections that occasion the formation of ulcers or suppurating sores on the inner or outer walls of the larynx, like tuberculosis, typhus, variola, ulcerous laryngitis, perichondritis, croup, diphtheria, etc.; or it may occur in a few cases as a continuation of an ulcerous angina to the larynx, as in scarlatina. Sometimes the disease seems to assume an epidemic character; this may be nothing more than we observe, for instance, in epidemic scarlatina, which causes characteristically violent and usually purulent anginas. Considering the manner in which the disease originates, the most correct explanation seems to be that a suppurative process in the neighborhood of the glottis causes œdema in the same manner in which a chancre causes within a few hours an excessive œdema of the prepuce. Our statistical tables so far show that the disease attacks men much more frequently than women.

Symptoms. The anatomical changes in œdema of the glottis consist in a more or less considerable puffy swelling of the mucous membrane, more particularly at and close to the root of the epiglottis. This swelling may become so considerable that the swollen parts protrude behind the root of the tongue like a stuffed pad or sausage. Usually the color is not bright-red but pale, and, on cutting into it, the swelling discharges a serous or sero-purulent fluid.

The phenomena of œdema glottidis sometimes develop themselves with an extraordinary suddenness, and at other times very slowly; moreover they are modified by the locality where they occur. In the course of one of the above-mentioned affections, hoarseness, pain and burning in the larynx set in. The hoarseness very speedily increases to complete aphonia accompanied by a cough which has all the characteristic signs of croupy cough. These symptoms are accompanied from the outset by a continually increasing dyspnœa which, in severe cases, may rise to a fearful height. The inspiration, in consequence of which the puffed-up and infiltrated lips of the glottis are forced towards each other and towards the rima glottidis, becomes more and more prolonged, hissing and labored, and the patients very often have a feeling as if a foreign body were moving around in the larynx. If the infiltration remains moderate in quantity, the respiratory process may go on without life being in immediate jeopardy; a condition of this kind may continue unchanged for many days, although an exacerbation may take place at any time. However if the respiration is seriously impeded, all the symptoms, which we have described when speaking of croup as characterising a poisoning by carbonic acid, set in and the patients die in a state of sopor. There is no fever unless it was present previously; it is only in case the infiltration becomes purulent that the phenomena peculiar to the formation of an abscess, manifest themselves; on the bursting of the abscess the inspirations may suddenly be restored. In such cases an œdematous swelling of the neck in the region of the larynx can almost always be seen.

The affection may last from twelve hours to upwards of a week. The most common termination is death by suffocation, and the prognosis is consequently that of inevitable death.

It is important to notice the features which distinguish the disease from croup with which it is most easily confounded. Many cases of so-called relapses in croup are probably nothing else than œdema glottidis resulting from croup and becoming manifest after the croupy process had run its course. The distinguishing characteristics are: In the first place, the swelling itself which, in severe cases, is noticed at the root of the tongue; the appearance of the disease subsequently to and during morbid processes which are scarcely ever associated with croup; the occurrence of the disease among adults, whereas croup attacks children almost exclusively; the peculiar sensation as if a foreign body were moving about in the larynx.

The prospect of a successful treatment is very slim, especially if the patient is a child. Our literature does not offer any positively successful cures of this disease, and, since it is one of the rarer kind, all we can do is to indicate the remedies which it may be necessary to use in a given case. We are acquainted with only one remedy which has œdema of the glottis among its physiological effects; this remedy is *Iodium*. For particular indications we refer to our remarks in the chapter on croup. Another remedy which offers some resemblance is *Phosphorus;* in this case, however, the resemblance is limited to a single symptom. If we consider the nature of the pathological process which results in the production of œdema glottidis, independently of the symptoms superinduced by the mechanical closing of the rima glottidis, we are more particularly led to three remedies that act similarly to the general disease, we mean: *Apis mellifica, Lachesis,* and *Rhus toxicodendron.* Lachesis especially has the peculiar serous infiltration of internal as well as external parts of the body which sets in without any symptoms that might properly be called inflammatory, and which reaches its full development in a few hours. However, since in this disease we cannot fall back upon experience for a positive knowledge of the curative action of drugs, it would be criminally indiscreet to depend exclusively upon internal treatment. In this disease, much sooner than in croup, success may be expected from tracheotomy, for the reason that the trachea is not usually involved; only the operation should be performed so soon as the symptoms of poisoning by carbonic acid begin to manifest themselves; otherwise the paralysis of the respiratory organs might have progressed too far for the operation to be of any use. An incision into the visible swelling has some advantage and cannot do any harm. Compresses as hot as can be borne, may be applied to the throat, whereas cold applications can only prove injurious. We should not forget that we have no inflammation to deal with, and it seems absolute folly to treat œdema of the glottis with copious depletions which are so generally recommended. [The following interesting case of œdema of the glottis occurred in the practice of Jacob Reed, jr., M. D., of this city, as reported by himself:

"Marth 16th, 1867, evening. Called to see Miss B., æt. 20, who had for some days "had a bad sore throat," and was reported as choking to death.

"When seen, the patient was evidently suffering from an acute œdematous inflammation of the larynx, there being high fever, pain in the region of the larynx, difficulty of swallowing and breathing, voice almost inaudible, every effort at speaking causing great pain, inspirations prolonged and stridulous, being effected only by violent effort; there was but little cough. Frequent spasmodic exacervations of these symptoms rendered suffocation imminent.

"Ordered inhalations of steam, medicated with Opium, cold pack to region of larynx, Aconite and Kali bichrom.; of the Aconite three drops of the tincture of the root were given in a half glass of water, of which she took a teaspoonful every twenty minutes.

"This appeared to afford relief which, however, proved but temporary as, upon paying my morning visit, I found the patient much worse in every respect. The leaden hue of the skin, with the intense anxiety of the countenance, showing that she had to fear the results of deficient aëration of the blood.

"This condition of affairs rendering bronchotomy necessary, I returned to the office for the necessary instruments and assistance, but in the mean while ordered two drops of the tincture of the Aconite root to be given every ten minutes.

"Upon returning, after the lapse of an hour, the patient was so far relieved as to render surgical interference unnecessary, and from this the convalescence was steady, although slow and imperfect. There remains, after many months, a cough with hoarseness, owing to constitutional tuberculosis." H.]

5. Spasmus Glottidis.
Spasm of the Glottis.

Spasmodic conditions of the glottis sometimes accompany other acute or chronic diseases of the larynx as severe complications. In this chapter we do not speak of these conditions, but of the purely nervous spasm of the glottis which occurs without any material alterations, and which is described in pathological treatises under the names of Asthma thymicum Koppii, Asthma Millari, Asthma periodicum infantum, or Laryngismus stridulus. All these conditions are essentially alike.

Spasm of the glottis affects pre-eminently children of a tender age; among adults it only occurs as an accompaniment of other pathological processes; or as an idiopathic disease it may attack females of exceedingly irritable nerves. Among children the larger number of those who are attacked by the disease, are boys; among persons of a more advanced age, the case is exactly the reverse. Ardent discussions have been carried on regarding the real cause of the disease; a retarded involution of the thymus gland, tuberculosis of the bronchial glands, a rhachitic affection of the occiput, the non-closure of the ductus Botallii, etc., have been accused as the exciting causes of the disease, until finally pathologists have concluded that the real cause of this peculiar spasm is as yet unknown. An hereditary disposition cannot be denied in many cases; not unfrequently the children of tuberculous mothers are attacked by the disease; so are children who are brought up by hand. Among adults, spasm of the glottis is undoubtedly a form of hysteria. Among children the disease occurs almost without an exception in the first year of their existence.

Symptoms and Course. The disease consists of paroxysms separated from each other by complete intermissions of various durations. The first paroxysm mostly occurs at night while the children are asleep, very rarely during a vehement crying spell. After sleeping quietly for a few hours, they are suddenly roused from sleep with a peculiar cry, as the parents describe it; or rather with a difficult, hissing inspiration of an unusually ringing sound; at the same time the faculty of breathing is either entirely suspended, or else the inspirations become rapidly more labored and in a few moments quite impossible. The children are lying as if dead, at most performing a few anxious movements with the arms; the face assumes a bluish pallor, the features become pendulous, the countenance looks bloated, the eyes are distorted and fixed. The breathing is entirely suspended. If the attack lasts any length of time, the skin becomes cool and the head is covered with a cold sweat. The pulse is of course very small and accelerated, and may even cease entirely. An attack of this kind which naturally enough fills the relatives with indescribable anguish, lasts a few seconds to several minutes, ending with an inspiration entirely like the one with which the attack commenced, which is followed by normal respiration, and, if the attack did not last too long, by perfect recovery; in the opposite case the patients feel anxious and languid, but only for a short time, after which they do not show any signs of discomfort. If an older child is attacked, the symptoms vary somewhat; the child makes great efforts to overcome the impediment to inspiration, and the loss of consciousness sets in more slowly. If the attacks return frequently and are very intense, clonic convulsions often supervene.

The very first attack may terminate fatally, but this is not often the case: as soon as general convulsions set in, the danger increases greatly, likewise if the attacks follow each other in rapid succession; if the patients are not asphyxiated, they perish by inanition.

The recurrence of the attacks is not governed by a fixed rule, not even in the case of the same individual. It is very rare that the disease is confined to a single attack, but a second attack sometimes does not take place until months have elapsed. The first attack almost always occurs during sleep; subsequent attacks may take place in the waking state. The more frequently they occur, the more dangerous they become. Recovery mostly takes place gradually, with a gradual decrease of the intensity and frequency of the attacks; it may drag along for months and may only be apparent, since another attack may break out again after a short interval of repose.

The prognosis is always more or less uncertain; neither the vigor of the little patients, nor the weakness of the first attacks is a guarantee against sudden death.

The diagnosis is not always easily made, more particularly if the spasm sets in in the course of laryngeal catarrh or of some other affection of the larynx, or if the patient does not lose his consciousness, in which case a deceptive croupy cough may set in. The fact should be kept steadily in view that a spasm of the glottis can only be thought of, if all the other symptoms of a disease of the larynx are wanting. A spasm of this kind can never be converted into croup or catarrh. The sudden dyspnœa without a sign of cough, the complete suspension of the respiratory movements, the subsequent complete intermissions constitute safe diagnostic marks in most cases.

As regards treatment, it will have to be directed against the disease as a unit rather than against a single paroxysm which never lasts long enough to admit of medical aid in every case; hence the treatment will have to confine itself to a few not altogether unessential arrangements. In the first place the child has to be laid in a proper manner; the best posture is to one side, with the head slightly bent forward. A sponge dipped in hot water and applied to the region of the larynx sometimes renders as effectual aid in this disease as a warm cataplasm in a case of vesical spasm. Sprinkling the parts very forcibly with cold water, is likewise a very efficient remedy in some cases.

For the totality of the pathological process we possess the following remedies which of course have to be given at long intervals:

Ignatia amara has an eminently characteristic symptom, it is the dyspnœa, the difficulty of drawing in breath, whereas the expirations are easy; such a difficulty is suddenly experienced about midnight. This remedy is very much praised, if the children suddenly lose their breath, which may be the lowest degree of spasm of the glottis; we have already stated under hysteria that Ignatia is likewise useful for many nervous complaints of females; but whether it will prove a proper remedy for spasm of the glottis, has not yet been verified. It may perhaps prove most appropriate if the spasm occurs as a symptomatic manifestation in croup, catarrh or whooping-cough.

Ipecacuanha has been mentioned as a remedy; indeed the symptoms justify this recommendation. We should not, however, overlook the fact that asthmatic difficulties do not really occur in this disease. Relief is easily afforded if a remedy is given at the outset, but it does not last, and we cannot recommend a remedy as a specific unless it controls the whole disease. We admit, however, that Ipecacuanha may have an excellent effect, for the time at least, in a catarrh accompanying spasm of the glottis.

The same remark applies to Belladonna. We refer to the few cases mentioned in Rückert which clearly show that Belladonna is only adapted to spasm of the glottis when occurring as a secondary symptom in other diseases.

Veratrum album and **Arsenicum album** deserve our attention if, as is often the case, the disease attacks feeble children with marked symptoms of cerebral anæmia.

Moschus is variously recommended in this disease, but we cannot see its homœopathicity to it. We are not acquainted with any decided cures that Moschus has effected in this disease, Hartmann's statement to the contrary notwithstanding.

Sambucus is represented by Hartmann as one of the leading remedies; he has noticed its good effect in a striking case which, however, does not, in our opinion, represent a high degree of spasmus glottidis. According to Hartmann, the following are the more important symptoms: The patient suddenly wakes from his slumber with his eyes and mouth half open, he has to sit up erect in order to catch breath; he can only make short, hissing inspirations, mingled with paroxysms of suffocation, during which he throws his hands about, and the face and hands look bluish and bloated, with dry heat all over, no thirst, an irregular, small and intermittent pulse; the patient cries at the approach of a paroxysm. All this occurs without cough about midnight. Hartmann commends *Menyanthes trifoliata* without having seen any curative results from this drug. We consider these indications very vague and of little practical value.

The remedies above named are either appropriate only in a simple attack of symptomatic spasm of the glottis; or else they are recommended on account of their marked resemblance to a single paroxysm; Veratrum and Arsenicum form exceptions. In our opinion, a successful treatment implies a special consideration of all the most trifling accessory circumstances without laying much stress on the particular paroxysm; and likewise a careful consideration of the etiological causes. Among these causes rhachitis, a deficient involution or hypertrophy of the thymus gland, swelling of the bronchial glands are undoubtedly the most frequent and most probable, and it is with particular reference to these etiological causes that we recommend the following remedies:

Iodium is undoubtedly a very excellent Simile, and is likewise adapted to all three above-named causal morbid conditions. With this remedy alone, given every other day at the fourth or sixth attenuation for four to eight weeks, we have cured five undoubted cases of spasm of the glottis, which evidenced their malignant nature by the fact that every subsequent attack was more violent than the preceding one. The patients were children not yet a year old, but only one of them showed an enlargement of the thymus gland. Supported by such striking curative results, we cannot be accused of hazardous speculation if we prefer this remedy to all others as long as the general organism has not become too much reduced.

Cuprum was already mentioned under croup on account of its peculiar influence over the rima glottidis. It is particularly appropriate if, during the local spasm, general convulsions have supervened and the children have become very much prostrated. Among the significant symptoms indicating this remedy, one is particularly noticeable, we mean vomiting after the attack.

Plumbum is very closely related to Cuprum in every respect, except that the general strength is still more reduced. The symptoms of a spasmodic closing of the rima glottidis are more distinctly marked in the pathogenesis of this drug than in that of any other. We are amazed that Plumbum should not yet have been recommended for this disease which, however, can only be cured by remedies that exert a deeply-penetrating, long-lasting influence over the whole organism. In this respect, *Sulphur* may deserve attention, although, we shall take the liberty of doubting the homœopathicity of its asthmatic symptoms to spasm of the glottis until this fact has been corroborated by experience. [We have cured more than one spasm of the glottis radically with nothing but the first attenuation of *Aconite-root*. H.]

Several other affections of the larynx have been left out, for the reason that they are either not accessible to treatment and are, therefore, only of a purely pathological interest to the physician, like laryngostenosis, for instance; or because they occur very rarely and mostly only as complications, like perichondritis. To devote a special chapter to hoarseness or aphonia, seemed to us inexpedient; for cases of this kind, if they present a peculiar character, a Repertory is the best guide. Nor have we devoted a special chapter to ulceration of the larynx. The therapeutic chapter of this affection is essentially the same as that of laryngeal catarrh, in which ulcers of the larynx occur as a complication with but few exceptions.

[Ulcers of the larynx are of so many different kinds and differ so greatly as respects their origin and treatment that we have deemed it expedient to devote a special chapter to this subject. We transcribe the following from Kafka's late work:

6. Ulcers of the Larynx,
Helcosis, seu Ulcera Laryngis.

All ulcers of the larynx are accompanied by catarrh of the laryngeal mucous membrane; it attends them from the start and remains while they last. A number of morbid processes predispose to ulceration; if a laryngeal catarrh arises during the existence of the ulcers, we are required to diagnose the ulcers that are peculiar to the particular disease. It is only when a laryngeal catarrh is present that we are justified in inferring the presence of ulcers. Ulcers on the epiglottis deprive it of its elasticity, whence laryngeal ulcers so frequently give rise to the so-called "swallowing wrong."

The sputa constitute another criterium for the existence of an ulcer in the larynx. The sputa are frequently streaked with blood, contain blood-disks or pus-globules, and are more particularly coughed or hawked up after eating or drinking.

The ulcers occur most frequently on the posterior wall of the pharynx and on the laryngeal mucous membrane, in front of, and between the arytænoid cartilages.

The local symptoms occasioned by the ulcers, do not essentially differ from those of chronic catarrh; only they are more violent and persistent. They consist in hoarseness even to the degree of aphonia; in continual dyspnœa, with labored, hissing, wheezing, panting respiration, especially after an exertion, such as a good deal of walking, talking, etc.; in cough which generally sets in in paroxysms, is always short and dry, and does not become loose till towards the close of the paroxysm; the sputa are scanty, in small lumps, not frothy, streaked with blood, purulent; in constant hawking occasioned by the accompanying catarrh and the quantity of mucus accumulating in the fauces; in various painful sensations and dryness of the throat; finally in swallowing wrong, as it is called, and in the return of liquids during deglutition, if the epiglottis is the seat of the ulcer.

The following kinds of ulcer are most frequently observed:

1) *Catarrhal ulcers.* They arise in consequence of chronic laryngeal catarrh, commence by the epithelium being detached, are flat, irregular, and often run together.

2) *Aphthous ulcers.* They emanate from the diphtheritic process; the mucous lining becomes infiltrated, is rapidly destroyed, and a small, generally round ulcer arises, which is surrounded with a red areola. They most commonly are present during pulmonary tuberculosis, and likewise occur on the pharyngeal mucous membrane.

3) *Follicular ulcers.* They are a result of the inflammation and ulceration of the mucous follicles, and form small, rounded, deeply penetrating ulcers. They generally break out in the pharynx, whence they spread to the larynx. If follicular ulcers in the pharynx are accompanied by constant hoarseness, the existence of such ulcers must likewise be suspected in the larynx.

4) *Tubercular ulcers.* They always accompany tuberculosis. Like tuberculosis they appear in two forms, as tubercular infiltration and as miliary tuberculosis. They are most commonly seated on the posterior wall of the larynx, less frequently on the epiglottis. During infiltration the infiltrated portion of the mucous membrane dies, leaving an ulcerated surface behind. During granular deposition, we first notice small, gray, little tubercles, which form little ulcers that not unfrequently run together and give rise to ulcerated surfaces of larger extent. Both these kinds of tubercular ulcers may spread in width and depth, invade the vocal chords and cartilages, and lead to perforations and destructions.

The so-called laryngeal phthisis is only a partial manifestation of a general disease. Most frequently it is tuberculosis that leads to laryngeal phthisis. This form of causative relation can only be adopted as long as the phenomena of the laryngeal affection are perceived, while the tubercular process in the lungs is either arrested or has not yet broken out. As a rule, tuberculosis of the larynx is connected with tuberculosis of the lungs or other organs.

In a case of continual hoarseness, we diagnose tubercular ulcers, provided we have become satisfied of the simultaneous existence of pulmonary tuberculosis. If the destructive process invades the vocal chords, complete aphonia sets in. The painful sensations in the larynx and the painfulness to contact are seldom very considerable; the violent cough comes mostly in paroxysms and is frequently accompanied by vomiting and gagging; the sputa are often streaked with blood. The presence of emaciation, fever which sets in every day almost at fixed hours, night-sweats, muscular debility, a certain degree of anæmia entitle us, if the objective signs are still doubtful, to conclude with a high degree of probability that a tubercular disease is developing itself in the lungs; perfect certainty can only be obtained if the presence of tubercles in the lungs can be demonstrated.

5) *Typhous ulcers.* The typhous ulcer arises from a typhous infiltration of the mucous follicles and of the surrounding mucous membrane by necrosis; the ulcer is shaggy, irregular and surrounded by badly-colored borders. It is the same process as takes place on the intestinal mucous membrane. These ulcers are seated on the sides of the epiglottis, and on the mucous lining in front of, and between the arytænoid cartilages. They are mostly flat; but if they dip down to the subjacent tissues, they may expose the cartilage and by necrosis lead to perforation into the œsophagus.

The typhous ulcer usually breaks out in the second or third week. Hoarseness or a hoarse cough announce a localization of the typhous process.

According to Dr. Maurice Haller the voice of the patient, as soon as the typhous process becomes localyzed in the larynx, is raised to a higher pitch; this higher pitch of the voice is not lasting, but it continues until the typhous process is terminated. The paroxysmal hoarse cough is mostly dry, the pains are slight.

The typhous ulcers are dangerous on account of the frequently supervening œdema of the glottis, and on account of the perforation which may even take place during the period of convalescence (perichondritis).

As soon as the typhous process becomes extinct, the ulcers in the larynx disappear.

6) *Syphilitic ulcers.* They almost always break out on the pharyngeal mucous membrane, whence they extend to the epiglottis and thence to the larynx. They are small, shaggy, with raised edges and a lardy base. If they penetrate to the subjacent tissues, they may cause necrosis of the cartilages. On healing they form cord-shaped cicatrices whose contraction causes stenosis of the larynx and aphonia. The syphilitic character of the ulcers is diagnosed by the simultaneously-existing or a previous attack of syphilis.

7) *Lupous ulcers* sometimes spread from the pharyngeal mucous membrane to the larynx, contracting the larynx and causing stenosis and aphonia.

8) *Variolous ulcers* arise by the spreading of variola pustules from the pharynx to the larynx where they change to small ulcers. Usually this process disappears as soon as the smallpox has run its course; in severe cases, however, the respiration is interfered with as in croup, and the symptoms of œdema glottidis may set in.

Course, Terminations, and Prognosis. Catarrhal, aphthous, follicular, typhous and variolous ulcers depend upon the disease which occasions them; as soon as this disease is cured, the ulcers heal likewise. They may easily terminate fatally by the sudden development of œdema of the glottis; or the destruction which they occasion, may lead to premature marasmus, or they may result in death in consequence of pyæmia.

Syphilitic ulcers can only be healed, if the cartilages have not already been destroyed, or stenosis has taken place.

Tubercular ulcers often run a very protracted course; they may cause very little destruction, and yet they scarcely ever heal. It is only if the tubercular process is arrested in its course that these ulcers can be healed for a time.

Lupous ulcers are generally incurable.

Treatment. The ulcers are treated with the same remedies as the diseases from which they result. Catarrhal ulcers require *Hepar, Phosphorus, Iodine, Spongia, Pulsatilla.* Aphthous ulcers require: *Sulphur, Borax, Mercurius, Nitri ac.*, also *Hydrastis can.* Follicular ulcers: *Alumina, Plumbum acet., Argentum nitr, Cuprum sulph.* Tubercular ulcers: *Oleum jec. aselli, Calcarea, China, Iodine, Sulphur, Stannum, Silicea;* the treatment is generally unsuccessful. Syphilitic ulcers require: *Kali bichrom., Mezereum, Phosphoric acid*, and the mercurial preparations: *Mercurius jod., Mercurius rub., Cinnabaris,* and *Mercurius corr.*, also *Mercurius sol.* Stenosis has to be treated surgically by tracheotomy. Typhous ulcers require the remedies given for typhus. For variolous ulcers we recommend principally *Tartar emetic,* also, in form of a gargle, one grain to three ounces of distilled water.

For the excessive cough caused by the ulcers, we recommend *Sulphate of Atropine,* second attenuation, ten drops in half a tumbler of water, a dessertspoonful every hour or two hours. *Cannabis indica* 2, given in the same manner, has likewise a soothing effect. For the diet and general management, we refer the reader to the corresponding diseases. H.]

B. DISEASES OF THE LUNGS.

The diseases of the lungs are some of the most important of the whole body, both on account of their frequency as well as on account of the disturbance of the most important function, the oxygenation of the blood. The importance of these diseases has induced pathologists for the last forty years to devote special attention to them, on which account this chapter may be regarded as the most complete and thoroughly cultivated in the whole domain of Pathology.

Pulmonary diseases are of essential importance to a homœopath, for the reason that he has it in his power to watch them objectively throughout all their phases and, thus, to become acquainted with the effects of his drugs beyond the possibility of deception. These diseases constitute most generally the battle-field upon which the struggle for supremacy between Homœopathy and her opponents has to be fought; a number of publications bearing upon this point have already shown that the importance and decisiveness of this struggle are fully appreciated.

One point of importance has to be carefully kept in view. We cannot expect that our older Colleagues, who fancy themselves rulers in medical Israel, should acquire a thorough knowledge of all modern means of diagnosis; the thing is much too arduous an undertaking; but no young homœopath should shun the trouble of availing himself both in his practice and in his reports of cases of the most refined minutiæ of an objective diagnosis. Unfortunately we cannot say that this is the universal rule. It is only by this means that we can convince our opponents with irrefutable arguments of the advantages of our System of Therapeutics. They brag of the exactness of their diagnosis and yet they have not as yet derived the least advantage from it for their own method of treatment. Here we have a point of attack, provided we prepare ourselves for the combat with arms that even the most redoubtable hero in diagnosis would stand in fear of, and provided we show at the same time that we do not study diagnosis as an intellectual entertainment, but as an addition to the science of Therapeutics, as a means to effect a cure of a given case of disease with more positive certainty. More than one homœopath has tried to cast a slur on physical diagnosis as a subject of no importance to Therapeutics, because, as is alleged, we have no physiological pathogenesis to contrast with the results obtained by means of a physical exploration of the chest. This, however, is entirely incorrect, for in respect to a number of drugs we are acquainted with the material changes with which the physical symptoms correspond; but even if this were not so, the objective diagnosis would still remain invested with the highest importance, for the reason that it often interprets the frequently obscure symptoms and traces them to their origin, and likewise because it enables us to determine with reliable certainty the effect of the medicine we have administered in a given case.

It is, therefore, our belief that there are not many homœopathic practitioners who do not attach great importance to physical diagnosis and declare it a thing of indispensable necessity. We should not have been able to refrain at the outset of this Section from expounding, as we have done at the commencement of our chapters on renal and hepatic diseases, the most important points in the diagnosis of diseases of the thoracic viscera, if we had been able to spare the necessary space for such an extensive undertaking. We should not only have had to deal with percussion and auscultation, but likewise with the measurement of the thorax, with spirometry, with the rhythm, frequency and fulness of the respiratory movements, the relation between inspirations and expirations, cough, expectoration, vocalization, etc. Any one who is acquainted with percussion and auscultation, must know that even the most necessary details in these departments are sufficient to fill a number of pages. Hence we take it for granted that every physician is fully posted in these branches of medical knowledge, and shall confine ourselves to interpolating particulars whenever necessary, while treating of the various affections; by pursuing this course we shall best fulfil the object of this work.

1. Hyperæmia of the Lungs.
Congestion, Plethora of the Lungs.

Considering the extraordinary quantity of blood which, in comparison with other organs, goes to the lungs; considering the dilatability of the pulmonary parenchyma and of its enveloping membrane, we at once not only comprehend the possibility of pulmonary engorgements, but that this possibility is even very great; if we devote some space to a consideration of this subject, it is because all pulmonary hyperæmias, primary as well as secondary, are of the greatest practical importance.

Pulmonary hyperæmia is of two kinds; it is an active hyperæmia or active congestion when caused by an afflux of blood to the lungs; and a passive congestion when resulting from an obstructed efflux of the blood from the lungs. Active hyperæmia presupposes in most cases an increased activity of the heart, hence constitutes an essential symptom of all cardiac anomalies attended with increased functional activity of the heart, but may likewise be occasioned by a temporary excitation of the heart's action by violent bodily efforts, such as running, dancing, singing, lifting, ascending a hill; or by powerful mental emotions, or by substances which cause a sudden acceleration of the circulation, more particularly spirits, wine, beer, coffee; it may likewise occur as a symptom of a general plethoric condition of the system occasioned by the suppression of habitual hemorrhages. Pulmonary hyperæmia is less frequently caused by irritants striking the lungs directly; very cold or very hot air, irritating gases, rarefied air, etc. Hence lively, sanguine, irritable individuals between the ages of twenty to thirty-five and forty years, during the prevalence of great heat or severe cold, or when residing on high mountains, are much more liable to pulmonary hyperæmia than persons of different temperaments and living under different influences. Various morbid conditions of the lungs, especially tuberculosis, engender a strikingly great disposition to pulmonary congestions.

Passive congestion is never a primary affection, but always a consequence of other morbid processes obstructing the return of the blood from the lungs. This result is more especially brought about by various anomalous conditions of the heart. In the proper place, passive congestion will be discussed more fully when we come to speak of the different pathological states of the lungs; in this place we shall speak of it only so far as may be necessary to discriminate between the two kinds of congestion, active and passive.

Symptoms and Course. The symptoms of pulmonary hyperæmia vary greatly, according to the condition of the lungs and the degree of engorgement. The lower grades of acute congestion only cause a sensation of oppression with shorter and more hurried breathing, at times passing away rapidly, at other times more slowly, or having remissions but being otherwise painless. In the higher grades the breathing suddenly becomes oppressed to an extraordinary degree, so that the patient seems on the point of suffocation. The respiration is hurried, superficial, noisy; the pulse increases in frequency and fulness, the face looks flushed. Most commonly these symptoms are associated with a desire to cough, and the frothy sputa are tinged with blood. There is no pain if the lungs are otherwise sound, whereas tuberculous individuals experience a great deal of pain. In the highest grades of hyperæmia the dyspnœa increases so rapidly and the sanguineous engorgement becomes so great that the patients die of asphyxia, sometimes so suddenly that an accident of this kind has been termed pulmonary apoplexy.

The lesser grades of the affection generally terminate sooner or later in complete recovery, whereas in the higher and more protracted grades of the disease, œdema of the lungs may develop itself, which may continue for a long time, even after the hyperæmia is entirely removed. It is questionable whether a simple hyperæmia can ever pass into pneumonia, notwithstanding that pneumonia is very commonly initiated by symptoms of hyperæmia.

Passive hyperæmia has almost the same symptoms as the active form, great oppression of breathing, turgescence of the countenance, accelerated action of the heart. The resemblance is sometimes so great that passive hyperæmia is treated in the same manner as the active form, to the great detriment of the patient. In such cases a correct diagnosis can only be determined by the anamnestic circumstances of the disease and a careful exploration of the condition of the heart; for passive hyperæmia never sets in without being preceded by considerable morbid derangements. Hypostasis of the lungs or, in other words, an accumulation of blood in accordance with the law of gravitation, is scarcely ever any thing else than a partial manifestation of other diseases; it occurs almost exclusively among old people, and is generally destitute of any symptomatic appearances.

The prognosis in acute congestion is almost always favorable; congestions caused by violent emotions are the least promising. A frequent repetition of the attacks is always a very bad sign; they show that either the heart is intensely diseased, or else that pulmonary tuberculosis is their exciting cause.

Treatment. The main remedy for all active congestions of the lungs is undoubtedly *Aconite*. We are amazed that Hartmann should have omitted any mention of this remedy. Aconite is particularly appropriate in hyperæmia depending upon cardiac affections, or indicating and accompanying tuberculosis; such individuals have a delicate skin, bright complexion and sanguine temperaments. Even a cursory review of its symptoms will satisfy any one that Aconite is homœopatic to acute hyperæmia of the lungs. If the disease was caused by a fit of anger, or vehement chagrin, or mortification, Aconite is indicated so much more fully. *Belladonna* has likewise many symptoms pointing to pulmonary congestion, but it is not so easy to determine the conditions for which Belladonna is indicated; they likewise occur less frequently. Belladonna is preferable if not only the lungs, but likewise the cephalic organs are involved in the congestion, and it is less depending upon cardiac disease than upon some other affection. Leading symptoms distinguished from those of Aconite are: turgescence of the cephalic vessels, with dark redness of the face, bluish redness of the lips, glistening eyes; anguish and restlessness; a constant dry, hacking cough, or else a spasmodic and dry cough. *Nux vomica* is an excellent remedy for certain kinds of pulmonary congestion, if the following conditions prevail: The attack is occasioned by sedentary habits, excessive mental efforts, the use of coffee, ardent spirits, in the case of sanguine, robust individuals who are free from cardiac disease; after a copious meal, in the night. The symptoms resemble those of Belladonna more than they do those of Aconite. *Digitalis purpurea* is, in our opinion, inappropriate in an isolated attack, but is, on the other hand, indicated if the congestions occur very frequently or evidently point to tuberculosis. In such affections, however, there is every reason why the medicine should be given very cautiously. It is not absolutely necessary for the heart to be the starting-point of the disease or to be considerably involved in the pathological process, for uncomplicated, tubercular hyperæmias of the lungs are likewise most easily relieved by Digitalis; *Bryonia* is the next best remedy to this latter drug. In very acute cases which may become dangerous to life by the premature supervention of an acute œdema of the lungs, no time should be lost unnecessarily by awaiting the effect of the first-named three remedies; if they act at all, they will show their curative influence after the very first dose. If they do not afford speedy relief, *Phosphorus* should at once be used, or, in case of cardiac affections: *Arsenicum*.

These remedies may suffice; after all, in most cases the selection of the proper remedial agent depends upon the nature of the case before us. We cannot refrain, however, from calling attention to *Ferrum* and *Pulsatilla* in the case of anæmic and tuberculous individuals, and likewise to *Veratrum album* and *Sepia*. [*Veratrum viride*, if given in comparatively larger doses, has often cured, without the use of any other remedies, hyperæmia of the lungs as well as pneumonia. H.]

We sometimes have great trouble to persuade such patients to desist from the frequent use of sanguineous depletions. It is true they afford a momentary relief, but in exchange they help the disease on its course, and are particularly dangerous to drunkards and to persons afflicted with incipient tuberculosis. There is scarcely any affection where it is as necessary to abstain from the use of coffee as pulmonary hyperæmia, which is caused by the action of coffee not only directly, but likewise through an increased excitability of the functional activity of the heart. Frequent deep and protracted inspirations are exceedingly useful in regulating the action of the lungs. Vigorous, but not excessive bodily exercise is useful rather than otherwise; the good results of careful ascensions of mountains by tuberculous patients afford the best evidence that this statement is founded upon facts.

2. Pneumorrhagia,
Pulmonary Hemorrhage.

If we consider the delicacy of the pulmonary tissue and the quantity of blood which is collected in it, we have no difficulty in comprehending that one of the pulmonary vessels may readily tear, and must cause a more or less considerable hemorrhage. For this reason pulmonary hemorrhage is one of the most frequently occurring morbid phenomena which of itself is not so very important, because the bleeding scarcely ever amounts to an excessive quantity, and does not threaten life with immediate danger.

Etiology. As we stated in the previous chapter, a high degree of pulmonary hyperæmia may easily result in effusion of blood into the air-passages. The effusion differs in quantity according as the affected lungs are naturally sound or otherwise morbidly affected. The causes of pulmonary hyperæmia are therefore in a certain sense the causes of pulmonary hemorrhage. The main reason, however, why pulmonary hemorrhage is invested with such ominous importance to every layman, is the circumstance that it implies the existence of morbid conditions which result in the destruction of the pulmonary tissue, among which tuberculosis occupies the first rank. It is difficult to explain why the same influences should occasion pulmonary hemorrhage in one individual and not in another. We know that sanguine, florid, irritable individuals are more liable to hemorrhages than phlegmatic and torpid persons; but we cannot decide whether this liability is owing to an accelerated flow of the blood, or to an excessive delicacy of the walls of the vessels. Diseases of the vessels themselves, atheromatous degenerations, aneurysms, etc., lead to the most profuse and most threatening hemorrhages. The not unfrequent occurrence of considerable pulmonary hemorrhages during pregnancy or after a suppression of the menses is difficult to account for. As regards age, it is self-evident that the age where the pulmonary activity is heightened and where the development of the pulmonary tissue is most active, is the age where pulmonary hemorrhages occur most frequently; this is the age between the years of fourteen and twenty-five. Whether one sex or the other is more liable, is not certain.

Symptoms and Course. Pulmonary hemorrhage either takes place into the bronchia or into the pulmonary tissue. It is either copious or scanty, in accordance with which we have in the first place hemoptysis, the evacuation of small quantities of blood together with the sputa; next: pneumorrhagia, the evacuation of large quantities of blood; the formation of clots or sanguineous deposits, by which the tissue of the lungs is not destroyed and the blood is not discharged externally; pulmonary apoplexy during which the blood is likewise effused into the pulmonary parenchyma, but with destruction of the tissue. These distinctions are, however, of very little practical use, and for practical purposes it is sufficient to distinguish hemoptysis and hemorrhage, according as a larger or smaller quantity of blood is expelled from the lungs. The formation of circumscribed coagula as well as apoplexy offer too many difficulties for a correct diagnosis in order to justify a therapeutic management based upon the latter.

Of itself hemoptysis is not a very important disease. It often occurs without any disturbance of the constitutional equilibrium, after violent exertions, in consequence of unimportant catarrhs, very often in the case of pregnant females, and sometimes consists of mere streaks of blood mixed with the mucus, at times in small detached portions of pure blood. As was said before, tuberculous individuals are most commonly affected, on which account the chest should be carefully examined at every ever so trifling hemoptysis. Slight pulmonary hemorrhages are not unfrequent accompaniments of a chronic catarrh of the bronchial mucous membrane, as is so commonly met with in emphysema of the lungs. If the quantity of the expelled blood is somewhat more considerable, the hemorrhage is usually preceded by various indefinite phenomena, such as palpitation of the heart, oppression, sensation of heat in the chest, stitches in the chest, congestions of the head; these symptoms generally disappear again after the hemorrhage has set in.

Pneumorrhagia is almost always preceded by a short preliminary stage. For several days previous the patients often feel excited, uncomfortable, oppressed on the chest, hot in the head, disposed to fainting fits; the pulse is somewhat accelerated, the beats of the heart are stronger. Real pains in the chest are seldom felt, and, if felt, are not attributable to the hemorrhage, but to the morbid conditions that gave rise to it. Shortly before the hemorrhage the symptoms of a violent pulmonary hyperæmia become manifest. While a feeling of increased warmth in the chest is experienced, the respiration becomes at the same time oppressed, after which an irritation and urging to cough are felt; with the first turn of cough a frothy, bright-red, pure blood is thrown up in various quantities, which is soon succeeded by a larger quantity attended with a cough like vomiting; or else the second hemorrhage may only occur after a longer paroxysm of cough. The patient has a distinct sensation that the blood is bubbling up in the chest; the râles can be heard even without the ear being applied to the chest.

As soon as the hemorrhage sets in, the hyperæmic symptoms abate at once, after which the patient feels very weak and experiences a disposition to faint. The fainting is not so much the result of the quantity of blood lost, but is more commonly owing to the moral impression which every hemoptoë makes even upon the most robust individual.

The disease is scarely ever limited to a single attack. After the trouble seems fully ended, generally in twenty-four hours, less frequently after several days, another attack sets in as suddenly as the former; a number of attacks may take place in this manner at indefinitely succeeding periods. In such a case anæmic symptoms may make their appearance; in severe cases the patient may even die of exhaustion.

At first sight it may seem as though the diagnosis of pulmonary hemorrhage could not well be a difficult task. Nevertheless deceptions occur nowhere more frequently than in this disease, on which account we shall explain the distinctive signs of pulmonary hemorrhage a little more fully. Nosebleed, especially when the blood is discharged from the posterior nares or during sleep, is easily mistaken for pulmonary hemorrhage, because the blood, the larger quantity of which is undoubtedly discharged into the pharynx, likewise gets into the larynx, where it causes a desire to cough which results in the expulsion of blood. At the same time blood is blown from the nose, and the posterior-superior wall of the pharynx is seen streaked with blood. If these signs are wanting, perhaps the circumstance that after the first bloody expectoration no more bloody mucus is brought up, may shed light on the nature of the attack. The absence of all local symptoms in the lungs is alone insufficient to justify the supposition that the hemorrhage is not pulmonary, but nasal. It is sometimes equally difficult to discriminate between hemorrhage from the lungs and stomach. In hæmatemesis the gagging and vomiting likewise easily excites cough; moreover in hemorrhage from the lungs a quantity of blood, before any is coughed up, is sometimes swallowed and vomited up. As a rule, the following points may serve as diagnostic signs: In hæmatemesis the symptoms of an intense affection of the stomach are almost always present for some time previous, and these symptoms likewise accompany the attack itself. The blood is always dark-red, even black, unless it should emanate from an artery. This could easily be determined by an exact diagnosis; whereas in pulmonary hemorrhage a bright-red blood is coughed up, although the blood that had first been swallowed and then vomited up, may likewise be black. A discriminative diagnosis is the most difficult in a case of hæmatemesis of tuberculous individuals, or if the physician is called upon to give an opinion derived from the report and description of the patient or his attendants. If the stools are tinged black for some time, this symptom should not be overlooked. It is likewise important to investigate the circumstance whether the blood was first coughed or vomited up.

It is much more difficult and most generally impossible to determine the precise spot in the lungs whence the blood is discharged. If the blood emanates from the trachea or larynx, the quantity will not be as large, nor will it be as large in bronchial hemorrhage as when the hemorrhage proceeds from the cavern; but a perfectly sure diagnosis will always be very difficult, and it is our opinion that this is of very little consequence in a practical point of view.

The prognosis is of particular importance to a physician for the reason that pulmonary hemorrhage is supposed to be such a frightful thing in the eyes of lay-people. We have already stated that the hemorrhage scarcely ever threatens life with immediate danger.

Even copious and rapidly recurring hemorrhages destroy life only exceptionally. The result is different if the importance of the hemorrhage to the general organism is inquired into. The scanty expectoration of blood which many persons, even without being affected with pneumonia, raise during every acute catarrh of the respiratory organs, is of very trifling significance, although it is proper that a careful exploration of the chest should be instituted with a view of determining the presence or absence of tubercular deposits. No more attention need be paid to the slight hemorrhages of pregnant or menostatic females, as long as no tubercular deposits are at the foundation of the bleeding. Persons afflicted with cardiac diseases, are very often attacked with pulmonary hemorrhage which, however, does not imply any particular danger. In general, however, we have to admit that in by far the larger majority of cases pulmonary hemorrhage points to the presence of tubercles in the lungs and to the progress of the tubercular disease; and that hence it is justly regarded as a dangerous symptom even if a physical exploration of the chest does not yet reveal the presence of any alarming disorganization. If the hemorrhage is very profuse, a return may indeed be apprehended, for a disposition to the disease remains, and cannot even be denied in cases where no tubercles exist. The meaning and importance of pulmonary hemorrhage in cardiac affections will be examined more fully when we come to treat of the affections of the heart.

To these paragraphs we have to add a few remarks concerning internal pulmonary hemorrhage, we mean infarctions and apoplexy, which frequently complicates pneumorrhagia and determines its most disastrous sequelæ.

Infarctions in the lungs have their foci. At times there is one, at other times several, varying in size to that of a walnut and even larger. They occur much less frequently near the periphery than the base of the lungs. Infarctions occur in the lungs as sharply defined dark-red or black spots of a granular appearance on their cut surface, without much firmness; a grumous, black fluid can be squeezed out of them. The surrounding parts are either œdematous or inflamed. In real apoplexy the infarcted spot is always of more considerable size, and the pulmonary parenchyma is partially destroyed.

Infarctions mostly take place where the pulmonary circulation had met with considerable obstructions, hence in cardiac affections, less frequently in tuberculosis. Apoplexy arises by the laceration of a larger vessel, either because the vessel is diseased, or in consequence of external violence.

Symptoms. Smaller and detached infarctions may form without any marked disturbances; blood will not often be coughed up in consequence. Infarctions of larger size or greater number scarcely ever exist without a group of tolerably characteristic symptoms. The precursory symptoms resemble those of pneumorrhagia, and are scarcely ever wanting. The occurrence of internal hemorrhage is marked by a sudden oppression on the chest, sometimes attended with tolerably acute, but not always definitely localized pains. The pulse is always hurried and is always small and weak. A copious spitting of blood may take place, but it may likewise be entirely wanting, nor is it generally very considerable. Nevertheless important general symptoms soon make their appearance, such as fainting, pallor of the countenance, cold sweat; it is the appearance of such symptoms that justifies the supposition of internal hemorrhage, although very little blood is lost externally. Only in acute and severe cases death may result very suddenly; otherwise the final result is determined by other circumstances: whether the extravasation is simply re-absorbed, which it takes weeks to accomplish; whether a reactive pneumonia or pleuritis sets in; whether the pleura is broken through and hæmathorax is developed; whether the infarction terminates in inflammation, abscess or gangrene; or whether an œdema of the lungs of sufficient importance will result.

It is very seldom possible that pulmonary infarctions can be diagnosed with certainty. Their occurrence, most commonly near the base of the lungs, renders them very seldom accessible to physical diagnosis; and if occurring near the periphery, they frequently develop uncertain symptoms. A circumscribed dulness not covering the extent of a pulmonary lobe, nor situated in the region where tuberculosis is usually localized or pneumonia exists, if the respiratory murmurs are either absent in that locality, or mucous râles are heard, of course suggests the supposition that infarctions may have formed. Of more value are the general symptoms, great dyspnœa and oppression of the chest, with pallor of the countenance and syncope, even sopor, without an opportunity being given to account for these symptoms by the presence of other morbid processes, more particularly if these symptoms affect persons afflicted with heart-disease.

It is easily conceivable that pulmonary infarctions must modify the course of pulmonary hemorrhage in a specific manner. The symptoms accompanying pulmonary hemorrhage will not suddenly disappear after the hemorrhage ceases, but the above-described sequelæ and anatomical lesions occasioned by the infarction will now step into the foreground together with all their characteristic phenomena. This circumstance has to be well weighed, lest the hemorrhage should be regarded as resulting from the pneumonia occasioned by the infarction, and we should be led to imagine that those sequelæ had only been covered up by the hemorrhage, and in reality represent the primary disease.

The treatment has to aim in the first place at arresting the hemorrhage, and after that at removing the subsequently remaining consequences of the hemorrhage. We commence with indicating a number of medicines that have been practically tested in pulmonary hemorrhage which is of frequent occurrence, and add to this list a few general considerations of more than ordinary importance.

Aconitum: If it were practically possible to draw a line of demarcation between active and passive pulmonary hemorrhage, we could not mark off the therapeutic sphere of Aconite more accurately than by saying that it is specifically adapted to the active form of pulmonary hemorrhage. This would, however, give rise to many errors, since many hemorrhages arising from an obstructed circulation, symptomatically resemble almost entirely an active hemorrhage. Hence the selection of the drug should be conducted very cautiously. In all active hemorrhages we meet with marked preliminary congestive symptoms; even while the hemorrhage is going on, symptoms of pulmonary hyperæmia still continue to exist, and, as we stated in the preceding chapter, no remedy is more appropriate for such states of hyperæmia than Aconite. Hyperæmia not only causing but likewise maintaining the hemorrhage, Aconite in this case effects a radical cure, and after its exhibition we sometimes see the hemorrhage arrested with wonderful rapidity. The following range of symptoms constitutes more particular indications for Aconite: The accident happens to animated individuals with a plethoric habit of body, bright complexion, disposition to palpitation of the heart, incipient tuberculosis; after a violent fit of passion, or severe exertion of the lungs. The blood is raised in small quantity, associated with a dry cough which is not violent, but torments the patient all the time; or else the blood is expectorated after a slight paroxysm of hacking cough, both in larger quantity and of a bright-red color. The patients are very restless, their countenances are at first flushed and hot, the pulse and beats of the heart very much excited; they complain of a burning or stinging pain in the chest. After commencing with the Aconite, the symptoms of febrile excitement very soon abate, after which the hemorrhage likewise ceases in almost every case. As a rule, it is well to continue the use of this drug for some time longer at more extended intervals.

Belladonna has already been mentioned in the previous chapter; it is one of the principal remedies for pulmonary hemorrhage, except that its indications are less positively defined. It is particularly applicable in the case of robust and plethoric individuals and for congestions towards the head, without any cardiac irregularities being complained of; also more particularly if the hemorrhage was the result of an incipient catarrh. A constant and tormenting desire to cough points to this remedy, the choice of which depends much more than that of Aconite, upon the general symptoms. In tubercular hemorrhage, this remedy has never had the least effect in our hands; on the contrary, it has been found very efficacious in vicarious menstrual hemorrhages and in those of pregnant females, or in the hemorrhages occurring at the critical age.

Arnica enjoys a high reputation in pulmonary hemorrhage, which it deserves much less, however, than Aconite. Hartmann gives the following characteristic indications: The hemorrhage is caused by some mechanical injury, or by severe bodily exertions; the expectorated blood is dark-red and lumpy, and is raised without cough and without much special effort; attended with stinging, burning, contractive sensation in the breast, rush of blood, palpitation of the heart and striking heat in the chest, loss of strength, fainting fits. A bright-red, frothy blood which is sometimes mixed with mucus and small clots, and which has to be hawked or coughed up, does not counter-indicate Arnica. In addition we have to observe that Arnica is particularly suitable for nervous, plethoric, not very robust individuals; the respiration is very much oppressed; during the bleeding, the patient is very much disposed to vomit; the patient is evidently tuberculous, or the heart may be somewhat affected; an attack is caused by every slight bodily exertion. Arnica is particularly suitable for young people.

Digitalis purpurea which used to be a favorite remedy for hæmoptysis in the hands of allopathic physicians, does not deserve the slight that is put upon it by homœopathic practitioners. It affords distinguished aid in pulmonary hemorrhage depending upon ob-

11

struction of the pulmonary circulation caused by heart disease, and is preëminently indicated if tuberculosis is present at the same time. The most essential indications for this drug which should be used much more frequently by homœopaths than is the case, are: engorgement of the veins about the head; a pale and livid complexion; coldness of the skin with cold sweats; irregular pulse and beating of the heart; extraordinary oppression of breathing apparently without any infiltration; great anxiety and restlessness or even a soporous condition with disposition to faint.

Pulsatilla is recommended by practitioners for the bloody cough excited by menostasia, not so much on account of its direct action upon the bleeding lungs as with reference to the causal indication, suppression of the menses. It is likewise an, excellent remedy in some forms of pulmonary hemorrhage in the ease of phthisicky persons, where the selection depends more, however, upon the rest of the symptoms than upon the hemorrhage.

Ipecacuanha will not often be found indicated where pulmonary congestions are evidently present. It is indicated by the following symptoms: Spasmodic, suffocative cough with shortness of breath, as in asthma, even unto vomiting; not too copious hemorrhage, the blood being very dark and mixed with mucus; pale or bluish-red complexion. In many respects Ipecacuanha acts very similarly to Digitalis, except that Ipecac. has none of the symptoms caused by obstructions in the pulmonary circulation.

Ledum palustre has yielded some practical results in pulmonary hemorrhage. Its local symptoms, however, are so indefinite that the homœopathicity of the drug cannot possibly be determined by means of them. It is said to be most useful in case of obstructions in the portal circulation.

Millefolium is much praised, although we have no very special indications for this drug. We find the following in Hartmann: "In almost every variety of hemorrhage, and likewise in pulmonary hemorrhage, Millefolium is an indispensable remedy, more especially in the case of robust and fleshy persons; the spitting of blood is unattended with cough, or the cough is very slight and is caused by the newly accumulating blood; at the same time there is a bubbling up in the chest, with a sensation as if warm blood were ascending in the throat, gradually increasing in intensity until blood is raised. More recently I have found that a condition of this kind yields to Aconite more promptly than to Millefolium of which we do not yet possess a sufficient number of reliable provings." Others are of a different opinion; they recommend Millef. especially in incipient phthisis.

Arsenicum album competes with Digitalis in some respects. We would give this remedy only if a high degree of weakness and irritability is associated with an extraordinary degree of cardiac excitability, together with all its accessory ailments. It is only in exceptional cases that we shall be able to use it in phthisis.

Phosphorus which was formerly a favorite remedy for pulmonary hemorrhage, is used much less by the homœopathic practitioners of the present day. We infer from its symptoms that only the lesser grades of hemorrhage are suited to its therapeutic range. Upon the whole no marked results can be expected from it; hence it ranks below all the other remedies mentioned for pulmonary hemorrhage. If it is to be used, the dose must not be too high, for even the fourth attenuation may still cause real, and therefore inconvenient medicinal aggravations.

In addition to these remedies we might complete the list by mentioning a number of others; but let it suffice if we simply name the following: *Nux vomica* and *Opium* (for the pulmonary hemorrhage of drunkards), *Drosera*, *Hyoscyamus*, *Cocculus*, *Staphysagria*.

Corresponding with our pathological data, the medicines may be ranged as follows:

For hemorrhage from active pulmonary congestion: *Aconite*, *Bellad.*, *Millef.*, *Nux vom.*; from passive congestion: *Digitalis*, *Arsenicum*; if caused by mental excitement: *Aconite*, *Nux vomica*, *Opium*; by exertions: *Aconite*, *Arnica*; by mechanical injuries: *Arnica*, *Bryonia alba*; if depending upon tuberculosis: *Acon.*, *Arn.*, *Puls t.*, *Millef.*, *Ledum*, *Phosphorus*; if depending upon heart disease: *Acon.*, *Digit.*, *Arsen.*; upon menostasia: *Pulsat.*; upon catarrh: *Bellad.*, *Hyoscyam.*, *Mercurius*; upon emphysema: *Arsen.*, *Digit.*, *Carbo veg.*; portal obstructions: *Ledum palustre*.

Regarding the effect of pulmonary hemorrhage upon the organism, it is the same as that of all other kinds of hemorrhage, and has to be treated in the same manner; this effect will never be very extensive. The consequences of hemorrhage to the lungs themselves, which are the most to be dreaded, often require different remedies from those that might perhaps be chosen without regard to the local process. If extensive infarctions have become localized in the pulmonary tissue, and the restoration of health is retarded by them, our first choice may have to be *Arnica*, afterwards *Bryonia*, *Digitalis* and finally *Phosphorus*. Pneumonia depending upon infarctions, frequently requires, beside the above-mentioned remedies, *Mercurius*, and the supervention of œdema of the lungs: *Arsenicum, Tartarus stib.*, and *Phosphorus.*

Beside attending to the present attack and its consequences, we have likewise to try to neutralize the evident tendency to pulmonary hemorrhage. Although the general conduct and mode of living of the patient are subjects of the utmost importance in this particular, yet we are in possession of a few remedies which are capable, independently of meeting other functional derangements, of preventing the frequent return of the hemorrhage; these remedies are: *Calc. carb., Ferrum, Sepia* and *Silicea*, whose special indications we cannot well enumerate in this place. *Carbo veg.* and *Conium* are often likewise adequate to this purpose.

The dietetic measures to be adapted in pulmonary hemorrhage and to meet a constitutional tendency to it, will suggest themselves without any advise from us. All we wish to say is that coffee and all other stimulants, even smoking, must be strictly forbidden.

[The following medicines have likewise been found useful in pulmonary hemorrhage; for particulars concerning most of them we refer the reader to Hale's New Remedies, 2d edition.

Erigeron canadense, when the blood is expelled in the shape of dark coagula; it is likewise recommended for passive venous hemorrhage generally.

Hamamelis, recommended for passive venous hemorrhage, although it has likewise been found an efficient remedy in active arterial hemorrhage.

Senecio aureus may be given for vicarious hemorrhage when occurring in the place of the menses.

Trillium, in tincture or infusion, is an excellent remedy for pulmonary as well as uterine hemorrhage.

Veratrum viride may afford aid in cases of hemorrhage resulting from uncomplicated, but severe pulmonary hyperæmia; the medicine has to be given in larger doses than usual.

Scilla maritima is excellent in hemorrhage from neglected catarrh; the blood bubbles up with a pricking sensation at the place whence the hemorrhage proceeds. H.]

3. Bronchitis Acuta.
Acute Bronchitis.

Concerning the affections of the bronchial mucous membrane, we find in our pathological treatises, especially if we combine both the older and more modern treatises in one Series, such a large number of names and corresponding categories, that it is only with difficulty that we succeed in mastering them. If we would adopt such a complicated course, we should have to devote a number of chapters to what we intend to present in one. We need not hesitate to adopt this course, since every homœopath is well satisfied of the necessity to individualize his cases. We shall afterwards, when decribing the symptoms, have abundant opportunities for showing the most essential forms of bronchitis.

Etiology. Acute bronchitis is one of the most frequent diseases of the human kind generally, and it is next to impossible to decide that a special age or sex is more particularly liable to it. Whereas it is not generally a dangerous disease when attacking middle-aged persons, it is on the contrary very dangerous to children and old people, and therefore constitutes one of the most important diseases of these two periods of human existence. It is undeniable that the first years of childhood are peculiarly predisposed to this disease. A predisposition of this kind likewise exists among persons of a more advanced age, and may almost always be attributed to the following circumstances: An effeminate mode of living, without adequate exercise in the open air, and not admitting of a free and easy respiration; constitutional diseases, even such as do not emaciate and debilitate the system, more especially scrofulosis and tuberculosis; irritability of the mucous membranes in consequence of frequent attacks of bronchitis; acute and chronic diseases of the lungs.

The exciting causes cannot well be traced with positive certainty. A cold and consequent suppression of the perspiration is undoubtedly one of the most ordinary causes, but not quite as common as is generally supposed. The atmosphere doubtless exerts a powerful influence not only in consquence of rapid changes in the temperature, but principally through the changes in atmospheric electricity and, as modern investigations seem to have confirmed, through consequent changes in the amount of ozone in the atmosphere. This becomes so much more probable, if we observe that a large number of cases of bronchitis are not so much caused by a damp and cold, as by a dry and cold wind, such as prevails in our region of country in the summer-season, when the wind blows from the northwest and north. If the temperature of the wind were the main cause of the trouble, an east wind would cause bronchitis most easily, which is certainly not the case. An epidemic bronchitis spreading over a large tract of country and being even considered contagious, the so-called influenza or grippe, depends upon conditions which we designate as miasmatic, but of the true nature of which we are as yet ignorant. Secondary bronchitis develops itself secondarily in persons afflicted with heart disease, emphysema of the lungs, or during the presence of acute exanthems, or various intensely acute constitutional diseases.

Symptoms. We may dispense with a description of the anatomical changes occurring in bronchitis; all we need do is to remind the reader that hyperæmia of the mucous membrane is always accompanied by a more or less marked swelling of the same; this statement is of essential necessity for a comprehension of various phenomena. In order to afford a general view of the disease, we will describe several forms of bronchitis which, however, are not essentially distinct from each other.

a) The lighter form of bronchitis, generally designated as bronchial catarrh, frequently sets in without any fever; at any rate most generally it is scarcely perceptible; sometimes no fever at all is present or the fever is at most indicated by a succession of creeping chills. This form of bronchitis scarcely ever exists isolatedly, but is almost always attended with catarrh of the nose and larynx. After experiencing a feeling of malaise for several hours, and a marked sensation of languor, the patients are attacked with a dry and spasmodic cough attended with a raw or sore feeling on the chest; at the same time the breathing is somewhat oppressed and there is no expectoration at the outset of the disease. The appetite is less but not gone, the tongue is not always coated; the patients are able to remain up, but feel drowsy and often complain of violent headache. Very often the cough remains dry for a long time, but more frequently a tenacious, greenish-yellow scanty expectoration commences already on the second day, which it is very difficult to hawk up. Auscultation yields no particular results, percussion none at all. At the end of three to nine days, very rarely at a later period and then only if the patients neglect themselves, the expectoration becomes more copious, whiter, lumpy, and is raised more easily, the normal feeling of health is restored and, while the cough is gradually decreasing, the disease passes off. The attack seems so slight, that many patients go about as usual, but, by pursuing this course, expose themselves to relapses which are very apt to take place and beget a tendency towards the inflammatory form of bronchitis or else originate the consequences that will be more fully described in a subsequent paragraph.

b) Bronchitis inflammatoria, inflammatory or acute bronchitis. This form of bronchitis which is marked by much more violent phenomena, is not by any means a purely simple form of bronchitis of a higher degree of intensity. It does not ordinarily result from an existing catarrh of the upper respiratory organs, unless the catarrh is suddenly and violently increased by severe neglect; but most generally it occurs as a primary disease. It generally commences with a violent chill which is distinguished from the chill that initiates acute inflammations, by the circumstance that it is not followed by as high an increase of temperature and that there is a frequent recurrence of the chill, especially on motion. The patient feels very weary and languid, complains most generally of a violent headache, exhibits frequent changes of complexion, experiences a rheumatic drawing in the limbs and great restlessness and is scarcely ever capable of remaining out of bed. Very soon these general symptoms which do not point out more particularly the locality of the disease, are followed by a burning, sore pain in the chest under the sternum at every deep inspiration, which is felt more severely when coughing. The cough sets in at the same time as the pain is felt; it is more or less violent, sometimes spasmodic, at first dry but not hoarse, but very soon accompanied by the above-described expectoration. There is no dyspnœa properly speaking, but the breathing is more labored, less full and hence somewhat more hurried. The pulse is accelerated, but it is only in the severer grades of the disease that it exceeds one hundred pulsations. In this form of bronchitis the digestive organs are always involved, the appetite is entirely gone, the bowels are constipated, there is seldom any vomiting. Percussion does not reveal any abnormal changes, but auscultation reveals a more or less prolonged expiration over the whole chest, less frequently a more prolonged inspiration, accompanied by wheezing. These auscultatory results are very much modified, if bronchitis becomes associated with a pulmonary emphysema, etc. as a secondary affection. Even in simple bronchitis, when not complicated with tubercles, the expectoration is easily tinged with blood, whereas raising a quantity of pure blood is a rare occurrence and always points to a more dangerous and more deep-seated constitutional disease. All the phenomena, especially the cough, exacerbate in the evening and about midnight. The further course of the disease is governed by a variety of circumstances. The importance of bronchitis of any degree in the case of tuberculous patients will be more fully inquired into when we come to treat of tuberculosis; and when speaking of pulmonary emphysema, we shall likewise discuss more fully the acute exacerbations of an existing bronchial catarrh which likewise assume the form of bronchitis. In favorable cases uncomplicated forms of bronchitis terminate in four or five days, or exceptionally at an earlier period, in simple bronchial catarrh. The general symptoms moderate in intensity, the fever abates almost entirely, the expectoration becomes more profuse, more fluid, of a whitish-gray color and is more easily raised by the cough which is now much less painful. Instead of the dry wheezing, auscultation now reveals coarse râles. The patients do not often feel well again before the tenth day. If the course of the disease is less favorable, its different phases are either more protracted, or else other morbid conditions become associated with it. In the former case the dry, spasmodic, distressing cough may last beyond the seventh or even to the fourteenth day, after which the period of a more profuse secretion of mucus lasts equally long. Although this longer duration of the disease shows as a rule that it is of a secondary nature, yet a purely primary form of bronchitis may run an equally long course, an occurrence peculiar to old age. The course of the disease is still more unfavorable and threatening, if the inflammation of the bronchia spreads to the more delicate ramifications, or if pneumonia and an acute œdema of the lungs supervene. The latter may set in with so much rapidity that the patient whom we had left comparatively comfortable, is found dead on our return. Generally this change develops itself more slowly and is at first recognized by a striking and rapid increase of the dyspnœa.

The patient's age exerts a greatly modifying influence over the course of the disease as well as over its danger to life. Of the bronchitis of children we shall speak hereafter. Among old people, or only somewhat advanced in age, the danger is quite considerable, and seems to depend more particularly upon the increased liability of the bronchial mucous lining to swell, upon the profuse quantity of the secretion at the same time as the respiratory process becomes feebler, and upon the consequently increased danger of œdema of the lungs. At the same time we should not overlook the fact that old people are scarcely ever without some degree of emphysema and that, where no emphysema is present, it is very apt to break out in an acute form.

Bronchitis Acuta.

Hence the bronchitis of old people differs greatly from that which we have described in the preceding paragraphs. The disease originates in the same manner, only the febrile symptoms seem to be less violent. With the appearance of the râles in the chest, which are generally very prominent, the strength of the patient diminishes instead of increasing, and dyspnœa rises to a high degree of intensity. The pulse soon becomes smaller and weaker, the skin becomes moist and cool, the tongue dry and brown, and the sensorium is powerfully affected by the disease: sopor, delirium and grasping at flocks setting in. In this manner the patient may succumb to the disease in a few days, the increase of the mucous râles and the decrease and final and total cessation of the expectoration constituting the most ominous signs of approaching dissolution.

One of the most common terminations of bronchitis is chronic bronchial catarrh which succeeds the acute form the more rarely, the younger and healthier the individual.

c. *Bronchitis capillaris.* We apply this name to an inflammation of the finest bronchial ramifications in the lungs. An inflammation of this kind frequently sets in as a continuation and still more frequently as a sequel of the inflammation of the larger bronchial tubes, and occurs much less frequently as an idiopathic primary disease. We here give only the symptoms peculiar to capillary bronchitis; the other forms of bronchitis suggest themselves to the reader, if he will simply associate the following description with a simple bronchial catarrh. This affection scarcely ever attacks middle-aged persons; it is most apt to occur among children, and very seldom befalls old people.

Capillary bronchitis commences like the acute form with the symptoms of a so-called catarrhal fever; but it is an insidious disease which, when occurring idiopathically, scarcely ever betrays its local focus by pain. At an early stage the patient is oppressed for breath, this oppression being determined by the extent of the portion of the lungs that is invaded; with a distressing cough without any expectoration at first, which, even if it should become very copious at a subsequent period, can only be raised with a great deal of difficulty. The breathing is accelerated, the inspirations being very much embarrassed and prolonged. Percussion yields no results; auscultation in this affection alone at first reveals a shrill wheezing which is afterwards mingled with fine crepitations and râles. If complicated with inflammation of the larger bronchia, the coarse râles of the latter are apt to disguise the more delicate râles in the finer bronchial ramifications, at any rate, the latter are heard much more indistinctly.

The constitutional symptoms soon assume a serious and threatening aspect. The fever ordinarily increases, yet the skin is not dry, but inclines to perspire very profusely; the feet and hands are apt to feel cold, and the face looks pale. The pulse soon becomes small and feeble, and the anxiety and restlessness of the patients generally increase in a corresponding ratio; the tongue is not unfrequently brown and dry. The paroxysms of cough sometimes become so severe that after each paroxysm the patients seem completely exhausted. In the case of a strong adult the pathological process seldom reaches a height where the respiration is impeded to the extent of inducing poisoning of the blood by carbonic acid. This is most characteristically revealed in the persons attacked by the supervention of cerebral symptoms, such as sopor, coma, delirium; in the case of adults these symptoms are of rare occurrence, in children and old people they are often met with. The capillary bronchitis of the latter is very much like the above-described inflammatory bronchitis, except that the typhoid character of the pathological process shows itself in the case of old people at a much earlier period, is much more intense, and the danger is much greater.

This form of bronchitis at times runs a very rapid course and then generally terminates fatally, at other times the course is more protracted. Robust individuals may recover already in the second week, very seldom before this time, whereas a duration of one month is a very common thing. Sometimes the affection continues unchanged for weeks in all its severity, and the patients sink under the terrible paroxysms of cough rather than from any other cause. It is always a good sign if a quantity of fine, filiform sputa are expectorated. This is most easily found out by receiving the sputa in water, when these fine threads are most easily distinguished. Among old persons in whom this process resembles almost entirely an attack of pneumonia notha, death sometimes takes place on the third day, very rarely after the second week. Independently of the circumstance that the disease is of itself a dangerous malady, the simultaneously existing pathological disturbances and the possible and ready occurrence of threatening complications are likewise of great importance. Among the latter the pneumonia which develops itself in the neighborhood of the bronchial inflammation may result so much more disastrously, as the existing bronchitis alone determines a most damaging interference with the respiratory act. Acute œdema of the lungs is equally dangerous. Acute emphysema is of a less threatening character. The most important complication is the presence of tuberculosis. Many assert that bronchitis is very often the cause of tubercular deposits; others, on the contrary, are of opinion that bronchitis only excites the suppurative process in tubercular deposits. This is not the place for a farther discussion of this subject. What is certain is that in tuberculous individuals capillary bronchitis is very apt to pass into a chronic form with a long-lasting, dry, paroxysmal cough. Relapses in capillary bronchitis occur much more easily than in any other form of this disease.

d. Croupous bronchitis is characterized by an exudation on the free surface of the bronchial mucous membrane, which, in the larger bronchia, assumes the shape of a tubular lining, and stops up the smaller bronchial ramifications like a plug. It is most frequently a secondary disease, a result, and an almost always fatal complication of a croupous inflammation of the larynx and trachea; or else it may originate as a primary disease. As such the acute form occurs very rarely, but it does occur sometimes. In such a case it presents the picture of an acute bronchitis, but with aggravated symptoms. The fever is very violent, mingled with chills, the pulse is very frequent, the prostration is disproportionally great from the very beginning. The degree of dyspnœa is determined by the fact whether the larger bronchia are alone affected or whether the smaller are involved in the disease. The cough is tormenting, the expectoration difficult, lumpy, tenacious, and, in water, assuming the form of fine tubes or arborescent ramifications. If a large portion of the bronchia is involved in this process, cyanosis, œdema of the lungs and death by poisoning with carbonic acid are the speedy terminations of the disease. The chronic form occurs almost exclusively in tuberculous individuals, and will be discussed more fully in the chapter on tuberculosis. Cases that seem idiopathic primary diseases, are likewise caused by a less extensive and hidden deposition of tubercular matter. The chronic form is distinguished by the violent cough that accompanies it. In this form of bronchitis the exudation is not secreted in the larger, but in the smaller bronchia, and is not only difficult to expectorate, but likewise acts as a most intensely irritating cause of cough.

e. After having described the other forms of bronchitis, we here devote a few lines to a description of infantile bronchitis which, as regards its course and importance, differs most essentially from the corresponding bronchitis of adults.

An inflammation of the larger bronchia, be it slight or severe, has almost the same phenomena in the case of children as in that of adults, except that the fever is much more violent and the breathing is in almost every case interfered with very considerably at an early period. The importance of this process in the case of children is much greater than in that of adults, for the reason that in the former it is apt to spread to the smaller bronchia, after which the children who at first gave no cause for alarm, suddenly appear attacked by a dangerous disease. Capillary bronchitis does not often occur as a primary affection; it is almost always the continuation of an inflammation of the larger tubes. The symptomatic development generally takes place as follows: After the children have had for some days a simple catarrh, attended with severe fever, the breathing becomes more hurried and progressively more oppressed, and the children become more and more restless and anxious. Whereas a physical exploration of the chest had so far revealed nothing abnormal, the respiration, during inspirations as well as expirations, now becomes wheezing, more especially during an inspiration, accompanied or not by distinct vesicular murmurs. The cough continues to increase in vehemence, without anything being expectorated; or, if anything is raised, it is only with great difficulty a small quantity of mucus which is swallowed again as soon as raised. The general organism, in such a severe disease, is of course correspondingly affected. The dyspnœa now increases from hour to hour and soon reaches a degree of intensity that is in no respect inferior to the worst attack of croup, and becomes still more distressing in consequence of the unceasing efforts on the part of the children to obtain relief by coughing. The pulse becomes frequent and small, the skin on the extremities and head is covered with perspiration, the face is pallid or livid, becomes bluish during an attack of cough, the anxiety and restlessness reach the highest degree of intensity. If at this stage of the disease there is no improvement by an increase of the expectoration and a relief from the dyspnœa, the disease presents the same picture as in the last stage of croup, only the hissing sound caused by the stricture of the glottis is wanting. The children become calmer, pallid and cool, they are lying in a state of unconsciousness or sopor, the respiration becomes very superficial, the paroxysms of cough abate more and more, and the children die comatose. This fatal termination sometimes takes place already in the first week of the disease, less frequently after the fourteenth day, provided no adventitious influence causes an exacerbation of the disease. Recovery always takes place slowly, the liability to relapses is very great; the strength does not easily return, and the cough sometimes continues for many weeks. The diagnosis is only difficult in the case of very small children; here the characteristic cough is almost always entirely absent, in general the reaction against the disease is either slight or non-apparent. The prognosis is the more doubtful the younger the patient. That dentition complicates the prognosis, cannot be taken for granted. The greater liability to the disease at this period is probably owing to the increased susceptibilities of the infantile organism.

In describing the treatment of bronchitis, we commence with the treatment of the previously-described forms, in order not to crowd too much material into one chapter, although influenza and chronic catarrh really belong in this category of disease. These two forms, however, cannot well be treated from the same point of view as a simple acute bronchitis. Let us first consider the leading remedies for the more important forms of bronchitis, to which afterwards, when we come to enumerate the remedies for the different forms singly, the less essential forms can be added. We place

Aconitum at the head of the list, not so much because we consider it as one of the more important remedies, but because it seems to have become a matter of routine to recommend it for incipient catarrh. We have on several occasions expressed our doubts concerning the propriety of recommending Aconite for catarrh. A common catarrhal fever is not the province of Aconite, and if we should be told that Aconite has moderated this fever in so many cases, we suggest that the improvement might likewise have taken place spontaneously without Aconite. How many catarrhs commence in the first twenty-four hours with a feeling of anxiety, a frequent pulse and an extraordinary rise of temperature, and yet run their course afterwards without any fever. This should not be attributed to the action of Aconite. A remittent fever is least suitable to this medicine. Where the fever, as is often the case in acute bronchitis, is continuous, the skin is dry and the heat is not mingled with chilly creepings, Aconite is in its place. The symptomatic indications are most fully met with in the incipient bronchitis of children. If the objection is raised that the diagnosis may be doubtful at first and that hence Aconite ought to be opposed to the general febrile symptoms, we meet it with the assertion that in every attack of bronchitis the fever has at first a catarrhal, not an inflammatory type.

Belladonna has among its symptoms all those that characterize the milder as well as the severer forms of bronchitis. In bronchitis setting in with a violent fever, it moderates the latter much more certainly than Aconite. When speaking of Angina we have had occasion to remark that we consider Belladonna a very efficient remedy in acute catarrh of the respiratory organs. The single diagnostic of a disposition to perspiration while the skin is very hot, constitutes a decidedly characteristic indication. Prominent symptoms, of which we only mention the local symptoms, are the following: A dry, continual, distressing and sometimes spasmodic cough; short paroxysms of cough, but very violent, especially towards evening; no expectoration, or else a yellowish, tenacious, blood-streaked, scanty expectoration. The respiration is oppressed, irregular, and hurried, especially while the patient is sleeping. Sensation of great fulness in the chest, without any real pain; determination of blood to the lungs. This shows that Belladonna is indicated in the lighter as well as in the severer and severest forms of catarrh, but ordinarily only in the first three or four days, very seldom at a later period.

Mercurius corresponds with the whole course of a severe attack of bronchitis, even better than Belladonna. It is particularly adapted to children and robust adults, but not so much to old people. There is a violent fever, the temperature is very high, there is great disposition to perspire without obtaining any relief from it; in contradistinction to Belladonna there is a constant alternation of chills and heat, with a remarkable sensitiveness to the most trifling changes of temperature. If the stomach and the digestive organs are likewise affected, the tongue has a thick yellowish coating, whereas under Belladonna there is only a thin whitish coating in the middle of the tongue; or if diarrhœa is present, Mercurius is indicated so much more positively. The most prominent and most important local symptoms are: Feeling of dryness, roughness, and soreness down the middle of the chest, burning in the side; dry, violent and wearing cough, especially in the evening and until midnight, with tenacious, yellowish, sometimes blood-tinged expectoration, every paroxysm of cough is preceded by anxious oppression, dyspnœa. Another characteristic which distinguishes Mercurius from Belladonna, is an unquenchable longing for icy cold drinks, although they always make the cough worse.

Bryonia alba will not often be found indicated at the commencement of bronchitis; if indicated, it will most likely be in the case of old people in whom the catarrhal fever assumes at the outset the form of an adynamic disease. This remedy is most commonly suitable after the fever has been allayed by one of the previously mentioned remedies, and the expectoration begins to become loose enough to enable the patient to cough up mucus. The cough is violent, spasmodic; it is excited by titillation low down in the chest; by every irritating impression, especially by tobacco-smoke, after eating, in the afternoon and after midnight; the expectoration is scanty, yellowish and tinged with blood. When coughing, there is violent determination of blood to the head, turgescence of the face. Paroxysms of oppressed breathing, but no constant dyspnœa.

Spongia is characterized by a hollow, barking, dry, seldom moist cough, continuing all day, and likewise all night in long-lasting distressing paroxysms; at the same time labored, crowing, wheezing inspirations, sometimes accompanied by râles. The remedy is most appropriate for children, more particularly if the disease set in as laryngitis and gradually extended to the lungs. It is an excellent remedy in croupous bronchitis.

Veratrum album is not often enough made use of in bronchitis. It is not suitable in the first stage, but on the passage into the second stage, if mucus is secreted in copious quantities which cannot yet be coughed up. This causes a constant titillation deep in the chest, with desire to cough, wheezing and coarse râles, but no expectoration, the distressing paroxysms of cough occur principally at night, with violent determination of blood to the head. The general failing of strength, the increased frequency or even irregularity of the pulse constitute additional indications for Veratrum, which is evidently suitable to old people rather than children.

Tartarus stibiatus of all other remedies enjoys the largest sphere of action in pulmonary catarrh, and is preëminently characterized by a profuse secretion of mucus which it is difficult to raise, with or without fever. This range of action is distinctly pointed out by the not very numerous, but significant lung-symptoms of Tartar emetic. Hence both the lighter and severer cases are adapted to this drug, fine curative results of which are reported in our Periodicals. The lighter cases are not often met with among persons of middle-age, more frequently among children and old people. In capillary bronchitis Tartar emetic is sometimes the only remedy from which help may yet be expected, only it must not be given in too small doses nor large enough to produce emesis. Symptoms of incipient poisoning by carbonic acid, such as sopor, delirium, coma with pallor and bloat of the countenance and an unequal temperature of the body are appropriate indications for Tartar emetic, so is œdema of the lungs when similar symptoms prevail. Profuse sweats without relief, disposition to vomiting and diarrhœa, paroxysms of a rattling cough ending in vomiting, likewise indicate Tartar emetic. All this shows that it is really the second stage of the catarrhal process which is adapted to the curative action of this drug which acts very similarly to Veratrum album. These two drugs differ principally in their phenomena of reaction which are very striking and active under Veratrum, but very feeble under Tartar emetic. Hence Tartar emetic will often be found useful after Veratrum.

Ipecacuanha bears great resemblance to the two last-mentioned remedies. The most essential symptoms for this remedy are: Loud mucous râles in the chest with wheezing respiration, great dyspnœa mostly in paroxysms especially in the evening and at night, convulsive suffocative cough during which the face becomes blue, sometimes ending in vomiting of mucus, or else dry cough in spite of the mucous râles, spasm of the glottis, convulsive twitchings, unequal temperature of the body, severe gastric ailments and intestinal catarrh, pallid or bluish and bloated countenance. Ipecac. is likewise suitable for a dry, spasmodic cough, but certainly not according to its physiological symptoms. The remedy is principally adapted to the bronchial catarrh of children; adults do not seem to be favorably affected by it, and its good effect upon old people is very questionable. The above stated symptoms show that the fine curative virtues of Ipecac. do not reside in its emetic properties, but in its specific adaptation to the bronchial disease. Allopathic physicians would soon become convinced of this fact, if they would give the remedy in doses small enough not to cause nausea. It cannot be denied, however, that the act of vomiting in suffocative catarrh may exert an expectorant and alleviating influence, and we could not find fault with a homœopath who, from this stand-point, were to prescribe massive doses of this drug. At any rate we know from experience that a smaller dose than a grain of the second trituration does not produce a reliable effect.

Nux vomica is recommended for bronchitis, but we must confess that we have never witnessed any curative results from this drug in the acute form of bronchitis, however much we may value it in the lesser degree of laryngotracheitis. We shall scarcely ever discover a real symptomatic similarity between Nux and bronchitis; if existing, it will only be found to apply to the more trifling forms of the disease.

Chamomilla may be found suitable for the bronchitis of children, not so much of adults; it is indicated if the larger bronchia are inflamed, with an urging to cough, the cough being excited or aggravated, by the least attempt to use one's voice. It is particularly violent at night, and accompanied by wheezing, and by coarse râles. Bad cases are not adapted to this medicine.

Pulsatilla is only indicated in the lighter forms of inflammation of the large bronchia, if there is no fever or the fever is already passed. We shall revert to this remedy again under chronic bronchial catarrh, to which the reader is referred.

Rhus toxicodendron seems to us very seldom indicated in simple bronchitis, but may prove of importance in the epidemic forms of this disease. On this account we refer the reader to the treatment of influenza. We have to recommend this remedy, however, in the first stage of the malignant forms of the bronchitis of old people. At an early stage already the symptoms resemble those of typhus; the danger is more particularly determined by the character of the fever which deprives the already exhausted frame of all power of reaction. Under these circumstances Rhus will be found eminently suitable, since it corresponds very strikingly with the exceedingly threatening constitutional symptoms.

Hepar sulphuris calc. is most nearly related to Spongia in bronchitis as well as in laryngitis. A characteristic indication for Hepar is a dry, spasmodic, barking cough with a wheezing sound over the whole thorax without any real mucous râles; it is a steady cough, only at intervals increasing to frightful paroxysms with danger of suffocation; it is excited by every attempt to draw a long breath, and only results in the expectoration of a yellowish, tenacious mucus. Hence Hepar is an important remedy in croupous bronchitis, likewise in the less acute or even chronic form of the disease; in capillary bronchitis its applicability is questionable. [We do not agree with Bæhr in this statement; we have used Hepar in this form of bronchitis with striking benefit, giving the third to the sixth attenuation. H.]

Iodium may be ranged side by side with Spongia and Hepar. However it is not by any means ahead of these agents, since it affects the larynx and trachea much more energetically than the bronchia. It has no particular symptoms that distinguish it from other remedies.

Bromine has not been sufficiently proved to secure it a prominent place among the remedies for bronchitis. The recommendations of this drug by homœopathic physicians are too vague and indefinite to deserve any further notice at our hands. Its practical results are exceedingly meagre and indecisive.

Baryta carbonica is not much used in bronchitis, although it deserves some consideration in at least one form of this disease. We allude to the bronchitis of old people during its transition from the acute to the chronic form; there is a constant desire to cough, with loud mucous râles, yet the expectoration is very difficult and scanty. In such cases we have seen this remedy act with decided benefit. In bronchitis with threatening symptoms we should never depend upon Baryta carbonica,

Arsenicum album is scarcely ever indicated in simple bronchitis; for particulars we refer the reader to the chapters on influenza and chronic bronchial catarrh.

Phosphorus is not, in our estimation, a remedy for bronchitis unless the disease is complicated with other affections. Hahnemann himself pronounces Phosphorus not only not suitable, but even hurtful in this disease; this statement certainly rests upon practical observations, although it does not seem confirmed by the physiological data of the Materia Medica. In his treatise on Phosphorus, Sorge does not allude to this agent as a remedy for bronchial diseases. In our further considerations of pulmonary affections we shall frequently have occasion to revert to Phosphorus. On this occasion we will merely state that if œdema of the lungs or pneumonia should supervene during the course of bronchitis, Phosphorus will be found one of the chief remedies from which help may yet be expected.

Let us now in conclusion consider the above-described forms of bronchitis in their relation to the remedies we have indicated to which a large number might be added, if we desired to present an absolutely complete list. To those who object to such a cursory review of remedies as favoring a tendency to dogmatic systemization, we reply that by this means a knowledge of the remedies is more easily obtained and an opportunity is afforded for mentioning a number of others that had been omitted in the preceding list.

In the milder form, the so-called simple bronchial catarrh, no remedy is required, since it most commonly passes off without any medication. Nevertheless, considering how easily this simple form may prepare the way for the more dangerous forms of bronchitis, it is advisable to get it out of the way as soon as possible. If fever is present, *Belladonna* should first be given, if not, *Nux vomica*. [*Aconite* or *Mercurius* may be required. H.] In the case of children, Belladonna is principally suitable, to which *Chamomilla* may be preferred under certain circumstances, especially if the children are very young. As soon as the cough is loose, *Tartarus stibiatus* or *Pulsatilla* may be required, less frequently *Bryonia* or *Ipecacuanha*. These few remedies will almost always be found sufficient.

In the inflammatory bronchitis of adults *Belladonna* will have always to be given first; *Mercurius* if the above-described symptomatic indications prevail, more particularly if gastric derangements or diarrhœa are present. If under the operation of these drugs the fever has abated and the cough has become loose, *Stibium*, *Bryonia*, *Bromine*, *Hepar sulphuris*, likewise *Hyoscyamus* or *Conium* may be required. *Bryonia* deserves a preference if the trouble seems disposed to run a very protracted course, in which case *Digitalis* may have to be resorted to. It is not our object to indicate all the different cough-symptoms; they can be found in any good Repertory. If the inflammation spreads to the finer bronchial ramifications, *Bryonia* will still be found most appropriate. In cases with typhoid symptoms and violent fever, *Rhus tox.* may have to be given. If the dyspnœa increases to a high degree, *Veratrum* or *Stibium*, or according to some, *Ipecacuanha* may be indicated. For a supervening œdema of the lungs *Phosphorus* and *Arsenicum* are mostly required; *Tart. stibiatus* will seldom be found indicated; *Carbo veget.* may have to be fallen back upon. *Iodium*, *Spongia* and *Bromium* may be indicated in capillary bronchitis, also *Ammonium muriat.* and *carbonicum*, [also *Hepar sulphuris*. H.]

In the bronchitis of old people we have in the first place to moderate the fever, for which *Aconite* or even *Belladonna* will but seldom be found suitable; *Bryonia* and *Rhus tox.* may do much better. If there is but little or no fever, *Tart. stib.* will be found most appropriate. If bronchitis is complicated with emphysema, the whole group of symptoms is best met by *Arsenicum*, which is likewise to be resorted to, if the fever should become complicated with dyspnœa. In the case of old people *Phosphorus* will not often be found suitable for the threatening terminal stages of bronchitis; *Tart. stib.* and *Veratrum* will be much better. We have recommended *Baryta* for light attacks during the stage without fever.

The bronchitis of children tends greatly to assume the form of capillary bronchitis; for this reason it behooves us to watch an attack of bronchitis in children with the utmost care. At the commencement of the attack, the symptoms generally point to *Aconite*, not, however, with such perfect regularity as to admit of Aconite being regarded as an invariable specific. *Belladonna* often competes with Aconite in this disease, in the further course of which, even in slight cases, the same remedies may have to be used that suit the case of adults. In the more dangerous forms *Mercurius* may generally deserve a preference at the outset; it is indicated if by nothing else than the thick, yellowish coating of the tongue, and the frequent alternation of chills, extreme heat and exhausting sweats. If the symptoms increase in intensity, *Spongia* is indicated; if there is a violent, dry, suffocative cough, *Hepar;* if the cough sounds loose, and there are mucous râles but no expectoration, *Ipecacuanha;* for excessive secretion of mucus, with severe dyspnœa and convulsive phenomena, *Tartarus stibiatus* may be required, but it will seldom act with as much benefit as Ipecacuanha.

Croupous bronchitis as a partial development of laryngeal croup does not require any other treatment than the latter. Even if bronchial croup should break out as a primary disease, which is seldom the case, *Iodium, Spongia, Hepar* and perhaps *Bromine* would have to be used. In subacute and even chronic cases *Arsenicum* is one of the most efficient remedies to prevent and mitigate the paroxysms of cough, which, considering their violence, must be considered a very satisfactory result.

In conclusion we call attention to a remedy which, so far as we know, has never yet been employed in bronchitis. We mean *Opium*. Latterly we have witnessed good results from *Opium*, which, doubtless, are not exclusively due to its palliative or narcotic action. We were led to its use by the description in an English Journal of a chronic case of poisoning with Opium, according to which a spasmodic and dry cough is one of the most common phenomena of this agent. We have to revert to this remedy more fully when we come to treat of influenza and pneumonia. To judge by the physiological symptoms of Opium as we find them in the Materia Medica, and considering the energetic action of this drug upon the childlike organism, Opium must be an excellent remedy in the capillary bronchitis of children.

The general management of the patient occupies a conspicuous place in this disease. It is unfortunately a wide-spread custom to endeavor to obtain an increase of cutaneous perspiration even in a case of incipient bronchial catarrh, without discriminating by what means this object is attained. We cannot encourage a proceeding of this kind. In lighter cases, where this proceeding seems to have had little effect, the question may be asked whether the case would not have turned out equally favorably without sweat; the rapid recovery of patients who do not resort to such means, shows that exciting a perspiration is not absolutely necessary to a cure. In bad cases an artificial perspiration is decidedly injurious. The object is obtained more promptly and more safely, if the patients are kept in their beds with but little covering, and the temperature of the room increased to about fifty degrees F. At the same time water should be allowed to evaporate in the room, by which means the irritating urging to cough is very much diminished. If the mere act of sweating were beneficial to the patients, they ought to feel better in summer. It is well known, however, that the bronchial catarrhs of the hot season are more obstinate and distressing than those of the cold. However, if we are anxious to avoid all conflict with the inveterate habits of the people, perspiration can be excited by drinking in bed a glass of hot water and sugar with a few drops of lemon-juice in order to make it more palatable; children may drink a glass of very much diluted warm milk, sweetened with a little sugar. If these simple means do not excite perspiration, other means will not excite any either, or, if they do, it will be to the patient's prejudice. There is another powerful reason against copious perspiration. It considerably increases the disposition to take cold, which is anyhow very great, and causes exacerbations and relapses; rising to void the urine or evacuate the bowels may be sufficient to superinduce a fresh cold, nor will the patients after recovery be able to go out again as soon as they otherwise might, without apprehending a new attack. An effeminate mode of life which is one of the main causes of catarrh in healthy persons, is likewise the cause of frequent relapses. This remark applies to little children in whose case every thing is often done to render them unfit for the least exposure to open air. The general strength of the patients is the best indication whether they can safly be permitted to go out of doors; if they feel strong again as usual, a little remaining loose cough need not deter them from going out, provided the temperature of the atmosphere and the weather generally are sufficiently inviting. In a case of tubercular bronchitis other considerations will have to govern the general management.

In matters of diet, the instinct of the patient may safely be taken as a guide. In bad cases the functional activity of the digestive organs is completely prostrated, and there is no necessity of forbidding the use of any kind of food; whereas in the more unimportant cases the choice of food is of very little particular consequence. All we have to do is to see to it that the nourishment which is introduced into the stomach, does not cause any catarrhal irritation of this organ. As soon as the appetite returns, a simple, but nourishing diet is the best. As regards drinks, it may be well not to implicitly gratify the desire of the patients who have a great longing for cold water. Drinking cold water is apt to excite or increase the cough, whereas it is diminished and moderated by warm beverages. As a matter of course, whatever might irritate the lungs, has to be avoided, such as continued or loud talking, mental excitements, dust, smoke, dry heat, the use of coffee, spirits, etc. For further details we refer to the article on diet in the chapter on pulmonary tuberculosis.

4. Influenza.
Grippe.

Influenza is not by any means a simple catarrh of the respiratory organs, though the anatomical changes indicate such a condition; but a peculiar, complicated and combined catarrh which in point of importance and treatment differs essentially from simple bronchitis. This instance shows most conclusively that it is wrong to undertake to determine the character of a disease by the anatomical lesions it occasions.

The etiology of influenza is completely enveloped in obscurity. It is an epidemic disease which may prevail in any season, and is frequently associated with other epidemic affections. Most commonly it spreads over a large extent of country and attacks anybody, although individuals who are affected with pulmonary diseases, more particularly tuberculous individuals, are most liable to its visitations. The most extensive influenza-epidemics have spread from east to west. We again call attention to the connection between influenza and the amount of ozone in the atmosphere.

Symptoms. If latterly every bronchial catarrh with typhoid symptoms has been designated as influenza, this appellation is no more proper than it is proper to refuse this name to larger or smaller epidemics for no better reason than because they do not come up either in extent or fatality to the epidemic of 1833. We apply the name grippe or influenza to every bronchitis invading a large surface of country and involving with marked symptoms of illness the whole organism, more especially the nervous system, attacking a number of individuals in the same epidemic with very similar symptoms, although these may differ ever so much in different epidemics.

The phenomena referring to the respiratory organs are altogether those of an acute bronchitis, such as we have described in previous paragraphs, and which easily changes to the capillary form; they are accompanied by catarrh of the nose, larynx and trachea, and are distinguished by the obstinacy and slowness of their course, at times being very intense and at other times so completely disguised by the constitutional disturbance that they are easily overlooked.

Influenza is generally preceded by a preliminary stage where the local symptoms of catarrh of the respiratory organs are still wanting, or are but imperfectly developed, whereas the patient complains already very much of an extreme languor, with nervous excitement, sleeplessness and loss of appetite, without or with only slight fever. As the fever increases, the local symptoms become generally more marked and more intense. At times a coryza is the only prominent symptom, at other times the mucous lining, from the nose to the finest bronchial ramifications, is inflamed. At the same time a violent and constant headache is complained of, which is commonly located in the forehead and is marked by all the peculiarities that so commonly characterize the headache in an incipient typhus. This headache is accompanied by rheumatoid pains in many parts of the muscular system, accompanied by a degree of debility that almost amounts to paralysis. After a gradual, very seldom sudden increase the disease reaches its full height. The catarrh is at times violent, at other times very slight. The fever is intense, but so plainly remittent that the remissions sometimes appear like intermissions. The debility is excessive. The headache is agonizing, and is either complicated with sopor or with violent delirium. The digestion is entirely prostrated; the tongue is thickly coated white or yellow, at times it exhibits a sickly redness with disposition to dryness; nausea and even diarrhœa are often present; the bowels are confined, diarrhœa is less frequent. The symptoms exacerbate in the evening and at night, the patient being very much distressed by the cough which aggravates the headache a great deal. Thus the more violent attacks of influenza simulate an acute typhus, milder cases a so-called nervous gastric fever. Death may take place in the second week amid symptoms of general exhaustion; sometimes it takes place at a later period in consequence of the peculiar secondary diseases which frequently break out as sequelæ of influenza.

In the case of sound, robust individuals the disease mostly terminates its course in a fortnight, but always leaving an extreme weakness which may last for weeks. In the case of old people the danger is always great and recovery takes place very slowly. An abatement of the fever is always the surest sign of an improvement.

The disease very often leaves very threatening results. If the patient had tubercles, their suppuration is an almost sure consequence of the bronchial affection, although we do not choose to hold to the opinion of many that influenza is itself capable of causing tubercular deposits. In opposition to this doctrine we might say that scattered tubercular deposits very often escape our notice. Influenza is very apt to leave in its track various affections of the respiratory organs, such as an obstinate hoarseness or even loss of voice and a long-lasting bronchial catarrh. The stomach likewise frequently remains disturbed, nor is a disturbance of the hepatic functions an uncommon event.

Thus we see that the prognosis in influenza is uncertain, even if the disease sets in favorably at first, and the patient had been in the habitual enjoyment of good health. If the individual had pulmonary disease, or in the case of decrepit subjects, a fatal termination is not uncommon. The peculiar nature of the actually existing epidemic may likewise exert a great influence; whereas one epidemic scarcely destroys a single life, another epidemic, on the contrary, claims a great many victims.

The reason why a description of the treatment of influenza is a difficult task, is the diversity of forms under which the epidemic appears. In influenza, as in other epidemics, remedies whose practical value had been tested by abundant experience, often have to be abandoned as unreliable, and other remedies have to be substituted in their stead. In influenza one or two remedies sometimes prove specifics in all cases, so that the epidemic might, after Rademacher's example, be conveniently named after the medicine that acts as its universal curative. To find out these remedies, persevering investigations are often indispensable, and we shall, therefore, confine ourselves to indicating the remedies whose practical value has been tested in a variety of cases.

One of the most dangerous cliffs, on which our treatment so often strands, is the frequent change of remedies for the purpose of meeting this or that symptom. The peculiar nature of the disease sometimes presses the local symptoms of an affection of the respiratory organs entirely into the background, whereas the symptoms of cerebral congestion, typhoid symptoms, or the symptoms of gastric or intestinal catarrh appear much more prominent. If, in such cases, we only direct our attention to the apparently most important complication, we shall often err in the choice of a remedy. It is only by weighing every circumstance of the disease that good results can be obtained by treatment; at the same time we are free to add that this task is not often easily accomplished, and that its accomplishment demands a persevering study of the Materia Medica. As a matter of course, such therapeutic investigations are very much facilitated by the presence of a prominent complication. In cases of cerebral hyperæmia, we will, of course, search for other remedies than in cases with prominent symptoms of liver-complaint, or with violent diarrhœa or gastric catarrh.

We repeat: let no one be content with the indications which we add to each of the following remedies. Guided by existing observations we only point out general landmarks, we do not give details.

Aconitum is particularly suitable to children in whose case this drug often suffices to effect a cure, whereas, in the case of adults, other remedies may be required in connection with Aconite. It is suitable if the fever has the inflammatory type, or the bronchial affection tends to develop pneumonia, and the patient is tormented by a distressing, violent, dry cough. *Aconite* will probably never acquire the rank of a specific adapted to a number of cases.

Regarding **Belladonna** we refer to the preceding chapter. It acts well in cases with violent congestions about the head and furibond or at least active delirium, as long as these symptoms have not assumed the characteristic appearance of adynamia.

For particulars concerning **Mercurius** we likewise refer to the previous chapter. In addition we offer the following remarks. Mercurius is one of those remedies which, according to experience, are all-sufficient as antidotes to some epidemics. Some reporters of cases even profess to have cut some cases of influenza short with this remedy. Special consideration is due to the existing coryza, which often is a valuable diagnostic sign in contra-distinction to the Arsenic-coryza. Mercurius is, moreover, indicated, by violent pains in the joints, angina, a sudden failing of the muscular strength, profuse sweat having a sour or foul odor and not affording any relief, thick coating of the tongue, severe gastric catarrh, diarrhœa. We add to these indications the following from Clotar Müller's treatise on pneumonia: "During epidemic influenza a kind of pneumonia occurs which is easily overlooked, because its subjective symptoms differ but little from the symptoms of the prevailing influenza. This form of pneumonia ordinarily sets in without much fever, its symptoms are not very violent and apparently of not much importance. Common symptoms are: a tearing and aching pain in the head, especially in the forehead, coryza, a slimy mouth and tongue, and dry lips; among other symptoms we distinguish the following: Loss of appetite, bad taste in the mouth, dry stools, urine mixed with a white mucus, a racking and dry cough, painfulness of the whole thorax, afterwards expectoration of frothy mucus, tearing pains in the joints, disproportionate weakness, tremulous nervousness, aggravation of the symptoms at night, with heat, sleeplessness at night, constant exhalations from the skin, or else copious and fetid sweat. On exploring the chest, we generally discover a not very considerable exudation. If overlooked or neglected the disease runs a very protracted course, sometimes occasions exhausting pulmonary blennorrhœas, or, if the exudation remains undissolved, phthisicky symptoms may be developed. These peculiar morbid conditions are very much abbreviated by *Mercurius*, so that a complete restoration of health takes place and, if the patients otherwise keep comfortably warm, no other remedy is required."

Bryonia alba is very closely related to Mercurius and it will be found difficult to discriminate very precisely between their respective symptomatic indications. Some facts regarding this point have already been stated in the preceding chapter; in this place we will add a few other details. The affection in the respiratory organs is confined to the larynx, trachea, and bronchial tubes; the nose remains unaffected, whereas coryza is a significant indication for Mercurius. The fever is less violent, but more continued; if there is sweat, it is copious and constant; the tongue is white, but has no thick coating on it, the bowels are constipated. The symptoms exacerbate in the day-time, not at night. The disease has an adynamic character, with deficient reaction, whereas Mercurius has a very decided reaction. Thus Bryonia may be frequently suitable after Mercurius, but Mercurius is never suitable after Bryonia. The supervention of pneumonic symptoms does not contra-indicate Bryonia, a supervening affection of the pleura indicates this drug very positively. If influenza attacks tubercular lungs, Bryonia is always appropriate, and is always preferable to Mercurius. Bryonia is one of those remedies that is calculated to become a specific for epidemic influenza.

Rhus toxicodendron is another important remedy in epidemic influenza which often corresponds to the whole character of the disease. Rhus is in its place if the local affection is so disguised by the constitutional disease that we rather seem to deal with typhus complicated with a bronchial catarrh. The use of this remedy is suggested by great debility, a prostrate condition of the whole organism, symptoms of violent reaction, such as a rapid pulse, burning heat, dry skin and tongue, delirium, sopor. Among the local symptoms, the most prominent indication is a short, distressing, dry cough, mostly at night, and excited by motion and by every little cold current of air.

Of **Nux vomica**, Hahnemann relates in his preface to Camphor that a very small dose often removes an attack of influenza in a few hours. We refer to the preceding chapter where we have expressed our doubts regarding the appropriateness of Nux; we have to repeat these doubts here in much more emphatic language. There are, of course, many who profess to have seen good effects from it even in influenza; but it is not so very easy to speak of curative results in this disease with positive certainty; as far as we ourselves are concerned, we never have been able to obtain any striking curative results with this agent.

Phosphorus is of all other remedies most positively indicated in influenza by distinct and fixed symptomatic manifestations. It is suitable if, in addition to severe constitutional disturbances, the disease is chiefly localized in the larynx; it is likewise appropriate in influenza with tendency to develop pneumonia, or if the influenza attacks tuberculous individuals in whose case the medicine has to be given with great caution; and finally in cases complicated with severe intestinal catarrh. Among the secondary diseases, such as aphonia or hoarseness, it is particularly Phosphorus that is characteristically indicated.

Arsenicum album is suited to an affection of the upper portion of the respiratory tract, the nose and larynx; it is less suited to bronchitis, except when it attacks individuals afflicted with emphysema. A violent coryza with copious watery, excoriating secretion, a burning pain in the frontal cavities; dryness and burning in the larynx and trachea, with hoarseness and a few violent paroxysms of cough are paramount indications for Arsenic. The constitutional symptoms are still more characteristic: excessive debility, with a rapid pulse, continual restlessness and sleeplessness, regular midnight exacerbations. Arsenicum is particularly efficient in cases where the conjunctiva is strikingly involved in the catarrhal process and where the disease has an unmistakable tertian type.

Opium is only mentioned once in our literature for influenza; it was successfully given for paroxysms of a distressing and tight cough, the paroxysms being always followed by yawning. According to our own experience, Opium controls paroxysms of a dry cough with congestions to the head and chest, it drives the patients to despair and breaks out particularly in the night. Opium will seldom afford help at the outset of an attack of influenza, but will afford speedy and substantial aid if such a cough remains after the departure of the fever.

Sabadilla is said to have helped in two epidemics, the symptoms of which we transfer from Rückert's "Klinischen Erfahrungen": "Excessive drowsiness in the day-time; chilliness, especially towards evening; shudderings with goose-flesh, the chills creeping up from the feet towards the head; lachrymation, with redness of the eyelids; pressure on the eyes, especially when moving them or when looking up. Headache, especially frontal; sore tongue, thick yellow coating on the tongue, the pain extends as far as the throat; painful deglutition; sensation as if a piece of loose skin were hanging in the throat; bitter taste in the mouth; complete loss of appetite, with nausea; dryness of the mouth without thirst; constipation with flatulence; in some, brown frothy diarrhœic stools which floated on the water; yellowish and turbid urine; cough with vomiting, headache, sharp stitches in the vertex, pain in the region of the stomach; cough of a peculiar, muffled kind; many cough up blood; painful lameness in the joints, especially the knee-joints. All the symptoms get worse in the cold; they exacerbate about noon, but worse towards evening; flashes of heat in the face, with chilliness and coldness of the extremities; the flashes of heat in the face are mingled with chilly creepings over the back from below upwards at intervals of ten minutes; the skin is dry as parchment; restless sleep, full of anxious dreams; the cough appears as soon as one lies down."

For the indications for **Ipecacuanha** and **Veratrum album** we refer to the preceding chapter; the latter is certainly an important remedy in influenza. In general the remedies, which we have recommended for simple bronchial catarrh, may likewise be required for influenza.

In order not to indulge in too many subjective indications in a disease where practical experience plays a most important part, we transfer from Hartmann's Therapeutics the passage concerning influenza with slight additions of our own, which will afford us an opportunity for briefly mentioning a few important remedies.

"Smelling of *Camphor* several times, as soon as the first symptoms of the disease became apparent, had the effect of suppressing the disease, but a few days later it broke out nevertheless, which was not the case in a subsequent epidemic where Camphor was given internally in the first attenuation and proved a sovereign remedy for the disease." Hahnemann says in his preface to Camphor: In influenza, if the heat has already set in, Camphor only serves as a palliative, but as a valuable one, if given in frequent but more and more attenuated doses; it does not shorten the course of the disease, which is not very much protracted any way, but moderates the vehemence of the attack a great deal and conducts it, shorn of its danger, to the end.

"If the thoracic organs were the chief seat of the inflammation, *Nux vomica* always did good service if given after *Aconite*. *Mercurius solubilis* or *vivus*, of which several doses were given every day, was particularly calculated to cure the disease or even cut it short in its very germ, if the following symptoms prevailed: the head, throat and chest were principally affected; there was a dry and racking cough which afterwards became loose and was attended with pleuritic pains; the patient was troubled with profuse sweats which did not afford him any relief; there were symptoms of an inflammatory fever, dull pain, not very hard pulse. If the trachea was much irritated, and the irritation almost bordered on inflammation, so that the intense pain made it impossible to speak, and the voice was very much altered, *Phosphorus* was an excellent remedy."

"Very often the disease broke out in the form of sporadic cholera; in such a case the catarrhal symptoms were unimportant, but the prostration was very prominent. Here *Veratrum* helped in every case. If an attack of this kind was followed by nervous symptoms, if the patient became delirious, had a wild and staring look, complained of great sensitiveness of the abdomen, and the pulse was full and hard, a few doses of *Aconite* were given with great benefit and the rest of the symptoms were removed by *Pulsatilla*, which likewise proved a remedy for the pappy and insipid taste that sometimes remained for a time, together with a mucous coating on the tongue and loss of appetite." We cannot yield our assent to this passage. The delirium occurring in influenza, and all the other so-called nervous symptoms, are always of a typhoid type and do not yield to Aconite, but require much rather *Belladonna*, *Bryonia*, *Rhus*, also *Stramonium* and *Hyoscyamus;* after the exhibition of such remedies symptoms indicating Pulsatilla will not often remain.

"An exceedingly distressing symptom in this disease was the violent, pressing frontal headache which, together with the accompanying cough and the loose and slimy expectoration was relieved by *Bryonia*, which likewise proved an excellent remedy, if the liver was enlarged and painful on contact, or during a coughing fit or a deep inspiration; if the cough easily ended in vomiting or caused a pain in the epigastric region, in which case Bryonia competed with Nux, or if the pain was felt under the short ribs as if the parts had been bruised so that the patient, when coughing, had to press his hands against them; *Bryonia* likewise proved efficient if the influenza attacked old people with great distress in the chest and coldness of the limbs, in which case the disease often destroyed life by paralysis of the lungs; the Bryonia was given in alternation with *Carbo vegetabilis*." In such cases *Tartar emetic* may deserve attention. "If the cough was dry and spasmodic, if the headache became unbearable and was aggravated by walking, talking, bright light and by every least motion; if the look became staring and the patients were troubled with fancies whenever they closed their eyes, *Belladonna* always afforded relief, so that in a few hours already this condition which seemed like an incipient meningitis, disappeared."

"*Rhus* was indicated if the attack had been caused in consequence of the patients getting soaking wet, and they were greatly oppressed on the chest, anxious, they frequently drew involuntarily a long breath, were very restless and had to change their position quite often."

"**Sabadilla** was given if the attack seemed like an inflammatory affection of the thoracic organs, with severe chills and external coldness." This indication corresponds but little with what was said concerning Sabadilla in a previous paragraph.

"**China** relieved the cough that was excited by a rattling under the sternum as if mucus had accumulated there." This indication is of very little importance and of no particular value in influenza. Independently of the cough which cannot be regarded as a characteristic symptom, China will be found suitable if the disease assumes the character of a nervous fever or the appearance of pulmonary phthisis.

"The alcoholic tincture of *Sulphur* was prescribed with good effect at the termination of the disease, after the fever had abated, the stitches in the chest were only felt indistinctly during a deep inspiration and a violent coughing fit, and the patient complained of oppression on the chest as from a heavy weight." In general *Sulphur* is a valuable remedy for pulmonary affections remaining after an attack of influenza and not traceable to tubercular infiltration.

"The spasmodic cough which remained for some time after an attack of influenza and sometimes tormented the patients for hours, was almost always relieved by one or more doses of *Hyoscyamus*, in some cases by *Belladonna;* but if the coughing fit did not cease until a mass of frothy mucus with a yellowish purulent nucleus had been raised, *Conium* proved the main remedy; if the cough broke out after a meal and the food was vomited up in consequence of the cough, *Ferrum aceticum* was found to be the specific remedy."

"If the influenza left the patient with a troublesome cough and a gray, sweetish-salt expectoration, wheezing and rattling in the chest, *Kali hydriod.* proved an admirable remedy." This medicine is likewise excellent for the remaining hoarseness or even aphonia, but should not be given in too small doses. *Iodium* itself is of no use for these symptoms, but may be resorted to in the febrile stage.

"In cases of a previously-existing disposition to phthisis, which the influenza threatened to develop more actively, a few doses of *Stannum* in alternation with *Carbo veget.* were often sufficient to prevent the further spread of the tubercular disease." In the sequelæ of influenza Carbo veget. is very closely related to *Phosphorus* and *Kali hydriodicum.*

"In some cases the influenza was succeeded by obstinate ophthalmia with ulcers of the cornea and violent photophobia, for which *Arsenicum album* seemed almost the only efficient remedy; repeated doses of *Belladonna* were likewise useful, but did not effect a permanent cure."

With reference to this long quotation we confess that Hartmann's indications seem to us rather vague and unprofitable; others may, however, not share our opinion.

A number of other remedies that might be mentioned in this place, would be directed against the various complications such as pleuritis, pneumonia, hæmoptoë, diarrhœa, and more particularly against the sequelæ; concerning the former, we refer the reader to the respective chapters on pleuritis, etc.; the sequelæ will generally yield to the above-described group of remedial agents.

The dietetic management depends a good deal upon the condition of the digestive organs. If the patient's appetite is good, there is no reason why he should not be permitted the use of nourishing and substantial food. But if the long duration of the disease has caused great debility, a great deal of caution has to be observed in gradually increasing the patient's allowance, because the stomach very often continues for a long time in a condition of atony. The same caution has to be used in allowing patients the enjoyment of open air; the sensitiveness of the lungs often becomes excessive during an attack of influenza, and it behooves us to ascertain and moderate this condition of the lungs with proper care and discretion. There is no reason of considering influenza contagious as many do; and every measure tending to counteract this contagion, is an useless torture. The only preventive measure which we advise with a good deal of success, consists in avoiding all those exposures which are generally apt to cause catarrhs of the respiratory organs. [In epidemic influenza our physicians depend a great deal upon Tartar emetic which is regarded by many as a sort of specific for this epidemic. We cannot do better than by transcribing Doctor John F. Gray's interesting note on this subject from my Symptomen-Codex, published by W. Radde, New York, in 1848. "In the first stage of influenza (generally of itself a fugitive state), I think it by very much the most strictly indicated, and on that account as well as from my own observations in many hundreds of cases, by very far the most efficacious means we can apply. The state against which I give it, is: lassitude with great sensitiveness to cold, with chilly feelings, headache, pasty tongue, inflammation of the throat (tonsils, arches of the palate or pharynx), short turns of nausea, achings in the bones, especially of the lower extremities, yellowness of the skin, slight hoarseness, more or less fever-heat and sweats.

The Antimony often acts as a perfect remedy in the stage of incubation, especially in those cases which would of themselves close this stage by profuse watery diarrhœa with some vomiting and cramps.*

---

* This stage, of which the angina faucium, the chills and the bone-pains, are the prominent sufferings, subsides of itself in twenty-four to forty-eight hours, and the physician is very apt to be deceived as to the efficacy of his treatment.

The second or bronchial stage of the true influenza having been successfully managed by *Phosphorus* or *Bryonia*, with the aid of *Aconite* or *Hyoscyamus*, I complete the cure by a return to the *Antimony*; that is to say, when the air-passages are loaded with mucus, the cough being frequent and the expectorations copious. H.]

5. Tussis Convulsiva, Pertussis.
Whooping-Cough.

We understand by this name a peculiar form of catarrh of the respiratory mucous membrane from the nose to the pulmonary vesicles, where the cough sets in in distinctly detached paroxysms.

Etiology. Whooping-cough is an epidemic disease which sometimes occurs in the form of very extensive, and sometimes circumscribed epidemics, in which latter case the few cases of whooping-cough might even be designated as sporadic. So far the real cause of the epidemic has not yet been determined. It cannot be the peculiar nature of the wind, for the reason that the disease breaks out without the least regularity in disconnected portions of country; all we know is that the outbreak of an epidemic occurs more frequently in the spring than in the fall, very rarely in the summer. A connection with other epidemic affections, especially measles, and likewise with variola and scarlatina cannot well be denied. Whooping-cough frequently precedes or succeeds epidemics of the last-named diseases, and in rare cases accompanies them.

As regards the spread of the disease by contagion, opinions differ a great deal; a number of observers favor the doctrine of a contagium; on the other hand we should not overlook the fact that during an epidemic all the individuals of one place and the inhabitants of one house are exposed to the same influences. As for ourselves we have not yet been able to satisfy our minds that whooping-cough is contagious; yet we are willing to admit that in its highest stage of development, this cough may give rise to a product which, when grafted upon susceptible organisms, may in its turn reproduce the disease. This is no idle question, as might appear at first sight, since it may lead to the adoption of measures that may prove exceedingly oppressive to a family having a number of children and

---

The allopathist praises his atrocious lancet and heroic purgatives, and the homœopathist his Mercurius, Belladonna or Nux, and the patient in either case thinks a wonder has been done for him; but the disease, if it be a real influenza, is not removed; it has only advanced a step beyond the process of incubation, towards the stadium of bronchitis, with its concomitant cough, dyspnœa, fever-sweats and prostration.

living in straightened circumstances. In spite of every isolation we have seen all the children of a family attacked by the epidemic.

The immediate causes which determine the outbreak of the disease during an epidemic are the same as those that occasion an ordinary catarrh of the respiratory mucous membrane. A special predisposition to the disease has not yet been traced; if it seems an established fact that girls are more liable to whooping-cough than boys, the same relation holds true in all other spasmodic affections which attack girls more frequently than boys. Every trifling catarrh may, under the influence of the epidemic assume the form of whooping-cough. As regards age, children between the second and eighth year are more commonly liable. Children under one year are seldom attacked by whooping-cough, although we have seen a severe case of whooping-cough in a child of four weeks. Children upwards of eight years old are likewise seldom attacked; whereas, during an epidemic, adults are frequently attacked by a spasmodic cough in the place of the light catarrhal cough.

Symptoms and Course. In the management of whooping-cough the fact must not be overlooked that the anatomical changes it occasions are simply those of an ordinary catarrh, to which the changes which are determined by the not unfrequently-occurring complications, have of course to be added. The supposed changes in the vagus are altogether hypothetical, although certain changes have indeed been discovered in a few isolated cases, but not sufficiently numerous to enable us to build a reliable theory upon such post-mortem phenomena.

In the majority of cases whooping-cough commences as an ordinary catarrh of the nose or of the larynx, trachea and bronchial tubes. This introductory catarrh which does not, properly speaking, form a component part of whooping-cough, may break out in all degrees of severity and extent without this circumstance justifying a conclusion regarding the approaching attack. Hence the most proper course would be to regard this preliminary catarrh as connected with the epidemic only in so far as it furnishes a soil or a susceptible spot upon which the whooping-cough miasm can be grafted, and in which it can germinate. This is shown by the cases where the whooping-cough breaks out without being ushered in by a simply catarrhal stage, or where a simple catarrh exists for weeks before it is converted into whooping-cough. At any one period of this first stage, in a few days or even after the lapse of weeks either a harmlessly-sounding cough sets in, or else an actually-existing cough becomes more severe, and sooner or later assumes a paroxysmal character which constitutes it whooping-cough. After this form of cough has reached its full development, the simple cough ceases entirely; only in a few instances violent paroxysms and simple turns of cough occur mingled together. A single paroxysm has the following characteristic symptoms: The children who had hitherto been bright and cheerful, shortly before the setting in of a paroxysm, become restless and anxious, or, if old enough, they complain of titillation in the larynx or under the sternum, or of oppression of breathing; it is very seldom the case that a violent cough sets in without any preliminary symptoms, which, after a short lapse of time, is succeeded by a wheezing and labored inspiration taking turns with the single paroxysms without admitting of a full expiration for the reason that all the respiratory muscles and more particularly the glottis are affected by the spasm. While the exertion to cough is constantly increasing and the spasm of the glottis is gradually abating, the children finally succeed in raising or vomiting up a more or less considerable quantity of a tenacious, white mucus, which terminates the attack. During the attack the children express great anguish and restlessness; in consequence of the impeded respiration the face and tongue become blue-red, the eyes weep, a watery mucus is discharged from the nose, even blood is spit up sometimes and flows from the nose to the terror of the parents. The vomiting either brings up mere mucus or the contents of the stomach. Involuntary discharge of stool and urine is a rare occurrence if the children are otherwise robust. After the termination of the paroxysm the children continue for some time in a state of confusion and languor, after which they play again as if nothing had happened. Only in the case of feeble or very small children the paroxysms are succeeded by real attacks of eclampsia, or else by a state of sopor or even complete catalepsy. In the above-mentioned case of the little infant only four weeks old, the cataleptic condition was so perfect and lasting that the patient lay for two minutes without pulse or breathing. Under such circumstances the intermissions are not free from morbid symptoms, whereas vigorous children seem perfectly sound between the paroxysms.

These paroxysms sometimes set in quite frequently and at other times at more protracted intervals. Generally their frequency increases up to a certain point where the affection remains stationary for some time, after which it gradually decreases in violence. In the space of twenty-four hours the children may have upwards of thirty paroxysms of cough; they occur more frequently in the night, and at this time likewise last longer and are more intense. A paroxysm lasts seldom longer than three minutes; if the parents assert that the paroxysms last longer, they are deceived by the anxiety which the mother particularly experiences, to whom a minute may possibly seem a quarter of an hour. The paroxysm is excited by talking, eating, screaming, or by violent exercise, likewise by a violent fit of passion; the cough may likewise occur without any apparent cause, for instance, during sleep.

The constitutional state of the little patients is variously affected by the cough, even if there are no complications. Strong children bear this cough for months, without losing flesh, or without their general well-being being interfered with. It may, however, be accepted as a rule that, if whooping-cough lasts longer than four weeks, children begin to lose their strength and flesh, and that this loss goes on increasingly in proportion as the cough lasts longer. Sick and very small children are speedily and threateningly affected by the cough, even if none of the foregoing complications are present. The children grow pale and languid, they lose their appetite, but are not often attacked with diarrhœa.

The course of the disease is generally for several months; but when we come to speak of the treatment, we shall show that this period is considerably abbreviated in homœopathic hands.

Of particular importance are the complications and sequelæ of whooping-cough, which alone constitute the dangerous features of this disease.

The most frequent of these complications are inflammatory affections of the lungs. The catarrh of the respiratory passages, which was inconsiderable at first, invades the more delicate ramifications of the air-passages more and more until a more or less intense bronchitis sets in, which easily assumes the capillary form and becomes readily associated with pneumonia. This pneumonia almost always assumes the lobular form and can scarcely ever be determined by auscultation and percussion. The presence of such a pneumonia is suspected if the bronchitis steadily increases in intensity and the intervals between the paroxysms are no longer free from a hacking cough and a constantly increasing dyspnœa. Even if bronchitis sets in violently at the outset, it never changes all at once to capillary bronchitis and pneumonia,—which may, at the same time, serve as a proof that an incipient catarrh, which happens to exist before the whooping-cough, does not necessarily constitute the preliminary stage of this disease,—but the signs of this untoward change do not set in until the cough has lasted for days and even weeks. In such a case the little patient does not entirely recover from the attacks, he grows languid and feverish, has a short and dry cough, he does not wish to rise from bed, the pulse is hurried, the respiration becomes more and more incomplete, more hurried; he feels drowsy and tosses about. If these symptoms manifest themselves in the later course of the disease, they always augur danger and very commonly lead to a fatal termination.

A severe bronchitis as well as lobular pneumonia very commonly lead to a more or less extensive deterioration of the pulmonary cells; if this deterioration is quite considerable, percussion yields an unmistakably dull sound, and auscultation yields bronchial respiration. But these symptoms must not be attributed to pneumonia, for in such a case their importance would be much less.

Cerebral diseases are scarcely ever caused by the direct action of whooping cough; existing diseases of this kind may become fatally aggravated by the cough. The convulsions which often attack little children during the course of whooping-cough, are more correctly attributed to the influence of whooping-cough over the whole nervous system, and, on this account, may become lasting. The apparently violent congestions of the head during the paroxysms are of very little importance to the brain of a perfectly healthy child, but they prognosticate trouble, if the brain was diseased before the cough set in.

Acute heart-disease is seldom one of the complications of whooping-cough. On the other hand, the development of tuberculous pulmonary affections is a very common thing. Usually, however, these affections existed before the cough set in, although many cases occur where the cough occasions the deposition of tubercular matter in individuals predisposed to this disease.

Emphysema does not occur as frequently as is generally supposed. A deterioration of the air-cells is very often mistaken for emphysema. Post-mortem examinations have, however, frequently confirmed the fact that emphysema may set in very suddenly.

Spasm of the glottis is a tolerably rare occurrence in whooping-cough, at least it does not occur in a high degree of intensity; if it does, it is always a very ominous complication which may suddenly terminate fatally.

Beside the complications the frequently occurring sequelæ may prove very dangerous to the patients. Among them we distinguish chronic bronchial catarrh, bronchiectasia, emphysema, deterioration of single parts of the lungs, with consequent malformation of the thorax, pulmonary tuberculosis, heart-disease, although the last-named rarely and then involving mostly the right heart; eclampsia, occasionally mental derangement, and lastly hernia which is of comparatively frequent occurrence. If the disease lasts a long time, complete marasmus is not an unfrequent occurrence; it is not attended with other morbid conditions and seems to result from the exhausted condition of the nervous system caused by the excessive paroxysms of cough.

The prognosis is always uncertain. Although the cough does not endanger the lives of healthy children, nevertheless, the supervention of one of the above-mentioned complications at any period during the course of the disease may occasion death or a life-long infirmity; thus it happens that we often see vigorous and healthy children come out of an attack of epidemic whooping-cough like wretched invalids. We claim for Homœopathy the advantage that such pitiable results are scarcely ever witnessed under homœopathic treatment, except perhaps in the case of children with deteriorated and rickety constitutions.

Treatment. We consider the homœopathic treatment of whooping-cough calculated to demonstrate the value of homœopathic therapeutics to obstinate sceptics, and deem this a good opportunity for premising a few general remarks.

Considering the extraordinary frequency of whooping-cough epidemics and the universality with which children are assailed; and considering moreover the greatness of the danger to which children are exposed during the prevalence of such epidemics, and the insufficiency of the ordinary mode of treatment, it seems quite natural that extraordinary efforts should have been made to lay bare the causes of this disease. It is an established fact that whooping-cough is the result of a noxa diffused through the atmosphere. But how is it that this noxa to which every body is exposed, engenders this peculiar cough only in the case of children? To adopt the theory of a specific affection of the vagus, does not harmonize with this exclusive invasion of the infantile organism whose pneumogastric nerves are certainly constructed in the same manner as those of adults; moreover this theory is not corroborated by the numerous post-mortem examinations. On such occasions these nerves were scarcely ever found altered, but most commonly unchanged. This hypothesis, like all other hypotheses that are not based upon the evidence of facts, has now been abandoned.

Nevertheless since a theory of the pathology of this disease must necessarily have an important influence on the treatment, we cannot refrain from recording our views on this subject. During the prevalence of epidemic whooping-cough, violent and obstinate catarrhs are likewise very common among adults. It cannot well be denied that the quality of the mucus secreted at such a time differs from an ordinary catarrhal mucus; the former is very tenacious and glassy, ropy, firmly adhering to the mucous membrane, whereas ordinary mucus is lumpy and globular, and frequently causing even in the case of adults a peculiarly spasmodic cough. Now we would ask, are there not conditions in the infantile organism sufficient to account for the convulsive nature of the cough? It is a demonstrable fact that the urging to cough caused by the secretion of mucus, is much less in children than in adults, and so much less the younger the children are. Whereas an adult expectorates every little quantity of mucus by a voluntary attempt to cough, the child does not expel the mucus until the urging to cough has reached an extraordinary degree of violence. This fact is evidenced in the case of children who sleep quietly in spite of a rattling respiration and mucous râles in the trachea and bronchia that can be heard at a distance. The child only coughs if compelled to do so by the dyspnœa and the urging is very great. This condition will necessarily give rise to a corresponding reaction, the cough will be so much more violent. Moreover the child has not sufficient strength of will to overcome the irritation which induces the cough; at any rate, this attempt is only noticed among larger children, and thus it is, that a violent struggle arises where an energetic resistance might have given rise to a moderate turn of cough. The evidence for this statement is derived from the circumstance that the older the children the less violent the cough. Again, robust children are attacked with less violent paroxysms than nervous children. Finally the spasmodic character of the cough is accounted for by the decisive disposition of the infantile organism to convulsive affections; this is likewise confirmed by the fact that among adults only such individuals are attacked by whooping-cough as exhibit a disposition to spasm, namely females.

It is therefore our opinion that the peculiar form of whooping-cough can be explained by the child's evidently feeble reaction against the urging to cough, by the insufficient energy to control the irritation and urging, and by the disposition to spasmodic affections generally.

These points, if applied to epidemic catarrh which not only causes the secretion of a peculiar mucus, but most probably determines essential changes in the irritability of the trachea and larynx, afford sufficient reasons for the paroxysms of cough which otherwise might appear inexplicable.

In this manner a number of symptoms that otherwise would seem incomprehensible, can be made intelligible. The continual increase of the violence of the paroxysms, for instance, for months at a time, cannot be accounted for by referring it to the simple action and development of the miasm, since we do not observe a similar feature in other miasmatic affections, which are generally most intense at the commencement of their course. The continual increase of the whooping-cough can be easily accounted for by the increase of irritability in consequence of the cough, and by the decreasing amount of resistance. Chorea exhibits a similar feature in its course. Niemeyer advises to abbreviate the paroxysms by exciting the children to make an effort to control the cough. An advice of this kind would seem foolish, if it could not be shown to harmonize with the explanation we have furnished. Our theory likewise accounts for the circumstance that the paroxysms mostly break out at night during sleep, or that they are easily excited if, in addition to the irritation in the air-passages, another irritation is caused by crying or laughing.

In making these statements, our aim has been to show that the spasmodic character of whooping-cough is not owing to the peculiar nature of the miasm, but to that of the organism upon which the miasm acts. We may as well observe in this place that, in our opinion, whooping-cough does not commence until the convulsive stage has set in, and that the previous simple catarrh is not by any means a sign that the miasm has now begun to affect the organism.

A glance at the Therapeutics of the Old School is in so far important as a comparison of results is best calculated to place the advantages of our own treatment in a more conspicuous light. Physicians as well as lay-persons are apt to express the opinion that there is no remedy for whooping-cough, and that it has to run its course for months. Wunderlich, who generally tries to enumerate the medicines that may cure a disease and who is not apt to be in favor of a purely negative treatment, declares that any treatment is absolutely powerless in the spasmodic stage and that all that can be done is to moderate the violence of the paroxysms by narcotics. In the case of children, however, the use of narcotics is attended with a good deal of danger for the reason that they are apt to develop dangerous cerebral congestions. No class of physicians knows how to appreciate such facts better than homœopaths who derive the most brilliant results from small doses of such drugs.

We care not to inquire why, we simply state the fact that the ordinary treatment of whooping-cough is quite ineffectual; that both physicians and lay-persons have lost all faith in it; that the former give nothing for the cough, and the latter allow the cough to run its course without giving any medicine at all, and that both parties declare themselves satisfied if the cough gradually disappears in three to five months; that finally under this routine-management a number of children succumb to the disease or its consequences. Whether Oppolzer's treatment which essentially consists in keeping the children in the same temperature, is as successful as Niemeyer would have us believe, is very questionable to our minds. We doubt whether a majority of the little patients recover in the promised space of four to six weeks.

In opposition to all this, Homœopathy can boast of favorable and speedy results without having to resort to such a rigorous mode of living as Oppolzer recommends. By means of the treatment which we have now been in the habit of pursuing for a number of years, we have succeeded in restoring at least ninety per cent. of our little patients, provided we had charge of them from the beginning, within the space of five and usually even four weeks, so far that all convulsive paroxysms ceased entirely, although a slight catarrh might have hung on for a short time longer. Yet among the large number of children whom we have had under treatment, there must have been a good many feeble and sickly ones to whom our statement applies nevertheless with equal force. The greatest merit, however, Homœopathy can boast of is, the freedom from secondary diseases· which do not occur under homœopathic treatment and generally result from whooping-cough when it lasts too long. The malignant complications likewise, though not entirely excluded under homœopathic treatment, yet are comparatively rare occurrences.

Before passing to the medicinal treatment of whooping-cough we have to offer some remarks about the preventive measures recommended for adoption during the prevalence of this epidemic and which impose such a heavy burthen upon families. The communication of the cough by contagion is at most questionable; we know from experience that in families where an infected child was kept strictly isolated from the rest of the family, nevertheless one child after another was gradually attacked by the disease. We are emphatically opposed to all such methods of solitary confinement which we would not recommend under any circumstances. The only sure preventive is the early removal of children from the district where the epidemic prevails. Few, however, will consent to such a step previous to the general spread of the disease; and then a change of locality is of doubtful value, or is of use only in so far as the children exchange city-air and artificial city-customs for the pure air and the more natural mode of living in the country. Another preventive is to guard children against every possible exposure to catarrhal influences. It is certainly true that a child scarcely ever has whooping-cough without first taking cold; but, on the other hand, this perfect freedom from exposure cannot possibly be secured unless we choose to deprive children of their most necessary nutriment, open air.

We have already stated in a previous paragraph that we do not consider the catarrhal stage an essential ingredient of whooping-cough, although the treatment of this stage is of importance to the whole course of the disease. It may be considered a rule that the sooner and more completely the premonitory catarrh is cured, the shorter and less intense will be the course of the convulsive stage. Hence we have every reason, during the prevalence of epidemic whooping-cough, to treat the most trifling catarrh with becoming care and attention. The remedies to be employed for this purpose are the same as those that have been recommended in former sections for catarrh of the nose, larynx, trachea and bronchia, all of which may come into play, though *Belladonna* will probably be found the most efficient at the commencement. The much vaunted *Drosera* is of very doubtful value in this as well as in the subsequent stages. At this stage it is of course indispensable to guard children against further exposure and consequent increase of the catarrh, for which purpose they had better be kept in the room, in an uniform temperature. In the case of lively and quick children this proceeding is undoubtedly of difficult execution. For a goodly portion of our success in the treatment of whooping-cough we are undoubtedly indebted to the comparative certainty with which we succeed in controlling this first stage without impairing the general strength of the little patient. Even a violent bronchitis at the commencement of the disease may not aggravate the symptoms of the spasmodic stage, which cannot be asserted of any other treatment.

As soon as the peculiar paroxysms of cough show that the convulsive stage has set in, an entirely different series of drugs have to be selected. We feel some embarrassment in giving a description of the treatment of this stage inasmuch as we are conscious of a marked difference in this respect between our own views and those of most of our colleagues. Hartmann gives a number of remedies that may be useful in whooping-cough but are suggested by groups of symptoms that render a differential diagnosis between one drug and another impossible and nugatory. His symptomatic arrangements are supposed to be in accord with the law of similarity, but the practical efficiency of the treatment is sadly impaired by such a course. However in order to avoid even the appearance of partiality, we shall afterwards mention single remedies and their most essential indications.

What are, in a case of whooping-cough, the characteristic indications which point most directly and positively to the correct remedy? This is an important inquiry. Is it the particular circumstances which, if the statement of the relatives may be believed, have caused the attack? We cannot accept a theory of this kind, notwithstanding that this chapter has been exhausted by the coarse symptom-coverers among us to the dregs. The same child has on the same day an attack of cough from laughing, crying, eating and drinking; this alone would require four different remedies. Shall we select a remedy in accordance with the specific symptoms of each particular paroxysm? In this respect we discover indeed symptomatic differences that ought not to be overlooked; but in ninety cases out of every hundred the paroxysms are mostly alike, and only differ from each other slightly in intensity. Hence it is only in exceptional cases that the nature of the paroxysm will prove a sufficient guide for the selection of a drug. Can we depend upon the symptoms between the paroxysms for light in selecting a remedy? Here too we shall be disappointed, for where no complications exist, the apyrexia is generally free from symptoms; one child may at most feel the immediate consequences of an attack a little longer than another.

In our opinion the simple, uncomplicated whooping-cough of healthy children does not present any salient points upon which the selection of a remedy could be based. Hence it will always be exceedingly difficult to select the right remedy from among a large number. We are supported by experience in believing that the number of remedies which are adapted to whooping-cough, is very small, for the reason that the characteristic effects of the whooping-cough miasm manifest themselves in almost every case in the same uniform manner: Excessive irritability of the respiratory mucous membrane with an extreme increase of reflex-action. By removing this increase, we cure whooping-cough, so that only a simple catarrh remains which would at most be distinguished by a somewhat more violent cough. That this is no hypothesis, but a fact, results from the decided effect obtained by exciting the energy of larger children; from the favorable influence of powerful external stimuli applied to various parts of the body as soon as the paroxysm threatens to set in, for instance the application of a sponge dipped in cold water to the pit of the stomach; from the circumstance that individuals who are not endowed with a marked degree of reflex-action, are not liable to attacks of whooping-cough, and finally from the abundant confirmations of experience.

The remedy of which we make use for the purpose of moderating reflex-action, is *Cuprum metallicum*. By continuing the use of Copper for two or three weeks in the sixth attenuation, a few drops morning and night, commencing as soon as the spasmodic character of the cough becomes apparent, we have succeeded so well in the treatment of whooping-cough that we have scarcely ever been obliged to resort to any other treatment. Many of our colleagues, on reading this statement, will of course accuse us of a crime against Homœopathy, of an attempt to perpetrate an extreme generalization. In spite of their censure we should have to continue our course, because it leads to success, and success cannot only be obtained in mild, but likewise in malignant epidemics. That *Cuprum* is homœopathic to the disease, may be learned by a mere glance at the Materia Medica. Instead of metallic Copper, Hartmann recommends the *Acetate*, which, however, has not yielded us as satisfactory results. After what we have said, we deem a detailed description of the whooping-cough to which Cuprum is adapted, unnecessary. Be the attacks violent or comparatively slight, whether they occur at night or in the day-time, or whatever other differences prevail, *Cuprum* will not fail us so long as no complications exist or the general condition of the organism does not greatly deviate from the normal state. Cuprum is really an antidote to the whooping-cough miasm. If the antidotal effect is to be obtained, the use of this remedy must not be discontinued in a few days; in general, a frequent change of remedies in whooping-cough can only result in injury to the patient.

We now pass to the other remedies for whooping-cough and expect to satisfy our readers that Cuprum is not regarded by us as the only remedy for this disease.

Belladonna has probably been better tested as a remedy for whooping-cough than any other medicine. Experience, however, has shown that Belladonna does not so much act favorably upon the spasm as that it limits the catarrh and brings it more speedily to a termination. Belladonna occupies the first rank when the disease first breaks out, and at this stage its good effects are most decisive; but to continue its use in the convulsive stage, would be a mere loss of time. It again becomes an important remedy if fever sets in in the course of this stage, the patients become restless and after that too quiet, the apyrexia is not free from cough, in short if the catarrhal symptoms again increase and spread towards the bronchia. In most cases, however, all that Belladonna accomplishes is to remove the threatening symptoms, after which the cough again sets in in all its vehemence. The congestive symptoms which may occur during a paroxysm, should never mislead one to employ Belladonna on this account.

Drosera has been recommended as a specific for whooping-cough, and the most diversified indications for its use have been enumerated by our earlier writers. Hahnemann says that a globule of the thirtieth potency cures a species of whooping-cough, which probably never occurs in practice. Many physicians are of Hahnemann's opinion, although they may not have seen any great results from this drug; others, on the contrary, deny its vaunted efficacy. The dispute cannot be decided as long as the discussion revolves around unmeaning symptoms. It is certain that Drosera is not made much use of at the present time, and scarcely ever against the fully developed convulsive stage.

Ipecacuanha is one of our best remedies in this disease; its indications are tolerably precise and unmistakable. If, instead of the usual tenacious and scanty mucus, a large quantity of simple catarrhal mucus accumulates, so that the cough is preceded and accompanied by loud râles; if every paroxysm of cough is attended with vomiting, not at the end, but at the commencement; if a paroxysm is excited by the ingestion of every trifling quantity of food or drink: Ipecacuanha deserves a preference over every other remedy.

We shall scarcely ever meet with suitable indications for Ipecacuanha at the beginning of the attack; more frequently if the cough had already lasted for some time and had been neglected. We have scarcely ever had occasion to use this drug, if we conducted the treatment from the start.

Tartarus stibiatus has an excessive secretion of mucus in common with the former drug, but is preferable if the strength had suffered a great deal and the stomach and intestines are affected with catarrhal symptoms, so that frequent and tormenting vomiting and diarrhœa set in. This remedy will have to be given for the complications rather than for the cough itself. On this acount we refer the reader to the last chapters.

Veratrum album acts very similarly to the two last-named remedies. Here, too, we have an excessive secretion of mucus, râles between and during the paroxysms, a marked disposition to vomit water and mucus, and, at the same time, the patient is troubled with diarrhœa. In addition we have the symptoms of a catarrh approximating more and more a malignant bronchitis: anxiety, restlessness, a short and superficial respiration, pains in the chest, accelerated pulse with disposition to cool perspiration alternating with a burning heat, pallid countenance, sopor; the paroxysms become feebler, but the general condition of the system deteriorates more and more. Veratrum is calculated to become a specific in epidemic whooping-cough, if an intense intestinal catarrh sets in as a complication.

Arsenicum album is no real remedy for whooping-cough, but of great value if the organism has become very much enfeebled by the long duration of the disease and the violence of the paroxysms. The patients become sensible for some time previous of the approaching paroxysm, become exceedingly restless, seem tormented by anguish; owing to their great prostration, stool and urine are passed involuntarily. Arsenicum deserves particular consideration, if the pulmonary tissue has become atrophied, or acute emphysema has set in.

Cina. It seems to us absurd that this remedy should be recommended for whooping-cough, if helminthic symptoms either precede or accompany the attack; they will hardly influence the nature of the paroxysm. A better indication is, if the children become convulsed during a paroxysm, as if they had an attack of eclampsia; another indication is, if a gurgling noise is heard after every paroxysm from the throat into the abdomen. In some epidemics other physicians have employed this remedy with a good deal of success.

Conium maculatum is said to be an excellent remedy, if the paroxysms set in principally at night, especially in the case of scrofulous and anæmic children. *Ledum palustre* is said to be the right remedy, if every paroxysm is preceded by a convulsive condition which is again succeeded by an exceedingly violent paroxysm. Numerous records of cures by this drug are not to be found in any of our publications.

We might enumerate a pretty long list of remedies that have been used for whooping-cough; but we not only doubt their specific adaptation to the disease, but cannot refer to any practical demonstrations of their efficacy. These remedies are: *Arnica, Hyoscyamus, Ignatia, Nux vomica, Lactuca virosa, Laurocerasus, Ambra, Sepia, Pulsatilla, Carbo vegetabilis, Iodium, Spongia, China* and others. Carbo vegetabilis deserves special consideration in cases where Arsenic might seem indicated, except that Carbo has a more copious secretion and expectoration of mucus. China is variously commended, but no available indications are given.

This list of remedies would have to be increased a good deal, if we would include those that may be required to meet existing complications. In this respect we prefer referring the reader to their respective chapters, for it amounts pretty much to the same thing whether capillary bronchitis or catarrhal pneumonia sets in as a complication of whooping-cough or as a primary idiopathic disease. Unless the whooping-cough claims special attention on account of inherent features of a threatening character, it is our opinion that in all complicated cases the cough itself had better be ignored and the complication attended to above everything else. This course will facilitate the choice of a remedy and will prove advantageous to the patient. The whooping-cough will certainly disappear as soon as the catarrh is removed.

Of particular importance and involving a good deal of danger is a combination of whooping-cough with tuberculosis, whether the latter was caused by the cough or existed previous to its occurrence. Naturally enough the paroxysm of cough irritates the diseased lungs in a most dangerous manner and invests the cure with immense difficulties. In such cases *Iodium* and *Silicea* prove excellent remedies.

The catarrh remaining after the convulsive stage is not distinguished in anything from an ordinary catarrh, provided it is not complicated with emphysema. If this is the case, a cure can be expected from scarcely anything except the persistent use of vegetable charcoal; in the case of young people a cure is not only possible, but probable.

The sequelæ are too numerous to admit of an extensive notice in this place. If whooping-cough is treated homœopathically from the outset, they will scarcely ever happen, except perhaps tubercles which, however, are never engendered by whooping-cough, but are at most converted into centres of suppuration. As regards the characteristic whooping-cough marasmus, we have never yet come across it in our own practice.

If the homœopathic treatment only commences at a later stage of the disease, the prognosis of course differs greatly from the prognosis under full homœopathic treatment; for at that stage we often meet with structural changes which it may be difficult or even impossible to remove.

Another important point is the patient's mode of living. In this respect physicians differ in their opinions more perhaps than in any other disease. As regards nourishment, it has to be of a nature not to cause any irritation of the stomach or intestinal canal that might exert a pernicious influence over the course of the cough. It is likewise an indispensable precaution that children should not be stuffed with food, lest a paroxysm should so much more readily occasion vomiting; it is a good plan to keep the children quiet after eating, in order to keep off an attack until the digestion is completed. If food is vomited up too easily and too often, a small quantity of Tokay will prove an excellent means of steadying the stomach. If opinions concerning the food and the beverages of patients cannot reasonably differ, they are so much more antagonistic as respects the balance of the management. We have already stated that Oppolzer, and with him a number of other physicians, prescribe a uniform temperature for the little patients, and even keep them in bed. By this means the catarrh is to be removed in the shortest possible manner. In one respect the usefulness of this proceeding may not admit of any doubt, but in other respects the general well-being of the patients is injuriously affected by it. In the absence of other efficient remedial agents, the usefulness of this confinement is undoutedly undeniable. Under homœopathic treatment, however, it becomes a useless deprivation. Of course the children should be kept in their rooms until the fever is passed; but if the whooping-cough sets in with a simple coryza, the children may safely be allowed the use of the open air, of course with proper precautions. As soon as the convulsive stage has set in, we enjoin upon the parents the duty of sending the children every day out of doors for a couple of hours, provided the weather is tolerably fair. We have never observed any injurious effects from this proceeding, even in winter; the disease does not, on this account, last longer than five weeks, and the children retain a fresh appearance and preserve their strength and regular appetite. Moreover another advantage should not be overlooked: the children remain in good spirits, whereas continued confinement in a room usually begets an irritable and headstrong temper which has the effect of promoting the frequency of the paroxysms. Regarding a change of residence, we have already hinted in a previous paragraph our doubts of the propriety of such a measure. We have never known the children of country-people to be favorably affected by such a change, only city-children gain by it sometimes, and in their case it is not the removal from the influence of the whooping-cough miasm, but the healthier mode of living that produces the good results. If city-children are sent back to the city, no good effects are perceived. Indeed, such aids are not necessary. Many lay-people, even physicians, object to washing the children with cold water, or to allow them their usual bath. This, too, is an useless precaution, and may even become injurious for the reason that the skin is made unnecessarily sensitive and its functional activity is forced into an unwonted mode of action.

In conclusion we offer a few words regarding the dose of the appropriate remedy. In this respect the partisans of large and small doses are diametrically opposed to each other, some regarding whooping-cough as an acute, others as a chronic disease. It may be possible to cure whooping-cough with the thirtieth potency; we have never attempted such a thing; at all events low potencies are not necessary to effect a cure, nor is it necessary to resort to frequent repetitions of the dose. Our own experience has led us to prefer the middle potencies, giving a dose morning and evening. A frequent change of remedies should be strictly avoided; rapid success can never be achieved by such means.

[We would call attention to two remedies which Bæhr has omitted to mention, we mean *Coffee* and *Mephitis putorius*. The former, if given in dessertspoonful doses of a strong infusion, sweetened with sugar and without milk, will have a tendency to shorten and moderate the paroxysms; the latter has been frequently used by homœopathic physicians with good effect; Doctor Neidhard of

Philadelphia has reported a number of successful cases treated with Mephitis in our various Journals. H.]

6. Bronchitis Chronica.
Chronic Bronchitis, Chronic Pulmonary or Bronchial Catarrh.

In the majority of cases chronic bronchitis owes its existence to one or more attacks of acute bronchitis out of which it arises by gradual development. Even as thus arising as a secondary disease, the affection is exceedingly frequent, but this frequency is still more increased by the circumstance that it accompanies most of the material changes of structure in the lungs, particularly tuberculosis, bronchiectasia and emphysema, and that it likewise occurs as a complication of diseases of other organs. The latter occurs more particularly in diseases of organs that obstruct the return of the blood from the lungs, such as heart-disease and affections of the liver. As a primary disease, chronic bronchitis is more particularly met with among persons who are upwards of forty-five years old; every chronic pulmonary catarrh of young people excites a well-founded suspicion that it emanates from some other pulmonary disease as its source. Men are much more frequently afflicted with chronic bronchitis than women; children are seldom attacked. In Northern districts chronic pulmonary catarrh becomes much more frequent; in countries with a damp and cold climate it is almost endemic; it likewise prevails among individuals whose business confines them to damp and cool places. Persons who have to inhale a good deal of dust during their work, such as stone-cutters, millers and sculptors, are likewise exposed to frequent attacks of chronic bronchitis. Smoking is likewise a frequent cause of this disease. This use of tobacco causes chronic catarrh of the bronchial lining membrane much more frequently than one imagines, without any acute attack having preceded the chronic form.

The symptoms and course of the disease are easily understood if we keep the anatomical changes which the bronchial mucous membrane undergoes, steadily in view. For this reason we will describe these changes before going any further. The bronchial mucous membrane is hypertrophied over a more or less considerable extent of surface; it is unequally raised up, is of a deep dark-red color and traversed by distinctly engorged vessels. It is covered by a massive layer of gray or even purulent mucus, of various thicknesses, or else the secretion is more scanty, but in that case very tenacious, transparent, ropy. The puffiness and thickening of the mucous membrane, as well as the infiltration of the submucous and muscular tissues diminish the elasticity and occasion a consequent dilatation of the bronchia which is mostly diffuse, but may likewise be partial. Emphysema may likewise result from these anatomical changes. If a bronchial tube becomes closed anywhere, atelectasia of corresponding parts of the lungs takes place. True pus is seldom formed on the bronchial mucus membrane; hence ulcers, which occur so frequently in chronic catarrh of other mucous membranes, are seldom seen on the mucous lining of the bronchia.

Considering our mode of living, and when affecting persons beyond the age of fifty, the milder cases of chronic bronchial catarrh do not present any marked symptoms. The patients cough a little, most generally in the morning, and after that they expectorate some, but assimilation is not affected by the disease, nor is the respiratory process interfered with, and the condition sometimes remains unchanged for years. The more violent cases, on the contrary, cause constant and most commonly increasing trouble.

After the termination of an acute bronchi..' catarrh,—for chronic catarrh seldom sets in gradually without any preliminary acute stage,—cough and expectoration remain and continue with slight variations until made worse again by another acute attack. The cough is marked by two essentially distinct features. If the bronchial secretion is scanty, tenacious and firmly adhering, the paroxysms of cough occur less frequently, but in such a case the cough is mostly severely spasmodic and not unfrequently leads to gagging and vomiting. The paroxysms occur most frequently at night, less commonly in the day-time. After violent exertions, some of the above-described mucus is expelled; sometimes a little mucus is not hawked up till some time after the cough. If the secretion is more copious, the cough sets in chiefly in the morning-hours or after the use of warm food; it may continue for a long time, but is not spasmodic, for after a few energetic spells of cough, the mucus is detached and expectorated.

Sooner or later the cough becomes associated with more or less violent oppression of breathing, which may even creep along without being perceived and corresponds with the increasing hypertrophy of the bronchial mucous membrane, a diminution of its elasticity and the copious quantity of the secretion. At first this oppression is only perceived by the patients when making an effort, during a rapid walk, going up hill; soon, however, it is felt even during an ordinary walk, even during rest, and causes a great deal of annoyance. In the higher grades of the disease, the patients are threatened during the paroxysm of cough with danger of suffocation; even between the paroxysms the nature of the existing affection is revealed at first sight by the elevated thorax and the consequent shortening of the neck. The most intense pain, however, is endured by the patients if an acute aggravation of the disease takes place. Under such circumstances they exhibit such a perfect picture of distress that it seems as though they could not possibly live longer than twenty-four hours. These acute exacerbations occur almost certainly once at least every spring and fall, even if the patients have not knowingly been exposed or have not even left their room.

The structural changes, superinduced by chronic catarrh, render the disease, if it lasts any length of time, almost constantly unbearable. Emphysema which often is produced by, but seldom engenders catarrh, usually accompanies the latter and occasions permanent dyspnœa corresponding with the extent of the emphysema. Dyspnœa is likewise occasioned by bronchiectasia and by the anomalous conditions of the heart excited by chronic catarrh. The worst is that the morbid conditions occasioned by the disease, in their turn feed and aggravate the exciting cause.

In unimportant cases the physical diagnosis does not reveal any abnormal changes. The percussion remains normal as long as the catarrh has not given rise to any material changes such as atelectasia, emphysema, etc. In a violent attack, auscultation always yields abnormal results. If the secretion is scanty and auscultation is instituted immediately after, or during a paroxysm of cough, a loud inspiratory murmur is heard over the whole thorax and a prolonged and loud expiration with wheezing; râles are very seldom heard, or, if they are heard, the bullæ are fine; between the paroxysms, the respiratory murmur may be normal over the larger portion of the thorax; crepitation or a fine wheezing is only heard in detached spots. If the secretion is copious, coarse as well as fine râles, with sibilant and buzzing sounds, are heard all the time, most loudly previous to a paroxysm of cough.

In the beginning the general organism is not affected by the complaint; even tolerably severe forms of this disease are borne for a long time without any perceptible detriment. Very seldom, and only if the secretion is very profuse, emaciation gradually supervenes, in spite of which the patients may live, however, for many years. The greatest danger is occasioned by the influence exerted by the impeded respiration over the circulation. The functions of the heart become abnormal; the deficiency of blood in the lungs and its imperfect aëration either cause passive hyperæmias of the liver and a corresponding chronic intestinal catarrh, or disturbances in the functions of the spleen or kidneys, or passive hyperæmia of the brain with its inherent dangers, so that it is not without reason that a raised thorax and short neck are designated as an apoplectic habit.

If the catarrh has become an inveterate disease, it is apt to last to the end of life; but that such a noble organ as the lungs should be capable of bearing for so long a time even a severe degree of an apparently dangerous disease, is indeed remarkable. It is not marasmus the patient need dread, but the constant succession of acute attacks which indeed are rarely immediately fatal, but may easily superinduce œdema of the lungs; most patients die of this disease amid symptoms of general dropsy. If an acute attack assumes the form of capillary bronchitis or pneumonia, the lives of such patients are indeed in extreme peril.

In recent cases the prognosis is not altogether unfavorable so far as a cure is concerned; life is very seldom endangered by such a disease. The chances of course depend upon what structural changes have taken place, and to what extent. The worst omen is heart-disease, which almost always terminates in dropsy in a very short time.

Treatment. Even under homœopathic treatment inveterate pulmonary catarrhs are very seldom cured; nor will this treatment ever succeed in effecting the retrograde metamorphosis of emphysema or bronchiectasia. But even though the homœopathic Materia Medica has only palliatives to offer against the totality of the disease, yet we are possessed of many more excellent means towards the limitation and complete cure of the exacerbations, and for the stoppage of the further progress of incipient alterations of tissue; and in this way we are able to afford a relief that may be called extraordinary if compared with what is accomplished by other methods of cure. Hence we earnestly advise every physician who treats chronic bronchitis, to keep these two last-mentioned points steadily in view, and never to lose sight of them in the effort to effect a radical cure.

With a view of affording a general view of the treatment, we will first describe the chief remedies in a few short paragraphs.

Tartarus stibiatus has already been mentioned when we treated of acute affections of the mucous membranes, but is perhaps of greater importance in chronic bronchial catarrh to which it is so characteristically adapted. In bronchitis with a violent, spasmodic cough, loud râles in the chest, a copious, white expectoration, dyspnœa occasioned by the quantity of the secreted mucus, *Tart. stib.* is a sovereign remedy; it speedily diminishes the quantity of mucus and thus affords much relief to the sufferer. Very seldom, however, a favorable effect will be witnessed in cases where emphysema has already set in; for this reason the remedy is better adapted to chronic catarrhs of recent origin, that had taken the place of the acute disease, than to inveterate cases.

Pulsatilla is much more useful in chronic than in acute bronchitis, if the following symptoms prevail: Cough, principally at night, excited by tickling in the trachea, with copious expectoration of mucus; the mucus is mostly white, but frequently mingled with yellowish or greenish lumps that impart to it an oily, offensive taste. There must not be any emphysema, whereas the presence of tubercles as cause of the disease points to Pulsatilla. Pulsatilla is next to indispensable in the bronchial catarrh of chlorotic patients which almost always, although not in every case, depends upon tuberculosis. If, in the case of children, an acute catarrh gradually changes to the chronic form, Pulsatilla is a remedy of the first importance.

Sulphur is undoubtedly the most important remedy in this disease because it corresponds to the worst and most inveterate cases. If emphysema is present, this remedy may never yield any marked results; even its palliative effect is questionable. Brilliant results may, however, be obtained, in cases of chronic catarrh of long standing, if the mucus is secreted in large quantities, or is very tenacious, and the symptoms point to a decided thickening of the mucous membrane. An eminent indication for Sulphur is the excessive sensitiveness of the skin, so that every trifling change of temperature causes an exacerbation and that, even if the patient remains in his room, he is still powerfully affected by changes in the weather. Only this hyperæsthesia must not be caused by pulmonary tuberculosis, the tubercles at least must not be in a state of suppuration. What we have said shows that the symptoms may be distinguished in two series. The cough is either loose, the mucus easily detached, but only at times, so that at night, for instance, there is a good deal of dry cough, whereas in the morning and during the day the cough is moist, the expectoration is mostly white, compact, but mixed with a number of yellowish or greenish lumps showing that the mucus had been secreted in the bronchia for some time before being coughed up; it has a foul taste and even a bad odor, and the accompanying hoarseness and sensation of rawness show that the larynx and trachea have become involved in the pathological process. Or else the cough sets in in more violent paroxysms with considerable dyspnœa, is dry and spasmodic, with wheezing in the chest; it occurs most generally late in the evening and in the night, and it is only towards morning or after rising that a tenacious, glassy mucus is brought up after a slight coughing spell. The digestive symptoms and the condition of the liver which generally appears very much enlarged in chronic catarrh, confirm the selection of Sulphur. It has always seemed to us as if the triturations of Sulphur did not act as well in this disease as the attenuations prepared from the alcoholic tincture, and that, as a rule, the higher potencies act better than the lower. We do not insist upon this point, for a comparatively small number of observations do not authorize the resort to apodictic assertions. Finally we have to observe that in the case of decrepit, and more especially old individuals, Sulphur seldom does any good.

Nux vomica acts in many respects similarly to Sulphur and, according to our experience is, like Pulsatilla, more efficient in chronic than in acute bronchitis, if the following symptoms prevail: The cough sets in with particular violence between midnight and morning, is dry, spasmodic, very persistent and racking, so as to cause pains in the bowels; it is easily excited by a change of temperature, and is associated with a continual titillation in the chest and trachea; only in the morning, mostly after, very seldom before rising, a loose cough sets in, with easy expectoration of a simple mucus. While coughing a sensation of soreness and roughness is sensibly felt down the middle of the chest. The condition of the digestive organs greatly facilitates the selection of the right remedy. In contradistinction to Sulphur, Nux vomica is much better adapted to comparatively recent cases without any serious complications and is otherwise more particularly suitable for patients with vigorous and otherwise sound constitutions.

Phosphorus, although variously recommended for chronic catarrh, is, in our opinion, only adapted to acute attacks of bronchitis setting in during the course of the malady, and when exceedingly acute and threatening. Particulars may be found in the chapter on acute pulmonary affections.

Belladonna, though not exactly a remedy for chronic bronchitis, renders excellent service in the continued, distressing titillating cough, excited by a tickling in the throat-pit, by cold air and long talking, without any or a very scanty, tenacious expectoration, and generally with a marked feeling of dryness in the respiratory organs, exacerbating during the last hours before midnight. This form of chronic bronchitis is not very frequent.

Calcarea carbonica is used in this disease much less frequently than it deserves. It competes in some respects with Sulphur, but is likewise fully adapted to emphysematous chronic catarrh, if the cough is dry and tormenting, sets in principally at night with a violent irritation in the respiratory organs, and if, after coughing for some time, a tenacious and frothy mucus of a saltish or offensively sweetish taste is expectorated. We shall revert to this drug when speaking of the catarrh of tuberculous individuals. Next to *Silicea* it is the most important remedy in the so-called stone-cutter phthisis.

Spongia is one of the principal remedies for chronic croupous bronchitis. The patients feel quite well for days; it is only occasionally that they cough once and then only very little; all at once, after an increasing shortness of breath, and excited by cold, a violent emotion or some other irritation, and attended with wheezing throughout the whole chest, a violent fit of spasmodic cough sets in, by which the distinctly-perceived murmurs in the lungs are continually increased, accompanied by a high degree of dyspnœa which lasts for several hours and mostly occurs in the night; the cough is quite dry, or else there may be a scanty, frothy expectoration which sometimes has to be vomited up, and not till several hours after, a glassy, hard, clear mucus of a globular or vermiform shape is easily hawked up in small pieces. Very commonly these symptoms point to tuberculosis, but not as a rule.

Sepia may claim our attention in a similar cough as Spongia, but we must confess that we have never derived very striking results from its use. The numerous symptoms in the pathogenesis of Sepia which point to bronchial catarrh, give evidence that Sepia must be a remedy for this disease. Only it is difficult, owing to the multitude of symptoms, to present a characteristic group. The leading symptoms of the group are: Dry, spasmodic cough, or cough with a copious, saltish expectoration, which is apt to set in during the late morning-hours. Sepia is not adapted to bronchial catarrhs accompanied with bronchiectasia, emphysema, etc.

Iodium is related to Spongia; perhaps it acts more readily than the latter; the paroxysms of chronic catarrh to which Iodine is adapted, occur irregularly during the day; the expectoration is glassy and hard or tenacious, but shapeless; the paroxysms are always accompanied by a violent asthma which does not entirely cease during the intervals. Iodium is probably never suitable in cases of old people.

Lycopodium is suitable for old people, if emphysema and marked changes in the bronchial mucous membrane have taken place; there is constant tickling in the throat, loud râles with scanty or unfrequent expectoration of a gray color and saltish taste, nightly exacerbations.

Manganum is suited to a spasmodic cough with difficulty of raising the phlegm; the cough is only in the day-time; only hard lumps are brought up after hard coughing, of a yellow or green color.

Baryta carbonica has acted very favorably in several cases of catarrh of old people, with excessive secretion of mucus and difficulty of expectorating it, and with paroxysms of a spasmodic cough during the period immediately following midnight. Two days after using the drug the mucus generally decreased in quantity and the patients felt relieved.

Silicea, although symptomatically indicated in many forms of catarrh, yet has only proved efficient in our hands in a very severe form. We are often called upon to prescribe for the common stonecutter bronchitis which is such a common cause of death among this class of workmen. It is characterized by profuse secretion of mucus, great shortness of breath without any perceptible emphysema; this shortness of breath not only sets in after an effort, but without any cause. These people generally die of phthisis pituitosa, that is to say in consequence of an excessive secretion of mucus, associated now and then with distinct signs of bronchial suppuration. We have tried a number of remedies against this dangerous affection almost without effect, whereas *Silicea* has always acted with prompt benefit. We must add that we have never derived any advantage from alcoholic attenuations, but always from the higher triturations.

Stannum has been tried by us in many apparently suitable cases, without any result; we cannot recommend it, whatever others may say to the contrary.

Senega is adapted to chronic bronchitis when accompanied by laryngotracheitis, but likewise to chronic bronchitis without this accompaniment; the cough has no expectoration, or else the above-described tenacious, glassy expectoration, especially troublesome at night, and excited by every exertion of the respiratory organs, or by fresh air.

Bryonia alba is preferable in the acute form, and is very seldom adapted to inveterate chronic catarrh. It is particularly indicated by a spasmodic cough with a copious expectoration of yellowish mucus; the cough distresses the patient all the time and is so violent that it seems as though the thorax would fly to pieces; it is easily excited by smoke and dust. We have never seen Bryonia relieve a dry cough, or a cough with tenacious, scanty expectoration.

Hyoscyamus, of all the remedies here mentioned has the most precise and most prominent indications, which are indeed not often met with in chronic catarrh. The Hyoscyamus-cough is a nocturnal, spasmodic cough, excited by a recumbent posture and abating immediately after the vertical posture is resumed. This combination of symptoms occurs very rarely, but if it does, Hyoscyamus is the right remedy.

Opium must not be overlooked. It is erroneous to suppose that the narcotic effect of Opium suspends the desire to cough only for a short time, for there are many forms of cough where Opium only exacerbates, but does not afford any relief, or affords relief only when administered in very large doses to be followed afterwards by an increase of the cough. In our opinion *Opium* is admirably homœopathic to a spasmodic, dry, paroxysmal, titillating cough which is especially tormenting at night, and has but a scanty expectoration. The fact that we have often cured a cough of this kind permanently by means of a few doses of Opium, entitles us to the belief that Opium is something better than a mere palliative in this affection. But we warn our readers against giving Opium, if the cough is attended with a profuse expectoration of mucus, since a decrease of the cough must necessarily lead to great dyspnœa.

Digitalis purpurea is mentioned here as a remedy for pulmonary tuberculosis to which chapter the reader is referred. A special indication for this remedy are cyanotic symptoms in the face and the sensation of an excessive determination of blood to the lungs, by which the breathing is at times oppressed and suspended.

Arsenicum album is one of the most important remedies for chronic bronchial catarrh. However, it will rarely be indicated in simple, uncomplicated, chronic, bronchial catarrh, but so much more frequently if emphysema has taken place, and if the symptoms which we have indicated as peculiar to Digitalis, prevail. The cough is always attended with more or less considerable asthmatic distress which does not entirely cease even during the intervals between the paroxysms; the cough is excited by a severe tickling in the trachea or under the sternum, by cold air and more particularly by changes in the atmosphere; it breaks out particularly in the middle of the night, has a dry and wheezing sound, and it is only with difficulty that a frothy and occasionally a tenacious, white mucus is raised. The symptoms indicating Arsenicum are only occasionally met with among young people, and only rarely among old ones. If the remedy acts favorably, it does so speedily; if Arsenic does not improve the case in the first eight days, no favorable change need be expected from the further use of this drug. Arsenic acts with particular benefit, if the catarrh has become associated with heart disease, though, in such a case, a radical cure can no longer be expected.

Carbo vegetabilis ranks with Arsenic in curative power. The symptoms of both drugs are very much alike. Carbo likewise acts best in old and neglected cases, with emphysema and hypertrophy of the mucous lining; the circulation of the lungs and heart as well as of the head and abdominal viscera is very much impeded; the patient is very sensitive to cold and to the direct action of irritants upon the lungs; the symptoms exacerbate at night, but the expectoration differs from that of Arsenic: Carbo affording help only if the expectoration is profuse, not when scanty. At times the expectoration consists of mere lumps of mucus; at other times it is purulent, or yellow and green, sometimes having a bad taste and a pungent odor, suggesting the possibility of an approaching pulmonary phthisis. If the larynx is very much involved, Carbo is indicated so much more. The drug must not be expected to act immediately, because patients for whom Carbo is suitable, are generally very much reduced and the lungs are so deeply implicated that a rapid improvement has become impossible.

Beside the remedies we have named, a number of other drugs may be ranged in this category; they are only of secondary importance, and we confine ourselves to giving their names: *Ipecacuanha*, *Antimonium crudum*, *Conium maculatum*, *Hepar sulphuris*, *Natrum muriaticum*, *Cuprum*, *Kali carbonicum*, *Ambra*, also *China*, and *Ferrum*.

A bird's-eye view of the therapeutic indications may facilitate the selection of the particular remedy appropriate in a given case. Starting from the mucous secretion which accompanies the cough, we have two principal kinds, one with copious, and the other with scanty or no expectoration. The remedies for the first kind, are: *Bryonia, Tartarus stibiatus, Pulsatilla, Calcarea carbon., Lycopodium, Manganum, Silicea, Sulphur, Stannum, Baryta carbon., Carbo veget., Digitalis, China, Ferrum, Antimonium crudum, Ambra.* For the second kind, the remedies are: *Nux vomica, Belladonna, Spongia, Iodium, Senega, Hyoscyamus, Opium, Hepar sulphuris, Arsenicum,* and, in so far as this second kind appears in the form of a spasmodic titillating cough: *Belladonna, Senega, Hyoscyamus, Opium.*

For chronic bronchitis of recent origin, when arising from the acute form, the following remedies are particularly appropriate: *Bryonia, Tartarus stibiatus, Pulsatilla, Sulphur, Nux vomica, Belladonna, Hepar sulphuris, Ipecacuanha;* if remaining after measle-catarrh: *Pulsatilla;* if after whooping-cough: *Cuprum, China, Ferrum, Arsenicum, Hepar.*

Among old people, chronic bronchitis requires: *Tartarus stibiatus, Lycopodium, Baryta, Carbo vegetabilis.* In their case only a palliative effect can be obtained, that is to say a limitation of the mucous secretion; we cannot expect to accomplish more by continuing the exhibition of these remedies.

For the so-called stone-cutter phthisis the leading remedy is *Silicea,* next *Calcarea carbonica, Carbo vegetabilis. Tartarus stibiatus* will seldom do much good, although the symptoms may seem to indicate this remedy. It is, however, indispensable that the respiratory organs be no longer compelled to inhale the stone or flour-dust, or the dust and delicate fibres of the wool. The best protection against this exposure is a moist sponge tied in front of the mouth and nose, or a thick woollen mask around the nose and mouth, which is continually kept moist. By adopting this course we have often succeeded in restoring stone-cutters who seemed irretrievably lost so as to enable them to resume their work and attend to it permanently. The difficulty is that such patients dread the derision of their fellow-laborers and that it is next to impossible to overcome this obstacle.

If the catarrh has either originated or is accompanied by organic heart-disease, a cure cannot well be thought of. *Arsenicum, Carbo vegetabilis, Lycopodium, Tartarus stibiatis* may be tried, but the most efficacious remedy is undoubtedly *Digitalin,* about $\frac{1}{100}$ or $\frac{1}{120}$ of a grain per day, and administered at intervals. Persons who do not smoke, will derive much relief for their asthmatic distress from moderate smoking. Old women know this well; they are very apt to smoke a pipe for the sake of easing their lungs.

For the passive cerebral congestions, with which organic diseases of the heart are so often associated, and likewise for the œdema of the lungs originating in a similar cause, *Digitalin* is likewise the best palliative; *Arsenic* or *Carbo vegetabilis* are much less frequently productive of any good results. If the disorganizations have progressed too far, it is no longer possible to save the patient, and all we can do is to palliate his sufferings.

In the intercurrent acute exacerbations, mostly of a threatening character and which, if the mucous membrane is considerably hypertrophied, cause extreme anguish and dyspnœa, and a blue-red or livid bloating of the face, the choice is between *Bryonia*, *Mercurius*, *Phosphorus*, and *Arsenicum*. These exacerbations are of a threatening import, for the reason that they are most apt to cause œdema and paralysis of the lungs. But even in lesser grades of chronic bronchial catarrh the exacerbations cannot be treated with sufficient care, because they so commonly increase the chronic trouble and originate bronchial changes of structure. Old people are more particularly exposed to danger from this source; during the transition-periods of the seasons they have to use great caution in exposing themselves to the deleterious influences of atmospheric changes.

In obstinate cases of chronic bronchial catarrh, if the patients are otherwise young and vigorous, we are forced to suspect the presence of tubercles, which will almost always be discovered on exploring the chest. For the remedies to be employed under these circumstances, we refer to the chapter on tuberculosis.

The general management of the patients cannot be made to conform to fixed general rules, but has to be adapted to the circumstances of the patient. The uncomplicated chronic bronchial catarrh of young and vigorous individuals does not require any particular caution; above all, the patients must not use any excessive care lest the acute exacerbations should occur so much more easily. With ordinary caution the patients may safely go out even if a tolerably high wind should be blowing; they should never be encouraged in the use of an inhaler. An inhaler is only admissible if every acute bronchial catarrh portends danger, as in tuberculosis, in which case attention has, of course, to be paid to wind and temperature. A measure of precaution, which is too much neglected, is the use of water-tight, warm shoes or boots; for nothing is more apt to give a cold which reacts upon the respiratory organs, than damp feet. We do not mean to advocate the use of India-rubber shoes which afford poor protection, for the reason that they prevent the proper action of the skin. On the other hand, double leather-soles with woollen stockings afford the most certain protection, without any incidental disadvantages; this foot-gear is doubly necessary to those who are troubled with sweaty feet. It is upon such apparently trivial circumstances that the success of our treatment sometimes depends.

In the case of children our measures of precaution have to be more complete than in the case of adults; even if a physical exploration does not reveal any abnormal changes, yet, in their case, the conditions which give the first impulse to tubercular disease, are much more easily developed.

For persons of an advanced age, it becomes imperatively necessary to guard against exacerbations and to submit to measures which would spoil young people and make them morbidly sensitive; we must not forget that the human body, after reaching the age of sixty, can no longer be prevailed upon to change its habits, dispositions or susceptibilities. Here it becomes necessary to provide as much as possible for an uniform temperature and for a supply of clothing corresponding with the deficiency of animal heat; by attending to these things, many have succeeded in prolonging their lives for years.

These general rules for different ages are not suitable for all individuals, and we must not insist, from preconceived notions, upon adhering to a regimen that may be prejudicial to the patient. Many young people cannot undergo the process of hardening, many older persons, on the contrary, do not feel well unless they go out in every kind of weather; one child is kept in the house for weeks and yet the catarrh of this little patient does not abate in the least, whereas it gets well very speedily if the child is allowed to be all day in the open air. These differences have to be found out while the patient is under our treatment.

Pure air which is the normal food of the respiratory organs, is of course an essential requisite for the cure of all pulmonary diseases. This circumstance is very much overlooked in the management of bronchial catarrh, for the reason that the influence of vitiated air is not so readily perceived and does not cause the patient any immediate discomfort. We know that the continued inhalation of dust will give rise to pulmonary catarrh; will not the same cause operate in feeding the catarrh that already exists? Let the patient, therefore, avoid dust and smoke, and let old people especially have their attention directed to the injurious effects of living in a room filled with tobacco-smoke. Wollen carpets in the rooms of such patients are objectionable, because the inhalation of the fine dust which detaches itself from the wool, may cause violent paroxysms of cough. Even lighting the rooms with gas is prejudicial to many persons, and does everybody some harm. The patients are not always aware of the fact that it is to the gas that they are indebted for some of their worst paroxysms of cough. [We think that these precautions are exaggerated; carpets, if kept clean and free from dust, have many advantages over bare floors, and oil or kerosene irritates the air-passages a great deal more than pure gas. H.]

As a rule food has no great influence over the course of the disease. Knowing, however, that the digestive organs become easily involved in the morbid process, we are bound to protect them with becoming care. It is only if the disease causes emaciation, that a nourishing diet is indispensable and that the cautious and moderate use of fat is quite proper, whereas farinaceous articles of diet should be restricted as much as possible. In the case of children especially the proper diet has to be prescribed with great definiteness; despite the prejudice that milk overloads the system with mucus, milk ought to constitute their chief nourishment; for chronic catarrh is really met with only among children with diseased constitutions, and it is in their case especially that the deleterious influence of catarrh upon the constitution is best perceived.

In conclusion we will add a few words regarding the use of particular places, the climate of which is supposed to exert a beneficial influence over the health of invalids. We do not deem it advisable to remove patients from their habitual home and climate so long as they may be able to recover their health at home; moreover a warm climate is not very favorable to uncomplicated bronchial catarrh. We may be able to do much better in our immediate neighborhood. The sojourn in mid-mountain woodlands is not only a palliative, but very often a genuine curative remedy for even very serious pulmonary diseases. This statement has been verified to us during the last years of our practice by so many irrefutable proofs that we do not intend to send away a single patient who has not first tried the influence of mountain-air in his own neighborhood. This air stimulates the lungs so powerfully that the result leads us to infer that even an existing emphysema may decrease under its agency, at the same time as the whole body seems to become invigorated by the change. More recently the results obtained by a sojourn in artificially compressed air have claimed the attention of the profession. Our own investigations and the results we have been able to achieve in our own practice, have satisfied us that this method of treatment has a distinguished future before it; we cannot with sufficient force urge upon our professional brethren the importance of acquiring a thorough knowledge of these new methods.

We cannot undertake to recommend particular spas for the reason that the curative virtues which are claimed for them are not expressed with a sufficiently definite scientific precision. The predilection of lay-people for the spas of Ems and others is undoubtedly very great, but the benefit derived from them is very questionable and is very frequently owing to the fact that the warm water which is drank early in the morning, promotes the solution of the mucus, but probably no more so than plain warm water would have done.

[Bæhr has included in the article on chronic bronchial catarrh a peculiar form of cough which is often described in pathological treatises as *dry bronchial catarrh* or *Catarrhus bronchialis siccus*, *tussis spasmodica* or *tussis titilans*, spasmodic or titillating cough. A special chapter has been devoted to this subject in Kafka's Therapeutics, which we transfer to this work, together with such remedies as have not been mentioned by Bæhr.

We designate, says Kafka, by this appellation a cough that sets in in paroxysms during which a titillation or tickling is continually felt in the trachea without any perceptible definite catarrhal affection of the bronchia. After the paroxysm the respiration, in genuine cases of such a cough, is again perfectly normal.

The appearance of the cough in paroxysms, the absence of a desire to cough and of any perceptible catarrhal process in the bronchia between the paroxysms, stamp this form of cough as a neurosis of the trachea.

The primary idiopathic titillating cough is *independent of any disease of the mucous membrane of the bronchia;* it is a disease during the course of which no sort of anatomical changes can be perceived in the mucous membrane of the trachea.

In the secondary form of titillating cough we observe an hyperæmia and hypertrophy of the mucous membrane which is readily seen by inspecting the fauces provided the titillation is located in that region. At the same time the mucous membrane is generally dry. The hypertrophy frequently spreads from the pharynx to the larynx and glottis, in consequence of which dyspnœa and spasm of the glottis frequently set in. If the hypertrophy extends to the more delicate bronchial ramifications, their contraction may cause asthmatic disturbances in the process of respiration.

If the titillation continues for a time, a muco-albuminoid substance, mingled with lumps of gray mucus, the *sputum margaritaceum of Laënnec*, is secreted and is coughed up without any rhonchus in the bronchia being heard.

Etiology. This form of cough is more frequently met with among children and women than among men. Primarily it is most commonly occasioned by irritants that affect directly the peripheral nerves of the bronchial mucous membrane. The inhalation of cold or damp air, an intense cold, a sudden change of temperature, cold winds, a draught of air, acrid gases or vapors, smoke, dust, very cold beverages such as ice-water, too long or too loud talking, especially during a walk or run; crying, screaming, singing, shouting, loud reading, especially if mixed up with a good deal of talking; exertions of the windpipe by the use of wind-instruments, whistling, by the blow-pipe, dancing, springing, etc., contribute greatly to the development of this form of cough. It is likewise excited by fits of passion, chagrin loud quarrelling, a sudden fright or surprise, etc. Sympathetically, this cough may attack hypochondriacs, hysteric women, children during the period of dentition, girls during the menstrual flow.

Secondarily this cough often supervenes during coryza, influenza, measles, acute or chronic bronchial catarrh, emphysema, tuberculosis.

Symptoms. The primary titillating cough generally sets in suddenly and without any preliminary symptoms; it occurs most frequently at night after one has laid down or during the first part of the night. The patients may spend the whole day or evening without being seriously troubled by the cough. Suddenly, after going to bed or being on the point of lying down, the patients are attacked by a violent irritation and desire to cough which does not allow them a moment's rest and prevents them from sleeping. The irritation is either experienced in the fauces, or in the larynx, throat-pit (in the region where the trachea bifurcates), or in the middle of the sternum or in the epigastrium; the irritation seems like a tickling and usually causes in the fauces a sensation as if little worms or insects were crawling about there; in the larynx and trachea a sensation of roughness is experienced, or as if the throat were irritated by dust, the vapors of Sulphur or Phosphorus, or by feathers or hairs; the titillation is sometimes so violent that it causes a spasm of the glottis. If the irritation is seated in the middle of the sternum, the patients experience a sensation of oppression on the chest and a more or less violent degree of dyspnœa which may even increase to asthma. The irritation in the epigastrium is sometimes very violent, causing considerable contractions of the diaphragm and an upward pressure of the abdominal viscera, which may result in nausea or vomiting. It is on this account that this form of cough has been dubbed "stomach-cough."

The cough is dry, continued, racking, *not hoarse;* sometimes it has a hollow sound; at times, if the titillation is located in the larynx, it is a dry cough; if spasm of the glottis supervenes, the inspirations are labored or accompanied by a peculiar panting sound, owing to which this cough is sometimes confounded with Asthma Millari (spasm of the glottis).

A titillating cough most generally sets in in single turns, sometimes two or three short paroxysms in succession; the subsequent inspiration is rendered difficult only if the glottis participates in the attack or if asthmatic symptoms supervene. Lighter grades of this cough are soon appeased; more violent attacks may continue for several hours or even the whole night. The patients are very much excited by the continual irritation and desire to cough; the face becomes flushed, the temperature of the body increases, the pulse is accelerated, a warm perspiration breaks out in the face or over the whole body; sensitive women and delicate girls are so violently shaken by the cough that the urine spirts out involuntarily during an attack.

After the dry cough has lasted for some time, a muco-albuminoid substance is usually secreted, mixed with a little saliva and containing here and there detached lumps of a gray, pearly mucus (sputum margaritaceum), which the most careful auscultation is unable to discover by the presence of rhonchi in the bronchia; that part of the trachea, where this little lump adheres, is stopped up and the respiratory murmur at this place is entirely absent; but as soon as the little lump is expelled, the normal respiratory murmur is again heard in this place, whereas the obstruction may again occur at some other spot. Percussion, at every point of the thorax, elicits a proper resounance. The expulsion of this little lump is sometimes a sign that the cough is going to terminate which, when violent, sometimes ends in vomiting.

After the paroxysm is over, the patients feel very languid, soon, however, fall asleep and wake with little or no cough; they remain almost entirely or altogether free from cough during the day, the respiratory mucous membrane likewise remaining unaffected, until at bed-time or in the first hours of the night they are again attacked by a paroxysm of cough.

The secondary form of titillating cough either supervenes during the course of acute catarrhal diseases, such as coryza, influenza, measles, acute bronchitis, and, in company with these diseases, runs an acute course, or else it accompanies, as a chronic cough, chronic bronchial catarrh, emphysema or tuberculosis. Even when associated with these diseases, the titillating cough is recognized as the result of a constant irritation which is felt, for a longer or shorter time, at different hours of the day as well as night, or even during the early morning-hours, and finally ceases and is replaced by a common catarrhal or tubercular cough which always has a catarrhal expectoration; whereas the titillating cough is generally dry, or is attended with only a trifling expectoration. The titillation is only experienced at the places indicated by the patient to whom it is a source of real distress.

Sometimes this titillating cough sets in with a sort of typical regularity.

Course, Terminations and Prognosis. The primary titillating cough generally runs an acute course, more especially if it was caused by a cold, by excessive exertions of the respiratory organs or by epidemic influences. The fever which accompanies it, is sometimes so violent that a speedy localization in one or the other part of the respiratory apparatus may be apprehended. This is particularly the case with children who are unable to explain themselves regarding the seat of the trouble. However the subsequent course of the symptoms, particularly the free intervals which often last for hours, and the return of the continual titillation after the cessation of these free intervals, soon disclose the true nature of the cough. Very frequently it sets in with but slight or even without any febrile motions, and the attacks continue until the causes or their immediate effects are removed. Sometimes only one or several attacks occur, sometimes they continue for several days, even from eight days to a fortnight, and they break out on the least provocation.

Most generally this titillating cough occurs in an uncomplicated form; sometimes, however, especially in the fall, winter or spring, during the prevalence of cold winds or in very cold weather, or when the weather is cold and damp, wet or foggy, or during the prevalence of an epidemic, the cough combines with one of the above-mentioned acute catarrhal diseases, and with them assumes an epidemic form and runs a similar course.

This disease always terminates in recovery; only when complicated with other diseases, these complications may superinduce threatening symptoms.

If the primary titillating cough lasts a long time and is very intense, emphysema or hernia may set in and may continue to the end of the patient's life.

Treatment. In treating this cough we have to aim at appeasing the existing paroxysm and preventing its return.

In the treatment we have to be guided by the exciting causes, the seat of the titillation, the phenomena developed by the cough in the general organism and more particularly in the organs of respiration, the consensual symptoms of the diaphragm, stomach and the upward action of the abdominal viscera, the circumstances by which the attacks are either meliorated or aggravated, the period when they set in, and the complications.

Above all we have to keep an eye on the causes that excite the titillating cough. To this end cold and damp localities, or localities containing acrid gases, vapors, dust or smoke, have to be abandoned, and every exertion of the respiratory organs by talking, reading, singing, blowing, etc., has to be avoided. The patients have to avoid with great care every sudden change of temperature, sudden cooling, draughts of air, cold or damp air, cold drinks, and every violent mental excitement; nor should they go out in windy, foggy, snowy or rainy weather. The room which the patients inhabit, must be kept at a uniform and moderate temperature; even in the night the temperature should not fall below 40° or 45° Fahr.; according to our experience, a lower degree of temperature in a room easily excites or exacerbates the cough.

Light cases of titillating cough, even if complicated with fever, do not require any medicinal treatment. A free perspiration by means of warm tea, warm lemonade, etc., and confinement in bed until the perspiration has ceased, is generally sufficient to restore the normal condition in the shortest possible space of time.

If the fever is severe, attended with dryness of the fauces and larynx and with a continual dry cough provoked by an unceasing titillation in the fauces or larynx; if the disease is the result of a cold, surprise or an excessive effort of the respiratory organs; if it is aggravated by excessive warmth of the room, by talking, drinking cold water; if the paroxysms set in in the forepart of the night during the first sleep, and if they are complicated with coryza, influenza, measles, acute bronchial catarrh, we give *Aconite* 3 in solution, after which the patient transpires profusely in two or three hours and all the symptoms improve.

Even in cases without fever or complications, *Aconite* acts with promptitude and efficacy, if the previously described symptoms are present.

If a troublesome feeling of dryness is experienced in the mouth, pharynx and trachea, attended with a continual titillation in the fauces and on the posterior wall of the larynx; if there is a sensation in the throat as if dust had been inhaled; if the cough is so violent that spasm of the glottis or asthmatic symptoms with flushed face, and heat of the head set in; if the nerves become irritable and sensitive to light and noise; if the disease has been occasioned by exposure to a draught of air, or by sudden fright or cooling off suddenly while the skin was covered with perspiration; if the paroxysm breaks out at the time when the patient wants to retire at night, and is made worse by talking, drinking or crying, *Belladonna* 3 is to be given, whether a fever is present or not, or whether the cough is complicated with coryza, influenza, measles, acute bronchial catarrh, hysteria or hypochondria, or not. For these symptoms Belladonna is always preferable to Morphine or the water of Laurocerasus; but it should be given in the form of tincture, the extract being less reliable.

If the titillating cough attacks teething children; if their mouths are hot and their gums red and swollen, with much saliva and redness of one cheek; if they start during sleep and are very peevish when awake; if the cough continues uninterruptedly after they have been put to bed, and if it is dry and short, we give *Chamomilla* 3. The same remedy is given if the cough is complicated with coryza, bronchial catarrh, when coarse râles and an audible rattling of mucus are present; or for cough accompanying influenza and acute intestinal catarrh, if the children cry violently previous to an evacuation, draw their legs up, and the passages look greenish or like stirred eggs. This remedy is likewise applicable in the case of sensitive women, if the titillating cough is caused by the inhalation of cold or damp air, by fits of anger, and is attended with a high degree of nervous erethism, and if the tickling in the trachea is associated with a constrictive sensation in the chest; if the cough is experienced at bed-time and torments the patient without ceasing. In our hands a single dose of Chamomilla has often sufficed in a vast number of cases to calm this cough, to quiet this cough during the night, which often keeps children, girls and women especially during the menstrual period, from sleeping.

Similar symptoms and complications likewise indicate *Mercurius sol. Hahn.*, especially in the case of teething children; it may likewise be used if the cough has a hollow sound, the titillation is experienced under the upper third of the sternum; if the cough had been caused by a cold, breaks out in nocturnal paroxysms, the patients perspire a great deal without being relieved by it, and if, after the attack, there remains an unconquerable disposition to stretch the limbs.

Conium 3 is used by us, if the titillation is felt in the middle of the sternum; if the cough is caused by exposure to rough weather and the paroxysms occur at night; if the cough is dry and so violent that it causes vomiting; if the use of acids and of salt food, or drawing a long breath make the cough worse; if during the cough the chest is spasmodically constricted and if, after the subsidence of the paroxysm, the patient complains of stinging pains in the head and a painful sensitiveness of the abdominal muscles. It deserves particular consideration in influenza, measles, acute bronchial catarrh and in the case of hysteric patients.

Rhus toxicodendron 3, for tickling and a feeling of dryness in the throat, down the trachea; the symptoms abate for a while after a swallow of warm tea or water and sugar, but soon reappear again in the same degree; accompanied by tearing pains in the extremities, especially if they set in at the same time as the cough in consequence of the patient being exposed to the influence of a damp and cold air, or getting soaking wet; the paroxysms occur in the night, attended with complete sleeplessness; the cough is complicated with coryza and frequent, spasmodic sneezing, or in cases of influenza with typhoid symptoms.

If the titillation and cough have set in after a walk in keen and cold air; if the tickling is chiefly felt in the larynx or extends down to the bronchia: if the cough is dry and so violent that it causes a spasmodic constriction of the throat and chest, and a more or less violent degree of spasm of the glottis, with an expression of anxiety in the face, cold sweat on the forehead and extremities, and the patients have more and more a cyanotic look; if the violence of the cough causes vomiting, and the paroxysms recur typically, we give *Ipecacuanha* 3 with decided benefit.

If the titillation is felt in the throat or pit of the stomach; if the cough is caused by rapid walking, running, mortified feelings or insulting treatment; if it is attended with dyspnœa and vomiting of the ingesta; if the attack sets in in the morning-hours and is aggravated by talking or eating; we give *Natrum muriaticum* 6, likewise if coryza is present, with entire loss of smell and taste, or if the cough is complicated with emphysema and tuberculosis. In the case of emphysematous women the titillating cough is usually attended with spirting out of the urine. This remedy is likewise valuable, if the titillating cough breaks out typically, or in the case of hypochondriacs or hysteric females.

We prescribe *Ignatia* 3 for a dry, constant, titillating cough which sets in more particularly at bed-time; the irritation is seated in the throat-pit, as from the inhalation of fine feather-dust, or the titillation is felt in the larynx or even in the epigastrium; the cough is of a preëminently nervous character and is caused by depressing states of the mind, or by humiliating treatment, grief, care; the cough is worse in the open air, after eating or drinking coffee. The disease may be primary and idiopathic, or attended with coryza and bronchial catarrh. Ignatia is particularly to be commended for hysteric women and for children inclined to spasms.

Ammonium carbonicum 3 is indicated by titillation in the larynx and a sensation in the trachea as of inhaled feather-dust, attended with dyspnœa; the paroxysms occur at night and are followed by a high degree of exhaustion; the cough is made worse by talking and open air; complicated with coryza, influenza and acute and chronic bronchial catarrh.

Acidum benzoicum 3 for a titillating cough caused by a cold, attended with a stinging sensation in the middle of the sternum which is worse during a deep inspiration; the cough is accompanied by asthmatic complaints and rheumatic pains in the joints.

Rumex crispus 3 is recommended by Kafka, if the titillation proceeds from the throat-pit or the middle of the sternum, attended with a sensation of soreness in the trachea; if the cough sets in at bed-time or after the patient has laid down, and is caused by the action of dry, cold air, especially in the winter-season; it deserves especial attention in bronchial and laryngeal catarrh. Doctor Carroll Dunham of New York has published a long and interesting article on the subject of Rumex crispus in the second volume of the Amer. Hom. Review, page 530, to which we refer the reader for full and correct information concerning the therapeutic uses of this drug in affections of the larynx, trachea and bronchi.

Graphites 6 for titillation in the larynx, with a feeling of soreness and burning in the throat; for nocturnal paroxysms of cough, with hard pressure on the chest; it is particularly useful in cough with chronic coryza or in the case of individuals who are at the same time attacked with a scrofulous eczema, or in the case of women when they have their menses.

We prescribe **Zincum metallicum** 6, if the titillation is located in the region of the sternum; if the cough is dry and exhausting, with stitches in the chest and oppression of breathing; if the respiration is labored and talking is quite an exertion, the attack takes place at night and deprives the patient of sleep; deserves particular attention for the cough of hysteric women and during the menses.

Kali carbonicum 6 is indicated by a dry titillating cough, with stinging in the larynx, pains in the chest, choking, violent headache, exhaustion after the attack which commonly sets in at night; is useful for titillating cough during the menses and in a case of incipient tuberculosis.

We have seen a very violent, acute titillating cough cured very speedily by means of a decoction of *Senega;* the patient was a lady and had contracted the cough during an ascension of the Rigi. This remedy is appropriate for cough, if the titillation is seated in the larynx, and the cough is attended with roughness in the throat and oppression on the chest; if the cough is made worse by the breathing of fresh air, and if the patient has to sneeze frequently and continually until the head feels heavy and giddy, without any coryza being present. It may be used during an attack of influenza and acute bronchial catarrh.

These remedies have enabled us to control every attack of primary titillating cough, no matter of what kind. (We remind the reader of the propriety of referring to the chapter on chronic bronchial catarrh for the other remedies not mentioned in this extract from Kafka.)

Even in the secondary form of this disease these remedies have always been found sufficient in our hands. In the titillating cough of tuberculous individuals, especially in the last stage of the disease, the best tried remedies sometimes remain without effect; in such a case we resort to empirical remedies from motives of humanity, such as *Cannabis indica* 2, *Atropin. sulph.* 2, or *Morphium acet.* 1.

(The *Spirits of Turpentine* on sugar and the *Balsam of Copaiva* likewise on sugar, or the alcoholic solution of the balsam have been found useful in chronic titillating cough.)

The selection of the proper remedy is often a very difficult matter, especially in the case of children who are unable to indicate the locality of the titillation or to furnish a proper account of their subjective sensations. The difficulty is likewise great in the case of hysteric females, because the consecutive, consensual and reflex-phenomena succeed each other with remarkable rapidity, and are exceedingly diversified. In such cases experience has taught us to *pay exclusive attention to the objective phenomena* which, to this end, have to be investigated with great correctness and interpreted with an enlightened knowledge of their character and meaning. After we have obtained an exact objective picture, we shall have no difficulty in picking out the remedy best suited to the case.

Having hit upon the remedy adapted to the present case by an arithmetical process as it were, we may rest assured that every subsequent paroxysm will yield to it. We exhibit the remedy during the paroxysm most commonly in solution, mixing four, six or eight drops in half a pint of water and giving one or two dessert-spoonfuls every quarter or half an hour, or every hour. Triturations like those of *Mercurius sol.* or *Hepar sulph.* are likewise ordered every half hour or hour in about grain-doses. After the termination of the paroxysm we continue the same remedy every two or three hours until the cough has entirely ceased. In order to prevent the return of the cough, we give two doses of the same drug every day, for some time longer. The patient's attention should be directed to the necessity of observing the dietetic and general hygienic rules which we have fully explained in previous paragraphs.

In a case of secondary titillating cough, we first stay the paroxysms and afterwards continue the treatment of the primary affection, such as coryza, acute or chronic bronchial catarrh, measles, influenza, emphysema, tuberculosis, for which we refer the reader to their respective chapters.

If the titillating cough occurs typically, we give, according to the symptoms, *Arsenicum, Ipecac., Nux vom., Natrum muriat.;* if these remedies prove insufficient, we give *Chinin. sulph.* 1, and in obstinate cases *Chinin. arsen.* 1, of which remedies we prescribe a dose every two or three hours during the apyrexia.

While the titillating cough lasts, the food should be salted or spiced as little as possible; mild nourishment containing a good deal of saccharine matter, is best. Even such articles of diet as contain a good deal of starchy matter, such as potatoes, chestnuts, peas, lentils, etc., should be avoided. Rancid fat, acids, cold and heating beverages are likewise hurtful.

Individuals who are liable to attacks of titillating cough, should observe the same precautions as those who are suffering with acute bronchitis, or are liable to attacks of this disease. H.]

7. Bronchiectasia.
Dilatation of the Bronchia.

We should not have mentioned this affection if it were not of particular importance to the correct appreciation of chronic bronchial catarrh.

A dilatation of the bronchia is of two kinds, a uniform or diffuse dilatation and a sacculated form. The former is always a consequence of an inflammatory acute or chronic disease of the bronchial mucous lining in which the elastic and muscular tissues have become involved, in consequence of which these tissues have lost their elasticity to a greater or less extent. This alteration of the bronchia is rarely confined to a small portion, but most commonly reaches over a large extent of the bronchial tubes. The sacculated form is caused by the closing of delicate bronchial ramifications above which it is located; this closing leads to atrophy of the pulmonary parenchyma and thus assists in restoring the space for a dilatation of the bronchia; or the dilatation may be a consequence of the closing of bronchial tubes occasioned by atrophy of the corresponding portion of the lungs.

Diffuse bronchiectasia, if not too prominently developed, is of no particular consequence; if occasioned by an acute attack, it is curable; but if resulting from chronic bronchitis, it may be difficult to repair the disorder. It has the same phenomena as chronic catarrh, or chronic catarrh in conjunction with emphysema which is scarcely ever absent.

Sacculated bronchiectasia is much more important, because it easily leads to suppuration and gangrene of the mucous membrane, and very frequently presents the picture of pulmonary phthisis, and generally modifies quite extensively the results of percussion and auscultation. Atrophy of the lungs superinduces retractions of the corresponding intercostal space, which, however, are not often observed at the apex of the lungs; the percussion-sound is dull, auscultation does not reveal any vesicular murmur, but bronchial respiration or else consonant murmurs, pectoriloquy, wheezing, coarse râles. The diagnosis is somewhat complicated, depending rather upon the absence of general symptoms of tuberculosis than upon the presence of any directly observed phenomena. In a case of severe chronic bronchial catarrh, bronchiectasia may be suspected with a tolerable degree of certainty if the expectoration has a very fetid odor. Otherwise the symptoms here are likewise the same as in chronic bronchial catarrh, very often associated with the phenomena resulting from the presence of emphysema which is very apt to supervene on such occasions.

Of course the treatment cannot aim at restoring the elasticity and contractility of the bronchia; hence it cannot be directed against the bronchiectasia, but the physician has to make the cure of the accompanying catarrh the chief object of his attention. Even a dilatation caused by an acute catarrh, if it should have been correctly diagnosed, does not require any special treatment. If we once have become satisfied of the presence of bronchiectasia, we feel convinced that the existing bronchial catarrh cannot be entirely cured, and we refrain from instituting fruitless experiments; at the same time as we may obtain light concerning the proper remedies to be prescribed which, of course, can only aim at a palliation of the symptoms. For all that, though bronchiectasia is an undesirable complication, yet it does not necessarily render the prognosis in a case of bronchitis more doubtful. Such patients may live to an old age, even if affected with sacculated bronchiectasia, if the expectoration is decidedly purulent, and has a foul odor.

8. Emphysema Pulmonum.
Emphysema of the Lungs.

Two essentially different kinds of emphysema have been described, an interlobular arising from the passage of air into the pulmonary connective tissue, and a vesicular representing an entirely different process, namely a dilatation of the air-cells. We have only to deal with the latter form.

Emphysema very commonly arises in consequence of processes in the lungs by which a portion of this organ is rendered inaccessible to the respiratory process; it may accompany atrophy or infiltration of portions of the lungs; it most commonly accompanies changes of structure which at the same time superinduce a diminution of the volume of the lungs. This form of emphysema can scarcely be regarded as anything morbid and will never become an object of treatment; it is termed vicarious emphysema. Vesicular emphysema has an entirely different origin and is of much higher importance; in a practical point it is essential that this origin should be known. We do not deem it necessary to recite the different theories regarding the origin of emphysema; we simply give what we consider the most correct explanation. Emphysema may be caused by morbid conditions of the air-cells which impair their elasticity more or less. This defect may arise in cases of violent bronchitis, pneumonia, etc., in which case the air-cells are affected similarly to the bronchia in diffuse bronchiectasia. This accounts for the frequent occurrence of emphysema in chronic bronchial catarrh Emphysema may likewise have another and different mode of origin. In consequence of an excessive but otherwise entirely normal exercise of the respiratory functions; or in consequence of the respiration being obstructed by organs situated outside of the thorax, the air-cells may become dilated to such an extreme degree that little by little they lose the power of resuming their former size, precisely in the same manner as an India-rubber bag that is often and excessively dilated, loses its elasticity.

In the former manner emphysema occurs principally in catarrhs of the bronchial mucous membrane, more especially in chronic catarrh with marked hypertrophy of the mucous membrane, and in an almost normal manner in old age where the walls of the air-cells, like most other tissues, lose their elasticity more and more.

In the second manner, emphysema is caused by excessive exertions in running, dancing, lifting, playing on wind-instruments, obstructed expiration by affections of the larynx, the closing of bronchial tubes, paralysis of the diaphragm, owing to which the expiratory act is performed in an incomplete manner; by occupations which leave one part of the lungs in a continual state of inaction. Very frequently both modes of origin combine, which is really always the case if chronic catarrh is sustained by lesser degrees of emphysema; at the same time chronic catarrh being an obstacle to respiration, and diminishing the elasticity of the air-cells, always increases the existing emphysema.

Hence the more special etiological causes determining the existence of emphysema are: catarrh of the mucous lining, especially chronic catarrh; various other affections of the lungs, whooping-cough, playing on wind-instruments, excessive bodily exertions, croup, stenosis of the larynx, paralysis of the diaphragm, tumors of the abdominal viscera, heart-disease, etc.

Emphysema may take place in every age, but occurs more particularly among persons beyond the age of fifty. Men are more liable to it than women, probably for no other reason than because they are more exposed to the causes producing it. Some individuals evidently inherit a disposition to the disease. Thin individuals contract the disease more easily than fleshy and robust persons.

The symptoms of pulmonary emphysema very naturally result from the anatomical changes it occasions. Some of the air-cells are excessively distended; hence, owing to their inability to contract sufficiently or at all, they no longer participate in the respiratory process, and consequently give rise to phenomena of dyspnœa. These are increased by the circumstance that the distended cells compress other neighboring cells and withdraw them from the process of respiration. The impeded respiration occasions passive hyperæmia of the lungs which again causes chronic catarrh, a deficiency of the heart's action, sanguineous engorgement of the abdominal viscera, the vessels of the head, and finally, in consequence of an abnormal composition of the blood, exudation of serum from the vessels and consequent dropsy.

These changes do not develop themselves all at once, nor do they all occur in the same sick individual; hence emphysema presents various groups of symptoms which we deem it unnecessary to delineate in this place. We prefer giving a more detailed description of the more prominent characteristic features of the disease.

Pulmonary emphysema runs an exceedingly chronic course, and the changes it occasions occur almost imperceptibly under the guise of a light chronic catarrh, but after some time progress with double rapidity since the existing emphysema necessarily originates additional emphysematous disorganizations. Patients may feel tolerably well for years, when suddenly the dyspnœa begins to increase steadily and imprints the true picture of emphysema upon the patient.

A physical exploration does not reveal at all times distinct phenomena. If on percussion, the pulmonary murmurs are heard beyond the liver and heart, we may safely conclude that emphysema is present; this circumstance, however, occurs only in high grades of the disease. Auscultation usually reveals only the symptoms of chronic catarrh which is in reality never absent, and moreover a very feeble, scarcely audible vesicular respiration which, owing to the extreme respiratory efforts of the patient, is indeed quite characteristic. If the emphysema has reached a high degree of development, the thorax assumes the shape of a tub. The ribs owing to the excessive action of the inspiratory muscles, retain the position which they assume during the act of inspiration, and thus it is that the upper portion of the thorax is dilated whereas the lower portion retains its normal width. Owing to the excessive inspiratory efforts the cervical muscles become very prominent, and the drawing up of the thorax gives to the patients their characteristic short necks. The influence upon the heart results more especially in abnormal changes of the right heart. Owing to the obstruction of the circulation in the lungs, the right heart is engorged with blood and finally permanently distended. It is only in the higher grades of emphysema that the heart is pushed out of its place. The effect upon the left heart is not constant. The change in the right heart explains various other phenomena of the circulation, the throbbing in the pit of the stomach, the venous hyperæmia of the thoracic viscera, the engorgement of the veins of the neck and head. From the deficiency of respiratory action and of the functional activity of the heart results a change in the composition of the blood which fluid finally assumes an intensely venous character. Usually the pulse is uncommonly small and feeble, frequently irregular or intermittent.

What torments the patients most, is the dyspnœa. If the catarrh is moderate, the dyspnœa is bearable, but it increases by every circumstance that interferes with the breathing, even by moderately filling the stomach, flatulence, but most permanently and most threateningly by an acute bronchial catarrh. It seems almost impossible that the patients should be able to bear this torture longer than a few days, and yet but few die of an attack of this kind. The most common cause of death is dropsy resulting from the above-described anomalies of the circulation. It most generally develops itself gradually, very seldom to a high degree, because ascites and œdema of the extremities are most commonly associated with œdema of the lungs.

The whole duration of the disease may be thirty, forty and more years. Emphysematous individuals, if pursuing a regular mode of life, may live to a high age in spite of all apparent danger. The constantly occurring variations in their state of health are not occasioned by an increase or decrease of the emphysema, but by an increase or decrease of the accompanying chronic catarrh. On this account summer and a dry and cold winter-air are most favorable to the patients, whereas the transition-periods from one season to another cause them frequently or almost regularly a violent distress; they commonly feel half a day in advance every approaching atmospheric change.

If we expect to effect a complete restoration of the patient, the prognosis is very bad; as far as longevity is concerned, it may be said to be very favorable. If emphysema has developed itself so far as to enable us to diagnose it, a retrograde metamorphosis can scarcely ever be thought of; all we can expect is to diminish the extent of the disease. The chances of a long life are mostly determined by the condition of the heart; as long as the heart preserves its normal state, we have nothing to fear. The renal functions likewise deserve our attention, since their condition generally first enables us to prognosticate the termination in dropsy.

If we mean to indicate a treatment of emphysema, we shall first have to inquire how far this disease can at all be treated. The elasticity of the air-cells is gone, they have become distended to such an extent that they cannot possibly recover their normal size; in many instances the walls of adjoining cells have disappeared, and cavities have formed in their places. Is it, under such circumstances, possible to restore the elasticity of the air-cells? From our stand-point this question, which a fanatical homœopath from the stand-point of his dogmatic faith, not from that of practical observation, may rashly answer in the affirmative, has to meet with a decidedly negative answer. Even if we admit that slight degrees of emphysema can be compelled to retrograde, by what method of investigation, what objective or subjective symptom will we be enabled to diagnose a trifling emphysema, and to demonstrate the fact that the improvement we had aimed at, has been achieved? After an emphysema has become evident to the senses it must have acquired an extent of development which renders a retrograde metamorphosis an impossibility. In our opinion a radical cure of emphysema of the lungs cannot be thought of, nor can any direct treatment be instituted; in other words, we declare this disorganization an incurable malady.

In saying this, we do not mean to assert that every treatment of emphysema is futile and useless; on the contrary, a physician can benefit his patients very essentially in two different directions. In the first place, a certain prophylactic treatment can be instituted, which of course cannot aim at preventing the disease altogether, but staying its further spread. Let every intense chronic bronchial catarrh be treated with the utmost care, especially in the case of old people and individuals disposed to shortness of breath, and let every contrivance or circumstance that might interfere with the respiratory functions, be avoided, more particularly tight clothes, continued stooping, violent bodily exertions. At the same time let the patients guard as much as possible against catarrh of the respiratory organs. That this cannot be accomplished in the most efficient manner by confinement in the room, by warm clothing, or in general by excessive care, has been shown by us in a previous paragraph. Suitable clothing does not mean very warm clothing; on the contrary, this is least appropriate. Strict attention to temperature, wind, rain or dryness of the atmosphere should be paid by every emphysematous individual; no one ought to dress more in accordance with changes in the temperature and weather than persons suffering from emphysema. Wearing flannel next to the skin, is undoubtedly beneficial, for the reason that extreme respiratory efforts easily excite a profuse transpiration even during a slight bodily exercise such as walking. Wearing flannel is indispensable, if the weather where the patient resides is habitually damp and cold. Much smoking is decidedly prejudicial, although we do not mean to assert that tobacco causes emphysema. The circumstance that the blood of such patients does not receive a sufficient quantity of oxygen, suggests the propriety of advising them to avoid localities where the air is vitiated by crowds.

Secondly we are obligated to try to meet the affections which inevitably accompany emphysema. At the list of these affections we place catarrh of the bronchial mucous membrane. Be it the primary catarrh as an exciting cause, or only a secondary affection, we should by all means endeavor to moderate or remove it, using for this purpose the remedies that have been recommended for acute and chronic bronchial catarrh. Some among these remedies are more valuable because the catarrhal symptoms in their pathogenesis, with which emphysematous individuals are most usually afflicted, have been confirmed by abundant practical applications. For the chronic form of catarrh we select: *Carbo vegetabilis, Arsenicum, Tartarus stibiatus, Baryta carbonica, Silicea, Ipecacuanha, Lycopodium.* The three first named again deserve the preference; any one who uses them in suitable cases, must be amazed at the improvement they achieve with so much promptitude. For particulars we refer the reader to the previous chapter, giving the following hints for these three remedies: *Tartarus stibiatus*, if there is a copious secretion of mucus which can only be raised with difficulty and then only scantily; *Carbo vegetabilis*, if a quantity of mucus is secreted and expectorated; *Arsenicum*, if the secretion of mucus is but scanty. In addition to these remedies we recommend *Causticum* and *Digitalis;* the former, if the action of the diaphragm is feeble, and the latter, if there are organic changes of the heart. These remedies will never achieve very striking nor very rapid results, on which account the frequent change of remedies should be condemned as an improper proceeding; such a proceeding simply tends to retard a favorable change still more. *Sulphur* has never effected in our hands any perceptible improvement.

Acute attacks of catarrh during the course of emphysema rank among the most severe affections, although more in appearance than as really dangerous to life. The main remedies for such an attack are: *Bryonia*, *Mercurius*, *Arsenicum*, *Phosphorus*, *Tartarus stibiatus*, also *Cannabis;* the last named acts only as a palliative. Bryonia and Mercurius are best suited when the febrile and general constitutional phenomena are most marked; the other three remedies, if the local symptoms are most prominent.

While attending to the thoracic organs, the condition of the abdominal viscera likewise claims our attention. It will scarcely ever be possible to do anything for the passive, almost mechanical hyperæmia of the liver. An intestinal catarrh with constipation of the bowels and flatulence is exceedingly distressing on account of the increased dyspnœa it occations. *Lycopodium* is indispensable for this condition of things; *Cocculus* is much less frequently applicable, but from *Nux vomica* which seems to be so frequently indicated, we have never derived the least benefit. As a matter of course, such a morbid condition of the digestive organs demands the most minute dietetic precautions which are unfortunately but too often neglected by the patients. Farinaceous food or flatulent vegetables should not be used in any considerable quantity, whereas nourishing food with a little wine is very much to be commended. By adhering to a proper diet patients can save themselves many distressing hours, for nothing increases their dyspnœa more than an interference with the movements of the diaphragm.

As regards the most important affection which accompanies

emphysema, we mean a change in the functions as well as the shape of the heart, our remedies are either powerless, or else their influence is, indeed, trifling. The exciting cause being permanent, the abnormal results, of course, cannot be removed. *Digitalis* is best calculated to palliate the distress, whereas *Arsenic*, *Lycopodium* and other remedies almost always leave us in the lurch. In one case *Natrum muriat.* relieved the truly frightful cardiac distress.

In conclusion we will make mention of an agent that exerts a decided influence over emphysema, we mean the pressure of the atmosphere. More recently we have become enabled to increase or diminish this pressure ad libitum to suit the condition of our patients; both the decrease as well as the increase of this pressure exert a wonderful effect upon emphysematous individuals. A diminished pressure of the atmosphere is procured by causing our patients to reside on high mountains. By this change the affection is improved in an uncommon degree, almost without an exception and in a very short time, the catarrh becomes less and the patient very soon gains in flesh. Any one who has resided on high mountains, must have experienced the great ease with which the act of respiration is performed, and what a pleasantly stimulating effect mountain-forests have upon the organism. Not only must the greater ease in breathing feel very pleasant to the patient, but the quality of the inhaled air must likewise afford a pleasant stimulation to his weary frame. Be this as it may, the best thing emphysematous individuals can do for themselves in the summer, is to live on high mountains.

How it happens that an increase of atmospheric pressure likewise exerts a beneficent effect upon emphysematous individuals, we are unable to decide, nor do we deem it essential to entangle ourselves in hypothetical speculations on this subject. That this effect is produced, is not only corroborated by experience, but likewise by the apparatuses contrived for the inhalation of compressed air. But few of such apparatuses are as yet in use, but we feel confident that in every large city an apparatus of this kind will sooner or later be introduced, and we deem it so much more our duty to direct the attention of our Colleagues to artificial contrivances of this kind, as our Materia Medica is utterly destitute of remedial agents for this disease, and the most we can do is to palliate the patient's distress. More detailed information concerning this subject may be found in the Essays of Dr. Vivenot, Jr., in Vienna, who has published several of them. The essential effect of inhaling compressed air for several hours is a decreased frequency of the number of respirations and the pulse. The relief obtained by emphysematous individuals must be owing to the circumstance that the inspirations become fuller and more oxygen is supplied to the lungs. We trust that all who have an opportunity of testing this method, or otherwise observing its effects, will take the trouble of directing their attention to it.

9. Pneumonia.
Inflammation of the Lungs.

By pneumonia we understand the effusion of a fibrinous exudation on the free surface of the pulmonary cells. This form of pneumonia is termed croupous in opposition to the interstitial and catarrhal form, the first-named of which, however, is the only one that is, strictly speaking, entitled to be classed among inflammations of the lungs.

On account of its frequency and the importance of the affected organ, pneumonia is one of the most important diseases. To the homœopath it becomes so much more important on account of circumstances which we shall endeavor to explain at the commencement of the paragraphs devoted to the therapeutics of pneumonia, although this proceeding may render us liable to the charge of inconsistency in not avoiding, according to promise, every species of polemics. But in the present instance the dispute about the first rank must be settled and is, therefore, unavoidable.

Etiology. An affection like pneumonia, which has at all times and more especially during the last decades, since the introduction of a physical exploration of the chest and the development of pathological anatomy, commanded the fullest attention and the most careful investigation on the part of all physicians, must necessarily have led to the most diversified views concerning its origin. To avoid prolixity we shall only mention the most important etiological causes. The two principal kinds of pneumonia are the primary and the secondary form.

Primary pneumonia may occur at any age, but attacks more especially individuals between the ages of twenty and forty years, very rarely children in the first years of infancy. No constitution is exempt from the liability to an attack; if a robust and plethoric constitution is generally regarded as more susceptible, it is, most probably, because robust men are more frequently exposed to the exciting causes of pneumonia. This circumstance is most likely the reason why men are so much more frequently attacked than women; the occupations pursued by men expose them more fully and more frequently than women to the deleterious influences productive of pneumonia. Infants at the breast, and children who have not yet passed through the first period of dentition, are seldom attacked with croupous pneumonia. The nature of the country does not seem to exert any palpable influence; for pneumonias occur in a level country as well as on mountains, in sunny districts as well as in exposed places. The seasons, on the contrary, exert a decided influence. Our statistical tables show to a demonstration that the transition from cold to warm seasons is the most fruitful source of pneumonia; the transition from warm to cold seasons is less productive of this disease, winter still less and summer least of any. That there must be other causes at work than the mere temperature, is self-evident. The great changes of temperature in April and May being at the same time attended with the most marked changes in the electric conditions of the atmosphere, it is concluded not without reason that these conclusions are correct, and that electricity exerts a powerful influence as one of the exciting causes of pneumonia. The influence of electricity likewise accounts in the most natural manner for the frequent occurrence of epidemic pneumonia which, though not always very extensive, yet is often very intense, and which, owing to the peculiar course it takes, has often very characteristic features. We doubt very much whether a mere cold is such a frequent cause of pneumonia; it unfortunately is very convenient to attribute pneumonia to it. In the absence of other constitutional predispositions it is only a very violent cold that is capable of causing pneumonia; even in such a case we would not regard the cold as a cause of the disease, unless it had taken place no later than eighteen hours before the commencement of the disease. Mechanical injuries, more especially a violent blow or kick, may likewise give rise to pneumonia; noxious agents acting directly upon the lungs, such as irritating gases, excessive cold or heat, may likewise excite the disease. A real predisposition to pneumonia will very seldom be met with; but it cannot be denied that the treatment of pneumonia with debilitating drugs, more especially by sanguineous depletions, always leaves an increased disposition to similar attacks. In the case of tuberculous patients a disposition cannot well be shown, they are more easily attacked with bronchitis. It likewise seems an established fact that individuals with a preëminently arterial habit are more liable than others, and that, for instance, emphysematous individuals with venous constitutions are not often attacked with pneumonia.

Secondary pneumonia is frequently an exclusively consecutive affection, originating in the spread of inflammatory affections to the lungs. It is particularly met with among children, much less frequently among adults, and occurs as a complication of all possible acute diseases, particularly exanthems. Pyæmia is one of the most frequent causes of secondary pneumonia. In chronic affections it is always a very dubious undertaking to show their connection with intercurrent pneumonia.

Pathologico-anatomical Changes. We give a description of these changes, because they facilitate a comprehension of the apparent symptoms.

For the sake of facilitating a methodical arrangement of the pathological changes, the pathological process has been divided into three different stages which, however, are not so rigidly distinguished from each other in reality, and often run a parallel course.

The first stage is that of bloody infiltration. On opening the thorax the affected part of the lungs does not collapse; the pleura covering this part is usually opaque, the elasticity at this part is more or less completely lost, and the color is sometimes much darker. On cutting into the lungs, only a feeble or no crepitation is heard. The cut surface is of a strikingly dark redness, usually in sharp contrast with the sound portion; on pressing upon it a dark-red or brownish, viscid, tenacious fluid is squeezed out. The tissue is dense. The weight of the affected portion is much more considerable than its normal weight, and in water this portion immediately sinks to the bottom of the vessel.

The second stage comprehends the period when the process of exudation is completed, and is generally designated as the stage of red hepatization. The affected portion feels dense and hard; the pleura over it has almost always lost its lustre and is thinly covered with exudation. It exhibits all the signs of the first stage pointing to a deficiency of air. The cut surface has the same color as in the first stage, or more usually it has the color of rust. When the light impinges upon it, the cut surface shows distinct granulations which are still more apparent on the surface adjoining the thorax and are caused by the firm exudation-plugs in the pulmonary cells. In spite of its density, the pulmonary tissue is much more easily torn.

The transition into the third stage does not, properly speaking, constitute part of the normal course, for by the normal course the resorption and exudation of the infiltration proceeds from the second stage. This third stage is designated as the stage of gray hepatization and purulent infiltration. The cut surface now has a gray color with a yellowish tinge, mingled with red or brown spots which often impart to it a mottled appearance. The granular appearance has disappeared or still exists very feebly. The tissue is quite friable. On pressure a turbid liquid is discharged from it consisting in most part of pus corpuscles. Gray hepatization of course arises from the red; the hæmatin is more and more decomposed or reabsorbed, on which account all transitions of color are commonly noticed, from a dark brown-red to a yellowish, rusty or gray color, and if the purulent transformation is perfect, to a straw-color.

The third stage may still be succeeded by the formation of abscesses, gangrene of the lungs, thickening of the exudation; we shall speak of this more fully hereafter, as well as of the less frequently occurring deviations from the general anatomical changes.

As regards the extent of the pathological process, in croupous pneumonia a whole lobe or at least a large portion of a lobe is commonly attacked; less frequently a lobe is attacked on both sides, still less frequently all the lobes together. If only one side is affected, it is most commonly the right lungs, less frequently the left. If only isolated, detached lobules are infiltrated in consequence of the pneumonic process, the inflammation is not usually a simple croupous pneumonia, but almost always of a secondary character.

Symptoms and Course. As yet we are not acquainted with any disease which, in the absence of any particular complications, runs its course in such fixed and stable forms as pneumonia and adheres as fixedly as this disease to definite critical days. In the chapter on the therapeutics of pneumonia we shall show how far the formerly customary treatment of this disease has been influenced by the discovery of a fixed typical course.

Pneumonia begins almost without an exception with a chill which is usually very severe and is in many respects of great importance. It is from this chill that we date the commencement of the disease and by it we determine the critical days. Moreover this chill which is sometimes of very long duration and is immediately succeeded by, but never alternates with fever, is in no other disease of such a peculiar nature, so that it may almost be considered pathognomonic, more especially if we consider that as soon as the chill sets in, the muscular strength vanishes so that the patient finds it almost impossible to stand erect. We will now first describe the course of pneumonia in the case of a robust and sound individual, and will append to it the description of various deviations.

As soon as the chill which almost always lasts several hours and scarcely ever only a few minutes, is over, a violent, dry fever-heat sets in, and the pulse becomes more or less accelerated, fuller and more tense, but very seldom exceeds the number of 100 beats. The temperature is always raised a few degrees. The face which during the chill has an almost cadaverous appearance, now becomes flushed, sometimes only on one side; the cheeks are bright-red, the eyes injected, and very commonly some headache is felt, and the patient generally feels thirsty, but is very seldom disposed to vomit. The appetite is at once gone, and owing to the intense fever, all the secretions are suspended. The patient feels more exhausted than he really is. This condition which is as yet free from all local symptoms, may last longer than twenty-four hours, but in such a case the local symptoms appear at an earlier period; in rare cases they precede the chill. The patient complains of unceasing stitching pains which he generally points out with tolerable accuracy as existing at the affected spot, very seldom far removed from it; they are aggravated by every unusual exertion of the respiratory organs, especially by coughing, and they sometimes increase to a high degree of intensity. The pain usually sets in associated with a short and at first dry cough, the respiratory movements are much less full and more frequent in number. The breathing is not only painful and accelerated on this account, but the violent fever likewise occasions an increased desire for breath which cannot be gratified and causes great restlessness and anxiety and a marked activity of all the other respiratory muscles which are not usually very seriously taxed in performing the respiratory movements. These exertions are generally so striking that pneumonia can be recognized from this very fact, more especially from the flapping of the alæ nosi during an inspiration. Vocalization is of course altered, feebler and shorter, and frequently interrupted.

Soon after the cough has begun to set in, the patient begins to expectorate; this expectoration is important as a diagnostic sign. It is scanty, very tenacious, and usually intimately mixed with blood from the commencement, which imparts to it the color of rust, or brick-dust; this color is scarcely ever absent in the case of young, robust individuals. At this stage the physical symptoms have so far advanced that they render the diagnosis perfectly certain. During the first days the fever gradually increases, showing but slight morning-remissions. Considering the high degree of temperature, the pulse is not so very frequent, scarcely ever exceeding 120 beats; however, in proportion as the parenchyma becomes more infiltrated, the fulness of the pulse decreases considerably.

The end of the inflammatory infiltration generally designates the period when a change takes place in the symptoms. The infiltration is seldom completed on the third day, sometimes not till the seventh, even still later. After this, the pains almost always cease, the breathing becomes more tranquil, the fever is apparently less, the pulse remains unchanged, the constitutional symptoms do not mend very perceptibly. The local as well as the general symptoms may remain unchanged in intensity, until a change takes place in the disease. Such a change seldom takes place before the fifth day, and, according to Traube, sets in on the odd days, which is denied by others. This critical change is very often preceded by the breaking out of herpes labialis which almost always authorizes the expectation of a favorable turn. Previous to the critical change, the intensity of the symptoms either rises to a great height by a gradual increase, or else it is often the case that after two to four quiet days a violent fever again rages for twelve to eighteen hours, after which the disease decreases very suddenly. This reappearance of the fever is most easily accounted for by the exudation of serum which is required for the reabsorption of the exuded fibrin. In uncomplicated cases the disease decreases with an uncommon suddenness and rapidity, sometimes in a few hours, and it is difficult to understand how the dyspnœa can decrease so rapidly since, as a rule, a copious expectoration does not occur and is sometimes entirely wanting. This shows that the exudation of serum which is alone capable of removing the exuded fibrin by a process of reabsorption, is chiefly concerned in disembarrassing the respiratory functions by the removal of this exuded material. In simple pneumonia, without abnormal deviations from a regular course, the so-called sputa cocta are only met with in small quantity and not by any means as a general rule. Convalescence takes place so rapidly that on the fourteenth day every trace of the disease has generally disappeared. As we shall see presently, the mode of treatment exerts a great influence in this respect.

In order to establish the diagnosis of pneumonia with perfect certainty in all dubious cases, it is absolutely necessary to resort to a physical exploration of the respiratory organs. We discuss this subject separately from the other symptoms of the disease, in order to afford a clearer and more connected view of the whole.

Pneumonia does not alter the shape of the thorax, or so little that no stress need be laid upon this symptom; nor are the intercostal spaces altered any more than the general capacity of the thorax. Very commonly, however, a more distinct vibration of the thoracic wall, corresponding to the diseased portion of the lungs, is perceived when the patient is talking. The most important positive signs are yielded by percussion which informs us with tolerable certainty whether a larger portion of the lungs is infiltrated or not. We speak, of course, of croupous pneumonia, for it is this alone that causes the infiltration of a considerable portion of the lungs, most commonly of a whole lobe. In the incipient stage of pneumonia, the sound either remains unchanged, or is only changed very slightly; hence, immediately after the occurrence of the chill, no changes can be discovered. But in proportion as the hyperæmia increases, the percussion-sound becomes more tympanitic, sometimes to such an extent that one might be led to believe, a piece of intestine had been struck. Hence, the tympanitic sound is really characteristic in pneumonia, and is only less marked, if the thoracic walls are very thick, or if the diseased portion of the lungs is separated from the thoracic wall by a normal layer of pulmonary parenchyma. In croupous pneumonia, this is very seldom the case. The more complete the infiltration, the more completely the air escapes from the lungs, and the more empty the sound becomes unless a layer, from which the air has not yet escaped, lies over the diseased portion of lungs On the sides of this normal layer, the dulness often first changes to the tympanitic and further on to the normal sound, the tympanitic sound is sometimes heard even in the non-affected portion of the lungs, most likely owing to the accompanying hyperæmia. A change in the infiltration is revealed by percussion if resolution takes place, in which case the tympanitic sound most commonly returns for a short time and soon after gives way to the full sound. The results of auscultation are equally valuable as diagnostic signs. At the commencement of pneumonia, the normal respiratory murmur is very often quite feeble, much less frequently increased. As soon as infiltration begins to set in, and the air is still able to circulate in the inflamed portion of the lungs, we perceive, especially during an expiration, the crepitation that is so rarely absent that it can almost be regarded as characteristic in pneumonia. It is less audible, if a co-existing bronchial catarrh hides it by râles. With the completion of the exudation, when the percussion-sound becomes empty, every murmur caused by the circulation of the air in the air-cells, necessarily ceases, and a bronchial respiration takes place, associated in the non-affected portions of the lungs with a more or less increased vesicular respiration corresponding perhaps with the necessary increase of the respiratory efforts in these portions. In the same manner as the air in the bronchia, when reaching the ear through the pulmonary parenchyma, sounds more loudly, so does the sound of the voice give rise to intense bronchophony and pectoriloquy, while the voice greatly increases the vibrations of the thorax. The resolution of pneumonia is indicated by râles. In the cells they are necessarily very fine, and on this account are sometimes described as crepitation, and sometimes are veiled by co-existing coarse râles in the bronchia. They often continue for a long time.

This most simple course of pneumonia is often modified by various trifling deviations which are of importance to a homœopathic physician and the more frequent of which we will now proceed to point out.

In the case of children, the invasion of the disease is often marked by convulsions, such as may occur in other acute affections; in the case of adults, spasmodic symptoms are seldom witnessed. A very severe intestinal catarrh sometimes constitutes the stage of invasion. In such a case the vomiting only lasts until the infiltration is completed, whereas the diarrhœa often continues throughout the whole course of the disease. In the case of children, as well as of old people, very seldom in the case of adults, pneumonia throughout its whole course is sometimes accompanied by such prominent cerebral symptoms that a physical exploration alone is capable of establishing the diagnosis upon a perfectly reliable basis; for even the cough in such cases is often wanting. These cerebral derangements are said to accompany the inflammation of an upper lobe much more frequently than those of a lower lobe. The patients sometimes remain unconscious during the whole course of the disease, which need not run a prolonged course on this account. Cerebral derangements of a lighter grade, a light delirium, mostly of a merry nature, sleeplessness or sopor, are very common occurrences. These happen most frequently in the case of drunkards. The tongue does not exhibit any regularly-occurring changes; at times it is quite clean, sometimes very much coated, at times humid, at other times quite dry. The last-mentioned appearance is not very promising; it is especially ominous if the balance of the symptoms impart to the affection a dubious character. The appearance of a slight icterus after the completion of the infiltration is very common, nor is it of any particular importance; but if icterus sets in together with symptoms of gastro-intestinal catarrh, it always indicates an unwelcome complication which threatens to delay the course of the disease. As a rule the skin remains pretty dry during the whole course of the disease; profuse or exhausting sweats occur much less frequently.

The symptoms specially appertaining to the lungs, vary considerably. The cough which is usually not very violent and occurs in single short turns, may assume a spasmodic character when, on account of the increase of pain, it becomes a source of great distress to the patient. It rarely is entirely wanting, or is quite dry. It is particularly old people who sometimes do not cough at all. The frequency of the respirations is sometimes but inconsiderably increased, and it is the insufficient depth of the inspirations that reveals the character of the disease. The pain varies more than any other symptom; in the case of old people it is generally very slight; in their case the admixture of blood in the sputa is generally missing.

In the case of young and vigorous individuals the resolution of the infiltration generally takes place very rapidly, sometimes in a single day, but it may likewise be more protracted, without on that account a transition into the stage of gray hepatization having necessarily taken place. Thus we find that the fever decreases on the ninth day and that the patient generally feels a little better; but there is no sudden decrease of all the abnormal phenomena, no immediate, but a scarcely perceptible, dragging commencement of convalescence. We seldom notice this condition of things in the case of robust men; it occurs quite easily among weakly persons and after an exhausting method of treatment. Sometimes, after convalescence has begun, an exacerbation with progressing infiltration sets in, in which case the fever is very apt to assume an asthenic character and the appearance of typhus, yet the course of the disease need not necessarily be very much protracted or unfavorable. But almost without an exception, important complications exist in such cases; such a form of pneumonia is very seldom the result of epidemic influences, but most generally of an exhausting treatment. Among the complications we notice more particularly pleuritis, bronchitis, peri- and endocarditis, all of which, without an exception, exert a disturbing influence over pneumonia.

Experience has shown that the seat of pneumonia is of great importance as regards the probability of a normal termination. As a rule pneumonia of the right side is much more favorable than that of the left, pneumonia of a lower lobe lighter than that of an upper one, which is apt not to terminate in resolution and to assume a tubercular form. Inflammations of the left upper lobe are especially obstinate and deviating from the normal course; they occur the least frequently.

The deviations of the infiltration are very essential, since the deviations in the course of the disease are mostly founded upon the former. One of the most common deviations is the tardy resolution of the infiltration. It occurs rarely in uncomplicated forms of pneumonia, but is a very common event if carditis supervenes during pneumonia. In such cases the deficient energy of the circulation seems to constitute the sole obstacle, for a purulent metamorphosis is not necessary to lead to such a result. We shall refer to this afterwards in treating of chronic pneumonia. No resolution of the infiltration need take place even for years; in one case, that of an apparently healthy man we discovered after a number of years over one or two pulmonary lobes, especially at their posterior border, marked bronchial respiration and a perfectly empty percussion-sound. Or else the infiltration may remain in some portions of the lungs, disappearing entirely everywhere else, and the patient may enjoy perfect health. If the infiltration remains, but changes to a tubercular deposition, the phenomena of the disease change entirely. We not only meet with this change in individuals who had been previously affected with tubercles, but likewise in individuals of whom we positively know that up to the time when they were attacked with pneumonia, they had enjoyed perfect health. On the critical days the fever indeed decreases, but some of it remains, and the patients are not able to recover their strength, or only slowly and imperfectly. There remain a dry and hacking cough and an imperfect fulness of the respiration, and sooner or later the symptoms of tubercular phthisis supervene, which in such a case usually runs a very rapid course. We should not, however, in every case of tardy reabsorption, infer a tubercular metamorphosis and express a prognosis corresponding with such a change. It often takes months before such a metamorphosis can be diagnosed with perfect certainty.

The most important, most frequent and at the same time most dangerous change of the infiltration is the transition into the stage of gray hepatization or purulent metamorphosis. It must always be apprehended if pneumonia continues beyond the ninth day with considerable febrile motions, and, unless we examine the symptoms very accurately, a progression of the pneumonia alone may deceive us for a short time. Upon the accession of this purulent metamorphosis the fever always assumes a marked adynamic character, and the process henceforward bears a striking resemblance to typhus. The fever increases very considerably, the number of pulsations frequently exceeds that of 120 beats which is the normal number for adults in a case of pneumonia, and at the same time becomes small and feeble. Not unfrequently the burning heat is mingled with short chills. The tongue which, even in a violent case of pneumonia, seldom becomes dry previous to the stage of purulent metamorphosis, resembles the tongue in typhus, and the supervention of delirium makes the resemblance to typhus still more striking, so that on first seeing the patient an error in diagnosis is quite easy, especially if diarrhœa is present. It is only the physical exploration of the chest, together with the previous history of the disease that affords certainty in such a case. Percussion does not yield exclusively an empty, but likewise a tympanitic sound. Auscultation reveals beside bronchial respiration, more or less extensive, consonant râles. The air passes through a fluid, but the general condition of the patient shows that no process of reabsorption is going on; this is likewise evidenced by the expectoration which is at times pure pus, at other times mixed with blood and has often a very offensive odor. If the pathological process takes this turn, life is always in great danger. Recovery always takes place very slowly, with frequent variations between worse and better days, and is frequently protracted for months. Death sometimes takes place already in the second week and at other times at a much later period. It sometimes sets in quite suddenly, while œdema of the lungs is supervening, and sometimes slowly in consequence of general exhaustion associated with the formation of abscess or gangrene, neither of which, however, can be diagnosed with reliable certainty during the lifetime of the patient; for foul sputa are no sure indication of gangrene, and an abscess cannot be recognized with positive certainty until it begins to discharge and the patient raises a quantity of purulent matter.

Another, not less important, but much less frequent form of the exudation-metamorphosis is *chronic pneumonia*. That a chronic, non-tubercular process of infiltration can take place in the lungs, cannot well be doubted; but it is a rare occurrence, and a reliable diagnosis cannot often be established in such cases. Hence, in this place, we simply speak of chronic pneumonia resulting from an acute attack. It exhibits essentially all the so-called metamorphoses of pneumonic infiltration, except in a less acute form, and, on this account, with less immediate danger to the preservation of the organism. Either we notice a simple infiltration at some particular spot, which had remained after an acute attack and which either does not affect the organism or else keeps it in a long-lasting state of debility, with disposition to a renewal of an attack of acute infiltration. Most likely it is owing to these remnants of non-absorbed exudation, that individuals who have had one attack of pneumonia, are so often liable to being attacked a second time. Or else only part of the infiltration remains consolidated; in one or several portions of the lungs we hear bronchial respiration; at the same time another portion of the infiltration undergoes the process of resolution, and cough with purulent expectoration sets in, in consequence of which the general organism necessarily suffers. Although fever is not always present, yet it is rarely ever absent, in which case it has more or less the character of hectic fever; hence the patient has a sick, yellow-gray appearance, and very speedily shows signs of considerable emaciation. If the exudation dissolves, and the pulmonary parenchyma is involved in this process of disorganization, an abscess forms distinguished from the above-mentioned abscess by nothing but the slowness of its course, for years sometimes pass away before the abscess finds an outlet through the bronchia. Several abscesses may form, but such a thing is not often the case. Where several abscesses form, the tendency to gangrene and ichorous dissolution is very commonly present. But the organism need not necessarily show severe signs of sympathetic suffering either from the presence of an abscess or that of gangrene. The patients look like tuberculous individuals in whose case the pathological process makes slow progress. They are not robust, but without fever, and emaciate very slowly. At various intervals which sometimes last for months, some fever generally sets in, the patients are attacked by great prostration, they have to lie down, and after this condition which is most easily brought about by a slight catarrh, has lasted for a short time, they suddenly discharge after coughing and gagging an enormous quantity of foul, badly-colored pus succeeded for a few days by a moderate expectoration that has likewise a very foul odor. At the same time the exhaustion continues to increase until the pus has been completely evacuated, after which the strength returns very rapidly, but not to the same degree as before the breaking of the abscess. A cure is possible, if the suppurating portion of the lungs is not too large and the strength is not too much reduced. Death either takes place in consequence of hectic fever or of the supervention of some acute process. Finally we must mention a termination of pneumonia which is of rare occurrence and exceedingly troublesome, we mean the evacuation of the pus through the walls of the thorax. This has occurred twice in our practice. The patients were young men, and the right lower lobe was inflamed. Although the profuse suppuration at first occasioned great exhaustion, yet both were completely restored.

Having said all we intended concerning croupous pneumonia, we will now add a few remarks concerning interstitial and catarrhal pneumonia.

Catarrhal pneumonia is scarcely ever a primary disease, but generally arises in consequence of the inflammatory process spreading from the bronchia to the pulmonary cells. It is almost without an exception confined to single lobules, and on this account the name of lobular pneumonia has been given to it. There may be many such scattered centres of inflammation, without the percussion-sound being altered in consequence; nor do they occasion bronchial respiration, so that it is scarcely possible to diagnose them with positive certainty. All we know is that capillary bronchitis is very apt to superinduce lobular pneumonia. Like capillary bronchitis, this form of pneumonia is preëminently a disease of infancy, and it has to be treated in the same manner as the worst kinds of bronchitis. Interstitial pneumonia is of no particular importance to us, because it does not require any special treatment; on the other hand it is of importance with respect to prognosis and as regards the diagnosis of other affections to which it resembles. It is always a secondary complication. The process is quite like the process in cirrhosis of the liver, on which account it has been termed cirrhosis of the lungs. An exudation takes place into the connective tissue of the lungs; this exudation first changes to connective tissue and afterwards to cicatrizing, shrivelling firm tissue, by which the air-cells become compressed, and a condition arises which is designated as induration of the lungs. Since this process may likewise set in as a consequence of croupous pneumonia, interstitial pneumonia is likewise a special form of the so-called chronic pneumonia. Its most important result is atrophy of the pulmonary tissue with caving in of the thorax and the development of sacculated bronchiectasia in consequence of which chronic bronchial catarrh assumes such a peculiar form.

Inasmuch as in pneumonia the prognosis depends more evidently than in any other disease upon the treatment that happens to be pursued, we have assigned to it a place in the section on the therapeutics of pneumonia.

Treatment. We have already stated at the commencement of this chapter that the treatment of pneumonia is well calculated to show the advantages of Homœopathy over other methods; hence it behooves us to devote some attention to the modes of treatment adopted by other Schools.

In the first place we have to consider the expectant method which Homœopathy has in truth created; for it is the success of homœopathic treatment which could not well be denied, although homœopathic doses were supposed to be equivalent to nothing, that emboldened the partisans of active treatment to try the treatment of diseases without any violent interference. We confess to our inability to comprehend a purely expectant treatment of pneumonia, for no conscientious physician will stand by quietly in a case of pneumonia, and allow the disease to run its course from beginning to end without doing something for his patient. This may do in cases of simple pneumonia, if the patients are otherwise endowed with sound health, and the disease runs a perfectly normal course; but what is to be done in regard to the more or less threatening deviations from the normal course? Will the physician remain idle? We do not believe it. But if we take the expectant method in a less rigorous sense of the term; if we allow the use of some mild adjuvants, the statistical tables of this method become at once vitiated. We admit, however, that this method of treatment leads to much more favorable results than the usual treatment with sanguineous depletions and a mass of powerful remedial agents.

The medicinal treatment of pneumonia is effected by means of a legion of remedies, which every physician admits are not so much given for the pneumonia, but for the inflammatory fever, or for single symptoms. The only remedy which years ago was used as a specific for pneumonia, is Tartar emetic. The use of this remedy as a specific has, however, been abandoned, for the reason that it was found impossible to determine the kind of pneumonia to which it was specifically adapted instead of using it indiscriminately for all kinds. Every homœopath is able to explain how it happened that Tartar emetic effected a cure in some cases of pneumonia, and proved a specific remedy even in whole epidemics, and yet left the physician in the lurch in so many other cases. The use of this drug in large doses has only yielded unfavorable results in respect to the whole duration of the disease. The other medicines in vogue are almost exclusively given for single symptoms of the whole group. Such medicines are mostly used as are supposed to have a depressing influence over the fever, such as Digitalis, Quinine, Veratrine, etc. We do not mean to say one word against these remedies, for we are well aware that under certain circumstances each one of them has its value as a remedy for pneumonia. But we cannot help giving utterance in a few words to our doubts regarding the propriety of prescribing these remedies for the fever in pneumonia. Fever in any disease is the manifestation of a reaction on the part of the general organism against a disturbance set up in its interior. Hence, fever is no disease of itself, although it is a necessary attribute of many diseases. At all events, pneumonia remains what it is, even if no fever should supervene. Hence, even if it were possible to combat the fever, in combating this fever we would not combat the disease. We even go so far as to maintain that, if the fever could be removed without the disease being acted upon at the same time, the treatment is sometimes without effect, and is usually hurtful and never of any use. For after the organic reaction has been depressed or even suspended, the morbid disturbance is either prolonged or does not disappear at all. In suppressing the fever, the natural curative agent would likewise become inoperative. It is different if Digitalis is given in order to diminish the impulse of the heart and depress the heart's action, and by this means to lessen the pressure in the pulmonary vessels. But in such a case Digitalis should only be given at the beginning of pulmonary hyperæmia, or might at most still be continued at the commencement of hepatization, which, however, is not done. In order to obtain a normal process of reabsorption, an undiminished action of the heart is indispensable ; its decrease may afford momentary relief to the patient, but cannot act favorably. Such an exhibition of palliatives may not always be hurtful and may not interfere with the course of the disease: it is certain, however, that this kind of treatment cannot be made the foundation for a true system of therapeutics in pneumonia.

A somewhat complete review of the common treatment of pneumonia would oblige us to exhibit the whole of the so-called antiphlogistic apparatus, from Calomel to the most harmless neutral salt. Inasmuch as the use of these drugs is based upon the same idea, they can be dispatched with the same arguments. A general antiphlogistic treatment is just as absurd as the exhibition of Quinine for the fever in pneumonia; the real disease is not met. It is not such a difficult thing to depress the organism by the copious use of cathartics and other remedies until an active reaction becomes impossible; of course, the theory has been complied with, the inflammatory fever is gone, but an adynamic fever has taken its place; and even if this is not the case, there is scarcely any doubt that the conquest of the local disease will not take place more rapidly.

At one time Chloroform-inhalations made a great noise, but seem to have been abandoned by modern practitioners. Todd's method of prescribing spirits, is nearly related to these inhalations. How happens it that Englishmen have not long ago stoned this destroyer of all faith in antiphlogistic treatment!

A proof how much pneumonia can endure without undergoing any essential modifications in its course, is cold-water treatment. Even Niemeyer is favorable to this method of treatment, but he is utterly unable to give any reasons for it; his only argument is that it helps. From a physiological stand-point we should reason in this wise: The wet bandage, frequently repeated, diminishes the amount of blood in the cutaneous vessels, hence superinduces in the interior of the organism a sort of engorgement, and at the same time acts as a stimulant, for it is followed by an increase of reaction; how can such an agent be said to act as a curative in a case of pneumonia? We consider this mode of reasoning correct.

Pneumonia being attended with pain, Opium has been made use of very liberally; this is all that can be claimed in its favor.

In conclusion we have to consider the chief remedy, we mean blood-letting. It constitutes the apple of discord in modern medicine, and because homœopathic practitioners have discarded it, even in pneumonia, they have been called murderers. How much has been said and printed on the subject of pneumonia, both *pro* and *con*, more especially after a physician had dared to treat a pneumonic patient without bleeding, in spite of which he obtained wonderfully favorable results. This change in the treatment of pneumonia would have caused less astonishment if physicians had paid some attention to Homœopathy during the last fifty years. Formerly pneumonia and blood-letting were as intimately united as the arm and hand. This is very different at the present time, and since we only deal with the present, we shall content ourselves with considering the modern developments of this question. Wunderlich and Niemeyer are sufficiently authoritative to permit us to present their views as the ruling opinions of their Schools.

Niemeyer gives three indications for a course of general depletion. First: Appearance of the pneumonia in a vigorous, healthy, young man, the temperature being over 92° Fahr., and the pulse over 120 beats.—Second: Collateral hyperæmia of the uninflamed portions of the lungs.—Third: Symptoms of pressure on the brain accompanying the pneumonia. Wunderlich gives the same indications, except that he adds to number one, that the patient should be bled on the first and second, or on the fourth and fifth day, not on the third, rarely after the fifth unless hyperæmia should still exist. The effect of bleeding, according to Wunderlich, is as follows, Niemeyer not attributing to bleeding a positive influence over pneumonia, but only a general influence or an influence over particular symptoms.

In the first place, venesection is said to shorten the course of the disease and to achieve the termination in recovery more rapidly and more completely. We ask any physician who has ever watched the course of pneumonia treated with blood-letting, whether this is true. We admit that immediately after the bleeding the fever abates quite considerably; but in twenty-four hours already the fever returns even worse than before. Every homœopath knows that pneumonic patients who are treated with blood-letting, even in accordance with the above indications, seldom finish their convalescence in a few days, but remain weak for several weeks. Even if we admit that Wunderlich's favorable prognosis is sometimes realized, yet, supported by our own experience, we cannot help affirming that the favorable change more frequently disappoints than meets our expectations, and that it is very often illusory.

Secondly, venesection affords the patient a sensation of relief. This is not always the case, but it is so commonly; but we would ask whether a mere sensation of the patient is more important than the regard for the general course of the disease, and whether the physician is not perpetrating a piece of quackery if he resorts to bleeding as a means to impress the patient with his power, when he must be well aware that the effect of this remedy passes away in a few hours, and the patient feels necessarily more exhausted than before.

Thirdly, the pulse decreases in frequency after bleeding; this can be accounted for, but it is not true that the former frequency does not return. It does return, but the quality of the pulse is altered; the pulse is feebler than it was.

Fourthly, the temperature declines, but the same thing happens as with the pulse. This mania of depressing the chief febrile symptoms has been commented upon by us in our review of the remedies that are used for such a purpose; we need not repeat our criticism in this place.

Fifthly, venesection moderates the dyspnœa and thus prevents acute emphysema. That this is not the case, can be affirmed by every homœopath; acute emphysema is a very rare occurrence in pneumonia and, if it does occur, it must have been the result of improper treatment.

Sixthly, venesection, by moderating the pulse and the temperature, prevents nervous exhaustion and acute consumption. How this is to be brought about, is an enigma which physiology does not solve. Nor does Wunderlich account any more explicitly for the possibility of such a process.

A few other points seem to us too unimportant to be mentioned here in detail; we shall interpolate them in our subsequent remarks.

Against the above-enumerated statements we will add to our previous remarks the following counter-propositions.

It is rather hazardous to declare an individual to whom we are called as a physician, positively robust and healthy up to the time when we are called. Every physician must have been deceived in this respect, and deceptions of this kind, if occurring in pneumonia, cannot lead to pleasant results. There are individuals who are very thin and pale and yet enjoy the most perfect health; on the other hand, we see weak persons who apparently look stout and florid. By what exact diagnostic signs are individuals suitable for the first indication, characterized?

Again we generally notice that robust men seldom have a pulse of over 120 beats, whereas such a pulse is very commonly met with in the case of weak persons. Why should not the latter be equally favorably affected by venesection? Have they a relatively less quantity of blood? The answer is that they do not bear venesection as well as robust persons who can bear a few venesections in pneumonia without any great disadvantage, whereas weakly persons cannot bear them. Where is the boundary, and how do those fare who occupy the line and in whose case we do not know whether they belong to one class or the other?

Blood is only to be taken from robust individuals. Since bloodletting is reputed one of the most powerful remedial agents, this phrase must be intended to mean that the pneumonia of robust men is much more dangerous than that of weakly persons, or that robust individuals find it more difficult to conquer the disease by the amount of strength on hand. This mode of reasoning is certainly not logical. The reaction of a robust man must naturally be more energetic and prompt than that of a person weakened by exposure, and that the strength of a vigorous person is capable of bearing a great deal more than that of a debilitated individual. Why should the more intense fever of vigorous persons entail more danger? We are at a loss to understand the anxiety caused by the presence of febrile symptoms; we admit, however, that the quality of the pulse is an excellent index of present danger, but not the number of the beats, or at least only to some extent.

Every homœopath can testify that collateral hyperæmia in pneumonia does not very frequently occur in a threatening form. If it exists, its intensity may be diminished by venesection; but this would be followed by the bad consequences to inflammation that will soon be enumerated. In such a case the question still is, which pathological process is worse, the hyperæmia which is a transitory condition, or the pneumonia which is liable to such unfavorable terminations. If, as is often the case, hyperæmia sets in after a venesection, it is very questionable whether the venesection is not in a great measure the cause.

The phenomena of cerebral hyperæmia are, at all events, the worst indication. They may be very marked and persistent, but they do not imply the presence of danger, and still less frequently of so great a danger that it has to be met by such an energetic remedy as blood-letting.

Let no one imagine that our views on blood-letting which are so directly antagonistic to those of other physicians, are mere vague assertions. No true homœopath will ever bleed either in pneumonia or in any other disease; hence only a homœopath is able to judge what course pneumonia takes with or without bleeding.

In the case of vigorous individuals, the course of pneumonia frequently remains unaffected by mild blood-letting, but full convalescence is always retarded by it. To many vigorous individuals, and the less vigorous the more so, venesection is decidedly injurious and superinduces one or the other unpleasant consequences that will be enumerated by and by. Niemeyer accounts for the rapid sinking of strength by the anæmic condition which is occasioned by a profuse exudation associated with an increase of waste by the fever, and a diminution of the supply; it is his opinion that most patients succumb to this acute marasmus. If this be so, nobody can comprehend how a sanguineous depletion and consequent increase of the loss of animal fluids can act favorably, and every body must see that the necessity of first repairing the waste, delays the complete restoration of strength.

The apparently or momentarily favorable effects of blood-letting scarcely ever last longer than twenty-four hours, and are very frequently succeeded by the transition of the fever to the adynamic form, or by an increase of the symptoms; the French method of excessive venesections has occasioned these results.

The exudation is never arrested by venesection, much less cut short or entirely prevented, but the possibility of œdema of the lungs is considerably aggravated by it. This results from the circumstance that the inflammatory exudation and the loss of blood diminish quite considerably the plastic portions of the blood, and that hence the blood contains much more serum and becomes much more disposed to serous exudations.

The resolution of the exudation is delayed, or is incomplete, or else it takes place by purulent dissolution, or not at all. If Wunderlich lays so much stress upon a diminution of the fever, that is to say of the pulse and temperature, we admit that a decrease of the fever on the critical days implies a disappearance of the local processes. Nevertheless it is not unfrequently the case that the exudation remains in spite of the defervescence; we have abundant evidence of such a fact. In such a case the re-absorption goes on slowly and uniformly, or else by fits and starts; but the patients scarcely ever recover their health very rapidly, but they remain for a long time feeble, although without fever. This result has only occurred to us after sanguineous depletions or, which deserves particular notice, after complications with inflammatory affections of the heart. The same remark applies to cases where remnants of exudation are left behind, not including the cases of tuberculous individuals in whom it is difficult to decide whether we have remnants of exudation or tubercles before us. The setting in of gray hepatization, the purulent dissolution of the exudation may sometimes be owing to peculiar constitutional or external atmospheric circumstances; indeed pus may form as the result of any inflammation; in such cases it is not likely that blood will ever be drawn, except perhaps in a case of pneumonia that runs its course under atmospheric influences and when one of the above-mentioned indications may indeed come into play. But if we mean the primary, uncomplicated pneumonias of persons who had hitherto enjoyed a vigorous and sound constitution, no pus will ever show itself under a strictly homœopathic treatment, but not very unfrequently after a debilitating, more especially after a depleting treatment. In view of the observation that the pneumonic exudation can be re-absorbed in a few hours under favorable circumstances, and seldom requires more than a few days for such a purpose, we must suppose that every reduction of the patient's strength, more especially by sanguineous depletions, causes a decrease of the reactive energy, consequently a diminution of the reactive exudation required for the business of re-absorption, and hence again a misdirection of the organic activity in the removal of the exuded fibrin. A proof for the assertions here made is furnished by the pneumonias that are associated with severe intestinal catarrh, in whose case the resolution takes place more or less abnormally. We account for this phenomenon simply by the excessive loss of animal fluids, on which account we consider the systematic use of purgatives in pneumonia as hurtful as bleeding. The tubercular metamorphosis of the exuded fibrin, if the patients were otherwise free from tubercles, has to be attributed to treatment. It is well known that tubercles and anæmia are closely related to each other, hence it is not difficult to suppose that an artificially excited anæmia may favor the formation of tubercles. All the cases known to us, where the pneumonic exudation had this termination, had all been treated with bloodletting.

These remarks show that chronic pneumonia is very commonly a consequence of debilitating treatment. We again call attention to the fact that carditis as a complication of pneumonia is apt to occasion a malignant metamorphosis of the exudation. In such a case it is not so much the perverse quality of the blood, whose influence we are, however, not disposed to deny, but the diminished energy of the circulation that exerts a disturbing effect upon the course of pneumonia. This is an additional proof how unphysiological is the theory of depressing the pulse in pneumonia.

The observation that individuals who have had one attack of pneumonia, are easily liable to a renewed attack, will scarcely ever be made by a homœopathic physician. If such frequent recurrences of pneumonia are witnessed even under homœopathic treatment, the former attacks had always been treated with depletions; we account for this susceptibility most naturally by the circumstance that the exudation had not been completely absorbed.

After this excursion into the therapeutic domain of the Old School, the length of which we beg the reader to excuse on account of the importance of the subject, we now enter upon a consideration of the prognosis of pneumonia. We might on this occasion avail ourselves of the existing statistics, if they were not calculated to mislead, and, on the side of Homœopathy, not sufficiently numerous. On this account we confine ourselves to short statements; if any one should feel disposed to doubt their correctness, we advise him, before pronouncing judgment, to first treat a few dozen cases of pneumonia homœopathically. An uncomplicated pneumonia, no matter whether the patient is robust or weakly, always terminates in recovery under homœopathic treatment, at the same time as an abnormal dispersion or alteration of the infiltration occurs very seldom. We can substantiate the correctness of this statement by upwards of two hundred and fifty cases of pneumonia from our own practice and that of other physicians. Accordingly pneumonia is one of the least dangerous diseases to a homœopathic physician. On the contrary, Wunderlich calls it one of the most frequent and most dangerous diseases that can befal man; in saying this he does not quote figures, but must have been lead by numerous deaths to make such a statement. Among the complications, carditis, intestinal catarrh, bronchitis and tuberculosis promise the least chances of a successful treatment. We have shown above why the first two complications present such ominous difficulties, although even in such cases we have never had to deplore a single loss. Bronchitis is dangerous on account of the dyspnœa being extremely aggravated by this complication; and a co-existing tuberculosis becomes dangerous on account of the probability of the metamorphosis of the exuded fibrin into tubercles, or of the hastening of the suppuration of existing tubercular depositions. Whether the seat of the inflammation exerts a peculiar influence during the presence of these complications, is not quite certain, but we may take it for granted that an inflammation of the apices, which are the most common locality of tubercular depositions, terminates in suppuration much sooner than an inflammation of any of the other lobes. It is frequently inconceivable why the pneumonic process should leave tubercles intact, whereas in other cases it leads directly to phthisis. We are almost without any data for a correct interpretation of these differences, and for this reason alone complicated pneumonias of this nature should be strictly excluded from all statistical tables. We shall have to revert to this subject when speaking of pulmonary tuberculosis. Whenever pneumonia meets with morbid conditions in the respiratory organs, its course generally deviates from the normal line, and its process is much more destructive. This remark applies principally to pulmonary emphysema, to stenosis of the larynx, to chronic heart-disease, especially of the right heart. The more these or any other affections aggravated the breathing before the supervention of pneumonia, the more dangerous they become to life on account of the existing dyspnœa. As regards constitutional conditions not of a morbid kind, old age and pregnancy are of particular significance with regard to the prognosis. Old people are often troubled with chronic catarrh and emphysema, to the presence of which the danger in pneumonia is principally to be attributed. For all that, we ought not to despair too soon; we can point to three old men between the years of seventy-eight and eighty-three, all of whom had chronic catarrh, and whom we cured of pneumonia after a somewhat protracted, but otherwise entirely favorable treatment. Pregnancy is exceedingly dangerous, the more so the more advanced it is. Whether the danger is owing to the obstructions in the respiration occasioned by the distended abdomen, or likewise to the altered composition of the blood, we are unable to decide. If a miscarriage takes place, which is not unfrequently the case, death is almost unavoidable, on account of the excessive exhaustion. Such cases likewise afford a striking picture of the effects of venesection, for it is evident what a deleterious effect the loss of blood exerts upon the parturient woman, whereas parturition ought to diminish the dyspnœa and consequently lessen the danger. In order to meet objections, we will state that we do not overlook the occurrence of two important processes going on in the organism simultaneously with pneumonia and that it is to these double functions that we attribute in a great measure the fatal termination.

Our opinion of the success of homœopathic treatment in complicated cases of pneumonia is to the effect that it is most commonly and preëminently favorable, especially when contrasted with other methods of treatment. We do not even except tubercular pneumonia. Thus we are able to assert without extravagance that pneumonia does not appear a very dangerous disease to a homœopathic physician, and that the disease may be considered comparatively devoid of danger, if we consider what an important organ the lungs are, and how intensely they are affected by an inflammation.

We pursue the same course on this occasion that we have pursued in regard to all other important pathological processes, and premise a list of the most important remedies.

Aconitum. All homœopaths admit the excellence of this remedy in pneumonia; their views only differ as regards the boundaries of its appropriate sphere of action in this disease. We cannot examine these views any further, since this would lead us too far. For particular information on this subject we refer to Müller's essay on pneumonia in the first volume of the Vierteljahrsschrift. According to Müller's arrangement, the following are the most prominent Aconite-symptoms in pneumonia: Intense fever preceded by a chill, with burning heat and dryness of the skin, quick and hard pulse and a deep, sometimes bluish redness of the face; accelerated, labored, incomplete respiration with restlessness, anxiety and palpitation of the heart; stitches in the chest during a deep inspiration and during motion, or dull pressure and weight on the chest, dry and racking cough, with a small quantity of a tenacious, slimy, blood-streaked or rusty expectoration; recumbent posture on the back; dullness and pain in the head; great thirst; scanty and red urine; evening exacerbation of the symptoms. The thorax is less movable, it is less depressed during an expiration; in other respects we have the physical signs that have been indicated for the first stage. By comparing toxicological post-mortem phenomena with these symptoms, we shall be able to determine the period up to which Aconite is suitable in pneumonia, with much more precision. Both in Müller's cases of poisoning by Aconite as well as in the cases, whether acute or chronic, which we ourselves have collected in the last ten years, the lungs were in every instance found engorged with blood, but in no case was a trace of croupous exudation to be seen. Although we do not expect that in our physiological experiments a drug that is said to be a specific remedy, will reproduce all the objective signs of the corresponding pathological series, yet the constancy with which a simple engorgement occurs as a post-mortem symptom of Aconite-poisoning, is remarkable. Experience has moreover satisfied us that this condition is the true therapeutic sphere of action for this agent. When speaking of pulmonary hyperæmia, we stated that in active pulmonary congestions Aconite is the leading remedy. In pneumonia the stage of red hepatization implies a most perfect hyperæmia; hence we consider Aconite best adapted to this stage where its specific curative virtues have been exquisitely confirmed by a multitude of the most favorable practical observations. On this account we do not, however, consider Aconite indicated in every case of pneumonia unless all the other symptoms correspond. Among these symptoms we distinguish more particularly the following: The disease attacks individuals with an active circulation; it is caused by a cold; according to many, by exposure to a dry, cold wind; it attacks robust individuals up to the age of sixty to seventy years, less frequently beyond this period where the characteristics of old age begin to creep along; there are no directly antagonizing complications, among which we number more especially an intense intestinal catarrh. Aconite alone will scarcely ever cure pneumonia, much less cut it short. On this account its importance in pneumonia should not be underrated. No one who has watched the striking effects of Aconite, will ever doubt its great virtues in this disease. Aconite diminishes the vascular excitement and reduces the pulmonary hyperæmia more brilliantly than the most copious bleeding; Moreover it diminishes the exudation to some extent and promotes in a corresponding ratio the favorable course of the disease. This favorable change which affords such great relief to the patient, sets in within twenty-four hours in almost every case. But as soon as the percussion-sound over the inflamed portion of the lungs becomes empty, as soon as the breathing becomes bronchial, Aconite in our opinion, which is shared by many, ceases to be indicated. There are, however, exceptions to this general statement. We stated in a previous paragraph that an excessive, collateral hyperæmia is one of the most common indications for venesection. This indication is specific for Aconite. If the exudation is completed; if the dyspnœa remains nevertheless considerable and out of proportion to the size of the inflamed portion of the lungs; if the sputa are thin, frothy and tinged with a bright-red blood, Aconite is decidedly appropriate and, even if it leaves the infiltration unchanged, relieves the extreme distress of breathing speedily and surely. Aconite is likewise indicated, if the pneumonia progresses by fits and starts, which is very seldom the case under homœopathic treatment. According to our previous remarks, Aconite will very often be indicated in the subsequent course of the disease, if it had been treated in the first place with the antiphlogistic apparatus of the Old School. In tubercular pneumonia Aconite has an admirable effect at the commencement of the treatment, the same as in the pneumonia of otherwise perfectly sound individuals.

Belladonna is, in our opinion, improperly commended in pneumonia. Toxicological appearances only show a more or less considerable engorgement of the lungs with dark blood. The pathogenesis of Belladonna does not point very strikingly to an inflammatory process in the pulmonary parenchyma, and, in a case of croupous pneumonia, we should find it very difficult to select Belladonna in accordance with its physiological symptoms. On the other hand certain anomalies in the symptomatic appearances of the disease point so unmistakably to Belladonna that no one who is acquainted with the pathogenesis of this drug, can hesitate to prescribe it. These anomalies refer principally to the manner in which other organs have become involved in the pathological process; it is more especially the cerebral hyperæmia that points to Belladonna. Inasmuch as Aconite may likewise be required by the same series of symptoms, we establish the following distinctions in favor of Belladonna: A dark-red, bloated and hot face, with evident turgescence of the veins; stupefying headache; drowsiness with delirium; sopor; convulsions. In such cases Belladonna is prescribed on account of the danger that threatens the brain, the pneumonia being left unnoticed for the time. Another series of cases that are frequently adapted to Belladonna, are the pneumonias arising from or accompanying acute bronchitis. In such cases Bronchitis is generally much more dangerous than pneumonia, and it is of importance that the former should be attended to with more particular care. Not unfrequently whole epidemics run a course of this kind, and they generally show typhoid symptoms from the commencement. In the case of very old people Belladonna is usually preferable to Aconite at the outset, likewise in the pneumonias of drunkards. In both kinds the symptoms have generally a typhoid character from the beginning. [During this first stage of hyperæmia, both of the lungs and brain, *Veratrum viride* is given with great success. It has been found sufficient in hundreds of cases to effect a radical cure of the disease. H.]

Bryonia alba is, like Aconite, indispensable in Pneumonia. The toxicological appearances described in the Viennese reprovings show that Bryonia is capable of occasioning exudations in the lungs. The pathogenetic symptoms do not furnish one constantly-recurring picture of the disease, but can be made available in various directions. This is evidenced by the different views entertained concerning Bryonia, all of which, however, are founded upon physiological provings. These indicate most commonly an acute pulmonary affection, with violent stitching pains, where pleuritis is manifestly indicated by a variety of secondary symptoms, on which account the remedy is very warmly recommended for pleuro-pneumonia. There are, however, numerous other symptoms which refer to the pleura much less than to the lungs; and it is upon these symptoms together with the general constitutional phenomena that the employment of Bryonia in pneumonia is founded. We find it inexpedient to enumerate the symptoms referring to the homœopathicity of Bryonia in this disease; moreover it is indispensable that such an important remedy should be known and remembered in its integrality. Nor do we deem it necessary to comment upon trivial differences of views in the use of this agent, since most of them harmonize in all the main points. Accordingly Bryonia is particularly indicated after the fever has abated and has no longer a decidedly inflammatory character, whereas the local process has reached its completion and appears to rest. This is the period when red hepatization is fully developed. The patients have passed through the excitement and constant restlessness of the first stage and are lying in a state of exhaustion but quietude; or they are in a condition when it is not quite certain whether the fever may not assume the character of adynamia. The skin now begins to show some moisture, a valuable indication for Bryonia. If Bryonia is given at this period, the inflammation generally runs a rapid and favorable course, and the remedy need not be left off until all the morbid symptoms have disappeared. However, if the resolution of the exudation is too tardy, and delays, may be, beyond the ninth day; if symptoms of a purulent dissolution make their appearance, Bryonia will be of no further use, even if the symptoms should still indicate this drug. In pneumonia running a normal course, such as we have depicted at the commencement of this chapter, we have never had occasion to use another remedy after Bryonia. As regards deviations from the normal course and from the ordinary symptoms, Bryonia is particularly adapted to cases where the tongue is covered with a thick white fur, the stomach is completely inactive and the liver is engorged and somewhat painful. But we have never obtained any good results with this drug when diarrhœa was present, which we regard as a positive counter-indication. In addition to these statements we have to direct attention to another indication, we mean pneumonia complicated with bronchitis, for which we recommended Belladonna in a previous paragraph. As we said before, pneumonias of this kind are generally epidemic, with the character of adynamia and typhoid appearances, without, on that account, taking a decidedly unfavorable turn, and are more particularly distinguished by the presence of a marked gastric catarrh. In Hanover we are just now in the midst of such an epidemic, and we become every day more and more convinced by experience what a splendid remedy Bryonia is, which has proved such an indispensable resource to the homœopathic physician in so many other epidemic diseases. If, guided by more recent observations, we have to deny in opposition to Hartmann, that dry and cold weather causes the kind of pneumonia to which Bryonia corresponds, we feel on the other hand bound to give prominence to another of his indications, namely the rheumatic and bruising pains in the muscles of the chest and back. In conclusion we wish to state, as evidence of the healing powers of this drug, that we scarcely ever notice under its administration a copious secretion of the so-called sputa cocta, and that the re-absorption of the infiltration takes place with very little, or perhaps without any expectoration, or, judging from the stand point of pathology, taking place in its most perfect form.

Mercurius is one of those remedies that is much more recommended than employed in pneumonia; we opine that this is an oversight. It is true an uncomplicated pneumonia has scarcely ever indications pointing to Mercurius; but they occur so much more frequently in complicated cases. We will not endeavor to show that Mercurius causes inflammation of the lungs in the healthy, and what special symptoms point to pneumonia. This can be learned from the Materia Medica. We are acquainted with one mercurial preparation which, in a case of poisoning, caused a fully developed pneumonia, we mean *Mercurius corrosivus*, to which we desire to call attention, thinking that a similar case may occur some time as a natural disease where this agent may prove curative. If, in addition to the existing physiological symptoms, we consider the whole manner in which Mercury affects the organism, its recommendation as a remedy for pneumonia seems perfectly justified. We cannot, however, agree with Müller, if he assigns Mercurius to the more chronic forms of pneumonia after the disease has run beyond the properly inflammatory stages. The third stage is undoubtedly adapted to Mercurius, but it is not the only one. Müller has the following more special indication for the third stage: The hepathization of a portion of lung continues and the critical sputa are entirely wanting; the cough is dry, not frequent and very rough and fatiguing, with violent irritation and urging to cough; the dyspnœa remains unaltered, the fever is rather continuous and lentescent, with profuse and exhausting sweats, the urine is scanty and dim, the color of the skin sallow, grayish; the patient is troubled with gastro-intestinal catarrh. Under these circumstances Mercurius is indicated so much more, if the disease is seated in a scrofulous, or generally dyscrasic organism. Nor can we agree with Müller when he asserts, in contrasting Mercurius and Sulphur, that the latter is indicated under similar circumstances as Mercurius, if the symptoms are more violent and tumultuous. We will afterwards account for our dissenting opinion. There are two forms of pneumonia where we consider Mercurius as a leading remedy. One is pneumonia complicated with bronchitis. Müller mentions this form; we have quoted his statements in our chapter on influenza, page 185. This form of pneumonia is almost always an epidemic disease; having at this very time had frequent opportunities in this district of testing the curative virtues of Mercurius in an affection of this kind, we cannot deem a short description of our epidemic superfluous. Under the modifying action of a widespread influenza, that is to say of catarrh accompanied by a deep irritation of the nervous system, the nose, larynx and trachea become affected with a slight catarrh which seems quite trifling for a few days; suddenly the fever becomes more violent, the catarrhal secretion ceases, dyspnœa sets in, together with a spasmodic, generally nocturnal cough, without any, or with a yellow-green, blood-streaked expectoration; the pulse is upwards of 120; in the case of a lady of upwards of fifty years, the pulse had 150 beats; it is small, has very little resistance, the skin is burning-hot, at times covered with copious perspiration, the tongue is yellow and very soon becomes dry, the sensorium is blunted, there is violent headache, the patient lies in a soporous condition, with light delirium; he has a great desire for cold drinks, after which the cough easily breaks out again. At the same time the patients do not complain of pain, and scarcely ever of pain in the affected side, on which account a careful exploration is very apt to be neglected. Such an exploration shows extensive hepatization, that is to say, complete dulness of sound with râles, and attended with bronchial respiration. This condition resembles typhus to such an extent that we do not wonder at hearing many physicians assert that influenza has changed to typhus. That this affection is of a serious character, is apparent from the fact that under allopathic treatment numerous deaths have taken place within a few weeks, and that even young and robust individuals have succumbed to the epidemic. We three homœopaths so far have not lost a single patient and, without having had any previous understanding on the subject, we have all of us commenced the treatment with *Mercurius* as the best and principal remedy. These favorable results have been obtained in an affection which, in opposition to Müller's statements, is attended with an exceedingly severe fever. The selection of Mercurius in broncho-pneumonia may be justified by its admirable action in bronchitis; for it cannot be denied that the greatest danger proceeds from this quarter and that, after the removal of the bronchial symptoms, the remaining pneumonia is comparatively insignificant. A third form of pneumonia, which is particularly adapted to Mercurius, is the catarrhal form or lobular pneumonia which has an entirely different meaning from the former. As soon as we have reason, in a case of bronchitis, whooping-cough, etc., to suspect the formation of small foci of exudation, Mercurius will first commend itself to our judgement as a remedial agent, and we shall have before our eyes an image of epidemic influenza, such as has been described in preceding paragraphs. In tubercular pneumonia we have never noticed any good effects from Mercurius. What mercurial preparation deserves a preference, we do not dare to decide. In the present epidemic we use *Mercurius solubilis;* although we do not object to the Sublimate by way of experiment, yet Hahnemann's preparation is so excellent in this disease that one hesitates to experiment with any other drug. As regards dose, we have found the third and fourth triturations the most useful; higher attenuations are of no use whatever.

Phosphorus. Fleishmann, of Vienna, the passionate advocate of Phosphorus in pneumonia, went so far as to assert that a pneumonia which cannot be cured with Phosphorus, cannot be cured homœopathically. He has been bitterly assailed for making this statement; yet we must admit that the period when Phosphorus ought to be administered in pneumonia, can easily be inferred from his arguments. We understand the case as follows. A simple croupous pneumonia in very many cases runs to a favorable termination without any medicine, and, even if not indicated, Phosphorus, when given in a very small dose, will not interfere with the normal course of the disease; but if deviations from the normal course take place, Phosphorus will most generally prove the correct remedy. We cannot, in this place, discuss the various views concerning this important remedy, and, for particulars, we refer the reader to Sorge's treatise on Phosphorus, where a full exposé of these views may be found. On the other hand, we cannot altogether share the opinions which Sorge has expressed in his brochure. Supported by at least a hundred and fifty cases of pneumonia, not one of which terminated fatally in our hands, we are bound to assign to Phosphorus a much larger sphere of action than Sorge seems willing to allow. Sorge only allows a therapeutic sphere for Phosphorus corresponding to its physiological action upon the lungs as far as this action has been determined by actual experimentation; we fancy, however, that this sort of exclusiveness will compel us to treat many cases of disease without Similia, and it is our decided opinion that practical trials, based upon suggestions derived from the Materia Medica, ought to have great and decisive weight. Among the symptoms of Phosphorus we find but few prominent kinds of pains, except vaguely localized stitches, a more or less marked embarrassment of the respiration, a bloody, muco-sanguinolent, or sanguineo-purulent, badly-colored, difficult expectoration, and a decided exacerbation of the symptoms towards evening and during the night. Adding to this the post-mortem results: Severe hyperæmia of single lobes, more or less extensive, hepatized portions of the lungs, and, according to Bibra, distinct tuberculization of the exuded fibrin, we are abundantly authorized to believe in the homœopathicity of Phosphorus in pneumonia. To these local symptoms the general symptoms of Phosphorus have to be added, these two are mostly full of meaning, but we shall have to leave their more particular examination to the reader's own judgment. Backed by the pathogenetic effects and by numerous practical, indisputable observations at the sick-bed, we recommend Phosphorus in the following more special cases:

If pneumonia sets in at the outset with the symptoms of adynamic fever and bears a close resemblance to typhus. Here *Aconite* would not even be suitable at the beginning of the treatment, *Belladonna* would do better, and *Rhus toxicodendron* still better, but even in twenty-four hours the symptoms will change so as to indicate Phosphorus, but even if the indications for Phosphorus should not be perfectly precise, let no precious time be lost with other medicines.

If pneumonia sets in as a partial manifestation of typhus, or if it has to be regarded as the exclusive localization of the typhoid process in the lungs. Pneumonias of this character leave us in doubt whether they are inflammations modified by the ruling typhoid type, or whether they are genuine typhus. We are disposed to incline to the former opinion as long as no signs of abdominal typhus are present.

If pneumonia does not set in with the characteristics of genuine typhus, but modified by the ruling epidemic. This condition is mostly met with in pneumonia setting in during epidemic influenza, and in general in all cases of epidemic pneumonia, but we have to observe at the same time that, according to our most recent observations, Phosphorus is so much less appropriate, the more fully and prominently bronchitis co-exists as a complication of the pneumonic inflammation.

If, after red hepatization is completed, on the third or fourth day of the disease, the fever increases instead of abating, the prostration becomes very great, the tongue dry, the sensorium blunted; in short, if phenomena set in, which lead us to suspect the supervention of an abnormal course of the disease.

If a purulent dissolution of the infiltration is evidently approaching; in such a case Phosphorus is, in our opinion, indicated only during the first twenty-four or forty-eight hours, and is no longer indicated if the suppuration is under full headway. Altogether, under such circumstances, Phosphorus is much less reliable than in the previously-mentioned conditions; but we have to observe that, whenever Phosphorus is employed in proper season, suppuration will scarcely ever take place.

If pneumonic infiltration supervenes during the presence of bronchitis, assuming the form of lobular pneumonia. In such a case, however, Phosphorus is not the principal remedy, at any rate, it should not be given at the outset.

If pneumonia is accompanied by marked and threatening hyperæmia, together with signs of adynamia, or if, after one lobe has become hepatized, the pneumonic process continues to spread from one portion of the lungs to the next.

If pulmonary œdema becomes apparent, as manifested by the above described symptoms. It is a very dangerous condition of things and the least significant manifestations of œdema have to be carefully watched. Phosphorus is possessed of extraordinary curative powers against œdema, and it alone is almost always sufficient to subdue this complication.

If pneumonia attacks tuberculous individuals, it is, with some exceptions, a distinguished remedy. Tuberculosis must not yet have assumed the form of phthisis, the patients must not manifest any great disposition to hemorrhage, and their strength must not yet have become too much reduced.

Among the complications, the presence of intestinal catarrh points very forcibly to Phosphorus. We stated above that this complication leads most easily and speedily to collapse, for which alone Phosphorus is such an excellent remedy. On the other hand, it is our opinion that a prominent gastric catarrh almost counter-indicates Phosphorus. The very common and sometimes threatening complication with hyperæmia of the liver and slight icterus is a decisive indication for Phosphorus.

To these indications we have to add a few considerations which are, in our estimation, additional recommendations for Phosphorus. One of them is the patient's age. Neither very young, nor very old individuals are best calculated for the favorable action of Phosphorus, nor are individuals with exhausted constitutions; robust, middle-aged persons are most susceptible to the restorative action of this agent. We should never employ Phosphorus in pneumonia running the above-described normal course; but the patient should be visited at least twice a day, for the symptoms sometimes undergo a most remarkable change in twelve hours, and the right period when Phosphorus ought to be given, is easily missed. If pneumonia is complicated with a higher grade of pleuritis (for it is almost always associated with some of the lighter grades of this disease), Phosphorus is, in our opinion, much less appropriate than other remedies, and we feel unable to accede to the opinion of some homœopatic practitioners who regard Phosphorus as peculiarly suitable to pleuritis. In the third stage, Phosphorus is apparently appropriate, but we deem it proper at this stage to recommend other remedies more urgently. In chronic pneumonia we have never seen Phosphorus do any good. Regarding the dose, we desire to state that we have never seen an aggravation caused by ten or tweve drops of the third attenuation in two ounces of water, given in dessertspoonful-doses; but that the second attenuation is very easily succeeded by the production of primary symptoms, especially an increase of hyperæmia, even hemorrhage, more particularly in the case of tuberculous individuals. As far as higher attenuations are concerned, we confess that we have never witnessed any effects from any above the sixth. [Some years ago we had an opportunity of witnessing a very beautiful and striking effect of Phosphorus. Some time during the summer, late in the evening, we were summoned by a farmer who complained of a severe stitch in the side. The patient was of a consumptive habit of body, forty-five years old; we found him lying on the sofa, with a high fever, short and panting breathing and a dry, racking cough with very scanty expectoration. It being very late, we made a rather hurried examination, and being satisfied that we had a case of pleuro-pneumonia before us, we prescribed *Aconite* 2, and left him with the promise of an early morning-visit. Next morning we found our patient worse, if any thing. Fever very high, skin dry, like parchment, complexion very sallow, dull headache, considerable thirst and extreme exhaustion. The cough was no longer dry, but muco-sanguinolent sputa were raised in some quantity. The patient complained of exquisite soreness at one spot in the left lower lobe of the lungs. The balance of the organ seemed to be in a state of hyperæmia; percussion still yielded some resonance, very little dulness anywhere, except in the left lobe. Prescribed *Bryonia*. Saw the patient again in the middle of the day; he was steadily failing. Saw him again in the evening and found him in a state of sopor, grasping at flocks, picking at the bed-clothes, and raising profuse quantities of a yellow-green pus having an exceedingly unpleasant odor. The pus was discharged from the first-named sore spot. The soreness now had reached a very high degree; the least pressure upon this spot caused the patient to moan; the cough was very short and the patient seemed to dread it; his tongue looked like parched leather, his complexion had a dark-brown icteric hue; the delirium was constant, bland; pulse about 140. It was evident that we had a large cavernous abscess before us, and that unless we succeeded in effecting a favorable change very soon, our patient would be a dead man in a very short time.

We now put him on *Phosphorus* 3d trituration. Half an hour after taking the first powder, a favorable change manifested itself. The medicine was continued through the night every hour or whenever the patient should wake. Early in the morning we found him with a moist skin, pulse down to 85, breathing much improved, symptoms of a general resolution apparent, passed water freely, the urine being thickly charged with decayed mucus; no headache, sputa muco-purulent, without any bad odor; the region of the abscess no longer sensitive, only a little sore but over a smaller surface. Continued the Phosphorus every two hours. In a fortnight after our first visit, the patient was able to resume his labor; every morbid symptom having disappeared. H.]

Sulphur. The symptoms which this agent causes in the respiratory organs are too numerous and varied to enable us to detach some of them from the whole list; the remedy has to be studied in its totality, more especially with regard to the respiratory organs for which it is of such extraordinary importance. If Müller says that the writers on sulphur agree in their views concerning the action of this agent, we cannot altogether agree with him, since the existing differences in their opinions are somewhat striking and of essential importance. The importance of this remedy must be our excuse, if we examine some of the details with more minuteness. In the first place and very generally Sulphur is recommended for pneumonias in dyscrasic individuals. Some authors mention psora by name, others undoubtedly had it in their minds. Is the existence of psora founded in reality? According to our own experience, we cannot admit this, especially in tubercular pneumonia where sulphur exerts curative effects only in very few cases. For this reason we believe with Müller that the indications for sulphur are chiefly set up á priori, and we cannot forbear taking this opportunity of again calling attention to the unprofitable part that psora has played in Homœopathy. Nor can we give our assent to the proposition that Sulphur should be given in the third stage when a purulent dissolution of the infiltration is already far advanced. Practical experience is against this proposition which is likewise contradicted by the results obtained in inflammations of other organs, where the completion of a purulent transformation constitutes a positive counter-indication to Sulphur. Hartmann likewise talks of a latent dyscrasia where the apparently best indicated remedies remain without effect; but we would ask how it happens that there are pneumonias almost all of which sometimes act in this manner in the same year among all those that are attacked by this disease? Of what use is it to at once jump at the doctrine of a latent dyscrasia? The same position is occupied by Watzke when he recommends Sulphur in pneumonia consequent upon the suppression or retrocession of an exanthem. With the access of almost any very acute inflammation exanthems disappear almost without an exception either for a time or for ever, which is of no more importance than the cessation of a coryza after the supervention of an inflammatory process. The more serious affection does not tolerate the simultaneous presence of a less serious one. Metastasis under such circumstances cannot be appealed to, nor can a definite influence over the course of the whole disease be determined beforehand. We transcribe Müller's chief indications: In the second and third stages of pneumonia, especially when the inflammation is deep-seated and extensive, Sulphur deserves particular consideration as an independent remedy. If after the removal of the first vascular excitement which generally results from the supervention of the exudation, an exacerbation of the febrile and other symptoms sets in again after the lapse of one to three days, as is frequently noticed in cases where no dispersion takes place, and the disease runs its course through the second and third stages, Sulphur is best calculated to meet this exacerbation, if characterized by vascular excitement, dyspnœa and intensity of the thoracic symptoms, and not by the so-called nervous symptoms, for which *Phosphorus*, *Belladonna*, *Bryonia*, *Rhus toxicodendron* and other remedies are indicated. Hence Sulphur must be indicated by extensive hepatization and suppuration (second and third stage) where not the nervous, but the synochal symptoms prevail, resembling those that indicate Aconite in the first stage of the disease. What we have to object to Müller's views is that we do not believe Sulphur ever meets synochal febrile symptoms. If we advance our own views concerning the indications for Sulphur, it is not so much in the expectation of uttering anything new, but of uniting existing opinions in one general series. In our opinion Sulphur is indicated, if pneumonia passes through its first two stages without any great deviations from the normal course, or without any striking changes, and then remains stationary without the supervention of any typhoid symptoms, such as occur in pneumonias to which Phosphorus is specially adapted. It is a period of anxious expectation to a physician, because he cannot decide whether re-absorption or a purulent dissolution of the exudation will take place. The patients do not seem extremely ill, the fever may be intense or may have commenced to abate; in this condition the disease has often continued for weeks. This is most frequently observed in pneumonias treated with venesections. Now is the period for the exhibition of Sulphur, and it is astonishing with what magical rapidity the organic reaction is sometimes kindled by this agent. It makes no difference whether the individual is otherwise diseased or not, whether dyscrasias, psora, tubercles are present or not. A deficiency of reaction and a simultaneous absence of such symptoms as point directly to the destruction of the organic powers, constitute in our opinion the best indications for Sulphur. But if suppuration has really set in, we feel disposed to doubt the curative virtues of Sulphur. The same relation obtains in chronic pneumonia; if it exists with symptoms of dissolution, Sulphur is most commonly capable of super-inducing the re-absorption of the atonic exudation, whereas in pulmonary abscess this remedy is altogether ineffectual. It is, however, conceivable that Sulphur may still have a beneficent effect in purulent decomposition. Suppuration frequently sets in on a limited scale, gradually invading the infiltrated portion of lung, and it is thus conceivable that Sulphur may occasion the normal re-absorption of the remaining firm exudation. From this point of view we agree with Wurmb when he advises not to delay the employment of Sulphur too long. The fifth or sixth day is generally the best time for this medication. After what we have said, we do not deem it necessary to institute special comparisons between Phosphorus, Mercurius and Sulphur. The relative position of these three remedies can be defined in a few words: All three are only suitable in a second stage; Sulphur in the absence of all signs of reaction; Mercurius, if there is a good deal of vascular excitement, and Phosphorus, if the reaction is excessive, and is necessarily followed by adynamia.

Tartarus stibiatus. It is well known what extravagant praise was bestowed, not very long ago, upon this drug as a remedy for pneumonia, and how soon it has been abandoned. These frequent changes in Old-School Therapeutics can only be accounted for by a homœopath who is acquainted with the fact that there are no general but only individual specifics, but that these latter, when applied to a large number of similar cases of disease, are very apt to be regarded as general specifics. Tartar emetic is undoubtedly one of the most important remedies in pneumonia, but only when it deviates from the normal course. We again forbear quoting symptoms and confine ourselves to the well established indications which the symptoms had first suggested. In uncomplicated pneumonia Tartar emetic is scarcely ever indicated in the first stage, not even at the beginning of the second stage. The sphere of action of this drug commences with the resolution of the exudation. If the resolution takes place rapidly, and the re-absorption is slow, the dyspnœa generally becomes quite considerable, because the lungs are unable to remove the copious contents from their cells. If great dyspnœa is present, and a spasmodic cough with expectoration that affords some relief; if the infiltrated portion of lung yields a tympanitic, not altogether empty sound, and loud and coarse râles over a large surface, Tartar emetic will have a fine effect. This termination of pneumonia is generally characterized by a sinking of the temperature with an increased frequency of the pulse, great anxiety and restlessness with copious, cool perspiration, cerebral congestions with a livid or at least a strikingly pallid complexion. In contradistinction to Phosphorus, the indications for Tartar emetic point to a deficient reaction; hence it is more suitable for old people than for vigorous and young persons. We doubt whether this remedy will ever be found appropriate in the stage of purulent dissolution. Among the complications it is particularly bronchitis that points to Tartar emetic. Here we meet most commonly with the above described condition, an excessive crowding of the bronchia, with insufficient ability to remove the secretion. It is this species of pneumonia, which is so apt to set in in an epidemic form, that has given rise to the commendations with which Tartar emetic has been honored as a remedy for pneumonia with unquestionable propriety; for in this kind of pneumonia the remedy displays extraordinary curative powers. It deserves particular attention in the more dangerous forms of bronchitis in the case of children, in pneumonia as a complication of whooping-cough, in pneumonia when supervening during the presence of emphysema. Not only by bronchitis, but likewise by an intense catarrh of the stomach is Tartar emetic indicated in pneumonia, and in this respect it may be properly given after Bryonia. We should never lose sight of the fact that when a large quantity of mucus accumulates in the lungs, the expectoration is difficult, but that, when it does take place, great relief is afforded. Regarding the dose, physicians agree most remarkably in the case of this remedy; so far as we know, a higher trituration than the third is not advised by any physician. The second trituration in grain-doses is probably the most appropriate, since it never gives rise to nausea.

Hepar sulphuris calcareum. We are amazed that this remedy is so little or rather not at all mentioned in the therapeutics of pneumonia; we would urge physicians to try Hepar in this disease. In making this request we are supported by several really brilliant cures, one of which we will relate very briefly. A boy of six years,

who had enjoyed good health up to that time and was otherwise
of a robust constitution, had been treated for pneumonia by an
allopathic physician for upwards of eight weeks, without recovering; he was allowed to languish in a diseased condition until a
rapidly increasing curvature of the thorax set it. Twenty weeks
after the first commencement of the pneumonia, the parents sought
our advice. The child was exceedingly emaciated, had a slight
hectic fever, was constantly troubled by a sometimes spasmodic
cough, with a purulent and fetid expectoration, diarrhœa, loss of
appetite. The right side of the thorax had caved in quite considerably, the left was abnormally bulging; on the right side the percussion-sound was perfectly empty, with intense bronchial respiration and slight râles. We diagnosed pleuro-pneumonia of the right
side, with absorption of the pleuritic exudation, but continued presence of the pneumonic infiltration in a state of purulent dissolution.
After various ineffectual remedies, the child was finally put on
Hepar, 3d trituration, with such excellent success that in eight days
already the caving in of the chest was considerably less. In about
four weeks the right lung had almost been restored to its normal
condition, and the curvature of the thorax had entirely disappeared
so that the child now looks perfectly straight and thoroughly sound
and healthy. A second pneumonia, with which the boy was attacked
four years after the former, was radically cured in seven days.
Since then we have often made use of Hepar and have arrived at
the following results: Hepar is preferable to other remedies after
the third stage has set in, provided the general symptoms are comparatively mild, a lentescent fever is present and the suppurative
process does not extend over a large portion of lung. It will act so
much more powerfully the younger and more vigorous the children
are. In pneumonia complicated with bronchitis there is scarcely a
better remedy after Mercurius than Hepar. The above described
case shows that chronic pneumonia is the best sphere for the therapeutic action of Hepar. In a case of pulmonary abscess, Hepar
effected a cure as far as the restoration of this patient was possible.

Rhus toxicodendron. Müller's statements regarding this remedy
in his Essay on Pneumonia seem to us so appropriate that we feel
called upon to transcribe his remarks: " Hahnemann's recommendation of Rhus tox. as a remedy for the typhus that devastated the
hospitals during the war of 1813, and the consequent employment
of this remedy in nervous and gastric fevers, and in typhus, seems
to have secured for it a predetermined part in the treatment of

pneumonia. It seems certain that nothing in the present pathogenesis of Rhus entitles this agent to a place among the remedies in the ordinary pneumonias of a lighter grade, and that the local chest-symptoms of Rhus have scarcely any relationship to this disease. What stamps it a remedy for pneumonia, are its general typhoid symptoms arising from a depression of the cerebral functions. These symptoms are undoubtedly very marked, placing the drug ahead of Belladonna and Bryonia, assigning it even a place by the side of Phosphorus and Arsenicum. Since these nervous symptoms occur in all three stages of pneumonia, Rhus need not be rigorously assigned to a definite stage, although the typhoid depression of the sensorium, as manifested by the symptoms of Rhus, is more particularly a characteristic of the later stages, and may not so much result from an obstructed circulation as from a deterioration of the blood in consequence of the purulent dissolution of the exudation and other causes; on which account Rhus may be more adapted to this stage, whereas Belladonna and perhaps Bryonia correspond rather to the cerebral symptoms occasioned by simple stagnations in the circulation and by cerebral congestions. Among the symptoms indicating Rhus, the following would, therefore, be the most characteristic: Loss of strength, sopor, hardness of hearing, subsultus tendinum, unconscious discharge of stool and urine, dryness and heat of the skin, dry, hard and sooty tongue. (Why Dr. Wurmb does not expect any marked effects from Rhus or any other remedy in purulent infiltration of the lungs, is difficult to comprehend; at any rate, this condition of the lungs does not legitimate doubts any more than any other condition; he seems to regard this stage as more unfavorable and dangerous than it really is, nor does he seem to consider that in every case of pneumonia, which is not cut short in the first stage, a purulent decomposition and resolution is the normal and almost the only favorable course.) Among the local symptoms one at least seems to deserve a more prominent place, it is a dyspnœa peculiar to Rhus and occasioned by distention of the pit of the stomach; however, even in this respect, it will only compete with other remedies, especially with Nux vomica and Phosphorus. Kreussler's recommendation of Rhus in case miliaria break out, attended with a general aggravation of the whole condition of the patient, is in our opinion, founded in nothing else than the marked tendency inherent in Rhus to cause exanthems, some of which resemble miliaria; nor can it be denied that it is in pneumonias complicated with miliaria, that the above-described nervous symptoms are most apt to prevail. Rhus might likewise be principally recommended for pneumonia occasioned by exposure to wet and cold, provided the power of Rhus to cure such catarrhal diseases, and which is now generally believed in, had a sure basis; it is evident, however, that this view has not been suggested by physiological experimentation, but rests upon an empirical basis; moreover, the definition of catarrhal disease is evidently too vague and indefinite to deserve very serious consideration. It might be replied that the reputation of Arnica in contusions has no better foundation; but here the case is a very different one. The virtue of Arnica in removing the consequences of contusions and blows, is not the result of empiricism, but a knowledge thereof has been obtained by physiological provings and could not have been obtained but for the circumstance that the symptoms occasioned by external injuries, are definite and fixed in their characteristic manifestations, and that their correspondence with drug-symptoms can very readily be established. The consequences of a cold, on the contrary, are not circumscribed within such narrow and precise limits, but are of the most diversified kind and meaning, so that, if we know a cold to be the cause, the connection between cause and effect can readily be suspected, but cannot, as in the other case, be inferred with perfect certainty from the existing symptoms." To this exposé we will add a few remarks. When speaking of Phosphorus, we stated that Rhus might be found indicated above every other remedy in cases of pneumonia setting in from the commencement with adynamic fever. We repeat this statement in this place. If in the first two days the diagnosis wavers between typhus and pneumonia; if the local process commences at the outset as if modified by a general deterioration of the mass of blood, Rhus will be found indicated, although, we have never seen the disease cut short by this remedy. In pneumotyphus Rhus ranks next to Phosphorus to which it may even be regarded as superior. Whereas Phosphorus is less adapted to pneumonia complicated with bronchitis, Rhus, on the contrary, is in its place in such circumstances, as we have latterly learned to know from abundant experience. Bronchitis is attended with a scanty secretion of mucus, it precedes pneumonia by a few days; the pneumonia itself supervenes almost imperceptibly and is only recognized by the increasing dyspnœa which becomes unbearable by exposure to stove-heat, and is accompanied by a characteristic dry and tormenting cough, by which sleep is disturbed particularly after midnight. As a rule, attention had better be paid to Rhus in epidemic pneumonia where it often renders excellent service.

Arnica. The value of this medicine has in some respects been impaired for having been so universally accepted as a remedy for the consequences of contusions and other mechanical injuries. Its use has almost been confined to this range, as the use of Aconite has been limited to inflammatory fever. But if our provings reveal such a decided, and we might almost say such a specific relation to definite organs, and more especially to the lungs, we must suppose that Arnica will prove an excellent remedy in pneumonia. In the first place, then, in pneumonia this remedy deserves a preference over any other in all cases where the disease is occasioned by mechanical injuries. We likewise recommend Arnica in cases where the pneumonic infiltration is associated with a marked tendency to hemorrhage. This coincidence generally occurs only in the case of plethoric individuals with sensitive and irritable nerves, for which Arnica is said to be preëminently suitable, and in whom the blood has undergone a peculiar alteration resembling the alteration in typhus, for which Arnica, if the results obtained by our provings can be accepted as reliable, is likewise a proper remedy as long as the strength of the patient is not in a sinking condition. Under these circumstances it competes with Belladonna, for Arnica has likewise symptoms of marked cerebral congestion. For this reason we commend Arnica in cases of pneumonia complicated with symptoms of meningitis. The first stage furnishes the most characteristic indications for Arnica; the second stage, and still less the third will scarcely ever afford a suitable sphere for a display of the curative virtues of this drug.

China will never be found suitable in pneumonia without any decided deviations; it may often be indicated for some of these deviations, but more on account of its general effect upon the organism, as on account of its specific action upon the lungs. Its recommendation for bilious pneumonia is suggested by theory rather than founded upon practical results; a slight degree of icterus is such an ordinary accompaniment of severe pneumonias that it cannot be regarded as an important complication; and if the stagnation in the liver is more considerable when the right lung is inflamed, the reason is simply because the circulation in the liver is obstructed by the impeded circulation in the lungs; as soon as the pneumonic infiltration is removed, the hepatic circulation will resume its normal course. To judge from the results obtained by means of our physiological provings, China is best suited where the course of pneumonia has been interfered with by sanguineous depletion, especially if hectic symptoms have set in with marked prostration of all reaction, or if, during the subsequent course of the disease, the threatening pulmonary symptoms become associated with hyperæmia of the liver, icterus, intestinal catarrh, violent distress in the stomach. For this reason China may be ranked among the principal remedies for chronic pneumonia, but its action is of limited extent, and it is scarcely ever the only remedy sufficient to effect a cure. Without doubt it often helps to kindle a reaction which is a necessary preliminary to the curative action of other drugs. Whether intermittent pneumonia can be reached by China, is not yet settled; this recommendation is very much like the Old-School recommendation of China for all typical or intermittent paroxysms. In pulmonary abscess it can only be depended upon for its general, not for its local symptoms.

Carbo vegetabilis. Few remedies in our Materia Medica exert such a marked and energetic action upon the lungs as Carbo; and will still prove efficient even in the most desperate cases. We cannot here transcribe the number of symptoms referring to the respiratory act, but we would urge upon every physician the propriety of making himself thoroughly acquainted with them in the Materia Medica. The general tendency of Carbo is to extinguish the reactive energies of the organism and to develop, at the same time, a tendency to decomposition and decay. From this stand-point the relation of Carbo to pneumonia can most easily be explained and accounted for. It is the third or suppurative stage that presents a symptomatic picture for the employment of Charcoal. The patients seem listless, covered with a profuse and cool perspiration, the pulse is very rapid and small, without resistance; the tongue is dry, yet the patients do not seem very thirsty; they pass foul, decaying diarrhœic stools; their breath has a foul odor, decubitus threatens to break out; the respiration is superficial, a loud rattling is heard in the chest, yet, in spite of the distressing cough, the patient does not raise the least particle of any thing. All the symptoms point to incipient paralysis. A bloated countenance, with injection of the facial veins, is a striking indication for Carbo. Such conditions are apt to set in among older people, to whom Carbo is an important remedy generally. If pneumonia assumes a chronic form; if abscess and gangrene set in; if the sputa become fetid and badly colored, no remedy is likely to afford the least help, if Carbo fails us. Of course, an immediate improvement must not be expected; the character of the disease renders such a thing impossible. Among the complications, Carbo is indicated by every process that interferes with the pulmonary circulation. Hence, we find it such an excellent remedy in the pneumonia of emphysematous individuals, where it is undoubtedly preferable to Arsenic; likewise in pneumonia complicated with defects of the right heart; and finally in pneumonia where the inflamed lung is suffering from chronic catarrh. In such cases the chances of a favorable termination are sometimes exclusively confined to the employment of Charcoal. It is likewise excellent in cases of pneumonia complicated with acute bronchitis. In such cases it is principally the dry and spasmodic cough, attended with mucous râles in the chest and occurring chiefly at night, with soreness and a burning pain, that points to Carbo, and makes it a valuable remedy in the malignant forms of influenza, especially of older people. The resemblance of Carbo to China is very great, extending even to the presence of bilious symptoms; nevertheless, in a given case, the selection is not so very difficult, provided the above-described general range of action is kept in view. From Tartar emetic to which Carbo bears likewise a great deal of resemblance, this drug is best distinguished by the circumstance that with Tartar emetic the expectoration is possible and affords relief, whereas Carbo has but a very slight expectoration which, moreover, affords no relief.

Lycopodium is recommended by Hartmann, if the patient feels very nervous, without heat in the head or flushes on the face, with circumscribed redness of the cheeks, great weakness, perspiration which does not relieve, redness and dryness of the tongue, frequent urging to cough with a little grayish expectoration which is raised with difficulty, after which the râles in the chest are not diminished in the least, and the dyspnœa is very striking. These symptoms seem to us very vague, and we doubt whether such a group has ever been seen in practice. Adding to the above the statements of other physicians, we assert that Lycopodium is only suitable in pneumonia after the acute symptoms have all passed away, whereas hectic symptoms have taken their place. Hence Lycopodium is very closely related to Carbo veget., even the local drug-symptoms are very much alike. As distinctive signs we point out under Lycopodium a deficiency of the symptoms denoting a general decomposition, the absence of colliquative symptoms in other organs, especially in the intestinal canal, and the absence or lesser degrees of passive congestion, and finally the copious expectoration which affords no relief. In pulmonary abscess Lycopodium may be tried, but it is not a leading remedy.

Regarding **Opium**, Müller, after quoting the scanty, literary material, has the following: "Despite the poverty of the homœopathic literature, Opium can be assigned a place in pneumonia with tolerable certainty. Excluding all acute inflammatory conditions of the lungs, Opium can be given with great success for paroxysmal obstructions of the respiration and for suffocative paroxysms that are occasioned by various disturbances of the pulmonary and cardiac functions (hence also in the course of a pneumonia where no resolution has taken place,) as well as when general cerebro-spinal affections are complained of. The following symptoms are especially characteristic: These symptoms originate during, or are aggravated by sleep; absence of pain, except a constrictive sensation on the chest; labored, rattling respiration, or very slow, almost imperceptible, even suspended breathing; sudden blueness of the face; staring, immovable, half-closed eyes; somnolence before or after an attack; trembling, twitching and jerking about the whole body, or else rigidity of the body, general coolness of the skin; irregular, intermittent pulse, constipation. Many give moreover the following symptoms as indications for Opium: Bad effects of fright and fear, likewise of wine-bibbings and ailments incidental to old age; general insensibility of the nervous system and deficient reaction after certain medicines." We do not consider these indications sufficiently clear and definite to be of much practical use in the treatment of pneumonia; for this reason we add a few detached observations, because we regard Opium as a really important remedy in pneumonia. That Opium causes pneumonic infiltration, is evident from a case of poisoning of a child of three months which is reported by Boyd-Mushet in the Med. Times and Gazette, March 20, 1858. It is remarkable that it is precisely in the case of children that the not simply narcotic effects of Opium are so prominently developed, on which account it is our opinion that it is only in infantile pneumonia that Opium ought to be exhibited, more especially in cases where the pulmonary inflammation is absolutely disguised by symptoms of cerebral congestion and oppression. In such cases the similarity between the pathological group of symptoms and those of poisoning by Opium is exceedingly great. Particular attention is due to the cyanotic color of the upper parts of the body with a slow, stertorous respiration which must evidently be regarded as a sign of paralysis proceeding from the brain. In old age a similar picture of pneumonia is not unfrequently met with. In general we account for the well-founded recommendation of Opium in cases where all medicines are ineffectual and where considerable cerebral symptoms are generally present, by the circumstance that the medicine brings the central nervous system back again to its normal activity and consequently secures a normal reaction. In the pneumonia and in many other diseases of drunkards the excellence of Opium is accounted for by a similar train of argumentation.

It now remains for us to mention a few remedies that have been recommended for pneumonia, but have neither been made use of very frequently, nor are they to be regarded as genuine and radical curative agents in this disease.

Nux vomica is not by any means an important remedy for pneumonia. This is our opinion as well as Müller's. Although we do not expect to see the therapeutic sphere of every remedial agent that we present as such, specifically marked out by pathologico-anatomical appearances, yet it must indeed seem strange that Nux vomica, of which we possess such a vast number of fatal cases of poisoning, has never yet occasioned a single decided hyperæmia, much less infiltration of the lungs. This one circumstance is a positive argument againt the employment of Nux in pneumonia. We do not even find the remedy indicated in pneumonia complicated with bronchitis; for such a bronchitis will greatly differ from that which comes within the curative range of Nux. In the pneumonias of drunkards Nux may influence the general disease, but it is exceedingly doubtful whether the local disease will ever be reached by it. For this reason we cannot recommend Nux for practical trials either á priori, nor upon the ground of experience.

To **Pulsatilla** the same remarks apply as to Nux. Of late years Pulsatilla has not been employed in pneumonia, and if the former success of this drug in pneumonia is appealed to, we beg leave to suggest that in those days the certainty of spontaneous cures of pneumonia was not nearly as well established as it is now. It is more especially in the pneumonia of anæmic and chlorotic individuals that Pulsatilla is principally recommended; in such cases it is evidently the general spasmodic condition of the organism, not the local affection that has been had in view.

Cannabis is considered by Hartmann a very valuable remedy in the subsequent course of the pneumonia, if the disease affects principally the lower portion of the thorax, or is localized in the left lung; if palpitation of the heart, oppression under the sternum with dull shocks in the region of the heart, frequent singultus, coldness rather than warmth of the whole body, with increasing heat of the face, are complained of as accompanying symptoms. It is in asthenic pneumonias that, according to Hartmann, the remedy deserves particular attention. It seems to us that these indications are not only vague, but useless. The symptoms of Cannabis do not by any means point to an inflammatory process in the lungs, but seem to result from the powerful action of Cannabis upon the heart. The remedy not having been employed to any extent in pneumonia, there do not seem to exist sufficient reasons why its use in this disease should be recommended.

Senega, according to its pathogenesis, is to some extent a remedy for pneumonia, but its therapeutic value in this respect is very much diminished by the accompanying remark that the painful sensations which Senega occasions in the thorax, are more particularly felt on the outside. In other respects Senega is particularly adapted to diseases of the respiratory mucous membrane, and, for this reason, to pneumonias complicated with bronchitis. Striking practical results by means of this drug have not yet been published.

Hyoscyamus. Toxicological post-mortem appearances determine the relation of this drug to pneumonia better than all its pathogenetic symptoms. The lungs exhibit marked hyperæmia, but they are filled with a black, fluid blood, and are infiltrated with serum. If, in addition to this, we consider that Hyoscyamus has no intense pains and that the cough is more particularly dry and breaks out at night, we have a right to declare that an ordinary pneumonia does not come within the curative range of this agent. On the other hand we consider Hyoscyamus, even with reference to its cerebral symptoms, a valuable remedy in hypostatic pneumonia when supervening during the course of other chronic affections; in pneumonia complicated with typhus; in the pneumonia of old people and when acute œdema of the lungs sets in. A violent delirium should always direct our attention to Hyoscyamus. As an intercurrent remedy, Hyoscyamus is often admirably useful in a nocturnal, spasmodic, dry cough, such as frequently occurs in pneumonia during the prevalence of influenza.

Arsenicum album. Howsoever much we may be disposed to regard Arsenicum as one of the most prominent remedies for pulmonary affections, yet it does not appear to us that it occupies a prominent rank among the remedies for pneumonia. Among the large number of toxicological post-mortem appearances, a decided fibrinous infiltration of the pulmonary parenchyma has never been noticed, but always only a marked hyperæmia and œdema. This circumstance could not possibly occur, if Arsenic were possessed of a specific power to excite an inflammatory action in the lungs. In an uncomplicated case of pneumonia we should therefore never resort to Arsenic. On the other hand, cases occur where the accessory symptoms indicate Arsenic so thoroughly that they entirely overshadow the fact of pneumonia; in such a case it is not prescribed as a pneumonic remedy. Wurmb gives the following more specific indications: Rapid and disproportionate prostration; tendency to colliquation and dissolution; marked periodicity of the more prominent symptoms; aggravation during rest and in a recumbent posture, with excessive restlessness and anxiety, and prevalence of the burning pain. It is at all events strange that Arsenicum should be so seldom mentioned in our literature as a remedy for pneumonia, whence we infer with tolerable certainty that it has only been found useful as an intercurrent remedy and not even then in a very striking manner. In our own opinion, Arsenic should be resorted to, if gangrene of the lungs develops itself with very marked signs of reaction; in the pneumonia of emphysematous patients and when complicated with cardiac affections; if œdema of the lungs sets in all at once, with passive hyperæmia of the lungs as not unfrequently occasioned by defects of the right heart; and finally in hypostatic pneumonia.

Sepia and **Silicea** both by their local as well as general symptoms are important remedies in excessively slow, purulent, as well as in true chronic pneumonia. The large number of important symptoms does not permit us to detach the most prominent from the series. These drugs have to be studied throughout. We likewise call attention to *Cuprum* which certainly deserves more particular attention in lentescent pneumonic conditions than has hitherto been devoted to it. We have the records of a case of poisoning by Copper where an abscess in the lungs was found. An observation of this kind should be treasured up with so much more care as our Materia Medica offers few, if any, similia for such a disorganization.

For the sake of completeness, we mention the names of a few other remedies which, so far as present experience goes, are of subordinate value: *Squilla, Zincum metallicum, Acidum phosphoricum* and *nitricum, Kali nitricum* and *Kali carbonicum, Camphora, Iodium.*

Spongia, *Digitalis purpurea*, and others. We have often given it as our opinion that too large a number of medicines for one class of diseases produces confusion and complicates the selection of a remedy; we have perhaps given too large a number of remedies in the present instance; our excuse must be that we consider pneumonia more important than any other disease as affording the best illustration of the efficacy of homœopathic treatment.

A condensed review of these remedies may not be superfluous in order the better to enable the physician in a given case, to hit on the specifically adapted agent; we shall adhere as closely as possible to the definitions we have presented at the commencement of this chapter.

In the first stage of pneumonia, *Aconite* is the chief remedy adapted to a vast majority of all the cases. If severe cerebral congestions are present, *Belladonna* is indicated together with Aconite (also *Veratrum viride*). If pneumonia is occasioned by mechanical causes, *Arnica* is given, which likewise corresponds to a co-existing cerebral hyperæmia. If the fever assumes from the outset the character of adynamia, *Rhus* is preferable, very rarely *Phosphorus* in the first place. Complications that will be stated by and by, may alter the choice of the remedial agent, so that other remedies may be required at the outset of the disease.

In the second stage *Bryonia* is the most essential remedy as long as the course of the disease remains normal and no exceptional changes set in; it likewise corresponds to the very common but slight co-existing hyperæmia of the liver. If, side by side with the infiltration, the congestion continues as collateral hyperæmia, *Aconite* is in its place; in such cases the alternate use of these two drugs may seem indispensable. If the reabsorption delays without the general symptoms changing alarmingly for the worse, *Sulphur* becomes the most important remedy. If the symptoms assume a typhoid character, *Phosphorus* should be given at once; in a few cases *Rhus* may be indicated. *Tartarus stibiatus* requires to be given, if the resolution of the infiltration takes place very speedily, but the reabsorption is very slow, and hence it becomes necessary to promote expectoration. If we are called upon at this stage to treat a pneumonia that had been managed with sanguineous depletions, *Phosphorus*, *Sulphur* and *China* may be suitable remedies.

In the third stage *Phosphorus* is commonly useful only at the commencement, and here competes with *Mercurius;* Phosphorus, and perhaps also Mercurius, are counter-indicated by excessive prostration. The last-named drug may come into play, if the disease exists in dyscrasic, especially in scrofulous individuals. If the suppurative process goes on without any marked febrile symptoms, assuming rather the form of a slowly-progressing hectic condition entirely confined to the lungs, *Sulphur* is often calculated to bring about a favorable termination; however we place more confidence in *Hepar sulphuris*. In such circumstances *Iodium* may likewise be prescribed with great propriety. If purulent dissolution takes place, and the whole organism seems to be affected by this change in a threatening manner, *China* deserves our first consideration, next to which we may compare *Lycopodium*, *Sepia* and *Silicea*. Pulmonary abscess, whether acute or chronic, requires the above-named remedies; in a case of chronic abscess, we would likewise depend in some measure upon *Carbo vegetabilis* and *Cuprum*. Gangrene of the lungs is always a very threatening change, and a cure can scarcely ever be expected. *Carbo veg.* and *Arsenicum*, and perhaps also *Lycopodium*, are probably the only remedies by means of which a favorable change can be wrought. To what circumstances *Terebinthina* owes its recommendation for gangrene of the lungs, cannot well be explained from the homœopathic stand-point, this remedy will most probably exert a more specific curative effect when administered by inhalation than when conveyed to the diseased organ by the stomach. On account of their general action more than on account of their special relation to the lungs, the mineral acids, more especially *Acidum phosphoricum* and *nitricum*, deserve particular attention during the whole course of the third stage, but only as intercurrent remedies.

The following constitute particular forms of pneumonia with reference to the circumstances which either occasion or accompany the attack, although they cannot be considered as complications.

Pneumonia of children assumes most commonly the form of lobular pneumonia, the more so the younger the individuals. In simple croupous pneumonia no other remedies are required than in the case of adults, although we would call attention to two remedies in such cases, namely *Mercurius* and *Opium*. The former is rarely suitable for adults in the second stage, on the contrary, it is often serviceable to children and is usually preferable to *Bryonia*. *Opium* is a very excellent remedy for the severe cerebral hyperæmia with which children are so often attacked. This condition of the brain very often makes *Belladonna* superior to Aconite even at the beginning of the pneumonia. Very seldom the symptoms in the case of children will point to *Phosphorus* which is aptly replaced by *Mercurius* or even by *Hepar sulphuris*. As a general rule, a simple uncomplicated pneumonia is neither a very important nor a very dangerous disease to the infantile organism; but it can easily be made so, especially by sanguineous depletions and cathartics. In the case of children the momentary effect of a debilitating treatment is greater; in the case of adults it is less instantaneous than persistent.

In old age pneumonia is almost always associated with catarrh of the bronchia, and hence much more dangerous. Simple pneumonia not unfrequently sets in with symptoms that call for *Belladonna* rather than Aconite; sometimes *Bryonia* is indicated by the symptoms from the very beginning. Here too the co-existing cerebral symptoms often call for *Opium* and *Hyosciamus*. The reabsorption is usually trifling; a crisis generally takes place by copious expectoration, and although *Sulphur* may be perfectly appropriate for a few days, the copious, but difficult expectoration requires without any further delay the exhibition of *Tartar emetic*, or *Carbo vegetabilis* or *Lycopodium*, also *Baryta*. We would not advise Phosphorus for the reason that all signs of an excessive reaction are wanting. The greatest danger to old people is the acute œdema and the paralysis of the lungs by which the œdema is often speedily followed. In order to obviate this event, the patient should be put on a nourishing diet and have a little stimulating wine given him, whatever the antiphlogistic theory may say against it. As far as medicines are concerned, help may be expected from Tartar emetic, Arsenicum, Digitalis, perhaps also from *Hyoscyamus* and *Squills;* even *Veratrum album* may have to be used in some cases. As a measure of precaution, which is of great importance to the patient, he should not be allowed to remain lying on his back too long at a time, but should be directed to change his position quite frequently, and to keep the upper part of his body in a more or less vertical posture, lest hypostasis should set in, which might otherwise easily occur.

Hypostatic pneumonia cannot, properly speaking, be regarded as inflammation; it represents a peculiar hyperæmia of the lungs depending upon a paralytic weakness of the circulatory and respiratory organs. It only occurs as a part of other pathological conditions, on which account no special treatment can be assigned to it.

Lobular pneumonia is likewise a co-existing and very serious complication of bronchitis, not an idiopathic affection, and it is still more difficult to point out for it a treatment based upon experience, for the reason that we are not in the possession of any means for obtaining an exact diagnosis. Knowing, however, that whooping-cough easily leads to lobular pneumonia, and the results of our treatment being uncommonly satisfactory, we may assert with good reason that we possess real remedies for this dangerous disease which will prove efficient in cases that did not originate in whooping-cough. If lobular pneumonia sets in with a decisive increase of the fever, or with a more violent fever generally, *Belladonna* will very often be found suitable, but still more frequently *Mercurius*. If the signs of cerebral hyperæmia prevail, we have in Opium a remedy that indeed does not cause the whole process to retrograde, but exerts an exceedingly curative influence by preparing the road for other more direct remedial agents. *Ipecacuanha* should be mentioned here side by side with *Opium*, because it likewise causes marked hyperæmia of the brain, but not sufficiently violent to cause sopor; convulsions, an exceedingly spasmodic cough with suffocative paroxysms and asthmatic complaints which even remain after the cough; loud mucous râles in the chest, coldness of the extremities and heat of the head are the chief indications. Still more important for this kind of pneumonia is *Veratrum album*, a remedy which, in the form of an alkaloid *Veratrine*, has found grace even in the Old School. Its most essential indications are: dyspnœa with slight rattling of mucus, dry and spasmodic cough accompanied by marked cerebral congestions, a hurried and small pulse, cold skin and cold sweat, together with excessive debility. This group of symptoms may sometimes require the use of *Veratrum album* in croupous pneumonia. Moreover *Phosphorus*, *Tartar emetic*, *Hyoscyamus* and *Cuprum* deserve to be mentioned in this place; in general, all the medicines that have been named under bronchitis, deserve attention in lobular pneumonia. The consecutive diseases have to be regarded with special care. A rapid termination in recovery is comparatively rare in lobular pneumonia; the patients remain feeble for a long time, hack a good deal or have to pass through frequent and severe paroxysms of cough; the assimilating functions are suffering, although diarrhœa need not necessarily be present; physical exploration reveals more or less distinctly a catarrhal condition of the most delicate bronchial ramifications. In such a case it would be a decided mistake to leave the further course of the disease to Nature, as it is perfectly proper to do with the remains of most other acute affections. In such cases *Sulphur* shows an extraordinary persistence of penetrating action; we advise, however, the use of high attenuations at protracted intervals. This action of *Sulphur* is most easily accounted for by the supposition, that the pneumonic exudation which, as was said above, takes place progressively from one portion of lung to the next adjoining, still exists either entirely or in part, keeping up the patient's illness, and that it is this exudation which is reabsorbed by the aid of this drug. *Calcarea carbonica* likewise has often a very excellent effect in this protracted course of the disease, especially if slight febrile motions or even hectic fever with intestinal catarrh supervene, or if infantile organisms are attacked. As for *Hepar sulphuris* we have not yet had an opportunity of trying this remedy in a pathological condition of this kind, but we deem it essentially adapted to it and worthy of a trial.

We shall discuss typhoid pneumonia when we come to treat of the typhoid process generally. Typhoid pneumonia is a partial manifestation of typhus, scarcely ever an idiopathic disease. The inflammatory processes in the lungs depending upon tuberculosis will likewise be discussed in the chapter on tuberculosis.

The pneumonia of drunkards is almost always characterized by peculiar phenomena depending upon sympathetic cerebral and cardiac irritation and a deficiency of reactive power. The cerebral symptoms mostly point to *Opium*, much less frequently to *Nux vomica*. In the second stage *Tartarus emeticus* occupies a prominent part, *Phosphorus* is less frequently useful, although it might seem so reasoning from analogy in other forms of pneumonia. If Tartar emetic is ineffectual, *Carbo veget.* may still be of eminent use. *Belladonna* and *Hyoscyamus* are on a par with *Opium*, whereas *Digitalis* and *Rhus* deserve our commendation in the second stage. Regarding *Ammonium carbonicum* we have no experience of our own to offer, but we consider this medicine worthy of a trial. *Sulphur* will be found of little use in this form of pneumonia, whereas *Arsenicum album* may render good service in the same circumstances that we have pointed out for Sulphur in simple pneumonia. [*Cannabis sativa* and the *Bromide of Potassium* may be important remedies in this form of pneumonia. H.]

Epidemic pneumonia either presents a characteristic group of symptoms, or else it has the peculiarity of not yielding to remedies that are apparently the most suitable, and of seeming disposed to run a perverse course. In naming the different remedies we have had in many respects regard to these exceptional characteristics. To hit the right remedy for epidemic pneumonia, the most persevering investigations in the domain of Materia Medica will often be found indispensable. According to present experience, *Bryonia*, *Rhus*, *Belladonna*, *Mercurius*, *Hepar sulphuris*, *Phosphorus* and *Tartar emetic* are the medicines that we shall have first to select from in epidemic pneumonia.

It is more particularly the complications of pneumonia that render the treatment difficult and the result doubtful. They determine in a great measure the selection of the remedy, and, on the other hand, present great difficulties in finding the true remedy for the reason that they often present a very confused group of symptoms. The most important complications are the following:

Pleuritis of a higher grade of course complicates the course of pneumonia in an eminent degree, in the first place because of itself it is a severe affection, and in the second place because it interferes with the process of reabsorption in the lungs. We shall refer to this complication when treating of pleuritis.

Bronchitis as a complication is perhaps equally important as pleuritis, and requires a more careful selection of the remedy than pneumonia itself; for a normal course of this disease can only be expected after the bronchitis has been moderated. In selecting a remedy, those have to be considered first that are suitable to both affections at once, but more particularly to the catarrhal process. From the reasons stated, and from our remarks concerning Aconite in the chapter on bronchitis, we shall commonly find that this medicine, which is such an excellent remedy for pneumonia, is generally ineffectual in pneumonia complicated with bronchitis. Hence we consider the very usual recommendation of Aconite as a remedy against the totality of the febrile motions as unfounded, and, in our opinion, its employment would imply a loss of time, without being of any advantage to the disease. At the commencement of the disease, the best medicine to be prescribed, is *Belladonna*, less frequently *Mercurius*. It is impossible to indicate characteristic distinctions of both remedies, for the reason that both have too many points of resemblance. In a given case these distinctions can be pointed out with more facility. A few valuable symptoms are: violent, remitting fever with sweat, for Belladonna; remitting fever with profuse, strong-smelling perspiration, mingled with creeping chills, for Mercurius. The latter has a thickly-coated tongue, the former a thickly-coated tongue, with free borders. Mercurius has intestinal catarrh, Belladonna constipation. Belladonna can only be employed for a few days, especially in the case of adults, whereas its use can be continued longer in the case of children. After Belladonna, *Bryonia* is generally suitable, which, in this complication, is undoubtedly one of the most important remedies. Mercurius sometimes corresponds alone with the course of this pathological process, especially in the case of adults, until nothing remains to be done but to accelerate the reabsorption of the pneumonic infiltration. For such a purpose, remedies like *Sulphur* and *Hepar sulphuris* will have to be chosen, one of which, we mean Hepar, is eminently serviceable. *Rhus toxicodendron* is particularly useful, if the catarrh is dry, and malignant fever-symptoms manifest themselves. The indications for *Tartar emetic* have been given above; it is only in rare cases that this remedy will be found indicated at an early stage, it is more commonly indicated in the subsequent course of the disease. This is likewise true with regard to *Carbo veget.* Of other remedies that may come into play, we mention *Nux vomica*, *Hyoscyamus*, and *Senega*, perhaps also *Pulsatilla* and *Veratrum*.

Chronic bronchitis and emphysema as complications of pneumonia are no less dangerous than acute Bronchitis. Previous to the acute attack setting in, the respiratory movements had become very much embarrassed, and these embarrassments are enhanced by the access of pneumonia, since the habitual expectoration of mucus is most commonly suspended as soon as the pneumonia commences. At the outset of such inflammations, if the fever is very acute, *Bryonia* and *Mercurius* are indispensable; *Rhus* will rarely ever appear suitable. Sometimes the symptoms indicate *Tartar emetic* from the start, or at any rate in one or two days; in affections of this kind, Tartar emetic often renders eminent service, provided the practitioner is not afraid of giving a sufficiently large dose. We have always found the second trituration necessary but sufficient. *Veratrum album* deserves attention in such a case, especially if marked cerebral symptoms are present, together with a rapid sinking of strength and marked febrile motions, the pulse being at the same time very changing. *Phosphorus*, which often seems indicated in such pneumonias, as well as *Sulphur*, will scarcely ever be of much use. In the further course of the disease, whether it shows a very slow and gradually progressing improvement or else an aggravation of the symptoms, *Carbo veget.* is a medicine of great importance which sometimes affords help even in desperate cases. But not too much must be expected in a short time, because the course of the disease is always very much protracted. *Lycopodium* may come into play, although we cannot recommend it from personal experience. Nor have we derived much benefit from the use of *Arsenicum* which apparently seems indicated in such cases; at any rate it is much inferior to *Carbo*. The tardy re-absorption of the infiltration is not specially accelerated by Sulphur, probably because the conditions are wanting which favor the action of this drug, namely a sufficiency of reactive power and a free action of the remaining respiratory channels; *Silicea*, on the contrary, promotes the course of the disease in a striking manner. If the symptoms of passive hyperæmia of the brain are very marked, the most prominent remedy is *Digitalis* which may have to be given at the commencement as well as at any other period in the course of the disease; it either removes or moderates the threatening symptoms of an imperfect return of blood from the brain.

If pneumonia supervenes during whooping-cough, it is generally lobular, and as such has to be treated with the same remedies that have been advised for the more malignant forms of this disease. Among them we mention more particularly *Tartarus stibiatus*, *Cuprum*, *Mercurius*, *Veratrum album*, *Ipecacuanha*. Owing to the uncertainty of diagnosing this pathological complication, it is very difficult to hit upon the most available remedy. No less malignant than lobular pneumonia is croupous pneumonia, if supervening during whooping-cough. In such circumstances the course of the disease will scarcely ever be normal. Nervous phenomena set in at an early period, the infiltration remains undissolved for a long time, and a long illness may be expected without doubt, during which the lives of the children are in the greatest danger. In the case of a child of eight months, which terminated favorably, *Tartar emetic* had the best effect, and next to it *Veratrum* and *Ipecacuanha*, whereas Hepar sulphuris, Phosphorus, Sulphur, and other medicines apparently had not the least influence over the disease. If we ever should have another similar case to treat, we should give two remedies in alternation, one for the whooping-cough, and the other for the pneumonia. It is true, after the inflammation has set in, the paroxysms of cough become less frequent and less violent, but they cause a horrid distress to the patient and they do not exert a good influence over the disease. It might be well, in such circumstances, to try to subdue the paroxysms by means of *Cuprum*. We do not mean to be understood as though we regarded these few remedies as the only ones suitable to this complication; they are the only remedies that have done us any good in such cases. Beside these remedies all those that have been recommended in previous paragraphs for whooping-cough complicated with acute bronchitis, may have to be employed, and for the sequelæ or secondary diseases another class of remedies may come into play, which it is impossible to enumerate in this place.

Pneumonia complicated with influenza, has to be treated according to the same rules that have been laid down for epidemic pneumonia.

Cerebral hyperæmia is a serious complication, although more frequently in appearance than in reality. Most commonly it can only be regarded as a disturbing symptom. But if, owing to its intensity, it should develop paralytic phenomena, sopor and coma, or if the patient is far advanced in age, this hyperæmia will require particular attention and treatment. Among children it is of much less importance. It has to be treated with *Belladonna, Opium, Hyoscyamus, Veratrum, Digitalis, Tartarus stibiatus*. The first three of these remedies are more suitable for children, the last three for old people. In the case of these cerebral phenomena we have to be careful in determining whether they originate in pure hyperæmia, or depend upon the process going on in the lungs, and a consequent alteration of the blood, and, therefore, belong to the category of typhoid symptoms. In the latter case, quite different remedies have to be used, such as: *Phosphorus, Mercurius, Rhus tox.*, and others. Sometimes a mistake is not easily avoided, especially in cases where the disease had a typhoid character from the beginning. The importance of cerebral hyperæmia is likewise to be measured by the locality of the pneumonic process; it is of much less consequence if it arises from an inflammation of the upper lobes, for in such a case it can be readily and directly accounted for by a disordered circulation, whereas, when the lower lobes are inflamed, the hyperæmia appears more in the light of an idiopathic disease whose connection with the fundamental inflammation is not easily explained.

Affections of the heart, whether they existed as chronic affections previous to the occurrence of pneumonia, or whether they occur as acute affections during the course of pneumonia, constitute most threatening complications. If chronic affections of the heart are present, the dyspnœa is extremely aggravated by their presence, an active as well as passive hyperæmia of the brain sets in much more readily, and the resolution of the exudation is much retarded and is rendered much more doubtful by such a complication. The selection of a remedy likewise becomes so much more difficult, since we cannot determine the degree of attention that the heart-symptoms may legitimately claim. *Tartarus stibiatus*, *Digitalis*, *Veratrum album*, *Cannabis sativa*, *Sulphur*, correspond most fully with both orders of symptoms; *Lycopodium*, and *Carbo vegetabilis* may likewise be included in the list. At all events, such complications render a most thorough investigation of our Materia Medica indispensable. Acute diseases of the heart, if considerably far advanced, constitute very dangerous complications, since they always interfere with the normal course of pneumonia. Of much more importance than that of bronchitis is the treatment of this complication, since the heart-disease has to be removed before the cure of pneumonia can be thought of. We therefore refer the reader to the therapeutics of diseases of the heart.

Hepatic hyperæmia is a very ordinary accompaniment of pneumonia, and is generally the most severe, if the lower portion of the right lung is affected. On account of the presence of icteric symptoms, a form of pneumonia, termed bilious pneumonia, has been adopted by pathologists; but it is our opinion that hepatic hyperæmia is too natural a consequence of an obstructed pulmonary circulation to deserve a very large share of attention. Quite recently we attended a man who had all the symptoms of a violent hepatitis, and yet was in reality attacked with nothing but a pneumonia of the right side. This combination is in the first place met by *Belladonna*, afterwards *Bryonia*, and *Mercurius*, and finally *Phosphorus* and *China* are the most suitable remedies. The hepatic symptoms only require special attention, if the flow of bile is completely suspended and the gastro-intestinal catarrh is kept up and aggravated by this stagnation of the biliary current.

Gastro-intestinal catarrh in a higher or lower degree is an almost constant companion of pneumonia. If violent, it contributes greatly towards impressing a typhoid character upon this disease. Gastric catarrh alone is not very important, although the modification of the symptoms superinduced by the catarrh, may render the exhibition of *Bryonia* or *Mercurius*, *Veratrum* or *Tartarus emeticus* indispensable at the very commencement of the attack.

Chronic pneumonia, which we will class in the same category as lentescent pneumonia, has very different symptoms and requires different remedies. If it consists mainly of the pneumonic infiltration, without any other marked morbid manifestations, the consistent use of *Sulphur* is alone calculated to bring about a cure. But if the infiltration is partially firm and partially dissolving into pus, without the general organism being perceptibly disturbed, we first recommend *Hepar sulphuris*, and after that *Silicea* or *Sepia;* and, in case of great prostration, *China* or *Carbo vegetabilis*. A very rapid improvement must not be expected from any of these remedies, on which account hasty changes in their employment must be avoided. *Cuprum*, *Lycopodium* and even *Arsenicum* may come into play, especially if the formation of an abscess threatens. Not one of these remedies, however, is a guarantee of success, and we, therefore, again call attention to the use of compressed air. We have witnessed most strikingly favorable results from the use of compressed air within the space of four weeks, results that would astonish any body who witnesses them. A similarly favorable effect is produced in chronic pneumonia by a sojourn on high mountains.

In conclusion we have to devote a few words to diet for the purpose of scattering the prejudices which still prevail in reference to this subject both among physicians and laymen, although, not by any means to the same extent as formerly.

Pneumonia being very generally regarded as the result of a cold, the fear of increasing this supposed cold is so great that at the very outset of the attack the windows are hermetically closed, and the patients are not only covered warm, but are kept in an artificial temperature of 65° to 75° Fahr. This shows to what erroneous measures a wrong and arbitrary hypothesis may lead, and how these measures in their turn afford sustenance to the hypothesis. The absurd method of keeping the skin too warm, makes it so sensitive to the least exposure that every draught of air must necessarily cause aggravations in the patient's condition. We cannot warn with sufficient urgency against such management. Let the temperature of the room be kept at an uniform point of 50° to 55° Fahr., rather less than more, and, if this degree of heat has to be reached by keeping a fire in a stove, let a vessel with water be kept on the stove in order that the dryness of the heat may be modified by the vapors ascending from the water. The patient should, moreover, be lightly covered with woollen blankets. This course will render the burning fever-heat more tolerable; at any rate, we enjoy the comforting assurance that the heat has not been unnecessarily increased. A copious perspiration during the course of pneumonia is never an agreeable circumstance. No less censurable is the dread that some people have of washing the skin for the purpose of keeping it clean. Any one who, during an attack of fever, has enjoyed the luxury of a rapid cold ablution of the face, neck, arms, will not hesitate to vouchsafe this blessing to a distressed pneumonic patient. A main point is the quality of the air in a sick room. No physician, not even a reasonable layman, will want to administer spoiled food to a deranged stomach; yet people have a dread of conveying pure and fresh nourishment to the lungs. Opening a window in the room where the pneumonic patient is confined, is regarded as a crime; yet it is absolutely necessary that fresh air should be admitted to the sick room, for the air is vitiated not only by the respiratory efforts of the patient and his attendants, but likewise by the cutaneous exhalations and the odor of excrementitious matter. Why should these odors be less pernicious in pneumonia than they are now universally admitted to be in typhus? The patient's own feelings may be taken as an evidence that fresh air is indispensable, for a larger number of persons in the room are always unpleasant to him and augment the difficulty of breathing, which can easily be accounted for upon physiological principles.

While the inflammation lasts, the patient will scarcely ever want anything else in the way of nourishment than some beverage; even the slightest desire for solid food is an exception to the rule. Cold, fresh water is the best drink and should be avoided only in cases where it excites the cough. Water sweetened with sugar, is not advisable; it causes acidity of the stomach, but water mixed with a little currant jelly, may occasionally be allowed. A small quantity of malt-beer, sweetened with a little sugar, and not drank too often, is exceedingly refreshing. The common prejudice against this beverage is entirely unfounded. Water-soups and dilute milk with a little wheaten bread, will be sufficient nourishment. But as soon as the fever begins to abate and the appetite returns, a more substantial animal diet will have to be allowed, for the reason that a considerable waste has to be repaired. A change in the course of pneumonia may render corresponding changes of this simple diet indispensable. If the patient feels very weak at an early period of the disease, good broth may be given him without fear; and the presence of adynamic fever may even require small quantities of some generous wine, especially in the case of old people; an undue stimulating effect need not be apprehended. In the case of small children it is a very common mistake to quench their thirst with wine. But if the stomach is again and again called upon to recommence the process of digestion, the catarrhal affection of this organ must, of course, be made much worse than it was in consequence of the pneumonic process; this conduct is reprehensible and should by all means be avoided. The avidity with which children drink cold water during their fever, is abundant evidence that it is in harmony with the wants of the infantile organism. Special cautions in regard to diet are only required by the presence of a complicating intestinal catarrh.

When the patient may again go out in the open air, will depend upon the weather, and likewise upon the fact, which has to be well ascertained by a careful exploration of the chest, that the pneumonic infiltration is completely reabsorbed. In this respect the superiority of homœopathic treatment is likewise apparent, for it scarcely ever leaves the lungs so sensitive to open air that from its action upon this organ any untoward consequences need be apprehended.

10. Gangræna Pulmonum.
Gangrene of the Lungs.
(According to Kafka.)

[This morbid process is distinguished from other similar processes in the organism by the circumstance that putrefaction associates itself with the death of the mortifying parts.

Anatomical Characteristics. Pathologists distinguish two kinds of gangrene of the lungs, circumscribed and diffuse gangrene.

Circumscribed gangrene occurs most frequently. Detached portions of pulmonary parenchyma of the size of a hazel or walnut, are transformed into a tough, brown-green, humid, horribly-smelling scurf which is sharply circumscribed and surrounded by œdematous tissue. The sphacelated portion of lung which is at first tolerably firm, soon dissolves into an ichorous fluid. It occurs most frequently at the periphery of the lungs and in the lower lobes. If a bronchial trunk opens into the gangrened portion of lung, the ichor often runs into the former, causing an intense bronchitis.

Gangrened scurfs may likewise form on the pleura. After softening, the gangrenous ichor runs into the pleural cavity, causing a severe pleuritis; if the gangrened portion of lung communicates with a bronchus, pyopneumo-thorax may result, and, if the vessels become corroded, hemorrhage from the lungs may take place. If interstitial pneumonia develops itself round the gangrened scurf, the latter is enclosed in a capsule as it were, and a cicatrix is formed; this termination is exceedingly rare.

Diffuse gangrene frequently affects whole lobes of the lungs; the parenchyma forms a decaying, blackish, fetid tissue, which is soaked with a blackish-gray, horridly-smelling ichor. The process is not circumscribed, but extends to the surrounding, œdematous or hepatized parenchyma. If the gangrene invades the pleura, this organ becomes involved in the process of destruction. The patients succumb to constitutional prostration.

Metastatic abscesses and embolia in the different organs are not unfrequently the consequences of gangrene.

Etiology. Diffuse pulmonary gangrene sets in, although rarely, at the height of pneumonia, if all renewal of the blood and the nutrient process have entirely ceased in the inflamed lungs; pneumonias arising from the clogging up of the air-tubes in consequence of the intrusion of particles of food, are very apt, owing to the putrefaction of these molecules of animal matter, to terminate in gangrene.

Circumscribed gangrene of the lungs may be occasioned by sanguineous clots compressing the bronchial arteries; the putrid contents of bronchiectatic caverns may give rise to putrid decomposition of the pulmonary parenchyma.

Diffuse gangrene of the lungs in the case of drunkards or of individuals whose constitutions are broken down by misery and starvation; the occurrence of pneumonia in the case of insane persons, without any foreign bodies having become lodged in the bronchia; and gangrene of the lungs setting in in the course of severe asthenic fevers like typhus, measles, smallpox, puerperal fever, etc., are difficult to account for.

Symptoms. A characteristic symptom of gangrene of the lungs are the cadaverous, blackish-gray, liquid sputa, and the cadaverous odor of the breath which, in some cases, precedes the sputa for a few days. The stench is often so horrid that neither the patient nor his attendants can bear it. The sputa, like the foul expectoration from bronchiectatic caverns, separate into three layers, namely, a superficial froth, a fluid, middle layer, and a thicker sediment at the bottom. The sputa contain elastic fibres, dark-brown masses resembling tinder, with a blackish tint, and soft plugs containing fat-aciculæ.

Diffuse gangrene in consequence of pneumonia manifests itself by sudden collapse, a high degree of debility, a small and irregular pulse, and by cerebral symptoms, with which phenomena the characteristic sputa and respiration soon become associated. If diffuse gangrene sets in without pneumonia, we perceive from the start symptoms of adynamia resembling the phenomena that generally accompany septicæmia with chills, stupor, delirium, singultus, etc.

Circumscribed gangrene sometimes cannot be recognized until the gangrenous ichor has passed into the bronchia and is expelled by the mouth.

Some patients bear this severe disease without much distress; their constitutional condition is not very much disturbed; they have no fever, walk about, attend to some light, domestic employment, and the disease often drags along for months.

If the gangrened portion of lung does not communicate with a bronchus, and has become isolated as within a capsule in consequence of secondary inflammation, the cadaverous odor may be altogether wanting.

To infer the presence of pulmonary gangrene alone from the cadaverous odor, would be an exceedingly superficial mode of reasoning, since this symptom may likewise occur in bronchiectasia and when tubercular caverns are present.

The physical signs during this morbid process are not very important.

In diffuse pulmonary gangrene consequent upon pneumonia, percussion at first yields a dull or tympanitic sound; auscultation reveals indistinct respiratory murmurs or râles; in the subsequent course of the disease percussion reveals cavities in the lungs, the same as in the case of tubercular caverns, and auscultation reveals bronchial respiration and cavernous sounds.

Circumscribed gangrene is very difficult to recognize by physical exploration.

Course, Termination, Prognosis. As has already been stated, even when affected with circumscribed gangrene, patients may seem apparently well for a long time, even for months, until hemorrhages set in sooner or later, which exhaust the strength, or else the patients perish in consequence of subsequent asthenia or tabes. However, a radical cure is not impossible; in such a case the fetor of the sputa gradually disappears; they gradually assume a yellow color and a purulent consistence, and, as soon as the gangrenous focus has become encysted, it dries up and the sputa cease entirely. This favorable termination may set in in consequence of an acute inflammation, or if the gangrenous process takes place in a bronchiectatic cavity or in some cavern in the pulmonary parenchyma.

Pulmonary gangrene arising in consequence of cachectic conditions, by hunger, poverty, misery, long-lasting diseases, etc., is mostly diffuse and almost always terminates fatally. Diffuse gangrene arising from any source, is almost always fatal.

Treatment. If, during the course of pneumonia, the patient's breath begins to spread a bad odor, we should at once think of the termination of pneumonia in gangrenous destruction. If large portions of the pulmonary tissue are destroyed, the externally-perceptible signs of this gangrenous decay become apparent, such as: great debility, collapse, delirium, sopor, decubitus, unquenchable thirst, fetid diarrhœa, etc., and death takes place in consequence of utter exhaustion of the vital power.

If pulmonary gangrene does not set in with rapidly developing and threatening phenomena; if the gangrene is limited to a definite locality; if the strength of the patient is sufficient to bear up against such a violent attack, and symptoms of adynamic fever set in, we give *Arsenicum* 6, or *China* 3 to 6, six, eight or ten drops in half a goblet of water every two hours.

If the course is more protracted, *Carbo veget.* 6, or *Camphor* 3 to 6, or *Kreosote* 3 to 6 may render efficient aid. The last named remedy is likewise useful as an external application for the purpose of neutralizing the fetid odor of the breath and sputa.

The horrid odor is likewise said to be neutralized by means of pulverized charcoal scattered in the spittoon; the best neutralizer is probably the Permanganate of Potash.

In obstinate cases *Secale cornutum* 3 to 6 may prove useful, especially if hemorrhage sets in accompanied by collapse, rapid prostration, coldness of the extremities, exhausting diarrhœa, delirium, vertigo, sopor. If this remedy does not produce an improvement, *Ergotin* 1 may be tried, which acts with more power and intensity.

Skoda recommends inhalations of turpentine, one drachm to two drachms of hot water, two to four times a day. Niemeyer thinks that these inhalations are only of use if the gangrene sets in in the neighborhood of bronchiectatic caverns.

Next to the internal remedies we must not forget suitable dietetic measures. To maintain the general constitution, we have to place the patient upon an invigorating diet and feed him on generous wines, Hock or Claret, good ale, provide for adequate ventilation of the sick-room, frequent fumigations with vinegar, purification of the air by means of Chloride of lime or Permanganate of Potash, and sprinkling the bed-linen, floor, etc., with vinegar or a solution of the Chloride of lime, Kreosote or Permanganate of Potassa. H.]

11. Œdema Pulmonum, Hydrops Pulmonum.

Œdema of the Lungs, Dropsy of the Lungs.

This consists in a serous transudation into the pulmonary cells and into the finer bronchial ramifications.

Anatomical Characteristics. We distinguish an *acute*, rapidly-developing œdema of the lungs, and a *chronic* œdema. Sometimes the œdema extends over a large surface, even over both lungs; at times it is merely local, circumscribed.

In the acute form of œdema the lungs are very much engorged, the parenchyma is very tense, so that an impression with the finger is at once effaced again; on the cut surface a fine-frothy, reddish or even dark-red, dim and not quite thin serum flows out, containing a good deal of albumen; the air seems to be entirely expelled, and the pulmonary tissue is easily torn.

In the chronic form of pulmonary œdema the lungs are not in a state of hyperæmia, but pale and tough, an impression with the finger remains; the serum is much less frothy, not at all so in the higher grades of the disease; it is of a yellowish-pale color, fluid, clear and contains but a small portion of albumen. Gradually the air leaves the pulmonary cells altogether; these cells and the fine bronchial ramifications are filled with a serous fluid.

On opening the thorax, the œdematous lungs do not collapse, they are puffed up and heavy. The larger the quantity of serum in the cells, the more air is expelled from them.

Etiology. Œdema of the lungs is generally only a secondary disease, arising in the course of other morbid processes.

Acute œdema, which is also designated as serous pneumonia or hydro-pneumonia, most commonly results from catarrhal fluxions or congestion. It sets in most frequently in the course of acute bronchial catarrhs, bronchial croup, acute exanthemata, such as measles, scarlatina, smallpox, etc., in the course of typhus; pulmonary œdema may set in in consequence of collateral congestion in the course of pneumonia, pleuritis, pneumothorax, emphysema, etc.

Chronic œdema of the lungs most commonly develops itself in consequence of passive hyperæmia in the course of diseases of the left auriculo-ventricular orifice, and hypertrophy of the right heart; in the course of pulmonary tuberculosis, carcinoma of the lungs, Bright's disease, infiltration of the bronchial glands, etc., chronic œdema of the lungs is almost always complicated with œdema of the lower extremities, or with hydrothorax, ascites. In such cases an apparently trivial cause, such as a cold, a physical exertion, a sudden outburst of passion, etc., is sufficient to give rise suddenly to a very general œdema of the lungs of which death may be the speedy result.

Acute œdema most frequently sets in during the death-struggle in the most diversified diseases.

Symptoms. The first important and striking symptom is the dyspnœa; it may attain a very high degree, is most commonly associated with the sensation of an oppressive weight under the sternum which does not abate by any change of position; at the same time the expression in the countenance is one of anxiety, and the *mobility of the thorax is less*, in consequence of which the patients at times sit up erect, at other times rest on their arms and again stretch their heads forward, in order to facilitate the breathing. The cough is spasmodic, the expectoration is exceedingly profuse, of a frothy-serous consistence, sometimes pale and at other times dark-red; moist râles are heard in the whole chest; cyanosis shows itself first in the face and afterwards on the extremities.

Gradually the sensation of suffocation increases in violence, the expectoration becomes less, the rattling becomes louder and is heard even at a distance; little by little, in consequence of the poisoning of the blood by carbonic acid, the patient becomes soporous, he is no longer able to cough up the sputa, because the muscular apparatus is semi-paralysed; the cough is less frequent, the breathing becomes more and more superficial and shorter. Finally collapse sets in, the cheeks become livid, a rattling is heard in the trachea, and the patients die of asphyxia.

If the œdema is extensive, and the air has been driven out of a large portion of the lungs, the percussion-sound is muffled or tympanitic; as long as air remains in the œdematous portion, the percussion-sound remains unaltered. The local or circumscribed œdema on percussion frequently yields no alteration of the sound; if the cells are entirely filled with serum, the percussion-sound may be dull and empty; if situated at the apex of the lungs, this condition of the cells may be confounded with tuberculous infiltrations. Auscultation generally reveals all sorts of râles, except consonan' râles.

The symptoms of acute œdema of the lungs sometimes set in with so much rapidity and violence that one symptom seems to chase the other.

If acute œdema sets in in consequence of collateral congestion in portions of lung that had hitherto remained free from the existing pneumonia, pleuritis, etc., new febrile motions generally appear, accompanied by a more or less high grade of dyspnœa and fine râles in the recently-invaded portions of the lungs which, unless speedily counter-acted, are soon succeeded by the above-described signs of pulmonary œdema.

In chronic œdema the above-described symptoms develop themselves much more slowly, and they are variously modified by the primary disease.

Generally the œdema is complicated with œdema of the extremities, sexual organs, serous transsudations into the pleura or peritoneum; percussion yields a dull sound in the lower portions of the lungs.

Course, Termination, Prognosis. Acute œdema generally develops itself with more or less rapidity, and if the symptoms are very violent, may soon terminate fatally. This is most frequently the case, if henomena of collateral congestion set in during the course of inflammatory processes in the lungs, pleura, heart, etc. This termination was designated by the ancients as apoplexia pulmonum serosa. In such cases the highest degree of dyspnœa very speedily develops itself; amid a constantly-increasing anxiety and restlessness the patients soon become cyanotic, cough a great deal, and expectorate a quantity of frothy serum, more or less tinged with blood; suddenly they become quiet; sopor and tracheal rattling set in, and they die very suddenly of asphyxia consequent upon poisoning of the blood by carbonic acid.

Chronic œdema of the lungs generally runs a slow course, and often has remissions; sometimes life is suddenly terminated by an acute effusion. If the constitutional vigor is well preserved, chronic œdema can be removed more easily than an acute attack which is generally very dangerous; for this reason the prognosis, as far as danger to life is concerned, is more favorable in a case of chronic than acute œdema.

Treatment. In all diseases in the course of which acute pulmonary œdema may set in, the supervention of a sudden dyspnœa with a characteristic cough and sputa, deserve our most serious attention. If a more or less violent fever supervenes during the dyspnœa, we at once give *Aconite* 3, every quarter of an hour, or every half hour or hour; the result is generally favorable. At any rate the exhibition of this drug secures us the advantage of moderating the violence of the œdema, and giving the physician time to arrange a suitable course of treatment.

As soon as fine râles are heard, and the dyspnœa is increasing, even without any sputa, we give at once *Phosphorus* 3, continuing this remedy even if a copious frothy serum, tinged with blood, is expectorated. This remedy sometimes has a brilliant effect; often in a few hours the whole trouble is ended.

If the cough is strikingly spasmodic, we very soon perceive a bluish color of the lips and tongue; in such a case there is great danger on account of the capillary engorgement that threatens to set in. In such a case we give *Ipecac.* 3; if no improvement has taken place in a few hours, we prescribe *Arsenicum* 3, or *Lachesis* 6. We have seen very fine effects from these remedies. If coarse râles are heard over the whole chest; if the characteristic sputa are very copious; if soon after the expulsion of the sputa râles are again heard with equal force and distinctness; if cyanotic phenomena are becoming manifest, and a high degree of dyspnœa and suffocative anguish torment the patient, we give *Tartarus emet.* 3, or *Veratrum* 3 every quarter of an hour. The result of these agents is of course very doubtful, on account of the air having already been in a great measure expelled from the cells owing to the vast extent of the œdema. If the strength begins to fail; if the cough grows less and the expectoration is more difficult, we again try *Phosphorus* which we now use as a restorative. Very frequently *Phosphorus* induces an increased desire to cough, with more copious expectoration and momentary relief; soon after all the former symptoms set in with more threatening intensity, and the patients are in danger of being suffocated by the mucus. This is the moment when an emetic may produce a marvelously favorable effect. Let not the use of an emetic be delayed until the strength is entirely exhausted and the patients have sunk into a state of sopor. As long as a certain degree of reactive power remains, we need not hesitate to give *Ipecacuanha* at the rate of five grains per dose, or *Emetin* half a grain per dose, every five minutes, until mucus is vomited up in copious quantities, after which many patients begin to improve.

As soon as we notice the first signs of drowsiness, we give *Ammonium carbonicum* 1 to 3; this remedy may prevent poisoning of the blood by carbonic acid.

A collateral congestion setting in during the course of pneumonia, scarlatina, pleuritis, carditis, etc., may become associated, beside the above-mentioned febrile and catarrhal pneumonia, with such a violent determination of blood to the brain, that cerebral apoplexy may be apprehended. In such a case we employ *Belladonna* or *Glonoine*, [also *Veratrum viride* in large doses, no less than five drops of the tincture every half hour, H.], together with applications of ice to the head; if these remedies have no sort of effect, we do not hesitate, as a last desperate resort, to bleed the patient. [We do not believe that under the use of Aconite, Belladonna and Veratrum viride, in appropriate doses, the necessity for bleeding will ever occur. II.]

If there is insufficiency or stenosis of the mitral valve, we give *Pulsatilla* or *Kali carb.* If œdema of the extremities, genital organs, etc., is present, we resort to *Arsenicum, Lachesis, Digitalis.* For serous effusions in the pleura or peritoneum we give according to the prevailing symptoms *Arsenicum, Helleborus, China, Scilla, Sulphur,* [also *Apocynum cannabinum,* H.], but without much hope of success. II.]

12. Asthma.

Under this name so many and such diversified pathological conditions have been comprehended from time immemorial that it would be difficult to write a treatise on this disease corresponding with the definition of asthma entertained by former pathologists.

If we omit the various conditions that develop asthmatic phenomena which have not generally the peculiar characteristics of nervous paroxysms, the etiology of asthma can be reduced to the following points: in the first place the affection is purely idiopathic, developing neither any special pathological alterations, nor traceable to any particular exciting causes. The patients are attacked at indefinite, much less frequently at regular periods. Asthma is likewise met with as a partial manifestation of other nervous affections, especially of hysteria and hypochondria, in which case it has likewise to be regarded as a primary affection occurring in peculiar circumstances. Finally asthma may be caused by topical impressions; we see asthma result with comparative fre. exposure to Copper, Arsenic, Iodine, Lead, and to the dust of Ipecacuanha. The most heterogeneous circumstances are assigned as the exciting causes of this disease; whether rightly or wrongly is difficult to decide in view of the utter absence of regularity in the occurrence of the paroxysms. It is certainly a supposable case that the attacks can be excited by the direct action of irritants upon the lungs, more especially by vapors and dust; but it is strange that this irritation does not seem controlled by any law. Intense emotions are undoubtedly one of the most frequent causes of asthma. Of undeniable influence is the condition of the atmosphere in a thermometrical as well as barometrical point of view; the attacks are most easily excited during a high state of the thermometer and a low state of the barometer. Electricity likewise plays an important part in regard to asthma, for the attacks are very apt to be excited previous to severe thunder-storms. Regarding a predisposition to asthma, it is certain that the male sex is most liable to it, and that most cases of asthma occur between the age of pubescence and the age of fifty. Constitutional influences seem almost null, thin as well as corpulent, feeble as well as robust individuals being attacked. In many cases we have undeniable evidence of the hereditary character of the disease.

Symptoms and Course. Asthma consists of a series of paroxysms separated from each other by intervals which at first are absolutely free from all symptoms of the disease. Hence, we have to consider first the paroxysm itself, and subsequently its effect upon the general organism.

The attack either sets in with distinct precursory symptoms, among which great exhaustion and an increasing oppression of breathing are the most common; or else, the attack sets in at once with great violence. It is remarkable, although it cannot be accounted for upon physiological principles, that the attack generally sets in at night, most frequently in the evening, scarcely ever in the day-time. This feature is, however, peculiar to all purely nervous affections, the cause of which may be the circumstance that the activity of the nervous system is constantly increasing towards night. Very often the patients are roused from sleep when the attack sets in like an attack of night-mare. They experience a constrictive sensation on the chest, with inability to draw a long breath; this sensation increases in proportion as the patient makes an effort to overcome it, and often leads to terrible dyspnœa during which he strains every muscle that can aid him in performing the act of respiration. At the commencement of the attack the cervical muscles are put upon the stretch, whereas the thorax is less called into requisition. This is owing to the fact that the expirations are less complete than the inspirations, in consequence of which the lungs gradually become filled with air to such an extent that the edge of the liver is felt considerably below its normal line. During the attack percussion yields a normal sound, whereas auscultation reveals before the paroxysm, and always immediately after its access, in the place of the vesicular respiratory murmur, wheezing, hissing, and occasionally rattling sounds, that sometimes are loud enough to be heard at a distance. That the patients look pale and sometimes have a bluish or livid appearance; that a cold perspiration breaks out on them; that the temperature of the skin is lower than usual; that the beats of the heart are much feebler and increase in frequency; and that the urine is frequently discharged involuntarily, is easily accounted for by the extreme dyspnœa. After the attack has lasted one to four hours, or even longer, its decrease manifests itself by a return of the vesicular respiratory murmur, and by a diminution of the wheezing and hissing sounds. The sensation of tightness sometimes disappears quite suddenly and at other times very gradually; a cough sets in accompanied by the expectoration of a small quantity of mucus; or violent eructations, or vomiting, with emission of flatulence, may take place, after which the patients often feel well again, except a lassitude that may continue for days. In other cases the paroxysm does not cease altogether, but abates for a longer or shorter period, which remission is again succceeded by a full attack of asthma, until, after several remissions and exacerbations, which may continue for weeks, a complete intermission takes place.

The course of such a disease varies according as the paroxysms set in at longer or shorter periods. In proportion as the disease lasts longer, the intermissions become shorter, the paroxysms increase in intensity, and structural changes in the lungs and heart take place which, in their turn, promote the disease. Emphysema, chronic bronchial catarrh, dilatation of the heart are very common results of asthma, which are easily mistaken for causes of the disease. A single paroxysm, no matter how violent, is not of itself dangerous, provided the paroxysm does not develop preëxisting conditions of apoplexy into a full attack. In the long run, however, asthma always becomes dangerous in consequence of the lesions which it occasions, and which are so much more certain, the more violent the single paroxysms are.

The termination of this affection cannot be determined beforehand. In many cases the paroxysms decrease at a more advanced age and finally disappear altogether; or else, they are replaced by pulmonary emphysema and its consequences. It is difficult to promise an early and complete recovery, for the paroxysms recur sometimes after the lapse of years. Death is a very unfrequent termination of this disease.

The prognosis, so far as the preservation of life is concerned, is very favorable; as far as a cure is concerned, the result of medical treatment must be considered uncertain. In contrast with Old Physic, which has no remedy for asthma, Homœopathy can at least boast of having achieved some brilliant results.

The *treatment* has to aim at controlling the present paroxysm and at curing the disease.

Respecting the possibility of shortening the paroxysm, it is doubtful whether, in view of the uncertainty how long an attack will last, any medicine can be relied upon for the accomplishment of such a result. If the paroxysms only last a few hours, it is immaterial whether we give any medicine; as regards paroxysms that have remissions and exacerbations before a complete intermission takes place, it would, of course, be desirable to relieve them. Our own experience compels us, however, to confess that, in this respect, we have no very brilliant results to brag of. The same remedies that seemed to have a good effect in one attack, did nothing at all in the next, although the symptoms seemed precisely the same. If we are called to a case, we give a little medicine to quiet the relatives, but for a cure we depend solely upon the treatment during the intervals. However, in order to avoid the appearance of a purely subjective exclusivism, we will mention some of the remedies that are most commonly used at the beginning of the attack, at the same time referring to the remedies that will be mentioned by and by, and which may likewise be used for a single paroxysm.

Belladonna, when the attack is accompanied by congestion of the head and an affection of the larynx, in the case of plethoric individuals, children and females of an irritable disposition.

Aconite, in the case of plethoric, active individuals, with severe cerebral hyperæmia, after mental excitement, the face being very much flushed.

Chamomilla, when the attack is caused by a severe fit of passion, with flatulence, particularly for paroxysms of hysteric asthma, or for children during the period of dentition.

Nux vomica, for attacks caused by nervous excitement, spirits, much eating, hysteria, hypochondria, inhalations of dust, with congestions to the head, distention of the abdomen, especially of the stomach, improvement by a change of position, night-mare; the attack is preceded by signs of congestion of the chest.

Pulsatilla, for asthma caused by the vapors of Sulphur, by uræmia, menstrual disturbances and hysteria, with copious vomiting of mucus, which affords relief, vertigo, sudden prostration with palpitations of the heart.

Moschus, for asthma without cough, with a violent feeling of constriction in the throat as if the glottis were involved in the attack, in the case of hysterical, hypochondriac, irritable individuals.

We might extend this list by adding other remedies; but since we believe that the indications for their use are mostly illusory, we will content ourselves with mentioning their bare names. *Cannabis, Colchicum, Tartarus stibiatus, Cocculus, Staphysagria, Nux moschata, Veratrum, Opium, Phosphorus, Nitri acidum,* etc. Many of these remedies owe their use to the mistaken notion that a catarrh or any other affection of the respiratory organs with asthmatic symptoms is real asthma. The remedies from which most may be expected during the attack itself, are *Belladonna, Cannabis, Moschus,* and *Opium.* Opium especially sometimes renders substantial aid without it being necessary to employ large doses on this account. *Morphia,* 2d trituration, two or three grains at a dose, exerts a sufficiently powerful effect, and if this dose is not sufficient, the remedy can only do harm. A copious secretion of mucus always counter-indicates Opium. *Cannabis* likewise only palliates by virtue of its narcotic properties, and hence will have to be given in a more massive dose; this remedy is altogether unreliable.

As we said before, we have no great confidence in the use of any remedy during the paroxysm which we compare to an epileptic paroxysm for which very little can be done by treatment. Nevertheless we should not remain idle spectators during an attack, since it is often possible to relieve the patient by all sorts of external applications. It is important, for instance, to regulate the patient's posture. Some people will not allow him to leave his bed; yet it is of great importance and affords great relief to the patient, if every respiratory movement is brought into play, as much as possible, by a change of position. For this reason the lower extremities should not be kept in a horizontal position, but should be placed vertically, and pressed against any object in order to facilitate the action of the dorsal as well as abdominal muscles. All tight clothing should be removed; if the patient is in his senses, he attends to this without being told. The temperature of the room must not be kept too low, for the reason that the paroxysm always excites a profuse perspiration; nor should it be too high, and, above every thing else, the air should be kept sufficiently moist. If we are called to a patient who has had a number of attacks, we shall find that he keeps every thing on hand which, by its direct action upon the lungs, may relieve a paroxysm; nor can it be denied that relief is often procured by such means during one and even several paroxysms. They are generally powerful domestic stimulants, such as the smelling and inhaling of the spirits of *Ammonia;* inhalations of the spirits of Turpentine or of Camphor evaporated on hot water; the inhalation of the fumes of burnt nitre-paper, feathers and Sulphur. We have tried the last remedy in our own case. That in such cases it is not the specific action of the inhaled substance, but the local stimulation that affords relief, is evident from the circumstance that the effect is only palliative and transitory and that inhalations of Chloroform, which have a direct narcotic effect, are scarcely ever borne by asthmatic individuals. Substances that are used for smoking, constitute another series of remedies. In this case, however, we deal with thoroughly homœopathic remedies, such as Tobacco, Iodine, Stramonium, Hyoscyamus. Tobacco can, of course, be useful only to persons who do not smoke, ladies, for instance, to whom we recommend for such purposes the small paper-cigarettes used by Russian and Spanish ladies. Smokers, on the contrary, mix the cut leaves of Stramonium or Hyoscyamus with their tobacco, sometimes with surprising effect; or they smoke Iodine-cigarettes. The use of these remedies is justifiable, because they afford relief to the patient, nor should they be discarded until we have better remedies to recommend in their stead. Very often we accomplish our purpose with the inhalation of simple vapors of water. The method of introducing appropriate remedies directly into the respiratory organs by means of an inhaler, has not yet been satisfactorily verified as a superior proceeding.

The main-point in the treatment of asthma is to meet the disease in its totality. As a matter of course, the selection of the remedy is not only governed by the symptoms between the paroxysms, but likewise by the paroxysm itself and by the constitution of the patient, and it is this indispensable consideration of so many and such varied conditions that renders the selection of the proper remedy exceedingly difficult. In the subsequent paragraphs we only furnish short indications for the selection of the most important remedies, since it is impossible to present these indications with anything like a satisfactory completeness.

Arsenicum album is undoubtedly the safest remedy for asthma; it not only corresponds to the simple spasmodic, uncomplicated asthma, but likewise to the secondary forms of asthma which owe their existence to the most diversified affections of a more primary character. Arsenic is even used a great deal in domestic practice and is highly commended by Old School practitioners. This remedy likewise shows very strikingly how the constant physiological effects of a drug can be employed with mathematical certainty as remedial agents when employed according to the law of similarity. In slow arsenical poisonings, asthma always occurs without an exception. We dispense with the enumeration of individual symptoms, since every somewhat violent attack of asthma corresponds to Arsenic. Nor can we particularize the cases where asthma occurs as a mere symptom, since in such cases the selection of the remedy is chiefly determined by the character of the primary affection. We will state, however, that, in the asthmatic paroxysms of tuberculous patients, Arsenic has always left us in the lurch. It is principally indicated by the following symptoms: The paroxysm always sets in towards midnight or shortly after; it seems to be governed by a tolerably fixed type, although asthmatic paroxysms occurring without any typical regularity do not exclude Arsenic; it reaches its acme with unusual rapidity. The more the patients seem on the point of suffocating; the more painful and distressing their restlessness; the more wheezing and louder their respiration, the more Arsenicum will be found appropriate. Accessory circumstances are: sudden access of a high grade of collapse with lividity of the countenance, cold perspiration and a very frequent and small pulse; palpitation of the heart; distension of the abdomen consequent upon the attack; involuntary emission of the urine; unconquerable dread of death; the paroxysm is excited by changes of temperature, atmospheric influences, talking or laughing, going up stairs. The consequences of the attack remain for a long time, among which excessive debility and nervousness are most prominent. When given during the paroxysm, Arsenic sometimes exerts a magical effect, so that the patients fancy they have received Opium; although Arsenic does not by any means help in every case, yet it had better be tried in every case that we are called upon to treat. During the apyrexia, the remedy had better be administered at long intervals and in the higher attenuations, although the success which Old School practitioners have obtained with Fowler's solution justifies the conclusion that massive doses are likewise conducive to a cure. The danger is that massive doses may affect the stomach injuriously. Whether Arsenic possesses specific antidotal powers against asthma caused by other metals has not yet been determined.

Cuprum is likewise one of the substances which, in cases of slow poisoning, develops asthmatic symptoms. However, it has not proved of such decisive practical value as Arsenic, for the reason that it has not the significant indications of this agent. In our opinion, Cuprum is indicated by the following symptoms: The remedy is suitable to individuals with nervous, irritable, enfeebled constitutions, who are, moreover, disposed to spasms, whereas Arsenic is suitable rather to vigorous and plethoric persons; or it is suitable to children, especially if the paroxysms set in at night, or in consequence of exerting the respiratory organs, as for instance, after a coughing fit; the paroxysm very speedily reaches the acme of its intensity; other muscular bundles are involved in the convulsive attack; the attack is accompanied by a constant hacking, which aggravates the asthma; the attack terminates by vomiting; pallor of the countenance, with cold perspiration. The apyrexia is not perfect, but a slight degree of dyspnœa remains, or violent paroxysms of an almost dry cough set in, which likewise end in vomiting. The action of Copper in whooping-cough is evidence of its general adaptation to spasmodic affections of the lungs. We have never known Cuprum to be of any use for the paroxysm itself, so that we now limit the use of this drug exclusively to the intervals between the paroxysms.

As regards **Plumbum**, it has not yet been sufficiently tried either physiologically or practically to present clear indications for its use in asthma. Nevertheless, the affections of workers in lead show that they are very commonly affected with a violent asthma. Upon the whole, it bears great similarity to the copper-asthma, from which it is not so much distinguished by its local as by its general symptoms. We recommend the remedy more especially in the severe paroxysms of tuberculous individuals, and likewise for the form of asthma, which is accompanied at the outset by a profuse accumulation of gas in the bowels.

Iodium is likewise one of those agents which, among its symptoms of slow poisoning, numbers asthma as one of its constant phenomena. In our Materia Medica these effects of Iodine are pointed out very imperfectly, and the reader is very much disposed to combine the symptoms pointing to asthma with the symptoms denoting inflammation. In the "Deutschen Klinik" of 1856, three cases of Iodine-asthma are recorded, which are of considerable interest: The asthma set in after a protracted use of Iodine, whereas an acute intoxication with Iodine never causes asthma; the paroxysm sets in towards evening or more commonly about midnight and lasts about half an hour; in one case it commenced with intense symptoms of laryngismus stridulus; the paroxysm was succeeded by excessive lassitude and an irresistible desire to sleep. Nothwithstanding the violent difficulties of breathing, every sign of a material change in the respiratory organs is wanting; there is emaciation without any increase of the secretions; great nervousness and restlessness during the intervals. Hence, Iodine corresponds well with the purely nervous asthma, for which it has been prescribed more recently by several Old School practitioners, of course, in enormous doses. Except a few not very striking cures, homœopathic literature does not offer any cases of asthma successfully treated with Iodine.

Stannum may be tried if the attack supervenes during the existence of chronic catarrh, and the decrease of the attack is attended with a copious secretion of mucus. We do not find any where reports of striking cures with this agent.

Under quite similar circumstances **Zincum metallicum** will be found a suitable remedy; an additional indication for this drug is a copious accumulation of gas in the bowels during the paroxysm.

Spongia has so far been found useful only in asthma depending upon tuberculosis, but it has never effected a complete cessation, but only a marked diminution of the frequency and intensity of the attacks. The paroxysm is characterized by a marked contraction of the glottis, a wheezing respiration, with complete loss of voice. In a few hours the patient hacks up a substance resembling soaked sago.

Aurum certainly deserves more attention than it has yet received. It is particularly indicated in cases where it is not quite certain whether the heart is primarily or secondarily involved in the attack; the attack sets in with violent palpitation of the heart, great anxiety, and marked symptoms of pulmonary hyperæmia.

Among the vegetable remedies there are but few that we would recommend for the totality of the disease; most of them are solely adapted to the complicated forms of asthma. We confine ourselves to mentioning their names: *Ipecacuanha, Belladonna, Lycopodium, Bovista, Lactma virosa, Bryonia, Pulsatilla. Lobelia inflata* is more adapted to emphysema than to asthma. Opium sometimes affords striking benefit in paroxysms that occur during sleep.

In a variety of cases we have witnessed remarkably favorable results from the use of **Digitaline**. With this remedy alone we have radically cured frequently-recurring paroxysms of asthma of less protracted duration; in inveterate cases all that we have been able to accomplish with this agent, has been to diminish in some cases, although to a considerable extent, the intensity and frequency of the paroxysms. It is, therefore, with a good conscience that we can recommend this medicine for further trials in asthma, provided the following circumstances are kept in view: The asthma is altogether a primary affection, it is the purely nervous form, a genuine spasm of the bronchia; in such a case Digitaline will have the best effect as long as no catarrh, emphysema or structural change of the heart supervenes. Digitaline is, however, suitable even if these complications exist, to which it is, indeed, preëminently adapted. more especially to structural alterations of the right ventricle. A high degree of sanguineous stasis in the veins of the head, especially a violent throbbing-pressing headache during and after the attack. Palpitations of the heart, especially if the attack is preceded by them. The asthma attacks irritable individuals with weak nerves, more particularly persons who have been guilty of sexual excesses. We do not simply mean persons who had been addicted to self-abuse, for we have known a married man who contracted asthmatic attacks in consequence of excessive sexual intercourse, and who was decidedly benefitted by Digitaline. The influence of Digitaline over the male sexual organs is extraordinary, and, in this case, we effected a truly radical cure, as is likewise evident from what we stated when speaking of the diseases of the male sexual organs. The influence of Digitaline over the female sexual organs, especially in its bearing upon the nervous system, is so difficult to define that we are as yet without any decided data regarding this matter. We always administer this remedy in the second or third trituration, giving never more than one grain of the former in the morning before breakfast, never at night, for the reason that sleep is generally disturbed by Digitaline. Nor is it necessary to give a dose every day; a dose every two or three days is sufficient. These precautions are important to avoid medicinal effects and homœopathic aggravations. Unless these precautionary measures are adopted, a remedy the great importance of which has not yet been sufficiently recognized, might easily fall into discredit.

Notwithstanding we believe that we have indicated the most important remedies for asthma, yet if the list of these remedies were to be exhausted, a great many other drugs might be added to it. In mentioning the following additional remedies, we recall to the reader's attention the fact that most of the remedies employed for asthma owe their recommendation to coexisting complications. The following remedies may be compared in particular cases: *Sulphur, Ferrum, Argentum, Bromum, Sepia, Calcarea carbonica, Carbo vegetabilis, Causticum, Lachesis, Asafœtida, Tartarus stibiatus.*

Beside medicinal agents a few other means to reach the disease, are at our command. These are remedies that invigorate the constitution generally and strengthen the tone of the nervous system specially, such as cold baths, cold ablutions, the wet sheet, living in mountainous regions or generally in the open air, etc. Of more importance are the means that have more particularly or even exclusively a local effect. Among these remedial means the movement-cure holds a prominent rank; it sometimes proves efficient where medicinal influences seemed entirely powerless, more especially in the case of women and likewise in the case of men who had broken down their strength by an effeminate and luxurious mode of living. The movement-cure has likewise the great advantage of acting favorably upon the constitution. The action of compressed air has likewise a surprising effect; however, it is as yet impossible to state what particular form of asthma is specially adapted to this curative influence. According to all probability this remedy is particularly adapted to shorten the protracted length of the paroxysms. Living on high mountain-tops has a favorable effect only in exceptional cases; the same statement applies to sea-air and surf-bathing.

C. DISEASES OF THE DIAPHRAGM.

We transcribe this chapter from Kafka. He only treats of inflammation, spasm and hernia of the diaphragm; atrophy, paralysis and tonic spasm of the diaphragm being generally partial manifestations of other pathological processes.

1. Diaphragmitis, Inflammation of the Diaphragm.

[It consists in an inflammation of the serous covering of the diaphragm, either on its thoracic or abdominal side.

This inflammation is never an idiopathic disease, but always occurs in the course of pleuritis (pleuritis diaphragmatica), or in the course of peritonitis (peritonitis diaphragmatica).

According to the statement of older authors the following phenomena are characteristic of diaphragmitis: continued, violent fever; burning, stinging, tearing and contractive pains all over the diaphragm, the pain encircling the body like a hoop; during an inspiration the pain is felt lower down, during an expiration higher up; it is aggravated by coughing, talking, and by every motion of the patient, rendering a deep inspiration impossible; the breathing is hurried, anxious, superficial; it is performed with the thorax, while the abdominal muscles remain passive; distressing singultus, vomiting of a green substance, great difficulty of swallowing, sometimes hydrophobia, delirium, spasmodic laughter, finally collapse, etc.

From the presence of these symptoms in the course of a pleuritis or peritonitis we may conclude that the diaphragm is involved in the inflammation. Idiopathic diaphragmitis has not yet been met with. The intensity of the symptoms is generally extreme; a physical exploration yields no result.

The course of the disease is generally very acute, the prognosis very unfavorable.

The etiology is the same as that of pleuritis or peritonitis. The treatment is likewise the same as that of pleuritis or peritonitis. It is only if out-of-the-way symptoms exist that they have to be met by special remedies.

The most troublesome symptom is the distressing singultus. For this symptom we recommend *Belladonna* 3, especially if complicated with difficulty of swallowing, risus sardonicus, delirium and vomiting. If, in a few hours, this remedy does not afford the desired help, we give the *Sulphate of Atropine* 3, or *Hyoscyamus* 3.

Bryonia 3 is an excellent remedy, if the inflammation proceeds from the pleura and is attended with considerable dyspnœa, violent pains during respiration, difficulties of swallowing, cerebral irritation.

If the vomiting is a prominent symptom, as is generally the case when peritonitis is present, we resort to *Belladonna*, *Nux vomica*, *Veratrum*. In obstinate cases we have recourse to *Opium*.

A very disagreeable symptom is the spasmodic laughter, for

which we recommend: *Belladonna, Hyoscyamus, Ignatia* and *Cuprum metallicum* 6.

2. Singultus, Hiccup.

This is owing to a spasmodic contraction of the diaphragm, during which the air is drawn in through the contracted glottis with a shrill and short sound.

The hiccup either originates in the nervous centres, as during a general erethism, neuroses, especially in the case of hysteric and hypochondriac patients; or when accompanying cerebral diseases, such as cerebral anæmia consequent upon long-lasting, exhausting diseases or upon considerable losses of blood and other animal fluids, as well as upon violent psychical impressions, such as fright, anger, etc.

Or else, it is simply a reflex-phenomenon, as during diseases of the pleura and pericardium.

Consensual singultus may occur during diseases of the stomach, liver, pharynx, intestinal canal, etc.

In the case of children it often occurs in consequence of a cold, or acid stomach.

Singultus occurring during cerebral anæmia consequent upon chronic diseases, such as carcinoma, Bright's disease, tuberculosis, etc., or upon exhausting diseases, such as typhus, cholera, or upon pleuritis with profuse exudation, likewise upon pericarditis and upon exhausting diarrhœa, is always a very dangerous symptom that may continue for days and finally increase to convulsions.

Treatment. A passing hiccup is scarcely ever noticed; only if it lasts too long and becomes too severe, medical treatment may have to be resorted to.

In cases of simple hiccup it may be arrested by stopping the breathing for some time, or by drinking a little cold water, by fixing one's attention upon a certain object, such as: holding a key in one's hand, by a systematic crossing of the fingers of both hands; by a sudden surprise, or such domestic remedies as eating a little sugar, magnesia, ice, etc.

Infants who have taken cold, have to be warmed, after which they should be put to the breast; if their stomachs are acid, we give them *Calcar.* 6 or *Nux vom.* 6; if they are affected with intestinal catarrh, we give them *Chamomilla* 3, or *Rheum* 3. A domestic remedy that is frequently made use of, is *calcined Magnesia*, as much as will cover the point of a knife morning and evening.

In one case, where not one of these remedies would help, a teaspoonful of recently prepared lime-water removed the spasm.

If the singultus is intense and lasts a long time, we have to select remedies that correspond to the co-existing pathological conditions or to the exciting cause. For the nervous singultus of hysteric or hypochondriac individuals, we give according to the symptoms: *Nux vomica*, *Ignatia*, *Belladonna* and *Hyoscyamus*, *Nux moschata* and *Natrum muriaticum*.

For singultus consequent upon a fit of chagrin, we give: *Chamom.*, *Ignatia*, *Pulsatilla*.

For singultus occasioned by diseases of the stomach and liver: *Bryonia*, *Nux vomica*, *Pulsat.*, *Natrum muriaticum* and *Sulphur*.

For painful singultus caused by inflammation of adjoining organs: *Belladonna*, *Hyoscyamus*, *Atropine*, *Opium* 1 or 2.

In a case of consensual singultus consequent upon spasm of the œsophagus, accompanied by nausea, *Veratrum* 3 has rendered us good service.

We are much less successful in the selection and use of remedies for singultus occasioned by exhaustion of the vital forces and cerebral anæmia. In such cases we have succeeded in relieving the patient by *Ammonium carbon.* 3, *Phosphorus* 3, and in desperate cases by *Moschus* 1.

As external remedies practitioners recommend: laying grated horse-radish upon the epigastrium, dropping ether upon the pit of the stomach, painting this region with the oil of chloroform, one drachm to two drachms of almond-oil, and in desperate cases the inhalation of ether or chloroform.

3. Hernia of the Diaphragm.

Accidents of this kind originate in rupture of the diaphragm occasioned by traumatic causes, or in strangulations of the thoracic or abdominal viscera in the natural openings of the diaphragm. They occur more frequently on the left than on the right side.

The phenomena in the thoracic range are: dyspnœa, cough, pain in the chest, singultus, suffocative paroxysms, fainting fits.

On the side of the abdominal organs we notice vomiting, colicky pains, obstinate constipation, sometimes symptoms of ileus.

If the strangulation is partial, the symptoms appear slowly and disappear equally slowly. If the constriction is very violent and sudden, the symptoms set in with equal violence, and life may be in the greatest danger.

The worst symptoms are those of ileus, which we meet with *Nux vomica* 3 and *Opium* 1. Tepid baths, and in severe cases frictions or inhalations of Chloroform are excellent adjuvants. H.]

D. DISEASES OF THE PLEURA.

1. Pleuritis, Pleurisy.

Inflammation of the Pleura.

Inflammatory affections of the pleura are not by any means rare occurrences; yea, the frequent adhesions of the lungs to the thorax revealed by post-mortem examinations, show that pleuritic affections are not only very frequent, but that they run their course unobserved. The more trifling inflammatory phenomena are without any practical value, nor do they ever constitute an object of treatment; for this reason we here treat only of the more acute forms of pleurisy with copious exudation.

Pleurisies of this character are scarcely ever really primary diseases; in the majority of cases they are of a secondary nature. The etiology of primary pleuritis is somewhat obscure, unless the disease is caused by some direct and mechanically acting agency. A most frequent cause is said to be a violent cold; but the case is here as in pneumonia, the connection is taken for granted rather than proven. The more frequent occurrence of pleuritis during peculiar states of the weather justifies the conclusion that atmospheric conditions exert a decided influence upon the origin of this disease. To designate such inflammations as rheumatic, is in so far justifiable to some extent at least, as acute rheumatisms occur epidemically at the same time. As a rule, primary pleuritis may, like peritonitis, be regarded as a rare disease.

On the other hand, pleuritis as a complication or secondary affection, is exceedingly frequent. All inflammatory pulmonary affections, even hyperæmia of more than ordinary extent, if occurring near the surface of the lungs, develop pleuritis which is generally confined to a very limited space, but may likewise be very extensive and violent. Inflammatory affections of the heart, more particularly of the pericardium, may lead to pleuritis. Acute rheumatism and peritonitis, and likewise acute exanthemata, easily result in the development of pleuritis. Among chronic affections the following may occasion the disease: Pulmonary tuberculosis, pulmonary abscess, suppuration of the vertebræ and ribs, Bright's disease. The occurrence of pleuritis during the stage of convalescence in severe acute affections, in pyæmia and generally in diseases characterized by marked signs of a septic condition of the blood, is a remarkable fact which does not admit of any further explanation. Like peritonitis, so pleuritis is superinduced in its worst and most extensive form by the intrusion of foreign substances into the pleural cavity, most commonly by the effusion of pus from a superficial cavern or from a suppurating bone.

Symptoms and Course. The peculiarity of certain phenomena in a case of pleurisy can only be understood by an anatomical analysis of this process, on which account we premise a concise sketch of the same.

By pleuritis we understand the deposition of an exudation upon the free surface in the cavity of the pleura. As in every other inflammation so we find here, at the outset, an hyperæmic condition of the cellular tissue situated under the pleura. This hyperæmia occurs most generally in striæ or clusters, scarcely ever over a large extent, and very frequently exhibits small ecchymosic spots. It is from these hyperæmic centres that the exudation proceeds over the free surface. According to its constituent principles the exudation is generally distinguished in four different forms which, however, cannot be rigorously separated from each other, but commingle in various ways. The first form is the so-called plastic form, where a small quantity of a highly fibrinous exudation is deposited upon the free surface of the pleura as a pseudo-membrane which, by coalescing with the membrane on the opposite side of the pleura, causes both sides of the pleural cavity to adhere without any further complications. This process occurs very commonly in pneumonia, but likewise on other occasions with so few symptoms that it is placed beyond the reach of therapeutic definitions. The second form is the sero-plastic form. The exudation consists of fibrin with which a more considerable quantity of serum is commingled. This form has the exuded membranes of the first form, but they are generally more extensive and thicker, and the pleural cavity contains an exudation of a yellow-green serum which sometimes weighs several pounds and in which more or less copious flocks of coagulated fibrin are seen floating. The copiousness of the plastic exudation increases the tendency to adhesions which are sometimes so extensive that they enclose the exuded fluid as within a capsule or sometimes as within a net consisting of a number of meshes and cavities. The third form is the purulent exudation, empyema or pyothorax. In this form the effusion may consist of mere pus, or serum may be mixed up with it in greater or less quantity. This form either characterizes an uncommonly acute pleuritis, as it is often observed in pyæmia, and where pus forms in a very short time; or else this third form is gradually developed from the second form in consequence of the solid constituents of this form being converted into pus. The further changes occurring in this form are absorption which is, however, scarcely ever as complete as in the other forms and generally leaves callous thickenings behind, or else enclosure of the fluid within a capsule which is a very common event, or finally invasion of the parts surrounding the suppurating process. In consequence of this invasion the pleura is perforated and the pus is discharged through the thoracic walls into the abdominal cavity or even into the bronchia. Recovery from such an accident is a very rare event. The fourth form, where scarcely anything but serum is effused, occurs very rarely, but is important for the reason that this serous exudation generally exceeds all others in quantity, exerts the most violent pressure upon the lungs and heart, and that its reabsorption is on this account exceedingly difficult. The hemorrhagic exudation does not constitute, strictly speaking, a distinct form, because a somewhat considerable effusion of blood in any of the above-described four forms may determine an hemorrhagic exudation. The ichorous dissolution of the exudation only takes place during the severest prostration of the organism as a consequence of general decomposition, less frequently if the pleural cavity comes in contact with atmospheric air.

It is absolutely impossible to draw a permanently and universally true picture of pleuritis; the symptoms characterizing an attack of pleuritis, vary greatly in intensity as well as extent; many symptoms are sometimes entirely wanting, whereas in other cases they are most prominently present. However inasmuch as the symptomatic differences of pleuritis are mostly depending upon the quality of the exudation, we subjoin a superficial sketch of these differences and shall discuss essential details in subsequent paragraphs.

The plastic exudation exists seldom as an idiopathic affection;

it generally accompanies other diseases, more particularly pneumonia. Inasmuch, however, as it is scarcely ever, even when existing as an idiopathic disease, accompanied by violent fever, we may suppose, that even where it exists as a complication, it does not contribute much to an increase of the fever. On the other hand it is precisely this form that causes the most violent pain which is very much increased by every somewhat more expansive movement of the thorax and of the body generally, more particularly by coughing, and which very frequently renders even percussion painful. After the lapse of at most a week the pain disappears again entirely; but the physical signs, of which we shall treat by and by, sometimes remain for some time after.

It is more especially the sero-plastic exudation that furnishes the picture of an idiopathic acute pleuritis. Like all other more extensive inflammatory processes, it almost always sets in with a severe chill followed by considerable increase of the pulse and temperature, attended with headache, intense thirst, loss of appetite, and almost immediately an intense pain in the inflamed region of the pleura. The pain generally decreases in proportion as the effusion increases in quantity. As the exudation increases the breathing of course becomes shorter, and a distressing cough sometimes sets in, with a thin expectoration which is tinged with blood, but is not to be regarded as a sign that pneumonia or bronchitis has supervened, but most commonly depends upon no other cause than the hyperæmia of the non-affected part, which hyperæmia is a necessary consequence of the pressure caused by the exudation, and for this reason does not show itself at the outset of the disease but only in its subsequent course. In favorable cases the termination in recovery may commence with the second week, and may lead to a complete restoration of health; or else, the process of reabsorption takes place very slowly, imperfectly, and the patients remain for a long time in a sickly, lentescent condition, where they are threatened with renewed attacks and exacerbations.

The third form, empyema, often develops itself, as was stated above, from the second form. That pus is forming, may be inferred from the circumstance that the fever does not abate, on the contrary, that in the subsequent course of the disease, and without any increase of the exudation, the fever increases in violence, mingled with chills, or assuming the character of an hectic fever, with a constantly increasing prostration of strength. If the purulent exudation is a consequence of pyæmia, of a septic state or a general dissolution of the blood, the exudation may originate and run its course without pain; it only aggravates the previously existing morbid phenomena. The course of the disease depends essentially upon the fact whether the exudation is re-absorbed or enclosed within a sac, or finally whether it escapes from the cavity, and in what direction.

The fourth form, where the exudation is chiefly serous, usually imparts to pleuritis a sub-acute or even chronic character. This form is very insidious, because it so often develops itself very gradually and without pain, and even commences without fever which does not generally supervene until at a later period. At first the patients only complain of lassitude, they lose their appetite, have a sickly appearance. Gradually the respiration becomes more oppressed and labored, but not by any means to a degree that might lead the patients to suspect the presence of a pulmonary disease. The quantity of the exudation occasions a displacement of the thoracic and abdominal organs. Recovery from such attacks always takes place slowly; it is only exceptionally that absorption takes place very rapidly amid a profuse diuresis.

Among the symptoms of pleuritis there is not one that could be pointed out as characteristic of the disease. It is true that in most cases of acute pleuritis we have the peculiar pain, but it varies exceedingly in character and intensity. At times the pain is simply a sensation of tenseness and constriction; at other times the pain is a seated, localized, stitching pain; at other times again the pain is spread over the whole side of the thorax, and is of a tearing or burning kind. Not unfrequently there is no pain at all; this happens more particularly in the most insidious cases. Because there is no pain, this is no reason why an exploration of the chest should be omitted. In genuine pleurisy there is very seldom any cough, especially at the commencement of the disease; if cough sets in at a later period, it may be occasioned by simple hyperæmia, or by pneumonic infiltration. At all events it causes the patient a good deal of distress, increases his pain to an extraordinary degree and complicates the course of the disease, since every additional obstacle must necessarily, in view of the existing dyspnœa, imply an additional amount of danger. The symptoms presented by other organs cannot be determined beforehand. Most generally it is the action of the heart, especially that of the right heart, which is altered; if any considerable amount of exudation is present, the beats of the heart become irregular, stronger and more rapid, the more so the more the heart is pushed out of its place by the effused fluid. A displacement of the liver is attended with pressure in the right hypochondrium, and slight symptoms of jaundice. Neither the intestinal canal nor the kidneys are involved in all cases. The brain becomes slightly engorged, if the effusion is copious and the circulation is interfered with. The position of the patients deserves particular notice, more especially as contrasted with their position in pneumonia. Pleuritic patients almost always lie on the painless and unaffected side, whereas, if the effusion is not attended with pain, they prefer lying on the diseased side. Very seldom the patient wants to lie on his back; if he does, the trunk has to be elevated a good deal.

All these objective as well as subjective symptoms, which we have described, are not sufficient to establish a reliable diagnosis. If a reliable diagnosis is at all possible, it will have to be based upon the results of a physical exploration, which is even more important in this disease than in pneumonia, for the reason that pleurisy often remains such a latent disease that the objective phenomena alone can shed light upon its existence and true character.

In pleurisy with simple fibrinous exudation or moderately extensive empyema percussion reveals nothing abnormal. As soon, however, as the quantity of the effused fluid becomes more considerable, it compresses the lungs, and a tympanitic sound is heard over the whole area filled by the fluid. If the whole or only a portion of the lungs is completely compressed, the sound is entirely empty, and the boundary of the effusion is indicated by the tympanitic sound. A dull sound is almost without an exception returned by the lower portion of the thorax, provided the effusion is sufficiently copious. A mistake may occur if the effusion is scanty and the lung is infiltrated as in pneumonia, or if the lower portion of the lung firmly adheres to the costal pleura and the lung can neither be pushed backwards nor upwards by the effused fluid. In pleuritis a change of position occasions very seldom a change in the dulness of sound. Generally the upper boundary of the exudation is formed by solidified exudation which resists all displacement. If a change of position induces a change in the level of the fluid, it is perfectly safe to infer the presence of an excess of serous effusion.

In pleuritis with plastic exudation auscultation reveals nothing abnormal at the commencement of the disease, sometimes not even during its whole course. The friction-sounds of the rough surfaces of the pleura, which, owing to the proximity at which these sounds are heard, cannot well be confounded with pulmonary murmurs, are not generally heard until the exudation has existed for some days, because the exudation requires this period of time to become sufficiently solidified for the production of those sounds. The pleuritic friction-sounds are wanting, if the effusion is very copious, but are often heard towards the termination of the disease, when absorption of the fluid takes place. If present, they constitute an infallible sign of pleuritis. Even if the exudation is scanty, the respiratory murmur is weakened, because the patients are afraid of drawing a full breath. If the exudation is copious, the respiratory murmur is often entirely absent at the lower portions of the thorax, whereas higher up bronchial respiration is heard more or less distinctly, and is more especially marked near the vertebral column. Bronchophony and ægophony are often heard together. In the free portion of the compressed lung, and generally likewise in the non-affected portion, the respiratory murmur is heard more loudly, and the symptoms of a more or less considerable catarrh are present.

Very seldom palpation discovers any peculiar changes during the presence of plastic effusion. A difference between the sound and the inflamed side is often noticed as far as the fulness of the respiratory movements is concerned, but the friction of the rough surfaces of both pleural laminæ against each other is perceived less frequently even by the touch. If there is a good deal of effusion, the thoracic wall over it does not vibrate from the voice, whereas this vibration is generally stronger at the borders of the exudation.

A view of the thorax shows very significant changes. During the presence of a plastic effusion, especially while the pains continue, the respiratory movements are much less distinct, and the patient mostly bends over to the affected side. If the exudation is copious, the affected half of the thorax enlarges in size; the intercostal spaces expand, and even become entirely effaced or bulge beyond the ribs, and the respiratory movements are either very slight or else entirely suppressed.

In measuring the thorax, the increase in its dimensions enables us to determine with great correctness the presence of a copious effusion.

Another important diagnostic sign are the displacements of the heart and liver occasioned by the presence of a large amount of effusion; the return of these organs to their normal localities is evidence of the fact that the effusion is decreasing.

As regards the *course* of pleuritis, we have already stated in previous paragraphs, all that is needful to observe on this subject. As a general rule, this disease comes less than any other within the possibilities of a reliable prognosis. It may have a scarcely perceptible beginning and, in its progress, assume a most malignant form; or else, from an exceedingly malignant and acute disease at the outset, it may run its course rapidly and completely to perfect recovery. These results cannot be determined beforehand; on this account, pleuritis has to be treated with great care, and every thing calculated to favor the progress of the disease, or to induce relapses, has to be carefully avoided.

The terminations of this disease are likewise various. The plastic form always leads to adhesions which, however, are seldom very extensive and do not interfere with the subsequent enjoyment of good health. It is usually the case, however, that afterwards the patients, during unusual bodily exertions, or during every trifling catarrh, complain of pain in the locality where the adhesions exist; this pain is, however, without any sort of importance. If the exudation is very copious, it may obstinately resist every effort of the organism to reabsorb the fluid and, by this means, a liability to relapses may be established. Or else pus may form; even then, a complete reabsorption may doubtless take place, but the pus likewise readily escapes externally, or into the lungs and abdominal cavity. In the former case, a thoracic fistula most commonly sets in, which generally terminates fatally in consequence of slow consumption, and very seldom heals in a very short time. The escape of the pus into the lungs and abdominal cavity is likewise dangerous, and holds out little hope of a complete recovery. An excess of serous exudation generally shows very little disposition to become reabsorbed, and very usually terminates fatally after a lingering period of suffering. Death scarcely ever takes place suddenly in consequence of asphyxia; most commonly it takes place in consequence of one of the above-mentioned changes. As important consequences of pleuritis, we have in the first place to keep in view the displacement of important organs which, during a long continuance of the exudation, is very apt to become stationary. A dislocation of the heart may become particularly pregnant with disastrous consequences. Next we have malformations of the thorax and consequent malformations of the vertebral column. Such malformations result if the lungs, which the effused fluid had compressed, are unable to expand again to their former size. If the malformation had not lasted too long, the prospect of a complete cure is not entirely unfavorable. An important consequence is the very common appearance of tubercles after the reabsorption of the pleuritic effusion.

To establish a prognosis in the higher grades of pleuritis is always a very hazardous thing, since unfavorable complications too readily annihilate the best founded hopes. As long as no pus has formed, we need not let our spirits flag; even empyema, if the patient has kept up a tolerable supply of strength, very often admits of a cure under homœopathic treatment. All complications, however, which diminish still more the breathing capacity of the lungs, are decidedly unfavorable to a successful treatment of the disease. In the front rank of such complications, we have pneumonia, whether it sets in simultaneously with pleuritis or supervenes during the course of the latter disease. Here the pleuritis interferes with the normal course of pneumonia, and the pneumonia prevents the rapid absorption of the pleuritic effusion. Even an ordinary catarrh, acute as well as chronic, is a serious matter, for the reason that it very much adds to the possibility of the supervention of acute œdema of the lungs. Inflammatory affections of the heart as well as chronic heart-disease constitute dangerous complications in pleuritis as well as in pneumonia. We need scarcely state that pleuritis arising from morbid alterations of the blood, from pyæmia, etc., is exceedingly unpromising.

It is sometimes impossible to arrive at a reliable diagnosis of pleuritis, more especially if the effusion only consists of coagulable lymph. The more the serous exudation preponderates, the more reliable becomes our diagnosis. What is of particular importance is to distinguish pleuritis from pneumonia with which, however, only the acute form of pleuritis with sero-plastic exudation, and which is of much less frequent occurrence, can be confounded. Pleuritis is diagnosed from the absence of the characteristic sputa of pneumonia, the different form of respiration, from the absence of all vocal vibrations which are considerably increased in pneumonia, from the dulness at the lower parts of the thorax with sharply defined boundaries. Bronchial respiration is an unreliable diagnostic sign; however it is to be observed that in pleuritis bronchial respiration is the weakest in the region where the dulness is the most marked and complete, whereas the reverse is the case in pneumonia. The dislocation of the heart and liver, the projection of the intercostal spaces and the expansion of the affected side taking place only after the exudation has become very copious, cannot be referred to at the outset of the attack as distinctive signs of pleuritis in contra-distinction to pneumonia. Nor is pain a safe indication of pleuritis; not only is the pain often absent, but a violent local pain may sometimes be characteristic of pneumonia. What is most difficult is a correct diagnosis of pleuro-pneumonia, since in this affection it is often very difficult to correctly determine the measure of the pleuritic effusion. Cases of this kind have such varied symptomatic manifestations, according as pleuritis is a primary or consecutive affection or a simple complication, that we do not deem it expedient to dwell upon them any further.

To indicate the treatment of pleuritis is not very easy if we mean to present it in a complete shape. Pleuritis being very seldom an idiopathic disease, we have to take into account so many accessory, causative and consecutive conditions, and the importance of pleuritis has withal to be placed in the foreground with so much care, that an exhaustive description of the treatment would become a very extensive task. For this reason we confine ourselves to the most important points in the following paragraphs, referring more particularly to pleuritis with copious exudation. The following are the leading remedies that may have to be resorted to in the treatment of this disease:

Aconitum. Regarding this drug we cannot communicate anything better than Wurmb's statement in the twelfth volume of the Hygea, which we transcribe from Rückert's Annals: "If the plastic elements prevail in the pleuritic effusion, or if, as the phrase goes, the disease has a marked inflammatory character; hence, if, as is usually the case, the disease sets in with violent febrile phenomena, no remedy deserves to be more frequently used at the outset of the disease than *Aconite*. We have never known Aconite to act upon the effusion itself; however, inasmuch as the curative process only commences after the fever has ceased, and inasmuch as it is consequently of importance that the fever should be removed as speedily as possible, and Aconite surpasses in this respect all other remedies, it is quite natural that the treatment should be commenced with this agent. Having observed that Aconite helps speedily, if it does help, I do not wait long for the result, and at once resort to another remedy, if I do not soon perceive a favorable change showing a decrease or a cessation of the fever. It is difficult to say how long, after giving Aconite, an improvement ought to be waited for; as a rule, however, we need not wait too long, since an improvement is often perceived already in a few hours; the fever abates, the stitching pains and the dyspnœa abate or disappear entirely, etc. The exudation still remains the same, but the circumstances of the patient now are such that Nature alone will be sufficient to complete the cure or will only require very little assistance for such a purpose. On the other hand, if the fever still continues, although in a slight degree, nothing further can be expected from Aconite and in order to prevent the disease from assuming a chronic form, other remedies will have to be chosen, especially such as act upon the exudation itself, among which I place *Sulphur* at the head of the list. If the effusion is more of a serous character, or hemorrhagic or purulent, Aconite will not do much for the fever, if any still remains. If, in a case of pleuritis with plastic effusion, the patient's carelessness or indiscretion brings on a relapse, the antifebrile power of Aconite will prove much less efficient than the first time; and, if repeated attacks take place, Aconite will do less and less for the fever, and finally, will prove entirely powerless." We have to dissent from the preceding remarks in one particular, namely, regarding the effect of Aconite upon the fever; it is our opinion that the remedy exerts its effect by diminishing the hyperæmia, by which means the pains are abated and the effusion is limited. Aconite is, moreover, a distinguished remedy at the outset of pleuritis supervening during the presence of tuberculosis, or for pleuritis complicated with pneumonia. It is without any effect if pleuritis is occasioned by marked decomposition of the blood, or by the onward spread of peritoneal inflammation, or by the escape of pus from the lungs or from carious ribs. Here Aconite cannot be depended upon even at the outset, if the fever is ever so intense. As regards waiting for a change after the exhibition of Aconite, we should never wait longer than twenty-four hours.

Bryonia alba is of all remedies more frequently used than any other in pleuritis and concerning which all physicians entertain an equally favorable opinion. Although we cannot help believing that many reported cures were due to the spontaneous efforts of Nature, and that the removal of a violent pleuritic pain has very often been mistaken for a recovery from a severe attack of pleurisy, whereas the pain alone is no adequate criterium of the extent and character of the pathological process. Bryonia could not possibly have been so often supposed to cure, if real cures had not been effected by this agent. Almost all practitioners agree that the period for the exhibition of Bryonia is the time when the fever has abated. In fixing this period, the comparatively rare form of pleuritis is thought of, that sets in as an acute disease and runs a similar course. Here Aconite is undoubtedly indicated first, and afterwards Bryonia. In a very large number of cases, however, Bryonia may be exhibited at the outset; they are the cases where the fever is not very high and the pain is severe but not intensely acute. We do not undertake to explain the action of Bryonia in such cases. It is certain that it has a very beneficial effect and generally accomplishes a speedy cure. Whether it acts directly upon the exudation and hastens its absorption, may be questioned; it is pretty well established, however, that under its influence the exudation scarcely ever progresses, and that the pains rapidly subside. A slight non-febrile, although very painful pleuritis, is rapidly controlled by Bryonia. Bryonia is likewise appropriate in the severer forms of a purely plastic pleuritis; in the first stage of the sero-plastic form it is the main remedy. If the exudation becomes purulent, the use of Bryonia is more questionable. If pleuritis complicates tuberculosis, the symptoms which very seldom point to Aconite, commonly indicate Bryonia. On the contrary we deem Bryonia indicated so much less, the more copious is the exudation; its sphere of action ceases if the inflammatory process is arrested and the effusion neither increases nor is reabsorbed. In pleuro-pneumonia Bryonia, after Aconite has been permitted to act for a short period, is almost an absolute specific. It is scarcely less specifically indicated in cases where bronchitis and pleuritis coexist.

Arnica. Hartmann's indications either occur very rarely in pleuritis, or else they are so little characteristic of pleuritis that they may be said to point to any form of this disease. Nevertheless, our Materia Medica Pura contains a sufficient number of symptomatic indications upon which the choice of Arnica can be predicated with great precision. Among these indications we range the stitching pain in the lower part of the chest, which is aggravated by pressure, motion and cough, shortness of breath, a continual day, hacking cough, or else a painful cough with expectoration of a frothy and bloody mucus. This last-mentioned symptom is particularly valuable, for it indicates Arnica in cases of pleuritis accompanied by hyperæmia of the non-affected side. We do not limit this remedy to the few cases of pleuritis occasioned by mechanical injuries. The excellent effect of Arnica in certain kinds of exudation is likewise verified in pleuritis, if the exudation is rather serous than plastic, or is copiously mixed with blood. In purulent pleuritis we should scarcely ever think of resorting to Arnica. An existing hyperæmia of the brain comes within the curative range of this drug as much as pneumonia within that of Belladonna. Old exudations are not acted upon by Arnica as positively as exudations of recent origin.

Digitalis purpurea. Wurmb writes concerning this drug: "There is a great difference between pleuritis serosa occasioned by an increased activity of the secretory functions, and hydrothorax occasioned by mechanical obstacles. This difference remained unknown to physicians who had been in the habit of confounding these two diseases, until more recently pathological anatomy directed our attention to the differences in the pathological appearances and a stethoscopic examination corresponding with these pathological appearances succeeded in clearing up the diagnosis. It is because these two different diseases have been confounded by physicians, that some of them report such favorable results from the use of Digitalis in watery accumulations in the pleural cavity, whereas others, on the contrary, report nothing but utter failures. An enlightened physician will certainly not expect any thing from Digitalis in hydrothorax occasioned by mechanical obstacles, such as an insufficiency of the valves of the heart; nor will he, on this account, entertain a less favorable opinion of the curative virtues of Digitalis, which renders such excellent service in pleuritis serosa where this remedy is really in its place. Dr. Fleischmann has noticed the best effects from Digitalis in pleuritis serosa, and I believe I may very properly recommend this remedy so much more urgently as I attach the highest value to the experience of this able practitioner. I prescribe this medicine in the first attenuation; higher attenuations have never shown any curative powers in this affection." If Wurmb recommends Digitalis only for chronic pleuritis serosa, we do not think he has done this remedy full justice. Its frequent employment by Old School practitioners, of course, in large doses, although only intended to depress the fever, is said to be crowned with good results in so many cases that it might likewise seem proper for us to experiment in the same direction. Most physicians are as yet deterred from pursuing this course by the idea that this remedy is not adapted to acute affections. This opinion is certainly erroneous and unfounded. It is particularly in pleuritis, for which we certainly do not possess too many remedies, that Digitalis deserves special attention on account of its specific relation to the rheumatic process. If this process spreads to the pleura, or if pleuritis is from the start a rheumatic disease, no remedy is next to Bryonia better adapted to this form of pleuritis than Digitalis.

Hepar sulphuris calcareum. No more than we were guided in our first trials with Hepar in pneumonia by the few corresponding symptoms of this drug, has Wurmb been guided by the symptoms alone when he says of Hepar: "To my knowledge, Hepar has never been employed in pleuritis, yet few remedies render such eminent service in this disease as Hepar. If the effusion is rather of a plastic nature, and if the disease has lasted for some time, or if a slow, lentescent course is to be apprehended from the commencement of the attack, I know of no better remedy than Hepar. Under its use I have seen copious exudations, which had already existed for a long time, disappear in a comparatively and incredibly short period of time, nor have I ever observed a case where, under such circumstances, it did not exert some influence upon the exudation. A complication with pericarditis or bronchitis demands its exhibition so much more urgently; if the effusion is rather more serous, Hepar is of little use." We share this opinion, adding at the same time that empyema, provided it is not too old, is above all calculated to substantiate the favorable action of this drug, and that the evident passage from the sero-plastic to the purulent form of pleuritis points more especially to Hepar.

Squilla maritima is much more talked about than actually used in pleuritis. We believe, however, unjustly, for the physiological effects of this drug show that it is in special rapport with the pleura and likewise with the lungs. Squilla is decidedly one of the medicines that it is proper to try in the treatment of pleuritis. It is more particularly adapted to pleuro-pneumonia, and is more especially indicated by a copious exudation of serum and even in serous pleuritis where the curative action of this drug manifests itself by a profuse diuresis. In former times Squills enjoyed a great reputation in this disease, and have fallen into disuse in the old system of medicine probably for no other reason than because the medicine did not help in every case, because its more special indications were either not sought or physicians did not know how to seek them.

We do not regard *Phosphorus* as a direct remedy for pleuritis although, having been mentioned as a remedy for pneumonia, it is very likely that it may be of some use in peripneumonia, in which case, however, the pleuritic exudation will be very scanty. On the other hand we deem it proper, from more general reasons, to direct attention to this drug in cases of pleuritis caused by or complicated with, pyæmia or septicæmia, and constituting from the start a state of purulent infiltration.

Mercurius is recommended by few physicians for pleuritis, and yet it is perhaps more appropriate in this disease than in pneumonia. We know from our Materia Medica Pura that quicksilver causes a number of symptoms pointing to pleuritis; hence its homœopathicity to this disease cannot be gainsayed. Moreover analogy justifies the conclusion that Mercurius has just as good an effect in pleuritis as in peritonitis, because we know that Mercurius acts upon definite systems rather than upon single organs. As in pneumonia so in pleuritis, Mercurius is indicated, if the exudation inclines from the start to change to pus, or if this tendency is imparted to it at a later period without, however, a special tendency to decomposition manifesting itself along with it. The following symptoms constitute essential indications: violent fever with frequent chills followed by a burning heat and exhausting, foul-smelling perspiration; considerable thirst; marked gastric catarrh with slight icteric symptoms; intestinal catarrh. In pleuro-pneumonia likewise, if the exudation is somewhat copious, Mercurius is one of the best remedies. In subacute empyema we do not consider Mercurius an appropriate remedy. Several reports in our literature show that Mercurius has often rendered distinguished services in epidemic pleurisy, both if the character of the disease was intensely rheumatic, or when the disease was complicated with bronchitis. Old School experience, according to which mercurial ointment is employed in exudative pleuritis with an advantage that cannot even be denied by the dogmatic adherents of the expectant method, can likewise be appealed to as an additional recommendation for the use of Mercurius.

Helleborus niger has not as yet been exhaustively proved; its local symptoms point, however, unmistakably to a pleuritic affection. Practical trials have led several physicians to recommend this remedy for the serous exudation in pleuritis, to which it is undoubtedly more adapted than to hydrothorax.

Arsenicum album is not, in our opinion, a remedy belonging in the category of anti-pleuritic medicines. Its exhibition in pleuritis as well as in pneumonia is determined by the general rather than the local symptoms. Wurmb expresses himself much more favorably concerning this drug in the following words: "In serous effusions Arsenic is probably the most important remedy; my confidence in this agent is so great that I doubt the possibility of curing a case where Arsenic does not effect the least improvement, as may possibly be the case with hemorrhagic effusions which defy all interference of art. The cases where Arsenic does not afford any relief, are not very frequent, whereas this medicine alone effects a number of cures or changes the form of the disease so that the cure can easily be completed by other remedies. The beneficent effect of Arsenic generally first shows itself by a change in the distressing asthmatic symptoms; afterwards dropsical swellings that may already have set in, together with the febrile motions, disappear, and lastly the absorption of the effusion itself is effected." We dare not decide whether Wurmb still adheres to these statements that were written down a good many years ago.

Sulphur holds the same relation to pleuritis as to pneumonia. Its employment depends more upon inferences drawn from its general effects than upon a rigid application of the law of similarity; its use is moreover substantiated by a vast number of practical successes. Here, too, we first transcribe Wurmb's views which seem to us strikingly correct in the main points: "In a case of seroplastic effusion *Sulphur* is powerless; if a plastic effusion has existed for sometime, *Sulphur* is less efficacious than Hepar; on the other hand, in pleuritis plastica, after first giving Aconite, or even without Aconite at the very outset of the attack, *Sulphur* is a truly specific remedy. If the fever is not sufficiently violent to require the use of Aconite, I commence the treatment at once with frequently repeated drop-doses of the *tincture of Sulphur* which is generally sufficient to remove the disease in a short time. If the fever runs high, and Aconite which seems indicated, does not very soon effect an abatement of the febrile symptoms, I at once resort to the administration of Sulphur and so far I have not yet had the least cause to regret this course of proceeding. If pleuritis is complicated with pneumonia, if the disease has already lasted a few days and the stage of hepatization has already set in, Aconite cannot do the least good although the fever may seem to indicate it; everything, on the contrary, may be expected from *Sulphur.*" This very warm recommendation which is indeed substantiated by practical results, seems to be liable to several objections. In the first place it is evidently too general. Taking the physiological effects of drugs and their applications in practice as our guide we are indeed authorized to draw conclusions far beyond the rigid boundaries of similarity; but Wurmb's mode of reasoning would lead us to general, not individual specifics, and our therapeutic opponents show us every day where the former would lead us. In the next place we are of opinion that all more violent febrile symptoms preclude the use of Sulphur, no matter whether the febrile phenomena arise from reactive endeavors of a more intense but normal character, or from reactive efforts that are excessive and incline to adynamia. Again, the symptoms of an incipient purulent metamorphosis are decidedly antagonistic to Sulphur. Finally, we think that *Sulphur* is adapted to every form of pleuritic exudation except perhaps an exudation depending upon septicæmia, because this agent is more than any other capable of stimulating the absorption of the plastic exudation. We know that in all more copious, even serous exudations, a thick plastic deposit very often lines the surface of the pleura, causing almost without an exception adhesions at the boundary-lines of the inflammation and enclosing the fluid as it were within a capsule. This newly-formed capsule is undoubtedly the cause why the fluid is not reabsorbed. Hence we see an exudation continue for weeks without change, after which it disappears very rapidly for the reason that the plastic fluid has disappeared and the pleuritic effusion is again undergoing a normal process of absorption. In such cases we have a right to expect a great deal from Sulphur because it materially hastens the disappearance of the plastic exudation.

Iodium deserves to be mentioned, because Old School practitioners have employed it in so many cases externally for the purpose of bringing about the absorption of the pleuritic effusion, which has often been accomplished with undeniable success. From its general effect as well as from its influence upon single organs we are justified in concluding that *Iodium* can be used for the absorption of a plastic pleuritic exudation, and that, indirectly, it may likewise, like Sulphur, aid in the removal of a serous effusion.

Beside the remedies we have named, many more have been recommended for pleuritis. But these recommendations are either based upon indications that we cannot accept as valid, or upon practical results where the diagnosis appears more than doubtful, or finally the remedies are recommended upon purely speculative grounds, and we, therefore, content ourselves with simply mentioning their names; they are: *Rhus toxicodendron, Nux vomica, Tartarus stibiatus, Carbo vegetabilis, Sabadilla, Spigelia, Acidum nitricum.*

For reasons mentioned at the beginning of this article, we do not deem it expedient to give a cursory view of the various remedies in apposition with the various forms and stages of pleuritis. The general management of an acute case of pleuritis is the same as in pneumonia. Here, too, the fear of relapses, the frequency of successive returns of the effusion, and our anxiety for a complete absorption of the exudation, should admonish us that suitable precautionary measures must not be abandoned too soon.

The consequences of pleuritis are of importance in two respects. In the first place, remaining adhesions of the two pleuras may cause great anxiety on account of the violent pain which such adhesions may occasion in subsequent diseases of the respiratory organs, and may likewise lead to the use of incorrect remedies. Another consequence emanating from the suppurative process, is much more important, and requires the application of direct therapeutic measures. In a case of thoracic fistula, the above-mentioned remedies have to be applied to in the first place; beside these we have moreover *Silicea*, *Lycopodium*, *Ferrum*, *China*, and more particularly *Calcarea carbonica* and *phosphorica*. Under the use of these drugs, each in accordance with the corresponding pathological indications, we need not all at once despair of a cure, as Old School practitioners indeed have to do with their means of treatment.

2. Hydrothorax.
Dropsy of the Chest.

Hydrothorax in the pleural cavity represents the same process as ascites in the cavity of the peritoneum. On this account we would pass this process over in silence if a few points did not make a more special allusion to it desirable.

Hydrothorax is either originated by all the various circumstances that cause an engorgement of the veins in the lungs, or else it is a symptom of general dropsy and depends upon an altered composition of the blood. In no case is hydrothorax a primary affection, but is occasioned by heart-disease, defects of the lungs, more particularly a high degree of emphysema, in which case the dropsical effusion is sometimes an isolated condition without any co-existing œdema in other parts; or hydrothorax is caused by affections of the spleen, kidneys, liver, etc., in which case it most generally constitutes the final development of general dropsy.

If hydrothorax arises from a sanguineous stasis in the lungs, its symptoms, independently of the results of a physical exploration, are scarcely ever of a nature that will enable the physician to infer the presence of this process with reliable certainty; for this sanguineous stasis is of itself accompanied by great oppression of breathing which is only more or less increased by the dropsical effusion. In a case of general dropsy, a gradually occurring dyspnœa indeed justifies the conclusion that water has accumulated in the pleural cavities. The following objective phenomena render the diagnosis perfectly certain: Complete dulness of the percussion-sound, from below upwards, as far as a line which, when the patient is in an erect posture, is exactly horizontal; when in a recumbent posture, is only felt posteriorly, or much lower down anteriorly; corresponding with this dulness the respiratory murmur is either entirely absent or very feeble; if the lungs are very much compressed, there is bronchial respiration posteriorly; the vibrations from the voice are missing; the thorax is expanded, but the intercostal spaces are not effaced.

If hydrothorax is a symptom of general dropsy, the treatment is the same as that of the latter disease; if it occurs as a more idiopathic disease, the treatment is chiefly determined by the nature of the existing cause. As a rule, it is beyond our power to effect a cure or even an improvement, although we succeed in a few cases to arrest, and even to diminish, the extent of the disorder. We may try to accomplish this result by means of *Arsenicum, Lycopodium, Aurum, Carbo vegetabilis* [also by *Digitalis* and *Apocynum cannabinum.* H.] For a description of the operation of *Paracentesis thoracis* for the removal of pus or water from the cavity of the pleura, the reader is referred to Surgical Works or to special treatises on diseases of the Thoracic Organs.

3. Pneumothorax.

This disorder is likewise in all cases a consequence of other pathological conditions. The entrance of air into the pleural cavity is most commonly the result of a perforation of the pulmonary pleura occasioned by ulcerous or other destructive processes in the lungs, or by the escape of pus from the pleural cavity into the lungs; much less frequently by a separation of the external walls of the pleural cavity. Tuberculosis is the most common cause of this accident; the next most common cause is purulent pleuritis, and the least common is gangrene of the pulmonary tissue.

Pneumothorax is always a terminal disease which very speedily ends in death unless the opening through which air penetrates into the thorax, closes in good season. This, however, is very seldom the case. The excessive apnœa which generally sets in all at once, and is attended with symptoms of the most marked interference of the circulation; the great expansion of the intercostal spaces of the affected side; the very full percussion-sound which changes its location with the posture of the patient and is generally associated with the metallic tinkling, without any respiratory murmur being audible; the amphoric resonnance and the metallic tinkling during auscultation render the diagnosis certain beyond all reasonable doubt.

That a cure of this dangerous condition is possible, is undoubtedly an established fact; but such cures are extremely rare. But it is likewise certain that medicinal treatment is utterly powerless in such cases. [This statement is too sweeping. It may be necessary to puncture the chest-walls for the purpose of relieving the patient from the excessive dyspnœa and the displacement of the viscera. Otherwise palliative treatment by means of stimulants for the purpose of overcoming collapse, diminishing the dyspnœa and relieving the pain, is not only proper, but indispensable. Small doses of Morphia and alcoholic stimulants, even pure alcohol, may be of great use. If the subsequent reaction is of an inflammatory character, with heat of the skin, a hard and strong pulse, soreness and pain of the affected side, the same treatment is to be pursued that has been indicated for pleurisy. H.]

NINTH SECTION.

Diseases of the Organs of Circulation.

A. DISEASES OF THE HEART.

The diagnosis of diseases of the heart as well as an intelligent appreciation of the phenomena characterizing and occasioned by these diseases, presupposes a correct knowledge of the physical properties as well as the physiological functions of the heart. Nobody will expect us to dispatch such a vast subject in a few brief paragraphs; on the contrary, we shall take it for granted that a physician is possessed of this knowledge, and confine ourselves, by way of introduction, to a few practical statements of particular importance.

Starting exactly from the mesian line of the thorax, the heart is situated about one-third to the right and two-thirds to the left of this line, behind the sternum and the cartilages of the right and left ribs, namely between the third and fifth on the right, and the third and sixth on the left side. The upper border of the heart is situated between the sternal margin of the right and left second intercostal space; the apex of the heart in the fifth left intercostal space close to the inner side of the nipple, or behind the cartilage of the left sixth rib close below the nipple. The anterior surface of the heart is mostly covered by the right and left lung, so that only a portion of the anterior surface of the right ventricle is in contact with the thoracic wall, within a space which is bounded on the right by a line from the sternal extremity of the sixth right rib to the sternal extremity of the left fourth rib; superiorly and on the left by a line curving in an upward direction and drawn from the sternal extremity of the left fourth rib to the left nipple; inferiorly by a line from the nipple to the insertion of the right sixth rib. It is only within this space that percussion returns complete dullness.

The various sections of the heart which it is important to know when exploring this organ, are situated as follows: The right auricle is situated farthest to the right, almost entirely to the right from the mesian line, from the sternal margin of the second right intercostal space to the insertion of the fifth right rib. The right ventricle, from the right auricle towards the left, occupies almost the whole of the anteriorly visible side of the heart. The left auricle is situated to the left of the mesian line behind the origin of the large vessels, so that it is almost entirely covered by the latter. The left ventricle is situated posteriorly behind the right; only a narrow portion of its wall, when seen in front, constitutes the left boundary of the space occupied by the heart.

The orifices and valves of the heart are situated as follows: the left auriculo-ventricular opening with the mitral valve close to the sternal margin of the second left intercostal space, and partially close above, partially below the cartilage of third left rib. The left arterial orifice with the semilunar valves of the aorta immediately next to and to the right of the left auriculo-ventricular opening, below the sternal articulation of the third rib on the left side and the sternum. The right auriculo-ventricular opening with the tricuspid valve on a line drawn from the sternal margin of the third intercostal space of the left side to the sternal articulation of the fifth costal cartilage on the right side. The right arterial orifice with the semilunar valves of the pulmonary artery close to the sternal margin of the second intercostal space on the left side. From its origin the aorta courses to the right and from before backwards, and the pulmonary artery to the left and from before backwards.

The impulse of the heart is felt within a space not altogether an inch wide, close below and to the side of the left nipple in the fifth intercostal space.

Of particular importance to an exploration of the chest are the following points: Never percuss with the plessimeter, always with the finger; if exact results are to be obtained, the chest should be percussed with firm as well as light taps. Auscultation should be instituted with the stethoscope for the reason that it can be more exactly applied to a smaller portion of the chest-wall. If the results of two different explorations are to be compared, the explorations have to be instituted in the same position of the individual. When percussing the chest, it should not be struck at one time during an inspiration, and at another time during an expiration, but uniformly during one or the other. If murmurs exist in the lungs which make it difficult or impossible to hear the cardiac murmurs, or make them appear less distinct, we sometimes succeed in hearing these murmurs by requesting the patient to stop his breath. The heart should never be explored immediately after bodily or mental exertions or excitements, but, if possible, while the patient is in as quiet a state as possible; it is even well not to examine the patient until some time after a quiet conversation has been had with him; many become considerably excited by the act of exploration. Regarding the number of heart-beats, it is to be observed that it is smallest while the patient is in a recumbent posture, and highest while he is standing up, and that the difference between these two numbers increases correspondingly with the patient's loss of strength. A single exploration of the heart is not sufficient to base our diagnosis upon. This precaution is too often overlooked in practice.

1. Carditis.
Pericarditis, Endocarditis, Myocarditis.
Inflammation of the Heart, Pericardium, Endocardium, Substance of the Heart.

We include the three above-mentioned anatomically-distinct forms of an inflammatory process in the heart in one chapter, because they generally not only occur associated together, but likewise because their treatment is the same in all essential particulars.

Inflammations of the heart occur more particularly between the age of pubescence and that of full manhood, or between the ages of fifteen and forty years. Men are more frequently attacked than women. Although it may be sufficient to say that this somewhat unaccountable fact is undeniably substantiated by statistical data, yet some light may perhaps be shed upon it by the circumstance that most cases of this disease originate in acute rheumatic attacks, and that the peculiar occupations of the male sex expose its members more severely to acute rheumatic diseases. Primary inflammations of the heart constitute some of the least frequent affections, and where they do occur, their causes are generally wrapt in obscurity. They are said to be occasioned by colds, excessive muscular exertions, abuse of alcoholic stimulants, mechanical injuries of the heart, etc. We likewise know that carditis may be occasioned by various poisons which will be mentioned hereafter. Generally inflammations of the heart are consecutive or secondary affections arising either by a continuation of the inflammatory process from the lungs and pleura to the heart; or in consequence of the heart becoming involved in affections of more remote parts, especially of the kidneys, and likewise of the stomach and spleen; or else, they may result from the operation of constitutional diseases. Among the latter acute rheumatism occupies the first rank, for there is not a case of intensely-acute articular rheumatism that is not, at the same time, accompanied by an inflammatory affection of the heart. We mention, moreover, scarlatina, variola, measles, typhus, and two other affections which are so apt to occasion an inflammation in every serous membrane, we mean pyæmia and puerperal fever. As regards chronic constitutional affections, it cannot be shown that they act as exciting causes in inflammations of the heart. Like all other inflammatory affections, inflammations of the heart sometimes occur in such numbers that we feel disposed to trace their origin to telluric or atmospheric influences.

Etiologically the various forms of cardiac inflammation are distinguished so far as this, that myocarditis occurs least frequently as a primary disease, but generally develops itself out of one of the other forms, both of which occupy the same rank in all other respects.

An exact knowledge of the anatomical changes occasioned by cardiac inflammation is not only essential to an intelligent appreciation of the single symptoms, but likewise to a knowledge of the possible consequences of such inflammations. We can here only indicate the main points.

Pericarditis has all the characteristics of an inflammation of other serous membranes. It is very seldom diffuse and is most commonly limited to single spots. The pericardium at first looks injected, opaque, sometimes spotted in consequence of slight extravasations, it is loosely-adherent and easily torn; at a later period the pericardium appears covered with coagulable lymph, which may be disposed as a delicately-organized membrane, or may have the appearance of granulated fragments of exudation. An effusion into the cavity of the pericardium is scarcely ever entirely absent, but may vary considerably both in quantity and quality. It may be from a few ounces to several pints. The exudation either consists of plastic lymph, or of plastic lymph and serum, and is not unfrequently mixed with blood, or hemorrhagic; it very seldom consists of nothing but serum. The exuded fluid may undergo the following essential changes: A complete absorption may take place and the patient may recover entirely. Or else, the fluid portion may be absorbed, and the plastic portion may be transformed into connective tissue giving rise to a membrane of more or less thickness. Or else, the effused fluid may be transformed into pus, which is either absorbed or may assume an organized consistence. The more plastic the exudation, the sooner adhesions of both surfaces of the pericardium take place; they generally show the most firmness at the base of the heart, but frequently consist only in threadlike attachments and again cause large portions of the pericardium firmly to adhere to the heart. The exudation is the more copious, the less fibrin it contains; the hemorrhagic exudation occurs more especially in great abundance.

Endocarditis is almost without an exception met with in the left ventricle. It attacks less frequently than pericarditis large portions of the endocardium; most commonly it is limited to single spots and has its chief locality near the valvular apparatus of the left heart. The inflamed portions of the endocardium lose their brilliancy, have a dim-white, grayish or reddish-gray appearance; it is puffed up and easily torn and detached. This exudation into the tissue of the endocardium may be associated with exudation upon its free surface in the shape of fine fringes upon which fibrinous deposits are apt to form. Further changes are: Either a complete cure by absorption, which is a rare occurrence, or else inconsiderable thickening of the exudation not materially interfering with the functions of the heart. Or else, indurated deposits may occur on the valves, containing calcareous matter. The most important consequences are those resulting from the breaking down of the exudation. The softened endocardium tears, thus giving rise to laceration of the chordæ tendineæ or of the valves themselves, and becoming chiefly instrumental in originating numerous defects of the valves; or the tearing of the endocardium on the sides of the ventricle may give rise to acute aneurysm of the heart, in consequence of the muscular substance not being able to resist the constant pressure of the blood. The purulent decomposition on the free surface, during which the broken-down exudation is continually carried along by the current of the circulation, easily results in the plugging up of single arteries or in the formation of metastatic abscesses, especially in the spleen and kidneys. The purulent infiltration of the muscular tissue of the heart occasions the same changes as the next form, myocarditis.

Myocarditis generally occurs in conjunction with one of the

other two forms. It is never diffuse, but always limited to isolated regions, sometimes in the interior of the muscular tissue, at other times more on the internal and external surface of the heart. It is most commonly located in the wall of the left ventricle and in the ventricular septum. The inflamed parts first show a dark redness, even ecchymoses, afterwards the affected fibres decay, being transformed into a reddish-gray detritus; or suppuration sets in leading to the formation of abscesses in the heart. This inflammation admits of a perfect cure, which is not very uncommon, if the inflammation is not too extensive. In the other case a partial cure may take place by the insulation and inspissation of the pus, in consequence of which callous indurations and calcareous concretions may result. If the pus escapes into the cavity of the ventricle, an acute aneurysm of the heart, or, according as the pus escapes in certain localities, valvular defects may arise, or, as in purulent endocarditis, metastatic abscesses and plugging of the blood-vessels may take place. If the abscess is located in the interventricular partition, it may lead to a communication between both ventricles. Perforation outwardly results in pericarditis.

Symptoms. The fact that inflammations of the heart occur almost only as complicating and consecutive affections, and the characteristic peculiarity of the symptoms occasioned by these inflammations, render it not only difficult but almost impossible to draw even a moderately-correct and striking picture of the disease. In the following paragraphs we shall, therefore, confine ourselves to furnishing detached details, first, the symptoms that can be observed without any physical exploration, and afterwards the physical signs. If, by pursuing this course, we are not afforded an opportunity of furnishing a perfectly coherent description of inflammations of the heart, on the other hand, we avoid the much more serious mistake of either describing these pathological conditions incorrectly or delineating fanciful pictures of disease.

All these forms of cardiac inflammation not unfrequently run their course with such inconsiderable signs of disease, or even so entirely without any symptoms, that the patients either do not consult a physician at all or that, in case carditis supervenes during the existence of other affections, the physician does not suspect the heart-disease unless he institutes a very rigorous examination. We ought even to take it for granted that many cases of carditis escape the most minute physical exploration, since we so frequently meet with remains of which not a trace had been discovered during the life-time of the patient.

Carditis setting in most commonly during the course of some other disease, its commencement is very seldom marked by a chill, generally it is even impossible to determine from the patient's own statements where the disease has precisely begun. Only pericarditis commences very commonly with shooting, more or less violent pains in the region of the heart. Most generally the patients complain of an intense feeling of illness and great anxiety, which they describe as proceeding from the pit of the stomach. If the inflammation has fully set in, the following symptoms are perceived in different combinations and degrees of intensity: Extreme feeling of illness not corresponding with the affection that the patient was already suffering with, and not suspending muscular power. Lassitude with constant restlessness, weariness, yet the patient is unable to sleep. Alteration of the expression of the countenance; this symptom is often sufficient for the attentive observer to suspect the presence of carditis: the face generally becomes more pallid, seldom turgescent, the features assume an appearance of tension, the eye has a shy, wandering expression, and, what is characteristic of this disease, the lips tremble a little while the patient is talking, at the same time the speech is somewhat hurried and jerked out as it were, which is not owing to the dyspnœa. The posture of the patients has no particular significance; they do not by any means lie steadily on the left side. Headache, which is sometimes of a violent kind, is a usual companion of carditis, whereas severe cerebral symptoms, such as delirium, sopor, coma, are rare occurrences, except in very bad cases which bear great resemblance to the typhoid process. The patients are restless, appear anxious without being conscious of it themselves; in severe cases the anxiety and restlessness become extreme, the patients manifesting an extreme sensitiveness to all psychical impressions. If fever was present, it is very seldom increased by the supervention of carditis, the temperature is less than when most other vital organs are inflamed. Chills occur very frequently, but they do not last long and are not succeeded by a burning heat. There is very commonly an excessive disposition to profuse perspiration which has generally a peculiarly musty odor. At the beginning of the attack the pulse generally becomes more rapid, fuller, harder, and has a peculiar tension; afterwards it remains more rapid, but becomes small, feeble, and inclines to be irregular. In some cases, on the contrary, the pulse is remarkably slow; in a case of pneumonia with pericarditis and endocarditis, that came under our observation, the pulse had sunk to forty-two beats in the minute. We likewise notice that in the same case the pulse is sometimes very rapid and at other times slow. Upon the whole, the character of the pulse is of no special value as a diagnostic sign. Sometimes the patients complain of severe tearing pains in the left shoulder-joint, or in the whole of the left arm; rheumatic pains may even be experienced in other parts of the body. The digestive organs are not influenced by carditis in anything like a constant manner. The respiration is very usually disturbed, dyspnœa of the most varied degrees setting in. At the outset of the attack the respiration is quick and short, but, when requested to do so, the patients are able to draw a long breath. Cough is not a usual symptom; at times it is dry and tearing, at others attended with expectoration of mucus and blood. The secretion of urine is almost always considerably less, the urine is saturated, depositing urates; sometimes albuminuria is present. It is further to be observed that, if carditis supervenes during a pre-existing disease, recovery from the latter is much more tardy. Other characteristic symptoms are: Marked interference with the circulation; œdema of the face, ankles; cyanotic phenomena in the face; passive hyperæmia of the brain. Increased dyspnœa. Accompanying disturbances of the spleen and kidneys. The profuse secretion of mucus is apt to result in the development of miliaria, which has given rise to the most erroneous views concerning metastases. If miliaria breaks out about the time when cardiac inflammation is about to terminate fatally, and the miliaria disappears again with the fatal termination, death has been laid to the retrocession of the exanthem which thus became invested with a peculiar significance. The truth, however, is that what takes place with other exanthems, likewise takes place in the case of miliaria: all these eruptions disappear at death in consequence of the sudden decrease of the vital turgescence.

All the above-mentioned phenomena may be present during every form of cardiac inflammation. We will now proceed to designate the most common symptoms characterizing each form of the disease.

Pericarditis: The disease sets in with a chill; rapid increase of the frequency of the pulse; pains in the region of the heart, which may likewise spread towards the back and shoulder, and are increased by a change of position, a deep inspiration and pressure on the pit of the stomach; palpitation of the heart which is exceedingly distressing to the patient. Dyspnœa sets in in a few days, after the exudation has become more profuse. Continued singultus is a not unfrequent symptom.

The symptoms of endocarditis are much more vague. It always approaches in an insidious manner, without pain, or only with a disagreeable sensation of pressure and constriction in the region of the heart. On the contrary the action of the heart is almost always tumultuous, more rapid and generally irregular, assuming the form of palpitations. The pulse, however, does not diminish in frequency. The respiration is accelerated, but dyspnœa is scarcely ever complained of during the first days of the disease. A violent headache, delirium, typhoid phenomena, swelling of the spleen and nephritic pains only set in in the subsequent course of the disease.

Myocarditis is not distinguished by regularly-occurring symptoms. Its supervention during one of the other forms of the disease may be suspected if the pulse becomes suddenly weaker and the action of the heart generally exhibits signs of excessive weakness. Even rupture of the myocarditic spaces does not furnish a clear picture of the pathological process. There is no pain, but very commonly an intense feeling of anxiety which may be accounted for by the rapidly diminishing power of the heart to propel the blood.

In contrast with these changeable, exceedingly inconstant morbid phenomena, we have the physical signs which are so much more important since they are much less apt to deceive and are very commonly sufficient for the establishment of a correct diagnosis.

At the commencement of pericarditis, the shock of the heart is stronger and is felt over a somewhat larger surface. Friction-murmurs are heard at an early period of the disease, very seldom not till a few days have passed. They vary a great deal in intensity, they are heard first and loudest at the base, do not follow the rhythm of the sounds of the heart, very often differ according to the position of the patient, and are heard more distinctly if the stethoscope is pressed against the chest, but not too hard. If the exudation remains scanty and chiefly plastic, the friction-murmur likewise continues to be heard, whereas, with the accumulation of larger quantities of serum or other fluid, the murmur grows feeble and finally, especially at the base, disappears altogether. The distension of the pericardial sac by the exuded fluid occasions the following phenomena: The intercostal spaces on the left side become effaced or even bulge, the shock of the heart cannot be felt, but in its stead we sometimes notice an undulating motion. Percussion returns a larger extent of dulness within a triangular space, with its base downwards. On auscultation, the sounds of the heart in a recumbent posture are only feebly audible, whereas if the patient stoops forward, they are frequently heard very distinctly, at any rate much more distinctly than in the former position. At the commencement of the disease, a feeble systolic blowing murmur is often noticed in the region of the mitral valve, likewise in the region of the aorta, or a double aortic murmur. Occasional throbbing of the veins of the neck. If the left lung is compressed by profuse exudation, a tympanitic resonnance or even dulness results. The first consequence of a decrease of inflammation is that the dulness becomes less in extent; after which the friction-murmurs again become audible, and may yet continue for some time. An important diagnostic sign of pericarditis is that while the area of cardiac dulness increases in size, the sounds of the heart become less audible, and the impulse of the heart diminishes in force.

The physical diagnosis of endocarditis is much more difficult than that of pericarditis. Since the sounds of the heart constitute the most important criterium by which the presence of endocarditis can be determined, it is of the utmost importance that the anatomy and functions of the normal heart should be correctly known, otherwise valvular defects that had already been existing for a long time, might be mistaken for consequences of the recent endocarditis. On this account we should guard against a hasty diagnosis, and explore the chest once a day or at least as often as may be convenient.

As long as the valvular apparatus has not been invaded by the endocardiac inflammation, the disease may remain completely obscured. Although a bad case of endocarditis, with formation of abscess, metastatic phenomena, etc., may exist without any valvular disease, yet a physical exploration does not reveal the existence of such inflammation by any positive sign. At the outset, the impulse of the heart is generally stronger and felt over a larger extent; it is likewise more tumultuous, yet the pulse is not unfrequently strikingly small. Endocarditis attacking almost exclusively the left ventricle, the first changes are noticed in the region of the orifices, one of the first changes being an increased ringing or tinkling of the first sound. With the increase of the pathological process, with the softening or partial disorganization of the valves, or in consequence of their incapacity from any other cause to close the orifices, a murmur is heard, most distinctly at the apex of the heart, side by side with, or in the place of, the systolic murmur. Friedreich calls attention to the fact that the diagnosis can often be more securely established by the circumstance that this murmur changes its intensity, duration, etc., more or less rapidly or slowly. Diastolic murmurs from disease of the aortic valves, or from excrescences upon the auricular surface of the mitral valve, are, upon the whole, rare occurences. Of essential significance is the increased intensity of the second sound of the pulmonary artery, which is heard soon after the murmurs, and the increased extent of the cardiac dulness which almost sets in simultaneously. It is hardly possible to indicate the variations in the cardiac murmurs with anything like absolute correctness, since they must necessarily differ correspondingly with the various changes resulting from the disease.

Myocarditis is not recognized by any fixed physical signs; if such are present they belong to the accompanying endocarditis and pericarditis. The participation of the muscular structure of the heart in the inflammation is more particularly inferred from the great weakness of the pulse co-existing with a tumultuous action of the heart. This pathological change can only be conjectured; it can never be verified with positive certainty.

The course and terminations of cardiac inflammations show the greatest differences in degrees of intensity as well as in other respects. In describing these particulars we shall follow a very summary course, since particular terminations will have to be dwelt upon afterwards. Our object will be best accomplished by considering the three forms of cardiac inflammation each by itself.

Pericarditis of a middle degree, if attacking individuals of an otherwise sound constitution, is not a very dangerous disease, but generally terminates in complete or almost complete recovery. After exudation is completed, the patients are confined for a few days or weeks without being very sick, unless they are prostrated by some previously-existing disease, strength gradually returns to them, the friction-murmurs that had disappeared, again become audible, or the existing murmurs become less distinct. Termination in recovery never takes place rapidly or suddenly, and the friction-murmurs sometimes remain distinctly audible for months, during which period the patients continue to retain their suffering and feeble appearance. In acute affections where rapid changes take place, pericarditis sometimes disappears very rapidly. Most commonly, however, we shall find that the supervention of cardiac inflammation during a primary affection imparts a lentescent character to the latter. If the exudation is very copious, it may only be partially absorbed, the patients incline to shortness of breath, palpitation of the heart, and relapses easily take place, chiefly for the reason that the patients do not take proper care of themselves. These relapses either have an acute or chronic character, in which latter case they give rise to a condition which is described as chronic pericarditis. It is very seldom that fibrinous pericarditis suddenly terminates fatally. On the contrary, if the exudation is purulent or hemorrhagic, a fatal result may take place very suddenly, and is generally determined by paralysis of the cardiac functions which leads to acute œdema of the lungs. An excess of serous exudation most generally results very speedily in softening of the muscular tissue of the heart, consequently in œdema of the lungs and general dropsy, this end is to be apprehended if the cardiac dullness, which persistently remains the same, extends over a large area and the pulse becomes very small and increases in frequency. A copious emission of urine only seldom occurs as a critical change. Adhesions of the pericardium are of subordinate importance, although of frequent occurrence. Very commonly pericarditis results in more or less considerable hypertrophy of the heart. The quality of the exudation cannot be determined with certainty from the course of the disease, although this very desirable knowledge would exert a great influence upon the prognosis. As a rule it is safe to take it for granted that a purulent or septic exudation only occurs as the result of a general dyscrasia or in consequence of pyæmia or puerperal conditions.

Endocarditis always runs a tedious, sub-acute and even chronic course. Of itself the disease very seldom leads rapidly to a fatal termination, and, if it does, it is always in company with exquisitely typhoid symptoms. The commencement of the disease is mostly uncertain; hence its duration cannot well be determined, so much less since the affection, in cases where it is diagnosed with positive certainty, had already developed valvular disease. A complete cure is possible, if the valves have not been invaded; but we likewise deem a cure possible provided the valvular alterations do not consist of loss of substance or solutions of continuity. A partial cure is still possible if the valvular changes do not materially interfere with the functions of the heart. The most common termination of endocarditis is the development of valvular disease which gives rise to chronic ailments and a slow decay of the organism. If these valvular defects arise from such lesions as cicatrices in the substance of the valve, they may not manifest themselves until after the endocarditis has terminated without any apparent anomalies of the valvular apparatus. Purulent endocarditis often results in speedy death in consequence of the diseases which it develops in other organs, more especially by plugging up important arteries.

Myocarditis generally runs a latent course; but if it is extensive; if an abscess forms within the parietes of the heart, it may result very speedily in a fatal end; if it coexists with the other two forms of cardiac inflammation, the former becomes the chief cause of death.

A combination of the three forms of cardiac inflammation impresses a different character upon the course of the disease. A pericardial inflammation alone can be very rapidly reabsorbed, whereas, if it is associated with endocarditis, the course of the former is always retarded by such a combination and a complete cure is rarely ever effected. The hypertrophy which usually results even if no complicating disorders are present, is greatly increased by the valvular deficiencies; paralysis of the heart consequent upon serous infiltration of the muscular tissue of the heart, is likewise considerably facilitated by a complication of cardiac disorders, especially by valvular disease, and the reabsorption of effused fluid from the pericardial sac must necessarily be interfered with by the deficient action of the circulatory organs. Less prejudicial, although always sufficiently ominous, is the influence of pericarditis upon endocarditis. The more impeded the movements of the heart, and the greater the effort this organ is called upon to make, the more easily valvular lesions will occur.

What we have said must show that the prognosis of cardiac inflammations must be exceedingly uncertain. In a case of complicating pericarditis, the prognosis is most favorable, if the coexisting disease is not characterized by septic phenomena. In all other cases and forms the sequelæ which are almost sure to occur, forbid the assurance of a favorable prognosis, and although Homœopathy achieves much more satisfactory results than the Old School, yet it cannot boast of infallible success. Cardiac inflammation occurring in connection with chronic dyscrasias, more especially tuberculosis, is almost certain to terminate fatally, yea, may be regarded as the terminal and necessarily fatal result of a constitutional disease.

Treatment. Although we can boldly assert that the homœopathic treatment of cardiac inflammations has so far resulted much more favorably than the treatment of these diseases in accordance with the principles of the Old School, yet we do not mean to affirm that we possess a large number of reliable indications for the use of our drugs, or even a number of such drugs as we might term cardiac remedies. We ought to accomplish a great deal more than we do; yea, in the treatment of heart-affections we are much less successful than in the treatment of diseases of the respiratory or digestive organs; nevertheless our successes are decidedly greater than those of the Old School, were it for no other reason than because we have abandoned so many therapeutic follies that even the modern physiological School is guilty of. We should be carried too far, if we would indulge in special statements bearing upon this point, subsequently we shall find opportunities for offering various remarks on this subject. We must, however, even here, protest most emphatically against heart-affections being treated by bloodletting either by physicians of the Old or New School. We would enter this protest even if we had no other reason than because every bleeding diminishes the functional power of the heart and the regularity of its action.

Let us at the outset dwell a little more fully upon the reasons why the therapeutic chapter of heart-diseases in the domain of Homœopathy is as yet so incomplete and so ill-conditioned. In the numerous homœopathic publications bearing upon this subject, the reason is given that our provings are deficient in symptoms corresponding with the signs elicited by a physical exploration of the condition of the heart. This is undoubtedly a great defect which cannot be remedied by re-provings were they conducted with ever so much energy and devotion. Nobody will probably want to poison himself so thoroughly as to produce distinct cardiac murmurs. The only light we can obtain in this direction is by a careful study of accidental cases of poisoning and by means of extensive experiments on animals. It is strange that in cases of poisoning a careful exploration of the heart before and after death has been omitted.

If the possession of objective physiological symptoms of heart-disease is still the object of an unfulfilled desire, we must go to work and discover a method of arriving at a knowledge of the true remedy without such symptoms. It is our opinion that the only method is the practical experiment, by which we mean that our medicines ought to be applied in accordance with our existing, vague, unreliable and insufficient indications, and that the results should afterwards be registered in accordance with the most careful physical diagnosis. This has not yet been done, and this is the reason why the homœopathic treatment of cardiac affections is so much more defective than that of any other class of diseases. A pneumonia and even a pleuritis can be recognized with tolerable certainty without percussion or auscultation, but the special form of an affection of the heart, and sometimes the existence itself of an affection of the heart cannot be determined without resorting to a physical exploration of the chest. Now we ask, in how many reports of heart-diseases contained in our literature have the requisites of a physical diagnosis been complied with? And how far, in the presence of such glaring defects, do these reports deserve to be credited? In passing these remarks we do not mean to cast a slur upon the labors of our homœopathic veterans who could not possibly be acquainted with our present means of diagnosis; we deem it so much more necessary to point out these defects in order to stimulate the efforts of our rising physicians to acquire this indispensable and highly useful knowledge.

It is from these points of view that we request the reader to consider the following statements, and to excuse the defects he may discover in them. One or the other remedy may perhaps have been omitted, but we have stated more than once that we consider an enumeration of too many remedies embarrassing rather than useful to the practitioner. The following are the main remedies in cardiac inflammations:

Aconitum. We have already shown in several paragraphs of this work that great abuse is made of Aconite by being given contrary to the homœopathic law in inflammations of various organs and other febrile affections. This admirable remedy deserves to be pointed out so much more emphatically in cases where it is truly homœopathic, and where its curative virtues have been so often and so brilliantly verified. There is no doubt that the lungs and the heart are the main organs upon which Aconite exerts its chief influence; whatever objections may otherwise be raised against their method of proving, Schroff and Van Praag have earned our thanks for having shed more light on the relations which Aconite holds to both the lungs and the heart. We here only relate the symptoms pointing to cardiac inflammation, as developed by a deeply-penetrating and protracted poisoning. At first the beats of the heart become more rapid and more violent, and this increase lasts so much longer the less excessive the quantity in which the experimental dose was taken. At the same time the respiration is extremely accelerated, the temperature is increased, a feeling of sickness is experienced, and all the symptoms of a more or less considerable cerebral hyperæmia set in. The pulse is hard and strong. The pain in the cardiac region is not a constant symptom, but was often felt. In the further course of the proving the beats of the heart become slower, sometimes to a great extent; or else they remain quick and grow feeble, irregular, they seldom remain vehement. On the contrary, the pulse changes to a feeble and small pulse, not synchronous with the beats of the heart, intermitting or unequal; the temperature is lower while the number of respirations increases rather than decreases. This last circumstance alone would be sufficient to stamp Aconite as a cardiac remedy, for slowness of the pulse and a simultaneous and considerable decrease of the number of respirations are phenomena that only occur in diseases of the heart. As to the symptoms developed in the organism generally, we do not mention them in this place; they embrace all those that always accompany cardiac inflammation. These physiological results have been confirmed by practice in a most striking manner. In every pericarditis and endocarditis, whether primary or secondary, Aconite is the first and most important remedy whenever the inflammation sets in with febrile phenomena. We consider this remedy indicated even if the fever is moderate or is altogether wanting. Aconite is not only indicated at the commencement of the disease, but in many cases during its whole course, more especially in rheumatic cardiac inflammations, as long as the organic alterations do not result in paralytic or cyanotic symptoms. We would rather treat a case of cardiac inflammation with nothing but Aconite, than a case of pneumonia. Of course, we must not, as is the custom with homœopathic routine-practitioners, limit ourselves to synochal fever as a paramount indication, but keep the whole series elicited by a thoroughly-penetrating proving in view. It is in this manner only that the full therapeutic range of this great remedy can be determined.

Digitalis purpurea has been and still is regarded by many as inappropriate in acute diseases and more especially in acute cardiac inflammations. We cannot sufficiently protest against this view which has a tendency to restrict the usefulness of a drug that may exert such a beneficent influence over disease. If Digitalis were more frequently and more rationally used in acute heart-affections, we should be much less frequently called upon to employ it in chronic heart-disease. Since I have devoted, for years past, special attention to the use of this drug, I have found it much more frequently applicable in the treatment of disease than in former times, and I am now prepared to assert most positively what I was then only able to announce in rather dubious language, that Digitalis is an excellent remedy in acute affections of the heart, more particularly in pericarditis. Digitalis is not so much adapted to inflammations setting in with very violent symptoms, but to inflammations approaching in an insidious and scarcely observable manner, more especially without any local pain, but with a rapidly increasing embarrassment of the respiration. We should take a very one-sided view of the action of this drug, if we were to regard the irregularity and slowness of the pulse as the chief criterium for its application, since a rapid and very weak pulse constitutes an equally reliable indication. Even a violent excitement of the functional activity of the heart, as generally occurs at the commencement of cardiac inflammation, is in characteristic accord with the first symptoms of poisoning by Digitalis. Among all the various forms of cardiac inflammation, we consider the rheumatic form best adapted to Digitalis, and likewise if it is associated with a copious effusion of serum; less, however, to pericarditis if the friction-murmurs continue unchanged from the beginning of the disease. The sooner these murmurs disappear, the better is Digitalis adapted to the case. In endocarditis it seems almost impossible to indicate special heart-symptoms requiring the use of Digitalis; in such cases the constitutional symptoms will have to determine our choice. In myocarditis the doubtful character of the diagnosis will render it an especially difficult task to point out indications for the use of Digitalis that have been confirmed by experience; one circumstance speaks in favor of Digitalis which is, that in myocarditis the action of the heart is most suddenly weakened to an extraordinary degree. Among the general symptoms the following invite more particular attention to the use of Digitalis: Rapidly-increasing dyspnœa, with occasional symptoms of acute congestion of the chest; inflammation of the pleura or lungs; bronchitis; chronic catarrh of the bronchia; expectoration mixed, not streaked with blood; spasmodic cough. Livid, turgescent face with blue lips; headache, vertigo, delirium, sopor. Vomiting at the commencement or during the course of the disease; hyperæmia of the liver, slight icterus, catarrh of the kidneys. Excessive feeling of illness, not corresponding with the perceptible symptoms; great anxiety, but without any continual restlessness. Aggravation by the slightest motion. A drawing-tearing pain in the left shoulder.

Veratrum album is one of the choicest cardiac remedies, although this place has not yet been assigned to it by homœopathic practitioners; the stage of functional excitement of the heart is still more apt to rapidly change to a state of paralytic weakness; the pulse becomes very irregular, generally extremely rapid, small and feeble; this change takes place although the alvine evacuations may not be by any means excessive, so that the heart-symptoms have to be regarded as the effect of direct action, not as resulting from a highly acute anæmia. Veratrum is our first choice in acute cases, if the following general symptoms are present: Violent dyspnœa; constrictive sensation in the throat; constant short, dry, hacking cough. Bluish complexion, with an expression of deep prostration; sopor, stupefaction, excessive dulness and tightness of the head. Vomiting and diarrhœa. Considerable diminution of the urinary secretion. Convulsive motions, more particularly of a clonic character. Cool, dissolving perspiration, with icy coldness of the extremities. So far we have no clinical records confirming the homœopathicity of Veratrum to heart-disease.

Arsenicum album is frequently mentioned as a chief remedy in cardiac inflammations; we confess, however, that we have never seen any good effects from it in acute affections. It is a remarkable fact that among the large number of cases of poisoning by Arsenic, post-mortem examinations have never yet revealed a single symptom that might lead us to infer that Arsenic exerts a specific inflammatory action upon the heart. This shows that the heart-symptoms, which Arsenic occasions so constantly and exquisitely, have to be accounted for in a different manner than by means of an inflammatory process. Clinical experience leads us to trace these symptoms to dissonances of the cardiac nerves, or else to regard them as secondary symptoms. Myocarditis presents many points of resemblance to the symptoms of Arsenic, and it is more especially in this disease that we should try Arsenic, were it only for the reason that Arsenic exerts an intensely-paralyzing effect upon the muscular tissue of the heart. This effect of Arsenic determines its relation to the other two forms of cardiac inflammation. Hence we consider Arsenic indicated in the cases where Veratrum seems indicated, if the pulse very speedily loses its fulness and strength, and an excessive state of debility sets in at an early period. This is most generally the case with cachectic individuals, and Arsenic is one of the most essential remedies in most cachexias. Among secondary heart-diseases, chronic pericarditis is the only one where Arsenic would be appropriate, if a copious exudation is present. In valvular disease, we have never obtained any decided improvement by Arsenic; it only acts as an uncertain palliative.

Spigelia is an important remedy in heart-affections, but its provings have to be greatly improved. In accordance with what is published of this drug, Hartmann gives the following symptomatic indications: Undulating motion of the heart; indistinct beats of the heart running into one another; when laying the hand upon the heart, tumultuous beating of the heart in a recumbent as well as in a sitting posture, not synchronous with the radial pulse; spasms of the chest, suffocative complaints; tremulous sensation in the chest and temples; increased by motion; tearing sensation in the chest, when raising the arms over the head, and when touching the pit of the stomach; purring murmur during the beats of the heart; stitches in the region of the heart; pulsations of the carotids with a tremulous motion; great dyspnœa at every change of position; bright redness of the lips and cheeks, changing to pallor during every motion; the impulse of the heart raises the four last true ribs, the sternum and xiphoid cartilage, and displaces the dorsal vertebræ; audible beating of the heart, causing a pain that is felt through to the back; cutting pains from the heart to the shoulders as far as the head and arms; excessive dyspnœa, with a pressing-cutting pain in the abdomen, at the insertion of the ribs; arthritic pains and stiffness of the joints; dull stitches where the beats of the heart are felt, and recurring with the measured regularity of the pulse; the beats of the heart can be felt through the clothes, with anxious oppression of the chest; scraping in the throat, affection of the tracheal and bronchial mucous membrane; the beats of the heart are not synchronous with the pulse; purring murmur. As respects this enumeration, it is to be observed that these symptoms for the most part are not the result of physiological experimentation, but clinical symptoms observed upon the sick, and hence are of less value to us. At any rate these symptoms do not contain the symptoms of sero-plastic, nor of serous pericarditis. On the other hand we distinctly recognize in this complex of symptoms both the purely plastic pericarditis as well as incipient endocarditis. But upon what basis are we to prescribe Spigelia in cases where the disease is painless and has scarcely any symptoms? This shows that it is a great mistake to lay too much stress upon sensations of pain, which is not by any means a constant companion of cardiac inflammation. What invites more than all these theoretical statements to the use of Spigelia in heart-affections is the fact that it has been so often and so variously employed in practice with decided advantage. According to practical experience, Spigelia is particularly adapted to rheumatic pericarditis, likewise to sero-plastic pericarditis during its whole course, especially if the patient complains of an intense local pain, and the affection is evidently characterized by all the signs of cardiac inflammation; and to rheumatic endocarditis in its incipient stage, or to endocarditis generally before marked valvular changes have taken place.

Nitrum has so far commanded too little the attention of practitioners, nor are we in possession of any decided clinical testimony. Nevertheless we have every reason to recommend Nitre in cardiac inflammation, more particularly if it sets in in company with active pulmonary congestions, or as a symptom of Bright's disease, or associated with acute rheumatism. A striking participation of the kidneys in the pathological process going on in the heart, points urgently to the employment of Nitre.

Phosphorus is not usually numbered among the cardiac remedies, nor can it be denied that its relation to the heart is not by any means constant. But if the post-mortem examinations of individuals who had been poisoned by Phosphorus, so often reveal lesions about the heart, especially where death did not take place immediately after the ingestion of the poison, it seems as though we could not deny the fact that Phosphorus exerts a direct action upon the heart, and that the cardiac phenomena which Phosphorus occasions, are not merely of a sympathetic or secondary nature. The main post-mortem appearances as far as the heart is concerned, are: the muscular tissue is flabby and easily torn; opaque appearance and interstitial distention of the endocardium; bloody infiltration which in certain circumscribed spots penetrates the whole thickness of the muscular tissue. If, in addition to this, we consider the very feeble, small and exceedingly frequent pulse; the frequent observation that the sounds of the heart either frequently disappear or are replaced by murmurs, it seems to us that Phosphorus has more claims to be regarded as a remedy for cardiac inflammation than most other medicines, more especially in cases of secondary origin. We cannot deny, however, that the indications upon which its homœopathic application has so far been based, appear to us totally erroneous. In our opinion the following are the true indications suggested by physiological experimentation: Phosphorus is exclusively suitable for inflammation of the endocardium and the muscular tissue, never for pericarditis. The constitutional symptoms would lead us to recommend Phosphorus in endocarditis associated with Pneumonia, where it has rendered us the most signal service on two occasions, we mean against the cardiac inflammation, not against the pneumonia, for we have already stated when treating of pneumonia, that, when pneumonia is complicated with cardiac inflammation, the presence of the latter constitutes an absolute obstacle to the absorption of the pneumonic exudation. In the next place Phosphorus takes the precedence over every other medicine in cardiac inflammations when occurring as complications of such processes as lead us to infer a dissolution of the blood, like scurvy, puerperal fever, malignant exanthematous diseases, typhus, etc. Finally we possess few remedies that embody in their pathogeneses as plain a picture of nephritic and cardiac inflammation, as Phosphorus. And lastly Phosphorus is almost the only remedy of which we are sure that it occasions an infiltration of the muscular tissue, and that on this account it becomes a highly important remedy in myocarditis. We are not in possession of any clinical material to prove the correctness of these statements, but, with a view of substantiating them more fully, we will call attention to one circumstance. Phosphorus is employed by most homœopaths in pneumonia as well as in other inflammatory and exanthematic diseases with the best result, whenever the inflammation assumes a nervous or rather a typhoid type. In a vast majority of such cases a strict examination would undoubtedly show the presence of cardiac inflammation, for it is this that most frequently imparts all at once a typhoid character to pathological processes that generally run an ordinary course. It is our belief that Phosphorus has often cured cardiac inflammations without the physician being aware of it. Finally we have to point out a symptom which most decidedly indicates Phosphorus, we mean the dilatation which develops itself during endocardial inflammation with such surprising rapidity. After all these remarks we do not deem it necessary to criticise the indications offered by other physicians, for they are almost all of them vague and indefinite.

Colchicum autumnale seems to us to be improperly ranked among cardiac remedies. We are in possession of a large number of both rapid and slow cases of poisoning, but in no case does a post-mortem examination show more than a quantity of bloody coagula in the right ventricle and the venæ cavæ; only in one case the endocardium was found ecchymosed, and there was a complete absence of pericardial fluid. All the heart-symptoms are of a secondary nature and are founded in the excessive losses of fluids occasioned by Colchicum. Although Colchicum is highly praised for rheumatism of the heart; this may be owing to the general curative powers it manifests in acute rheumatism, though not by any means in a very striking or constant manner. According to Müller, Colchicum is more suitable as a remedy for pericarditis than for endocarditis. Hartmann's indications are utterly meaningless. One important point has to be well kept in view in selecting Colchicum, it is this: that Colchicum causes an extraordinary increase in the secretion of uric acid. It is precisely this circumstance which invests this remedy with importance in heart-affections during an attack of gout.

Bryonia alba is, next to Aconite, regarded by many homœopathic practitioners as the main remedy in pericarditis with sero-plastic effusion. In this case the exhibition of the drug is evidently not based upon the symptoms in the Materia Medica Pura, for the heart-symptoms in the pathogenesis of Bryonia are mostly unmeaning or at least very vague. The analogy of pleuritis and pericarditis has doubtless led to the use of the drug; nor do we intend to dispute the propriety of such a conclusion, since Bryonia has such an excellent effect in all inflammatory affections of serous membranes, and is altogether indispensable in acute rheumatism. We likewise admit that the pathological picture developed by the supervention of pericarditis during pneumonia or pleuritis, generally corresponds very fully with the pathogenesis of Bryonia. We would limit the use of Bryonia to such cases; for uncomplicated pericarditis we undoubtedly possess more suitable remedies.

Cannabis is undoubtedly one of the remedies that has a direct action upon the heart, but we do not yet know what is the precise nature of this action. More recently a number of investigations have been instituted concerning the nature of Indian hemp (haschisch), from which we have extracted the following group of cardiac symptoms: Violent palpitations of the heart, sometimes without any anguish, and sometimes attended with perfect agony or the most frightful restlessness; pulse small and sometimes intermitting for a minute, from 100 to 120 beats; constriction of the pit of the stomach; paroxysms of anguish; the beats of the heart are scarcely perceptible and extremely weak; fear of death, which is felt every time the pulse intermits. To judge by these few symptoms, which always set in after large doses of Cannabis, this drug would seem to be a powerful cardiac remedy; yet all secondary circumstances being considered, we shall find that this is not the case. The incipient exaltation of the heart's action coincides with great exaltation of cerebral action which is attended with phenomena of congestion. The cerebral exaltation very soon changes to extreme depression, even partial paralysis, (for instance of the nerves of the senses, skin,) and this depression is likewise accompanied by symptoms of diminished action of the heart, the latter lasting precisely as long as the cerebral depression. From this connection we can infer almost with certainty that the heart-symptoms do not arise from disease of the heart itself, but from a functional change in the brain. Otherwise it would be inconceivable how such marked alterations of the functions should pass off so speedily and without leaving a trace behind. Our opinion that Cannabis cannot be relied upon as a remedy in cardiac inflammations, is confirmed by the circumstance that the clinical trials that have been instituted with this remedy, have not in any respect substantiated the recommendations with which this medicine has been honored.

Opium might claim the privilege of being considered a cardiac remedy with as much propriety as Cannabis; but in its case the cardiac symptoms are likewise secondary results of a primary functional change in the brain. If one of these two remedies were to be employed in heart-affections, it would be in cases of endocarditis where the brain is very much involved; this scarcely ever happens in pericarditis.

Lachesis. It is a remarkable fact that the opinion of practitioners concerning this agent are diametrically opposed to each other. Many pretend to have effected extraordinary cures with this agent; others have always used it without any benefit. The reason of this is undoubtedly that one preparation was reliable and another was not; for that the serpent-poison has a powerful effect, is shown by every fresh bite of the reptile. Every case of poisoning by the bite of a serpent shows that this class of poisons exerts a specific action upon the heart. We have an unusual increase of the frequency of the pulse which becomes feeble and small, or intermittent; there is pain in the region of the heart, the pain being sometimes intense; palpitations of the heart, fearful anguish, bloody expectoration with constant hacking cough, marked symptoms of cyanosis, icy coldness of the extremities, with cold perspiration, retention of urine; paralytic sensation in the whole left side of the body, or a violent pain in the left shoulder and left arm, etc. Post-mortem examinations have always shown the heart more or less affected. The endocardium in the region of the valves is infiltrated and easily torn; ecchymoses cover its internal and external surface; exudations in the muscular tissue of the heart. According to these symptoms, Lachesis must prove a good remedy in very acute cases of endocarditis, not in pericarditis. As a matter of course, our clinical trials must be instituted with a good preparation, which ought to be readily obtainable, since the poisons of the different kinds of Viper act equally upon the heart. The fact that the blood is speedily decomposed after the Lachesis trigonocephalus has inflicted its bite, deserves special consideration. This circumstance indicates Lachesis very pointedly in typhus and acute exanthems.

[Bæhr has omitted the mention of **Naja tripudians** as a remedy for heart-disease. We are indebted to Dr. Russell, of England, for a proving of this snake-poison. Dr. Hughes, in his late Manual of Pharmaco-dynamics, confirms the therapeutic value of this agent in diseases of the heart. "To quiet," says he, "chronic nervous palpitation, to aid in the restoration of a heart recently damaged by inflammation, and to assuage the sufferings of chronic hypertrophy and valvular disease, it was ranked by Dr. Russell as the chief remedy: and I think I can confirm his estimate." H.]

Sulphur is not classed by us among the cardiac remedies, although its pathogenesis contains a number of symptoms referring to the heart; nevertheless, we consider it valuable for reasons that we have already stated when treating of inflammatory processes in former chapters. No remedy is better able than Sulphur to effect the reabsorption of an exudation that had already existed for a time, and in our opinion this proposition applies to all inflammatory processes. In a case of pericarditis, where uncommonly loud friction-murmurs and a rubbing of the pericardial surfaces against each other, that could even be felt by the hand, had already existed for upwards of three months, these symptoms disappeared entirely after Sulphur had been given for a fortnight. We only recommend Sulphur for pericarditis, especially the plastic form of the disease, after the inflammatory stage proper has run its course. In endocarditis there is generally no exudation to be removed; for its severe consequences are limited to losses of substance which it is difficult to replace.

Iodium likewise deserves attention where all that remains to be done, is to remove the exudation. Indeed, we cannot afford to overlook a single remedy of this kind, considering the small number of those that can be of any use in this direction. Besides, however, the pathogenesis of Iodium contains a number of useful symptoms referring to cardiac affections.

If we would here furnish an exhaustive list of our cardiac remedies, we should have to add a considerable number to those already described, more particularly if we were to include all the remedies referring to the remote consequences of cardiac inflammation, to which we have devoted a separate chapter under the heading of "Valvular Diseases." Many remedies among them we do not regard as cardiac remedies and consider their employment governed by peculiar complications. Such remedies are: *Belladonna, Pulsatilla, Tartarus emeticus, Mercurius, Rhus, Arnica.* Other remedies have not yet been sufficiently investigated in their relations to the heart, such as: *Bismuthum, Laurocerasus, Acidum oxalicum.* The effects of the last-named remedy upon the heart are certainly worthy of a careful study.

In order to facilitate the study of these drugs we here furnish a synoptical view of each drug, with reference to the special cardiac conditions, with which it is in therapeutic accord.

In pericarditis, if setting in as a primary affection, *Aconite* will always be the best remedy to commence the treatment with. How long this remedy is to be continued, will depend upon the course the disease takes, more especially upon the course of the existing exudation. As soon as a copious exudation has set in, both the pains and the fever generally abate, after which some other remedy may be chosen with great propriety. *Bryonia, Spigelia, Digitalis,* and likewise *Nitrum* may now claim our attention. *Bryonia* and *Spigelia* may be given when loud friction-murmurs are heard, and the patient complains of continual pain, the area of cardiac dulness is somewhat enlarged, and the pulse is accelerated and not weakened; *Nitrum* may be resorted to, if the lungs are intensely congested, and there is a good deal of cough with bloody expectoration. *Digitalis,* if the cardiac dulness is rapidly extending over a larger area, the friction-murmurs disappear very rapidly and collapse sets in, the pulse being either very quick and feeble, or else very slow or intermittent. *Veratrum album* acts similarly to Digitalis. These two remedies, in connection with Arsenicum, are most generally adapted to the violent dyspnœa with cyanotic symptoms. After the true inflammatory stage has run its course, the absorption of the plastic exudation is promoted by *Sulphur* and perhaps *Iodine*, and of the serous exudation by *Arsenicum, Digitalis*, and perhaps also by *Tartarus stibiatus* and *Colchicum*.

In the secondary or complicating pericarditis, the following remedies are of importance: For acute rheumatism, with increase of fever: *Aconite;* if rheumatism sets in without any special symptoms: *Digitalis;* if pains are present: *Spigelia*, moreover *Colchicum, Tartarus stibiatus, Rhus, Mercurius.*—If complicated with pneumonia: *Aconite, Iodine, Phosphorus, Bryonia;*—if with pleuritis: *Bryonia, Spigelia, Digitalis*, also *Nitrum*. In the malignant forms of pericarditis supervening during the presence of pyæmia or other septic forms of disease, *Arsenicum*, and above all, *Phosphorus*, will prove the most important remedies. Pericarditis, complicated with acute exanthemata, requires principally: *Aconite* in the case of measles; *Rhus toxicodendron* in scarlatina and measles; *Mercurius* and *Tartarus stibiatus* in small-pox; *Ammonium carbonicum* in scarlatina; it is questionable, however, whether the cardiac inflammation had not rather be treated first without reference to the exanthem.

It is only in rare cases that primary endocarditis will be of a nature to require Aconite exclusively. The chief-indication here is the quality of the pulse; as long as the pulse is hard and full, *Aconite* is undoubtedly suitable. We have shown above that *Aconite* may be indicated during the whole course of the disease. After Aconite, *Spigelia* may be required, Digitalis less frequently; *Nitrum* and *Veratrum album* may likewise have to be given. In very acute cases *Lachesis, Veratrum album,* or *Arsenicum*, may often be required from the first. If the brain is greatly disturbed: *Veratrum album, Cannabis, Opium.*

In rheumatic endocarditis with complications: *Aconitum, Colchicum, Spigelia,* less frequently *Digitalis;* if co-existing with pneumonia or pleuritis: *Phosphorus, Veratrum album, Nitrum,* also *Bryonia;* with typhus: *Phosphorus,* also *Rhus toxicod.* and *Arsenicum, Opium* and *Cannabis;* with nephritis: *Phosphorus, Nitrum, Arsenicum, Colchicum,* also *Cantharides;* when acute exanthems are present, the same treatment as for pericarditis:

In myocarditis we would depend upon *Phosphorus, Arsenicum*

and *Digitalis;* we likewise call attention to the importance of Plumbum in this disease.

[Of *Kalmia latifolia* which has likewise been recommended as a cardiac remedy, we have no reliable clinical reports worth mentioning.

Cactus grandiflorus is the last important cardiac remedy which has been introduced to the profession by Doctor Rubini of Naples. It seems to be particularly adapted to the organic defects consequent upon acute cardiac inflammations, especially rheumatic endocarditis. Hypertrophies and valvular deficiencies seem to come more particularly within its curative range. In the cases where we have tried it, we have seen better effects from it in the tincture than in the attenuations. The case of hypertrophy of the right ventricle reported in the May number 1866 of the British Homœopathic Review, presents a very fair illustration of the curative effects of Cactus in heart-disease. It is likewise recommended for chronic nervous palpitation. According to Dr. Hughes, the feeling as if the heart were grasped and compressed as with an iron hand, is very characteristic of Cactus in these cases of nervous palpitations. If this be so, it rivals Digitalis which causes this feeling in a most marked manner. See my Materia Medica. H.]

If the three forms of cardiac inflammation occur together, our chief attention should, in our opinion, be first devoted to pericarditis, the presence of which always favors the progress of the other two forms of inflammation and retards their retrograde metamorphosis.

Dietetic and hygienic measures are of the utmost importance in cardiac inflammations, especially if the disease runs a rather latent course, which might throw the patients off their guard and even make them believe that a little exercise will hasten their cure. Our chief attention should be directed to avoid every thing that might have a tendency to stimulate the heart's action; hence mental as well as bodily exertions are entirely out of place. This point must never be lost sight of, even if all signs of inflammation have disappeared, especially in a case of endocarditis. The stomach being generally involved in the cardiac disturbance, the patients generally reject all kinds of nourishing food; but even if this should not be the case, the most rigid diet should be advised as a matter of precaution, at least at the beginning of the disease. This is all the more advisable since cardiac inflammations do not of themselves exhaust the system. Coexisting affections, of course, may render dietetic modifications necessary. As soon as the febrile symptoms have been subdued, a more invigorating diet may be advised. However, if in the case of other inflammatory affections we have not hesitated to recommend a glass of wine or beer during convalescence, we would with equal emphasis advise against the use of these stimulants in convalescence from cardiac inflammations. The smallest quantity of such stimulants has a tendency to excite the functional activity of the heart. This remark applies even to malt-beer, which contains a sufficient amount of carbonic acid gas to excite the circulation in many persons. The fact that cardiac inflammation often runs a latent course, is undoubtedly the reason why, in such circumstances, stimulants often have an injurious effect upon convalescent persons, and so greatly predispose the minds of physicians against their use. The severe diet observed during the period of convalescence should be pursued some time after, for the reason that the inflammation very often leaves remains that escape our observation and entail a tendency to relapses or to organic alterations, such as hypertrophies and valvular diseases, that can only be prevented by the utmost care from increasing to a fatal termination.

2. Hypertrophia Cordis.

Hypertrophy of the Heart.

By this name we designate a condition of the heart, where its volume is considerably enlarged by the increased thickness of its muscular tissue, and by a more or less considerable distention of its cavities. The formerly current forms of hypertrophy of the heart are no longer accredited before the tribunal of modern pathology. An increase of the size of the heart by adventitious formations within the tissue of the heart, is no longer regarded as a genuine form of hypertrophy.

This disease is caused by conditions which sooner or later determine an increased activity of the heart, on which account hypertrophy is generally to be regarded as a secondary or consecutive affection. Since the whole heart does not become hypertrophied at once, but the hypertrophy generally begins with one particular cavity, we find that hypertrophy arises from the following pathological changes:

Hypertrophy of the left ventricle: stenosis and insufficiency of the aortic orifice, stenosis of the aorta itself, aneurisms of the aorta, atrophy of the renal parenchyma, amputation of the thigh and consequent ligation of the femoral artery. The same causes most commonly lead to hypertrophy of the left auricle and stenosis of the mitral orifice.

Right ventricle: Stenosis and insufficiency of the orifice of the pulmonary artery; insufficiency of the mitral valve and stenosis of the left auriculo-ventricular orifice consequent upon the obstruction offered by this insufficiency to the complete emptying of the pulmonary veins; diseases which restrict the capacity of the lungs and considerably diminish the lesser circulation, such as emphysema, atelectasia, tuberculosis, pleuritis, caries of the vertebræ, curvatures. Hypertrophy of the right auricle alone scarcely ever takes place; on the other hand this auricle always participates in the hypertrophy of the ventricle.

Every attentive observer must have noticed that primary hypertrophy arises in consequence of hereditary disposition without any apparent cause; or it may develop itself in cases where a peculiar mode of living stimulates the heart to a constant and severe action, as may take place in consequence of severe manual labor, continued running, excessive gymnastic exercises, fencing, abuse of strong coffee, wine, beer, spirits; or finally, hypertrophy may arise if the heart is kept in a constant state of tumultuous action by strong psychical impressions, hence in the case of individuals with intensely sanguine temperaments.

Hypertrophy of the heart may occur at any age between the years of fifteen and forty. Males are decidedly more liable to it than females, especially to hypertrophy of the left ventricle; this, however, is probably owing to the circumstance that men are more frequently exposed to the causes giving rise to such structural changes.

The anatomical changes consist in a thickening of the walls of the heart and of the inter-ventricular partition, in a more or less considerable dilatation of the cavities, very commonly in a darker color of the muscular tissue, in displacements of the heart and changes in its external shape. If the hypertrophy is general, the heart assumes the shape of a triangle with obtuse angles; if the left ventricle alone is hypertrophied, the heart becomes elongated and somewhat conical, and the apex is turned more towards the left side; if the right ventricle is hypertrophied, the shape of the heart becomes more rounded, its diameter in breadth is longer, and the heart approximates more to the right side. The base of the hypertrophied heart generally reaches a little below the normal line.

Symptoms and Course. Only two forms of cardiac hypertrophy can be described symptomatically, because they alone occur as primary diseases, we mean hypertrophy of the whole heart and that of the left ventricle; whereas hypertrophy of the right ventricle is almost always of a secondary character, and its symptomatic manifestation is essentially depending upon the nature of the primary disease. So far as hypertrophy of the right ventricle is concerned, we shall therefore have to confine ourselves to indicating the general consequences of this disorganization.

Whereas primary hypertrophy of a certain grade always represents a really morbid condition of the heart, secondary hypertrophy can at the commencement only be regarded as an endeavor of the organism to restore the disturbed equilibrium. This is the reason why the lesser degrees of this structural change exist without any morbid symptoms, or are only accompanied by disturbances, such as are called forth by accidental stimulations of the heart's action. The more frequent and violent such stimulations and the longer their duration, the more they contribute to increase the existing hypertrophy and to complicate it by the production of valvular disease and dilatation of the cardiac cavities.

In moderate hypertrophy of the left ventricle, without any marked dilatation, the arterial blood is driven with increased power into the arteries of the systemic circulation and likewise through an increased frequency of the contractions of the heart. The impulse of the heart is stronger and generally visible, and extending over a larger area, so that it can be felt even in the fifth and sixth intercostal spaces, and even beyond the nipple. A larger extent of dulness is not always traceable on account of the overlapping portions of lung. While in a state of rest, the patients generally feel well, they complain at most of a slight feeling of pressure in the præcordial region. Every rather violent and continued motion, every mental excitement not only causes a troublesome and even distressing palpitation of the heart, but along with it an oppression and feeling of anxiety in the chest, a sensation as if the clothes were too tight, dyspnœa. The increased excitement in the arterial circulation gives rise to congestions of the head, the face looks flushed, the eyes glisten and are injected, the margin of the lids often looks as if inflamed, there is buzzing in the ears, vertigo, etc., the congestion is less frequently met with in the tract of the aorta descendens, because the situation of the arteries it supplies renders them more yielding to its impelling power.

A high grade of hypertrophy of the left ventricle scarcely ever exists without valvular defects, most generally stenosis of the aortic orifice; it very soon becomes associated with dilatation of the left ventricle. As long as the mitral valve remains intact, such a hypertrophy is characterized by the same phenomena as those described above, only in a more intense degree, and with shorter, or without any intermissions. But if, owing to the excessive dilatation, the mitral valve is no longer sufficient to close the auriculo-ventricular orifice, the consequence is that the more forcible expulsion of the blood into the aorta becomes associated with a stasis in the lesser circulation and more immediately in the function of the right ventricle, in consequence of which the whole heart becomes hypertrophied in the most dangerous acceptation of this term. The impulse of the heart is perceived over a large extent by the eye, ear and touch; it is even heard without the ear being applied to the chest; the concussion of the thorax is extreme; the dulness extends further on to the left, and is returned over a larger area, the heart descends below its normal line, the ribs even bulge. The sounds of the heart are either muffled, or else ringing, and, if the valves are diseased, murmurs are heard. Other symptoms can easily be inferred by any one who considers that the arteries are extremely engorged, and that the lungs are in a state of hyperæmia. All these conditions will be dwelt upon more fully when we come to treat of valvular anomalies.

The phenomena emanating from the hypertrophied right ventricle, are very frequently entirely disguised by those of the affection which had given rise to the hypertrophy. Anxiety, dyspnœa, oppression, palpitation of the heart, may be caused by pulmonary affections alone. Simple hypertrophy merely results in a greater accumulation of blood in the lungs, and a consequent catarrhal affection of the lungs, with hemorrhage, hyperæmia of the lungs. The physical signs are: Increased extent of dulness on the right side, even beyond the right border of the sternum; pulsation in the pit of the stomach, perceptible raising of the lower border of the sternum; accentuation of the second sound of the pulmonary artery.

Hypertrophy with dilatation may be very considerable without superinducing any serious derangements. It implies a sort of uniform compensation of functional power, and the patients only perceive a dirturbance of equilibrium if they undertake to undergo severe bodily exertions. In hypertrophy with dilatation the heart often thumps very violently, without causing the patient any great trouble; the impulse of the heart often raises the head of the auscultating physician, and is felt over a much larger extent; the cardiac dulness is returned over a longer and wider area; the sounds of the heart are stronger and more sharply accentuated, and have very often a metallic ring.

The course of hypertrophy is more especially determined by the consequences resulting from it to the general organism. Under favorable circumstances such patients may live to an old age provided they live within the bounds of moderation, prudence and frugality. If other morbid dispositions exist, the cardiac disease may give them a fatal start. Cerebral as well as pulmonary apoplexy of young people is preëminently a consequence of cardiac hypertrophy. If hypertrophy coexists with, or is depending upon aneurism or an atheromatous condition of the vessels, it acts both as a compensation to the obstructed circulation and as a cause of the rupture of the vessels. We should always bear in mind that simple hypertrophy is not, of itself, a dangerous condition, but that it becomes dangerous as soon as valvular defects arise. We, therefore, refer the reader to the chapter on valvular diseases where all these complications will be explained and accounted for.

Professor Niemeyer furnishes the following excellent diagnostic details: For eccentric hypertrophy of the left ventricle: Visible pulsation of the carotids; loud systolic murmur in the large arteries, full pulse which is visible even in the smaller arteries; increased impulse of the heart, felt much higher up from the apex; the apex of the heart reaches lower down than normally; larger extent of dulness from the apex upwards; increase of the sounds of the heart in the left ventricle and in the aorta, and sometimes a metallic ringing.—For the hypertrophy of the right ventricle: Stronger impulse of the heart, extending to the sternum and sometimes even to the left lobe of the liver; displacement of the apex outwards, scarcely ever at the same time downwards; greater extent of cardiac dulness in breadth, increase of the sounds of the heart, in the right ventricle and in the pulmonary artery, the second sound of which is most important.—For hypertrophy with dilatation: The arteries and the pulse as in hypertrophy of the left ventricle; the impulse of the heart is considerably stronger and extending more in length and breadth; the apex of the heart points lower down and outwardly; cardiac dulness is felt over a larger area in every direction; all the sounds of the heart are louder.

The prognosis becomes in the long run unfavorable, for the reason that the disorder bears within itself the conditions of growth.

Treatment. That cardiac hypertrophy is a curable disease as long as the disorder is not too far developed, is admitted on all sides, although the chances of a cure are not very great. Most pathologists, however, doubt whether a cure can be effected by the direct action of medicine. Before indicating the drugs that require to be used in the treatment of this disease, it may be well to offer a few suggestions that may be of importance in conducting the treatment.

If hypertrophy is a necessary and compensating consequence of other morbid conditions, it would be wrong, by removing the hypertrophy, to disturb the equilibrium which the hypertrophy had restored. Fortunately, this is not well possible; nevertheless, attempts are too readily made to depress the apparently excessive energy of the left heart more particularly, and it is this proceeding which we consider injurious. In such circumstances all we can and should aim at, would be to remove the primary pathological cause, and, if this is not possible, to leave the condition intact and at most to treat a few incidental troublesome symptoms. The physician will have enough left to do in supervising and regulating the patient's mode of living, and in controlling intercurrent conditions that might result in an increase of the disorder. If the hypertrophy is a primary disease, either congenital or imperceptibly acquired, there is still a prospect of the disease being overcome, provided the physician is made aware of it in time. As long as the body continues to grow, we deem it possible to remove the hypertrophy, or at least to reduce it to scarcely perceptible dimensions. For this reason, it is of the utmost importance that, if there is the least suspicion of heart-disease in the case of children or growing people, their hearts should be examined with the utmost care. Young people addicted to the practice of onanism, are very apt to be afflicted with hypertrophy of the heart; when excited by such a cause, the disease can undoubtedly be arrested or even completely removed.

In our opinion the following points ought to determine the treatment of cardiac hypertrophy.

In the first place, if possible, the cause should be acted upon. This will be difficult if the circulation is obstructed by some material obstacle, such as an aneurism, an atrophied kidney, constriction of the aorta, valvular defects. A possibility of this kind, however, exists, in the case of young people, if the hypertrophy is caused by onanism, premature mental exertions with their necessary attendant consequences of nervousness, excitability, chlorosis, anæmia. The remedies adapted to this purpose are numerous and have already been mentioned in the chapter where the corresponding pathological diseases were treated of. A second causal indication requiring particular attention is the patient's mode of living.

The dietetic management has to aim at two objects, in the first place the avoidance of every thing in the patient's mode of living that might aggravate the disorder; and secondly, to surround the patient with influences that will have a direct tendency to ameliorate his condition. As regards the first point, spirits, coffee, strong spices, the excessive use of salt, very substantial and more particularly fat food will have to be avoided. The patient should be governed by the nature of his business in the quantity of food he consumes. Overloading the stomach is very hurtful; frequent and small meals are preferable. A person afflicted with cardiac disease should never go to sleep immediately after dinner, or go to bed with a full stomach. Every bodily motion occasioning a sensation of increased action of the heart, is too great a tax on this organ; all mental excitement is likewise strictly to be avoided. As regards the second point, we would call attention to the fact that we very often succeed, by changing the patient's mode of living, in avoiding or diminishing the violent congestions of the head. A business that compels the patient to lead a sedentary mode of life, or exposes him to much excitement, should be abandoned. If icy coldness of the lower extremities is accompanied by heat of the head and a flushed face, this trouble might perhaps be remedied by rapid walking which, by exciting the action of the heart, would, on the other hand, prove a source of mischief, whereas gymnastic exercises with the feet alone might often render the best service, without causing palpitation of the heart. An exhaustive development of these rules would occupy too much space in a work of this size. What we have said will suffice to show in how many ways a patient with heart-disease claims our attention.

In the third place, it is a matter of essential importance that all morbid conditions as well as isolated symptoms, which occasion an increased action of the heart, should be remedied as speedily as possible by appropriate remedies. Here, too, all we can do is to simply mention the leading remedies that we may have to resort to in meeting complicating disorders of this kind, the most important of which we will now proceed to point out.

Palpitations of the heart, that is to say: a very violent increase of the action of the heart setting in without any fixed order, with irregularity of the beats of the heart, and always of short duration, are generally met with only in the case of very irritable, nervous individuals. We have obtained the best success in such cases from the use of Digitalis or Digitalin, which we recommend as the best remedies to begin the treatment with. The paroxysms being short, we cannot expect to do much for a single paroxysm, on which account the remedy has to be continued for a time at rather long intervals. *Ferrum* may likewise be tried, of course very cautiously, especially if the affection is complicated with tuberculosis and chlorosis. *Pulsatilla* and *China* may be classed in this category, but we cannot speak in their favor from personal experience. In one case we have seen good effects from *Argentum nitricum* and *Platina*. *Sepia* may prove useful to women, but will not do much in the case of men.

Palpitation of the heart is one of the most common and most distressing complaints in cardiac hypertrophy, but is at the same time so intimately connected with this disorganization that it is impossible to apply to it remedies that will have an infallibly curative effect. If the palpitation takes place at altogether irregular intervals, or if it only lasts a short while, or even if it continues all the time, we advise the remedies that will be found indicated in the following chapter, and which may be given with a view of treating the whole disease, not merely a single symptom. If the paroxysms set in frequently, or at definite periods, or last some time, we have remedies that have a decidedly soothing effect. If the attack is excited by severe mental labor, by the abuse of coffee or spirits, or by some unpleasant emotional excitement, *Nux vomica* may be resorted to; with this precaution that it as well as the remedies to be named hereafter, must not be given in strong doses. If the palpitation attacks robust, full-blooded, excitable individuals with bright complexion, disposition to changes of color in the face, glistening eyes, injected conjunctiva, headache, stinging or shooting pains in the præcordial region, *Aconitum* is the most appropriate remedy. It is likewise suitable for palpitation caused by a sudden or intense emotion, and more especially if the individual is afflicted with tuberculosis. *Arnica* is indicated very nearly by similar conditions. If the palpitation is excited by a fit of anger or vexation, in the case of very nervous persons and children, we give *Chamomilla*. If excited by a violent fright, or if attended with sopor and restlessness, the face being livid or pallid, we give *Opium* in a very small dose. *Coffea* is indicated by nocturnal palpitation of the heart, with great weariness and a constant change of position, with a peculiar anxiousness, after too copious a meal, or after imbibing ardent spirits. Chlorotic individuals require *Pulsatilla*. If the patients do not smoke, or to female patients, smoking often affords rapid and essential relief, and constitutes one of the best palliatives. Little paper-cigarettes are best adapted to such palliative purposes. If any one should be disposed to doubt the homœopathicity of this drug, let him read one of the many published essays on the effects of tobacco.

Pulmonary hyperæmia or rather pulmonary congestion does not occur very frequently, but is very distressing. If emanating from the left heart, *Aconitum* will most generally relieve it completely. *Belladonna* has never seemed of much use in this complaint; *Arnica* and *Cannabis* may do some good. [Likewise *Veratrum viride*, H.] If the pulmonary congestion is traceable to the right heart, *Digitalis* generally proves a sovereign remedy to which *Belladonna*, *Pulsatilla*, *Carbo vegetabilis* are essentially inferior.

Cerebral congestions which are sometimes excessive, are likewise frequent accompaniments of cardiac hypertrophy, especially hypertrophy of the left ventricle. Here, too, *Aconite* is one of the most efficient remedies. We prefer *Opium* if the head feels excessively constricted, the complexion is dark-red, and the anxiety and restlessness extreme. We should never resort to *Belladonna* in such a case. If the congestion originates in hypertrophy of the right ventricle, *Belladonna* is sometimes useful; *Digitalis*, however, affords relief more efficiently and promptly.

The characteristic headache accompanying hypertrophy of the heart, and resembling hemicrania, can scarcely ever be relieved. If such a headache is attended with, and perhaps caused by, hyperæmia, the remedies which we have indicated previously, will have to be depended upon. If the headache is unaccompanied by congestive symptoms, we advise *Digitalis*, *Arsenic* or *Spigelia*.

In the fourth place we must try to meet the hypertrophy by all proper remedies. We are aware that to many the abatement and still more the cure of an hypertrophy of the heart seems an impossibility; indeed we ourselves should not feel anxious to rashly and unhesitatingly promise a favorable result from our treatment. Nevertheless we have often found that, after using proper remedies, the dangerous phenomena consequent upon hypertrophy of the heart became less, and that in young individuals the hypertrophy yielded so far as to become inaccessible to the usual means of diagnosis. Hence we would, by all means, advise to treat such a case, were it only to make the patient believe that he is taking something, and thus to keep him from using strong and generally deleterious drugs, or to continually remind him, by the use of a little harmless medicine, of the necessity of avoiding every kind of excess and even the least violation of the rules laid down for him by his medical adviser. The medicines which we deem the best adapted to such purposes, are almost all of them metals or inorganic substances, no vegetable drugs. At any rate, we have never obtained any permanently good results from a vegetable drug. We recommend *Arsenicum*, *Aurum*, *Argentum*, *Cuprum*, *Plumbum*, *Platina* and *Ferrum*. It would be useless to undertake to assign to each of these remedies definite limits in the treatment of hypertrophy; we only recommend in general terms *Arsenicum*, *Plumbum* and *Ferrum* for hypertrophy of the right ventricle, and the other remedies, including likewise Arsenicum, for hypertrophy of the left ventricle. In a given case, the selection of the remedial agent will have to be governed by the nature of the existing general symptoms. *Sulphur*, *Natrum muriaticum* and *Petroleum* may be added to our list of metals. If we desire to obtain good effects from our drugs, we must guard against too strong and too frequently repeated doses, and against changing the remedy too often.

Considering the mischief which is so often done by the abuse of large doses of Digitalis, we repeat with decided emphasis that the effect of this drug in hypertrophy of the heart is never permanently curative, but only palliative, and that, if it is given for sleeplessness, it will act so much more like Opium, the more it is homœopathically indicated by slowness of the beats of the heart.

3. **Dilatatio Cordis.**

Dilatation of the Heart.

We mention this condition here so as to avoid incurring the reproach of incompleteness and rendering the pathological statements in other numbers unintelligible. As regards treatment, the treatment of dilatation of the heart coincides with both hypertrophy and fatty degeneration.

Dilatation of the heart may arise, if the heart or the respective ventricle or auricle is exposed during diastole to an increased pressure of the inflowing blood which overcomes to a certain degree the resisting power of the walls of the heart. Inasmuch, however, as the blood flowing in during the diastole of the heart is driven by a proportionally feeble *vis a tergo*, it is easily understood why the thick walls of the left ventricle and auricle are so rarely dilated, and why this dilatation is so much more commonly met with on the side of the right ventricle and auricle. Since, in such circumstances, the ventricle makes greater efforts to free itself from its contents which have become excessive, a dilatation is almost always succeeded by hypertrophy, giving rise to eccentric hypertrophy.

In another series of cases the cause of dilatation is not an increased pressure of the blood, but a diminished energy of the muscular structure of the heart, and here we meet with a genuine dilatation without any compensating, consecutive hypertrophy. This diminished energy of the muscular structure of the heart either originates in exceedingly debilitating constitutional diseases, such as typhus and a high degree of anæmia; in which case dilatation of the heart is merely a symptom of these pathological processes whose disappearance generally implies a complete disappearance of the dilatation; or else this defect originates in a disease of the muscular tissue itself, most generally fatty degeneration, less frequently serous infiltration, such as may take place during inflammation of the muscular tissue of the heart, in which case this form of dilatation and fatty degeneration become more or less identical.

From these reasons we have deemed it unnecessary to devote a special chapter to the treatment of dilatation.

4. Adipositas Cordis.

Fatty Degeneration of the Heart.

Fatty degeneration either consists in an abnormal increase of the normal quantity of fat about the heart, or in the adventitious formation of fat within the muscular tissue of the heart.

In the former case, the fatty heart proper, the disease can be traced to all those causes that determine a general increase of fat; hence fatty heart is generally met with among persons inclined to grow fat; fatty heart is likewise the result of an excessive use of ardent spirits. On the contrary and in defiance of all physiological explanations, a fatty heart is sometimes, although rarely, met with in cachectic individuals or in persons tainted with a constitutional dyscrasia.

The second kind, fatty degeneration of the muscular tissue, not unfrequently results from the former. Other more or less reliable causes of this disorganization are: All pathological processes that impair the assimilative power of the muscular structure of the heart, myocarditis, adhesions of the pericardium, largely developed hypertrophy of the heart, valvular defects, more particularly obliteration or degeneration of the coronary arteries.—All other causes that result in morbid fatty metamorphoses in other organs.—Dyscrasia of drunkards.

In fatty heart, the normal quantity of fat covering the sulcus and apex of the heart, etc., is sometimes increased to such a degree that the whole heart seems surrounded by a thick cushion of fat. The layer of fat deposited on the right side of the heart, is always more considerable and is formed sooner than on the other side. Not unfrequently the fat dips into the interstices of the muscular fibres, impairs their nutrition and either results in atrophy or a fatty degeneration of the muscular tissue.

In fatty degeneration which affects more particularly the left heart, as the other form, fatty heart, affects more particularly the right heart, the affected parts of the heart have a pale, yellowish color, are flabby and easily torn. Commonly the degeneration is confined to striated portions of the muscular tissue, is apt to affect the columnæ carneæ, and, if very extensive, is always accompanied by considerable dilatation of the heart. The single muscular fibrils, when seen under the microscope, are seen filled with fat-globules, and have lost their transverse striæ.

Symptoms and Course. The lesser grades of fatty heart and fatty degeneration of the heart may run their course without any morbid phenomena; there may even exist a considerable deposition of fat, and yet the general health of the patient may be perfectly sound. Morbid symptoms may not take place until the pressure of the fat causes atrophy or fatty degeneration of the muscular tissue. The first symptoms of this disease consist in functional deficiency of the heart: peculiar feelings of weakness, dyspnœa from the least exertion. In addition to this we have disposition to vertigo, fainting fits or paroxysms resembling syncope and sometimes even apoplexy. Except a distressing sensation of pressure the patient does not experience any pain. In the higher grades of this disease the skin becomes cool, disposed to perspire profusely, it assumes a pale and sickly appearance, œdema sets in, and the excessive weakness of the circulation may result in dropsy. The physical signs are the following: Increasing weakness of the impulse of the heart; feebleness of the sounds of the heart, especially of the first ventricular sound; increased extent of cardiac dulness, only in far advanced cases; blowing murmurs in the region of the orifices, owing to the circumstance that the diseased columnæ carneæ no longer permit the valves to completely close the orifices; easily compressible, soft, unresisting pulse which may show every possible irregularity and is often extremely slow.

This affection only runs an acute course if the fatty degeneration sets in rapidly and very extensively in consequence of inflammatory processes; otherwise the disease runs a very chronic course and depending upon the following conditions. If the fatty degeneration affects an hypertrophied heart with valvular disease, dilatation and finally paralysis of the heart result, or else rupture of the heart takes place. This may likewise result from a less extensive fatty degeneration, after partial dilatation has occurred. The disease is very commonly characterized by marked remissions or even complete intermissions. Death takes place, although not in a majority of cases, either by general marasmus with dropsy, or by œdema of the lungs or paralysis of the brain, or, which is most commonly the case, very suddenly by acute anæmia of the brain, rupture or paralysis of the heart.

In treating this disease, we have to aim in the first place at arresting its progress by the avoidance of every hurtful influence generally and every dietetic indiscretion in particular; next, at stopping the paroxysms of distress as soon as possible; and finally at effecting a retrograde metamorphosis of the disorganization.

In a curative point of view, the dietetic treatment is really applicable only to fatty heart, not to fatty degeneration. There is no doubt that we are sometimes able to remove an excessive tendency to fatness, and most probably to influence by similar proceedings, the excessive deposition of fat about the heart. In this respect, the extraordinary efficacy of the Karlsbad springs is so well known that we could not help censuring a physician who would refuse to send his patients to Karlsbad from no higher motive than a fanatical adherence to a therapeutic system. Unfortunately the fat which had disappeared under the influence of Karlsbad, but too often and rapidly returns even in an increased quantity after the patient has gone back to his home. This is sometimes and perhaps most commonly the patient's own fault; but not unfrequently it is the fault of the improper dietetic instructions emanating from the physician. We should be led too far, if we were to go into full particulars regarding the diet; all we shall do is to present the following general propositions to the reader's attentive regard. The production of fat is owing to an excessive supply of food, the supply considerably exceeding the waste. The quantity of fat produced will be so much greater the more the supply consists of substances that are known to make fat, principally animal and vegetable fats and starch-containing food. Beer generally promotes the formation of fat either directly or indirectly. Meat, if constituting the chief article of diet, scarcely ever makes fat. These few points suffice as general dietetic directions. Let the supply and waste be properly balanced by bodily and mental occupation, and let whatever excess remains be done away with. The patients should principally use lean meat, not starch-containing vegetables or fruit, and but little bread and wine; and they should be directed never to overload their stomachs as so many people do from mere habit, not from necessity. By pursuing such a system of diet and hygiene, the patient will be able to do without a resort to Karlsbad. Starvation-cures are the more condemnable in the case of such patients, the more the heart has already become diseased. At the same time, it must be admitted that there are many persons who, most generally in consequence of abnormal changes in the functions of the liver, deposit such quantities of fat, even under the simplest and most cautious diet, that it seems impossible to suggest any further changes in this respect.

Fatty degeneration may sometimes, but assuredly only in rare instances, have its primary origin in a constitutional tendency to fatness; otherwise we are unacquainted with any other cause of this disease that might suggest special dietetic preventive rules.

If the presence of the cardiac disease is substantiated beyond any doubt, the patient's mode of living has to be regulated with a view of preserving his strength as much as possible. Substantial nourishment, so far from being forbidden, should be recommended; the moderate use of wine is generally attended with the happiest results. In the case of drunkards, spirits should be withdrawn gradually, not all at once. A sudden and complete abstemiousness might lead to dropsy; indeed the frequent occurrence of such an event should be a warning to us. The prostration which follows every considerable exertion, admonishes the patient never to use his strength to the point of exhaustion. This precaution likewise applies to mental efforts. The frequent paroxysms resembling syncope or simulating apoplexy are very apt to lead to the adoption of measures which, by depressing the strength, are at the same time calculated to aggravate the patient's condition for the reason that these cerebral phenomena do not depend upon anæmia, but hyperæmia. Venesection is of course out of the question; patients with whom we are not yet sufficiently acquainted, should have their attention directed to the pernicious consequences of blood-letting, lest they should feel disposed to resort to it without the advice of a physician.

Of the intercurrent morbid phenomena these pseudo-apoplectic paroxysms and those resembling angina pectoris deserve most attention and should by all means be met by some appropriate remedy. In the former, *Camphora* will be found most efficient, more particularly on account of the rapidity with which it acts. Beside Camphora we may try *Veratrum album* and *Pulsatilla*. As soon as a fainting sensation comes over the patient, he must be laid in a horizontal position, with the head on a level with the rest of the body. If the syncope lasts too long and life seems to be endangered by it, *Ammonium carbonicum* and even *Ether* may be resorted to without fear.

In paroxysms attended with an increase of the heart's action, *Digitalis* is the most homœopathic and therefore the most efficient agent, provided it is given in a small dose. *Opium, Cannabis, Laurocerasus* may likewise be administered with some chances of success.

The disease in its totality will have to be acted upon both by means of medicines that exert an influence over the excessive formation of fat, such as *Ferrum, China, Calcarea, Arsenicum,* and likewise by such medicines as are in special rapport with the heart. First in rank we have undoubtedly *Digitalis* whose pathogenesis presents the most striking image of excited and yet powerless, extremely irregular action of the heart. Whether it is of much or any use in adiposis, we dare not either affirm or deny; but in fatty degeneration its influence is as great as that of any other remedy. Of course, the dose has to be proportioned to the quantity of reactive power with the utmost care. *Iodium* is likewise of considerable importance. It has an extreme tendency to palpitation of the heart during the least motion, improved by a horizontal posture; it has the peculiarity inherent in inflammatory exudations to undergo an abnormal metamorphosis; it has a disposition to an abnormal deposition of fat. Hence *Iodium* is one of the few remedies that corresponds to the morbid process in question in every direction. On a former occasion we have already once denied the power of *Arsenic* to influence structural changes of the heart; we here repeat this statement, although it is undoubtedly true that the pathogenesis of Arsenic has many symptoms which, when detached from their connected series, can be referred to fatty heart. We have two other remedies which we cannot recommend with sufficient emphasis in heart-disease generally and more especially in fatty degeneration, we mean *Cuprum* and *Plumbum*. Both remedies act similarly, except that the action of *Plumbum* is more persistent and penetrating. We would only use either of them in cases of uncomplicated fatty degeneration. Since their provings do not contain a single heart-symptom, we will indicate those that may be found in cases of poisoning. *Cuprum* has: Pulse irregular, small, easily compressible, intermitting, accompanied by excessive muscular debility; the beats of the heart are scarcely, or not at all perceptible; the sounds of the heart are indistinct; dyspnœa, feeling of anxiety, disposition to faint. *Plumbum* has: The impulse of the heart is very feeble, or even imperceptible, intermitting; sounds of the heart indistinct; palpitations attended with excessive dyspnœa; pulse very soft, easily compressible, intermitting; irregular, fifty to sixty in the minute, less frequently over a hundred, after which it is scarcely perceptible; heart flabby; sudden paralysis of the heart; fainting fits during every exertion, also attended with slight convulsions; extreme muscular debility and oppression from the least motion; despondency and dread of death; nightmare; œdema of the skin. As for *Sulphur*, we should not expect any favorable effects from it in these disorganizations; its pathogenesis does not indicate it in this disease, nor can it be referred to it by a process of analogy; for even if fatty degeneration were to be regarded as the expression of a perverse metamorphosis of some inflammatory exudation, we cannot show from analogy in other organs that *Sulphur* is capable of antagonizing a metamorphosis of this kind. *Aurum*, on the contrary, is a remedy well worthy our attention, more particularly if the heart-disease causes great depression of spirits; usually the local symptoms are insufficient to legitimate the choice of this agent; and clinical testimony is entirely wanting.

5. Anomalies.

Abnormal Conditions of the Orifices of the Heart;
Valvular Diseases.

Although every alteration of the orifices might be designated as an abnormal condition, yet, in pathology, this term is applied in a therapeutical aspect to such alterations only as really interfere with the functions of the heart. In view of our powerlessness in the presence of such disorganizations, nobody will find fault with us for only mentioning the most essential characteristics of these disorders.

The etiology of these abnormal conditions of the orifices is very obscure, and in very many cases no definite cause can be assigned to them. All influences that occasion acute endocarditis, may likewise be considered as causes of valvular diseases; among these causes rheumatism occupies the most prominent rank. This applies particularly to anomalies affecting younger persons. Among persons of a more advanced age it is the still obscure process of chronic endocarditis, the atheromatous deposition and degeneration which affects the valves as well as the arteries. Other causes which, however, are extremely rare, are: Dilatation of the heart, external pressure or a severe strain, excessive exertions, ruptures. Sex does not seem to have any influence in this direction, except that repeated observations have shown that women are more frequently affected with anomalies of the venous, and men more frequently with anomalies of the arterial orifices. Beyond the age of twenty-five a liability to every kind of anomaly sets in, which seems to increase in proportion as persons grow older. Corresponding with the prevalence of endocarditis, acute as well as chronic, in the left heart, it is only exceptionally that orificial anomalies are met with in the right side of the heart.

The following are the more particular alterations to be met with in the different orifices respectively:

a. *Insufficiency of the Mitral Valve.*

During the systole the mitral valve closes the ventricle more or less imperfectly against the auricle, either because its lappels are shrunk or torn, or the tendinous chords and the coulmnæ carneæ are abnormally altered. Hence, during the systole blood regurgitates into the auricle. This causes a gradual dilatation of the auricle, the flow of blood from the pulmonary veins is impeded, the vessels constituting the lesser circulation, become engorged with blood, finally, the right heart is overcrowded with blood, giving rise to eccentric hypertrophy and, as an ultimate result, causing a stasis in the peripheral veins. If the insufficiency is but little, the left ventricle remains unchanged; the higher degrees of insufficiency lead to dilatation and hypertrophy of this ventricle. Physical signs: Greater extent of cardiac dulness in breadth; impulse of the heart stronger and over a larger area; undulatory movements of the right ventricle. Systolic murmur, most distinct at the apex, sometimes like a purring murmur; second sound of the pulmonary artery louder, sometimes so loud that it can be felt; pulse either normal, or, if the insufficiency is considerable, very much weaker, sometimes irregular.

The consequences of this anomaly to the whole organism are: hyperæmia of the lungs; sanguineous clots in the lungs; catarrh of the bronchial mucous lining; hæmoptoë; dyspnœa; emphysema; hyperæmia of the brain, liver, spleen, kidneys, stomach, with chronic gastric catarrh; subsequently œdema and serous effusions in the different regions attacked by hyperæmia.

The prognosis of this affection, of itself, is not entirely unfavorable. Although a cure is scarcely ever possible, yet patients may, with care, live to an advanced age. This depends upon the compensation established by the right ventricle and auricle; as long as this compensation is sufficient, the patients are not in any very great danger. But if an increase of dyspnœa, a stasis in the peripheral circulation, or œdema show that the compensation is incomplete, an approaching termination of the patient's sufferings may be safely prognosticated. The prognosis is still worse if valvular insufficiency becomes associated with stenosis of the left auriculo-ventricular orifice, as is most frequently the case. Before speaking of the treatment, let us dwell a little further on the stenosis of the left auriculo-ventricular orifice.

b. *Stenosis of the Left Auriculo-ventricular Orifice.*

A constriction of this orifice interferes with the passage of the blood from the auricle into the ventricle, so that a portion of the blood remains behind in the auricle.

This result is superinduced by the following anatomical changes: The valves are thickened, especially at their insertion or base, or their segments or lappets are more or less completely soldered together or variously distorted in shape, or the chordæ tendineæ may be contracted, shrunk and deprived of their elasticity, so that the valves are drawn down into the ventricle, and their segments assume a funnel-shaped appearance. In this way, an ostium naturally large may be reduced to the condition of a mere slit or to the diameter of a goose-quill or pea.

The consequences of stenosis are the same as those of insufficiency of the mitral valves: Imperfect emptying of the left auricle, stasis of the blood in the pulmonary vessels, overcrowding of the right ventricle followed by eccentric hypertrophy as a means of compensation, which may increase to such an extent that the tricuspid valve becomes insufficient to close the right auriculo-ventricular orifice. The left ventricle receives a smaller supply of blood; hence, the flow of blood through the arteries becomes less active, the pulse grows very small and feeble. In the course of time the capacity of the ventricle becomes reduced and its walls become atrophied. These changes do not take place if the stenosis is associated with conditions in the aortic system inviting increased exertions on the part of the left ventricle. Even in more remote organs the stenosis results in the same phenomena of stasis as are consequent upon valvular insufficiency, and generally more rapidly and more extensively.

This lesion is characterized by the following physical signs: Cardiac dulness very extensive in breadth, owing to the often extraordinary distention of the right ventricle; the impulse of the heart is heard over a more extensive area both to the left and to the right, even as far as the right sternal border, and powerfully shakes the thoracic wall; the præcordial region is sometimes arched; the flapping of the tricuspid valves is sometimes sensible to the hand; diastolic purring is very commonly perceived at the apex of the heart. Auscultation returns a diastolic murmur at the apex of the heart, and the first sound is considerably feebler; or if the stenosis is associated with valvular insufficiency, a murmur is heard instead of the sound. The aortic sounds are weaker, the sounds of the pulmonary artery, especially the second sound, are considerably stronger.

From what we have said, the subjective symptoms may be readily inferred. The patients always suffer more from stenosis than from valvular insufficiency; the untoward consequences set in sooner and more intensely, and hemorrhages of the most varied kind accompany stenosis much more commonly. Accordingly the prognosis is of course much more unfavorable, since in the long run a compensating equilibrium cannot possibly be maintained.

The treatment of these two anomalies can never aim at a complete cure. Even if we were to concede the possibility of curing orificial defects that had but recently arisen from an attack of acute endocarditis: yet these defects do not become an object of treatment until they have existed for a long time without being noticed. Hence we shall have to confine ourselves in any event to a purely symptomatic treatment, and even then shall have to abandon all hope of achieving any permanent improvement.

In selecting a remedial agent for these abnormal conditions, we have to limit our choice to remedies characterized by insufficiency and weakness of cardiac action, not allowing ourselves by an occasional appearance of functional excitement of the heart to be led to the adoption of remedies that are only adapted to an augmentation of cardiac activity. However, the mischief which an improperly selected remedy might do, would only be of a serious nature in case disproportionately large doses of the remedy were given; for the loss of time which a mistake of this kind might involve, would be of very little importance considering the slow course which such disorganizations generally run. In other respects the selection can never depend exclusively upon the cardiac symptoms which are almost always the same, but will have to be determined by the locality and quality of the consecutive affections. In the following series of remedies we mention after each remedy the main consecutive or secondary symptoms requiring its use.

Digitalis purpurea claims undoubtedly the first rank. No remedy corresponds by its physiological symptoms more fully than Digitalis with the group of pathological phenomena evolved by disease of the mitral valves. In the heart we have the deficient action of the arterial half, with increased action of the venous half; the tumultuous movements of the heart in spite of its diminished energy; the irregularity of the rhythm, etc. All the other organs likewise exhibit the most significant phenomena. The urinary secretion is considerably less. We have passive hyperæmia of the brain with its consequences. We have likewise pulmonary hyperæmia, sometimes as a passing congestion, and at times in the form of a chronic bronchial catarrh with hemorrhage, dyspnœa. There is hyperæmia of the liver, even to the extent of giving rise to icteric phenomena. We have symptoms of intestinal and gastric catarrh; moreover a tendency to serous effusion. In short, the whole complex of the pathological phenomena points to *Digitalis* as our first choice in the treatment of these disorganizations. Digitalis is even indicated by the peculiar pneumonia which is not unfrequently favored and even excited by the stenosis of the left auriculo-ventricular orifice. Only let the remedy be administered in a small dose; this is of paramount importance. Even if large doses seem to agree at the beginning, yet in the long run they exert a decidedly pernicious influence.

We advise the use of **Belladonna** in all cases where Aconitum seems indicated by the symptoms. In this kind of disorder Aconite never exerts a favorable influence. Belladonna is especially indicated by the paroxysmally increasing pulmonary hyperæmia and the headache which sometimes reaches a terrible degree of intensity. It is less frequently efficacious in the resulting hepatic derangements.

Pulsatilla cannot be numbered among the prominent remedies; we would at most employ it in the higher grades of bronchial catarrh.

Veratrum album competes with Belladonna as far as the affected organs are concerned; yet there are symptomatic differences. It is suitable for cerebral and pulmonary congestions setting in with pallor and coldness of the outer skin, or with a decidedly cyanotic tinge.

Opium, in small doses, in the case of drunkards is a main remedy for celebral hyperæmia, less for the respiratory difficulties. In such cases it often acts with wonderful rapidity and completeness, although the effect does not last.

Tartarus stibiatus is indicated by bronchial catarrh with profuse secretion of mucus, and by a gastric catarrh the symptoms of which may be compared in the Mat. Med. Pura.

Arsenicum which seems indicated much more frequently than it really is, has only shown a decisive effect in our hands against the sleeplessness which is a not uncommon symptom in these disorders; it has never seemed to be of any use in affections of the respiratory organs for which it seems such an excellent remedy if these affections are not occasioned by valvular defects. Nor does it ordinarily seem to have any effect in dropsical difficulties.

The remedies we have named so far, are in general adapted only to overcoming single ailments either acute or subacute; to this list we will add the following: *Phosphorus, Squilla, Secale cornutum, Iodium, Ammonium carbonicum.* Another series of drugs has to be opposed to chronic secondary affections which, although necessary consequences of the cardiac disorganizations, very often admit of a diminution, or at least of an arrest of the symptoms.

China and **Ferrum** here occupy the first rank; the former more especially, if the anæmic phenomena which are an inevitable consequence of the deficient activity of the left ventricle, are associated with frequent paroxysms of passing congestions of the brain, and if the hepatic functions are greatly interfered with. *Ferrum* is indicated rather by a tendency to pulmonary congestions and to hemorrhage from the bronchia, by prominent symptoms of gastric catarrh, and, like China, by enlargements of the spleen. *Ferrum* is not very suitable to old people; *China*, on the contrary, is eminently so.

In chronic ailments **Arsenicum** deserves more attention than in acute complaints. It may be tried in liver-complaint as well as in renal affections; sometimes it renders good service, but more frequently it leaves us in the lurch.

Baryta carbonica has already been mentioned in the bronchial catarrh of old people; we likewise recommend it, if the catarrh is occasioned by valvular deficiency.

Carbo veget. may still afford help, if every other remedy had left us in the lurch. This remedy embodies in its pathogenesis all the consequences of the anomalies here treated of: a disposition to atonic hemorrhage; the anæmic symptoms in cyanosis; œdematous swellings, pulmonary œdema; passive hyperæmia of the brain, lungs, liver, spleen; chronic bronchial catarrh in every stage, pulmonary hemorrhage; gastric catarrh. There is scarcely another remedy that represents so clearly a definite morbid condition. Clinical results have substantiated the truth of this similarity.

Beside these remedies, those that have been named for fatty degeneration may likewise be ranked here, especially *Plumbum*, *Cuprum* and *Aurum*. For single symptoms: *Lycopodium* and *Natrum muriaticum* are particularly efficacious. The last-mentioned remedies likewise embrace within their curative range, if help is at all possible, the last link of this series of consecutive disorders, namely: local and general dropsy.

The mode of living has an influence upon the final result that must not be underrated. Bodily motions and exertions are regulated without the least difficulty; proper dietetic precautions are easily violated. Inasmuch as the whole tendency of the anomalies, of which we have treated, is to change the blood to venous blood, since the interference with the lesser circulation only admits of an imperfect oxygenation of the blood: our whole aim should be to furnish the patient with such nourishment as will not require the assistance of the pulmonary circulation, and likewise in an easily assimilable form on account of the gastro-intestinal canal being generally very much disordered during the presence of these anomalies. Hence, fat food and starch-containing substances have to be avoided, whereas good meat and beef broth should be recommended as chief articles of diet. The use of wine which seems to be counter-indicated by the tumultuous action of the heart, is not only very useful, but even necessary, especially in the case of old people. We likewise call attention to the inhalation of compressed air which deserves particular recommendation in this disease; a great deal depends upon rendering the act of respiration easier to the patient by furnishing him a larger supply of oxygen, which is accomplished by this proceeding.

c. *Insufficiency of the Aortic Valves.*

The semilunar valves are no longer sufficient to effect a complete closure of the aorta during the diastole of the heart. This may be owing to a shrinking, laceration, rigidity, adhesions and distortions of the valves. Disorganizations of this kind very seldom result from mechanical force or from acute endocarditis, but commonly from chronic endocarditis and from atheromatous degeneration. On this account aortic insufficiency is generally met with in older persons.

Insufficiency results in a regurgitation of the blood during the diastole of the ventricle from the aorta into the ventricle. In consequence of this overcrowding, the ventricle becomes abnormally distended; hence, if the valves are insufficient, the left ventricle becomes more distended in consequence of this anomaly than from any other. The increase of the ventricular contents invites an increased contraction of the muscular fibres, thus giving rise to eccentric hypertrophy which becomes the more excessive the greater the valvular insufficiency. If at the same time the left auriculo-ventricular orifice is normal, the insufficiency shows no further consequences in the lungs, nor does it react upon the right ventricle. On the other hand, the consequences are visible in the arterial system; the arteries, being exposed to a considerable increase of pressure or a force acting *a tergo*, dilate and, in the further course of the disease, very commonly undergo an atheromatous degeneration.

The objective symptoms of aortic insufficiency are generally very plain as soon as the affection has acquired a certain degree of importance. Corresponding with the extensive hypertrophy of the left ventricle, the cardiac dulness extends over a much larger area, more to the left side and even as far as the seventh intercostal space. Palpation discovers a much more forcible and more extensive impulse of the heart, which sometimes shakes very violently the whole of the anterior wall of the chest; a purring murmur is not unfrequently heard at the upper end of the sternum, and a peculiar whir or buzz during the systole of the heart. Auscultation returns over the ostium of the aorta, at the place of insertion of the third costal cartilage, a diastolic murmur which is most commonly heard as far as beyond the sternum and vanishes the more completely the more the ear approximates to the apex of the heart. The second aortic sound is at times entirely absent, or else is faintly audible at the commencement of the murmur. The first aortic sound is either normal or associated with a murmur. The sounds of the right ventricle are normal, the second sound of the pulmonary artery is at most somewhat louder. The changes in the arteries yield the following exceedingly characteristic phenomena: The pulsation of the arch of the aorta is sometimes felt in the jugular. The carotids pulsate so strongly that their vibrations are distinctly seen and that the whole neck and head are sometimes shaken by the motion. A distinct murmur is likewise easily heard in the carotids in the place of a feeble second sound. The arteries at the periphery are dilated and pulsate visibly. The pulse is large, hard, and bounds against the finger in a peculiarly short and rapid manner; sometimes it vibrates, especially under soft pressure.

The subjective symptoms differ greatly according as the insufficiency is more or less considerable or the hypertrophic compensation more or less complete. As long as the hypertrophy equilibrates the insufficiency, the patients feel quite well and do not even complain of palpitation, no matter how much more forcible the impulse of the heart may seem. But as soon as the compensating equilibrium is disturbed by an excess of hypertrophy, constitutional derangements begin to become manifest. These consist at first in more or less violent congestions especially in the brain which, if accompanied by considerable atheromatous degeneration of the arterial walls, easily result in rupture of the vessels and apoplexy. Attacks of vertigo, luminous vibrations before the eyes, highly flushed face with a violent throbbing sensation, throbbing headache, sleeplessness, etc., if occurring during insufficiency of the aortic valves, are always unwelcome phenomena which show that the compensating equilibrium which Nature had set up, is disturbed. In other organs, likewise, we notice a tendency to bloody extravasations, especially from the genital organs of young women. If the opposite takes place in the course of the disease; if the hypertrophied ventricle is unable to compensate the valvular insufficiency, which is apt to be the case if a process of fatty degeneration is at the same time set up in the muscular tissue of the ventricle, the morbid picture assumes an entirely different aspect. The vessels which had been very much dilated previously, now receive too scanty a supply of blood, and, in consequence of having lost their elasticity, are not even able to completely propel this smaller quantity; hence, symptoms of cerebral anæmia supervene, and even in the veins the blood courses more slowly. At this stage, the discharge of blood from the left auricle is likewise interfered with, and all the consequences of stenosis of the mitral orifice develop themselves in this case, although in a less degree and less rapidly.

This shows that the prognosis of aortic insufficiency depends greatly upon the equilibrium between the action of the heart and impediments to the circulation. As soon as this equilibrium is disturbed the danger increases the more, the more considerable the disturbance. The older the patient; the greater the probability of an extensive atheromatous degeneration of the arteries, the more seriously is the patient's life threatened which generally ends with a sudden attack of apoplexy. If symptoms of disturbance in the pulmonary circulation supervene, the final catastrophy is undoubtedly at hand. If valvular anomalies at other orifices are simultaneously present, our previous remarks will of course undergo considerable modifications.

As regards treatment we may refer to our statements when speaking of hypertrophy, since it is hypertrophy that invests valvular deficiencies with threatening danger. The general conduct of such patients has to be regulated with much more care than in simple hypertrophy, for the reason that every unusual exitement of the action of the heart may result in what is so much to be dreaded, a rupture of the vessels. Every sort of bloodletting is exceedingly pernicious; even now this is sometimes recommended by physicians, or resorted to by the patient without the physician's advice, for the purpose of preventing or removing intercurrent congestions.

d. *Stenosis of the Aortic Orifice.*

The aortic orifice is constricted and does not admit of a free passage of the blood. The narrowing is occasioned by a thickening of the semilunar valves consequent upon endocarditis, which incapacitates the valves from adjusting themselves to the walls of the aorta. This constitutes an insufficiency the force of which is in inverse ratio to stenosis.

The necessary consequence of an impeded emptying of the left ventricle is an increased activity of its walls to propel the blood, hence hypertrophy. It is to be observed that, if stenosis is the only difficulty, the hypertrophy does not become eccentric, or at least only very little so, whereas, if insufficiency is present at the same time, hypertrophy becomes associated with dilatation. Stenosis does not exert a marked influence over the other parts of the heart until the hypertrophy is no longer sufficient to keep up the compensating equilibrium. In such circumstances the pulmonary circulation is disturbed, the right ventricle becomes hypertrophied, but never in such a high degree as from stenosis of the left auriculo-ventricular orifice. The influence of stenosis upon the motion of the blood through the arteries is manifested by the incompleteness and feebleness of the arterial current.

The objective symptoms of this disorder are: All the symptoms which have been previously indicated as characterizing a considerable hypertrophy of the left ventricle. Auscultation over the aortic orifice usually returns a loud systolic murmur which frequently reaches a good ways laterally and downwards, disguising the sounds of the heart more or less, and being most commonly audible even in the arteries of the neck. The first sound of the aorta is absent, the second sound is generally feebler, more indistinct, or likewise replaced by a diastolic murmur if the stenosis is complicated with insufficiency. The sounds of the right side of the heart are normal. As long as the stenosis is properly compensated by hypertrophy, the pulse is indeed somewhat small but hard, and only becomes small and even soft after the compensating equilibrium is disturbed. The pulse generally constitutes an excellent means of obtaining a correct judgment of the condition of the heart.

In cases where the stenosis is completely equilibrated by ventricular hypertrophy, the subjective symptoms are generally of no importance; the patient may feel quite well, only his countenance is somewhat pallid. If the compensation becomes insufficient, symptoms of a deficient supply of blood to the brain and of real anæmia first become apparent, after which symptoms of stasis in the lesser circulation and in the veins slowly show themselves.

It is impossible to indicate a definite mode of treating this stenosis, for the simple reason that the character of this anomaly varies too much and that it is always complicated with other abnormal alterations. As long as the patients feel well, medicine is useless or even hurtful; the stenosis cannot be cured and all that the medicine might possibly accomplish, would be to disturb the functional cardiac equilibrium. If the compensation becomes insufficient, we have to resort to the remedies that were recommended for fatty degeneration: *Veratrum, Iodium, Arsenicum* and especially *Digitalis*, and with reference to the deficiency in the process of sanguification: *Ferrum, Calcarea carbonica* and *China*. If symptoms of venous stasis make their appearance, we have to choose such remedies as have been recommended for mitral stenosis. The regimen to be pursued differs of course from that recommended for aortic insufficiency, since in view of the deficient supply of arterial blood the process of assimilation is of course rendered more difficult. Hence our chief aim should be to give the body a chance to make good blood, by furnishing it a supply of easily digested and nourishing food and an abundance of fresh air. Even the use of wine need not be forbidden; on the contrary, it is often to be recommended, both in order to promote the process of digestion and as a direct stimulant for the heart. If the stenosis is at the same time associated with insufficiency of the semilunar valves, the treatment becomes much more difficult, because it is often difficult to decide, the consequences of which of these two anomalies ought to be met first. Generally one anomaly will probably be more marked than the other, in which case the course to be pursued in the treatment is naturally indicated.

The combinations of valvular diseases of the left heart, as they generally present themselves, complicate the treatment by presenting difficulties for which it is, however, impossible to arrange definite therapeutic rules and practical applications of drugs. Since conditions of this kind fortunately never require the immediate intervention of remedial agents, there will always be time enough in a given case to consider what treatment had better be pursued, and what remedies are most adapted to the case. Any special presentation of the symptoms characterizing such combinations is not called for, since anybody may construct such a series in his own mind.

e. *Defects of the Orifices and Valves of the Right Heart.*

They occur so seldom, especially as isolated affections, that we will condense all we may have to say on the subject, in a few brief remarks.

Insufficiency of the tricuspid valve is the most frequently occurring defect on the right side of the heart, and originates in the same morbid processes as insufficiencies in the left heart. Its consequences are: eccentric hypertrophy of the right ventricle and stasis of the blood in the veins of the systemic circulation. If the anomaly is considerable, it gives rise to venous pulsation. Defects of the mitral valve and of the consequent excessive eccentric hypertrophy of the right ventricle may lead to a so-called relative insufficiency of the tricuspid valve which is of special importance to a proper diagnostic appreciation of the whole condition, for the reason that, on the appearance of this insufficiency, the stasis in the venous system reaches an extraordinary degree, and dropsy is eminent. The diagnosis is determined by a systolic murmur which is most distinctly audible in the region of the tricuspid valve. The treatment has to be conducted in accordance with our remarks on mitral insufficiency, since the consequences are entirely the same as those of the latter anomaly.

The rest of valvular diseases as well as stenoses are exceedingly rare; no special remarks can be offered regarding their treatment.

6. Nervous Palpitation of the Heart.
Palpitatio Cordis.

Palpitation of the heart, by which we mean a momentary, more or less continuous increase of the frequency and strength of the beats of the heart, is not only met with in a large number of morbid conditions beside the cardiac affections of which we have treated in the preceding numbers, but likewise in persons of sound health, after violent mental and bodily exertions. This is not the kind of palpitation that we wish to consider in this article, but those detached paroxysms of increased cardiac activity which set in without any demonstrable alterations in the substance of the heart, and without any definite exciting cause.

The etiology of this affection, as far as regards a knowledge of the physiological connection between cause and effect, is exceedingly obscure. All that we know is, that this palpitation frequently, but not by any means constantly, sets in after strong emotions either of an exciting or a depressing kind; that it may result from all such circumstances as weaken the nervous system and consequently render it more irritable, such as anæmia, chlorosis, onanism, venereal excesses, excessive mental exertions; that it may likewise result from certain nervous affections, such as hypochondria, hysteria, spinal irritation, softening; that it may likewise result from the condition which is designated as general plethora; and that it finally may occur as a reflex effect of certain morbid conditions, especially of the abdominal cavity, such as helminthiasis, cholelithiasis.

The symptoms of this affection vary in the main in two directions, according as the increased action of the heart is only felt by the patient, or is likewise perceptible as an objective phenomenon. In neither case is the paroxysm preceded by distinct symptoms; it arises all at once after a trivial exciting cause, or even without any evident reason. Paroxysms where the patient alone is conscious of the palpitation, are by far the worst and attended with the greatest distress. The heart feels as if it were hanging loose, trembling or falling down, without any external change being observable; the single beats even are feebler rather than stronger. At the same time the patient experiences a fearful anguish and restlessness, and with every new paroxysm imagines that his death is at hand. The face is pallid, covered with a cold perspiration, the eyes stare, the extremities are cool, the consciousness sometimes seems to vanish for a time. The pulse is always small, compressible, sometimes intermitting. Paroxysms of this kind seldom last for a long time, perhaps only a few minutes, seldom longer than an hour. Paroxysms of the second kind are characterized by an externally perceptible increase of the cardiac activity, the impulse of the heart is a good deal stronger, the beats succeed each other more rapidly, the patient experiences a painful throbbing in all the arteries, the pulse is full and hard, and even in this case not unfrequently unrhythmical. The face is turgescent, highly flushed, the eyes glistening and staring, the body is at times cool, at other times hot. The patients complain of headache, buzzing in the ears, luminous vibrations before their eyes, dyspnœa which interrupts speech and obliges them to sigh frequently, and of vertigo which may even be very violent. Nothing abnormal is perceived at the heart, only the sounds of the heart are considerably stronger. These paroxysms at times are only of short duration, at other times they continue for hours.

The course of this affection varies; often it is very obstinate, at other times it disappears together with the complaint occasioning it. Very seldom the paroxysms show any regularity. If the affection is incidental to the period of evolution, it generally disappears of itself and gradually.

The affection is not a very serious one, provided life is not directly threatened; this could only be the case if other complaints should assume a dangerous character in consequence of the abnormal increase of the heart's action. The disorder being a source of torment to the patient, the physician must necessarily desire to free him from it completely. We can certainly promise a cure unless the palpitation depends upon an otherwise incurable affection.

The diagnosis must never be based upon an examination instituted during the paroxysm, but should be derived from the condition of the patient during the free intervals.

As regards treatment, it is of importance that the previously established distinction between subjective and objective palpitations should not be lost sight of, if possible. Cases do occur where the objective increase of the heart's action is associated with subjective palpitation, although not always to the extent that the patient's distress and lamentations might lead us to suppose. For this reason the remedies contained in each of the two following series respectively ought not to be considered as belonging to either of them exclusively, but we have resorted to this arrangement simply with a view of facilitating the selection of the appropriate remedial agent.

Another point deserving special consideration in selecting a remedy, are the influences which excite the attack and the affections, if any, of which the palpitation constitutes a particular or the most distressing symptom. We can neither afford time nor space to dwell upon this point more fully, since this would lead to repetitions, and the appropriate remedies are, moreover, specially mentioned when the different pathological processes are treated of. In treating the palpitation of a chlorotic female, for instance, our first endeavor will certainly be to find a remedy that shall correspond with the totality of the chlorotic symptoms.

We do not wish to incur any censure if we mention the following remedies very briefly; it is our opinion that in a difficulty, which is so entirely local, the suitable remedy can be just as easily found in the Materia Medica as if we here compiled a repertory of all the remedies bearing upon such a case. For the sake of completeness we should likewise have to indicate the various accessory circumstances, which would plunge us into a maze of details.

For the objectively perceptible palpitation, which is particularly characterized by congestive symptoms, we recommend the following remedies:

Aconitum in the case of robust, plethoric, young individuals, likewise in the case of persons with excitable temperaments and who are subject to rushes of blood from every trifling emotion; likewise in the case of tuberculous individuals, where pulmonary congestions and palpitation of the heart exist together. Aconite is not indicated unless the column of blood is in a general state of excitement and increased movement. The action of Aconite is not governed by any particular time of day, but it is particularly suitable if the paroxysms occur more habitually towards evening. The movements of the heart are stronger, more rapid, but not by any means irregular.

Spigelia: The action of the heart is increased, but it is irregular both in rhythm and impulse, which is more like an undulating motion; the paroxysms occur at indefinite periods, but more especially in the morning; the patient's temperature is unequal, the extremities are cold to the touch; Spigelia is indicated for palpitations arising from worms.

Arsenicum: The heart beats much more forcibly and rapidly, seldom irregularly or indistinctly; the paroxysms occur principally at night during sleep, or about midnight, and are attended with excessive anxiety and restlessness; the skin does not feel cold, but burning hot; at most the extremities may feel cool. *Arsenicum* is particularly suitable if the paroxysms set in with typical regularity, or more particularly at the time of the menses; it is likewise suitable for chlorotic and asthmatic individuals, and for drunkards.

Ferrum is adapted to chlorotic and anæmic individuals, if the palpitation is attended with frequent changes of color in the face, and if the face looks flushed at the beginning of the paroxysm; it is likewise adapted to tuberculous individuals, likewise to individuals with excitable nerves, or with nerves rendered irritable by excessive excitement; it is adapted to females more particularly if the menses are scanty and the patients are suffering with uterine catarrh.

Nitrum as well as **Acidum nitricum** are characteristically distinguished by violent, but short-lasting pulmonary congestions without any real pain, they either precede the palpitation, or else set in simultaneously with it.

Nux vomica deserves particular consideration, if the palpitation is occasioned by irregularities in the digestive process, never lasts long, is attended with cerebral congestions or nausea; also if the palpitation is caused by abuse of spirits, in the case of drunkards; or if caused by abuse of coffee, or depending upon spinal irritation.

Platina, if the palpitation is attended with menstrual irregularities or retention of the menses; likewise if it is attended with a good deal of sexual excitement.

Belladonna is indicated under similar circumstances; it may likewise prove suitable for palpitation generally.

Phosphorus, Veratrum album, Aurum, Argentum likewise belong in this category.

In the second series we class the remedies that have a debilitating influence over the action of the heart, which the patient imagines is only excited momentarily or transitorily by these drugs.

Pulsatilla, if the palpitation is excited by the least irritation, is attended with great anxiety which seems to be out of all proportion to the slight objective symptoms; there is a rapid change of color in the face, the patient feels chilly; if the palpitation is relieved by motion, especially by exercise in the open air, or by a little pleasant social entertainment; if the palpitation rouses one from sleep at night. Pulsatilla is excellent in chlorosis if the nervous symptoms prevail, and is likewise suitable for palpitation during the menses.

China: Palpitation of the heart, with external coldness, soft and small pulse; after losses of animal fluids; in the case of individuals with great nervous prostration, hypochondriacs, persons addicted to self-abuse.

Camphora, for irregular palpitation, with unusual oppression of the chest evidently not arising from determination of blood, with very feeble pulse, general coldness of the body.

Ignatia, Sepia, Asafœtida, Nux moschata have very similar cardiac symptoms; they all have a small and weak pulse during the palpitation and a variable irregularity of the heart's action. They are chiefly adapted to hysteric palpitation of the heart.

In hypochondria where the heart's action is as frequently disturbed as in hysteria, the main remedies are: *Natrum muriaticum* and *Lycopodium*, moreover, *Cocculus, Aurum,* and *Nux vomica.*

Cannabis is next to Digitalis the surest remedy for palpitations occasioned by self-abuse and by an erethic weakness of the male organs.

Chamomilla and **Opium** are regarded as specific for palpitation caused by fright. [Also *Aconitum.* H.]

A third series is composed of drugs that may be classed indiscriminately in one or the other of these two series.

Digitalis is here the most important remedy. We have given its characteristic symptoms on former occasions, and here again point out a marked excitement of cardiac action associated with evident weakness of the muscular tissue, and likewise the irregular movements of the heart. *Digitalis* is the surest remedy for palpitation caused by self-abuse, in general for palpitation arising from some cause in the male sexual sphere.

Coffea. The palpitation is at times strong and visible, at other times is only felt by the patient; a characteristic symptom is great restlessness with weariness, yet the patient has no sleep, more particularly after a copious meal and late in the evening. Every one who drinks coffee, has experienced the good effects of coffee in this direction after a copious meal. For evening-palpitations *Coffea* generally affords relief to such only as do not use coffee as an habitual beverage. As a rule, the excitement of cardiac action occasioned by coffee is not associated with an increase of temperature or flushed face, even if the patients experience a sensation of increased warmth.

Calcarea carbonica is an excellent remedy, not for a single paroxysm, but for the affection generally. It is particularly adapted to chlorotic females, without pallor of the face, and with great tendency to rush of blood; it is especially adapted to children and young women, whose habitual palpitation it very often cures without the aid of any other drug.

Sulphur likewise is eminently useful in obstinate cases, where it often effects a radical cure. It holds the same relation to male persons of a somewhat advanced age, that Calcarea does to women and children.

Whether in a given case the treatment ought to be conducted with reference to the single paroxysm or to the whole disease, is sometimes difficult to decide. If the palpitation is excited by definite causes every day, or at least very frequently, the best course to be pursued is, not to prescribe for the single paroxysm, but to continue the suitable remedy at somewhat extended intervals and for some time, as we do in other chronic cases. This course has, of course, to be pursued if the palpitation is caused by some other pre-existing affection. If the paroxysms occur at indefinite periods and continue for a long time, the patient must have his medicine always handy, for it is of the utmost importance, with a view to shortening the existing paroxysm, that the remedy should be taken as soon as possible after the commencement of the attack. Or else a suitable remedy may be prescribed for the special paroxysm, and afterwards another medicine for the disease generally.

The diet and mode of living that have to be recommended, vary according to the origin of the trouble, but can easily be inferred from the nature of the case. We should, however, strenuously guard against the mistaken notion that invigorating nourishment, vigorous bodily exercise, even gymnastics or the use of wine must be avoided by those who are liable to palpitation of the heart. This disorder is but too frequently symptomatic of great weakness, hence requires invigorating nourishment and a strengthening mode of living.

If the palpitation arises from sexual disturbances, cold sitz-baths of a moderately low temperature and not persisted in too long at a time, will prove excellent auxiliaries. General cold baths very seldom agree with a patient thus afflicted, nor do cold shower-baths.

7. Angina Pectoris, Stenocardia.

This upon the whole very rare affection has not yet been accounted for in such a manner that any explanation that has been given of it, might not be objected to for a variety of reasons; nevertheless all attending circumstances justify the classing of this disease among the neuroses. Whether the cardiac plexus is the seat of this disease, or not, cannot be determined with any degree of certainty.

The etiology is obscure and vague; we only know from statistical data that males are infinitely more subject to this disease than females, and that fat individuals, or such as incline to make fat, are principally attacked. Persons beyond the age of forty are mostly liable to the disease, and they generally belong to the higher classes. Its frequent combination with cardiac anomalies, especially with atheroma or ossification of the coronary arteries, does not justify the opinion that the disease originates in such disorganizations, for it is known to occur without any material alterations of the heart. All exciting causes are very often entirely absent; but the attacks are usually provoked by a bodily effort giving rise to an augmentation of cardiac activity.

It is only exceptionally that a paroxysm does not set in suddenly; generally it takes place after very short and altogether vague preliminary symptoms. The patients suddenly experience a peculiar pain in the præcordial region, which is sometimes extremely severe and at other times dull, yet of such a peculiar kind that the sufferer is scarcely ever able to describe it either according to its quality or extent. With the pain a sensation of prostration and fainting sets in; all patients agree in describing this sensation as if death were at hand. What is remarkable is that not a sound of pain escapes the lips of the sufferers, probably however owing to their dread of increasing the distress by the least exertion. They carry this precaution so far as to arrest the breathing which gives them the appearance of great dyspnœa, although they are perfectly able to take a long breath, if they choose. Generally the patients remain immovably erect or in a sitting posture, a recumbent posture suits them very seldom. The action of the heart is at times normal, at other times slower than usual, and again hurried and irregular, especially if the patient is afflicted with heart-disease. Very seldom the pain remains confined to the præcordial region; most commonly the pain radiates to the left shoulder and arm, less frequently to the neck and nape of the neck, or to the lower extremities, or even the right side. The pain very seldom increases gradually; it mostly sets in immediately in its greatest intensity.

A single paroxysm generally lasts only a minute or two, it scarcely ever exceeds one hour. As the paroxysm generally sets in in all its intensity, so it generally ends all at once. It is only if the paroxysms are slight, that the patient's health is at once completely restored or at least very soon after the cessation of the paroxysm; whereas in this as in most other paroxysmal nervous affections great lassitude and sleeplessness remain for some time.

The course of this whole disorder varies greatly. Very seldom a paroxysm is succeeded by a complete feeling of health. It more commonly happens that the paroxysms commence slightly and increase in intensity with every succeeding attack. Except in cases of heart-disease, the intervals are quite free from all morbid symptoms, the patients do not show a single trace of the insidious disease, they often have even a very florid appearance. The single paroxysms, as well as the whole disease, are of an indefinite duration; a paroxysm seldom occurs more than once on the same day;

ordinarily they are separated by days, months and even years. Many doubt the possibility of curing this disease; we, however, believe in the absolute possibility of the contrary, although a violent paroxysm may suddenly terminate in death. It is questionable whether the disease ever changes to some other form of heart-disease, for the reason that the heart-disease most likely was already in existence when the angina first broke out.

The prognosis is decidedly bad, if the angina is associated with organic heart-disease, and likewise in the case of older individuals, whereas the purely nervous form in the case of young persons very possibly admits of a cure. We must always keep in mind that this insidious disease sometimes remains quiescent for a long time before it suddenly breaks out again in all its former, or with an increased violence.

Treatment. A treatment for a single paroxysm cannot well be arranged; we might even inflict injury if we would violently interfere with the position the patient may have selected instinctively for his relief. Even the use of local applications, especially severe cutaneous irritants, to which we might feel tempted, may prove dangerous; in no case is the people's rule, not to touch an individual seized with a nervous spasm, more appropriate than in angina pectoris. Such precepts as may be found in every therapeutic treatise, are unpractical, for the reason that the attack does not last long enough to test their clinical value. This remark likewise applies to the use of remedial agents which we might not even be afforded sufficient time to procure before the attack is ended. If the attacks last long enough, we may try *Arsenicum*, and next to Arsenic *Laurocerasus* and perhaps *Ignatia*.

We have a number of remedies that seem homœopathic to the disease, but we confess that our clinical records are exceedingly scanty and unreliable; in view of the great rarity of this disease, the scantiness of our clinical cases cannot well surprise us.

The only case which we have ever been called upon to treat in our own practice, and which had already been going on during a number of not very violent paroxysms, we have cured with not very often repeated doses of *Digitalin*, 2d and 3d trituration. The patient has now been free from the disease for the last six years. It was a purely nervous angina pectoris. It would not be safe to recommend a remedy upon the strength of a single experiment, if the symptoms and the whole therapeutic range of the drug did not correspond with the disease. Whether *Digitalin* and the *Tincture of Digitalis* would have an equally favorable effect in angina pectoris accompanied with heart-disease, we are unable to decide. Hartmann recommends *Digitalis* and bases his recommendation upon the ground of practical experience in the use of this drug.

Next to Digitalin *Arsenicum* undoubtedly promises the most successful results in the treatment of this disease. Hartmann has the following remarks: "Not only the actual paroxysms, but the disease generally finds in Arsenicum its appropriate remedy, provided the disease is not complicated with structural changes of the heart and the large arteries, or other extensive disorganizations. It is indicated if the patient can only breathe very gently with his chest stooping forward, and if the least motion causes a complete loss of breath; if oppression and stitches in the præcordial region are associated with anxiety and a fainting sort of weakness; if the breath gives out even while the patient is getting into bed, and it takes him a long time to recover his breath; if the paroxysm is excited afresh by a simple change of position in bed. In my opinion, and according to the experience I have had, *Arsenicum* is the chief remedy, more especially if the angina is a pure neurosis; its curative power is of course problematical, if the angina is complicated with disorganizations which we can never expect to cure and where we can only exert a palliative influence. In this respect no remedy can be more certainly relied upon than Arsenic." We will add a few suggestions bearing upon the dose. There is not the remotest doubt that in purely nervous affections Arsenic, if given in a low trituration, either does not show any curative effect at all, or else causes severe aggravations. Our urgent advice therefore is that in angina pectoris only the higher attenuations should be used, both for the actual paroxysm as well as during the intervals.

Although the frequent occurrence of angina pectoris in conjunction with atheromatous degenerations of the larger vessels and the heart itself, suggest all the different remedies of which mention has been made in the paragraph on fatty degeneration, yet we call particular attention to *Plumbum;* for particulars we refer to what we have stated at the end of the fourth chapter.

We have not a word of commendation to offer in favor of *Sambucus, Augustura, Lactuca virosa, Veratrum album, Asafœtida* and *Sepia,* which are likewise recommended by Hartmann. Our dissent is of course based upon theoretical reasons, but Hartmann has no clinical proofs to offer any more than we have. *Asa-*

fœtida and *Sepia* might be tried if the angina seems an hysteric affection.

Regarding the dietetic treatment but little can be said. If the causes which give rise to an attack, are well known, they have to be carefully avoided. That the mode of living exerts otherwise a decided influence, cannot well be maintained. Nor can we expect much good from a course tending to a general invigoration of the nervous system, for most patients of this kind are in general men of robust constitutions. All that the patient can do, is to observe a regular, quiet and prudent mode of living and to avoid every thing that might excite the heart's action.

TENTH SECTION.

Derangements of single Systems.

A. DISEASES OF THE BONES, MUSCLES, AND ARTICULATIONS.

1. Ostitis, Periostitis, Pott's Disease.

Inflammation of the Bones and Periosteum.

Inflammations of bones occur in every age, less frequently, however, before the second and after the fiftieth or sixtieth year. In most cases they originate in mechanical injuries or mechanically-acting deleterious influences, they are less frequently owing to the extension of inflammation from the soft parts. In the great majority of cases the mechanical is associated with a constitutional cause, very frequently the latter existing alone. Among the constitutional diseases it is more particularly scrofulosis, tuberculosis, syphilis and hydrargyrosis that give rise to ostitis. Very often it is very difficult to trace the cause with anything like certainty, especially so far as an inflammation of the substance of the bones is concerned, because it generally develops itself with scarcely perceptible symptoms and in a very insidious manner, hence too long a period of time may have elapsed since the cause first began to act, to permit of the disease being traced to a definite origin.

Bones that are but thinly covered by soft parts, are particularly exposed to inflammation from mechanical causes; inflammation arising from more dynamic or constitutional causes may attack any bone; nevertheless inflammations of the mastoid process, of the inferior maxilla, of the vertebræ, the bones of the hands and feet and of the ribs, occur most frequently and are of particular importance.

Periostitis occurs more particularly on the fingers, on the bones of the lower extremities and on the skull-bones.

The symptoms and course of ostitis differ very remarkably in extent as well as intensity. It is very often found that at the outset the disease is entirely without any symptoms until the disease is finally revealed by the process of suppuration. It very seldom runs an acute and rapid course; this is generally the case, if the inflammation attacks the outer surface of the bone and the periosteum. In such a case the intensity of the pain depends upon the extent of the inflammation; the fever is high, delirium sometimes sets in, slight chills are common and the patient very soon begins to lose his strength. Cases of this kind, which run a rapid course, always terminate in suppuration, and the artificial removal of pus is in most cases a matter of absolute necessity. After the pus is evacuated, a cure does not always take place immediately; the bone divested of its periosteum becomes more or less carious before a cicatrix has time to form.

If the periostitis runs a slow and somewhat chronic course, the inflammation of itself is not very painful; but very violent pains can be excited by contact; here too the exudation may be transformed into pus, but is likewise apt to result in osseous growths and to form extensive flat or tuberous bony indurations.

If the inflammation is located in the interior of the bone, the latter is generally distended in its whole length, is not very sensitive to pressure, but the patient is tormented by paroxysms of peculiar dull boring pains which, even in the absence of any specific cause, are particularly apt to set in, and to become aggravated at night. These pains are usually felt for some time before the bone commences to swell; they interfere with the mobility of the limb more or less, generally the less the more remotely they are felt from the articulation.

Ostitis of this central character always runs a chronic course. Its terminations are suppuration or ossification of the exudation. The pus is seldom reabsorbed, nor does it often become transformed into a tubercular mass; most generally it escapes outwardly and, unless the disease is cured, caries and necrosis result. The ichorous dissolution of the exudation generally determines a more rapid course of the disease. If one of the large bones is invaded by the suppurative process, death almost always results, although in some cases not till the patient has lived through years of suffering. An important diagnostic symptom is the presence of albumen in the urine; it almost always occurs if the suppuration is extensive and augurs very badly for the final result.

The importance of inflammations of bones varies a good deal. Age exerts a characteristic influence; whereas children and young people generally recover from such inflammations, even if these should last a long while, unless they originate in inveterate, constitutional maladies; older persons, especially when on the other side of forty, generally fall victims to such inflammations. Children very often recover when the second period of dentition sets in, or when they enter upon the period of pubescence. The seat of ostitis is of no small importance; inflammation of the bones in the upper part of the body is less dangerous than inflammation of the pelvic bones, or the bones of the lower extremities. It is likewise important to determine whether the inflammation is so located that vital organs may become involved; on this account inflammations of the skull-bones and ribs are more threatening on account of the danger of meningitis or pleuritis resulting from them. What renders the prognosis in every case of non-traumatic inflammation doubtful, is the uncertainty concerning the transformation and extent of the exudation. Sometimes the inflammatory symptoms disappear entirely for a time, and then suddenly reappear again from some cause or other, or without any cause; or else, in one portion of the bone the inflammation runs a favorable course, and then all at once takes a new start either continuously in the tissue of the bone or in separate portions. Every inflammation involving more than one bone, renders the prognosis so much more unfavorable.

Among the terminations of ostitis we have to mention two of particular importance, caries and necrosis.

Caries represents a process where the purulent transformation of the inflammatory exudation involves the destruction of the bony substance; hence it always implies a loss of substance of bone. It occurs more particularly in scrofulous and tuberculous, but may likewise take place in perfectly healthy individuals. It most commonly involves the spongy portion of the bones.

The symptoms of caries vary greatly like those of ostitis. In rare cases, if the pus has no escape or the carious portion of bone is very small, it may remain a latent disorganization. In other cases the pus finds an outlet outwardly, and the rough surface of the bone can be felt with the sound; the detached particles of bone can even be discovered in the pus between the fingers and certainly under the microscope. But if the carious process takes place deep in the interior of the bone, the pus may gravitate downwards, may form fistulous canals and finally break forth in some remote locality.

The disease always runs a chronic course, sometimes extending through a series of years, unless, owing to the presence of some other disease, a radical transformation into ichor brings about a rapid termination.

Terminations: Recovery by means of granulations, resulting in a firm, tense, retracted cicatrix, or else death amid symptoms of slow, hectic consumption, or in consequence of the inflammation extending to other vital organs; in less frequent cases bones continue to suppurate for years without the organism being much affected by the loss. After the bones are healed, the destructive nature of caries, in case the loss of substance is great, very often leaves deformities and other derangements depending upon the nature of the bone affected. Among these deformities the most important are: Cyphosis in caries of the vertebræ, and impaired mobility of the lower extremities from caries of the head of the femur.

The prognosis is very doubtful. If the patients are otherwise sound, and the pathological process is limited in extent, a cure can be depended upon with tolerable certainty; otherwise it is, after all, questionable whether the disease will not sooner or later result fatally. If the carious process takes place very near the serous covering of important viscera, we have at all times to expect an extension of the inflammation to these parts.

Necrosis is the gangrenous destruction of a bone or part of a bone. It is a frequent consequence of ostitis attended with sclerosis, and a frequent accompaniment of caries. It is a well known fact that Phosphorus may cause necrosis of the inferior maxilla. A medicinal treatment of necrosis is of course out of the question, except in so far as secondary ostitis may be present; all that can be done, is to remove the necrosed portion of bone.

Treatment. The frequent occurrence of ostitis in individuals whose constitutions are tainted with some constitutional dyscrasia, invites a careful inquiry into the presence of such a constitutional taint, even though not manifested by any outward signs; and, in the second place, to employ such remedies as not only correspond with the constitutional affection, but likewise aim at remedying the local disease. A mere comparison of symptoms will scarcely ever answer the purpose, for the reason that the localities may differ too much; it is only for a few definite localizations of ostitis that we possess real similia. In general we advise therefore that the general, not the local symptoms be taken as our guide; on this account we mention the following remedies with a few short comments.

Mercurius is a medicine of whose specific and almost constantly definite relation to the osseous tissue we may always rest satisfied. It is indeed suitable in most cases of ostitis and periostitis provided they do not originate in mercurial poisoning. It is particularly indicated by: Violent bone-pains, distention, swelling, redness of the integuments, and in general by the more acute symptoms of the disease. However, we do not mean to deny its usefulness in chronic cases of ostitis, and even in caries. The infantile organism is more rapidly and certainly affected by Mercurius. The dose had better be as small as possible; the slow course of the disease would seem to point to small doses and given at comparatively long intervals, as preferable to large doses of this agent.

Mezereum antidotes Mercurius in the bone-range; this alone shows that both remedies must be homœopathic to ostitis. *Mezereum* is particularly adapted to periostitis, less to ostitis, and is particularly appropriate at a period of the disease when no complete suppuration has yet set in. With this remedy we have cured an inflammation of the tibia, where a portion of the bone, several inches in extent, was considerably and painfully distended; the patient was a boy in whom there could not have existed the remotest suspicion of some specific cause. We cannot point out a special locality for Mezereum; according to Hartmann, it is particularly the superficially situated bones to inflammatory conditions of which Mezereum is best adapted. [This may have been a case of scrofulous rheumatic inflammation; in the course of our practice we have cured quite a number of such cases by means of *Aconite, Belladonna,* the *Iodide of Mercury,* likewise *Iodine* and *Iodide of Potassium.* H.]

Acidum nitricum is indeed chiefly indicated in mercurial ostitis, [and in ostitis originating in syphilis and abuse of Mercury, H.]; yet this recommendation must not be understood too literally; for this agent may likewise be of use in other forms of ostitis, especially of the lower extremities, and in periostitis generally.

Phosphori acidum is generally preferred to Acidum nitricum in non-mercurial ostitis; it is indicated in the inflammatory bone-affections of children, especially in inflammations of the vertebræ, if there is an evident disposition to caries and ichorous dissolution. In fully developed caries with symptoms of slow hectic fever, *Phosphori acidum* is one of the most important remedies.

Phosphorus is inferior to Phosphori acidum for the reason that the latter acts more specifically and more penetratingly in chronic affections. In other respects the therapeutic sphere of both remedies is very similar; we would accord the preference to Phosphorus, if consumption with unceasing colliquative diarrhœa has set in.

Staphysagria is indicated, if the ostitis runs its course with severe pains, and the bone and its periosteum are affected at the same time; in the case of scrofulous individuals; if the facial bones or those of the legs and feet are involved.

Manganum is recommended by Hartmann for painful periostitis, and for inflammation of the articular extremities of the bones.

Baryta carbonica is eminently adapted to a slow and almost painless scrofulous inflammation of the bones of the extremities, after suppuration has begun to set in.

Aurum is, like Nitric acid, an exquisitely anti-mercurial medicine, and hence deserves special attention in cases of mercurial ostitis. It has likewise an excellent effect in non-mercurial ostitis with caries, and violent pains, especially at night. Aurum is a specific remedy for inflammatory ulceration of the nasal bones and facial bones generally. In affections of this kind we prefer *Aurum muriaticum* to the common gold.

Silicea is one of the most important remedies in caries from any cause and at any age, as soon as the inflammatory stage has run its course; it is adapted to every constitution, but may not have a very favorable effect in acute ichorous suppuration. We must not forget that Silicea acts very slowly; we recommend small doses at long intervals.

Sulphur, in our hands, has never had a permanent effect in caries, nor have we ever been able to effect with it a return towards recovery. It can at most be of use only in the latter stages of the disease, not at the beginning.

Calcarea. This agent is not so much indicated in uncomplicated ostitis, as in ostitis depending upon scrofulosis; in our opinion it does not act directly as a curative, but by virtue of the favorable change it effects in the scrofulous disease. On this account its use should be deferred until the suppurative process is fully established. We will not decide whether Calcarea carbonica or phosphorica is preferable; we consider it a wrong theory, however, to employ the Phosphate of lime because it is a constituent of bone. In caries of the vertebræ Calcarea is superior to any other drug; often at least, it arrests the destructive process.

For further comparison we recommend: *Hepar sulphuris, Iodium, Kali bichromicum, Graphites,* also *Rhus toxicodendron* and *Lycopodium.* Rhus is particularly recommended for periostitis. The use of Aconite, Bryonia and Pulsatilla as recommended by Hartmann, seems to us to involve a loss of time; we do not consider these drugs adapted to ostitis. On the other hand, *Belladonna* is appropriate in the ostitis of scrofulous children with florid complexions.

2. Rhachitis.
Rickets.

We treat of this affection here, instead of deferring it to the chapter on constitutional anomalies to which it really belongs, because it is exclusively localized in the bones.

The causes of rhachitis are upon the whole involved in obscurity. It is certainly not correct to describe rickets as a consequence of scrofulosis, for not all children who are afflicted with rickets, are scrofulous. With respect to rickets the following are established facts: Rhachitis can only be diagnosed with reliable certainty between the first and second period of dentition; it is preëminently an affection of the lower classes, and more particularly of children that were brought up by hand; sometimes it seems hereditary. The almost constant coincidence with more or less intense digestive disturbances justifies the inference that the main cause of this disease is an abnormal condition of the assimilative functions.

Symptoms and Course. Manifest symptoms of rickets are with few exceptions preceded for some time by precursory symptoms. The children are afflicted with diarrhœa which is at first more slimy and afterwards watery; they lose their appetite or, which is still more common, they have perverse tastes, craving black rye-bread and potatoes; the abdomen is distended, the complexion sickly, the desire to move about is less, and yet, intellectually, the children are more matured than their age would seem to indicate. This lack of disposition to move about, which is particularly prominent in the case of children that had already commenced to walk about, is the first suspicious symptom which is very soon, and sometimes almost immediately followed by pains in the bones and articulations. That these pains exist is evident from the cries which the children utter, whenever an attempt is made to have them move about. This circumstance is often interpreted as naughtiness, more especially since the children already commence to cry at the mere approach of their parents whom they suspect of an intention to make them move about. Soon the characteristic changes in the articular extremities of the bones become manifest, more particularly, on account of the thin muscular covering, at the lower articulations of the radius and ulna, at the lower articulation of the tibia, and at the sternal extremities of the ribs. These articular extremities are enlarged, sometimes unequally bunchy, separated from the shaft by a more or less deep fold of integument. The disease is almost always accompanied by emaciation, especially of the lower extremities, which causes the swelling of the articular extremities and the distention of the abdomen to become still more prominent. The painfulness of the articulations is generally very great, scarcely ever hardly perceptible; hence not only the pain, but direct weakness seem to be the cause why children absolutely refuse to walk.

In the further course of the disease all those changes take place which depend upon the softness of the bones. The lower extremities bend outwardly, if the children attempt to walk, whereas they remain straight, if children are attacked who are not yet able to walk and have to remain extended in a recumbent posture. The bone often looks as if bent at an angle. The ribs are pressed in and the sternum protrudes, giving rise to the so-called chicken-breast. The upper extremities are less crooked, but bent a great deal more, if the child crawls about on all fours. The vertebral column at times assumes the form of cyphosis, at times that of scoliosis or lordosis; the form of the pelvis is likewise altered. The closing of the fontanelles and sutures delays for several years.

It is remarkable that the rickety bone does not show any disposition to inflammation with suppuration and caries; nor is such a bone as liable to fracture as a bone normally constituted. The consequences to the general organism which are sometimes inconsiderable even with fully developed rhachitis, consist in impediments to the respiration owing to a narrowing of the thorax and deficient mobility of the ribs, with chronic catarrh of the air-passages. Excessive emaciation, with greatly distended abdomen. Delayed, irregular, sometimes perverse dentition. Great tendency to spasm, especially eclampsia, sometimes setting in in consequence of the least pressure on the fontanelles.

The affection always runs an exceedingly chronic course, sometimes extending over many months. The disease may heal spontaneously at any stage of its development; we see this in cases where no physician had been employed, and where the true character of the disease can be inferred from the still remaining articular swellings. The first sign towards an improvement is the restoration of a normal digestion. The articular swellings seldom disappear very rapidly; the curvatures never disappear entirely, but usually diminish very materially.

The common termination is in recovery; if death results, it is mostly in consequence of the supervention of other complaints, and is the result of actual marasmus only in cases where the patient is utterly neglected.

So far as danger to life is concerned, the prognosis is extremely favorable, whereas the curvatures may give rise to many secondary affections in after-life; a rickety pelvis, for instance, may materially interfere with the process of labor.

The treatment of rachitis has to be, above all, strictly prophylactic or hygienic. It is certain that in almost all cases the disease depends upon abnormal assimilation, and hence first manifests itself by disturbances in the assimilative sphere. On this account we often succeed in arresting the development of the disease, if we see to it that the children are properly fed, kept clean, their skin is well washed and rubbed, and they have an abundance of fresh air. A compliance with these dietetic rules is a primary duty not only at the commencement, but likewise in the further course of the disease. It is moreover of great importance that the children should be prevented from moving about, and more particularly from sitting, since they avoid motion anyhow. By pursuing this course, very considerable curvatures are often very much improved, their further increase is checked, and the development of new curvatures is prevented. The most appropriate position is a recumbent posture upon an uniformly stuffed, not too hard mattress with a slightly raised pillow, or no pillow at all. Sea-weeds or fine chips, corn-husks are excellent material for the stuffing, likewise on the score of cheapness, since such patients generally belong to the poorer classes. Concerning the diet, we have already stated our views when treating of the intestinal catarrh of children, and shall refer to this subject again in the chapter on scrofulosis.

The medicines which we require for the cure of rickets, are few in number, but so much more reliable in their effect. After attending to the main requisite for a cure, namely the regulation of a suitable mode of living, the next business in order is to remove the intestinal catarrh as soon as possible, for which purpose the most rigid diet is often insufficient. All the medicines that have been recommended for the intestinal catarr of children, may be called into use, but *Calcarea carbonica* undoubtedly heads the list. It is well known that the partisans of the Rational School account for the use of this agent in rickets upon chemical grounds, namely as a compensation for the excessive loss of the salts of lime in the urine. This excretion of the salts of lime is not the cause, but an effect of the disturbed nutrition of the bones, nor is it borne in mind by "rational" physicians that substances like lime, when given in their crude shape and in a massive dose, have no effect, or even act injuriously. On this account the use of such agents is soon discontinued again. Nevertheless Calcarea is the surest remedy for rhachitis, and we can present it to our opponents as a striking illustration of the efficacy of small doses. When given in the higher attenuations, it shows curative effects very promptly, even if there is no change in the mode of living; we have noticed this on many occasions. We have never witnessed such rapid results from the lower triturations; hence we advise everybody to first try the sixth and higher attenuations before resorting to the lower attenuations and triturations. The diarrhœa often ceases after the first dose, and this change implies a positive victory over the disease. Having almost constantly succeeded with the *Carbonate of Lime*, we scarcely ever venture to change to the *Phosphate* or *Acetate*. A copious, watery, sour-smelling diarrhœa is the surest indication for *Calcarea*.

A second remedy which is likewise extremely beneficial in every suitable case, is *Arsenicum*. As regards the dose, we apply to it the same remarks that we have to Calcarea. The Arsenic-diarrhœa is less copious, less watery, of a foul smell as of decomposing matter, attended with a good deal of flatulence, hectic fever, great restlessness, sleeplessness, also vomiting, loss of appetite, whereas Calcarea is characterized by a great craving for certain inadmissible kinds of food.

Sulphur is seldom indicated in rickets. Its chief indication is seldom present, namely a slimy or muco-purulent diarrhœa, with discharge of pure bile or a copious admixture of bile. It is asserted by many that a few doses of Sulphur administered previous to Calcarea, renders the effect of the latter more reliable and prompt; we have no experience of our own to offer on this point.

These three remedies are sufficient to a cure in by far the larger number of cases. For other remedies we refer the reader to our chapter on intestinal catarrh. [In this disease the continued use of small quantities of Cod-liver oil is decidedly appropriate. H.]

3. Enchondroma.

Pædarthrocace ; Spina ventosa.

Enchondroma represents a disease of the bones where cartilaginous substance is formed within the bone, in consequence of which the substance of the bone is more or less destroyed.

The causes of this affection are quite obscure; assigning scrofulosis as the origin of the disease, does not shed much light on the subject. It occurs most commonly among children and during pubescence.

The enchondroma is most commonly located in the metacarpal bones and in the phalangeal bones of the fingers, much less frequently in the bones of the feet, but may likewise occur in other bones and organs. It either commences without any pain, or else with indefinite sensations in the affected bone, very seldom with marked pains like ostitis. The swelling of the bone is generally the first symptom. It seldom spreads uniformly over the whole bone, but has mostly a spherical or conical shape. The swelling is of slow growth; the soft parts by which it is covered, retain for a long time their normal appearance, until finally, after the swelling has reached a considerable size, the skin reddens and breaks in one or more places. The sound now penetrates into the opening without any difficulty, and is easily passed around in the swelling which is commonly found to consist of a very soft, spongy mass. There is very little discharge from the opening, very seldom any pus, but rather a serous liquid resulting in the formation of a crust that closes the opening. At this stage pains are generally entirely absent.

The disorganization runs a very chronic course. If adults are attacked, the general organism is much affected by the disease; in the case of children a cure may be promised with perfect safety.

For this disease we do not possess any specific, properly speaking, but have to select our remedies in accordance with the rules of analogy. Practically *Silicea* has so far yielded the best results, next to which we rank *Graphites*. Besides these two, the following remedies are recommended: *Calcarea, Staphysagria, Mezereum, Cuprum, Sulphur, Ledum palustre*. There is no clinical experience recorded with these agents. We should always bear in mind, in treating a case of this kind, that enchondroma can never be cured with external means, and that the knife never need be resorted to.

4. Psoitis.
Inflammation of the Psoas-muscle.

Of inflammations of muscles this is the only one that is proportionally of frequent occurrence, and is of very great importance.

If psoitis sets in as a primary disease, its causes are involved in great obscurity; excessive exertions, a cold, rheumatism, etc., are assigned as probable causes, most likely because no better causes are known. Mechanical injuries seldom result in psoitis. Secondarily psoitis may supervene during inflammation and caries of the lumbar vertebræ.

At first, the disease is often quite painless and develops itself very slowly; sometimes, however, it sets in in an acute form. In such a case the patient experiences a sudden or rapidly increasing violent pain in the lumbar region, which he finds it difficult to define; it often radiates upwards or downwards; as soon as the pain is felt, the motion of the limb is interfered with, especially flexion and rotation inwards. Under such circumstances a violent fever is always present, the pulse being remarkably rapid. The patients lie with their thighs semi-flexed and somewhat turned inwards. Pus forms sometimes rapidly, and at other times slowly, and sometimes in such profuse quantity that its first appearance is indicated by creeping chills. The fully-formed abscess can be reabsorbed, which is, however, seldom the case; or else, it bursts in the lumbar region, the pus escaping inwardly and immediately threatening life; or the pus burrows downwards following the course of the psoas-muscle until it finds an outlet, generally on the anterior surface of the thigh, rarely posteriorly by the side of the vertebral column. The pus thus forms a fistulous canal, which is always the case if the lumbar vertebræ are carious.

If suppuration sets in, the course of the disease is always slow; it is only in rare cases that the inflammation does not terminate in suppuration; the organism may become involved in consequence of a profuse suppuration gradually consuming the patient's strength, or in consequence of the escape of the pus into the abdominal cavity, or of the inflammation communicating itself to the vertebræ. For these reasons the prognosis is always doubtful.

The treatment is not surgical, except in so far as it may be necessary to open the abscess. Homœopathic physicians have a higher duty to perform. In the first place we have to try to scatter the inflammation before suppuration sets in; even if this cannot be accomplished in all cases, it is at all events certain that the spread of the inflammation can be prevented by appropriate internal treatment. For this purpose we commence the treatment if a violent and continuous fever is present, with *Belladonna*, especially if the fever is accompanied by copious perspiration and every motion aggravates the pain extremely. *Rhus* should be given if the fever consists of a burning, dry heat, with intense thirst, if the trouble seems to have originated in a cold and the pains are worse at night, and when the patient is lying down. If these two remedies do not effect an improvement, and the fever is mingled with chilly creepings, the pulse becomes very much accelerated, and the skin is at times burning-hot and at other times drenched in perspiration, we should at once give *Mercurius*, which is the only remedy that can arrest the suppurative process, if such a result can at all be accomplished. If an abscess forms, we give *Hepar sulph.* in order to promote the suppuration; for the main point now is to evacuate the pus as rapidly as possible and by this means to heal the sore as soon as the pus is discharged. Hartmann names a number of drugs, such as *Bryonia, Nux vom., Pulsatilla, Cantharides,* etc., without any practical testimony, and, in our opinion, without practical value. *Staphysagria* may be tried if the disease runs a slow course, without much fever. After the abscess bursts, and the patients are free from caries, we advise the continued use of *Hepar sulph.*, by which means a rapid termination of the formation of pus is most speedily effected. If the opening becomes fistulous, we must be prepared for an exceedingly tardy recovery. If the pus is of good quality and the patient preserves his strength, *Silicea,* and next to it *Sulphur,* are most calculated to promote a cure, although we confess that we have never seen any decided effect from their employment. If the pus becomes watery, sickly-looking, acrid; if the strength begins to fail and hectic symptoms set in, we still may succeed in arresting the bad turn by *Phosphorus, China, Ferrum,* or by *Calcarea carbonica.* If the smell and the general quality of the pus show that the continuance of the purulent discharge is due to caries of the vertebræ, we can scarcely expect any change from any medicine and the patient must be prepared to die of slow consumption.

5. Lumbago.

This affection being commonly regarded as rheumatism of the dorsal muscles, it ought to have had its place assigned to it in the

Lumbago.

chapter on rheumatism; however, inasmuch as we have several reasons for questioning the rheumatic nature of this affection, we will describe its character and point out its treatment in this place.

The affection is supposed to originate more particularly in a cold attended with a severe exertion. That this explanation is improbable, is evident from the circumstance that lumbago is commonly an isolated affection, not attended with catarrh and extensive rheumatic symptoms; yet, if a cold were the real cause, this would be a very strange localization, so much more as scarcely a trace of fever is present with the attack.

The difficulty arises suddenly almost without an exception; it is rarely preceded by vague pains in the lumbar region. The patient, while stooping, or making an attempt to raise anything or to rapidly turn about, suddenly experiences a fearful, racking pain in the back, which makes it almost impossible for him to raise himself again, and which may even be so intense that he tumbles forward as from a blow. The pain continues, is fearfully increased by every movement of the trunk and even the extremities, even by coughing and sneezing; it is suspended for a short time while the patient is lying quiet, but then returns again and compels him to make a painful attempt to change his position. Sometimes walking is utterly impossible, or else the person has to walk with the trunk rigidly erect, or stooping forward, with an unsteady gait, because the least misstep causes a horrid pain. No constitutional disturbances are experienced unless they are occasioned by the excessive pain. If the affection is left to itself, it lasts at least three days, but may continue for several weeks, after which the pain leaves gradually, mostly with great tendency to relapses.

We do not see upon what ground Hartmann proposes so many remedies for a strictly local affection. In all cases the symptoms are alike and differ only in degrees of intensity. On this account two or three remedies have always sufficed in our hands for a cure. *Tartar emetic*, second or third trituration, a dose every three or four hours, helps more rapidly than any other remedy. In twenty-four hours the pains generally disappear, except a little stiffness. *Rhus* is preferable if the lumbago originates in a sudden cold and the pain, so far from being mitigated by rest, is, on the contrary, aggravated. *Arnica* is indicated if the attack is caused by a severe exertion. Beside these three remedies we have never been obliged to employ any other; it is only in order to be complete that we add the medicines mentioned by Hartmann: *Bryonia, Nux vomica, Sulphur, Ledum, Pulsatilla, Rhododendron, Colchicum, China.*

Kneading and pounding the affected locality is of undoubted use, so is the application of humid warmth. This application is made by dipping a towel in cold water, wringing it well, folding it four to six times and then applying it to the painful locality, after which a dry cloth folded together several times, has to be laid over the wet compress, and a hot flat-iron pressed upon the whole, so that the heat penetrates through the whole and imparts to the skin an intense sensation of warmth. These applications only palliate, but never remove the pain entirely. [We have cured numbers of cases of lumbago by rubbing a moderately strong liniment of the tincture of Aconite-root upon the back, and at the same time giving the first or second decimal attenuation of Aconite-root internally. H.]

6. Progressive Muscular Paralysis.

The origin of this very peculiar affection is involved in great obscurity. We are not acquainted with any really constant cause of this disorder, and such causes as have been assigned to it, a cold, excessive exertions, hereditary descent, are at all events doubtful. What is certain is, that men are more particularly liable to this disease.

An essential characteristic of this disease consists in a gradual atrophy of one or more muscles attended with fatty degeneration of the affected part. It first invades the muscles of one hand, especially the right, less frequently those of the arm, shoulder or face, and never those of the lower extremities; and even when invading the muscles of the hand, it almost always first affects a limited portion of them, after which it gradually spreads further. Generally it sets in without pain, seldom with an intensely acute pain, and almost imperceptibly, the affected muscles losing more and more their functional power and at the same time becoming atrophied. Not till the atrophy is complete, does the palsy reach its acme; until then the muscles retain their sensibility, reflex-action continues and the sensitiveness to the electric current is preserved more or less.

The affection may remain confined for years to the starting-point without making headway, but this is a rare circumstance. It more frequently happens that the muscular affection gradually spreads from one muscle to the other, successive portions of the body become involved in the paralysis, and, after having suffered for years, the patient finally perishes if the muscles of deglutition and respiration become paralyzed.

This disease can be distinguished from ordinary nervous paralysis by the circumstance that in progressive muscular atrophy the susceptibility to the electric current remains intact for a long time. With scarcely an exception, the prognosis is unfavorable, especially if the disease rapidly progresses from the start.

As for the treatment of this disease, we are as yet unacquainted with reliable specific remedies. It is characteristic of this disease never to invade the muscular fibres of the heart, so that fatty degeneration of the heart and muscular atrophy seem to be very distinct diseases. In the therapeutic range we can only recommend *Plumbum* and *Cuprum*, both of which have paralysis with emaciation; but it is not certain whether the emaciation is not altogether the consequence of the palsy. At all events *Plumbum* is more appropriate than Cuprum. *Arsenicum* may likewise give rise to expectations of success. Beside these three remedies we still recommend *Sulphur*, *Causticum* and *Lachesis*. Gymnastic exercises, with a careful avoidance, however, of all active exertions and a strict limitation of the exercise to passive motions, and likewise a resort to electricity by induction, or faradisation, are said to have occasionally yielded favorable results, and to have effected an arrest of the palsy and even an increase of muscular volume. [This disease is also described by English pathologists as wasting palsy. Doctor William Roberts, of Manchester, published the first systematic treatise on this subject, in 1858. In France, the disease has been described by the name of "*atrophie musculaire progressive*," or "*paralysie graduelle du mouvement par atrophie musculaire.*" There are several other forms of progressive paralysis, one of which is described as progressive locomotor ataxia or the *ataxie locomotrice progressive* of Duchenne. We transcribe the following description of the disease from Aitken's Science and Practice of Medicine: "Pains like rheumatism first attract attention, rather than failing power. Paralysis of the sixth or third pair of nerves, giving rise to temporary diplopia, with unequal contraction of the pupils, are early symptoms; and another distressing harbinger of the disease is incontinence of urine, associated with spermatorrhœa during the night, with a great proclivity to sexual congress, which is no mere impotent desire but results in effective sexual intercourse. In the erect posture, the muscles may sustain a heavy weight; and general paralysis does not supervene after these extremely anomalous symptoms until a period of months or even years. There is then a gradual and progressive loss of the power of co-ordination in the acts of volition. An awkward, unsteady gait is the earliest indication of such progressive paralysis." "At first the feet are moved in a slatternly manner, the heels lounging on the ground before the toes; and then, as the disease advances, they are thrown involuntarily to the right or left without purpose, and without the power of restraining their irregular movements..... The act of turning round is performed with great difficulty. The sensation of the feet is apt to become blunted during this period of the disorder, so that the patient feels as if he were always walking on a soft carpet, and is therefore so much the more insecure.... The bladder and rectum are also frequently implicated.... but electro-muscular contractility is retained throughout the whole disease (see Meryon, Medico-Chirurgical Transactions, vol. 35, page 194). The duration of progressive ataxia is from six months to ten or even twenty years. If the patient is put on his legs with his eyes shut, and his feet close together, it is seen that, although he has the muscular power, he has not the muscular sensibility to preserve his body from falling, or to guide him in taking even a few steps forward with his eyes closed. He will reel and tumble about like a drunken man (see Trousseau, Meryon). It is a disease of middle age and affects males rather than females; and is apt to be hereditary." H.]

7. Inflammation of Joints.

The articulations composed of a number of essentially different tissues, are variously exposed, both by their functions and their situation, to inflammatory affections which differ greatly in their natures, for the reason that several of these tissues may be attacked together and in various combinations. Moreover, an articular inflammation, wherever it may be located, is always of special importance, on account of the organism falling such a ready victim to its consequences. Homœopathy has given abundant evidence that it is possessed of means to modify the course of these inflammations and to impress upon them a favorable change. It has no specific remedies for articular inflammations generally, but for each special form thereof. We call attention to this point, because we cannot dwell upon every special form of articular inflammation and request the reader to select the proper remedy for himself in a given case.

Among these inflammations we single out the following as the most important:

a. *Coxalgia, Coxarthrocace, Inflammation of the Hip-joint.*

This inflammation, the chronic form of which is designated as luxatio spontanea or "voluntary limping," cannot be traced to any definite cause. It affects principally children and young people during the first years of pubescence. Its extremely frequent occurrence during the years fourteen to seventeen, and in persons of rapid growth, leads us to infer that a rapid growth of the bones constitutes a disposition to this inflammation, and that an exertion, a cold or other scarcely apparent circumstances simply act as exciting causes. A connection between this disease and some constitutional affection cannot be traced with any positive certainty.

Acute coxarthrocace sets in suddenly even with a violent chill, like all other acute inflammations, with which severe pains are associated. The patient locates these pains at times in the small of the back, at other times more in front, very seldom in the hip-joint; they are extremely acute, tearing, burning, stitching, shooting, aggravated by every motion of the lower extremities, not altogether, and sometimes not at all, relieved by horizontal posture. At the same time a high fever accompanies the pains, the pulse being not unfrequently upwards of 120; this circumstance distinguishes the disease from lumbago with which it is easily confounded. Amid symptoms of this kind which may become sufficiently intense to simulate typhus, the following objective phenomena become manifest in one, two or more weeks: The affected hip and the buttock of the same side swell, so that the fold between the nates is much deeper; the thigh is somewhat rotated outwards and slightly drawn up towards the abdomen; the knee is half bent; extension and rotation of the thigh are very painful, nor can these movements be executed completely. Walking is not entirely impossible, but can only be performed with the greatest pain. It is very seldom that an improvement begins at this point; as a rule an extensive suppuration sets in, amid frequent chills and burning heat of the skin. After this, a short intermission seems to take place in the further development of the disease, until the abscess reaches the skin and bursts. This may take place posteriorly, laterally or in front. After the pus is discharged, the patient feels much better, and then worse again, provided the suppuration becomes very profuse and continuous. Upon the whole, the prospect of a speedy closure of the cavity is very slim; most generally fistulous openings result. The articulation itself is variously affected according as one or the other tissue is most involved. If the inflammation was originally located in the bone, this is partially destroyed together with the acetabulum, and caries is the result; if the inflammation emanates from the fibrous tissues or from the synovial membrane, the bones may remain intact. Thus the terminations of the disease are: Very rarely a complete and rapid restoration; long-lasting suppuration with final recovery and a total or partial destruction of the articulation; long-lasting suppuration with caries which may end in hectic fever and death. The prognosis is always very uncertain.

Chronic or subacute coxarthrocace presents a very different group of symptoms. The disease commences with vague symptoms in the hip-joint resembling rheumatic pains and alternately exacerbating, remitting, or even intermitting for some time. These pains may be absent and in their stead the patient may only complain of a stiff joint which is more especially felt during motion. Sensible pressure on the hip-joint generally causes more or less pain, and the thigh is usually rotated outwards to some extent as soon as the disease commences. With such trifling symptoms it may go on for some time, before more serious changes become manifest. The pains increase in intensity and cause the patient to limp, the thigh is slightly flexed and turned inwards, being at the same time, however, rotated outwards. Almost without an exception a more or less violent pain is at the same time felt in the knee, very generally surpassing the pain in the hip-joint in intensity. The affected limb becomes elongated, its muscles become relaxed and flabby, the glutei muscles of the affected side become depressed, the gluteal fold is much deeper, the trochanter is somewhat turned outwards. In the further course of the disease suppuration supervenes, the pus escaping on the outside and destroying life by caries and hectic fever. A cure at this stage is a rare occurrence; or else no suppuration sets in and the head of the femur and the acetabulum adhere together; or finally the head of the femur slips out of the acetabulum, in which case adhesions occur with a greater or less degree of immobility of the thigh, or with suppuration outwardly.

It may take several years before the disease exhausts the different phases of this course. The prognosis is always doubtful, and, so far as a final cure is concerned, generally very unfavorable. The younger the individuals the more hope we may entertain of a final cure; the older the patient the greater the danger of hectic fever succeeding the suppuration.

Although the number of homœopathic remedies for coxarthrocace is but small, yet the success with which they are used in this disease, is a source of pride to our practice. In view of the almost positive certainty of a correct diagnosis in most cases of hip-disease, the clinical results that have been obtained in the treatment of this disorder, may be regarded as absolutely reliable testimony. In the following paragraphs we give the treatment of the different varieties of coxarthrocace and their stages.

At the outset of acute coxitis with violent fever and accelerated pulse *Belladonna* or *Rhus tox.* may be required, but only as long as no pus has yet formed. For the distinctive symptoms of both drugs the Materia Medica may be consulted. If the symptoms are not very violent, *Bryonia* may deserve a preference. If symptoms of suppuration have plainly set in, no remedy can compete with *Mercurius* which of itself is capable of moderating and even arresting the suppurative process. Only if the abscess threatens to break, we advise a resort to *Hepar sulphuris*. After the bursting of the abscess, the selection of a remedial agent will depend upon the constitutional symptoms. If the patient gains in strength and the symptoms point to a rapid healing of the sore, *Calcarea carb.* renders excellent service in so far as it promotes the nutritive process. *Acidum phosph.* is likewise appropriate under such circumstances. If the suppuration is profuse, and a laudable pus is discharged, the continued use of *Sulphur* will bring about a diminution of the secretion or, if Sulphur should fail us, *Silicea* will achieve this result. If the pus becomes thin, smells badly and the patient loses strength, we have to select in accordance with the constitutional symptoms: *Phosphorus, Acidum phosph.* and *nitric., Calcarea carbon.* and *phosphor., Arsen., Lycopodium.*

We have a few remedies which, when given at the outset of chronic coxitis, have often succeeded in decidedly arresting the further progress of the disease. *Rhus tox.,* if the pains are chiefly felt during rest, affect the whole thigh, and the lameness is very great. *Belladonna* in the case of young, robust, plethoric individuals, if the pains are severe, limited to circumscribed localities and set in more particularly towards evening and after exercise. *Arnica,* if the disease is traceable to some mechanical injury, with a burning and frequently shifting pain which causes a great deal of restlessness. *Colocynthis* for very severe and constant pains resembling ischias and increasing or decreasing independently of external circumstances.

Even in the second stage of the disease, *Colocynthis* is still indicated, and is very much commended by physicians. If we are satisfied that suppuration has set in, *Mercurius* will of course be our choice, more especially in the case of scrofulous individuals. *Calcarea carbonica* and *Hepar sulphuris* are likewise variously recommended at this stage.

If pus is formed and the abscess has burst, the same treatment has to be pursued as in a case of acute coxitis.

The following remedies are recommended in isolated cases, and may be investigated more particularly in the Materia Medica: *Conium, Lycopodium, Pulsatilla, Petroleum, Digitalis purpurea, Aurum.*

The rest of the treatment may be condensed in the following points which it would lead us too far to account for by a special train of reasoning. The patients should not remain in a state of absolute rest, on the contrary, they had better move about by means of crutches. If pus forms, warm poultices may be applied; they not only promote the formation of pus, but very often favor its reabsorption. Only if carious destruction of the joint has taken place, the patients will have to remain quiet lest spontaneous luxation should result; in such circumstances a suitable extension-apparatus may be resorted to, which will have to be applied, however, with a great deal of caution. The diet should be at all times plain and strengthening; the use of fat is to be rigidly prohibited.

b. *Gonarthrocace, Tumor Albus Genu, Gonitis, Inflammation of the Knee-joint.*

This is one of the most frequently occurring inflammations of joints; owing to the exposed situation of the knees, this might indeed be expected. Its etiology is no less obscure than that of the inflammation of any other joint; it is certain that a mechanical injury is the least frequent cause of this inflammation. Very often gonarthrocace seems to be the expression of a constitutional affection. As regards age, young people are indeed more disposed to this disease, which is likewise, however, met with after the twenty-fifth year of age, and occurs, it appears, more frequently among females than males.

A simple inflammation of the knee, to which the name of tumor albus should never be applied, and which is generally the result of some mechanical injury or of excessive use, is an unimportant affection as long as the inflammation is confined to the integuments. It is scarcely ever attended with fever, is never ushered in by a chill, and runs its course within a few weeks. However, inasmuch as we can never be sure whether such an unimportant disease may not result in the more dangerous tumor albus, it ought to be managed with all due precaution.

Tumor albus never runs an acute course, at most subacute and usually very chronic. While using the joint, the patient complains of pain and impaired mobility; in more rapidly progressing cases the temperature of the joint is higher than usual. If the inflammation emanates from the soft parts, the pains are generally less than when the bones constitute the starting-point. Sometimes the knee swells rapidly, at other times more slowly, and most slowly if the bones receive the first shock of the disease. In the latter case the knee preserves its form for a long time, whereas in the other cases the swelling soon modifies any former shape of the knee. As the swelling increases, which generally has a very white appearance, it grows progressively softer, elastic, and finally shows symptoms of fluctuation. The cutaneous veins become very much enlarged. The pains generally increase with an increase of the swelling. Sometimes not till after the lapse of years, and, in a few cases, after that of weeks, distinct fluctuation is perceived in one or more places; here the skin reddens, breaks, and a pus which is mostly thin and mixed with flocks, is discharged. In spite of this evacuation of pus, the swelling remains almost unchanged.

The suppuration in a case of tumor albus is generally very tardy. The openings may close for a short time, after which they generally open again, so that, in a fortunate case, suppuration may cease after many months, and the swelling may grow smaller, but the joint remains stiff and thick, and the leg somewhat bent. A cure of this disease is witnessed only in the case of young people. If the case terminates less favorably, the suppuration gradually superinduces hectic fever, and finally ends in death.

The prognosis is always bad, for no one escapes from such an attack without some permanent injury; the difference in favor of young and robust individuals is that death needs not be apprehended in their case, which is generally sure to occur in individuals of upwards thirty years of age.

Treatment. We cannot boast of possessing many similia for

gonarthrocace whose clinical value has at the same time been tested by an abundance of practical observations. Moreover, it is unfortunately a difficult matter to select a remedy for a given case in accordance with the symptomatic records of the Materia Medica.

The simple, rapidly terminating and benign inflammation of the knee, without any affection of the bone or any marked tendency to suppuration, readily yields to *Arnica*, if the trouble originates in a mechanical injury. If the trouble proceeds rather from internal causes, *Belladonna* will generally be found sufficient, if there is much pain, and *Bryonia*, if both pain and swelling are considerable; *Conium*, *Pulsatilla* or *Rhus toxicodendron* will be required less frequently. [We think *Pulsatilla* is not sufficiently appreciated by Bæhr; we know of no remedy that has a more specific relation to the synovial lining of the cavity of the knee than *Pulsatilla*; hence in gonitis, if the inflammatory process is primarily and chiefly located in the synovial membrane, *Pulsatilla* is undoubtedly the leading remedy. In chronic gonitis of this character we should depend chiefly upon *Silicea*, higher attenuations, with intercurrent doses of Pulsatilla. H.]

If tumor albus begins as a subacute disease, with severe pains, slight febrile excitement, rapid increase of the swelling, *Bryonia* is the main remedy as long as the inflammation is confined to the soft parts; if the trouble is primarily located in the bone, if the pain is excessive, although the swelling is only slight, *Mercurius* will have to be employed. In the case of young and robust individuals *Belladonna* is preferred by many physicians, even if the bones are affected primarily. If the swelling progresses without much pain, *Conium* is indicated. Beside these remedies the following deserve attention at the outset: *Ledum* for severely-stitching nocturnal pains; *Mezereum* for nocturnal, tearing pains; *Rhus tox.*, if the pain is very much increased in a recumbent posture; and *Lycopodium*. We shall seldom be able to arrest the swelling with these remedies; as a rule, it will progress to the stage where we have to dread the advent of suppuration. At this stage a favorable change may yet be effected by one of the following remedies: *Mercurius, Iodine, Hepar sulphuris, Sulphur*. Their special indications cannot well be stated *a priori*, because they generally result from the constitutional symptoms which the disease happens to have evolved; all we can here say is that *Mercurius* and *Sulphur* are more adapted to very hard and not very extensive swellings; *Iodine* and *Hepar sulphuris* to large and soft swellings, with symptoms of fluctuation. If pus forms notwithstanding, and the abscess bursts, a remedy has to be selected, with reference to two conditions, namely: whether the suppuration threatens to speedily superinduce consumption, or whether the patient's strength bears well up under it. In the former case *Calcarea carbonica* and *Phosphorus* will have to be given; in the latter, *Silicea*, *Graphites* and *Baryta*; *Arsenicum* may likewise be of eminent use in the case of scrofulous individuals.

External applications are not always appropriate in this disease. Poultices are injurious if they increase the pains; in most cases they not only relieve the pain, but likewise exert a favorable effect upon the reabsorption of the pus in the diseased joint. An uninterrupted recumbent posture is to be avoided as long as the patients remain capable of moving about; only the diseased limb must not be used for a walk. A moderate and constant pressure by a starched bandage is only borne if the bones are not too much diseased; it has the double advantage of antagonizing the swelling and protecting the limb during motion. It has the best effect, if the abscess has already broke, for, in such a case, the bandage most decidedly promotes the course of the suppurative process. Amputation is only advisable if the joint is utterly disorganized and the constitution begins to show signs of failing under the constant pain and loss of fluids.

c. *Inflammation of the Tarsus.*

The inflammation is either seated in the bones or where they articulate with those of the metatarsus; or else in the articulation of the tarsus and tibia, or in both localities at the same time. Here, too, mechanical injuries are rarely the cause of the inflammation. An inflammation of the metatarsus is particularly met with among children and during the age of pubescence; an inflammation of the tibio-tarsal articulation occurs more frequently among adults.

The symptoms are most commonly the following: At first a pain is felt in walking, particularly during certain positions of the foot; in a state of rest the pain subsides almost entirely. Gradually the joint begins to swell, the swelling increasing more and more and gradually extending over the whole foot; at the same time the pains increase, become continuous, and walking is entirely out of the question. At last the pus finds an outlet in one or more places. In favorable cases the suppuration now decreases, the strength keeps up, the fistulous openings close, although sometimes not till years have elapsed. Or else, the swelling continues to increase even after the bursting of the abscess, the foot becomes completely distorted, and hectic fever is the unavoidable consequence.

The course of the disease always exceeds one and even more years, until the pus escapes outwardly. At all times life is in danger even in the case of children; adults succumb almost always with scarce an exception.

A peculiar form of tarsal inflammation is a flat foot. Sometimes it affects already small children, although it is only slightly developed at that age; it mostly shows itself after pubescence, most generally among males if they suddenly grow up in height. Every time after the foot is perseveringly used, violent pains are experienced in the joint, which becomes stiff after walking, with inability to stand upon the affected limb. On the inside a little swelling is perceived under the malleolus. Little by little the foot loses its arched shape, the os naviculare is turned downwards, away from the heel, and the patients generally walk on the inner edge of the foot. The malformation of the foot may become very considerable, and may materially interfere with its use. Sometimes the trouble does not cease spontaneously until after the patient is thirty years old. This form of inflammation which, under similar circumstances, may likewise occur at the knee, never results in suppuration.

The treatment involves difficulties for the reason that we are entrusted with it at too late a period, and likewise because we can never expect to accomplish a rapid success. At the outset of the inflammation we may still hope to accomplish something by means of *Staphysagria*, *Ledum*, *Sabina*, *Ruta*, *Mezereum*; but it is only in few cases that we succeed in preventing suppuration. If the bones are the starting-point of the inflammation, *Belladonna* and *Mercurius* are preferable to the previously-named remedies. Suppuration generally sets in slowly and amid signs of an apparent improvement which, however, should not deceive us. Suitable remedies are: *Calcarea carbonica*, and especially *Hepar sulphuris*, besides which we have *Graphites*, if the metatarsus is likewise involved. If the abscess bursts on the outside, the same remedies have to be employed that have been recommended for tumor albus under similar circumstances, to which *Aurum* may still be added. Poultices are out of place in an affection of such slow growth. The abscess should never be lanced; a tight bandage scarcely ever agrees with the patient's feeling of comfort.

For flat foot *Staphysagria* and *Graphites* seem to us to be the best remedies; their effect is, however, questionable, for the reason that in all the cases that we have had to treat, we have always resorted to a firm bandage, most generally a starched bandage, in order to afford the joint the necessary support; indeed we have often cured this disorder radically by means of such a bandage. Shoes firmly laced beyond the ankles, and with only moderately high heels, are indispensable.

Articular inflammations of the upper extremities are less important, because they are less dangerous to the organism. Suppuration is borne for years without any great inroad upon the general health. The remedies to be employed are mostly the same as those mentioned for inflammations of the lower extremities; other remedies can be found in the Materia Medica, which is so much more practicable as the disease does not require any immediate medicinal interference.

B. DISEASES OF THE ARTERIES, VEINS, LYMPHATICS,
AND
LYMPHATIC GLANDS.

1. Diseases of the Arteries.

The various diseases of the arteries are, indeed, of a very high pathological value, but of very little importance in a therapeutic point of view, for the simple reason that they cannot be treated medicinally.

Arterial inflammation, mostly only a symptom of other diseases, is scarcely recognizable with positive certainty, even in the case of larger arterial trunks. Of course, an inflammation of the larger arteries is highly interesting, because the closure of an arterial trunk near the heart may give rise to cardiac hypertrophy.

Aneurisms are not exactly pathological diseases, but consequences of other influences. We do not see how medicines are to accomplish anything in such cases, either in the uniformly developed arteriectasia or in the aneurism resulting from partial laceration of the vessel. It is only the disturbances which such arterial lesions cause in the heart, that suggest the propriety of medicinal interference, and we regard it as downright absurdity to recommend medicines for the cure of aneurisms, as has indeed been done. [There is no reason why *Aconite* and *Digitalis* should not be tried for aneurism. We know of a case of aneurism of the subclavian artery that was to be operated on by a celebrated Professor of one of the Philadelphia Colleges. Previous to the operation the patient was placed on the alternate use of tolerably large doses of *Aconite* and *Digitalis*, for a week. When the patient presented himself for the operation, the aneurism had so far disappeared that the Professor was unable to trace it and concluded to wait; what became of the case afterwards, I am unable to say. H.]

2. Diseases of the Veins.
a. *Phlebitis. Inflammation of Veins.*

Phlebitis, the correct diagnosis of which is a recent triumph, is, so far as its consequences are concerned, one of the most important of all known morbid processes. The veins of the lower extremities and of the cavity of the skull are particularly liable to inflammation, besides all the veins whose sides do not collapse, such as, above all other veins, those of the gravid uterus.

The causes of phlebitis are: Direct injuries of the vessel; coagula arising from impediments to the circulation occasioned by dilatation of the vessel; introduction of foreign substances resulting in a decomposition of the blood. This last-named explanation is applicable to phlebitis which sets in in an epidemic form in limited localities; or else the disease may arise secondarily from inflammatory affections of neighboring parts, or of remote parts, but lying in the tract of the vein; or from puerperal conditions, pyæmia, suppurations of bones, especially caries of the bones and ossicula of the ear.

The symptoms of phlebitis vary according to its extent and intensity. The most intense forms of phlebitis originate in pyæmia, to which we therefore refer; in this category belongs especially epidemic phlebitis, where the local process is rapidly extended through the whole organism. The less intense cases very usually set in with a chill recurring either irregularly with more or less frequency or otherwise, or else setting in typically, like an intermittent paroxysm. The diseased vein is often indicated by a seated, circumscribed, burning pain, but is quite often altogether painless. The chill is succeeded by a feeling of illness, usually so severe that it is entirely out of all proportion to the objective symptoms. The pulse is accelerated and very much reduced in volume, the digestion is interfered with, a tendency to perspire sets in, the tract of the vein becomes œdematous. If the circulation in the vein is restored, all these symptoms may disappear as rapidly as they came. If pus forms in the vein, the inflammation gradually ascends towards the heart, and the picture of pyæmia becomes more and more marked. If the vein remains closed, œdema develops itself beyond the closure and, if a collateral circulation can be established, may last only a short while, or else remain permanent. In such a case lassitude, chills at irregular intervals, irregular flashes of heat sometimes continue for weeks.

The terminations of phlebitis depend upon the changes going on in the inflammatory exudation. If no purulent decomposition takes place, life is not exactly in danger; if pus forms, it may be carried along with the current of blood, and a most malignant phlebitis may suddenly arise notwithstanding the trifling character of the symptoms at the outset of the inflammation. It is in this manner that lying-in women and persons that had been operated upon, often perish quite suddenly although not a single symptom existed at first that could have given rise to the least apprehensions of danger.

The prognosis is uncertain. If the chills recur but seldom and with increasing weakness, the danger is less; whereas frequent chills, prostration and sopor, the supervention of icterus and petechiæ, are decidly ominous signs.

Treatment. Phlebitis is one of those diseases that can scarcely ever be treated in accordance with the rules of a rigorous symptomatic similarity, and where, if we do not mean to commit grave mistakes, we have to keep constantly and clearly in view the whole internal process not manifested to the senses by a single symptom. Thus a purely symptomatic similarity can only have a secondary value, and the drugs whose special action upon the veins we have become acquainted with from cases of poisoning, necessarily occupy the first rank in the treatment of this disease. Their number is not great, and a portion of those we shall name, is still very little correctly known, and, what is worse, the clinical applications of these drugs are still exceedingly unsatisfactory and insufficient. Among these remedies we distinguish: the *serpent-poisons*, the *poison of the honey-bee*, *Curare*, *Secale cornutum*, *Phosphorus*, *Mercurius* and *Arsenicum*. Of all these, *Phosphorus* is undoubtedly the most important remedy, corresponding with the most diversified forms of phlebitis, from the most trifling form to that accompanied by icterus and petechiæ. *Apis* is particularly indicated, if the veins of the cavity of the skull are inflamed; it is less homœopathic to phlebitis of the lower extremities. *Lachesis* and *Secale*, as well as *Arsenicum*, are particularly indicated by the heart-symptoms, the anxiety, dyspnœa, etc. *Mercurius* is especially appropriate if the phlebitis remains more localized and is attended with external inflammation and suppuration. We do not dwell upon these remedies more in detail, because they will have to be referred to again under pyæmia. In lighter cases the following remedies have been found practically useful: *Bryonia*, *Staphysagria*, *Rhus toxicodendron; Bryonia* if the inflammation was not very painful, but attended with marked constitutional disturbances; *Rhus tox.*, for local symptoms radiating from the inflammatory centre like erysipelas; *Staphysagria*, for phlebitis of the lower extremities. [*Belladonna* and *Hamamelis virg.* are eminently useful in phlebitis; we have cured a very severe and threatening case of inflammation of the femoral vein, where the inflammation spread rapidly as far as the hip, by means of tolerably large and frequently repeated doses of *Belladonna*, without the aid of any other remedy. H.]

The subsequently remaining and very prominent œdema of the parts which lose their normal circulation in consequence of the obstruction of the vein, cannot be removed by treatment. It does not disappear until the collateral circulation is restored, which it sometimes takes years to accomplish; the uniform pressure of a bandage, if it can be applied, may, if it does not effect a cure, afford at least a good deal of relief.

b. *Phlebectasia. Varices; Dilatation of Veins.*

In most cases the causes of these very frequent dilatations can be determined with perfect certainty; in other cases, however, they are involved in obscurity. These are the cases where the disease cannot well be traced to some mechanical obstruction in the circulation of the blood. At all events, these cases are the least frequent. But even in cases where mechanical causes undoubtedly co-operate, they cannot be regarded as the sole cause of the disease, since individuals who are exposed to the same deleterious influences remain free from any such trouble. Hence, the existence of a peculiar predisposition in the walls of the veins, or else the subsequent supervention of a morbid change in those walls, will have to be taken for granted. The most frequent causes are: Obliteration of the vein owing to which the portion beyond the obliterated vein dilates in its whole extent; dilatation or contraction of the venous trunk, which has the same effect as obliterations, only in a less degree; every pathological change that interferes with the flow of blood to the heart, such as dilatation of the right ventricle, affections of the liver, emphysema, tumors compressing the vein, tight clothing. In all such cases, phlebectasia is of a secondary character; it may likewise occur as a primary disease in a manner that we have not yet been able to account for, in the case of men who have to be continually in a position that interferes with the reflux of the blood, persons for instance who have to be continually in a sitting or standing posture. In a sitting posture, the dilatation of the vessels can often be accounted for by the pressure exerted upon the abdominal viscera in the stooping posture; in the standing posture, on the contrary, the dilatation is entirely owing to the circumstance that the vertical position of the body embarrasses the course of the blood onwards through the veins. In very many cases another influence exists of whose mode of action we have no definite idea, namely bad nutrition and living in damp, unwholesome dwellings. That these circumstances are of importance is shown by the frequent occurrence of varices on the lower extremities among the lower strata of the population, more particularly among weavers and washerwomen.

Every vein in the body may become dilated; dilatations occur most frequently in the veins of the rectum, lower extremities and spermatic cord. We will briefly dwell here upon varices of the lower extremities. They occur more frequently among women in whom the cause of the dilatation is traceable to the impregnated uterus, whereas primary dilatations are decidedly of more frequent occurrence among men. What we have said just now concerning the originating causes of dilatation is particularly applicable to this form. At first one of the larger cutaneous veins of the leg is most commonly affected, whence it does not usually extend to the thigh, but involves very regularly the larger as well as the more minute veins of the foot, especially the veins situated around the ankles where they give rise to a considerable swelling covered with a bluish net of both delicate and coarser vessels. In most cases these varicose veins are painless. In other cases the leg pains for a short time, after which the pain again disappears. Very often the pain is felt while a portion of the skin assumes a bluish redness, swells and becomes quite hard; the pain increases continually, finally the skin suddenly breaks at the place of infiltration, without this lesion being caused by mechanical injury as most of these patients fancy, and an ulcer of the size of a pea forms, which is at first round and provided with thin, somewhat undermined edges. Without proper management and hygienic precautions the pains increase all the time; the ulcer spreads, its edges gradually swell, the surrounding skin becomes hypertrophied, the ulcer secretes a watery and sometimes exceedingly fetid fluid, and its base has a sickly color. If the same mode of living is continued, during which walking hurts only a little, but standing hurts a great deal, the ulcer may spread over the whole surface of the leg from the ankle to the calf, and may even penetrate to the periosteum. Ulcers below the ankle and on the anterior portion of the foot are of rare occurrence. The fetor of the ulcer increases in proportion as the ulcer spreads over a larger surface. In one of our cases, during the summer-season, a crowd of worms of half to three quarters of an inch in length, were seen in the ulcer whenever the dressing was removed. Persons go about with such ulcers for years, and it is inconceivable that the constant drain of their vital fluids does not result in speedy emaciation. If a fever or some other constitutional disease breaks out during the existence of the ulcer, it seems to heal spontaneously, in which case the disease is very commonly, but improperly, regarded as the consequence of the healing.

If the patients are so situated as to be able to remain at once in a recumbent posture, the little sores heal very speedily, but break open again very easily if the person has to stand a great deal, so that the existence of such ulcers at any previous period leaves a constant liability to their returning again at a subsequent time.

In the higher walks of life, where every measure is taken from the start to prevent the formation of ulcers, a peculiar cutaneous affection is witnessed in their stead. The skin assumes a very dark and bluish color, and scattered and violently itching pustules form very frequently, or else the skin peels off in scales, leaving the surface moist. This form of the varicose affection is by far the most malignant and distressing.

With an entire change in the mode of living the varicose ulcers may heal of themselves, but this is undoubtedly a very rare occurrence.

Treatment. Painless varices, without ulceration, cannot be regarded as an object of treatment, nor do we believe that anybody can imagine the feasibility of removing them by means of medicines. If pains are felt, and the subcutaneous cellular tissue becomes infiltrated, it would seem as though medicines might be useful; at any rate we have seen a rapid improvement take place after the use of *Staphysagria*, *Lycopodium* and *Graphites*. These are the only remedies which we can recommend as long as the ulcers are painful. Of other remedies, of which we have had abundant opportunities of trying a large number, such as *Sulphur*, *Sepia*, *Silicea*, *Mercurius*, *Aurum*, *Rhus tox.*, etc., we have never perceived the least effect. [*Hamamelis virg.* is frequently used by American physicians. H.] If the ulcer has become atonic, even the three first-named remedies are no longer of any use, and a mechanical treatment is the only treatment that can prove of any use. These three remedies are likewise the only ones that we can recommend for the peculiar cutaneous affection, but we must confess that they too will often leave us in the lurch. Our main resource in treating these varicose disorders are external or mechanical means. The dilatation of the veins being chiefly a passively mechanical change, it is evident that moderate compression by means of a good bandage will moderate and finally remove the varicose dilatation altogether. If individuals with marked varicose dilatations constantly wear a bandage, they will never be troubled with ulcers nor with any other cutaneous affection. Existing ulcers heal very rapidly under a carefully-applied bandage, so much more rapidly if we first cover them with strips of adhesive plaster and a layer of cotton wadding over these, so as to protect them from all contact with atmospheric air. By pursuing this course we have never known ulcers of any size or of upwards of twenty years' standing to remain uncured; but we have never shunned the trouble of applying the bandage ourselves. The longest time it has taken us to heal these ulcers, is six months. In this case the ulcer was about a quarter of a square foot in size, the subjacent periosteum was considerably infiltrated, the skin was hypertrophied from the toes to the knee as in a case of exquisite elephantiasis, and had the appearance of an enormous wart. All these deep-seated alterations yielded to the exclusive use of the bandage. If the excessive sensitiveness does not admit of the immediate application of a bandage, the patient must be kept for a short time in a recumbent position with his leg raised; in such a case warm cataplasms afford a good deal of relief.

3. Diseases of the Lymphatic Vessels and Glands.

a. *Lymphangioitis and Lymphadenitis Acuta.*

Acute inflammations of lymphatic vessels occur so seldom alone; lymphangioitis especially occurs so seldom without inflammation of the lymphatic glands, that we will treat of both these conditions together.

These inflammations exist very seldom as primary diseases; even if they seem to be of this character, yet a careful examination shows even in such cases that the inflammation is a secondary occurrence. Secondarily the affection most commonly supervenes during the course of pathological processes that depend upon some special infection, such as syphilis and variola, or during the course of diseases depending upon or occasioning septic processes, such as puerperal fever and typhus. Any, even ever so trifling suppuration on the skin may inflame the adjoined lymphatic vessel and its glands; sometimes this may not take place until the primary suppuration has healed, so that the inflammation in such cases may seem to have originated as a primary disease. We may finally observe that some constitutions show a striking predispositon to inflammations of lymphatic vessels, whereas others are scarcely ever attacked by them.

Lymphangioitis, so far as it is an object of observation, if the inflamed vessel is situated near the periphery, sets in suddenly, sometimes after an injury of the primarily inflamed parts, and appears like a fine, sharply circumscribed, rose-colored cord which is very sensitive to contact, and interferes with the free motion of the limb. This lasts very seldom longer than two days. Sometimes even a few hours after the appearance of the red cord, at times not till hours have elapsed after its disappearance, one or more of the lymphatic glands in relation with the inflamed vessel begins to swell, becomes painful, and very speedily shows an inflammatory redness. It is more particularly the inguinal, axillary and posterior cervical glands that are liable to becoming thus inflamed. Sometimes no kind of pain is felt at the commencement, which may not set in until the swelling of the gland has reached a very high degree and suppuration has begun to make its appearance, owing to which circumstance we feel very much disposed to regard such inflammations as primary. After the gland has reached the size of a hazelnut to that of a hen's egg, the pain may disappear again without the gland having softened, and the swelling may very gradually go down again and the gland return to its former size, or else one portion of the gland may resume its normal condition, and the balance remain indurated. Most commonly, however, the inflammation terminates in suppuration, the pus escaping outwardly and leaving the skin round the opening undermined, a closure of which generally takes place very slowly.

We have occasionally noticed a very peculiar form of lymphangioitis, more particularly in the case of women, and about the head. With this inflammation a violent fever breaks out very suddenly, accompanied by tearing pains in the scalp and nape of the neck. The abatement of these pains is attended with the simultaneous appearance of several nodes and hard cords about the head, which, however remain seldom longer than forty-eight hours. After a short interval of ease another attack takes place, and this may be going on in this manner for several weeks. We have never been able to trace such an occurrence to any definite cause.

The treatment has to be in conformity with the exciting cause. Of syphilitic inflammations of the lymphatic glands we shall speak in the further course of this work. If the inflammation is caused by the introduction of poisonous substances into a wound, the best remedies are *Ammonium carbonicum, Acidum nitricum* and *muriaticum,* and likewise *Apis*; the last-mentioned agent more particularly in cases running a rapid course. If an important constitutional derangement supervenes during the local affection, *Arsenicum* and *Rhus tox.* are likewise indicated. In such cases remnants of inflammation usually remain, that have to be treated precisely like any other case of chronic lymphangioitis, of which we shall treat hereafter.

If the inflammation of the lymphatic vessel is not caused by a specific virus, the first requisite of the treatment, if suppuration or inflammation is still present, is to direct our chief attention to this condition of the gland as the starting point of the whole disease, in order, by this means, to deprive the pathological process in the lymphatic system of its nutriment. If the inflamed vessel and its gland are very painful, and no suppuration has yet taken place, a few doses of *Belladonna* are frequently of much use; this treatment, especially in the case of children, will sometimes secure the retrogression of the inflammatory process. If the gland is very much swollen, *Mercurius* is the only remedy capable of still preventing suppuration. In many cases, where fluctuation is already distinctly perceptible, and a raised and very red spot shows the point where the pus will escape, *Mercurius* still effects a cure. As a rule we hold that it is best to give *Mercurius* at the onset, more particularly in the case of individuals in whom every little wound is disposed to suppurate. If the suppuration progresses unceasingly in spite of all treatment, *Hepar sulphuris* undoubtedly hastens the suppurative process, but is only suitable until the abscess begins to discharge. Considering the circumstance that *Mercurius* so very often acts favorably even in cases where pus has already begun to form, we may sometimes be disposed to doubt the propriety of giving *Hepar*. We may be guided by the rule that, if the cellular tissue round the gland is very much inflamed, and suppuration cannot be prevented, *Hepar* should be given at as early a period as possible; if the gland alone is inflamed, the use of Hepar should be postponed as late as possible. The subsequent suppuration need not be assisted by treatment as long as the pus has a healthy appearance and shows a normal consistence. If the pus becomes thin, assuming the consistence of serum, *Sulphur* at protracted intervals is appropriate to this condition. On the other hand, if the suppuration proceeds sparingly, and the bottom of the ulcer is filled in with whitish flocks of cellular tissue, which, when touched with the sound, show the consistence of lard, we advise decidedly the employment of *Iodine*. As regards the other consequences of such an inflammation, they coincide entirely with chronic lymphangioitis.

In the above-mentioned form of lymphangioitis of the head neither *Bryonia*, nor *Belladonna*, *Rhus tox.* or *Mercurius* has been of the least use to us; *Apis* showed a marked effect, so that no more paroxysms took place.

As regards external applications, we do not deem them necessary, although they need not be rejected, for they very often alleviate the pain and enable the patient to enjoy longer intervals of rest. But we only recommend warm poultices which not only favor absorption on the one hand, but promote suppuration on the other. We are not in favor of any premature lancing of the abscess; the abscess should only be lanced, if, owing to the depth at which the gland is situated, the spontaneous escape of the pus meets with difficulties, or if the pus can be distinctly seen shining through the integuments.

b. *Lymphadenitis Chronica, Chronic Inflammation of Lymphatic Glands.*

This affection either develops itself out of the acute form, or else it is a primary disease depending upon constitutional peculiarities, such as characterize scrofulosis; or else, in infectious diseases, it takes the place of an acute inflammation. Chronic lymphadenitis sometimes occurs as a phenomenon of marasmus with typhoid characteristics. Childhood and the period immediately after pubescence furnish most cases of this disease.

If chronic lymphadenitis develops itself out of the acute form, the swollen gland either remains unopened, or else, if the pus had found an outlet on the surface, the opening closes again at an early period, and the gland which had been reduced in size by an incomplete suppuration, remains as a firm and hard swelling that gradually becomes quite painless but may continue to grow by subsequent turns of inflammation and finally suppurate. In cases where chronic lymphadenitis sets in as a primary disease, it first attacks only one gland, but soon invades a number. The swelling is generally without pain and takes place very gradually; most commonly such swellings reach a much larger size than in acute lymphadenitis. The swollen gland may remain unchanged for years, after which it may gradually disappear spontaneously, the swellings that had originated in childhood, commonly disappearing immediately after pubescence; or else further degenerations of the gland may take place. It is a common occurrence for a torpid glandular swelling that had remained painless for a long time, to suddenly become painful, and to inflame and break. Such a swelling always discharges a thin, badly-looking pus, the swelling decreases very slowly in size, the bottom of the abscess is filled with a whitish, elastic, lardaceous substance. Very commonly several openings exist at the same time. The suppurative process is always very slow, and, if the patient is unfavorably situated in life, may develop an hectic state of the system; or else the sore may heal with a badly-colored, radiating, retracted cicatrix, under which remnants of the indurated gland are very commonly still felt. It often happens that after one gland is healed, another adjoining gland swells and passes through the same process; this may be the course of the glands for years. An affection of this kind is at a later period very generally followed by tuberculosis.

There is another form of lymphadenitis where the glands are likewise swollen and where a row of such swellings extends along the tract of a lymphatic vessel, but the glands are soft and fluctuating, generally painful even if not red. There is not always an escape of pus, in consequence of which the swelling rapidly discharges and heals to return again in some other locality; absorption sometimes takes place in spite of the evidently considerable accumulation of fluid. We have noticed a phenomenon of this kind in the case of a child one year old which was affected with an intense anæmia and—we state this incidentally—exhibited the peculiarity that blowing murmurs were heard over the whole extent of the skull-cap; in this case the whole body was covered with these swellings; they fluctuated, became inflamed, disappeared and then showed themselves again in other places. The child died of hydrocephalus at an age of eighteen months. Another chronic form was observed in the case of a man fifty years old. In this case the swellings appeared in company with the symptoms of a general marasmus, every swelling broke, but was perfectly painless, and the patient's strength was rapidly consumed by the suppurating process. The most ordinary localities for chronic lymphadenitis are the neck and the upper extremities including the axilla, much less frequently the lower extremities, without mentioning the non-suppurating glandular swellings in the abdominal cavity.

The manner in which the swelling originates, is of considerable importance in a therapeutic point of view, exclusive even of specific glandular swellings to which no reference is made here. If the swelling remains as a rest of acute lymphadenitis, *Sulphur* is a sovereign remedy to disperse the swelling. This agent will seldom leave us in the lurch, and compel us to look for other remedies, such as *Aurum, Iodine, Silicea, Calcarea carbonica.*

For a primary glandular swelling *Baryta* is one of the most efficient remedies; in many cases this agent alone has enabled us to avoid the suppurative process and to effect a complete absorption, especially of glandular swellings on the neck. *Conium* has never shown any marked effect. If suppuration has set in, *Iodium* and *Calcarea carbonica* render the most reliable aid. Beside these two remedies we mention *Graphites, Sulphur, Phosphorus, Silicea, Kali bichromicum* and likewise *Aurum,* not the metallic Gold but the

Muriate. We should never lose sight of the fact that a rapid disappearance of the swelling is among the impossibilities.

If the swellings constitute the expression of an intense hectic constitutional affection, *Calcarea* deserves a preference among children and *Arsenicum* among adults. In such cases a cure is a thing of very doubtful possibility.

In other respects the treatment is very plain. If the patient's mode of living is improper and the constitution is likewise tainted, the first thing to be done towards a cure is to regulate the diet and to prescribe an abundance of out-door exercise. This is more effectual than medicine. We are acquainted with a family where the children, three in number, were all of them suffering with extensive lymphadenitis in consequence of occupying an unhealthy dwelling in town and being restricted to an improper diet. The youngest child succumbed to hectic fever and marasmus, the other two children who were sent into the country, have regained their health and have grown stout and fresh, although both, at the time when they moved out of town, were afflicted with at least a dozen glandular abscesses.

We ought not to omit mention of the Iodine springs of Hall which are an admirable remedy for these glandular abscesses. Unfortunately most of our patients are too poor to visit these springs, and the bottled water is not by any means what it should be and leaves a good deal to be desired.

C. DISEASES OF THE NERVES.

The nervous system as immediately connected with the brain and spinal cord, having been considered in a previous chapter where all its general morbid alterations were treated of, it remains for us here to devote a few paragraphs to two other abnormal conditions of the nervous system. We did not deem it expedient, from many reasons, to treat of all the different neuralgias generally in one chapter.

1. Ischias.

Neuralgia of the ischiadic nerve constitutes one of the most frequent, and at the same time one of the most distressing forms of neuralgia. Its causes are generally involved in uncertainty; a cold, excessive exertions, abdominal affections, stagnation of habitual hemorrhages, etc., are mentioned as such causes, but it is difficult to trace a distinct connection between these two orders of phenomena as cause and affect. It is of course true that ischias attacks healthy and robust individuals much less frequently than persons of a sickly frame.

At times the affection commences very suddenly, at other times the pain arises gradually from sensations that resemble a slight attack of rheumatism. The pain is generally located between the ischium and knee, so that the course of the nerve can be determined very exactly by the pain. It is very seldom that the pain radiates upwards, more generally downwards below the knee as far as the foot, on the internal or external surface of the leg. We distinguish two kinds of pain; either the pain is constant, somewhat remittent, but never entirely intermittent, and usually following very exactly the tract of the nerve without the patient being able to define the quality of the pain; or else peculiar tearing-darting pains may supervene, resembling electric shocks, setting in paroxysmally and being excited by motion or by making a wrong step, sneezing or coughing. At the same time one or more places in the course of the nerve are generally sensitive to pressure. Although the pain does not seem to exacerbate at definite periods, yet all patients complain that it is worse in bed, and that this exacerbation is sometimes so great that they dare not go to bed. Inasmuch as the pains are very much increased by an extension of the leg, by pressure or by the nerve being put on the stretch, the patients generally keep the limb slightly flexed, using it as little as possible during a walk or for the performance of any other motion. This is generally the cause why the diseased limb, after the ischias has lasted for some time, grows thin, although the emaciation may likewise be caused by a gradually-developing paralysis. The diagnosis being sometimes extremely difficult, it is important to know that ischias always attacks only one limb.

In ischias antica the pain follows the tract of the crural nerve; this form of ischiadic neuralgia is very scarce, nor is the pain near as acute as in ischias postica.

This disorder runs a chronic course. The attack is supposed to at first set in with a fever, but these are exceptional cases. A spontaneous cure only takes place with a gradual abatement of the pains, but not till months have elapsed. The general health is very much disturbed by the constancy of the severe pains and by the sleeplessness; the appetite becomes impaired and the bowels are torpid.

The treatment of this affection constitutes one of the shining features of Homœopathy, not so much because we cure every case of this kind as because our opponents admit that they have no means of doing anything for this disease and have to let the patient suffer for months; whereas we homœopaths never fail of a cure in the course of a week or two at latest. Yet even we ought not to boast of being absolutely certain of success, for the reason that this affection has but few symptoms, and only a few of them are entirely local; hence the selection of a remedy is always invested with difficulties, and a successful result is often defeated on this account. However, in order not to wrong Homœopathy, if no cure is effected, or is effected very slowly, we call attention to the fact that ischias sometimes depends upon causes that cannot be removed, such as exostoses in the pelvic cavity.

The four leading remedies for ischias, the effect of which has been verified in many instances, are: *Colocynthis*, *Rhus tox.*, *Arsenicum* and *Lycopodium*. Colocynthis is more particularly adapted to recent cases, the pain sets in suddenly in all its fierceness, it is a constant pain, becoming intolerable only in paroxysms excited at once by cold and motion; at the same time a feeling of numbness is experienced in the whole extremity.—*Rhus tox.* is very seldom adapted to quite recent cases, but comes into play in the further course of the disease, if the following symptoms are present: Stinging or burning-tearing pain, increasing during rest, and alleviated only for a short time by motion; heaviness, lameness and even actual paralysis of the affected limb; frequent paroxysms of cramps in the calves.—Lycopodium in more chronic cases, the pain is chiefly a burning or fine stinging pain, with complete intermissions, aggravated by rest and somewhat alleviated by motion, with lameness of the extremity, disposition to painful muscular twitchings; especially if the bowels have become very much constipated in consequence of the distressing affection.—*Arsenicum*, if the pains are marked by complete intermissions, break out with typical regularity, exacerbate every night even to an unbearable degree of intensity; they are a burning-tearing distress, seem to be seated close to the bone, are increased by vigorous, and alleviated by gentle movements, excited at once by cold, and momentarily moderated by warmth. At the same time the patient feels sick, the paroxysms are characterized by an extreme restlessness and an inability to remain long in the same position.

These four remedies do not, however, constitute the whole of our curative means for ischias; they only correspond with the most frequently-occurring forms. Other important remedies are: *Chamomilla* in recent cases, for a drawing-tearing pain which becomes intolerable at night and is especially aggravated by the warmth of the bed. *Arnica* for a burning-tearing, or stinging-tearing pain, with a numb and bruised feeling in the affected limb, with great sensitiveness to any kind of touch; for the ischias of lying-in females.— *Pulsatilla* for a drawing pain which is worse at night, compels the patient to move the diseased limb continually; the pain is much improved by movement, and is sometimes increased by warmth, not by cold; the cause of the attack is menstrual suppression. — *Carbo vegetabilis* in protracted cases; the symptoms are like those indicated for Arsenic. — *Causticum* for ischias antica and for the paralysis caused by ischias. — *Ferrum;* the pain is at first increased by motion, but improved by the continuance of motion, more particularly suitable for worn-out individuals with extremely irritable nervous systems.

We might mention a number of other remedies, but those we have named will suffice. In special cases a suitable repertory may be consulted.

We do not advise the employment of external applications; they generally weaken the patient still more. The vaunted application of strips of fly-blister is very seldom of any use; if it is, it is most probably because its action is in homœopathic rapport with the symptoms. We may not often be obliged to send a patient afflicted with this neuralgia to the springs; if this should be necessary, we would recommend Teplitz and Sulphur springs.

2. Neuralgia Intercostalis.

Intercostal Neuralgia.

This species of neuralgia is still more frequent than ischias; it attacks principally females, and occurs very seldom before the age of pubescence, and subsequently to the critical age. The physical constitution does not seem to influence this affection; nor can it be traced to definite causes. This affection succeeds very frequently an attack of herpes zoster; it much less frequently precedes this exanthem. The intercostal nerves of the left side, and more particularly the nerves between the sixth and eighth intercostal spaces are most frequently attacked.

As in ischias, so in intercostal neuralgia, the pain is very seldom felt all at once in all its intensity, but most commonly develops itself progressively; it is generally located in one intercostal space, is at times tearing, at other times lancing or jerking, and always mingled with a burning sensation; every more violent movement of the thorax excites or aggravates the pain. A characteristic peculiarity in this affection is that three spots are uncommonly sensitive to contact; namely one spot close to the vertebral column, in the middle of the intercostal space, one half way between the sternum and vertebral column, and a third spot towards the front, close to the sternum or mesian line of the abdomen. These points are very seldom missing; they are well known to the patients, and the extreme sensitiveness of these points, which is very much increased by the least attempt at percussion, easily suggests the presence of inflammation. This suspicion is set at rest by the circumstance that hard pressure is generally borne without trouble. The affection is unaccompanied by fever, its course is mostly chronic and may last for years. The more gradually the pain arises, the more obstinate it is as a rule. The paroxysms of syncope, palpitation of the heart, dyspnœa and the like, which are often caused by the intensity of the pain, are very apt to mislead one in the diagnosis.

In treating this affection we shall find it difficult to hit upon a remedy, if we depend upon the symptoms in the Materia Medica. In selecting a remedy, we may lay great stress upon the circumstance that the pain is semi-lateral and likewise that the kind of pain, the time of its appearance and other features, are characteristic indications. The favorable results which have so far been obtained by the use of *Pulsatilla*, *Rhus toxicodendron*, *Arsenicum* and *Mezereum*, speak very much in favor of these drugs. [*Cimicifuga racemosa* is likewise excellent. H.] *Mezereum* is undoubtedly the chief remedy, and is especially indicated if the neuralgia sets in after zoster. The general indications, as stated above, are easily verified by corresponding symptoms in the Materia Medica. The following remedies are indicated *a priori*, although they have been very little used in practice: *Ranunculus sceleratus*, *Rhododendron*, *Ledum* and *Spigelia*. Many circumstances speak in favor of the latter, more especially the efficacy of Spigelia in neuralgia of the trigeminus. We will here repeat the advice which we have repeatedly given on former occasions, namely not to give too large doses which are apt to superinduce homœopathic aggravations; nor to repeat the dose too frequently, for the reason that a favorable effect is never obtained very suddenly.

D. DISEASES OF THE SKIN.

In treating of diseases of the eyes, we have pointed out several inconveniences which render even an approximatively satisfactory arrangement of the therapeutics of ophthalmic diseases a very difficult task. In regard to cutaneous affections, it is likewise all but impossible to present them from the stand-point of homœopathic Therapeutics. In order to render such a presentation profitable, it would have to be very extensive and take in a good deal that is purely hypothetical. The space that is allotted to us, is too limited for such a purpose. For this reason we have confined ourselves to the most essential points, and have only stated practically verified facts. Before, however, passing to the consideration of the special cutaneous affections, we deem it proper to briefly expound the reasons why cutaneous diseases are a sore point in the homœopathic Materia Medica.

Cutaneous diseases are not, like the affections of other organs, spread over several parts of the body; they only offer us a single symptom, namely the cutaneous efflorescence, as a means of diagnosing the cutaneous disease and selecting the appropriate remedy. This symptom is of course accompanied by a variety of general symptoms, but we would go too far if we were to allow these variable companions of the cutaneous affection to decide the selection of the remedial agent; at all events these accessory symptoms are only of secondary importance. Hence we only have ONE objective symptom of disease, but where do we find a corresponding symptom in the Materia Medica? The leading symptoms of our drugs are, moreover, indicated in such a superficial and vague manner that their true meaning can hardly be deciphered from such a text. In making this assertion, we expect to incur the censure of those who deem it a crime even to think of the possibility of amending the Materia Medica. Well, we will endeavor to pocket the censure, but we desire to be convicted by logical evidence. Until then we shall stick to our text that it is impossible to treat cutaneous diseases with certainty if we take the Materia Medica for our guide.

We will now consider another expedient which might be resorted to in this case, as it is in other cases, for the purpose of supplying or covering up the defects of our Materia Medica, we mean the practical result, the experience gathered *ex usu in morbis.* But what else do we meet with in this direction but endless confusion? If our literature exhibited the richest treasure of really useful practical observations, it would either have to be left untouched, or else the use of it would involve a great deal of trouble or expose us to numerous mistakes. For the last fifty years, cutaneous diseases have constituted an arena for those who were anxious to subserve the purposes of Science by manufacturing names or making an ostentatious display of their erudition. In this manner we have obtained a brilliant nomenclature which, however, is unintelligible to those who have not devoted years to its study. This circumstance has reduced the value of clinical cases almost to zero.

In the presence of so much uncertainty and want of clearness in our Materia Medica and of confusion in the department of cutaneous diseases in the literature of our School, a therapeutical arrangement of cutaneous diseases is certainly a hazardous task. Many preliminary labors are required before we can think of perfecting a tolerable system of therapeutics of the cutaneous diseases; above all, we recommend uniformity in our nomenclature, coupled with a rigid precision in diagnosis.

The febrile exanthemata which have been excluded from the following list, have been transferred among the constitutional diseases, for the reason that their importance is determined by the accompanying derangements of functions rather than by the form of the exanthem. The series in which the special forms are successively presented, has been arranged in accordance with the pathologico-anatomical changes; we have simply avoided the custom of distinguishing special sub-divisions in each form.

1. Erythema.

Erythema occupies a middle rank between hyperæmia and inflammation of the skin; it is easily confounded with a benign form of erysipelas.

Its causes are: Mechanical injuries of the skin; the influence of a high temperature, of various medicinal agents; continual moistening of one part of the skin by urine, liquid stool, perspiration, tears and even the constant use of moist compresses; constant irritation of the skin by rough clothes. In the case of children, erythema seems to be likewise caused by hearty and fat food. Erythema seldom occurs as a wide-spread affection, to which the designation of "epidemic" might be applied. Chronic erythema breaks out chiefly in the face, and more especially on the nose; its causes sometimes seem to be purely local, and at other times constitutional.

Erythema is characterized by a more or less diffuse redness of the skin, not separated from the normal redness by sharply-drawn outlines, assuming a yellowish, not a white tint under the pressure of the finger, and continuing for some time and, finally, terminating in desquamation. These characteristics belong to all forms of erythema. Erythema caused by external irritants, most generally breaks out on the scrotum, at the anus, between the thighs, in the axillæ, face, and in the deep integumentous folds of fleshy persons, or at the place where the irritating cause exerts its influence. After the cause ceases to act, the erythema generally disappears of itself in a few days. If the irritation continues, the epidermis may become detached (intertrigo), and ulcers may form, or the skin may even become gangrenous, as in decubitus. Erythema arising from internal causes, is almost exclusively located on the dorsal surface of the hands and feet, where it is never absent, even if other parts are likewise affected. At first the place exhibits a redness, and in a few days darker-colored papules of various sizes spring up, which remain even for some time after the diffuse redness has disappeared; the affected spot likewise retains a yellowish tint for some time after. In particular circumstances subsequent crops of this eruption break out on its borders, by which means the affection runs a very protracted course. This form of erythema is generally attended with a little fever, and at the diseased spot a darting-burning pain is generally experienced. The former variety, on the contrary, has no fever as long as the erythema is of the simple kind, whereas the intertrigo of sensitive children may be attended with fever. The second variety, without any subsequent crops, lasts from one to two weeks.

In treating the first variety, all that it may be necessary for us to do, is to remove the exciting cause. In some individuals the disposition to erythema is so great, and it leads so easily to more serious consequences that we are led to suspect behind the local irritation the existence of some constitutional disposition. This is particularly the case with the intertrigo or soreness of children. Since this soreness is often caused by improper diet, the first thing to be done is to regulate it with care; if the soreness continues in spite of this change, a few doses of *Mercurius vivus* or *solubilis* will cure the trouble very speedily. If this remedy should fail us, *Lycopodium* will effect a cure. Among local applications, finely pulverized starch is the best and most harmless; frictions with grease must be avoided, they are very apt to give rise to the formation of pustules.

For erythema from internal causes, *Mercurius* is likewise a specific remedy, if the redness is intense, the red spot raised and sensitive, and the erythema is accompanied by fever. *Rhus tox.* has always proved ineffectual in such cases. If the erythema is confined to the leg, *Mezereum* is the more appropriate, the more the affected spot itches and burns. *Ledum* likewise deserves our attention; so does *Staphysagria;* this remedy is especially indicated if the erythema is seated on the upper extremities. We advise *Lycopodium*, if the eruption runs a protracted course in consequence of successive crops breaking out for a time.

2. Erysipelas.

Erysipelas proper is altogether a primary affection the cause of which it is difficult to trace in every case. The disease occurs almost exclusively between the age of pubescence and that of sixty, and is of less frequent occurrence among old people than among children. Atmospheric influences are generally regarded as the cause of erysipelas, but this theory is not justified by the evidence of fact. All we know positively is that erysipelas often sets in as a sporadic disease, and that sometimes it breaks out in the form of a limited epidemic which never assumes a very extensive range and has given rise to the erroneous view that erysipelas is a contagious disease. It is a characteristic feature of this disease that every new attack of erysipelas increases the patient's liability to other attacks, which only becomes extinct at an advanced age. The cause of successive attacks of erysipelas is very often to be found in violent emotions, gross errors in diet, and in colds, more especially in the action of severe cold upon a heated skin. We have known a lady who was several times attacked with erysipelas simply because she suddenly went from the kitchen-stove into the cellar.

The origin of wandering erysipelas is involved in complete

mystery; it is to be observed that it inclines to set in previous to the age of pubescence.

Traumatic erysipelas is regarded by many persons as a simple form of dermatitis. It arises in consequence of injuries if suppuration ensues, or even at the start, soon after the infliction of the injury; or it accompanies suppurating inflammatory processes, such as gum-boils. It may be looked upon as an excess of reaction against the inflammation from which it proceeds. Erysipelas neonatorum is altogether a form of traumatic erysipelas. The introduction of septic substances undoubtedly exerts a prominent influence over the origin of this disease. This circumstance likewise accounts for those cases of erysipelas that supervenes during typhus and other constitutional diseases as a malignant complication or as a terminal disease.

Symptoms and Course. True, or the so-called exanthematic erysipelas really only breaks out in the face, whereas erysipelas on other parts of the body is, properly speaking, erythema. The appearance of the exanthem upon the skin is generally preceded for a few hours or even days by a preliminary stage consisting of a severe fever with marked gastric symptoms, with which symptoms of cerebral hyperæmia, and more especially a violent headache, sometimes become associated at an early period. During a first attack these precursory symptoms are scarcely ever absent; but they do not usually occur with a return of the disease. While the fever is on the increase, the face feels hot and tense, and sometimes rheumatic pains in the nape of the neck are complained of, a vivid redness breaks out at a certain circumscribed spot in the face, which spreads rapidly and causes a burning pain. In proportion as the redness becomes more intense, the swelling likewise increases and the skin assumes a glistening appearance. Erysipelas generally breaks out on one cheek, whence it spreads to the nose, the eyelids, forehead, ears, less frequently to the lips, and scarcely ever to the chin. Within two or three days, and sometimes in thirty-six hours the erysipelas reaches its acme at the spot where it first appeared, amid febrile symptoms which are sometimes exceedingly severe, attended with a foul-smelling catarrh of the mouth, vomiting, and most generally delirium; these symptoms, however, are not constant, whereas the headache and soporous stupefaction are exceedingly annoying. The face is now very much swollen, the features are disfigured to such an extent that they are no longer recognizable, the redness has a bluish and even brown-red tint, and vesicles of various sizes sometimes spring up upon the inflamed surface, which always indicate an intense degree of illness. The inflammation decreases very rapidly; the redness disappears after the existing vesicles had dried up previously and had become transformed into thin and flat crusts, and very soon desquamation commences first in large patches and afterwards in very small scales. But inasmuch as the disease never terminates with its first appearance, and usually spreads over the whole head, we find erysipelas in full bloom close to the original spot in process of healing, and find the redness gradually diffusing itself into this spot, whereas it forms a sharp contrast with the surrounding normal parts of the face. In this manner erysipelas gradually wanders over the whole face, even beyond the ears, invading a portion of the nape of the neck, and spreading over the forehead and the hairy scalp. In this latter case the patients suffer severe local pains, even after the fever abates. The intensity of the fever, as it first breaks out at the commencement of the disease, does not keep pace with its gradual progression. Whereas at one spot the inflammation runs its full course in five to six days, yet, on account of its progressive appearance in different localities, the whole course of the disease lasts from ten days to a fortnight. The process of desquamation may last much longer, and the most severely affected parts often exhibit for a long time a yellowish tint with signs of serous infiltration.

Deviations from this course are not unfrequent. The whole face may be covered so rapidly that it would seem as though the exanthem had broke out all over at once. These are cases of intense virulence, where one ear, however, commonly remains uninvaded. Moreover, the inflammation may communicate itself to the cerebral meningæ; generally, however, this does not take place until the local process has reached its height. In such a case the redness very soon assumes a dingy and livid look; the skin becomes lax and wrinkled, a most violent delirium sets in, and coma and death speedily supervene. This course has been mistaken for a metastasis of erysipelas; whereas in such a case the same changes take place as in other similar cases, namely that, with the appearance of a violent disorder, the previously-existing lesser disease abates and disappears. Erysipelas seldom becomes associated with diseases of other important organs. Attacks of erysipelas succeeding the first attack are very apt to show deviations from the normal course. These attacks are very seldom preceded by precursory symptoms, the less so the more frequently the attacks have occurred. Nor is the fever as severe, the swelling is less, and the spread of the disease over the face takes place more slowly. It not unfrequently happens that in subsequent attacks the patients are not obliged to lie down and that their appetite remains the same as in their normal condition. Subsequent attacks are more like erythema than erysipelas. The frequency of the attacks differs greatly in different individuals; sometimes there are several attacks in a few weeks and, after a short time, cease entirely; or months and even years intervene between the attacks; in such cases a spontaneous cessation is much less frequent.

Among the consequences of true erysipelas the following deserve particular mention: Swelling of the skin, especially that of the lids, nose and lips; the swelling is mostly œdematous, the epidermis having a pale look and being disposed to the formation of comedones; if the attacks are very frequent, the swelling may reach a considerable degree of thickness, and is very obstinate. Loss of the hair, which almost always falls out if the scalp had been intensely affected by the disease; in most cases the hair grows again, but there are exceptions to this rule.—Subcutaneous abscesses in the lids, lips, ears.—Severe catarrh of the external meatus, with obstinate hardness of hearing.—Catarrh of the conjunctiva, which is generally very obstinate.—Disposition to neuralgia of the trigeminus.

Wandering erysipelas, or erysipelas ambulans or erraticum, attacks the face less frequently than the extremities. On one of the extremities an erysipelatous spot appears which heals exactly like the above-described spots, only there is very little tension and pain, and the general organism is not so much involved. From this spot the erysipelas spreads towards the trunk; the spot which is attacked next, being either in close contact with the first, or else all subsequent spots being more or less remote from each other.

Symptomatic erysipelas, as an accompaniment of inflammatory processes, is of no great importance, except when it covers a large extent of surface and depends upon septic causes. Generally it disappears of itself as soon as the cause that occasions it, is removed. If it is very intense, it may result in suppuration or gangrenous destruction of the skin. If the erysipelas sets in in the course of serious, constitutional febrile diseases, it is always a bad omen. In such cases the redness is never very vivid, rather dingy, having a bluish tint; the swelling is not excessive and yet the disposition to form blisters is very great; these blisters do not always dry up, but often become transformed into badly-looking ulcers which are apt to become gangrenous. The fever accompanying this form of erysipelas, always increases to a high degree, but speedily assumes the character of an adynamic fever, the pulse becomes very small and frequent, the temperature increases considerably, the cerebral phenomena become very marked, and sopor and coma set in at an early period, and death sometimes takes place so rapidly that life becomes extinct already on the third day after the appearance of the inflammation.

Erysipelas neonatorum generally sets in in the first week after the birth of the infant, very seldom after the first month. It almost always proceeds from the umbilicus, on which account it has been traced with great probability to the consequences of an improper management of this organ, more especially to a purulent inflammation of this organ which can easily be accounted for by bad management.—As a rule the erysipelas spreads from the umbilicus over the abdomen, the sexual organs, thighs, less frequently over the thorax and back. The redness is not very vivid, the swelling, on the contrary, is very considerable. The children are exceedingly restless, feverish, and incline greatly to spasmodic affections and sopor. The dermatitis is very apt to become associated with peritonitis. Death is the most common termination.

Treatment. In speaking of the efficacy of a medicine for erysipelas, it is in the first place important to inquire whether the course of the erysipelatous inflammation is shortened by the medicine. It is well known that erysipelas of the face, if the whole face is covered with it, never disappears, spontaneously under nine days, and that the course is limited to five or six days if only one side of the face is invaded; this last-mentioned circumstance has often led to the supposition that a case had been cured by medicines, whereas the cure was altogether spontaneous. In a first attack of primary erysipelas it is very seldom the case for only one side of the face to be affected. At all events, we should be very guarded in claiming curative virtues for some of our remedies for erysipelas, and should only believe after repeated and successful trials in the treatment of analogous cases that they were cured by means of drugs.

Simple, smooth erysipelas of the face, as long as fever is present, is best combated by *Belladonna*, and, under this treatment, generally runs its course in six days. Nevertheless, although *Belladonna* responds completely to the symptoms of violent cerebral hyperæmia, yet it is not suitable for the meningitis which may supervene during the course of erysipelas. Here *Rhus tox.* is preferable. This remedy is generally more particularly adapted to the higher grades of the disease, more especially if copious vesicles spring up upon the inflamed skin, if the fever, although intense, yet assumes an adynamic type, if the tongue becomes dry and the nervous excitement is superseded by a soporous stupefaction. Even the color of the affected part affords a decisive hint for the selection of one or the other drug; *Belladonna* is indicated by a bright-red, and *Rhus tox.* by a bluish or yellowish-red tint.—If we may credit recent reports concerning *Apis mellifica*, this remedy is preferable to either *Belladonna* or *Rhus tox*. *Apis* is said to be a specific remedy not only for smooth, but likewise for vesicular erysipelas, and to be suitable even if the brain is affected. We have not yet had an opportunity of verifying the pretended virtues of this drug in our own practice. A special indication for Apis is an inflammation of the mouth and fauces accompanying erysipelas. Although these remedies are sufficient in all ordinary cases, yet other remedies may be required to meet exceptional deviations from the normal type. For the excessive cerebral phenomena, while the exanthem is still out and hence no meningitis had yet set in, *Ammonium carbonicum* and *Camphora* are important remedies; *Opium* likewise is often an important intercurrent remedy, when the patient is lying in a state of sopor. True erysipelas, especially erysipelas of the face, very seldom terminates in gangrenous destruction; if this should be the case, *Arsenicum album*, *Carbo vegetabilis* and *Secale cornutum* would have to be administered. An incipient suppuration cannot be cut short by *Mercurius;* it is much better to at once give *Hepar sulphuris* and thus to promote the suppurative process. For the erysipelas of old people *Lachesis* is said to be superior to either *Belladonna* or *Rhus tox.* Here too we would advise to keep an eye on *Ammonium carbonicum*, [also on *Arsenicum*. H.]

For erysipelatous attacks without fever, we have never found either *Belladonna* or *Rhus tox.* suitable; they are not homœopathic to this condition. On the other hand we cannot recommend *Lycopodium* with sufficient emphasis, and if the local process is strikingly marked, *Hepar sulphuris*, were it for no other reason than because both these remedies prevent the frequent return of the disease. In such cases *Borax* may be a reliable remedy which Bœnninghausen recommends for erysipelas on the left side of the face; for it is only in this non-febrile form of erysipelas that the inflammation is generally confined to one side.

The sequelæ generally deserve particular attention, for the reason that they are mostly very obstinate and because it is in them that the disposition to relapses is generally founded. Some redness and a doughy, not œdematous swelling generally are some of the most common sequelæ of erysipelas; the swelling is apt to be increased by extreme cold or heat, in which case a stinging and tensive pain is experienced in it. As long as this swelling lasts, the use of remedies must not be discontinued. The remedies which will effect the removal of this swelling, are *Graphites*, *Sulphur*, *Aurum*, and if the swelling is frequently painful, *Lycopodium* and *Hepar sulphuris*. These remedies are the only ones capable of counteracting the extensive œdema of the face which sometimes baffles all treatment for years, or yields only very slowly.—Swellings of lymphatic glands do not often remain; if they do, *Baryta* is most efficient in removing them. After erysipelas of the hairy scalp, the hair is apt to fall out; in the case of older individuals, this kind of baldness can scarcely ever be arrested, much less cured; in younger persons, on the contrary, the hair grows again without anything being done for it. For chronic conjunctivitis after erysipelas, we advise principally *Graphites*, and likewise *Arsenicum*. A subsequent deafness or hardness of hearing is very difficult to cure, it generally remains unchanged. *Sulphur* and *Baryta* may be tried for it.

If the erysipelas is not seated in the face, some other remedies may have to be resorted to, more particularly if the erysipelas breaks out on the lower extremities. *Nux vom.* is recommended as a specific remedy in such cases; we prefer, however, *Staphysagria* and *Graphites*, and if there is a great deal of pain, *Mercurius*. [*Arsenicum* may likewise be very efficient. H.] If erysipelas develops itself as a consequence of debility, or attacks old people, so that a gangrenous destruction of the skin has to be apprehended, *Secale cornutum* may render efficient service.

Symptomatic erysipelas, if caused by external irritants or by a suppurating injury or sore, does not require any special treatment; the use of such remedies as are recommended for it, is very problematical. If it arises from general causes as a terminal affection of a most threatening character, we have of course every reason to hunt up efficient remedies. *Rhus tox.* and *Apis* will be very often found indicated in such cases; likewise *Phosphorus*, *Carbo vegetabilis* and *Arsenicum*. The selection, of course, will be governed by the character of the disease in whose soil the erysipelatous inflammation has taken root.

In a practical point of view, it is best to regard erysipelas neonatorum as a form of phlebitis and to treat it with the remedies that have been recommended for phlebitis. Hence we are in doubt whether *Belladonna* will ever be capable, as Hartmann thinks, of arresting the mischief; in the place of Belladonna we should at once give *Mercurius* or *Hepar sulphuris*, and, if icterus has supervened, *Phosphorus* or *Bryonia*.

Wandering erysipelas is generally a very obstinate disease, for which it is very difficult to select remedies from the Materia Medica. *Graphites* has furnished practical evidence of its curative powers in this disease, whereas *Pulsatilla*, *Lycopodium* and *Cocculus* are unreliable.

As regards other points in the treatment of erysipelas, we desire to deprecate the common practice of resorting to an excess of warm covering which can at most only increase the intensity of the inflammatory process going on on the skin, as well as the disposition to relapses by superinducing an extreme sensitiveness of the skin. There is neither use nor reason in covering the inflamed skin with cotton wadding, nor is there any reason why the patients should not remain in a uniform temperature, without any extra amount of covering.

[It is well known to every physician and nurse that the distressing itching and burning of the inflamed skin is very much relieved by sprinkling a thin layer of fine flour or pulverized starch upon it. In erysipelas of the extremities I have likewise resorted to a weak watery solution of the *Sulphite of Soda* as an external application. The effect has been to blanch the skin, alleviate the itching and burning, and, in conjunction with proper internal treatment, to shorten and moderate the course of the disease.

Traumatic erysipelas of the face, in the case of habitual drunkards, is very apt to involve serious consequences, especially under allopathic treatment. If the inflammation invades the meningæ, which it is inclined to do, death under this treatment is all but certain.

Some years ago, a case of traumatic erysipelas occurred in our city, which speedily terminated fatally under Old School treatment. The patient, a very stout man, had been on a bender for a day and a night, and was very much under the influence of liquor. A fall on his face lacerated the skin near the left temple. Erysipelas set in, and he died in two days.

Inasmuch as I may not have another opportunity in the course of this work, of offering the present remark, I desire to avail myself of the present chance. Delirium tremens is the ultimate result of alcoholic poisoning. Can such a condition be removed in every case with such small doses as we are in the habit of using in our practice? This is questionable. In my opinion there are cases where we cannot do our patient justice without treating him with large doses of the proper antidote. We remember a case of delirium tremens where the patient complained of vermin crawling over his bed and hands. *Arsenicum* 30 cured him entirely. In other similar cases this treatment utterly failed. A stout young man had drank thirty-nine glasses of whisky on a wager in one night. We found him cold and the skin dry and husky like parchment. He felt numb all over. Pulse scarcely perceptible. He was in great agony of mind and expected to be utterly paralyzed. He was unable to sustain his own weight. I gave him six globules of *Nux vomica* 30, in half a cup of water, a dessertspoonful every five minutes. The patient sank visibly under this treatment. Being satisfied that Nux was his remedy, I now mixed five drops of the strong tincture in six tablespoonfuls of water, of which mixture I gave him a dessertspoonful every five minutes. After the second dose he began to perspire. The perspiration seemed to be pure alcohol; he was literally drenched with alcohol. He had to be changed seven times during the night; next morning he felt quite well, except a little weak. I have treated a number of cases of delirium tremens with variable doses. Upon the whole, small doses have not proved very effectual in my hands. Doctor Reed, Jr., of this city, has treated a number of cases; proceeding upon the principle of curing the patient as speedily and effectually as possible, he treated his patients irrespective of dose. A few of his cases will show that delirium-tremens patients sometimes bear unusually large quantities of medicines. To illustrate this fact I will take this opportunity of relating a few of the cases which he has related to me from his note-book.

G. L., forty years of age, a butcher and confirmed drunkard, precipitated an impending attack of delirium by falling and breaking three ribs; he suffered but little from pain or prostration. The tremor was severe, but the case was remarkable in the character of the delirium, and as showing the immense quantity of Opium necessary to overcome the obstinate wakefulness.

For two days the delirium was evidenced by the most delightful visions, he saw angels hovering over his bed, and held delightful interviews with the saints. Not being properly watched, he at night escaped from the house, and after the lapse of some hours returned to relate how he had been upon another Mount of Beatitude, having held sweet converse upon a neighboring sand-hill with our Saviour and the Blessed Virgin, returning after the holy interview much edified, to demand more whiskey. His hallucinations were all of this religious character, and this before the Opium had been given.

Within twenty-four hours there was given him in divided doses at least three ounces of Laudanum, he being carefully watched for the result, and it was only after the last half-ounce dose of the quantity stated, that he showed any effect from the drug. This effect, however, was a good and in all respects natural sleep, lasting thirty-six hours and followed by an entire relief from all the symptoms of his disease.

C. C., laboring under his fourth attack of delirium tremens, under the care of a Doctor who had treated him in the old-fashioned way, with Opium and Digitalis, had passed seven nights without sleep.

On visiting the patient on the morning of the eighth day, I found him quietly brushing the vermin from his clothing, and occasionally ordering the nurses to clear the room from the strange animals which were in every corner, and under every chair. His pulse was fair, tongue but lightly coated, skin moist and warm, appetite good, face somewhat flushed. The attack, and all former attacks had commenced with severe vertigo. His eyes were injected, bowels loose, owing to purgatives. I ordered rest from all medicines, strong soup, and oysters with an abundance of Cayenne pepper through the day; at 8 o'clock at night I administered one drachm of the Bromide of Potassium to be followed, if necessary, every hour by one half the quantity. The dose had to be repeated but once, a quiet sleep being obtained for twelve hours.

Five months subsequently C. C. again suffered for the fifth time, and for three days I used every endeavor to obtain sleep. The Bromide which had before acted so effectually, failing entirely. On the fourth night, however, sleep was obtained after the use of large doses of Opium and Tartar emetic; recovery followed immediately.

An habitual drunkard of great capacity, having already suffered from many attacks of delirium tremens, after, according to his own and his friends' accounts, abstaining from food for some weeks(?), subsisting entirely upon liquors of which he took a great variety and an incredible quantity, was attacked with a very severe form of delirium tremens. The prostration was extreme, the tremor excessive, but the delirium bland, the chief hallucination being that the ceiling was about to fall and crush him, rendering it necessary for him to jump from the bed and hop around the room with as great activity as his weak condition would allow. His tongue was heavily coated, pulse small and irregular, skin moist, the forehead being constantly bedewed with a cold, clammy sweat. His voice was feeble, husky and tremulous, he had had no sleep for three nights. The treatment was directed principally to sustaining his strength, but all efforts to obtain sleep were for fifty-two hours unavailing. At the end of this time two boluses containing each one scruple of Cayenne pepper, were given, and within two hours the patient was quietly sleeping, the skin, feet and hands for the first time being warm. After fourteen hours of quiet sleep, he awoke with a desire for something to eat, and from this made a fair recovery. During the treatment Digitalis acted very satisfactorily in ten-drop doses of the tincture in strengthening the heart's action.

A tailor of intemperate habits, aged about forty, after a protracted debauch became delirious, imagining that he was pursued by demons. I was first called owing to his having jumped from a third story window. His fall having been broken by a shed, he sustained no severe injuries.

He complained of seeing horrible phantasms, struggling with his attendants that he might escape from them. However, he answered intelligibly to inquiries, complaining of pain in the head and stomach; his tongue was heavily coated, face pale, pulse small and quick, skin dry but cool, had eaten nothing for some days, and had had no sleep for two nights. I prescribed the tincture of Nux vomica, three drops every half hour. Upon calling within three hours, I found the patient sweating profusely, relieved from pain in the head, and from the phantom which had been troubling him. Under the use of supporting measures his recovery was rapid and uninterrupted. H.]

3. Roseola, Rubeolæ.

This exanthem is characterized by spots of the size of lentils and of a bright-red color, more or less scattered and rarely appearing in groups; they are not attended with fever, or else the fever is very slight, and does not result in any perceptible desquamation.

Roseola sometimes accompanies severe catarrh, in which case the exanthem lasts at most twenty-four hours; if it is preceded by a slight catarrhal stage, the exanthem disappears at the latest on the third day. In this last shape roseola sometimes appears epidemically, but not over a large extent of country, in which case the eruption looks very much like a mild form of scarlatina to which it is related like a sort of transition-link. In the same house we have seen two children laid up with the mildest form of roseola; another child, on the contrary, was attacked so violently that it seemed perfectly justifiable to diagnose scarlatina, so much more as distinct desquamation took place, and a slight degree of œdema was noticed over the whole body. Roseola never involves any danger.

The disorder may originate in catarrh or in a marked change of temperature, as a rule it is owing to such atmospheric conditions as favor epidemic diseases. A species of roseola which is apt to supervene during the course of dangerous constitutional diseases, more particularly of typhus, does not belong in this category

Owing to the trifling character of this disease, the employment of medicines is generally unnecessary; if catarrhal angina is complained of, a few doses of *Belladonna* may be administered. The fever is scarcely ever sufficiently severe or generally of a character to require *Aconite*. [A few doses of Aconite are very serviceable in this eruption, even if the fever is ever so slight. H.] If this exanthem is confounded with a mild attack of scarlatina, the poor patients suffer from such a mistake in consequence of being kept in the room for an unnecessary length of time; we shall dwell upon such a proceeding more fully when treating of scarlatina.

4. Urticaria.

Nettle-rash, Hives.

Blotches or wheals may be caused by the direct action of irritants upon the skin, such as extreme heat alternating with cold (ladies at a ball often expose themselves to such influences), mosquito-bites, flea-bites, bed-bug bites, bee-stings, the stings of gad-flies, contact with nettles and other plants; or else by the action of irritating substances which, after being introduced into the stomach, react upon the skin. This, however, is not generally the case, but the result of peculiar idiosyncrasies, as from strawberries, raspberries, crabs, oysters, etc. Urticaria proper is for the most part depending upon individual predispositions which it is impossible to account for with any certainty; a very common exciting cause is gastric catarrh from indigestion, and likewise catarrh of the female sexual organs, chronic as well as acute. In acute constitutional diseases blotches sometimes break out, but they are not of any special significance.

Urticaria very commonly commences with febrile symptoms sometimes of a considerable degree of intensity, and which may continue during the whole course of the eruption. It is a question, however, whether the urticaria does not result from the fever instead of the fever from the urticaria. Generally the digestion is very much affected, symptoms of cerebral hyperæmia are less commonly present. The appearance of the exanthem is generally immediately preceded by great restlessness and an oppressive anxiety. In other cases the eruption comes out suddenly after a short feeling of indisposition, without any fever. Amid a burning and violent itching of the skin a diffuse redness or rather large red spots, without sharp outlines, make their appearance, upon which soon after risings or elevations start up, of a white or red color, but more generally with white tops. Their size varies from a quarter of an inch to one inch in length and breadth; most commonly they are isolated, less frequently they appear in clusters on the same spot. The warmth of the bed seems to promote their appearance. A single wheal does not remain out very long; it disappears even in a few hours, without leaving a trace, but other wheals may break out in other places, by which means the whole process may be very much protracted. The localities where the exanthem most commonly breaks out, are the extremities, and the anterior surface of the trunk, less frequently the face. The urticaria from gastric causes likewise originates in this manner, except that it scarcely ever lasts longer than twelve hours; on the other hand, its first appearance is often attended with an intense fever, anxiety and restlessness. Even the urticaria caused by the stings or bites of insects, is often attended with fever.

A first attack generally superinduces an increased disposition to the disease; this disposition increases in proportion to the frequency of the attacks, and may continue for years under the designation of chronic nettle-rash. In such circumstances the fever is less with every new attack, whereas, on the other hand, the most trifling error in diet, the least cold may excite a new crop of wheals. In the case of women the eruption often seems to have some connection with the menses. In chronic urticaria the wheals are always scattered, and the surrounding redness is trifling or entirely wanting; the wheals generally look red. This chronic urticaria is a very obstinate disorder, but often remains uncured for the reason that the constitutional anomaly in which it originates, is not regarded.

A single attack, if not very violent, does not require any treatment; medicines may have to be resorted to on account of the constitutional symptoms, not for the exanthem. For decided symptoms of indigestion, *Pulsatilla* may be given; for a severe gastric catarrh, *Antimonium crudum*. If the fever is intense, *Rhus toxicodendron* is a chief remedy; the severe rheumatic pains, which sometimes accompany the eruption, require *Bryonia*, the acompanying diarrhœa, *Dulcamara*. If the affection becomes obstinate, and new wheals continue to break out, or if a first attack is soon followed by a second or third, the speediest possible interference with suitable remedial agents is eminently proper. The selection will have to be chiefly determined by the constitutional symptoms. If no such symptoms are present, and if every attack is occasioned by the most trifling changes of temperature, without fever or any other derangement, *Urtica urens* is a very excellent remedy. This remedy is likewise appropriate in cases of urticaria complicated with renal and urinary difficulties. In the case of children, *Calcarea carbonica* is suitable for urticaria without any constitutional symptoms. Of the *Balsamum copaivæ*, which is recommended by many physicians, we have no special indications, and should, therefore, not use it until Urtica urens had been tried in vain. If the urticaria breaks out with the menses, *Pulsatilla* may be given if the menses are scanty, *Belladonna* if they are profuse. If a chronic uterine catarrh is the cause of the eruption, *Apis* is an excellent remedy, which may be associated with *Lycopodium*. It is not necessary to mention more remedies for such a trifling affection, the different combinations of which it is, after all, inexpedient to point out. [We have almost always succeeded in controlling our cases of urticaria with *Aconite* and *Ipecacuanha*. H.]

In habitual urticaria the diet plays an important part. In the first place, if the skin is excessively irritable, we have to aim at hardening it; this object is more easily reached by vapor-baths than by cold bathing and cold ablutions. In the next place the diet itself has to consist of simple articles; fat, spirits, acrid and stim-

5. Miliaria.
Rash.

Miliaria is mostly a secondary, symptomatic affection; as a primary and more particularly as an epidemic disease it is a rare occurrence among us. Symptomatic miliaria may break out during the course of all kinds of severe acute diseases.

Primary, epidemic miliaria runs its course after the fashion of all other acute exanthemata. The eruption is preceded for one to three days by febrile symptoms characterized by the presence of rheumatoid pains in the limbs, frequently shifting from one locality to another; excessive perspiration, great anxiety and oppression, and finally by peculiar prickling, burning pains in the skin. Afterwards small vesicles break out, first on the neck and subsequently on most other parts of the body; they are of the size of millet-seeds or lentils, are seated upon a red base, and at times are filled with a clear, at other times with a dim fluid.—*Miliaria rubra* and *alba.*—These vesicles generally spread in clusters.—The violent symptoms of constitutional disturbance disappear with the breaking out of the vesicles which separate in bran-shaped scales within five to seven days. Inasmuch as the same period of time is required for every new crop, the duration of the disorder may be protracted to a fortnight and longer. The usual termination is recovery, except in epidemic miliaria where the disease sometimes assumes a malignant type and frequently results fatally.

Symptomatic miliaria is regarded by some as a symptom of the highest import, whereas others view it as resulting from the action of certain external influences, and not deserving any special attention. We are decidedly inclined to share this opinion. Symptomatic miliaria generally attacks individuals who perspire a great deal from excessive covering, as in the case of lying-in women, rheumatic patients, likewise in cases of measles and scarlatina if mismanaged in the old fashion, and in other febrile or even non-febrile affections. Except in acute rheumatism, we shall always find that miliaria is caused by excessive external heat. This circumstance will easily account for the symptoms preceding the eruption, such as restlessness, anxiety, dyspnœa, even delirium; the bad management still rendered worse by the anxiety caused by the appearance of the exanthem, explains why miliaria may give the disease a bad turn. That our explanation is founded, is evident from the fact that miliaria is scarcely ever seen in hospitals, but is a very common occurrence in private practice, and that it never breaks out on patients who are constantly kept in a mean temperature under a moderate amount of covering.

In view of the frequently dangerous character of primary miliaria, medical treatment in all such cases is indispensable; the rare occurrence of the disease has not yet, however, afforded sufficient opportunities of positively determining the remedies that are in specific curative adaptation to it. The most suitable remedy which corresponds with the whole course of this pathological process, is *Aconitum*, more particularly if the eruption is not so much accompanied by anxiety as by great nervous excitement. If there is much anxiety and restlessness and a burning feverish heat, *Arsenicum* is the remedy; if the patient is lying in a listless condition, with typhoid symptoms, *Bryonia* is best suitable. *Mercurius* may likewise deserve attention in this disease, and if the patient perspires to excess, *Sambucus*.

Regarding the propriety of instituting a treatment for symptomatic miliaria, it is our opinion that it is unnecessary and that all efforts to prevent the appearance of miliaria by medicinal agents, are of very doubtful utility. Moreover, the selection of a remedy in all acute diseases depends rather upon the more important symptoms of the disease than upon the appearance of the vesicles. Nevertheless, in order not to slight the views of our Colleagues, we mention the remedies recommended by Hartmann for this exanthem: *Ipecacuanha* (for the precursory symptoms in diseases where the miliaria may be expected to break out); *Bryonia* (under similar circumstances); *Arsenicum* (for restlessness and anxiety); *Aconitum* (for violent rush of blood); *Belladonna* (for accompanying congestive symptoms of the brain); *Coffea, Chamomilla, Valeriana.*— Hartmann further remarks: "Chronic miliary eruptions which partially disappear in one spot in order to reappear sowewhere else, and cause a good deal of itching and burning, are most safely and reliably removed by such antipsoric remedies as *Mezereum, Clematis, Sarsaparilla, Staphysagria, Arsenicum, Ammonium carb., Sulphur,* and *Carbo vegetabilis.*"

6. Pityriasis.
Dandruff, Dandriff

This exanthem consists in an exfoliation of the skin either in thin scales, or in larger patches: it may be unaccompanied by any other cutaneous symptoms and the exfoliating skin may to all appearances be perfectly sound; or else, the process may be accompanied by trifling local or more extensive symptoms of hyperæmia of the cutis. According as the skin is unchanged or looks red under the scales, the affection is designated as pityriasis simplex or rubra.

The causes of this affection are very obscure; in some cases the disease can be traced with some certainty to a derangement of the functions of the liver and of the female sexual organs.

Pityriasis rubra, when spread over more extensive portions of the skin, not unfrequently sets in with slight febrile motions which may break out at every renewed appearance of the exanthem. On portions of the skin, which itch and burn very fiercely, large red spots of indefinite and irregular shapes make their appearance. Accompanied by a peculiar feeling of tension, the cuticle on these spots very soon begins to exfoliate. The eruption first manifests itself on the trunk, and only invades the face if exceedingly severe. The almost inevitable itching may cause a moisture to ooze from the otherwise dry spots on the skin. This itching which is absolutely agonizing, very commonly interferes with sleep. The affection is very obstinate, but at the same time one of the rarer forms of cutaneous diseases.

Pityriasis, confined to isolated spots, is much less frequently of the character *rubra* than a general pityriasis; it is most commonly met with on the hairy scalp, in the palms of the hands, on the soles of the feet, and in the face. The itching is much less distressing, but is still very violent on the hairy scalp. By scratching the skin until it tears, a moisture is secreted from the irritated spot, resulting in the formation of superficial scurfs and crusts and agglutination of the hairs.

In treating a case of general pityriasis, we must not forget that we are dealing with a very chronic affection which never promises rapid success, and where it would be consequently improper either to make a frequent change of medicines, or to repeat the dose too often. The most important remedies are *Graphites* and *Arsenicum*, with which it is most likely that a cure can be best effected. The good effects of *Lycopodium* are questionable, and *Sulphur*, in spite of its symptomatic similarity, scarcely ever acts with sufficient persistence.

In partial pityriasis we never depend upon Arsenicum, whereas in pityriasis capitis *Graphites* renders excellent service. Beside these remedies we may compare the following: *Sepia, Thuya, Calcarea carb., Ledum pallustre*, also *Phosphorus*. *Sepia* is particularly indicated in the case of females, if the spots break out in consequence of menstrual irregularities, or at definite periods of the year.

7. Psoriasis.
Scaly Tetter.

This is pre-eminently an affection of the male sex; in the case of females it is never attended with sexual disorders. It attacks individuals between the seventh and fiftieth year, and occurs most frequently in the cold season. It cannot be traced to constitutional derangements, since persons who are afflicted with this disease, otherwise enjoy the most perfect health. With the appearance of some constitutional disease, the psoriasis disappears at once, but returns again as soon as the disease is removed.

Psoriasis begins in this wise: at various, more or less numerous, scattered spots, the detached epidermis forms a small, white rising—psoriasis punctata. These spots gradually spread from every point of the periphery until they reach the size of drops—psoriasis guttata; on removing the scales, we find the skin underneath slightly red and bleeding. In proportion as the circumference continues to expand, the original spot becomes cleansed of its scales, and a ring forms surrounding a healthy-looking skin—psoriasis annularis; in the further progress of the exanthem, this ring opens, losing its roundness—psoriasis gyrata—and finally disappearing altogether. All these stages, or most of them, coexist side by side in almost every case of this disease. Psoriasis is not attended with itching, or at most only at the commencement, but in no case if it has become an inveterate disease. It may remain stationary, though breaking out in new places, or it may intermit in its manifestations for months and even years.

Treatment. In selecting our remedies, we must not overlook the fact that psoriasis is not an itching eruption. This seems to have been ignored by many practitioners; Hartmann's delineation of the disease is especially untrue to Nature. The selection of remedies is rendered particularly difficult by the circumstance that the patient enjoys perfect health, and that on this account we are without any co-determining symptoms. It is wrong and unscientific to try to get symptoms out of a patient by persistent questioning and to hunt them up even among his ancestors in order to realize our dreams about reliable remedies. For this reason we content ourselves with giving merely the names of the remedies that have already been employed in this disease with some advantage, or that may seem adapted to further trials. We arrange the series in accordance with the practical value of each drug: *Sulphur, Phosphorus, Sepia, Petroleum, Calcarea carbonica, Acidum nitricum* and *phosphoricum, Arsenicum* and *Tellurium.*

Among external remedies the only application which is never hurtful and usually efficient, is the vapor-bath accompanied by frictions with castile soap, or, if the affection has already existed for a long time, with brown soap. Cold bathing is of decided use, although its effect may not be perceived immediately.

8. Ichthyosis.
Fish-skin, Porcupine Disease.

According to Hebra, ichthyosis is an hereditary or, at any rate, congenital disease, never acquired; where acquired ichthyosis is spoken of, the eruption has been mistaken for psoriasis or some other cutaneous disorder. It occurs most frequently among males, so that even in its hereditary descent the disease is confined to the male branch of the family, leaving the female branch intact.

Ichthyosis is characterized by an hypertrophied condition of the papillæ of the skin, with excessive development of the epidermis; the function of the sebaceous follicles seems to be entirely extinct. This disease does not show itself plainly until after the first year of infancy unless the children are frequently and carefully washed. Until then the patients only show a remarkably harsh and tough, dry skin which often has a deep-yellowish tinge. The scales never form in the face, nor on the flexor-surface of the joints or on the scrotum; they form most copiously on the extensor surface of the arms, thighs and legs, and on the knee. In this affection the skin is not infiltrated; where the scales are seated, the skin has a natural color. In the lesser grades of the disease the scales are thinly scattered over the skin; in the higher grades they form a thick, horny covering exhibiting cracks and furrows in all directions and, on account of the dirt which adheres to them, having a dingy-brown color. Scales that fall off, or are picked off with the fingers, are constantly replaced by new ones.

The disease is considered incurable; it does not endanger life.

Treatment. We are not acquainted with a single case of cure of this disease by means of homœopathic remedies; nor have we ever had an opportunity, in our own practice, of trying the effect of homœopathic treatment. In our part of the country the disease is of very rare occurrence. If we had a case to treat, we should in the first place depend upon *Silicea, Sulphur, Calcarea carbonica* and *Lycopodium;* and in the next place upon *Arsenicum, Aurum* and *Petroleum.* Knowing that cleanliness and attention to the skin generally can keep the disease at a very low stage of development, we urgently recommend the daily use of warm baths and frictions with castile soap, likewise vapor-baths. If we desire a speedy removal of the scales, we have to rub the affected portions of the skin with oil a few hours before bathing.

9. Lichen, Strophulus.
Tooth-rash.

This exanthem appears in three distinct forms, as strophulus, lichen simplex and agrius.

Strophulus is in reality nothing else than lichen simplex in the first period of dentition. It is caused by a continued irritation of the skin, or is a consequence of bad nutrition, catarrhal irritation of the intestinal canal, or else it seems to be exclusively occasioned by the process of dentition. Beside the derangements which such causes necessarily occasion, the appearance of this eruption seems very seldom preceded by fever and restlessness. On one or more places, sometimes only in the face, and at times over the whole body, scattered papulæ or pimples break out which either have a reddish or else a natural color like the rest of the skin. If the children are sufficiently advanced in age, they show by their manner that the papulæ itch, especially in the bed. A single papule heals in three to four days, but successive crops of papulæ are apt to occur, protracting the whole process for weeks.

Lichen simplex arises from similar causes as strophulus; it may likewise be occasioned by a high degree of temperature and occurs in every age. Its appearance is very seldom preceded by distinct fever. The papulæ come out unperceived, mostly in the face, have the same color as the skin or look a little redder; they generally form clusters and itch pretty severely; the destruction of their tops by scratching gives rise to very small scurfs. Single papulæ disappear within ten to twelve days; this form of lichen may likewise be protracted by successive crops for months, so that the originally acute disorder may assume a very obstinate, chronic form.

Lichen agrius often represents a higher degree of the former, but it may likewise break out as a primary disease. Its appearance is always preceded by febrile symptoms which sometimes do not entirely and speedily disappear even after the eruption is fairly out. The pimples are surrounded by a red halo and cause a burning pain. The unavoidable scratching not only increases the cutaneous hyperæmia, but likewise changes the eruption to that of eczema. The pimples sometimes, though seldom, scale off already in ten days to a fortnight, and without leaving any alterations. New crops of pimples generally break out in rapid succession, in consequence of which the skin becomes infiltrated to such a degree that even long after the disappearance of the pimples the skin remains hard and callous, and even chappy. Lichen agrius constitutes one of the more obstinate exanthems; if the whole body is covered with it, the eruption may even involve danger to life. In such a case the patient emaciates very rapidly and a general cachexia is the consequence.

Treatment. Strophulus, if unaccompanied by other derangements, does not require any special treatment; the most that is required is that every attention should be paid to cleanliness and to the clothing of the children. If it sets in as a consequence of other morbid conditions, the medicines administered for the latter will likewise remove the strophulus.

Nor is lichen simplex, when it first breaks out, of sufficient consequence to require medical treatment. If it is spread over a considerable portion of the skin, and the itching is intolerable, *Staphysagria* or *Mercurius* may be given. If it increases to lichen agrius, or becomes chronic, the medicines indicated for this form of lichen will have to be used. [*Aconite* is an admirable remedy to control the hyperæmia of the skin and to afford material aid in removing this distressing eruption. H.]

In a case of lichen agrius *Mercurius* is most appropriate to the paroxysms of acute exacerbation [also *Aconite*, H.], and next to it *Rhus toxicod.* and *Staphysagria*. *Cocculus* is likewise recommended. To eradicate the disease, other remedies are required, such as: *Graphites*, *Lycopodium*, *Arsenicum*, *Sulphur*, also *Nitri acidum* or *Conium;* the selection of a particular drug depends a good deal upon its homœopathicity to the accompanying constitutional symptoms. External applications, even baths when indulged in too freely, most generally prove injurious.

10. Prurigo.

According to Hebra, genuine prurigo is only met with among the lower classes; it never shows itself previous to the second period of dentition, and gradually disappears again after the fiftieth year. Sex does not exert any modifying influence over the disease. Bad nourishment and want of attention to cleanliness and the condition of the skin generally, are the main causes of the disorder.

The first symptom of prurigo is a violent itching as from the sting of an insect; at the itching place a small induration is soon after perceived, which rapidly rises above the skin in the shape of a papula. The color is the same as that of the adjoining cuticle. If pricked, this pimple discharges a small quantity of a clear fluid. New pimples keep constantly breaking out, whereas the former ones, owing to the scratching, impart a changed appearance to the skin. The top of the pimple or papule being lacerated by the scratching, a small quantity of blood oozes out, which dries up on the pimple and forms a small dark scurf, a number of which may be seen on the skin of persons afflicted with prurigo. As the disease lasts longer, the papulæ and crusts increase in size, and not unfrequently the effused fluid suppurates, causing pustules which form larger crusts and, by running into one another, undermine portions of the skin, and give rise to lymphangioitis and swelling of the lymphatic glands. In this manner prurigo assumes an exceedingly variegated appearance. If the scurfs and crusts fall off, they leave colored marks which, by their number, impart a spotted appearance to the skin. At the same time the skin usually becomes hypertrophied, especially in the folds of the larger joints. The lesser grades which occur among young persons, are generally confined to the lower extremities, and are designated as *prurigo mitis;* the more fully developed form as *prurigo formicans.* The disease remits in the summer or fall; in the winter and spring it generally reaches its acme.

The consequences to the general organism are less severe than the constant and distressing itching, which is worse in bed, would lead one to suppose. Nutrition is not perceptibly impaired. On the other hand, it not unfrequently happens that the disease becomes so intolerable as to drive persons to suicide. The higher grades of the disease have a peculiar disposition to rapid effusions of serum, especially into the pleural cavity and the meningæ; in this way many patients fall victims to the disease, or become mentally deranged. According to Hebra, these not unfrequent terminal affections of prurigo represent the itch-metastases of the ancients, and there is no denying the fact that this view has great probabilities in its favor. Patients afflicted with prurigo most commonly die of tuberculosis, which might likewise suggest the idea of metastasis inasmuch as with the increase of phthisis the itching disappears completely. The disease is never contagious.

As regards diagnosis, prurigo is distinguished from scabies, with which it is most easily confounded, by the circumstance that in prurigo most of the efflorescences and scratched places are found in localities where they are either wanting, or else very sparse in scabies, namely on the extensor surfaces of the extremities, more particularly on the leg and back.

What is otherwise called prurigo, such as prurigo senilis, prurigo pedicularis, etc., has nothing in common with true prurigo except a very violent itching.

In regard to prognosis, Hebra considers the affection altogether incurable; nevertheless by timely and uninterrupted management it is possible to maintain the disease in the form of prurigo mitis, and thus to avert its worst consequences.

Treatment. We are not acquainted with a single case of prurigo that has been cured by homœopathic treatment; however, we do not mean to assert that such a cure is impossible, or that it has not already been achieved. Hebra is the first who has given a reliable and accurately defined diagnosis of prurigo. Physicians having formerly been entirely unacquainted with the genuine characteristics of this disease, it was very easily confounded with scabies. Owing to the great rarity of the disease, it will be a long time before we have a comparatively sufficient number of cures recorded in our published writings. Among the remedies for this disease we have to rely solely upon such antipsorics as will meet the dyscrasic and exceedingly chronic character of the disease; we name: *Sulphur*, *Sepia*, *Arsenicum*, *Calcarea carbonica*, *Plumbum*. A few other remedies may be required for acute exacerbations and complications which arise in the course of prurigo more frequently than in that of any other exanthem. The vapor-bath and frictions with brown soap should never be omitted; by such means the skin is properly cared for, and the relief to the patient is speedy and lasts a pretty long time.

In conclusion we request every practitioner who has treated prurigo with success, to publish his cases, not omitting a specific as well as differential diagnosis of each case. We have already shown in previous chapters that a careful examination of prurigo is calculated to annihilate the whole theory of psora and the itch-metastases, and it is time that this stain should be removed from the fair escutcheon of Homœopathy.

11. Acne.
Stone-pock.

Acne is situated in the sebaceous follicles of the skin; it depends upon the quality of the sebaceous secretion, and is not, or at least very seldom, determined by the narrowness or closure of the excretory duct. If the sebum secreted by the follicle is too thick, it naturally reaches the surface with more difficulty, solidifies near the external opening, and closes the follicle by means of a plug which has generally a black color. These blackish points are called comedones, or acne punctata. In certain circumstances the disease may not progress any further; on some portions of the skin, as for instance on the nose, this condition becomes habitual. Under other circumstances that will be stated below, the glands thus closed show a disposition to become inflamed. That this is not alone owing to the pressure of the sebum upon the follicular walls, is shown by the circumstance that in persons of a more advanced age the comedones scarcely ever inflame, or that they enlarge to the size of small bursæ without any symptom of inflammation whatsoever. The inflamed follicle either changes to a small pustule, discharges and sometimes forms small scurfs, or else the inflammation does not terminate in suppuration, the follicle retains for a time the shape of an indurated, somewhat painful and red papule, and gradually the exudation is reabsorbed. If the inflammation is severe, if the irritation is increased by the pressure and friction of the clothes, the subcutaneous cellular tissue becomes involved, giving rise to a furuncle of a larger or smaller size. These different changes or processes come under the designation of acne simplex. This form of acne appears principally in the face and on the neck, on the back, buttocks, thighs, less frequently on the chest, sometimes on the skin of the penis and scrotum. No other consequences are involved in this affection, except that the places of the acne-pustules remain red for some time. Considering that a number of follicles sometimes become diseased while others are at the same time in full bloom, the face must become considerably disfigured.

Acne scarcely ever makes its appearance except between the age of pubescence and the twenty-fifth or thirtieth year. After this period, a few single follicles may become inflamed, but not a whole number together. Males are more subject to acne than females. All the circumstances connected with this eruption show that acne has its essential origin in the sexual sphere. In corroboration of this statement we will allude to the circumstance that on many ladies a few acne-pustules break out during the menses, and that almost every individual who is addicted to onanism, is afflicted with an excessive breaking out of acne. We do not mean to say that acne only breaks out in the faces of onanists. Among the young people of the city acne seems to be general, whereas among country-youths it is comparatively a rare disease. If a predisposition exists, acne may be developed under the operation of a variety of causes, such as overheating, washing a heated skin with cold water, partaking of boiled and roasted or fried fat, more particularly the fat of geese; indigestion, the excessive use of wine or spirits. Among us, for instance, acne prevails in the winter-season, because so much pork or gooseflesh is eaten in winter; jews are likewise troubled with acne, for the reason that they replace the fat of swine by goose-fat, and for the additional reason that they are generally fond of very fat eating.

It follows from these remarks that the first thing to be done when treating a case of acne is to prescribe a careful and appropriate diet. This task, however, is very difficult of accomplishment, for the reason that acne-patients generally enjoy the sensation of perfect health, and that a rigid diet, if only persisted in for a short time, effects very little improvement in the disease. The next point is to see to a proper management of the skin generally. Cold bathing and washing is of no use; on the contrary, the trouble seems to get worse in consequence. For acne on the trunk, frictions with soap and the use of the flesh-brush in a vapor-bath are the best remedy; for acne in the face the following proceeding is better than all cosmetics: Every morning, or, if the patient has to leave his home early in the morning, then every evening, the face should be gently rubbed for a few minutes with a soft piece of flannel moistened with warm water and greased over with soap, after which it is washed with warm water, and subsequently again with water that is almost cold. The best soap for such a purpose is the so-called Venetian soap made of vegetable fats. By means of these washings the disorder is reduced to its minimum proportions. The formation of pustules is, moreover, best prevented by the comedones being squeezed out. The nails must not be used for such an operation, but a small watch-key, the opening of which must neither be too narrow nor angular, is placed upon the spot so that the black point of the comedo is exactly encompassed by the opening of the key which is firmly and vertically pressed upon the skin. This had better be done previous to washing. By resorting to such simple proceedings, the face can be kept tolerably clean.

A treatment of acne with internal remedies is undoubtedly possible, but likewise superfluous in most cases. In very bad cases we have derived very satisfactory results from Arsenic, but a cure has never been achieved. Hartmann and others likewise recommend: *Cantharides, Sulphur, Staphysagria, Antim. crudum, Dulcamara, Mezereum, Natrum muriaticum, Acidum nitricum, Capsicum, Sepia,* etc. In our opinion, however, internal remedies need not be resorted to as long as a non-medicinal external management will accomplish all that can be desired.

12. Sycosis, Mentagra.
Barber's Itch.

This is exclusively a disease of the male sex, and occurs about the age of twenty-four or twenty-five years, when the hair of the beard grows thick and hard. If persons who do not shave are attacked by it, which is a very rare occurrence, its causes are very obscure. In cases where the beard is shaved, the eruption may be caused by bad or irritating soap or by a dull razor, and, although generally so frightfully obstinate, yet may, under such circumstances, heal spontaneously even without much loss of time; all that need be done is to omit shaving the affected parts. Dirt and snuff likewise seem to occasion sycosis.

The disease generally sets in, like herpes labialis, with a sensation of burning, heat and tension; most commonly we first notice on the chin a small cluster of isolated, red tubercles of a pretty large size, each of which is perforated by a hair. Some of these tubercles in a few days change to pustules, break and form dark crusts, without the infiltration which forms the little tubercle, disappearing on that account. In spite of all care, and generally in consequence of continued irritation, the number of tubercles increases slowly but uninterruptedly, the former ones growing larger; the skin upon which they are seated, becomes more and more infiltrated; after breaking, the pustules change to ulcers; deep, ulcerated rhagades and finally bulbous infiltrations of a pale-red color are perceived.

The patients do not complain of much pain, but their ugly appearance fills them with anxiety. The disease is extremely obstinate and may last for years. It is true that it not unfrequently abates in severity, and at times even disappears altogether; but it breaks out again with renewed fierceness, and in such a case in more than one spot simultaneously. Its first appearance is almost always on the chin; it is here that the disorder exists most commonly in its fiercest intensity, but it likewise invades every other bearded portion of the face, and in severe cases even the eyebrows.

Treatment. Although sycosis, when it first breaks out, sometimes heals spontaneously, yet a spontaneous cure, after the disease has existed for some time, is a rare event, and the higher grades of the disease obstinately resist every attempt to cure it. However, we have seen cases where a mentagra of many years' standing permanently disappeared after an attack of typhus.

In treating this affection, success depends upon commencing the treatment as early as practicable. The first and most important measure is to investigate and remove the cause of the disease. We would not advise the use of internal remedies until we are satisfied, after having pursued this course for a short time, that it leads to no satisfactory result; otherwise we might easily be deceived regarding the effect of our remedies. We have cured three cases of this disease permanently and radically with *Graphites* 4th and 6th trituration; two of these cases had lasted for several years, and two of these patients, moreover, never shaved. This statement shows that *Graphites* deserves our attention in sycosis. *Acidum nitricum* is another remedy that is often very useful; its symptoms bear the greatest resemblance to this disease. However, we ought to state that we have never achieved a cure with this remedy alone, although the cases improved considerably under its influence. We make the same remark of *Aurum muriaticum*. *Silicea*, *Oleander*, *Carbo animalis*, and a few other remedies, are indicated by the symptoms, but we have no clinical evidence to adduce in their favor. Hartmann mentions a few other remedies; but it is evident, from a perusal of his description of sycosis, that he classes under this denomination all sorts of heterogeneous eruptions.

We must not omit to mention a few external remedies that may be of great use. In recent cases of mentagra it is undoubtedly of use to pull out the single hairs that perforate the tubercles. This being a painful proceeding, it must be carried out gradually. However, it is of very little, if any, use if the whole cutis is hypertrophied and infiltrated. Among the caustics *Acidum nitricum* occupies the first rank, probably because it is eminently homœopathic to the disease. *Aurum muriaticum* is likewise a good caustic in some cases. Hebra advises to pull out the hairs before cauterizing; this proceeding undoubtedly increases the effectiveness, but likewise the painfulness of the cauterizing process. Hebra's mode of treating this disease deserves being mentioned so much more as he professes having cured every case by means of it. First the hairs are pulled out, and afterwards a paste of Sulphur, Glycerine and Alcohol is rubbed upon the diseased skin every morning and evening. A cure is very rapidly effected. *Sulphur* is the only medicinal ingredient in this case. We shall revert to the external application of Sulphur in the next chapter. All other external applications of corrosive substances, except *Nitric acid*, are utterly condemned by Hebra.

13. Acne Rosacea, Gutta Rosacea.
Copper-nose, Bottle-nose.

Acne rosacea is an exanthem consisting of tubercles with some disposition to suppurate, suppurating tubercles; and, moreover, of continual venous hyperæmia.

It almost always commences at the tip of the nose, whence it spreads over the dorsum of the nose and over both cheeks, finally over the forehead and the rest of the face. First we notice an erythematous spot of small extent, painless, and distinctly traversed by dilated cutaneous veins. Upon this erythematous base single tubercles start up, which sometimes suppurate at an early period, but likewise spread in size after the pus is discharged. New tubercles keep constantly forming, new erythematous spots keep constantly breaking out, the skin becomes more and more hypertrophied, the veins become more and more varicose, the isolated little blotches change to large tubercles, cracks and deep rhagades, and even ulcers make their appearance, and the face looks very much disfigured in consequence of this extreme development of the nasal exanthem. At first the affection has remissions, but the dark redness never disappears entirely; at a later period the disorder keeps growing all the time.

Abuse of wine and spirits is the cause of the disease in by far the larger number of cases; but it likewise breaks out on individuals of very moderate habits and where the disease cannot be traced to any apparent cause. Among women the disease is of rare occurrence and most generally associated with menstrual anomalies. The disease is not often seen previous to the twenty-fifth year; its most frequent occurrence is after the fortieth. Overheating the system and immoderate drinking are very apt to cause a renewed outbreak of the disease. It is exceedingly obstinate and, in its higher grades, is considered incurable.

Hartmann recommends the following remedies for this disease: *Carbo animalis, Kali carbonicum, Arsenicum, Veratrum album, Cannabis, Acidum nitricum* and *phosphoricum, Thuya, Phosphorus, Euphrasia, Silicea, Ledum, Ruta, Aurum, Kreosotum, Sepia, Petroleum, Plumbum, Sulphur, Acidum sulphuricum, Capsicum, Clematis, Psoricum.* We cannot be blamed for not attaching any sort of importance to so many remedies for a morbid condition that is so characteristically marked by definite and unvarying symptoms, and so little involves the general health. Among the above-mentioned remedies, *Carbo animalis, Arsenicum, Acidum nitricum, Aurum, Sepia* and *Sulphur* are the only ones that promise partial success in the treatment of this disease; *Carbo animalis* and *Arsenicum* in the case of drunkards, and *Sepia* in the case of females. The treatment is always protracted and the results uncertain or imperfect, for the redness most generally remains. More recently we have witnessed a marked improvement after the following treatment: We mix two drachms of the washed flowers of Sulphur with two ounces of distilled water, and after vigorously shaking this mixture, we cause a linen rag to be dipped into it and have the affected parts of the face moistened with this rag every evening before bed-time, allowing the liquid to dry upon the skin, which is washed clean again in the morning. By means of this simple proceeding the tubercles are made to disappear in a surprisingly quick period of time, and the redness likewise becomes less intense. The success of this proceeding never fails, and this instance again shows what an excellent effect the external application of a specific remedy will sometimes have, whereas the internal use of this same specific would either have no effect whatever, or else develop its curative results in a very tardy manner.

14. Lupus.
Wolf, Jacob's Ulcer.

Lupus is preëminently a disease of the lower classes; it occurs more frequently in some parts of the country than in others, but it attacks individuals indiscriminately any where, without distinction of sex. Lupus has not yet been known to occur previous to the tenth and after the fortieth year; it is most frequently seen between the tenth and twentieth years of age. It is said to result from scrofulosis and congenital syphilis; this, however, is problematical, the more so since lupus likewise attacks persons of sound health and vigorous constitutions. It is never infectious.

In describing this disease we will distinguish four different forms, namely : Lupus exedens, hypertrophicus, exfolians and non exedens.

Lupus exedens commences with the formation of a few, rarely of a number of dark-red or brownish spots, or of dark, small papules resembling acne and seated upon a cuticle rendered smooth by infiltration. The spots slowly enlarge in size, the papules never increase rapidly in number; some even, which are situated in the centre of the affected spot, disappear, but are immediately replaced again by new ones starting up at the circumference. The epidermis on the affected spot continually exfoliates in small scales. After the papules have lasted for an indefinite length of time, and while the cutaneous hyperæmia and infiltration are increasing, the tops of the papules ulcerate and become covered with scurfs which are constantly growing in size and thickness and hide somewhat funnel-shaped ulcers that gradually unite in one and destroy the skin over a large extent of surface. The healing of the sore always commences in the centre, while the ulcerative process is being renewed at the periphery; this constitutes the lupus serpiginosus. Lupus exedens is chiefly located in the face, but not unfrequently spreads to the neck and ears, and may likewise break out on other parts of the body. If the lupus is situated on the nose, it not unfrequently happens that the ulceration destroys the integuments, cartilages, and even bones. This seems to be a particular form of lupus that sometimes commences on the mucous membrane of the nose. Lupus exedens is the most frequently occurring form of lupus.

Lupus hypertrophicus likewise breaks out more especially in the face; the papules increase to the size of large tubercles and the subcutaneous cellular tissue becomes strikingly hypertrophied, absorbing the tubercles in such a manner as to give rise to a prominent, deep-red elevation of the skin, which is soft to the feel and at whose periphery new papules keep constantly forming, some of which suppurate but never to any considerable extent. After a time a retracted cicatrix may be seen, traversing the diseased surface. Gradually the affection may invade the larger portion of the face, the ears, and may even spread below the chin; it is most commonly associated with considerable eversion of the lids.

Lupus exfolians, which Hebra is unwilling to regard as a form of lupus, begins, like the former species, with a dark-red, superficially infiltrated spot upon which very flat or no papules are seated, and where the epidermis is constantly passing through a process of exfoliation. This spot never heals spontaneously, neither does it increase in size, the only alteration it exhibits, is a more marked paleness of the skin. It is more particularly seen among females, is easily confounded with nævus, from which it may be distinguished by the circumstance that this form of lupus does not break out until persons have reached an advanced age, whereas nævus is a congenital affection.

Lupus non exedens commences like lupus exedens, except that the papules and tubercles do not ulcerate, but become dissolved and are reabsorbed, leaving a retracted cicatrix with atrophy of the skin at the affected spot, which looks like the scar from a burn.

The different forms of lupus are exceedingly chronic; it is a rare event for lupus exedens to pass through its stage of ulceration rapidly and as it were subcutaneously. The disease is not painful, nor does it impair the general health; but it may easily bring on a very severe attack of conjunctivitis and by this means endanger the visual power.

Treatment. In view of the great obstinacy of this affection, the first requisite towards a successful treatment, both on the part of the physician as well as the sick, is a good supply of patience, in order to give the remedies a fair chance to develop and exhaust their full effect. As far as particular remedies are concerned, we are still without a sufficient number of clinical cases to enable us to point to certain remedies as specifically adapted to lupus; on which account it is extremely desirable that every case of lupus should be made public in our Journals. *Lycopodium* is efficient in lupus exedens, if the disease has not yet existed too long, if the ulceration does not penetrate too far into the tissues, and if the disorder attacks feeble individuals of a sallow complexion. In lupus exedens as in acne rosacea, both of which conditions have a great deal in common, *Graphites* is one of the most important remedies; *Graphites* is particularly suitable for nasal lupus with deep-seated ulceration. Next to Graphites we recommend *Aurum*, more particularly *Aurum muriaticum*. This remedy has sometimes a surprising effect; it is indicated if the lupus starts from the Schneiderian membrane, or if it spreads from the skin, gradually invading the Schneiderian membrane, the bones and cartilages. In such cases *Acidum nitricum* or *Sepia* are likewise suitable. *Calcarea carbonica* is adapted to lupus in the case of scrofulous individuals.

For lupus hypertrophicus at an advanced stage all remedies prove ineffectual. At the commencement of this disorder we may recommend *Conium*, *Baryta*, *Graphites* and *Sulphur*.

Lupus exfolians is no less obstinate than the previous variety, and it is very difficult to pick out suitable remedies for this disease in our Materia Medica. We may try *Arsenicum*, next to which *Sulphur*, *Phosphorus*, *Kali bichrom.*, and perhaps *Thuya*.

Lupus non-exedens does not require any other remedies than lupus exedens.

Other remedies for lupus are: *Iodium*, *Carbo animalis* and *vegetabilis*, *Silicea*, *Alumina*.

The usefulness of external applications is sometimes evident, but not unfrequently questionable; cauterization sometimes does a great amount of injury. In a case of lupus hypertrophicus, cauterization is especially a proceeding of doubtful propriety; like carcinoma, it usually grows so much more rapidly afterwards. If cauterization is insisted upon, it should be done with the pointed extremity of a stick of the Nitrate of silver; it is important to remember that only the little tubercles must be cauterized, not the whole of the diseased surface. All liquid caustics irritate the infiltrated skin still more, and make the disease worse than before.

Cod-liver oil in large doses has sometimes an excellent effect; it might perhaps be sufficient to improve the constitution by good and substantial nourishment; for cod-liver oil is only useful to patients whose assimilative system has been very much impaired.

15. Herpes.

Tetter.

All forms of herpes are characterized by the formation of little vesicles, clusters of which are seated upon an inflamed, red epidermis; the vesicles of one cluster breaking out simultaneously and running an acute course. In obedience to the habitual nomenclature as well as on account of differences in the treatment, we will consider the main forms each by itself.

a. *Herpes Facialis, Facial Herpes.*

This form of herpes accompanies a large number of febrile and chronic diseases without exerting any specially modifying influence over their course; except in pneumonia where this form of herpes is said to constitute a decidedly favorable omen. As an idiopathic exanthem it seems to manifest itself when indicating the commencement of a catarrhal affection, provided the catarrhal irritation is not very intense. A first appearance predisposes most decidedly to relapses.

Herpes facialis (also hydroa febrilis, herpes phlyctænodes) most generally breaks out on the lips, less frequently on the cheeks, forehead, ears, eyelids. A tension, burning, and a marked sensation of swelling are experienced at a certain infiltrated spot, where the vesicles start up amid slight febrile motions and an unusual feeling of lassitude. In the face they are always of a tolerably large size, but there are not many of them clustered together, they incline to run into one another; the cuticle of the spot where they are located does not show a very vivid redness; sometimes they are pitted or cleft. They contain a clear liquid which soon becomes dim and changes to a rather dark scurf that soon falls off, leaving for some time a red, somewhat infiltrated spot; burning pains likewise remain for some time.

One attack does not render any treatment necessary, because it does not alter the course of the vesicles that are already out. But if new crops break out in rapid succession, at definite intervals, it may be well to give *Hepar sulphuris* or *Arsenicum* in not too frequently repeated doses. *Bryonia* is an excellent remedy if each succeeding crop of vesicles is accompanied by fever and great lassitude. If the affection is very obstinate and inveterate, *Graphites* may be given for it. [*Aconite* is better than any other medicine, if the eruption is acute, attended with fever; by using Aconite, the inflammation is speedily subdued, and the vesicles dry up, leaving small scurfs that fall off in a few days. H.]

b. *Herpes Preputialis.*

This is principally located on the prepuce, although it not unfrequently appears on the scrotum, penis, and on the female sexual organs. It bears a very close resemblance to herpes facialis, the single clusters are small, the vesicles not very numerous, and proportionally of some size. It breaks out without any symptoms of general disturbance; its appearance is accompanied by the burning peculiar to all forms of herpes. If the vesicles are seated on the outer skin, superficial, bright-yellow scurfs form on the fifth day; if seated on the inside of the prepuce, instead of vesicles we may have superficial ulcers which occasionally become covered with thin scurfs. The causes of this affection are unknown; what is positively known is that syphilis does not modify the course or character of this form of herpes; its frequent association with balanorrhœa has led this to be regarded as the cause, whereas the reverse is true, that herpes is the cause of a more copious secretion of smegma.

Herpes præputialis acquires its importance from the fact that it is easily mistaken for chancre, especially by lay-persons who had been infected with chancre previously, and are now living in constant dread of constitutional syphilis. By fixing one's attention to the following points, the diagnosis becomes quite easy: herpes always consists of several vesicles seated close together upon an infiltrated base, in a case of chancre we scarcely ever see the primitive vesicle which is moreover completely isolated. If properly guarded, herpes very soon becomes covered with a scurf, the syphilitic ulcer never.

The use of treating herpes præputialis that is fully out, with a view of shortening its course, is very questionable; we have thought, however, on some occasions, that this course is abbreviated, if the proper remedy is administered. The main point is to counteract the tendency to relapses which is just as great in this form of herpes as in that of herpes facialis. *Hepar sulphuris* meets both these indications, provided its use is continued for some time after the disappearance of the efflorescence. Hartmann, on the contrary, recommends the red precipitate and nitric acid. *Caladium seguinum* is likewise indicated, but more in the herpes pudendorum than in the preputial herpes of males. If balanorrhœa is present, a frequent and careful cleansing of the parts is of course indispensable.

c. *Herpes Zoster, Zona, Shingles.*

This form is characterized by the development of clusters of vesicles, of which there are generally several, along the tract of one or more spinal nerves, assuming on the trunk the shape of a zone or belt, but on the extremities breaking out in a more irregular form.

The etiology of this exanthem is involved in obscurity, but every physician of extensive practice must have noticed that at certain periods of the year several cases break out simultaneously or soon one after the other, as though epidemic influences were prevailing.

Zoster commences almost without exception with rheumatic pains in the parts where it is to break out, and is often attended with great lassitude and fever. The preliminary pains are not unfrequently like inflammatory pains. At the origin of one or more nerves, in company with a violent and painful burning, an efflorescence breaks out, after which papules arise, next, clusters of vesicles with tendency to run into one another. These vesicles remain out for four to six days, after which they change to flat scurfs. But inasmuch as a new cluster may arise after the first, and these successive crops may continue even after the first vesicles are entirely healed, the whole process may last even three weeks. It is very seldom the case that scratching or the friction of the clothes will cause a superficial ulceration. There may be no pain during the continuance of the efflorescences, except the slight burning attending the successive breaking out of new crops of vesicles; but the greatest distress to the patient is the burning itching which is especially severe in bed. After the falling off of the crusts all pain is gone, or the peculiar itching may perhaps continue for some time, or finally — and this is not by any means a rare occurrence — intercostal neuralgia of a very obstinate type may set in, apparently the more readily the less scantily the herpes was out on the skin.

Treatment. Although zoster is an entirely typical form of disease, and we have no certain sign whether our medicines have diminished the number of vesicles, and abbreviated their course, yet it is certain that intercostal neuralgia sets in much less frequently when zoster is treated with appropriate remedies, which alone is a sufficient reason why zoster should never be allowed to run its course without proper medicinal treatment. The remedies indicated by Hartmann, namely: *Mercurius, Rhus, Causticum, Graphites, Sulphur, Arsenicum, Acidum nitricum* and *Euphorbium*, with the exception of *Rhus* and *Euphorbium* do not correspond with the general features of the disease. So far as Rhus is concerned, we know positively that the remedy is usually given without any benefit, although its symptomatic similarity would seem to recommend it, and as regards *Euphorbium*, we have no clinical evidence of its curative influence in this disease. *Mercurius* sometimes seems to prevent the breaking out of new clusters of vesicles. *Mezereum* is a remedy that renders excellent service in some respects and which we cannot recommend with sufficient warmth, since intercostal neuralgia very seldom occurs after its use: We likewise suggest *Oleum crotonis* for experimental trials. The treatment of the subsequent neuralgia has been discussed in a former chapter.

d. *Herpes Iris and Circinnatus.*

Both these forms being essentially identical, we describe them together.

Herpes iris consists of a larger vesicle or bulla which is not unfrequently filled with a blood-tinged liquid, and is surrounded by a wreath of smaller vesicles round whose external border another and larger wreath may form. The course is the same as that of other herpetic vesicles. The efflorescences first appear on the dorsa of the feet or hands, spreading on the extensor-surfaces from below upwards, and the new clusters of vesicles appearing either in the same relative position as the vesicles of herpes generally, or else again assuming the form of herpes iris. This form of herpes most frequently occurs among women and children.

Herpes circinnatus which comes out in the same manner as herpes iris, is distinguished from the latter by the circumstance that the central bulla is missing, and that only the wreath of vesicles is present.

Essentially both forms represent a form of herpes zoster on the extremities, so much more as they are sometimes succeeded by a peculiar pain which is not quite as severe as intercostal neuralgia. This affection which is altogether of rare occurrence, scarcely ever requires any other remedies than those that have been indicated for zoster.

16. Eczema.

Eczema is one of those exanthems that has given rise to an immense amount of confusion. In the following sketch we reproduce essentially the views and statements of Hebra who enjoys the undisputed merit of having first cleared up this pathological process.

The causes of eczema are either external irritants acting directly upon the skin, or else substances that affect this organ through the general circulation into which they had been absorbed, or finally constitutional influences. Heat, for instance, causes the so-called baker's itch; and heat, intense cold, salt-baths, mercurial frictions, Croton-oil, etc., a number of medicinal agents taken internally, fat food or food giving rise to an unusual deposition of fat, scrofulosis, affections of the female organs of generation, varices, and in general all kinds of stasis in the venous system, and a number of other similar circumstances and influences uniformly occasion eczema. Among the direct cutaneous irritants we distinguish: neglect in attending to the skin, vermin, friction by the clothes, continued rubbing of a part, for instance between the thighs when riding on horseback, and by continued walking.

The reason why eczema has given rise to so much confusion is, because its various modes of origination were not properly considered, and an eye was only had to the various modifications which the appearance of an eczematous part undergoes in consequence of the formation of crusts or scurfs, scratching, dirt, hair of the body, etc. The typical form of eczema is obtained by rubbing Croton-oil upon the skin. Upon a red surface a number of vesicles or pimples shoot up which, if carefully guarded, heal in a few days leaving the affected portion of the skin injected. If the vesicles are not protected, if they are scratched or rubbed against by the clothes, the vesicles break, and crusts form, beneath which, if the irritation continues, the exudation continues likewise; or else the exudation may be so copious that no crusts can form, in which case the affected part always looks red and moist. If the irritation continues, the eczema spreads to the adjoining parts; scratching even communicates it to remote parts; beside the vesicles, pustules form likewise, the so-called eczema impetiginoides, and the original form of the exanthem is totally altered.

Three modifications have been distinguished more particularly. First the eczema simplex. Upon the cuticle, having a natural color, small vesicles spring up irregularly, without forming any definite clusters; they gradually grow in size, break, discharge a moisture, heal by desquamation, then reappear again at the same place, and, favored by circumstances, pass into the following forms: Eczema rubrum; upon an injected and infiltrated spot, vesicles or small pimples spring up whose tops are filled with a watery moisture. After the bursting of the vesicles, desquamation ends the process.— Finally eczema impetiginoides which is by far the most common form of eczema, consisting of vesicles and pimples or papulæ, some of which change to pustules ending in the formation of crusts; hence this form is properly speaking a combination of eczema and impetigo.

According to their locality we have several strikingly characterized forms of eczema, among which we distinguish the following:

Eczema of the face (crusta lactea, crusta serpiginosa, porrigo larvalis, melitagra) is almost always of the impetiginoid form, it may invade the whole face at once, in which case it usually spreads to the ears; or else, it may remain confined to single localities, especially the cheeks and chin. As a rule, the skin is seldom, and only inconsiderably, infiltrated. This form chiefly attacks children.

Eczema of the hairy scalp is likewise generally of the impetiginoid form; it makes the hair look and feel like felt, is very apt to spread a foul odor and to give rise to the formation of vermin, and is strikingly disposed to migrate beyond the hair, especially in the nape of the neck. This form of eczema is more particularly met with among adults.

Eczema of the male organs breaks out on the penis in an acute form as eczema simplex; on the scrotum, on the contrary, it develops itself in a very chronic form as eczema rubrum. The last-mentioned form causes a horrid itching, and is generally maintained by a dilatation of the cutaneous veins on the scrotum. It is almost always confined to the scrotum, and is one of the most obstinate cutaneous affections. It is very seldom attended with the formation of pustules, but is very apt to lead to hypertrophy of the scrotal integuments.

Eczema of the legs (salt-rheum) really depends almost exclusively upon varicose veins, more especially upon dilatation of the small cutaneous veins, whereas the larger vessels may continue in a perfectly normal condition. This eczema is extremely obstinate, itches most horridly, generally exacerbates in the spring and fall and is a species of eczema rubrum with occasional formation of pustules and an infiltration of the skin that makes it almost look like elephantiasis.

Eczema has a peculiar tendency to attack correspondingly situated portions of the skin, even though the morbific irritation originally only acted upon one side of the body.

Eczema seldom runs an acute course; the extremely acute form of "eczema universale" is very rare; on the other hand, it not unfrequently commences as an acute exanthem, with slight fever, but very soon assumes a chronic character. All the different forms of eczema itch more or less; scratching, which it is impossible to avoid, is a main cause of the onward spread and the protracted course of the disease. Every kind of eczema may heal and does heal spontaneously, provided the chief requisite towards a cure, namely rest in a horizontal posture, is attended to. Eczema of the leg and scrotum is the least promising of any.

Treatment. There is no cutaneous affection the cause of which is more easily discovered than that of eczema; nor is there any cutaneous affection where the removal of the cause is more essential to the success of our treatment. How the causal indication can be satisfied in every case, is difficult to determine owing to the diversity and number of the noxious influences giving rise to the eruption. Above all, local irritants giving rise to eczema, must be removed. In most cases eczema gets well of itself after the cause is removed; however, this is not always the case. Not unfrequently, after the exanthem has lasted for some time, the cutaneous disease acquires such a power of independent existence that a germ of inherent development has become ingrafted upon it. Eczema arising from constitutional causes, is of less frequent occurrence than any other.

In the next place we have to aim at removing the cause, which is the chief promoter of the spread of eczema, namely scratching. In some cases it is impossible to prevent scratching, not only in the case of children, but likewise in that of adults; the itching is too intense and the scratching may be indulged in by the patient while he is sleeping, when the scratching cannot always be prevented in the long run. Under such circumstances it is a good plan to protect the hands by means of gloves or linen-bags and to remove the possibility of the nails being used; for there is no doubt that the laceration of the exanthem with the nails may transfer the eczema to other parts of the body by a regular process of grafting. In other cases scratching may be prevented by appropriately covering the eczematous part; on the leg, for instance, by applying suitable bandages, and in the case of children by covering the head with a calf's-bladder from which the mucous lining has been removed, and beneath which the exanthem sometimes heals with wonderful rapidity. Finally, we will name a few external applications, after the use of which the itching abates with more or less certainty. We ought to state that the greatest amount of irritation, which superinduces the itching, proceeds from the fully-developed crusts, whereas a moist eczema itches much less. Hence, the great object is to limit the formation of crusts as much as possible, or to prevent their excessive adhesion and desiccation. This object is reached by frequent ablutions with cold or tepid water. We are aware that these are dreaded by many physicians and lay-people, but without any adequate cause if proper care is used. A shower-bath is still preferable to washing; but the water must not have a fall of more than two feet, nor should the temperature be below fifty to sixty degrees. For eczema of the body tepid baths with frictions with soap are eminently to be commended. Liquid fats are excellent means of softening the crusts. By moistening them with almond-oil, they break up into little fragments and can be removed more easily. Glycerine renders the same service. We must be careful, however, not to apply the oil too often, nor too much of it, otherwise it might result in the formation of pustules. Twelve to sixteen hours after the application of the oil the parts ought to be washed with soap. If very thick crusts are to be speedily removed, the surest means is the use of warm cataplasms which, however, must not be applied too long at a time, for the reason that cataplasms are likewise apt to lead to the development of pustules. Ointments, no matter what they are made of, can never be of any use, but are generally hurtful.

Regarding the medicinal treatment of eczema, we find a large number of medicines indicated in the books, most of them accompanied by all sorts of the most subtle and refined indications, which are not only of no practical use, but are not even substantiated by the symptomatic record of our Materia Medica. This subject affords us another opportunity of satisfying ourselves of the injury resulting from an inappropriate and vacillating nomenclature which positively defeats all the good that could be done by the accumulated records of clinical experience. Moreover, it is impossible to furnish reliable indications for every drug; the causative as well as the accompanying secondary phenomena are too varied and yet claim our chief attention, for the reason that the selection of a remedy that meets the cause of the eruption, is often exclusively determined by an investigation and knowledge of these phenomena. For this reason we have confined ourselves to merely naming the medicines, accompanying some of them by practical hints, and referring to the Materia Medica for special information, to obtain which the chronic nature of the exanthem affords abundant time. In order to facilitate the search of proper remedies we have associated them with the chief forms of eczema, each according to its locality.

Eczema in the face, which chiefly attacks children, is often made to dry up in a few days by means of *Oleum crotonis*, third trituration. This remedy shows its curative action so much more certainly, the more recent the cutaneous affection; moreover, it is most appropriate in eczema rubrum, and is so much less adapted to the case, the more nearly the eczema assumes an impetiginoid form. If the disorder is of long standing, and hence more inveterate and more extensive, *Lycopodium* often acts with surprising benefit. Next to this remedy comes *Sulphur*. For crusta lactea proper *Borax* is recommended; *Mercurius* and *Lycopodium*, and likewise *Hepar sulphuris* are more reliable. [I have cured the most horrid cases of crusta lactea with *Aconite* and *Belladonna*. H.] From *Viola tricolor* we have never obtained the least sign of a curative effect. For eczema impetiginoides the remedies we have just named, are likewise useful, but we have a much better selection among the following: *Mercurius, Hepar sulphuris, Antimonium crudum, Cicuta virosa, Baryta*. The last-named remedy has a specific action in cases where the eczema is accompanied by swelling of the lymphatic glands, and generally in the case of impoverished, scrofulous individuals.

[We once cured a baby that had been vaccinated with impure vaccine, of a horrid attack of *Crusta serpiginosa*, by means of a single pellet of *Arsenicum* 200. On the third day after vaccination a black pustule broke out on the arm, which grew very rapidly to the size of a big potato and was filled with a foul-smelling corrosive ichor. An ugly-looking sore formed wherever the ichor touched the skin. In the course of twenty-four hours the face, neck and upper arms looked like one mass of blackish, dark-brown ulceration. This disorganizing process spread almost visibly. The eyes could no longer be seen. The sides of the face and neck, ears and part of the scalp were covered with this horrid crust. The mother likewise had become infected. One pellet of *Arsenicum* 200 was placed upon the child's tongue at night. Next morning the sores had not spread any further, and those that existed were perfectly dry; they fell off in two days, and in a week after even the traces of the ulcers could no longer be seen. H.]

If eczema is exclusively seated on and behind the ears, it is very obstinate; hence, the remedies must not be changed too often. The best remedies are: *Mercurius, Iodium, Kali bichromicum, Baryta, Sulphur*.

Eczema of the hairy scalp, both when confined to the scalp and when the face is invaded by the exanthem, either runs its course rapidly, more especially in the case of children, and generally in the form of eczema impetiginoides; or else it assumes the form of eczema rubrum, most commonly in the case of adults, its course in such a case being very chronic. For the former acute form the best remedies are: *Hepar sulph.*, *Oleander*, *Lycopodium*, *Sulphur*, *Staphysagria*, *Mercurius* (when a tendency to acute lymphadenitis prevails), *Baryta carbonica* (when attended with a painless or, at any rate, not acute inflammatory swelling of the lymphatic glands), *Borax*, *Clematis*, and, according to Hartmann's urgent recommendation: *Dulcamara*. For the obstinate eczema of adults we cannot recommend with sufficient emphasis *Arsenicum* and *Graphites*. With *Arsenicum* alone we have several times removed an exceedingly humid and horridly itching eczema in the space of six to eight weeks. Quite recently we have cured eczema of seventeen years' standing with *Graphites*, the patient being otherwise in a state of perfect health. She had to continue the remedy for over six months in the fourth to the sixth trituration, but even the excessively hypertrophied ears finally resumed their normal shape. We do not mean to deny the possible adaptation of *Sulphur*, *Lycopodium*, or even *Phosphorus*, to this disease, but we are obliged to confess that we have never derived the least curative effect from either of these remedies.

Children passing through the second period of dentition are often attacked with an eczema that is confined to the lower border of the hairy scalp on the occiput, between both ears, and which, after being once cured, is apt to break out again, and is always accompanied by glandular swellings of considerable size. Hartmann recommends *Dulcamara* for this eruption; we have used for it with perfect success: *Rhus toxicod.*, *Calcarea carbonica*, *Oleum crotonis*.

Eczema on the scrotum occurs in very few cases as an acute impetiginoid eczema; for such cases no medicine surpasses *Croton oil* in efficacy, beside which we call attention to *Caladium seguinum*, *Rhus toxicod.* and *Hepar sulphuris*. In cases of chronic eczema great patience is required not only on the part of the physician, but likewise on that of the patient; it is an exceedingly obstinate affection. The remedies to be employed in such cases are: *Sulphur*, *Arsenicum*, *Lycopodium*, *Nitri acidum*, also *Graphites*, *Petroleum*, *Thuya* and *Anthrakokali*. A fact deserving special consideration is the very common co-existence of profuse hemorrhoids with this eruption; the scrotal integuments are likewise traversed by a number of varicose veins.

Eczema between the thighs is generally cured by means of *Mercurius* or *Lycopodium*; of course the cause has to be strictly avoided. Daily ablutions of the part with good soap are indispensable.

Eczema on the leg is likewise very obstinate, no less so than eczema on the scrotum; in order to cure this disease, we have to neutralize the effect of the varices by a carefully applied roller bandage. If the eczema has the impetiginoid form, it is advisable to place the patients for a short time in a horizontal posture, and to order flax-seed poultices to the part; at the same time *Rhus toxicod.* or *Carbo vegetabilis* may be given internally, and, if erysipelatous redness sets in: *Mercurius.* — Afterwards the chief remedy is *Staphysagria* which is often sufficient to eradicate the disease; we likewise call attention to *Graphites, Sulphur, Lycopodium.*

Beside the above-mentioned remedies the following are likewise more or less homœopathic to eczema: *Kreasotum, Aurum muriaticum, Sarsaparilla, Sepia, Silicea, Alumina, Conium, Ranunculuc socleratus,* also *Tartarus stibiatus.*

17. Impetigo.

By this term we designate the breaking out of small pustules on the skin, either scattered or in clusters.

This affection is traceable to the same causes that have been pointed out as causes of eczema; indeed, both these exanthems generally appear associated. Besides this, however, impetigo is generally the expression of a constitutional affection, more particularly of scrofulosis, the first symptom of which is not unfrequently the formation of pustules. Among adults the disease may be caused by an excessive supply as well as by an extreme deprivation of good and nourishing food. Owing to peculiar causes, a subacute impetigo may break out after vaccination over the whole body.

The appearance of the pustules is sometimes accompanied by symptoms of an inconsiderable febrile irritation, generally, however, without the general organism being involved. At a certain spot on the cuticle, seldom at several spots at once, an efflorescence makes its appearance, attended with itching and burning which, however, never equals in intensity the itching and burning of herpes or eczema; very soon the efflorescent cuticle appears covered with small vesicles of the size of lentils or peas, containing an opaque liquid; after having been out a few days, the vesicles break, and their contents change to yellowish, greenish and brownish crusts, which adhere with a tolerable degree of tenacity and, on falling off, leave for some time red and flat cicatrices. In the case of a single pustule this course is terminated in ten days to a fortnight. But new pustules keep forming ever and anon, adjoining the first pustule; they cover a large portion of the skin, and in this manner the whole process assumes a chronic form. While the new crops of pustules are developing, the exudative process generally continues at the previously-affected places, by which means the originally not very thick scurfs are changed to crusts of considerable thickness, beneath which a superficial ulcerative process may still be going on (impetigo rodens). With impetigo the lymphatic glands involved in the exanthem, almost always swell and become inflamed. In pursuing this course the exanthem may continue on for years, whereas, at other times, the whole course of the eruption may be ended in a few weeks. Scratching and the consequent grafting with the nails contribute a great deal to the spread of the pustules; by this means the eruption may easily be transferred to other individuals, as often happens in the case of children's nurses.

Impetigo-pustules, if not excited by local irritants, such as plasters or moist poultices, break out chiefly in the face (crusta lactea, melitagra, porrigo larvalis), upon the hairy scalp (porrigo, tinea), on the nape of the neck and on the lower extremities. The pustules at times appear isolated (impetigo sparsa), at times in large groups or clusters (impetigo figurata), and at other times upon a brightly inflamed base (impetigo erysipelatodes). The pustules generally involving a hair-follicle, the hair, in impetigo of the hairy scalp, is not only glued together in clusters, but is likewise dry and brittle; a good portion of it falls out, giving rise to bald spots of more or less size. Otherwise the constitutional condition of the patient is not impaired by this affection.

In treating a case of impetigo, the causal indication is just as important as in a case of eczema, especially if we deal with little children, and a suspicion is consequently excited in our minds, of the disorder being occasioned by a scrofulous taint. In their case it is necessary to attend closely to their diet, cleanliness, etc. A very common cause is not, as is often supposed, too fat milk, but the excessive and too frequent use of milk. We likewise not unfrequently see children attacked with impetigo whom their mothers, especially in the country, nurse until the little ones are two or three years old. Many occupations carried on in a high temperature, are likewise apt to induce impetigo, and all our efforts to cure the disease would be fruitless, if this circumstance were lost sight of.

Local treatment has to be conducted in accordance with the rules laid down for eczema; above all, the crusts have to be carefully removed and their return prevented; the further spread of the exanthem by scratching has to be limited as much as possible by appropriate barriers. In resorting to external applications, we must not overlook the fact that the skin of many individuals is exceedingly vulnerable, and that the application of oil or of water-compresses, etc., to such a skin may very speedily excite impetigo, or increase it where it already exists.

Medicines employed for this affection may deceive us regarding their curative powers, for the reason that such an exanthem often heals spontaneously within a few weeks. A spontaneous cure of this kind can never be determined beforehand, for it but too often happens that an apparently acute or subacute course is changed to a very chronic one, or that the disorder is continually oscillating between remissions and exacerbations. On this account it is proper that suitable medicines should be given at once at the commencement. In the case of children, and when the face or the hairy scalp is invaded, *Mercurius* renders the best service as long as the efflorescence of the cuticle continues. *Hepar sulph. calc.* sometimes arrests the disorder at the onset. If the affection has assumed a chronic character, *Antimonium crudum*, *Lycopodium*, *Arsenicum*, *Calcarea carbonica*, *Acidum nitricum* or *Clematis* have to be resorted to. *Lycopodium* and *Staphysagria* are particularly adapted to impetigo of the legs. According to our experience, *Sulphur* is utterly ineffectual in this affection; Hartmann, on the contrary, writes of this and other remedies as follows: "In impetigo *Sulphur* is undoubtedly one of the most distinguished remedies, provided it is not given in too scanty a dose; even a bright efflorescence of the base does not counter-indicate it. Among chronic cutaneous affections *Graphites* seems to be characteristically adapted to impetigo. *Acidum muriaticum* is useful for impetigo on the legs in the case of old people, with burning pain." He likewise mentions *Conium*, *Carbo vegetabilis*, *Sepia*, and a number of other remedies that are scarcely ever in homœopathic relation with the case. For impetigo rodens Hartmann recommends *Staphysagria*, *Kali hydriodicum*; however, his delineation of impetigo does not seem to us to represent an exact image of the disease.

18. Ecthyma, Rupia.

Both ecthyma and rupia (or rhypia), according to their general characteristic properties, are nothing else than forms of impetigo, that is: pustules upon the skin, differing only in size.

Both may have the same etiology as impetigo, and may likewise break out on individuals of apparently sound health; in most cases, however, both exanthems are signs of constitutional disease, and are more particularly met with among the poorer classes inhabiting damp and unwholesome dwellings, and not having a sufficient supply of nourishment. The ecthyma-pustule is very often a symptom of neglected itch, rhypia a symptom of constitutional syphilis.

The ecthyma-pustules are seated upon an injected and infiltrated base which is at times of a bright, and at other times of a dingy redness, the latter, if some constitutional cachexia prevails. They are always distinct, very seldom close together; they are of the size of a large pea, semi-globular, and at the onset filled with a yellowish-turbid, or sanguineously-opaque fluid. Only a few pustules break out at once, generally only one at first, the other pustules following in successive crops. The eruption is sometimes preceded by pains in the joints and febrile symptoms. The halo of the pustule fades away with the desiccation of the vesicle, and a firmly-adhering incrustation forms, not very thick, but which may increase in thickness very considerably, if the suppurative process continues underneath it; this change usually, however, takes place only in a case of cachectic ecthyma. In consequence of a succession of crops this pathological process may become protracted for weeks and even months. The pustules are most commonly seated on the legs, much less frequently on the thighs and the rest of the body, scarcely ever in the face.

Rupia-pustules are large bullæ sometimes of the size of a modern penny; yet they ought to be ranged among the pustules for the reason that their contents though serous at first, yet soon change to a puriform liquid, and are very generally mixed with blood. They are seated upon a dingy-red base, are never very much elevated above the skin, but are loose blebs which, in a few days, change to brown incrustations raised in the middle, and sometimes separating very rapidly, leaving an ulcerated excoriation (rhypia simplex), or beneath which the suppurative process continues and causes the incrustations to grow to considerable thickness (rhypia prominens). If the incrustation is removed, a deep, sickly-colored ulcer is revealed underneath which obstinately defies every attempt to heal it, but upon which new crusts are disposed to form. Rupia, too, is most generally seated on the leg, never in the face, very seldom on the rest of the body. It is an exanthem of a bad character, but is generally curable; it is only when the ulcer becomes ichorous (rhypia gangrænosa) that it may lead to hectic fever and result in death.

Treatment. Ecthyma associated with scabies and the syphilitic rupia will be treated of when we come to speak of the itch and syphilis. If not accompanied by malignant symptoms, ecthyma hardly requires any medical treatment. Otherwise our best remedy is *Antim. tartar.*, which is suitable as long as the cutaneous disease has not assumed a chronic character. *Mercurius* is decidedly inferior to Tartar Emetic. *Arsenicum, Staphysagria* and perhaps *Lycopodium* may be tried to keep off the new crops of blebs. As long as rupia does not assume a gangrenous character, *Rhus toxicod., Acidum nitricum, muriaticum* or *phosphoricum* are sufficient to cure it; but if the affected parts are invaded by malignant ulceration, we meet this change with excellent effect by means of *Arsenicum* and *Secale cornutum*, to which *Carbo vegetabilis* and *Staphysagria* are decidedly inferior although they may at times be useful. The main object is to treat the general condition; both exanthems will disappear so much sooner and will be so much less disposed to break out again, the more carefully the skin is attended to, together with the internal treatment.

19. Pemphygus.

This affection which is likewise described under the name of pompholix, is characterized by the formation of large blisters. Its origin, especially that of the acute form, is involved in obscurity, whereas the chronic form is evidently traceable to a constitutional taint, which is so much more probable as the chronic form of this exanthem is so apt to terminate fatally.

Pemphygus may represent an acute affection, but, as such, is of very rare occurrence; we do not consider it necessary to devote any more space to it.

Chronic pemphygus most generally commences without fever; nevertheless in cases where the disease consists of several successive crops of blisters, with intermediate free intervals, it often happens that each special eruption sets in with some fever and pains in the limbs. The disease commences with the breaking out of lentil-sized red spots, attended with itching and burning; soon a white appearance is perceived in the middle of the spot, which increases rapidly in size, and forms the blister; this sometimes remains quite small, and at other times grows to one inch and a half in diameter. The blisters are filled with a clear fluid, very tense, break very easily, after which no incrustation forms, but the detached and dry epidermis separates, leaving for some time a moist excoriation, so that a blister runs its whole course in about a fortnight. Inasmuch as the blisters seldom cease to form after their first appearance, on the contrary new blisters form almost every day, the disease may become very much protracted and all the stages of the pemphygus-disease may be seen and observed on the same patient. Pemphygus is most frequently seated on the leg, blisters may, however, break out over the whole body. The course of the eruption varies greatly. Either the blisters come out in crops separated by intervals of weeks or even months;—this is a comparatively favorable sign;— or else the affection commences with a few or with only one blister, new blisters continuing to form, which involves a loss of serous plasma that may, after a lapse of time, lead to gradual emaciation, hectic fever and death. At all events pemphygus is one of the most obstinate and at the same time one of the most dangerous cutaneous affections. This statement, however, only applies to the above-described form, not to the pemphygus which, like the ecthyma-pustule, sometimes breaks out as a secondary symptom of other cutaneous affections and a variety of other acute diseases, and which has no particular significance.

Treatment. Considering the importance of this exanthem, we are not particularly blessed with reliable remedies for it. We may compare: *Cantharides, Causticum, Kreosotum, Lachesis, Dulcamara, Rhus toxicodendron, Ranunculus bulbosus* and *sceleratus, Secale cornutum*. These remedies are theoretically indicated by our provings, but, so far as we know, not one of them has yet cured a single case of this disease. We doubt very much whether *Dulcamara* is capable of doing any thing for such a deep-seated constitutional disorder. Lachesis of all other remedies has the best and most marked symptoms. *Mercurius* seems to be in curative rapport with pemphygus. Some years ago we saw in Vienna a woman who for several years had been a nurse in one of the sections for syphilitic patients, and who had rubbed up a good deal of quicksilver with her bare hand. Since then she was attacked with pemphygus, but whether her handling of Mercury was the cause, is of course problematical. In the subsequent course of the disease other remedies have to be employed for the general consequences of the exanthem rather than for the exanthem itself. *Arsenicum, China, Sulphur, Ferrum* may possibly keep off the threatening decline, but they are not homœopathically related to pemphygus.

20. Furunculus and Carbunculus.
Anthrax.

Although both furuncle and carbuncle are generally regarded as surgical diseases, yet we are perfectly satisfied that either of these pathological processes can be managed by internal treatment in such a manner as to make all surgical interference unnecessary.

A furuncle generally proceeds from a single cutaneous gland, or else from several in close proximity to one another, and the first deposition of the exudation takes place into the glandular follicle. The inflammation, however, is not limited to the gland, but spreads to the surrounding cellular tissue, enveloping the follicle in a firm exudation-plug. Amid severe pains, and sometimes in company with intense fever, pus forms in the space of three to ten and more days, and breaks through the skin. Usually the exudation-plug or core cannot be removed until some time after the opening has existed. Furuncles of some size generally break out singly, especially on the buttocks, but it very commonly happens for one furuncle to be followed by another; lay-people consider it an established fact that seven boils must break out one after the other, which shows how seldom a boil is without successors. The cause of boils is very often a local irritation; but there are real furuncle-epidemics which have to be accounted for by atmospheric influences. Boils very often occur during convalescence from severe acute diseases and after the excessive use of fat as an article of diet.

Carbuncle or anthrax is regarded by many as a combination of several furuncles; but in our opinion this theory is erroneous. A boil is never attended with gangrenous destruction; with a carbuncle this is the rule. Carbuncle, moreover, has its favorite localities, namely the integuments along the dorsal spine, especially in the nape of the neck; less frequently the sternum or the inguinal region. Carbuncle, moreover, is chiefly met with among older persons; boils, on the contrary, may occur at any age, especially among young people. Otherwise it is difficult to decide what are the causes of carbuncle, for it occurs among individuals with cachectic and deteriorated constitutions as well as among perfectly healthy and robust persons. Carbuncle begins and runs its course with great pain. At the painful spot a mere change is scarcely perceived at first; soon, however, it acquires a bluish and sickly look, but without any perceptible swelling. The pus seldom escapes before the sixth day, generally in several places at once, which afterwards unite and from which a thick, easily decomposed pus is discharged, mixed with a quantity of shreds of detached cellular tissue. This whole process is attended with fever which is apt to assume an adynamic type and, after the sudden supervention of cerebral symptoms, may terminate fatally. In a favorable case the cure takes place very slowly, because the loss of substance may be many square inches in extent. Further details about the course of the disease will be given in the next paragraph.

Treatment. Boils require very seldom any medicinal treatment; warm poultices bring the boil to a head in a few days. If the boil is very large, attended with considerable inflammation of the cellular tissue, and a good deal of fever, and if it breaks very tardily, a few doses of *Mercurius vivus*, to be followed by a few doses of *Hepar sulph. calc.* hasten the course. We do not advise lancing, because the pains and the suppuration generally last much longer in such a case, whereas, if the boil breaks spontaneously, it generally heals in a few days; however, we should see to the removal of the core at as early a period as possible, for the presence of the core keeps up the suppuration. To eradicate a tendency to a constant return of new boils *Acidum phosphoricum* or *nitricum* and still more *Arsenicum* have seemed to us useful remedies. As a matter of course it is very difficult to decide this point.

If we desire carbuncle to run a benign course, we have to treat it with medicines from the commencement. *Acidum nitricum*, *Silicea*, *Carbo vegetabilis*, *Secale cornutum* are recommended for carbuncle, but it is difficult to determine special indications for each of these remedies; nor are we acquainted with definite and permanent results in any case. *Arsenicum*, given at the onset, renders excellent service, and contributes greatly towards securing a favorable result. *Secale cornutum*, which is too little thought of in such cases, may be given if cerebral phenomena set in at an early period of the disease; *Phosphorus* may likewise be indicated under such circumstances. *Silicea* is suitable if the suppuration has fully set in. Here, too, as in the case of boils, we urgently advise against the artificial opening of the carbuncle, more especially if it is premature. An early access of atmospheric air favors the development of gangrene, pus is but too readily taken up by the cut vessels, and the inflammation is enabled to spread. We are fully aware that surgeons are of a decidedly contrary opinion; but we can only ask them whether they have ever attempted the cure of a carbuncle without a crucial incision. No opponent of our view will be able to answer this question affirmatively. After the carbuncle is broke, the shreds of cellular tissue have to be removed as soon and as completely as possible; the sore should likewise be cleansed very frequently. Warm poultices ought to be applied from the start.

21. Seborrhœa.

An excessive secretion of sebum on the hairy scalp is a regular occurrence during the first year of infancy. It may likewise take place among perfectly healthy and robust men up to the age of thirty; women afflicted with uterine diseases, and likewise pregnant women, often suffer from it.

Seborrhœa chiefly takes place on the hairy scalp, more frequently on the sinciput than on the forehead, nose and on the sides of this organ. On the hairy scalp the secreted sebum forms fine yellowish-white scales or, as in the case of children, incrustations which sometimes acquire considerable thickness. In the face the sebum either remains liquid, in which case the affected part looks somewhat injected and has a shining, greasy appearance, and the grease can be removed by means of blotting paper; or else the sebum coagulates very rapidly, forming a yellowish, scurfy, soft lining, beneath which the skin has a natural appearance, except a little redder than usual; numerous excretory ducts of the follicular glands are likewise seen.

This disorder, oscillating between more or less, always runs a very chronic course. It is of no great importance, for the general health is not affected by it, except that the patients experience in the affected part a disagreeable tension and prickling, or a violent itching on the hairy scalp. The seborrhœa of pregnant females almost always ceases after confinement. Seborrhœa is important in so far as it is easily confounded with pityriasis and eczema, a mistake that is apt to lead to erroneous and even injurious management. The diagnosis is secured by the circumstance that in seborrhœa the epidermis remains intact.

Treatment. Internal treatment is only necessary in cases where the affection is of a primary origin, or depends upon uterine disorders. In the last-mentioned case our chief and, indeed, sole object should be to remove the cause, for the cure of the uterine derangements involves the disappearance of the cutaneous affection. As a primary affection the disease is very obstinate; quite recently, in the case of a robust young farmer, we have employed in vain every imaginable remedy, more particularly *Aurum, Graphites, Lycopodium, Acidum nitricum, Calcarea carbonica.* The only remedy that improved the case, was *Arsenicum.* Tried remedies for this disease are as yet very scarce. [We have cured a case of seborrhœa where the patient, a young woman, looked as if she were enveloped in a coat of liquid and shining grease, with nothing but *Aconite* and *Sambucus;* the treatment lasted about two weeks. H.] Too much washing, either with cold or warm water, is hurtful. If soap is used, it must be very mild, lest it should prove disagreeable. Washing with spirits is sometimes useful. Fat food must be strictly avoided.

22. Favus.
Honey-comb Tetter, Scald-head.

This cutaneous affection, which is likewise described under the names of porrigo decàlvans or tinea favosa, is characterized by the accumulation of multitudes of fungi around the roots of the hairs, hence their exclusive appearance on the hairy portions of the skin.

Favus is a disease of the lower classes. It only attacks individuals who pay no sort of attention to cleanliness. In other respects such individuals may either enjoy the most perfect health, or else be of sickly and cachectic constitutions; favus may attack either class. This exanthem can be transferred to other persons by hats, caps and other head-gear, likewise by sleeping in the same bed; it has likewise been transmitted purposely from one individual to another.

A single favus-efflorescence has its origin in the orifice of a sebaceous follicle in the form of a small, imbedded, not painful papule, which is perforated by the hair and keeps constantly increasing in breadth and height, until the characteristic crust finally arises from it. This crust has the shape of a dish, with a rounded central depression and round elevated borders; it has a yellowish or gray tint, without any exudation underneath, and has a peculiar odor. If, as usually happens in old cases, the efflorescences are close together, they unite to an uneven incrustation, at whose borders the distinct crusts are never missing, so that the diagnosis is quite easy. The consequences of favus are: Partial atrophy of the skin in consequence of the crusts being imbedded in it; eczema occasioned by the scratching; destruction of the hair on the affected parts; on the other hand, this disorder has no influence upon the general state of the constitution. The disease runs a very chronic course, yet spontaneous cures occur, although very tardily and not without corresponding modifications in the hygienic circumstances of the patients.

According to what we have stated concerning the etiology of the disease, we deem an internal treatment of it useless and ineffectual; Hartmann's remarks in this respect have no reference to true favus. If constitutional disorders are present simultaneously with favus, they have, of course, to be treated with appropriate remedies; at the same time they must not be regarded as the originating cause of favus. This can only be cured by removing the crusts in which the fungi are imbedded, and by preventing their return. The surest means of accomplishing this result, is care and cleanliness. The removal of the crusts is secured by softening them with oil, and afterwards removing them together with the perforating hair. This is a very tedious, but sure undertaking. Every sickly-looking hair has to be pulled out singly, for the reason that the disease has already invaded the soil in which it grows.

[This eruption is treated with success in some cases by means of *Iris versicolor;* a cerate is applied to the scalp, and a few drops of the tincture, even as many as twenty, in half a tumblerful of water given internally, in teaspoonful doses, three or four times a day. See Hale's New Remedies. H.]

23. Scabies, Itch.

It is with a certain reluctance that we enter upon a discussion of this affection, since we are satisfied that our views concerning it differ from those of most of our Colleagues. We will, therefore, anticipate all objections by stating that the opinions which we promulgate in this chapter, are simply our own, not those entertained by a majority of our Colleagues, whose opinions we have not even sufficient space to refute.

The itch is caused by a parasite, the acarus scabiei or sarcoptes hominis. Any one who wishes to become specially acquainted with the natural history of this animalcule, is referred to an article by Gudden, in Vierordt's Archiv, 1855; series XIV, No. 1, from which we transfer the following leading points.

The female full-grown acarus is from $\frac{1}{5}$ to $\frac{1}{4}$ of a line broad, having an ovoid shape, with wavy lines; it is provided with eight limbs and a number of long hairs. To the bare eye it looks like a faintish-white or yellowish corpuscle. Each acarus contains from 40 to 60 eggs which are laid seriatim and from which the young acarus originates in about eight days. The male acarus is much smaller than the female, and is said to die soon after sexual converse. In the cold the acarus remains quiet, but in the warmth its movements become very lively; the young acarus especially shows a disposition to wander.

If an acarus is placed upon the skin, it very soon commences to burrow by placing itself in a vertical position, supporting itself by the bristles projecting from the posterior part of its body. Having perforated the hard layer of the epidermis, it lowers the posterior part of its body continuing to burrow horizontally and very soon beginning to lay eggs. At intervals it makes an opening in the canal towards the outside, probably to afford the young a passage to crawl out. The cuniculi of the male acarus are short, those of the female often one inch in length, generally with irregular curves; but the young acari soon again leave the spot where they had buried themselves, hence do not form cuniculi, but papules and vesicles. From ten days to a fortnight elapse between the time when the acarus first begins to burrow and when the characteristic itching is first perceived.

The places preferred by the acarus, are the hands, between the fingers and on the sides, the surface of the wrists, the inner sides of the extremities, the entrance to the axillæ, the abdomen, the inter-gluteal space, the region around the nipples, especially those of the mammæ, the penis and scrotum, and the feet around the tarsus. The acarus, however, may locate itself anywhere on the trunk, but is never met with in the face.

The cuniculi the presence of which is indispensable to establish a correct diagnosis, are most easily found on the hand, at the places indicated; they appear like fine, irregularly dotted dark streaks, owing to dirt having adhered to the orifices of the cuniculi; whereas on the trunk the cuniculi have a whitish appearance. The commencement of the cuniculus is marked by single scales of the epidermis which, being detached, afford an opening to the cuniculus which remains uninterrupted in its further course. The end of the cuniculus is recognized by a whitish-yellow, somewhat elevated point which hides the acarus. If the epidermis is carefully removed at this spot by means of a needle and the needle is firmly pressed against, and moved over the cuniculus, the acarus will readily adhere to the needle and can easily be recognized by means of a glass. With a little practice it will be found quite easy to catch an acarus. In the efflorescences occasioned by the young acari, one of them is seldom found for the reason that they wander about from place to place very rapidly. On individuals who do not wash themselves with care, a cuniculus is most easily discovered by lightly passing a finger moistened with saliva over it several times, in consequences of which the dirt penetrates between and adheres to the scales of the epidermis. In persons with callous hands the acarus has to be sought at the wrist.

A transmission of the acarus is most easily effected when it has the greatest desire to wander, hence in a warm bed; it takes place much less frequently by touching objects that had been handled by persons affected with the itch; but it is easily accomplished through wearing apparel.

The phenomena caused by the acarus upon the skin, proceed from it either directly or indirectly. The presence of the acarus upon the skin remains without symptoms except a slight itching which is not always present, and does not always become very troublesome even when, as is often the case, especially on the penis, the cuniculus is closed by a little exudation deposited below it and on its side. But immediately after leaving the canal, the young acari again bury themselves in its proximity, and small papules topped with fine vesicles break out close to the primary canal, itching violently, and being either speedily lacerated by scratching or, as in the case of children, changing to pustules and forming scabs and crusts of various sizes. The indirect phenomena, according to Hebra, owe their origin entirely to the scratching caused by the itching; as an evidence of this fact he refers to the circumstance that children and paralytic persons who do not scratch, remain free from these symptoms, and that in healthy persons they are only met with in localities that can be scratched. First papulæ, each perforated by a little hair, break out, less frequently vesicles or pustules. These papules are scratched, after which their tips become covered with fine, dark-looking scabs. After the cutaneous irritation has lasted for some time, pustules arise from the papules. On parts of the body that are exposed to constant pressure, or to constant pressure with friction, the skin soon appears infiltrated and is thickly covered with the above-mentioned efflorescences, as for instance round the waist in the case of females on account of the clothes being fastened around too tightly, or in the case of shoemakers on the nates. In these instances, as in any other persistent cutaneous irritation, eczema may break out.

After this explanation it behooves us to examine the question whether, in a case of what is called the itch, and where the above-described process takes place in its totality, the mechanical irritation of the acarus or some other coexisting agent is the cause of the disorder. The doctrine has been started that acari, like Cantharides, contain some corrosive poison which is communicated to the skin and becomes the origin of a chronic itch-dyscrasia. But many other irritations of the skin produce the same symptoms as the itch, without a virus having been their cause; we notice, moreover, that the itch is always confined to the localities occupied by the acari; that it spreads in proportion as the acari increase in number, and that it ceases to spread as soon as the acari are destroyed. In such a case the consecutive cutaneous phenomena may remain for some time, but the same thing takes place in the case of eczematous eruptions occasioned by other cutaneous irritants, and which, in the long run, had assumed the character of independent diseases. There is not a single symptom connected with the whole course of the itch, that might lead us to think that the consecutive phenomena in the case of the itch differ from those manifested by other kinds of vermin, such as lice or fleas. If we are asked whether all the old doctrines about the terrible consequences of the itch are false, we answer that we partially admit and partially reject them. They are unfounded in so far as they originate in the hypothesis of a specific itch-virus; on the other hand, they are founded in so far as the itch, especially if the disease remains for a long time uncured, and more particularly as it used to be managed in former times, may superinduce consecutive diseases. If the body is rubbed for a long time with ointments containing noxious substances, the organism undoubtedly suffers in consequence of such a proceeding, and no homœopath would want to deny this. The absurd bathing for hours, sweating for days in overheated rooms, and other similar measures, may make the healthiest person sick, and develop germs of sickness in an apparently healthy individual. Even the continued disturbance of the cutaneous functions by the itch may cause sickness, the more so, the more coexisting constitutional disturbances affect the exanthem unfavorably and *vice versa.*

The best proof that the itch is not a constitutional disease, is afforded by the circumstance that, if the destruction of the acarus is effected with all due caution, the equilibrium of the organism is never disturbed by such a proceeding. This view does not upset the formerly entertained doctrines of secondary diseases resulting from the suppression of the itch. Only if such secondary affections resulted, it was not the itch but prurigo. Those who had no knowledge of the acarus, must necessarily have mistaken prurigo for the itch, and it is the suppression of prurigo that leads to the most dangerous constitutional diseases and more particularly to tuberculosis.

After these remarks we need not say what we think of Hahnemann's theory of psora and of Psoricum as a medicinal agent. Psoricum might have had something in its favor, if it had been prepared from the acari themselves.

Treatment. Although we have tried in the course of this work, to be in accord with our homœopathic Colleagues in most things, yet in the matter of scabies we have to differ with many of them. We hold that all treatment of the itch, as long as the acarus is not extirpated, is downright absurdity. It is our opinion that the cures of the itch which are reported as having been effected by the exclusive use of internal remedies, are not compatible with correctly scientific observation.

The destruction of the acari is the causal indication which not only can, but has to be satisfied. The most simple, never hurtful proceeding and which never fails, if carefully carried out, is the following: First the patient is placed in a water-bath of about 92° F., in which he remains for half an hour. At the end of this period of time he rubs himself well with brown soap, more particularly at the places where the acarus is principally located. By this means the cuniculi are almost completely opened. After the bath the patient is thoroughly dried and enveloped in a woollen blanket for a quarter or half an hour, for the purpose of removing every particle of moisture from the skin and at the same time enabling the ointment to thoroughly penetrate the cuniculi. We now resort to frictions with the following ointment: Two ounces of lard, two drachms of the washed flowers of Sulphur, and half a drachm of the Sulphuret of Lime. These proportions are abundantly sufficient for every adult. The whole body, except the head and neck, has to be rubbed very carefully, especially the places that constitute the favorite haunts of the acarus. The rubbing is best done by two persons at once, one on each side. After the rubbing, the patient is again enveloped in the woollen blankets, in which he remains for an hour and a half. At the end of this period he is placed in a warm bath of a temperature of 92° F. and, while in the bath, thoroughly rubbed with brown soap. After the bath the patient may take a shower-bath, and be kept in the room for some time longer in order to guard against taking cold. After such a proceeding which we have employed in a number of cases, we have never seen a relapse. The best method of cleansing the clothes as well as the bed-linen is to boil them at a temperature of 200° F.

Under certain circumstances the proceeding here recommended may have to be somewhat modified. In a case of pustulous scabies which is so often met with among children, the pustules have to heal first, otherwise the soap would irritate the skin too much. According to their ages, children only require one-third, one-quarter or one-half of the quantity of ointment, and, on account of their skin being so much more tender, need not be kept in the baths, nor remain in the blankets as long as adults. If several members of a family are infected at the same time, they have to undergo the treatment simultaneously. Frictions with brown soap alone are hardly sufficient to kill the acari; still they may be resorted to twice a week in order to make doubly sure of the result.

After the cure which does not cause any marked irritation of the skin, this organ is allowed about a fortnight for its restoration to a normal condition. If, after this, any efflorescences remain, they are treated according to the principles laid down above. In most cases the daily use of a tepid or shower-bath is sufficient to complete the whole cure.

We have never known this treatment which can be easily pursued in a private family, to be followed by any of the terrible consecutive diseases described in the books.

Lest we should be accused of condemning what we know nothing about, we will here state that we have tried every remedy recommended for the itch by homœopathic practitioners, in the form of triturations, tinctures, attenuations, high and low potencies without the least benefit. The acari would not die and the pustules kept increasing in number. In one case, that of a child of six months, we fancied that *Sulphur* 6 did arrest very speedily the disposition to the formation of pustules.

We are satisfied that in making the preceding statements, we shall give offence to many homœopathic physicians, but we shall be happy to hear all condemnations and objections, and shall deem it a pleasure and a duty to answer them.

ELEVENTH SECTION.

Constitutional Diseases.

A. ACUTE AND CHRONIC CONTAGIOUS DISEASES.

1. Morbilli.

Measles.

Measles are not only a contagious, but a more or less universally epidemic form of disease. In most cases they arise by a transfer of the contagium. This is contained in the catarrhal secretions, and is transmitted by contact, and still more frequently by the air. It is not very susceptible of being indirectly transmitted by the clothing; this theory is probably adhered to with so much zeal for no other reason than because the doctrine that measles are contagious, is to be maintained at all hazards. The incubation-period of the transmitted contagium is eleven to twelve days, as anybody can easily determine for himself in any outbreak of epidemic measles. The contagium is most active shortly before the appearance of the exanthem upon the skin. We have observed this to be the rule in the epidemic that has now been raging among us for upwards of a year. An apparently mild catarrh is taken no notice of, the child is sent to school in spite of it, and next day the little one is down with the measles. Exactly on the twelfth day after, the nearest neighbors of the sick children are attacked. In this way schools become the true nurseries of the exanthem, whence it afterwards spreads to families. After the exanthem is once out, its infectious nature is decidedly less, and becomes entirely extinct as soon as desquamation sets in. Personally we hold that epidemic measles can spread without contagion, although this is not often the case. We likewise believe in this possibility in the case of scarlatina and small-pox. It would lead us too far, if we would corroborate this assertion by the evidence of facts; we bespeak so much more urgently the attention of our Colleagues to this fact in existing epidemics.

Measles attack individuals of every age and sex, but least frequently very old people and infants. Inasmuch as almost everybody has an attack of measles in his early youth, they are on this account seldom met with among old people. One attack of measles generally protects persons against a second one; exceptions, however, are not very rare, although it behooves us to guard against mistaking roseola for measles. [In the late war measles raged with great fierceness in many of our regiments, and, under allœopathic treatment, destroyed a number of lives. H.] No later than two weeks ago we treated two little girls in the same family who were down with the measles, one severely, the younger without any marked constitutional symptoms, but with the eruption in full bloom. Three weeks after desquamation had taken place, the younger child was again attacked with all the preliminary symptoms of measles; indeed, they again broke out with much intensity, attended with severe constitutional symptoms, but in other respects running their course regularly.

The ordinary season for measles are the months when catarrhs are common, from October till April; nevertheless measles raged here very extensively last summer, which, it is true, so far as the temperature was concerned, was more like winter. This circumstance alone ought to suffice to show that the measles are not exclusively propagated by a contagium.

Symptoms and Course. We have already stated that the incubation-period of the measle-contagium, until the efflorescences break out upon the skin, is eleven or at most twelve days. Whereas the general health does not seem in the least disturbed in the first eight to nine days of this period, definite preliminary symptoms show themselves in the last two or three days. These preliminary signs are falsely said to have been noticed at an earlier period; but inasmuch as catarrhal affections are very prevalent during epidemic measles, it is very likely that purely catarrhal symptoms have been mistaken for the prodromi of measles. The prodromi proper begin with a slight catarrh of the nose, lassitude and some fever. This fever increases considerably on the second day, frontal headache supervenes, the eyes look red, are sensitive to the light, but the conjunctiva is seldom puffed up. On the third day there is another increase of fever, the patients feel unable to sit up, the tongue is thickly coated, the appetite gone, and in the night from the third to the fourth day, immediately previous to the appearance of the exanthem, a hoarse, barking cough sets in resembling croup, which, however, is scarcely ever attended with the danger that generally characterizes croup, and never changes to true croup. These symptoms may increase to a considerable degree of intensity, may be associated with vomiting, delirium, sopor; at times, however, they are entirely wanting or so slight that it is not deemed necessary to confine children to the room. This is the reason why the measles spread so rapidly through the schools, for it is precisely on the day previous to the breaking out of the measles that the infectious principle is most active, and that hence the measles are most easily communicated. We account for this circumstance by the fact that in the last twenty-four to twelve hours previous to the appearance of the exanthem upon the skin, distinct, lentil-sized measle-spots are perceived in almost every case on the palate and on the sides of the fauces. We have noticed them in all our cases of the present as well as of last-year's epidemic. Without doubt, it is the extension of these spots to the larynx and trachea that causes the peculiar croupy cough, and we have always considered it an excellent diagnostic sign to find this cough associated with red spots on the palate, in which case we were able to positively predict the appearance of the eruption within twenty-four hours. In other respects the prodromi have no distinctive peculiarity from which the character of the exanthem might be inferred; it can at most only be suspected after several cases had already occurred in the place, or in its immediate vicinity. As a rule, adults suffer much less from prodromi than children, nor has, in the case of adults, the cough very often the croupy sound.

The measle-exanthem breaks out gradually, in one case more rapidly than in another. The first spots always show themselves in the face, most commonly on the cheeks and temples. They are of the size of lentils, of a bright redness and with rather sharp outlines; after being out for a short time, they become somewhat raised above the skin and harder to the feel than this organ. With more or less speed, generally within twenty-four to thirty-six hours, the exanthem comes out over the whole body from above downwards, and is fully out in forty-eight to sixty hours, so that no new spots appear, whereas, up to that time, new spots had continued to break out in addition to the first spots that were more or less scattered and isolated. The spots keep growing in size to such an extent that some of them run together, and the normal skin, in the place of spots, exhibits here and there irregular red patches. In proportion as the exanthem comes out more profusely, its color generally grows darker, sometimes with a bluish tint. With the fuller development of the eruption the constitutional symptoms most commonly increase in intensity. The catarrh of the conjunctiva and the cough especially grow much worse. The pulse sometimes increases to one hundred and forty beats. Sometimes the skin is dry, but at other times covered with perspiration. In very rare cases the constitutional equilibrium remains undisturbed even during the eruptive stage; however, in every considerable epidemic a child with measles is occasionally seen running about the streets.

If the exanthem runs a benign course, its decrease commences at the end of the third day, seldom before this time, and continues with great rapidity until the eruption has entirely disappeared. The spots grow smaller, assume a distinctly yellowish tint which is especially marked on pressure with the finger, and within twelve to twenty-four hours the spots have completed their disappearance without leaving a vestige of their existence. Very frequently, however, the yellowish tint remains for several days. The fever declines very speedily, the catarrh of the conjunctiva likewise abates, whereas the bronchial catarrh most generally continues for a few days longer, and resolution sometimes does not take place until a considerable quantity of mucus has formed. Not unfrequently the patient is at this period attacked with diarrhœa for one or two days. Profuse perspiration is not the rule, but is not by any means an anomalous occurrence.

Desquamation commonly commences on the seventh day, but may delay until the fourteenth. The epidermis comes off in bran-shaped scales, very seldom in larger patches; in the face and on the extremities the desquamation is most distinct. During this period the general health is generally good; except that the bronchial catarrh and still less frequently the diarrhœa may continue to some extent. In very few cases the irritation of the conjunctiva likewise continues some time longer.

According to the nature of the epidemic or other supervening disturbances this normal course of the measles undergoes various modifications which we now proceed to point out, classifying them as benign, that is such as do not complicate the prognosis, and as malignant. We ought to observe, however, that under certain circumstances every anomaly in the course of the measles may become a bad omen, and that we have to watch every case where deviations from the normal course occur, with redoubled attention.

Among the anomalies of a benign character we class the following:

The eruption does not break out in the face first, or comes out sparsely on the rest of the body.

The single spots are topped with little tubercles or vesicles.

The exanthem comes out more slowly than usual, and the spots remain much longer, sometimes beyond a week.

In the case of little children the appearance of the exanthem is attended with symptoms of severe cerebral hyperæmia or even convulsions.

The cough retains its croupy sound beyond the first day or even during the whole course of the exanthem.

Among the malignant deviations we number the following:

The spots, when first coming out, are of a pale-red color which does not increase in intensity, nor does it acquire the yellowish tint. Within the spots hæmorrhagic appearances are manifested, and between the spots ecchymoses are noticed. The spots fade away soon after their appearance, or else they fade very suddenly at the regular period or before.

In the case of children the pulse exceeds 140 beats, and in the case of adults 120 beats; moreover it is a small pulse. The tongue is dry. Angina tonsillaris. Diphtheritic membranes form in the buccal cavity. The respiration becomes hurried and superficial. Sopor and delirium after the second day of the eruption.

Of great importance are certain complications of measles, that are very apt to occur and which were formerly regarded as metastases, because the exanthem disappears with the appearance of these complications. Laryngitis with croupous exudation is of rare occurrence while the exanthem is still out; it is more commonly met with after the exanthem has left the skin. A slight bronchitis is an accompaniment of every case of measles; it only assumes a dangerous character if it continues beyond the stage of decline, or reappears again during the stage of desquamation, or otherwise assumes a very acute form. It is very apt to run into an exceedingly obstinate chronic catarrh. Pneumonia is not unfrequent; it is mostly lobular, much less frequently lobar, and may break out in every stage of the disease. It is most threatening, if setting in after the eruption has run its course. It does not usually terminate in complete resorption and, on this account, is very apt to lay the foundation for subsequent pulmonary phthisis. Pleuritis is a rare complication, so is pericarditis. Enteritis is a rather frequent complication in some epidemics; it excites legitimate apprehensions, for the reason that other consecutive diseases, more particularly scrofulosis, are apt to follow in its train. Affections of the brain are rare; their intensity is rarely such as to excite apprehensions; the supervention of sopor is a bad sign, because it may usher in a fatal general paralysis.

Of the highest importance are likewise the numerous and always obstinate sequelæ of the measles, which make this exanthem one of the most malignant, whereas its ordinary normal course and character entitle it to be regarded as one of the most harmless. Among these sequelæ we distinguish:

Cutaneous affections, especially impetigo and eczema, more or less extensive, but always very obstinate.

Chronic conjunctivitis, with impaired vision; chronic otitis, with deafness; chronic ozæna; chronic inflammation of the lymphatic glands, mostly without suppuration; chronic inflammation of the parotid and submaxillary glands.

Chronic bronchial catarrh, with which bronchiectasia easily becomes associated and which gives rise to a peculiar spasmodic cough; or real whooping-cough which is much more severe as a sequela of measles than when setting in at other periods, and which very often develops a most dangerous lobular pneumonia.

Anasarca with affection of the kidneys is a very rare sequela of measles; it is not exactly an occurrence of a threatening character.

Noma is likewise a sequela of rare occurrence; it is not without importance.

After the measles, children are very frequently attacked with scrofulous symptoms. It is very likely that, in the case of little children, the measles simply act as an exciting cause of scrofulosis; but it is likewise among larger children that, after an attack of measles, all sorts of phenomena make their appearance, which we are in the habit of designating as scrofulous and which go to show that a morbid change has been impressed upon the whole activity of the organism.

Tuberculosis likewise frequently breaks out after measles. We believe with Niemeyer that pulmonary phthisis after measles is most commonly a chronic lobular pneumonia, having nothing in common with tubercles, or else, a lobular pneumonia with suppuration. That tubercles not unfrequently do occur after measles, is shown to us by the circumstance that we have recently lost three children with acute hydrocephalus, in the neighborhood of Hannover, where the measles prevailed much more fiercely than in the city. In every one of these three children the symptoms of acute hydrocephalus set in soon after the measles.

Treatment. Measles are universally regarded as a typical disease, on which account the so-called rational physicians consider every interference with medicines in a case of measles running their normal course, as useless. From the stand-point of Homœopathy this negative treatment on the part of our opponents, is liable to several important objections. In the first place the measles do not constitute a fixed typical exanthem, for, as regards time, they vary greatly both with respect to the time it takes the eruption to come out, and to the duration of the stage of efflorescence. It is conceivable that this irregularity in the course of the exanthem may be modified by medicines, and every homœopathic physician will agree with us in the statement that, under homœopathic treatment, the measles very seldom run an irregular course. A second proposition the correctness of which has been demonstrated by an abundance of clinical experience, is that under homœopathic treatment complications are rare occurrences and that sequelæ are seen still less frequently. All our most excellent observers, of whom we number a great many, agree with us in this statement. It is, therefore, our advice to treat every case of measles, even the mildest, with a little medicine, although the action of the medicine may not always be distinctly perceived.

The preliminary stage of measles, if there is otherwise nothing abnormal in the existing symptoms, requires either *Aconite* or *Belladonna*. We prefer the latter if the fever is purely catarrhal, the skin is hot but moist, the tongue thickly coated, the pulse hurried but neither hard nor full. These symptoms were uniformly present in the preliminary stage of our last epidemic. We prefer Aconite if the skin is hot and dry, the catarrhal secretion scanty, the tongue is red and the pulse full and hard. We have never seen the much vaunted Pulsatilla do the least good at this stage of the disease, and we are at a loss to perceive upon what grounds the exhibition of this drug could be justified. The croupy cough is a good indication for *Belladonna;* at any rate, we have never seen it last longer than twenty-four hours after this remedy had been given. Others recommend *Spongia* or *Hepar sulphuris calc.*, either of which may be a suitable remedy according to circumstances. *Aconite* renders excellent service for this croupy, catarrhal cough. If the exanthem had begun to come out, the best course then is to continue the remedy that had been given last, for beside the spots no other symptoms generally make their appearance: the increased, but short-lasting intensity of the existing symptoms does not justify a change of remedies, for the reason that such an increase of the symptoms inheres in the normal course of the disease. As soon as the eruption begins to pale off, we advise the discontinuance of all medicine. If the spots have entirely disappeared, yet the cough continues, the treatment will have to be resumed; if the cough is attended with rattling and wheezing, and the expectoration is not very difficult, *Hepar sulphuris calc.* is to be given; if the cough is particularly troublesome at night, and is otherwise loose, not very hard, *Pulsatilla* may be required; for a dry, nocturnal, titillating cough we give *Hyoscyamus*, and if the cough torments the patient the whole day: *Nux vomica*. The general management of the patient is of great importance, for it is a certain fact that an irregular course of the eruption is sometimes attributable to hygienic neglect or to the enforcement of improper rules and measures. We forbear showing in this place how the poor measle-patients were formerly abused, and still are very frequently abused by insane nurses and practitioners. We pursue the following course from which we have never seen any bad consequences result. If the measles prevail, we have the children who complain of a febrile catarrh, kept at home, but do not confine them to their beds unless they themselves insist upon it. A measle-patient should never be covered too warmly, nor should he ever remain in a temperature above 50° Fahr. The room should be carefully and cautiously ventilated; pure air is of immense benefit to the patient. The room should never be obscured more than is desired by the patients themselves. The best beverage is fresh water in small quantities; if this should increase the cough, the water may be drank with the chill taken off, sweetened with a little white sugar. There is no danger involved in daily ablutions of the patient's face and hands with tepid water. Owing to the impaired appetite there is danger of the patients being treated to improper food. We never refuse stewed fruit; and we allow meat and broth if the patient craves it. After the spots have disappeared and the cough has ceased, or nearly so, we have the patient transferred every morning from the bed into a lukewarm bath, where he is thoroughly washed with soap and afterwards well rubbed dry in a woollen blanket. Next morning he is rapidly washed with cold water and again rubbed off in a woollen blanket. We now regard him as fully recovered and, if the weather permits, send him out into the open air, of course, with all suitable guarantees against taking cold. We have never yet seen any bad consequences result from this treatment.

We will now mention the treatment that ought to be pursued for some of the deviations from the normal course, and likewise for the complications and sequelæ, for it is these abnormal conditions that require a most thorough knowledge of the appropriate remedies.

If the eruption is unusually pale, we have to suspect the presence of complications, and if they cannot be traced, we give *Veratrum album* or *Ipecacuanha;* if the exanthem disappears all at once, without any apparent complication, *Arsenicum, Opium* or *Digitalis* will have to be given according to circumstances. If the measle-spots are hemorrhagic, *Phosphorus* and *Arsenicum* are suitable, sometimes also *Mercurius.* Angina, which is a rare occurrence in this disease, requires *Belladonna, Mercurius,* or *Apis.* Delirium and sopor after the exanthem is out, may require *Rhus toxicodendron, Zincum,* or *Opium; Ipecacuanha* may likewise have to be used. This last-named remedy likewise arrests the vomiting which sometimes precedes the appearance of the exanthem. A moderate diarrhœa does not require any treatment; if it becomes too copious and painful, *Mercurius,* or *Veratrum album,* or *Phosphorus* and *Ipecacuanha* may have to be given. Adults retain for some time a thickly-coated tongue, and an impaired appetite, for which symptoms *Antimonium crudum* is an excellent remedy, and, if the tongue is clean, *Ipecacuanha.* These remedies should be given at once if the appetite does not return immediately after the spots have begun to pale off.

Complications require the same treatment that is pursued if they occur without measles, hence, we refer the reader to the chapters on pneumonia, bronchitis, pleuritis, etc. But we must not forget that these complications are very dangerous and may easily adopt an abnormal course; pneumonia, for instance, may assume a chronic form, pleuritis may be transformed into pleuritis serosa.

Like the complications, so the sequelæ do not require any special treatment on account of the measles; for special conditions, however, certain remedies have become exceedingly valuable. A chronic bronchial catarrh is one of the most common sequelæ, and is generally very obstinate; not to mention other remedies that are specially indicated by particular symptoms, *Sulphur* is the regular curative remedy in such a case, which we deem, however, equalled by *Causticum.* If the cough is accompanied with hoarseness, *Carbo vegetabilis* as well as *Tartarus stibiatus* will meet the case, if an abundance of mucus is secreted. If the cough changes more and more to a croupy cough, *Cuprum* has to be given the sooner the better. The subsequent hoarseness or even aphonia constitute great impediments to a cure. With the exception of *Carbo vegetabilis, Iodine* is the only remedy that has shown any curative results in our hands for this affection; all other remedies have proved fruitless, and it has only been in the course of time that the natural voice returned. Phthisis after measles can only be regarded as tubercular, if no sign of pneumonia had been noticed either during the acute stage of the exanthem, or during the period of convalescence; if symptoms of pneumonia had existed, we may take it for granted that the existing phthisis is the result of chronic pneumonia. This point is important on account of the remedies that have to be used; for in the last-mentioned case *Sulphur, Hepar sulphuris,* and *Iodine* are the chief remedies, whereas in tubercular phthisis these remedies are of no higher importance than others. Chronic diarrhœa is likewise completely cured by means of *Sulphur,* likewise by means of *Phosphori acidum.* Catarrhal conjunctivitis, if setting in in the stage of desquamation, is exceedingly obstinate. The conjunctiva is not very much thickened, but very red and unusually sensitive to a glaring light as well as to intensely cold air. For this trouble *Arsenicum* does more than any other remedy; only it must not be discontinued too soon, because the result generally develops itself very tardily.

2. Scarlatina.
Scarlet-fever.

Scarlatina is unquestionably a contagious disease; at times it occurs in a sporadic, but more frequently in an epidemic form. What is the nature of this contagium, and what contains it, cannot be determined, but many circumstances argue in favor of the doctrine that it is transmitted through the air. It is often indisputable and certainly more probable than in the case of measles, that scarlatina sometimes breaks out spontaneously and sporadically without any infectious contagium, and likewise epidemically, in which category belong the cases where scarlatina is said to have been transmitted indirectly through the agency of non-affected individuals. It is difficult to determine the duration of the period of incubation; it is generally supposed to last eight days. The contagium is most fiercely active soon after the appearance of the exanthem, during the period of desquamation the contagious nature of scarlatina has most probably become extinct. The susceptibility to the influence of the scarlatina-contagium is much less general than that to the measle contagium; many persons escape scarlatina altogether. The largest number and the most malignant cases occur between the second and seventh year, a much smaller number between the eight and twenty-fifth year. At a later period, as well as during infancy, scarlatina occurs very seldom. One attack of scarlatina acts almost as an absolutely certain preventive against any subsequent attacks. Epidemic scarlatina most commonly prevails during the transition-seasons, less frequently in the summer, and least frequently in winter. Although certain atmospheric conditions may be supposed to exist during the prevalence of scarlatina, yet they are unknown to us; nor are we able to explain what circumstances render one epidemic so dangerous and leave another comparatively mild. Epidemic scarlatina very often occurs simultaneously with, or subsequently to epidemic measles; it likewise not unfrequently occurs together with small-pox; its relation to whooping-cough is less definite.

Symptoms and Course. No acute exanthem is so variable in its course as scarlatina, although certain fixed types are always recognizable. The various epidemics differ very particularly from each other. We have not space to consider all these particular differences and shall therefore content ourselves with describing the normal course of ordinary benign scarlatina, and shall afterwards mention the deviations from this course, as we have done when treating of measles.

The disease is undoubtedly ushered in by a precursory stage which has no characteristic symptoms any more than the prodromic stage of measles. The patients exhibit the symptoms of a severe catarrhal fever which, in contra-distinction to measles, is not attended with an irritation of the respiratory tract, but with inflammation of the fauces and catarrh of the stomach. This stage differs in no respect from a catarrhal angina, not even by the pulse which, in an affection of this kind, is generally very rapid. Only the skin of the patient is much less frequently moist.

After the prodromi have lasted for two days, the exanthem makes its appearance, generally with a marked increase of the fever and the other preliminary symptoms; children are attacked with convulsions. The exanthem always first breaks out on the neck, whence it spreads downwards over the rest of the body. First we notice closely-crowded red stigmata, generally of a much darker color than the measle-spots; these stigmata very speedily run into one another, causing an homogeneous, faintly dotted redness (scarlatina lævigata), or else they grow in size and, running together, form single spots of a darker color, seated upon a more faintly-red cuticle (scarlatina variegata), or, finally, small vesicles spring up upon the red surface, most generally in consequence of the intense character of the cutaneous affection, some of which are closely crowded together, others are more scattered (scarlatina miliaris). The exanthem is generally fully out in twenty-four hours, when the stage of efflorescence commences. The redness is most intense on the neck and on the extensor-surface of the extremities, likewise on the hands. Throughout this stage the constitutional symptoms preserve their intensity, but the fever begins to abate in the last two days; it does not pass away suddenly, as in the case of measles. The angina is very intense, the fauces are dark-red; the tongue, having got rid of its original coating, looks very dark, with prominent papillæ, imparting to it a strawberry appearance. The urinary secretion is much less. Sometimes a little bronchial catarrh makes its appearance at this time, but it scarcely ever assumes a violent form.

On the fifth or sixth day after the appearance of the exanthem, it commences to pale off, with considerable abatement of the fever and more particularly of the angina. Soon after, the process of desquamation begins. It always commences on the neck in small scales, whereas on the body, and more particularly on the hands, the epidermis most generally peels off in large patches. The appetite now speedily returns and the patients feel quite well. In a fortnight at the latest the desquamation is completed.

We will now consider the most important anomalies in the course of the disease, corresponding with the order in which the different stages succeed each other.

The preliminary stage may be so slight that it may seem as though no such stage had existed. This, however, does not justify the expectation that the disease will run a mild course. On the contrary, if the preliminary stage is considerably longer than usual; if an excessive lassitude is a marked symptom of this stage, we may almost expect with certainty that the disease will assume a comparatively malignant character. Occasionally the fever reaches even at this stage a height that gives to it the appearance of an intense typhus, so that the patients soon fall victims to its fury. At this stage the angina is never so violent as to cause any anxiety. The convulsions occurring at the breaking out of the exanthem are seldom of any particular significance, for an affection of the brain, except in so far as the excessive fever may cause an irritation of this organ, is a rare occurrence.

It is during the eruptive stage and the stage of efflorescence that the course of the exanthem can be watched and learnt. It varies in color, is at times bright-red, at other times of a violet-red, without these distinctions justifying any particular inferences being drawn from them. An extremely bright color is an inauspicious prognostic only if the fever has at the same time a marked adynamic type. A union of the smaller spots to larger patches of redness is of no great importance. The formation of petechiæ and larger hemorrhagic effusions on the skin always points to a severe type of fever. In some epidemics the exanthem remains quite rudimentary, the redness is very slight, is confined to small spots of a bright rose-color, remains only a few days upon the skin and is not attended with any marked constitutional symptoms. Such cases have been designated as roseola or rubeola, and an attempt has been made to view this exanthem as a special form of disease. The fact that roseola occurs in every mild scarlatina-epidemic, shows that it is nothing else than a very slightly developed case of scarlatina.

The angina is likewise liable to important deviations. It is generally of an erythematous character, but not unfrequently involves the parenchyma and shows an extraordinary tendency to invade the glands and cellular tissue of the throat and neck. Since this change does not occur until the exanthem has run its course, it has been supposed that it is the result of a metastasis, which is not the case. Whereas a parenchymatous angina seldom terminates in suppuration, an inflammation of the cervical cellular tissue, on the contrary, has this termination so much more readily; it is this circumstance which constitutes one of the most malignant sequelæ of the disease. What is still more dangerous is the supervention of diphtheritic ulcers during the inflammation. Although the diphtheritic ulceration very seldom spreads to the larynx, it communicates itself so much more frequently to the nose, the Eustachian tube and the inner ear, to the cervical cellular tissue and glands; if it does not destroy life by its direct action, the patients succumb slowly to the suppurative process, or are attacked with an incurable deafness. Not too much attention can be paid to this malignant angina, especially in the case of children, an examination of whose throats we are very apt to neglect in consequence of the difficulty attending such an operation. A discharge from the nose which is at first thin and has no smell, is almost always a sure sign that diphtheritis has set in; it should never be regarded as a favorable symptom, for the reason that a simple nasal catarrh never occurs in scarlatina.

Inflammations of the joints, pleura, pericardium most commonly only occur in cases of great intensity, and do not present any particular features, although they render the prognosis much more dubious and complicated.

Nephritis occurring at this stage, is never very acute, and is so much inferior to the other morbid phenomena that it is allowed to pass unperceived.

The most obstinate and most dangerous anomalies occur in the stage of desquamation. They do not always date from this period, but are most generally developments of former disturbances that had remained unnoticed during the violence of the fever. This applies to inflammations of the joints, pleura, pericardium, inner ear. Enteritis occurs very rarely; on the other hand, diarrhœa may set in, which, within certain limits, is not a dangerous occurrence. The worst symptoms are the suppurating inflammations of the cervical cellular tissue and lymphatic glands, to which allusion was made previously, and inflammation of the kidneys. During the process of desquamation nephritis becomes a more prominent complication, probably because a suspension of the cutaneous functions, as in extensive burns for example, excites the action of the kidneys in an extraordinary degree, in consequence of which a slight renal catarrh, during the stage of efflorescence, changes to a genuine croupous inflammation during the stage of desquamation. The various reasons which have been adduced to account for the supervening nephritis, do not stand the test of a rigorous examination; in some epidemics there is no nephritis at all, in other epidemics it occurs in every case, no matter how the patients were managed in hygienic and dietetic respects. What is certain is, that nephritis is more easily excited by excessive warmth, especially by too much clothing, which precludes the access of air, than by the patient being kept in a cool room and accessible to the influence of pure air. The renal affection sets in almost imperceptibly; the patients have felt quite well for several days; but, without showing any symptoms of fever, they do not seem properly to recuperate. The appetite does not return as it should; the discharged urine is dark, and the quantity is scanty; suddenly it shows a still darker, sometimes black or blackish-gray color, and contains a quantity of albumen, blood-disks, fibrinous cylindrical casts. The appetite is gone, the skin becomes œdematous first in the face, and afterwards over the whole body, and to a very high degree. If we do not succeed in controlling the renal affection, the patients die in two or more weeks of œdema of the lungs, or of cardiac disease.

In some rare cases œdema sets in as a post-scarlatinal complication without the signs of a marked renal disease; this affection is of infinitely less importance than that which we have just described.

All these deviations, complications, etc., vary with the character of the epidemic, both as regards intensity and danger. It is almost impossible, when the epidemic first commences, to establish a prognosis upon a reliable basis; apparently trivial cases sometimes take all at once a bad turn, whereas apparently severe cases run a very normal course. For this reason every epidemic requires to be specially studied; not one epidemic resembles another in every respect.

Treatment. In regard to treatment we apply to scarlatina the same rule that we have proposed for measles, which is, that the specifically-appropriate remedy should be given at the very onset of the disease, because this is the most efficient method of keeping the course of the disease within normal bounds. We infer this from the circumstance that the homœopathic treatment of scarlatina is undoubtedly superior to any other; for this reason we advise the exhibition of *Belladonna* at the very commencement of the disease, this remedy not only corresponding to the cutaneous affection, but likewise to the angina. This medicine should be continued, provided no particular anomalies set in, until the exanthem begins to pale, the angina disappears, and the pulse decreases in frequency. Under the use of Belladonna the fever generally runs a regular course, during which the special symptoms of course do not undergo any alteration; but this is not expected in the course of any typical affection. Whether *Belladonna* can be regarded as a prophylactic against scarlatina, we will not decide, although we are willing to admit that we doubt the prophylactic virtues of this agent for the simple reason that we do not believe in any kind of preventives. We have already stated that scarlatina does not infect everybody with the same facility, and we have known more than one family where one child was taken down with scarlatina, and the other children all remained well, without Belladonna having been given them. Before discussing the treatment of anomalies occurring during the course of scarlatina, we will first indicate the diet to be pursued during the normal course of the disease. Even at this time a great repugnance still seems to prevail against allowing scarlet-fever patients still less than measle-patients the blessing of pure air and cleanliness; the rule was to confine patients to their rooms full six weeks. Even Hirschel lays this down as a rule in his "Treasure of Medicine." This is evidently the result of erroneous views concerning the sequelæ. Since they apparently originate in the desquamative period, it was supposed that the sequelæ had to be traced to a disturbance of the process of desquamation. The most common disturbance was supposed to be a cold. We have endeavored to show that the commencement of all post-scarlatinal diseases is traceable to the stage of efflorescence, hence that they are continuations of previous beginnings, not new diseases; and we here add that the obstinacy of many a consecutive disorder is owing to wrong management during the disease itself and immediately after. From abundant personal experience we recommend the following rules. The patients should be kept from the commencement of the disease in an uniform temperature of from forty to fifty degrees F., and should only be covered with a linen sheet and blankets. If possible, the sick-chamber should be ventilated several times a day, of course with all proper precautions. The patient may be allowed to drink pretty large quantities of fresh water, because the fever deprives the body of a large quantity of moisture. The juice of fruit is a refreshing beverage, and may be allowed in moderation; if used too freely, it is apt to cause nausea and a bad taste in the mouth. Pure malt-beer we have never known to do any harm. The patients not desiring any food, gruels, milk, and wheaten bread or bread made of unbolted flour, are sufficient nourishment. As soon as the pulse has become normal, the redness has disappeared, and the desquamation is fully established, the patients may be allowed to rise, but the temperature of the room must be a little higher than while they were confined to their beds. A fortnight after the disease first broke out, a general ablution, as has been recommended for measles, may take place, and, if the weather permits, the patient may be sent out of the house, of course with all suitable precautions. No reason can be imagined why such a treatment should be injurious.

Scarlatina.

We will now devote some space to the treatment of the anomalies that may turn up during the course of the disease, but we shall not go into details concerning particular indications, for the reason that every epidemic has, after all, to be combated with specifically-appropriate medicines whose symptomatic correspondence will have to be studied out in the Materia Medica.

The excessive fever in the preliminary stage, which is often of a threatening character, has to be met by *Rhus toxicod.* or *Arsenicum*, as long as the brain remains free; but if delirium, sopor, etc., sets in, *Phosphorus* or *Opium* may be tried; we would likewise recommend Digitalis.—If convulsions set in previous to the appearance of the exanthem, *Belladonna* is entirely sufficient. If the fever sets in with an adynamic type, and the exanthem delays its appearance, *Bryonia alba* will meet this condition.

We do not dwell upon supposed distinctions between smooth scarlatina and purple-rash, because we believe them to be unfounded. We admit that in cases where the angina is very slight or entirely wanting, *Aconite* is better adapted to purple-rash than Belladonna. If the efflorescent surface is studded with miliaria, *Rhus toxicod.* is more appropriate than Belladonna. If petechiæ and ecchymoses break out, the fever generally has an adynamic character; *Phosphorus*, *Arsenicum* and *Kreosotum* are the remedies adapted to this change.

If the fever has an adynamic type during the stage of efflorescence, great danger is impending. *Bryonia* may be sufficient in the lower grades of this fever, but the higher grades require: *Rhus toxicod.*, *Phosphorus*, *Digitalis*, *Veratrum album;* the two last-named remedies correspond more particularly to the frequent and small pulse with cerebral symptoms resembling typhus. *Ammonium carbon.* may deserve a preference, if the pulse accompanying the cerebral symptoms is not excessively rapid. *Zincum* is likewise recommended in such cases. If a sudden disappearance of the redness is attended with ominous symptoms; if a general paralysis threatens, *Camphora* should be resorted to. The special symptomatic indications of these various remedies can be learnt from the Materia Medica Pura.

The angina, even if only of an erythematous character, is sometimes intense, and Belladonna does not seem to have the least effect upon it. In such a case *Apis* not unfrequently mitigates the severe pain. If we may judge by the provings, this agent must be an important remedy in scarlet-fever; the clinical record of this drug is still very scanty. Whether Apis will prevent the inflammation from penetrating to the deeper tissues, has not yet been decided. If the angina is accompanied by swelling of the tonsils, *Mercurius* should be given; this remedy often arrests all further progress of this feature of the disease. If the angina is confined to the tonsils, it will seldom be found necessary to give *Hepar*, for the reason that no suppuration generally sets in. If suppuration takes place, *Hepar sulphuris calc.* should be resorted to without delay. If the inflammation invades the cervical cellular tissue and the cervical glands, which it may do while Mercurius is being exhibited, in which case this remedy is no longer indicated, *Bryonia* may be given. We do not advise a premature lancing of the abscess, because such a proceeding would undoubtedly favor an ichorous decomposition. For chronic suppuration we recommend *Silicea*, for subsequent indurations *Baryta* and *Sulphur*.

A malignant form of angina requires the same treatment as diphtheritis. *Iodine* has frequently rendered excellent service in this affection; *Acidum muriaticum* is likewise commended; but, as we said before, such recommendations are not always to be depended upon in all cases, for the reason that one remedy will do better in one epidemic, and the very next epidemic may require a different treatment. A scarlatina-coryza sometimes requires a peculiar treatment; it often remains even after the diphtheritic angina is cured. *Aurum muriaticum* is the most reliable remedy for it; *Sepia* or *Calcarea carbon.* is less so.

Parotitis is very seldom an isolated affection in scarlatina; it is generally accompanied by a malignant or parenchymatous angina and requires to be treated with the same remedies that have been recommended for this disorder. If existing alone, we treat it with the remedies that have been recommended for it elsewhere.

Pleuritis and pericarditis as complications of scarlatina have no peculiar features requiring any special treatment; they are treated as idiopathically-existing, independent diseases; however, we may state that *Tartarus stibiatus* has been variously recommended in pericarditis, and *Mercurius* and *Rhus toxicod.* in pleuritis.

Articular inflammations in scarlatina have the peculiar feature of rarely terminating in suppuration and resembling almost entirely articular rheumatism. *Arnica*, *Phosphorus* and *Rhus toxicod.* deserve special attention in these affections.

Cerebral affections occur very rarely in scarlatina; isolated cerebral symptoms, although sometimes very marked, must not be all at once taken for inflammatory symptoms. If the symptoms denote congestion, with nervous excitement and restlessness, *Arnica* or *Ammonium carbon.* may be resorted to; if they occur accompanied by a cold perspiration and coolness of the trunk, *Ipecac.*, *Camphora*, *Veratrum album* may be tried; marked sopor indicates *Opium*, convulsions point to *Zincum.*—We should always endeavor to determine whether the cerebral symptoms are not altogether superinduced by the intense fever and whether our remedies ought not to be primarily directed against it.

For nephritis and dropsy *Helleborus* has acquired a well-earned reputation; it sometimes relieves these affections very speedily. However, it is not sufficient in every case. If the urine contains a good deal of blood, *Cantharides* and *Terebinthina* may have to be given; *Arnica* and *Nitrum* likewise deserve our regard in this direction. If threatening heart-symptoms supervene, *Arsenicum* should at once be resorted to, and if the renal inflammation has already run its course, *Digitalis* or *Lycopodium*.

Finally we wish to make mention of cold water in connection with scarlatina. The not unfavorable results of cold-water treatment while the exanthem is out on the skin, may serve to quiet anxious physicians regarding the danger which they imagine their patients would incur if they were not kept very warm or were not forbidden the luxury of a refreshing, although ever so carefully conducted ablution. We would not resort to the cold pack during the efflorescent stage, for we have remedies that surpass the cold-water treatment in efficacy. Whether cold water will still prove useful if the exanthem recedes from the skin, is not certain; it can only be resorted to as a last resort in such a contingency. During the period of desquamation cold-water treatment is decidedly in its place. If there is nothing abnormal in the course of the disease, the baths and ablutions which we have recommended for measles, are sufficient; but if œdema has set in, these means are not sufficient, for the skin has to be kept very active. In the case of little children who object to being packed, we sometimes accomplish our purpose by placing them every day in a warm bath of at least 92° F., leaving them in each bath for 15 or 20 minutes, after which we have the little patients carefully dried and wrapt in a woollen blanket for half an hour. Most generally, however, the wet pack is indispensable; of course it ought not to be used to excess and after each pack the patient ought to be rubbed down very thoroughly. In a few days already perspiration begins to set in, when the patient may be considered safe. Under this management we have not yet had to deplore a single loss from post-scarlatinal dropsy.

3. Variola.
Small-Pox.

It is with a certain timidity that we enter upon a discussion of this subject, because we are aware that our views in this respect differ greatly from the views ordinarily entertained by physicians; nevertheless space is wanting to enable us to substantiate our views by corresponding arguments. We shall have this privilege in due time, in a more appropriate place.

Small-pox is chiefly the result of infection. The contagium undoubtedly resides in the contents of the variola-pustules, probably also in the exhalations and in the secretions of the mucous membrane. Although it has been proven beyond a doubt that the contents of the pustules retain their infectious principle for a long time, provided it is kept from great heat and is not exposed to the action of atmospheric air, yet we cannot subscribe to the doctrine that the exhalations adhering to the patient's clothing retain for a long time the power of transmitting the disease; hence we believe in a spontaneous origin of variola as well as of scarlatina. The circumstance that small-pox at times only appears sporadically, and at other times breaks out epidemically, likewise speaks in favor of our views. The contagium is not very volatile. It is simple in its nature, that is to say, the same in each of the three species of the small-pox disease, so that varicella may cause variola in one, and varioloid in another. Hence these distinctions do not result from so many distinct contagia, but from the different susceptibilities of the infected individuals, as is likewise the case with measles and scarlatina. For similar reasons we do not attribute the malignant character of one small-pox epidemic and the mild type of another to differences in the nature of the contagium, but to different degrees of susceptibility in the individuals, as well as to other circumstances of a general or local character, upon which the malignant nature of the epidemic depends; precisely as we know similar results to take place during epidemic scarlatina. There is not an individual living of whom we can positively assert that he is inaccessible to the small-pox contagium; it is true, however, that at times the susceptibility seems to be considerably greater, and that it is unquestionably most intense in childhood and up to the age of forty-five years, beyond which it begins to decline. The same proportion obtains in all epidemic, and likewise in all non-infectious diseases. One attack of small-pox is a tolerably sure, but not an absolutely certain protection against another attack. This accounts for the apparent immunity of numbers of people; while young, they had an attack of varicella without the fact being noticed, and on this account enjoy a protection against small-pox, which is improperly attributed to vaccination, concerning which we shall give further details when speaking of the treatment. Epidemic small-pox breaks out most commonly in mid-summer, very seldom in winter; it is most generally accompanied by epidemic measles and whooping-cough; yet a connection or logical succession between these epidemics cannot be traced.

Symptoms and Course. For the sake of convenience and in obedience to custom, we adopt the division of the variolous disease in varicella, varioloid and variola, although these three forms generally exist in the most varied transitions to each other, so that, in a case of varicella, single pustules assume the form of varioloid-pustules and in cases of varioloid, some pustules adopt the form of variola-pustules, or that the whole exanthem runs a medium course between two of these forms.

Varicella or chicken-pox constitutes the mildest form under which the variola-disease with contagious pustules develops itself. Chicken-pox is infectious and may give rise to either of the other two forms. It infects more particularly children, although not exclusively. Quite recently we treated a case where a young man of eighteen years, who had varioloid, infected his sister, a child of six months, with variola, and his mother with a very mild form of varicella.

This eruption generally sets in without any precursory symptoms, perhaps with slight symptoms of gastric catarrh, but otherwise very seldom with precursory symptoms resembling those of varioloid. A few red stigmata break out in the face which grow rapidly and spread irregularly over the whole body; the largest number are seen on the chest and back. Each of these red stigmata changes in a few hours to an elevated vesicle, the contents of which grow dim in thirty-six to forty hours, and afterwards form thin scabs that fall off already on the seventh day. The vesicles sometimes breaking out in successive crops, the whole exanthem may require a fortnight to complete its course. Very commonly some of the vesicles grow to larger pustules, like variola-pustules, and leaving scars behind. At the same time the general health is often so little impaired, especially if the vesicles are not numerous, that the family have not the remotest suspicion of the child being sick. Fever, however, is very commonly present on the first days, even a mild delirium not unfrequently occurs, the appetite is gone, the patients feel languid, complain of headache and difficulty of swallowing caused by the vesicles having broken out in the throat and on the palate. The constitutional symptoms are never very important. The exhalations from such patients have the same odor as those of varioloid patients.

Varioloid, or modified variola, always commences with a distinct, but not characteristic precursory stage. The patients experience a violent chill, or most frequently chilly creepings which are at once succeeded by a violent febrile heat with increased temperature and a rapid pulse, and with such an intense feeling of illness, that the approach of a severe disease is unmistakable. With the gastric symptoms, a violent headache and even active delirium become associated, and likewise a somewhat pathognomonic, severe pain in the back and small of the back. As a rule, the fever remits in the morning and exacerbates in the evening, increasing every day in intensity until it reaches its acme on the third evening, when the eruptive stage commences. Shortly previous to the appearance of the exanthem, an hyperæmia, consisting of large spots, is sometimes perceived on various portions of the skin.

The exanthem in most cases first breaks out in the face, whence it spreads with tolerable regularity over the whole body, from above downwards. Red, scattered, lentil-sized spots break out. Each single spot passes through the following course of development. In ten to twelve hours it changes to a papula, which, in the next twenty-four hours, becomes transformed into a vesicle, the centre of which is perforated by a hair and correspondingly depressed. In the next twenty-four to forty-eight hours the contents of the vesicle grow dim, and a pustule forms surrounded by a narrow halo. About the sixth day after the breaking out of the exanthem, the contents dry up, giving rise to a brown scab which falls off in three to four days, leaving the spot somewhat injected. This course of development of one pock is not pursued by all the other pocks simultaneously, but occurs in the order in which the exanthem broke out, so that the whole process requires about eleven days or a fortnight until the scabs have completely formed. The general health shows the following changes while these phenomena are taking place upon the skin. During the eruption the fever abates somewhat, upon the whole the patient feels a little better, but is tormented by the breaking out of pustules upon the mucous lining, which cause difficulties of deglutition, photophobia, croupy cough, urinary troubles. After the eruption is fully out, the patient feels almost well, and only complains of the distress caused by the injected and tense skin. The suppurative process is generally attended with a mild fever which disappears entirely as soon as the pocks begin to form, and which gives place to a feeling of health. We will mention a few deviations from this course when we come to treat of true small-pox. The remaining red spots seldom disappear entirely under a month. Scars remain after varioloid, the same as after variola, only not in such large numbers, nor so deep; in varioloid the disorganizing process takes place most generally upon the external surface of the cutis, but does not penetrate beneath it.

True variola begins with the same precursory symptoms as the previous species; according to Hebra, the precursory stage of variola is often even less severe than that of varioloid. It lasts three days.

Without an exception, the exanthem first breaks out in the face, thence spreading over the whole body, from above downwards, within two, at most three days. The face always shows the largest number of efflorescences. Inasmuch as variola penetrates the cutaneous tissue more deeply, the course of each single variola-pustule differs somewhat from that pursued by a varioloid pustule. Within twenty-four hours the stigma changes to a papule, and in another twenty-four hours the papule to a vesicle, the contents of which assume a puriform consistence until the sixth day after the appearance of the stigma. The pustule thus formed is surrounded by a broad halo. Hence in variola the eruptive stage and the stage of efflorescence last at most ten, but never less than nine days.

The general health in these two stages is about the same as during a similar period in varioloid. The fever abates to a certain degree; the affection of the mucous lining is generally a little more intense.

On the ninth or tenth day commences the suppurative stage so characteristic of variola. The fever, which had almost entirely disappeared, breaks out again with frequent chills and an intense heat. Hebra accounts for this fever by the circumstance that pus has been absorbed, not by the intensity of the cutaneous affection, for it is not unfrequently absent, even during a most violent attack of variola and never sets in until the pustules had become filled for some time, but, on the other hand, is always present if ulceration takes place. The pyæmic nature of this fever accounts most easily for the dangerous character of this stage upon which we shall dwell more fully by and by when we come to treat of the complications. While the fever is gradually abating, the suppurative stage continues until the fourteenth day, when the desiccation and the scabbing process commence in the same order as the eruption had developed itself. The patients, during this time, are without fever, and feel quite well. The scabs very seldom separate before the seventh, sometimes not till the fourteenth day, leaving reddish-brown, pigmentous spots and scars which disappear very slowly.

It now remains for us to indicate several important anomalies in the course of the disease. In doing this, we shall confine ourselves to variola, varioloid having the same modifications except in a lesser degree.

In the first place the pustules, instead of remaining isolated, may run together (confluent small-pox). This confluence of the pocks may take place to some extent in every severe case of small-pox; but if it is extensive, the disease becomes much fiercer, the fever abates very little during the stage of efflorescence, the suppurative fever is very intense, because confluent pustules cause deeply-penetrating ulcerations. As a rule, this process only takes place in the face. In the suppurative stage the pustules not unfrequently become mixed with blood, giving rise to the so-called black pock which always constitutes the most dangerous form of the disease, because it sets in with an exquisitely adynamic fever attended with profuse nose-bleed, hæmatemesis, hæmaptoë. The filling of the pocks with an ichorous pus is a very rare occurence. The size of the pustules varies considerably in the same individual. Some only attain the size of a lentil and dry up very speedily; others resemble the bullæ of pemphigus, and some again do not even leave their papular form. A few single variola-pustules are met with in every case of varioloid; it is the universality of the suppurative process, and the longer duration of the disease that determine the characteristic nature of small-pox.

With regard to the whole course of the disease we distinguish small-pox where the fever preserves an adynamic type during the whole course of the disease, and small-pox with septic tendencies throughout its course. It not unfrequently happens that, after the disease has passed its first stage, the fever suddenly assumes an adynamic type. In adynamic small-pox the pustules may not reach their full development; in septic small-pox they are apt to become hemorrhagic and gangrenous. The phenomena accompanying a change of this kind, resemble altogether those of an intense typhus. Variola without an eruption is a speculative theory rather than a practically verified fact.

Complications and sequelæ occur much less frequently after small-pox than after measles and scarlatina, but are no less dangerous, for the reason that they have their origin in the suppurative process; hence, they occur almost exclusively during and after the course of variola, and very seldom after or during an attack of varioloid. As direct consequences of the variola-pustules we mention: diphtheritis, croup and œdema glottidis. The last-mentioned process likewise occurs as a complication of varioloid. The course of these complications and sequelæ does not essentially vary from that of other analogous diseases. The croupy sound is often heard already during the efflorescent stage of small-pox, but at this period it has no dangerous significance; it only becomes threatening during the stage of suppuration. Violent inflammations especially of the serous membranes, meningitis, pericarditis, pleuritis, inflammations of the large joints, deep-seated abscesses only occur after the suppurative fever has set in. They certainly do not arise from the intensity of the inflammatory process upon the skin, but from the absorption of pus. The eyes in consequence of an inflammatory process going on in their interior, are not unfrequently threatened with hypopyon, whereas it is immaterial in a case of varioloid whether a number of pustules have become seated close to the eye or on the conjunctiva. The danger is altogether determined by the supervention of the suppurative process.

In both variola and varioloid the prognosis is very uncertain; the most favorable appearances at the beginning sometimes give way very suddenly to the most dangerous symptoms, and *vice versa*, cases that set in with symptoms of great severity, turn out very mild at the end. Age is of great consequence in this disease; old people have to suffer a great deal more than young persons, evidently owing to the greater rigidity of the skin. As a matter of course, a vitiated constitution and unfavorable social circumstances, above all, pregnancy and confinement invest small-pox with a character of most threatening gravity.

Treatment. Before speaking of the remedial agents that may have to be used for small-pox, we will express our views concerning the great preventive of small-pox, vaccination. Without questioning the right of the State to require the individual citizen to make himself or his children sick; without meaning to inquire whether morbid matter can be transmitted by vaccination, for this might be avoided with due caution; simply looking at the fact whether vaccination is really useful or not, we feel bound, from this single point of view, to declare our opposition to this proceeding, for the reason that we do not believe the vaccine-virus possessed of the least prophylactic virtue against variola, by which we mean against the transformation of the pock into a suppurating pustule. If epidemic small-pox is so much less dangerous and extensive at the present time than it was a hundred years ago, this can be just as well accounted for by the undeniable fact that epidemics gradually increase and decrease in intensity, as by the universally practised process of vaccination. If persons who are not vaccinated, die at the present time more frequently of variola than those who are, the cause may be that only those remain unvaccinated at the present time, who, living in the worst conditions of society, are more apt to fall victims to epidemic diseases. The last epidemic among us has shown very satisfactorily that the danger of small-pox is derived from accompanying local circumstances, not so much from the fact that vaccination had been neglected. In the city of Hanover, where we have not had any malignant epidemics since the year 1846, we have had numerous small-pox cases for the least year, with only few deaths, whereas more northward, in our marshy districts, where severe epidemics have prevailed during the last few years, small-pox has likewise claimed a larger number of victims in spite of vaccination. We, therefore, have no hesitation in admitting that we belong to the number of those who repudiate vaccination, and we favor the more and more rapidly spreading movement that has been initiated against this measure. It may be difficult to entirely do away with this peculiar institution; but what can be accomplished is, that, if people insist upon being vaccinated, the operation should be performed under appropriate circumstances. We deem the following points essential to such a purpose: Frequent renewal of the lymph by cowpock-virus;—extreme precaution in selecting the children from whom the vaccine is taken;—a revision of the statute which makes it obligatory upon parents to have their children vaccinated in the first year of infancy;—insertion of the vaccine in only a few places with a view of diminishing as much as possible all unfavorable consequences to the organism. In this respect we maintain that, if vaccination has at all any protecting virtue, one pustule ought to protect as much as a dozen. Speaking of vaccination we cannot help raising the question whether the diminished mortality in small-pox epidemics may not be owing to a more enlightened management of the disease.

The preliminary stage which is not always recognizable as such at the beginning of the attack, will always invite the employment of remedial agents, although the usefulness or efficacy of such a proceeding is extremely questionable. *Aconite* is more than any other medicine recommended at this stage, but we do not altogether agree with our Colleagues in the propriety of this course of medication. Aconite is indicated in all inflammatory fevers, but not in febrile conditions that evidently owe their origin to toxication of the blood. For this reason we do not advise Aconite either in measles, scarlatina or typhus, still much less in small-pox. *Belladonna* will be found preferable, even after a most careful comparison of the symptoms, and ought to be continued until the eruption is fully out. *Bryonia* will be found much less frequently suitable at this stage of small-pox. Upon the whole we opine that any medicine is useless either totally or nearly so, for the reason that the first stages of small-pox are without any malignant symptoms, even if delirium should set in. As soon as the exanthem is out, the patient feels tolerably well; but now is the time to administer suitable remedies for the purpose of preventing the purulent metamorphosis which must now be expected, and of which we can never positively know how it will result; and, in general, for the purpose of maintaining the course of the disease within normal bounds. We have but one remedy that answers this purpose; this remedy is *Mercurius*. In any circumstances we would advise our Colleagues never to repeat the dose too often in this disease. It might be a difficult task to show its usefulness as long as we have not a number of comparative observations at our command. If medicine is to be given, it is certain that *Mercurius* is the most appropriate. Just as well as *Mercurius* will prevent suppuration in cases of abscesses and small boils,—and we know from abundant experience that it will do this,—we may likewise expect a favorable effect from it upon the suppurative process in small-pox, so much more as the symptomatic similarity between the pathogenesis of Mercury and small-pox in this special point extends to the minutest particulars. If suppuration does really set in, we may try *Hepar sulphuris* for the purpose of preventing the excessive development of this process. As long as no anomalies occur, these three remedies will be found sufficient in every case of small-pox or varioloid. Neither the frequently severe conjunctivitis, nor the difficulty of swallowing, nor finally the croupy cough demand any other remedies than the three above named; for these phenomena are simply occasioned by the exanthem running its course upon the mucous lining, and are, therefore, without any special significance. Upon what grounds a number of other remedies are recommended for small-pox, we are unable to conceive, and we, therefore, do not mention them lest their multitude should cause confusion in the reader's mind. *Antimonium crudum* and *tartaricum* have made more noise than any other remedy, nor can it be denied that the principle of similarity is in their favor; so far, however, it has not been shown that these remedies exert either a modifying or abbreviating influence over the disease, or that the suppurative stage is prevented by them.

Among the anomalies and complications we only mention a few, since it is impossible to furnish a complete list of such occurrences. Variola with an adynamic type of fever is always very threatening, and is characterized by an extraordinary tendency to decomposition and to an approach to typhus. At the commencement *Bryonia* will very generally be indicated, on the other hand, we think that it is under these circumstances that *Tartar emetic* is in its place, more especially if the brain is involved. After the pustules are formed, *Arsenicum* is most likely the most appropriate remedy, not only on account of the constitutional symptoms, as on account of the putrid decomposition which is so apt to set in at this period, attended with hemorrhagic effusions into the pustules and ichorous dissolution. We likewise call attention, at this stage, to *Secale cornutum*, and to the mineral acids, especially *Acidum muriat.* This last-mentioned remedy is particularly appropriate if the pustules become associated with symptoms of diphtheritis in the mouth and fauces, and the life of the patient is in the greatest jeopardy. Croup which sets in during the suppurative stage, is not controlled by the medicines usually recommended for croup; it is not the ordinary croup, but a symptom of diphtheritis. We would recommend *Hepar sulphuris* first, and afterwards *Phosphorus.* Œdema glottidis during small-pox requires the same remedies that have been suggested for this disease in a former chapter.

[I once saved a boy's life with *Arsenicum.* The child had never been vaccinated, or rather eight different attempts had been made to vaccinate him, but every attempt had proved futile. The boy was attacked with confluent small-pox. The disease was running as favorable a course as could be expected, when I was sent for one night in a great hurry because the disease had taken a bad turn. I found the boy in an undescribable state of apathy and lethargy. The pustules had suddenly receded and those that were still out upon the skin, looked black. Involuntary diarrhœic evacuations took place every fifteen minutes spreading a most horrid stench through the room. The skin was cold and clammy, the pulse filiform and could no longer be counted. I gave him *Arsenicum* second centesimal trituration, one half of a grain at a dose, repeating the dose every fifteen minutes. After the third dose the diarrhœa stopped entirely, the skin warmed up, the pulse returned, the remaining pustules resumed a normal appearance, and the disease went on its course very favorably. After the boy had been sick twelve days, and seemed all but well; after the fever had entirely disappeared, and the child expected to be dressed and play about the room, he was all at once taken with a severe angina, the fever returned with a severe chill, he was seized with partial convulsions and next day was covered with scarlet-rash. He had caught the scarlatina at school, but the variola kept it under until the severer disease had run its course. The boy made a fine recovery, and only showed one or two scarcely perceptible pits on the chin. H.]

Secondary inflammations, when occasioned by the absorption of pus, are generally very severe and obstinate; they require different treatment from what similar inflammations require when setting in as primary diseases. *Bryonia,* and above all *Mercurius, Phosphorus, Hepar sulphuris* and *Arsenicum* are most generally the most appropriate remedies. Among these five remedies to which we can add *Sulphur,* the proper remedy for a given case will undoubtedly be found. [*Tartar emetic* may likewise be added; a case of pneumonia supervening in the course of scrofulous periostitis, and which could only be accounted for agreeably to Virchow's theory of pus-globules having been deposited in the lungs by the current of the blood, yielded promptly and radically in our hands to the exclusive use of Tartar emetic, third centesimal trituration. H.]

As soon as the formation of the scabs is completed, all danger is over. Only in very exceptional cases deep-seated abscesses form, but in such a latent manner that they are only discovered after the desiccation is terminated. Hence the patient may be safely regarded as cured.

In view of the measures which it is common to enforce even at this time in the management of small-pox, a few rules for the external treatment of such patients seem to us of some importance. Experience has abundantly shown that the spread of small-pox cannot be prevented by even the strictest and most careful quarantine; hence it is useless to exile such patients from all human society, although it is undoubtedly proper that all unnecessary intrusions should be avoided. Above all, let the patient enjoy an abundance of pure air; the access of fresh air not only affords the surest guarantee of a successful result, but is likewise the most effectual means of preventing the further spread of the disease. It is entirely useless to cover the patients burning up with fever, more than they wish to be. Cautious ablutions never hurt, and are always refreshing. As soon as the patient is free from fever, and desires to leave his bed, let him be permitted to do so. The scabs are most speedily removed by softening them with almond-oil, and by frequently washing and bathing the patient as soon as possible. Ablutions and baths have the additional advantage of helping to restore the normal action of the skin. As regards diet, the patient's own wishes may be consulted as far as possible; as long as the fever lasts, he will not want anything, but the lightest fever-diet; every other kind of food causes nausea and indisposition. As soon as the fever has disappeared, a more substantial diet may be allowed. As soon as the scabs have come off, the patient may be permitted to go out. Nothing can be more unreasonable than to keep him confined in a room even after the exanthem has run its full course; an extreme irritability to catarrhal affections are the frequent consequences of such an unnecessary confinement.

4. Syphilis.

Venereal Disease.

Syphilis is a disease concerning which it is very difficult to make comprehensive and satisfactory statements in a few paragraphs. The disease is too varied, and undergoes too many modifications by constitutional influences; moreover the best mode of treating it, is not yet positively settled. We request the reader to receive our subsequent remarks with a good deal of forbearance; let it be understood above all things that we do not intend to present a monograph on the subject of syphilis.

Etiology. Syphilis is either communicated by a contagium, or else it is inherited; this last statement, however, only applies to a few forms; whether syphilis can break out spontaneously, is very uncertain, although there is no valid reason to deny it. The fixed nature of the contagium cannot be denied; it is most certainly contained in the primary ulcer, whereas its presence in secondary affections as well as in the blood is maintained by some, and denied by others. The adoption of a different contagium for simple and for indurated chancre depends upon observations, the correctness of which cannot be positively impeached. In the vast majority of cases the chancre-virus is communicated by sexual intercourse; in a few cases only the virus is communicated by a different channel. It is not absolutely necessary that the chancrous matter should be inserted at a spot where the epidermis is injured; inoculation can take place, even if the epidermis is intact; for this purpose it has to be very delicate, as the epidermis of the sexual organs generally is. Syphilis can be inherited from the father as well as from the mother; it would even seem as though it were more easily inherited from the former. Most observations show that constitutional syphilis is a protection against a second infection by the virus of an indurated chancre, as much as a first attack of variola is a protection against a second attack of this disease. The incubation-period is short and does not last beyond the second week, whereas secondary affections incubate for at least five weeks. A disposition to contract this disease, inheres in every individual; however, its ordinary mode of origination accounts for the circumstance that male adults are more generally affected with it. Some persons seem to possess a natural immunity from constitutional syphilis, whereas others manifest a peculiar susceptibility to this disease; this susceptibility seems founded in the so-called lymphatic constitution.

A description of the separate forms under which syphilis generally manifests itself, cannot well be given in one connected paragraph; we therefore prefer describing the various phases of the disease, each by itself, in the order in which they generally succeed each other.

a. *Primary Chancre.*

Syphilis always commences with the primary syphilitic ulcer. Except when the disease is hereditary, we have no evidence that syphilis can have any other beginning.

The soft, simple chancre is chiefly seated on the inside of the prepuce, on the glans, and in the transition-fold from the prepuce to the glans, more particularly on the frenulum; among women it is chiefly seated at the posterior commissure, at the entrance of the vagina, and on the lesser labia. But inasmuch as other parts of the body may either accidentally or designedly come in contact with the chancre-virus, a chancre may likewise break out on the integuments of the penis, on the scrotum, at the anus, on the lips, mammæ, and in the posterior parts of the vagina. Its course is generally as follows: at the place of inoculation a small vesicle starts up, surrounded by a red halo; or, if the virus was inserted in an open wound on the skin, an ulcer may form immediately which, when arising from the vesicle, develops in a very short time, so that the vesicle is very seldom seen. The ulcer is generally round, less frequently oval, never sharply angular, of the size of a lentil or pea; it has sharp, shaggy, not prominent borders and a lardaceous base. It gradually spreads, but never grows to a large size; it sometimes acquires a fungoid growth from its base, without, however, becoming indurated on that account. At first only one ulcer of this character generally breaks out, very seldom three, but in the course of the disease new ulcers break out in the immediate neighborhood of the former, so that the glans is surrounded by them as by a wreath; they may likewise become confluent. It is a noticeable fact that the more recent ulcers generally heal faster, very seldom more tardily than the primary sore. These ulcers heal between three and eight weeks. The healing process is manifested by the fact that the bottom of the ulcer loses its dirty color, becomes covered with usually readily-bleeding granulations, and that the edges lose their shaggy appearance. The cicatrix is generally radiate. If the soft chancre is seated in the urethra, it generally occupies the locality immediately behind the orifice, where it can be seen. If it is seated farther on in the urethra, its presence may be inferred from a seated pain when the part is touched, and which is likewise experienced during urination; and also from a scanty discharge of pus, whereas, if the chancre is complicated with gonorrhœa, the diagnosis is very generally impossible. The cure of this urethral chancre takes place in the same manner as that of a chancre seated in some external locality.

The indurated, so-called Hunterian chancre is chiefly located in the transition-region from the prepuce to the glans, and on the frenulum, but it may likewise break out on any other place, the same as soft chancre. Many look upon the virus of the Hunterian chancre as different from that of the soft chancre. This question is not, by any means, decided. This chancre often arises not from a vesicle, but from an induration in consequence of the dissolution of the inflammatory exudation. According to some, this is its only mode of origination. It has chiefly a rounded form; its appearance scarcely varies from that of the simple chancre; its base, however, has a less lardaceous and dirty look. If the induration occupies the bottom of the ulcer, the latter is raised, forming the elevated ulcer; if the borders are chiefly indurated, they form a wall round the funnel-shaped ulcer. The induration sometimes spreads to some distance round the ulcer, and is generally of a cartilaginous consistence. If the indurated chancre develops itself out of a simple chancre, which is very seldom the case during the first appearance of the latter, and generally not till after the latter has existed for some time, the appearance of the ulcer often changes very suddenly. The indurated chancre does not multiply on the surrounding parts; hence we seldom see more than one or at most two indurated ulcers. It heals much more slowly than simple chancre, and is almost surely followed by secondary phenomena if a slowly disappearing induration remains after the healing of the ulcer. The delicate scar of the indurated chancre is easily torn by friction, when a chancrous ulcer readily forms again immediately.

Phagedænic chancre is a chancre modified by the constitution of the patient. It only breaks out on cachectic individuals, arising more generally from the simple than from the indurated ulcer. If such an ulcer becomes phagedænic, it assumes an irregular form, with indentations; it shows a dirty-gray or greenish base, lined with diphtheritic exudations, is surrounded by a sickly-colored and livid areola, and secretes a quantity of thin, sickly and very fetid matter. The ulcer inclines to spread rapidly and to destroy the organic tissues, in consequence of which it may involve a considerable loss of substance and even result fatally in a short time. A phagedænic chancre most commonly arises in cases where Mercury had been very much abused; it is not difficult to understand that the abuse of Mercury should aggravate a phagedænic chancre very materially. A cure takes place by a separation of the infiltrated parts in the same manner as takes place in a case of simple chancre.

A gangrenous chancre may arise both from the simple and indurated chancre in consequence of the parts round the ulcer becoming considerably infiltrated; the ulcer acquires a sickly color and, together with its surroundings, changes to a scurf which is encompassed by a considerable serous infiltration. A cure takes place by means of the scurf becoming separated; or, in the opposite case, the disorganizing process spreads, but scarcely ever as far as in a case of phagedænic chancre. Death may very readily ensue. It is not always possible to trace the gangrenous change to its true cause.

Either directly caused by the primary ulcer, or in company with it, without any definite connection being perceivable, and sometimes outlasting the ulcer, we have:

The syphilitic bubo, that is, lymphadenitis occasioned by the syphilitic affection. The bubo is seated on the side nearest to the place where the infection was first communicated, more especially in the groin below Poupart's ligament. We distinguish acute and chronic buboes.

The acute bubo seldom develops itself in the second to the sixth week after the appearance of the primary ulcer, seldom at an earlier period, and likewise seldom after the cicatrization of the ulcer. It generally breaks out after simple chancre, and is most likely to make its appearance if the chancre is located close to the frenulum. Irritating the ulcer, most likely favors the development of a bubo. At a spot in the bend of the groin, the patient, especially when moving the part briskly, experiences a pain which is very much aggravated during contact, although the inflamed gland can scarcely yet be felt. It generally grows rapidly in size, is very painful and may reach the size of a goose-egg. It adheres to the integuments, hence is not moveable, and the integuments soon show a red color. Suppuration does not take place very rapidly; fluctuation is never perceived over a large surface, because resolution only takes place fragmentarily. The spontaneous breaking of the abscess takes place with much difficulty; after its discharge the truly virulent bubo forms an ulcer with all the characteristics of chancre, the secretion from which is infectious. A bubo very seldom arises from a simple sympathetic irritation of the lymphatic gland. In the latter case, a cure mostly takes place very speedily, whereas in the former case the healing process is very tardy, and the swelling may remain even a long time after the wound is closed. An extension of the inflammatory process to the surrounding cellular tissue, even to the peritonæum; the formation of fistulous canals and a descension of the pus are not unfrequent occurrences. These bad results generally occur if the bubo is lanced prematurely. We shall revert to this subject when we come to speak of the treatment of syphilis. There is no difficulty in diagnosing the true nature of a bubo, except after the chancre is healed without leaving a scar, or if the bubo develops itself without any previous chancre. A characteristic circumstance in the history of a syphilitic bubo is, that it almost always breaks out below Poupart's ligament.

The chronic, indolent bubo runs a slow course; it comes on without pain and is very obstinate; it is distinguished from an acute bubo by the circumstance that it only occurs in connection with an indurated chancre, and is not, like an acute bubo, confined mostly to one gland, but involves a number of them. The swelling progresses very slowly; a single gland does not attain any considerable size, but from several glands swelling close together, a large, hard, bunchy tumor is formed. Single glands very seldom terminate in suppuration; if this happens, pus forms very slowly, the sides of the abscess are very slack, and a whole gland is transformed into purulent matter. Very seldom the inflammation attacks the surrounding parts. Whereas an acute bubo does not justify the conclusion that secondary phenomena will certainly make their appearance, an indolent bubo is almost invariably succeeded by them.

A catarrh of the mucous lining of the urethra or vagina does not very frequently accompany the primary ulcer. Chancres in the urethra may run their course without a sign of gonorrhœa, or else the gonorrhœa may be very violent and painful. To account for the latter case, the doctrine has been started that there is a double infection with the chancre as well as the gonorrhœal virus. This is not necessary to account for the gonorrhœa, for a chancre in the urethra may very readily give rise to extensive urethritis; if it does not, the cause must be the different degrees of irritability of the mucous lining of different individuals. The secretion of a chancrous gonorrhœa is characterized by a strong, very offensive smell.

Condylomata are vegetations of the skin belonging to primary as well as to secondary syphilis, but they may likewise occur in combination with gonorrhœa without chancre. We will devote a few general remarks to them in this place.

There are two pretty essentially distinct species of condylomata, the soft, humid condyloma with a broad base, and the acuminated condyloma.

Soft condylomata very frequently accompany primary syphilis; secondary syphilis is almost always accompanied by them. They are seated on the integuments of the sexual organs, on the glans, thighs, scrotum, in the intergluteal fold, on the external pudendum and in the vagina, in general in localities where two folds of integument are exposed to frequent frictions against each other. They are flat risings, very little or not at all injected, covered by a very thin epidermis, very soft to the feel, and moistened with a scanty, muco-purulent, and most generally disagreeably smelling secretion. By growing the isolated condylomata may unite and rise to a considerable height. The exulcerations and the deep rhagades on their surface impart to the skin that covers them a peculiar ulcerated and split appearance, which is most strikingly noticed at the anus. The period when these vegetations break out, differs a good deal; they come most speedily with an indurated chancre, more particularly, if the primary ulcer is accompanied by profuse blennorrhœa.

Acuminated condylomata occur less frequently as accompaniments of chancre, more commonly as accompaniments of gonorrhœa; they grow more especially on places that are continually bathed by the poisonous secretion, hence in the same localities where the soft condylomata are chiefly seated, principally on the glans and prepuce, in the female urethra, and at the entrance of the vagina. Their presence does not always imply the existence of a general infection. As a rule, they have a cauliflower-shaped appearance, are covered with a hard epidermis, are seated on a narrow base, are sometimes pedunculate or, in consequence of being flattened by a pressure on both sides, have a cock's-comb shaped appearance. They often show a great tendency to grow like fungi, in which case they exhibit considerable vascularity; they may reach the size of a man's hand. If they are seated between the glans and prepuce, and of sufficient size, they may cause a great deal of suffering in consequence of being pressed upon and pulled at. They never suppurate, nor are they ever fissured, except by the action of direct force. When healing, they sometimes disappear quite suddenly, sometimes decline gradually.

b. *Secondary Syphilis.*

The phenomena of secondary or constitutional syphilis are all confined to the external skin, the mucous membrane and the higher organs of sense. They succeed the primary ulcer at different periods, very seldom, however, before the sixth week and after the sixth month. They are generally preceded by a period of rest or latent condition, but it likewise not unfrequently happens that secondary syphilis breaks out while the primary phenomena are still running their course. The mercurial treatment of primary syphilis is said to exert a modifying influence over secondary phenomena; whether for the patient's weal or woe, is a question that will be more fully examined by and by. Secondary syphilitic affections do not yield infectious matter. It almost always happens that an indurated chancre superinduces secondary phenomena, whereas a simple, soft chancre may run its course without any such result. Most observers maintain that secondary syphilis never gets well entirely, but that, on the other hand, it is a protection against constitutional symptoms. It is conceivable that these two conditions may coexist, but not one alone without the other. We have seen secondary phenomena break out more than once on the same person after repeated infectious intercourse; the phenomena following the last infection were undoubtedly milder, and lasted less long than the phenomena succeeding the first attack.

Constitutional syphilis is not unfrequently ushered in by vague constitutional symptoms which sometimes exist during the whole period that the disease exists in a latent state. These symptoms are: lassitude, ill-humor, vague rheumatoid pains, backache, pains in the throat, slight transitory febrile motions. Such symptoms are generally so vague and trivial that the patient does not consider it worth his while to complain of them.

Cutaneous affections occur in all the different forms that characterize such diseases; they are distinguished by one reliable diagnostic, namely the peculiar copper-color of the hyperæmia by which they are accompanied. The form of the exanthemata is a less reliable indication of their syphilitic origin. They generally represent circular or curvilenear figures always of the same style, especially the squamous exanthemata. Finally secondary exanthems reveal a tolerably constant predilection for certain localities on the surface of the body, more particularly for the hairy scalp, the frontal and nasal regions, the nape of the neck, the volar surface of the hand, the region around the sexual parts, the lower extremities and the soles of the feet. The most frequent exanthems are:

Syphilitic roseola, generally constituting the first stage of constitutional syphilis. It consists of small, rounded, bright-red spots which rarely run together, and are scattered about irregularly; they are immediately preceded by the above-mentioned symptoms of constitutional malaise. After the spots have been out a good while, they assume a yellowish, and soon after a copper-colored tinge which does not yield under the pressure of the finger. The spots break out in different crops, hence are present in various stages of development, which is an important diagnostic. They never itch.

In *syphilitic psoriasis* the scales form upon a very dark base; they are thin, nor are they massed on top of each other in thick layers; different from non-syphilitic psoriasis, it spares the elbows and knees, and is most fully developed in the palms of the hands, and on the soles of the feet. Under the scales the skin is considerably infiltrated, hard and callous, and superficially fissured.

The other forms, *lichen, impetigo, acne, ecthyma, rupia, pemphigus*, have no peculiar features except the copper-redness. *Exanthematic tubercles* constitute one of the more frequent and, at all events, more malignant cutaneous affections, since they evince a marked disposition to purulent dissolution, and to ulceration. They always exhibit an intensely red color, and break out chiefly on the forehead as the Corona veneris. They give rise to the syphilitic *lupus*. They usually form definite, most commonly circular clusters; the ulcers arising from them retain the same arrangement. However, they have a very different significance from real lupus, and very seldom involve any considerable loss of substance. Their place is really among the tertiary phenomena; they have been mentioned here simply for the sake of brevity.

The syphilitic exanthemata in one form or another generally exist throughout the whole course of secondary or tertiary syphilis, very often constituting the only symptom of the continued presence of the disease. This applies more particularly to acne syphilitica, and to the impetigo of the lower extremities, also to the psoriasis in the palms of the hands; the two last-named exanthems are very frequently associated with considerable callosities in the skin.

The hair very frequently becomes diseased, but not as a rule. It is certainly a mistake to suppose that the baldness of syphilitic individuals is always a consequence of mercurial abuse; we have seen this baldness occur in two cases where no Mercury had been taken. What is certain, however, is that after mercurial abuse the hair either does not at all grow again, or only very imperfectly. What causes the falling out of the hair, cannot well be explained, since the scalp not unfrequently has a perfectly normal appearance.

The affections of the mucous membranes are mostly seated in the lining membrane of the mouth and nose, less frequently of the larynx, and still less frequently of the rectum. In the mouth their favorite locality are the tonsils and the velum palati, and the region immediately back of the last molar tooth. Here a deep-colored hyperæmia is generally noticed simultaneously with the appearance of the roseola, attended with stinging pain and a difficulty of swallowing as after a cold, which, be it remarked incidentally, frequently excites the hyperæmia. This hyperæmia either remains, or else, it disappears for a short period to return again so much more intensely, until finally ulcers break out, having all the appearance of primary chancres. These ulcers may remain unchanged for a long time; sometimes they are very flat, causing very little trouble. In other cases they show a great tendency to spread to the nose and to the posterior wall of the pharynx and larynx. In such a case they may remain superficial, or else, penetrate even to the cartilages and bones. From the losses of substance thus occasioned, and likewise from the contracting cicatrices caused by the healing of the ulcers, great inconveniences may arise. The ulcers of the Schneiderian membrane are most commonly revealed by a fetid, puriform, sanguinolent discharge.

Syphilitic iritis is a phenomenon that cannot be accounted for. It occurs very frequently, and sometimes runs such a mild course, that it is entirely overlooked and is only recognized by its consequences. It only sets in after the appearance of the exanthems, never at the commencement of the secondary phenomena, and there is an evident connection between the iritis and the cutaneous affections; the more intense and extensive these affections, the more certainly we may expect the supervention of iritis. It most generally affects only one eye, very seldom both eyes together, sometimes one after the other. The iritis sets in with violent pains in the globe of the eye; these are scarcely ever absent and exacerbate at night, attended with more or less disturbance of the visual functions and severe illusions of light. The color of the iris seems changed, the organ looks specked, the pupil is all but immovable, angular or ovoid, the anterior chamber looks dim as if filled with pus, sometimes slightly and at other times more strikingly. Occasionally small excrescences are noticed at the border, or dark points on the surface of the pupils. This affection generally runs a chronic course, and is less painful in such a case; if the affection is very acute, it is attended with frightful pains, in which case the eye is apt to be destroyed. A complete cure without any disturbing remnants of disease, can scarcely ever be expected.

c. *Tertiary Syphilis.*

Under this collective appellation various alterations are comprehended involving a number of organs and being principally located in the osseous system. Sometimes they set in very soon after the appearance of the secondary symptoms, ordinarily, however, after the lapse of years. During the development of these tertiary symptoms the secondary phenomena do not disappear, but generally accompany the former in a greater or less degree of intensity. We cannot here undertake to examine the question whether tertiary syphilis is caused by a gradual spread of the infection, or whether it is indebted for its existence exclusively to the use of Mercury. This question it is certainly very difficult to decide in last resort. We are most assuredly of the opinion that tertiary symptoms only set in in consequence of the improper use of Mercury; our reason is that we are not acquainted with a single case of syphilis where tertiary symptoms showed themselves under homœopathic management. If, in reply to this statement, the objection should be raised that under homœopathic treatment syphilis is cured more rapidly, we are perfectly willing to throw in tertiary syphilis, for the superior value of our treatment would not be invalidated by such an admission. The various affections that will be enumerated in the following paragraphs, have the peculiar characteristic of either tending to the purulent metamorphosis and consequent destruction of the affected parts, or causing atrophy of the affected organs by the formation of adventitious areolar tissue.

Diseases of the bones and periosteum most commonly involve the skull, and facial bones, the bones of the lower extremities, and more particularly such bones as are not provided with a thick muscular covering, such as the sternum, ribs, etc. The disease sets in with horrid pains which have the peculiarity of exacerbating at night with terrible fierceness (dolores osteocopi). The pains sometimes precede the objective symptoms for some time. At the painful spot tumors are seen, which seem to be super-imposed on the bone and are of two kinds. Some constitute elastic-doughy, soft, flat swellings, called gummata; they contain a tenacious fluid, and either disappear again gradually, or else, become transformed into abscesses. The other class, called tophi, are infiltrations beneath the periosteum, having all the hardness of exostoses. If these tumors do not slowly disappear, they may become real exostoses; they suppurate only in a few cases. The substance of the bones itself is much less frequently the primary seat of inflammation, but is very apt to be invaded by secondary inflammation occasioned by the suppuration of the above-described swellings. It is more particularly in the bones of the nose and face that the disease develops malignant consequences. These bones are destroyed to a greater or less extent, in consequence of which the face becomes horridly disfigured. If the affection is located on the inner surface of the skull, the brain is exposed to great danger, partly in consequence of the pressure exerted upon the brain, and partly in consequence of the probable or at least possible extension of the disease to the meningeal membranes.

Gummata are not exclusively seated on the bones, but likewise occur in the interstitial areolar tissue of muscles; various peculiar tertiary affections of special organs seem likewise to be traceable to the existence of gummata.

Syphilitic sarcocele occurs pretty frequently; it generally attacks only one testicle, very rarely both at the same time, sometimes one after the other. It is seated in the substance of the testicle itself, without attacking the epidydimis. Its development takes place slowly and without pain; the testicle may gradually enlarge to the size of a goose-egg, becomes indurated and unequal on its surface. The termination in suppuration is a rare occurrence, and most probably owing to bad management. A retrograde metamorphosis takes place very slowly, and in a majority of the cases the interstitial infiltration leads to subsequent and sometimes extensive atrophy of the substance of the testicle. Among the viscera of the trunk the liver is first attacked by an inflammatory process that is exceedingly chronic and sometimes remains latent; as in the testicle so in the liver, this process may result in a contracting cicatrix, and consequent atrophy and callous degeneration of the substance of the liver. For the spleen, heart, lungs and kidneys we have no forms of disease to which a syphilitic origin might be attributed with positive certainty.

The contraction of the biceps muscle without paralysis, or with diminution but not entire suspension of its functions, is almost always a symptom of tertiary syphilis, whereas, if other muscles are similarly affected, a syphilitic origin is more questionable.

Upon the general organism tertiary syphilis exerts without exception a most deleterious effect, either in consequence of the disturbances resulting from the above-mentioned processes, or in a more direct manner. A very common consequence is a deep melancholy and hypochondria occasioned by depressing reflections concerning the obstinacy of the disease, and afterwards leading to the most intense derangements of the digestive functions. This result is most apt to take place in the course of sarcocele. Finally all these various complications and disturbances may lead to complete cachexia which, however, is not distinguished by any particular features.

In reviewing the pathological process of syphilis in its totality we have to offer a few suggestions that are not unessential in a therapeutic point of view; we shall avoid, however, all hypothetical propositions, so much more as a good many points in syphilis still require further examination. In our previous statements we have chiefly adhered to the views of Old School practitioners, with a view of presenting an uniform picture of the disease. Inasmuch, however, as the treatment of syphilis must necessarily exert a greatly modifying influence over the form of its manifestations, it behooves us now to review the changes taking place under homœopathic management.

The total course of syphilis is the more rapid, the more vigorous and healthy the affected individual otherwise is; its course is the more tardy, or inclines to chronic and dangerous developments the more, the more debilitated the constitution of the diseased person. In view of this general proposition it is undeniable that under the treatment with large doses of Mercury, the course of syphilis is not only much retarded, but is likewise more easliy forced into abnormal deviations.

The treatment of syphilis with large doses of Mercury keeps the syphilis latent for a longer period, and by this means prolongs its course. A complete cure takes place so much more speedily, the more speedily the secondary symptoms manifest themselves, for they have to be regarded as curative efforts of the organism. The greater the number of single chancres that break out on an individual, the more intense the cutaneous exanthems, the more speedily will a complete cure be effected.

Whether there is a secondary syphilis, is a fact susceptible of demonstration; but it is not so easy to decide what symptoms or modifications of secondary syphilis have to be charged to the action of Mercury. In this respect the judgment of Homœopathy is more reliable than that of any other method of treatment. From the stand-point of Homœopathy we assert that the spots and papulæ, the intense hyperæmia of the mucous lining of the fauces, the superficial ulcers of the fauces, and the condylomata are purely syphilitic; that, on the contrary, the impetigo, the scaly and more particularly the tubercular exanthems, the ulcerations of the fauces and nose, and likewise those of the larynx are unquestionably due to the treatment. Iritis is likewise a syphilitic phenomenon. The whole series of phenomena that are designated as tertiary, is undoubtedly the result of Mercury, not syphilis.

If syphilis is treated homœopathically from the commencement, and every objective symptom has disappeared under this treatment, it is safe to assume that the disease is completely cured, provided no new symptom breaks out in the space of five or six months. Under the old-fashioned mercurial treatment new symptoms may break out even after the lapse of years. It is not fair to infer that these mercurial symptoms are purely and simply the result of mercurial poisoning, for Mercury does not produce such effects when employed in other diseases; the truth seems to be that it is from the union of mercurial and syphilitic action that these phenomena result. The case is precisely similar to that of intermittent fever cured with massive doses of Quinine; the cure is simply apparent and altogether temporary.

Hence the total course of syphilis under homœopathic treatment is altogether different from what it is, when the treatment is conducted in accordance with the principles of the Old School. If we have availed ourselves of the course of syphilis under Old school treatment for the purpose of presenting a full picture of the disease, it is because homœopaths are but too often applied to for treatment by syphilitic persons who had been poisoned with Mercury. Under homœopathic treatment the course of syphilis is about as follows: The soft chancre heals between six or ten weeks, most generally by multiplying considerably; it is scarcely ever followed by secondary phenomena. The indurated chancre heals between nine to fifteen weeks, during which period the infiltration disappears; it is generally succeeded by secondary symptoms, but they break out while the chancre is still existing, and heal completely between two to four months. An acute bubo breaks only exceptionally, generally it retrogrades without any subsequent secondary symptoms, and is finally completely reabsorbed without leaving any particular infiltration. We have observed this course in the case of buboes that had already reached the size of a hen's egg, with intense redness of the integuments and distinctly-perceptible fluctuation. So far we have never treated a case of syphilis where, after a complete disappearance of all the symptoms, syphilitic phenomena again showed themselves at a subsequent period.

In conclusion we must not omit to state that in Schneider's treatise, entitled: "Syphilis and the methods of curing it," Leipsic, 1861, we possess a valuable work, where the pathological as well as therapeutical views concerning syphilis, are subjected to a lucid and exhaustive criticism. We here call attention to this work for the benefit of those who desire to become acquainted with the different methods of treating syphilis, and which we have not space to dwell upon more fully.

Treatment. The only remedy for all the uncomplicated forms of syphilis is Mercury. Every homœopath accepts this proposition the practical value of which has been verified in a large number of cases, as correct. Simple syphilis whose course we have indicated above, requires for its complete cure nothing but Mercury; but syphilis as manifested in the various forms, a description of which has been given in previous paragraphs, requires for its cure a number of other remedies in almost every case. With a view of simplifying the presentation of our subject, we will describe the treatment of the above-mentioned single forms in successive order.

The simple soft chancre heals in the time indicated, seldom within three weeks, under the exclusive use of *Mercurius solubilis.* If practitioners entertain different views concerning the dose, it is probably because no adequate allowance has been made for the course which syphilis takes; moreover, there is no doubt that one individual requires a larger, and another a smaller dose. In our practice we are in the habit of employing triturations, although many physicians profess to have effected cures with the sixth and even higher attenuations; we never give more than one dose a day, of one grain each, second or third trituration. Under this treatment the chancre never shows an immediate tendency to heal, but it increases in size, three, four or even eight new chancres break out, all of which heal within ten weeks at the latest, leaving a scarcely perceptible cicatrix. Hence the appearance of new chancres should never deceive us; on the contrary, it is a favorable sign, since secondary phenomena scarcely ever break out in such a case. For the last three years we have likewise applied the second trituration of *Mercurius solubilis* externally, dusting the ulcer with it every day by means of a little camel's-hair pencil. This proceeding seems to hasten the cure; the ulcer becomes a little raised, after which the cleansing takes place very rapidly. As soon as this change is beginning to set in, we discontinue the local application, and now give a higher attenuation less frequently, continuing it even for two or three weeks after the cicatrization of the chancre. The inflammation of the prepuce is less important than it might seem; an operation need only be resorted to, if the glans is too much constricted by an existing paraphimosis. However, since the circumstance that the cut surfaces are apt to become chancrous, does not involve any danger, and phimosis may cause a good deal of distress, our advice is to slit the prepuce whenever it becomes inflamed and swollen. In order to protect the chancre from all unnecessary friction, and at the same time prevent an adhesion between the prepuce and glans — an event of very rare occurrence — we cover the chancre with a thin layer of lint.

The indurated chancre likewise requires *Mercurius solubilis;* this preparation is, however, insufficient in very many cases; under its use the disease runs too protracted a course. However, inasmuch as we cannot fix a normal period for the curative action of Mercury, we should not lose our patience too readily. It is unnecessary to give larger doses than in a case of simple chancre; a dose need not be given more frequently than every other day. In these cases the local application of the remedy has seemed to us of decided benefit. Whether some other mercurial preparation is indicated, had better be determined by the nature of the consecutive phenomena. If an indolent bubo forms, we advise the use of the *red Precipitate.* For soft, flat condylomata we prefer *Corrosive Sublimate,* a weak solution of which we likewise apply externally. We have never yet found it necessary to give stronger doses of either of these two remedies than one grain of the second trituration a day, nor have we ever had to deplore the supervention of medicinal symptoms after either medicine. [We once prescribed half grain doses of the red precipitate, first decimal trituration for several Hunterian chancres on the labia majora; the disease was speedily cured, but a horrid salivation broke out, which it took a week to subdue. H.] Condylomata most generally last longer than chancre, but very seldom longer than the induration. Indolent buboes always disappear very slowly. In order not to be led by our impatience to the commission of mistakes, we should always remember that a rapid cure is only preferable to a tardy one, if it is at the same time safe; but that in an opposite case the latter is decidedly preferable. Syphilis can never be cured rapidly. If we are called upon to treat an indurated chancre after it had already been for a long time treated with large doses of Mercury, it is decidedly proper not to give any more Mercury even for three weeks, and to substitute Nitric acid instead. By pursuing this course we obtain so much more certainly an uncontaminated picture of the syphilitic disease, nor need we dread its progress near as much as the insidious development of a syphilitico-mercurial monster. Several physicians recommend for indurated chancre the *Iodide of Mercury*, and likewise *Cinnabaris*. It is very likely that these two remedies act well in this form of chancre; we have never yet employed them for the reason that we have always got along with the remedies above mentioned.

As we have stated previously, phagedænic chancre is determined by peculiar constitutional tendencies. It does not bear large doses of Mercury; if this is to be used, it has to be employed with great caution. The best mercurial preparations for this chancre are *Corrosive Sublimate* and the *red Precipitate*. Upon the whole, however, *Acidum nitricum* or *muriaticum* had better be substituted for Mercury until the ulcer spreads no longer, and the bottom of the ulcer becomes cleansed. In very bad cases *Arsenicum* is said to have had a good effect.

A gangrenous chancre should never be treated with Mercury until the gangrened parts have sloughed off and provided the remaining ulcer still shows the characteristic properties of chancre, which is not usually the case. *Arsenicum* is the only remedy capable of arresting the gangrenous destruction. It is a well known fact that this form of chancre is scarcely ever followed by secondary syphilis; hence the apprehension of secondary symptoms need never suggest a resort to Mercury.

An acute bubo does not require any other treatment than that of the simple chancre from which it had proceeded. Under the use of Mercury it generally runs its course without suppuration, and even, if pus has already been deposited, it is very often reabsorbed. *Acidum nitricum*, *Hepar sulphuris calc.*, the *red Precipitate* and *Carbo animalis* have likewise been recommended for buboes. Except *Hepar*, we cannot recommend a single one of these remedies as superior to *Mercurius sol.;* Hepar can only prove useful after the suppurative process has become fully established. Hepar is likewise indicated if, after the evacuation of the pus, or after a partial retrograde metamorphosis, the gland still remains for some time hard and swollen. *Sulphur* may likewise have to be employed in such circumstances, provided of course that no secondary phenomena have broken out.

An indolent bubo which is almost always a sure sign of so-called constitutional syphilis, never disappears rapidly; hence remedies ought not to be changed too rapidly. In such a case the *Iodide of Mercury* is decidedly appropriate and sufficient, unless the affections of the skin and mucous membrane which may be beginning to make their appearance, should require another remedy.

Gonorrhœa occasioned by chancre in the urethra, does not require any special remedies; *Merc. solubilis* cures the gonorrhœa at the same time as it heals the chancre.

For condylomata, *Thuya* is not a sovereign remedy; this fact is now established beyond a doubt by abundant experience. It is an excellent remedy for the acuminated, dry condylomata, but seems to have very little, if any, effect upon the soft condylomata, either when used internally or externally. In our opinion, these soft condylomata do not always require any particular medication. If they break out in company with a simple chancre, they generally disappear soon after the chancre is healed, and it is good policy, as long as the condylomata last, to continue the Mercury in smaller and less frequent doses. If they accompany an indurated chancre, they remain for a long time even after the latter is cured, for the reason that they constitute a sign of the more intense and more universal infection. But even in such a case we do not advise any special treatment on their account, because the other constitutional symptoms are much more important. What is certain, however, is that as long as condylomata are present that had come out after a chancre, the syphilitic disease is not cured. If they constitute the only manifestation of the disease, we advise both the internal and external use of *Corrosive Sublimate*. We have no personal experience to offer concerning *Nitri acid.*, *Cinnabaris*, *Sabina*, *Staphysagria*. [*Tartar emetic*, internally as well as externally, is an admirable remedy for soft or mucous tubercles. H.]

Among the secondary symptoms we first notice the exanthems. They are best managed with the more intensely acting mercurial preparations, *Corrosive Sublimate*, red and white *Precipitate*, and, according to our own very satisfactory experience, with our *Mercurius vivus* which, it seems to us, is not sufficiently appreciated. The violent action of the Napolitan ointment shows that quicksilver acts more rapidly, and even energetically, than most other mercurial preparations; we have found this statement corroborated in a number of cases. Of course not the first, but the third trituration has to be used. It is, moreover, certain that *Mercurius vivus* causes exanthematic phenomena more certainly and specifically than any other mercurial preparation. For this reason we cannot recommend Mercurius vivus with sufficient emphasis for experimental trials, so much more since it likewise corresponds so perfectly with the hyperæmia and ulceration of the mucous lining of the fauces. For the above-described uncomplicated affections of the skin and mucous lining, the remedies which we have pointed out will be found sufficient; however, a marked increase of the cutaneous efflorescences must not be regarded as a bad sign, for the more rapidly and numerously they break out, the more speedily and thoroughly they will be cured. The falling off of the hair is very often remedied by *Hepar.*

Iritis cannot well be treated without Mercury; but it has to be used cautiously; *Corrosive Sublimate* is the best mercurial preparation for this disease and the most efficient remedy to avert all immediate danger. After the Sublimate, the remaining symptoms are most effectually controlled by means of *Clematis;* we have cured two cases of iritis with this drug alone, although the pupil was already considerably distorted.

The next syphilitic forms which we shall describe, are a mixture of syphilis and mercurial poisoning, or, which is likewise possible, of syphilis and constitutional anomalies. The treatment of these forms is therefore very different, sometimes exceedingly difficult and always very tedious. It is of great importance that, even in regard to the forms that we have just described, we should know how much Mercury had been used in treating them; this knowledge is indispensable if we are called upon to treat mercurio-syphilitic combinations. We again call to mind a chief rule which is applicable to all these cases, namely: that a curative result must not be expected too impatiently, and that we had better commence the treatment with some indifferent substance, which will afford us time to decide upon the course of treatment that ought to be pursued. We would tender this advice to all those who fancy that a syphilitic patient cannot pass a day without suffering for the want of medicine. Drenching the patient with quantities of medicine is sufficiently destructive in the hands of Old School practitioners, it is likewise hurtful in homœopathic hands, were it only because such a treatment obscures the curative results obtained with our remedies. And we again suggest with all proper emphasis that the cutaneous efflorescences and most other syphilitic phenomena are curative endeavors that ought to be sustained rather than prematurely suppressed.

The remedies which homœopaths employ to combat the mixed forms of syphilis and mercurial poisoning, and whose value has been ascertained by clinical experience, are: *Mercurius bijodatus, Kali hydriodicum*, *Hepar sulphuris calc.*, *Sulphur*, *Aurum muriaticum* and *metallicum*, *Kali bichromicum*, *Acidum nitricum*, *Sarsaparilla*, *Lycopodium*. To undertake to give special indications for every single remedy would be a vain endeavor. In reality we have to be guided by clinical experience, without being able to act in full accord with the law of similarity. We shall rarely be able to effect a cure with any single one of these remedies; most commonly frequent changes will be found indispensable. For this reason we confine ourselves to giving the most necessary rules in the subjoined paragraphs.

Syphilitic exanthems, with the exception of roseola, scarcely ever require any Mercury; it is only if the improvement is tardy, or does not seem disposed to set in, and if we are certain that the patient had not yet been poisoned with this drug, that a few doses of Mercury can sometimes be given while the treatment is mainly conducted with some other leading remedy. Psoriasis yields most promptly to *Sulphur*, *Nitri acidum*, and, according to some, to *Sarsaparilla* and *Lycopodium*. The pustulous forms require the *Iodide of Mercury*, *Nitric acid*, the *Hydriodate* and *Bichromate of Potash*. Syphilitic pemphigus requires: *Hepar sulphuris calc.*, *Sulphur*, likewise *Graphites*. Tuberculous exanthems: *Aurum metallicum*, *Acidum nitricum*, and likewise *Graphites*; *Lycopodium* may likewise be appropiate.

The ulcers on the mucous lining are of a mercurial character, if they are deeply-penetrating and affect the bones; we have to avoid Mercury in treating them, and only resort to it, if we are satisfied that no improvement can be achieved by any other means. In such cases the red and white Precipitates are preferable to all other mercurial preparations. For ulcers in the mouth *Kali hydriod.* may be given alternately with *Kali bichromicum*; for ozæna, if the bones are yet intact, *Kali hydriod.* may be prescribed, and if the bones are invaded, *Aurum muriaticum*. If the patient had previously taken a good deal of Mercury, *Acidum nitricum* may be given every now and then for a few days at a time. Laryngitis requires above any other remedy *Hepar sulphuris*, moreover *Iodine* and the *Bichromate of Potash*, and according to Hartmann, *Lycopodium*.

The tertiary phenomena require throughout a cautious, but continued use of the *Iodide of Potassium*. It is only for single forms that other remedies are required, *Aurum*, for instance, for syphilitic lupus, for caries of the facial bones, the suppurating tophi, and finally for sarcocele. *Sulphur* scarcely ever produces marked results in tertiary syphilis, nor does *Hepar sulphuris*. On the other hand, the Iodine-springs of Hall deserve high praise; the water from these springs is the mildest and at the same time most penetrating form in which Iodine can be administered.

It remains for us now to make a few remarks concerning the diet of syphilitic patients. In this respect opinions differ even among homœopathic physicians to such an extent that they sometimes are in direct antagonism to each other. We have found the following rules uniformly substantiated by our own experience. Syphilitic patients should never be deprived of a sufficient supply of simple and nourishing food; they should not be allowed to eat to excess, nor should they indulge in fat and spiced articles of diet, spirits, heavy beer; light wines do not hurt; a beverage composed of wine and water may safely be permitted. The patient should be allowed to enjoy fresh air, but should avoid violent exertions, long walks, dancing, etc., until the chancre is healed. These rules are based upon the observation that, if the bodily strength is well preserved, the syphilitic disease runs through its different phases more rapidly; it is moreover a general principle in therapeutic science that the reactive energy of the organism should never be voluntarily depressed in any disease. Mercurial poisoning does not require a deviation from this principle, for it is in debilitated individuals that Mercury causes the most terrible devastation. Of great importance in protracted cases of syphilis is careful attention to the skin which is undoubtedly the most important organ for all critical endeavors of the organism. This is the reason why inveterate secondary and tertiary syphilis improves so rapidly under a rationally and methodically conducted cold-water treatment which should always be resorted to in such cases. Sulphur-baths are much less effectual; they may afford relief, if the patient is attacked with severe rheumatic pains; otherwise they have no other effect than to increase the sensitiveness of the skin to atmospheric influences.

B. EPIDEMIC AND ENDEMIC INFECTIOUS DISEASES.

1. Intermittent Fever, Fever and Ague.

Intermittent fever is now almost universally traced to the influence of malaria; any other origin of this fever is denied. What malaria is, and whence it arises, is either entirely unknown, or else our knowledge of malaria is very uncertain. Where a quantity of vegetable matter is exposed to rapid decay, intermittent fevers are a very common occurrence, and they are the more intense the more rapidly the process of putrefaction takes place, consequently their intensity is greatest in very hot weather. We should be led too far, if we were to dwell more particularly upon the nature of malaria, and we omit this so much more readily as no advantage accrues to the treatment from such speculations. It is well, however, that our attention should be kept fixed on one point, namely the decaying vegetation; for this will remind us of the prophylactic measures that it may be necessary to take. Where malaria prevails, intermittent fever is endemic. But this fever likewise breaks out in a more or less epidemic form, when it invades malarious districts with great violence, or when it visits regions that are generally free from intermittent fever, in a mild form, and does not spread over a large extent of country. Whether epidemics of this kind likewise owe their origin to malarious miasms that had been wafted over from their original locality, is questionable, for, after all, it is difficult to understand why in one year the infectious matter should be carried upon the wings of the wind, and not in another year. Nor are such epidemics confined to certain atmospheric relations. What is remarkable is that such fever-and-ague epidemics are very apt to precede epidemic cholera. Where intermittent fever is an entirely sporadic disease, its origin is still more obscure, as is the case among us, for instance, in the city of Hanover.

A special disposition to the disease is determined by age only in so far that middle-aged, robust individuals are more exposed to the exciting causes of the fever. In infancy intermittent fever is a comparatively rare disease. Tuberculosis is an almost certain guarantee against intermittent fever.

As regards the seasons, the disease occurs most frequently when the decay of vegetable matter is going on most extensively, namely in the months of April, May and June, in hot summers with copious showers of rain, likewise in very warm fall-months. Fever and ague is least prevalent during the winter-months, in very cold weather and likewise in very warm, dry weather.

Predisposing causes of fever and ague are: errors in diet, catarrh of the digestive tract, colds, working all the time in wet places. This last-mentioned circumstance is the reason why brickmakers are so readily attacked with fever and ague, even if the locality where they work is situated on high ground.

One attack of fever and ague undoubtedly increases the disposition to have a second one; persons who move from perfectly healthy into malarious districts are likewise attacked much more readily, whereas a protracted sojourn in a malarious district diminishes the susceptibility to the malarious miasm.

To picture intermittent fever as it really exists, is a difficult undertaking; in the first place, the disease of itself varies greatly in its manifestations; and in the next place the fever is greatly modified by the employment of remedial agents. Inasmuch as these deviations from the normal form will have to be mentioned more particularly when we come to speak of the remedies for this fever, we here confine ourselves to a short description of the most essential modifications.

Uncomplicated, genuine intermittent fever is characterized by paroxysms of chill, heat and sweat, returning at regular intervals and separated from each other by a more or less complete apyrexia.

The first paroxysm is very generally preceded by a more or less distinct preliminary stage lasting at times a day, at other times a week and even longer, and not presenting any phenomena that definitely point to intermittent fever. In sporadic cases especially, a gastro-intestinal catarrh with slight remittent fever is very apt to run into fever and ague.

The paroxysm is very frequently ushered in with a feeling of malaise, stretching and yawning, drawing pains in the extremities; these symptoms are soon succeeded by chills down the spine, and by a feeling of coldness in the extremities and whole body, attended with shaking of the body and chattering of the teeth. On the parts of the body most remote from the heart, the skin generally loses its turgescence, its temperature falls quite considerably, its color is bluish and as if dead. On the other hand, the temperature in the axillæ as well as in the mouth is considerably higher. The chill is very generally accompanied by violent headache and a distressing thirst, and, if any food had been introduced into the stomach shortly before the paroxysm, it is ejected when the chill sets in. The chill seldom lasts less than half an hour, nor more than three hours. The pulse is small and contracted, the urine has not much color, the spleen is somewhat enlarged.

The second or hot stage never sets in all at once; the chill abates gradually and is interrupted by local flashes of heat, until the heat finally becomes permanent and general. With the heat, the turgescence of the skin likewise returns, the temperature gradually increases to a considerable height, sometimes over 100° F., and the pulse becomes full and bounding. The headache, restlessness and thirst increase considerably, delirium is not unfrequent, the color of the face changes to a bright-red. The enlargement of the spleen continues during this stage which seldom lasts less than two to three, but frequently upwards of six or eight hours.

The sweaty stage likewise sets in gradually; perspiration first breaks out on some parts and gradually covers the whole body. At the same time the temperature sinks rapidly, according to Wunderlich, in regular stages, and a feeling of comfort is soon restored to the patient. As a rule, the urine at this stage is strongly saturated with urates. The sweat lasts from one to six and even ten hours; the apyrexia commences as soon as the sweat ceases. This period which is of the utmost importance to a homœopathic practitioner, always shows some, although sometimes very trifling morbid symptoms which differ in different individuals.

Fever-and-ague, in its uncomplicated form, generally follows the tertian type; in other words, forty-eight hours elapse between two successive paroxysms. If the intensity of the fever remains the same, the paroxysms generally return at the same period. In proportion as the disease decreases in intensity, the next paroxysm always sets in at a somewhat earlier period, and in a less degree of intensity; it is much less frequently the case for the paroxysm to set in with less force and at a later period. If the paroxysm sets in sooner and with more violence, a transformation of the tertian into the quotidian type may be expected; a change of this kind almost always takes place, if the fever lasts a good while. At the same time the affection shows a higher degree of intensity and obstinacy. The quartan type, that is, the return of the paroxysms at intervals of seventy-two hours, only sets in after the disease has lasted for a long time, at times developing itself directly from the tertian type, while the paroxysms postpone, and at other times from the quotidian fever. This quartan type implies the highest degree of tenacity in the disease.

The other types, double-tertian, sub-tertian, and whatever their names may be, occur too seldom to deserve special mention.

It is difficult to say what constitutes the normal course of intermittent fever, for the reason that it is always modified by treatment. The following may be regarded as tolerably fixed: In a favorable case the paroxysms scarcely ever cease suddenly; they decrease gradually both in intensity and duration, and are apt to discontinue entirely at the end of seven days, the apyrexia being more and more prolonged and gradually becoming permanent. In unfavorable cases, either under the influence of improper management or under the continued action of the malarial poison, but never, or at least very seldom, under homœopathic treatment, we have a gradual development of the so-called malarial cachexia which we shall dwell upon more fully after having previously described a few deviations from the normal type.

Upon the whole, these anomalies occur very seldom at the commencement of the malarious infection, but they become the more frequent, the more the disease approximates to a malarial cachexia. One of the three stages may be entirely wanting, or, if it exists, it may be scarcely perceptible. It is generally the chill and sweaty stage that remain suppressed, the hot stage is almost always present. Some of the stages, more particularly the heat and the sweaty stage, may be separated by an apparent apyrexia of a few hours' duration. Among children, convulsions are not unusual in the first two stages, but they are not of a dangerous import, except when violent and long-lasting. An intermittent fever of long duration and under the continued action of malaria, changes to the remittent type; this circumstance, however, points without an exception to malarial cachexia. In simple intermittent fever, the spleen never enlarges to any very great extent.

One of the characteristic effects of malaria is intermittent neuralgia; the paroxysms set in with all the typical regularity of fever-and-ague paroxysms, but without any marked febrile symptoms. During these attacks, the temperature of the body is generally considerably higher than usual. [There are other intermittent paroxysms which take the place of fever and ague and may be regarded as masked forms of the intermittent disease. Some of the more common forms of masked fever and ague are: Intermittent neuralgia, dysentery, pneumonia, articular rheumatism. We have never been able to get along in the treatment of these masked forms of fever and ague without *Quinine;* it is not necessary to give large doses, but Quinine is indispensable. H.]

The most important anomaly is the intermittens perniciosa or comitata. Most commonly intermittent fever adopts this form in the subsequent course of the disease, very seldom at the beginning. Intermittens perniciosa is a form of fever where a simple increase of the ordinary symptoms becomes dangerous to life. This malignant increase often takes place in the first stage, more particularly in the case of children, but more commonly during the hot stage; the danger arises either from the brain being paralyzed, or else from paralysis of the heart in consequence of the excessive vascular excitement. If the brain is threatened with paralysis, the attack is characterized by delirium, sopor, coma, likewise by paroxysms of excessive maniacal exaltation; if paralysis of the heart threatens, the chill increases to icy-coldness, like the coldness in cholera. Many a case of fever and ague assumes the pernicious type simply because the paroxysms are of an extraordinary duration. [This form of intermittent fever is designated in our country as "Congestive chills;" it acts precisely as Hufeland's febris apoplectica or perniciosa. We have seen a great deal of it. During the chill we give *Aconite* or *Gelseminum,* as the case may be, and we sometimes resort to the spirits of Camphor to hasten reaction; during the hot stage we continue the Aconite, or substitute *Belladonna;* and when the sweaty stage has fairly set in, we give *Quinine* in sufficient quantity either to keep off the next attack, or at least to secure a modification of the paroxysm. We do not believe that congestive chills, such as we see them in our malarious countries, can be arrested without Quinine; we believe that Quinine is the specific remedy for this form of chills, although other remedies may likewise be required. When the late Dr. Channing was still practising in the city of New York, he had a case of congestive chills to treat, for which he gave the patient, a Western gentleman, a dose of tolerably highly-potentized *Nux vomica.* A second chill, of course, took place much more violent than the first. The Doctor, with his large brain crammed brimful with the doctrine of homœopathic aggravations, being perfectly satisfied that the Nux had aggravated the symptoms, gave him a drop of Alcohol to counteract the terrible mischief the harmless little globule of Nux had done; a third paroxysm occurred, which destroyed the patient. II.] The febres comitatæ are characterized by the supervention of other threatening symptoms during the paroxysm, more particularly a severe attack of intestinal catarrh like cholera, rupture of the spleen, excessive hyperæmia of the brain, inflammatory affections of vital organs, hemorrhages, apoplexy.

Malarial cachexia in its severest form is most usually met with, if a quantity of Quinine is administered to the patient while he continues to be exposed to the action of the malarious miasm. This action alone, without Quinine, never produces a malarial cachexia of the same degree of intensity. Individuals who had taken a great deal of Quinine, after moving out of the infectious district, are very apt to be attacked with malarial cachexia. According to the observations that have been made by a number of practitioners, the close connection between malarial cachexia and Quinine cannot be denied. We will now proceed to describe the course which fever and ague takes when mismanaged by Quinine.

With large doses of Quinine we generally succeed in effecting a sudden cessation of the paroxysms; but the period following such a suppression is not free from morbid symptoms; the patients complain more or less. A fortnight, or more commonly three weeks, less frequently four weeks after the suppression, another paroxysm breaks out very suddenly. This paroxysm likewise yields to Quinine, but after this second suppression the patient generally complains more than after the first; for a third paroxysm, which generally breaks out after a short apyrexia, Quinine now proves ineffectual. The paroxysms either assume the quartan type, or else they break out with great irregularity, and combine with constitutional symptoms that gradually increase in intensity. The spleen is sometimes so large that it fills one-half of the abdominal cavity; the liver becomes enlarged and after a while shows symptoms of fatty degeneration; the digestion is entirely deranged, the appetite is gone, the bowels are excessively constipated, or else, the patient is troubled with a diarrhœa as in hectic fever. The patients seem to be attacked with a deep-seated anæmia and have a strikingly sallow complexion. The changes in the abdominal viscera may sooner or later lead to ascites. If, as we have often noticed, a catarrhal affection of the lungs sets in, we obtain a complete picture of florid phthisis. The emaciation of the patients soon reaches a high degree, and, under improper treatment, death now is an almost inevitable result.

The prognosis in intermittent fever revolves around the following points: If the attack is recent, the prognosis is quite favorable; the longer the disease had lasted; the more irregular the paroxysms had become; the more strikingly the blood had become altered, the more protracted will be the recovery of the patient. Sporadic cases in a healthy district are of very little importance. Diseases breaking out while the patient continues to be exposed to the influence of malaria, get well very slowly; but even if the patient is removed from the further action of the miasm, the cure takes place very slowly. An advanced as well as a very young age; a dilapitated organism, and more particularly alcoholism, render the prognosis very uncertain.

To treat fever and ague according to the homœopathic law is a task which is undoubtedly invested with great difficulties even for the most experienced practitioner. The homœopathic treatment of fever and ague has undoubtedly led to many errors, for the reason that spontaneous cures were too often overlooked and appropriated as the results of the medicine that had been administered for the fever. In consequence of this, the number of our remedies for fever and ague has been very much increased, to the great inconvenience of the physician who is in need of a remedy for a particular case. For this reason we furnish in the subsequent paragraphs a limited number of remedies with definite indications; of the more unreliable medicines we shall only give the names.

In treating a case of fever and ague a few points should never be lost sight of, since attention to these points will save the practitioner from many mistakes.

In the first place, it is an important point in the treatment of fever and ague that the totality of the symptoms should never be lost sight of; in other words, not only the symptoms characterizing the paroxysm, but likewise those that are perceived during the apyrexia, or new symptoms, should be carefully noted. A remedy should never be chosen exclusively according to the symptoms of the paroxysm or the apyrexia. It is evident, however, in view of the great similarity of the paroxysms, that the appropriate remedy will more especially be determined by the symptoms during the apyrexia.

Higher potencies are undoubtedly sufficient to effect a cure, although a preference is generally accorded to the lower. If a remedy that is evidently homœopathic to the case, does not cure it, it is perfectly proper to try a lower attenuation before parting with this drug.

If possible the remedy should never be given during the paroxysm, but as soon as possible after the paroxysm is terminated.

If, under the operation of a medicine, the paroxysms decrease in duration and intensity, it should be continued as long as the good effects of this medicine last; by pursuing this course we obtain the most reliable information concerning the use of special remedies in fever and ague.

If an epidemic breaks out in a non-malarious district, it will be found that one or two remedies are generally sufficient to cure every case.

The following are the most efficient remedies for simple fever and ague:

China or **Quinine** is undoubtedly the most important remedy for fever and ague, but its value is very much impaired by the fact that it is employed as a sovereign remedy not only for fever and ague itself, but likewise for all intermittent diseases. We need not dwell any further upon the manner in which this remedy is abused; this fact is too well known to the Profession. All we can say is that *China* is the most effectual and reliable of all anti-typical medicines, but that it only helps when it is homœopathic to the case. *China* is suitable in a majority of all cases of endemic and epidemic fever and ague, even during the whole course of the disease, whereas in sporadic cases it is generally of very little use. China is particularly indicated by the following symptoms: Precursory symptoms consisting in nervous excitement, anxiousness, headache, nausea, general irritability; the chill is of short duration, very soon mingled with heat, without thirst which is only experienced at the commencement of the hot stage, and is never very intense. Sensitiveness and excessive irritability especially during the chill; the sweaty stage lasts a long while and the perspiration is exceedingly profuse. During the apyrexia we have: great debility with restlessness, loss of appetite with canine hunger, bitter taste and thickly-coated tongue. We do not attach an extreme importance to these indications, for they are often deceptive. As a rule, it is true that *China* cures every case of fever and ague originating in malaria; the case must be of recent origin and attended with nervous irritability and gastric-bilious symptoms. In inveterate cases, with marked hypertrophy of the spleen and liver, anæmia, dropsy, *China* will seldom be of much use; such patients have always been dosed with this medicine to excess. If they have not, *China* is indicated by: anæmia, a yellowish-gray complexion; occasional attacks of diarrhœa, palpitation of the heart, congestions of the head, back-ache, œdema; irregularity of the paroxysms, the single stages not succeeding each other immediately, and not being completely developed. [We have frequently met with such symptoms under the symptom-treatment of high potentialists, where a few small doses of Quinine would wipe out the whole disease, after the patient had been kept sick and sicker for weeks. H.] Upon the whole, a tertian type is most adapted to the curative range of China, the quartan-type much less frequently. As regards dose we advise the use of the lower preparations in all recent cases, but it will scarcely ever be necessary to go below the second trituration of *Quinine* or the first attenuation of the tincture of *Cinchona*. Fevers that do not yield to such doses, are not amenable to the curative action of Quinine, and can only be suppressed, but not cured, by more massive doses of this drug. In the genuine malarial cachexia, China will very seldom render much service.

Ipecacuanha is decidedly adapted to epidemic fever and ague; if it cures one case, it will undoubtedly cure most of the other cases. This circumstance at one time procured for it the inordinate praises of the Old School; afterwards it fell into disrepute, because it was not found adapted to all epidemics, its opponents not being aware that fever and ague epidemics differ amongst each other in character. *Ipecac.* is only suitable in the milder forms of intermittent fever, scarcely in any other than the tertian type; the different stages run their course without much intensity and the chill is most marked; it is particularly indicated, if the fever is accompanied by gastric symptoms, such as loss of appetite, loathing of food, nausea, vomiting, diarrhœa with very little bile in the evacuations, or if the paroxysm is caused by dietetic transgressions. Intermittent fevers of this character are generally epidemic in non-malarious districts.

According to Hartmann **Nux vomica** is indicated by the following symptoms: Fever, with constipation, gastric-bilious symptoms; it breaks out after gross violations of diet, and is characterized by nervous symptoms proceeding from the spinal cord. [We once cured a case of fever and ague of nine months' standing with a few doses of Nux. The patient had been in one of the Nashville hospitals for nine months, and had taken Quinine by the ounce. He was very fond of liquor and a paroxysm broke out after every debauch. Nux cured him so perfectly that the paroxysms did not even return after he had been drinking. H.] Quotidian and tertian-fevers, setting in in the afternoon, evening or night, with alternation of heat and chills, enormous craving for beer, frontal headache, vertigo, nausea, bitter taste and eructations, cardialgia, great weakness.—In congestive chills *Nux* is likewise indicated by the following symptoms: Paralysis of the extremities at the onset, prostration, weariness, trembling, fainting, vertigo, dyspnœa, palpitation of the heart, heat of the head with coldness of the body, delirium. *Nux* is undoubtedly one of our more important fever-remedies; it will not be difficult to determine its homœopathicity in given cases. In inveterate cases *Nux* would not often be our choice. It is likewise an important remedy if the fever is complicated with bronchitis.

Veratrum album is likewise one of our most important fever and ague remedies; marked chill which is slowly followed by heat, with convulsive symptoms and great thirst, vomiting or retching, quick, feeble and small pulse; stupor during the hot stage, with bland delirium; the third stage is not strikingly marked. In febris comitata *Veratrum album* is an important remedy if the cerebral symptoms, the pulmonary hyperæmia and the profuse intestinal catarrh are prominently developed.

Arsenicum, in our estimation is still more important than China; its range of action is still more extensive. In recent cases it is indicated by the following symptoms: Intensity and long duration of the paroxysms, especially burning heat; unquenchable thirst during the whole attack, and extreme anxiety and restlessness except during the sweaty stage, attended with palpitation of the heart, and a subdued, accelerated pulse; moreover functional derangements of single organs. *Arsen.* is indicated the more specifically the cleaner the tongue remains in extremely violent paroxysms, the more rapidly the strength is exhausted by the single paroxysm and the sooner the characteristic sallow pallor makes its appearance. For this reason *Arsen.* is an important remedy in endemic fever and ague. In congestive chills the imminent paralysis of the heart points to *Arsenicum* beside Verat. alb.; *Arsen.* is likewise indicated if the fever is complicated with severe cholerine. In fever and ague cachexia *Arsen.* is a sovereign remedy. Its effect is truly marvellous. With a single dose of *Arsenicum* 30 we have cured a cachexia of thirteen weeks' standing. The patient, a very robust man, presented the picture of a complete phthisis florida; he was cured even without leaving his home situated in a truly malarious region of country. Another case of nine months' standing was cured by means of a few doses of *Arsen.* 30, so completely that even the hypertrophied spleen was reduced back again to its natural size. The patient was a Hollander who brought the disease with him; after residing in our very healthy city for four months and swallowing large quantities of *Quinine,* all the symptoms of phthisis florida had developed themselves.—*Arsen.* is not only a fever-remedy, but likewise an antidote to *Quinine.* We need not point out special symptoms, for cachexia is amenable to *Arsenicum* in all its manifestations, which, it is true, generally resemble each other very closely; it is least reliable when the anæmia is extreme and the reactive powers of the organism are very much depressed. In the above-mentioned cases we have stated the dose, because we are satisfied that in cachexia small doses exert the most curative influence; on the other hand we are equally satisfied that in more recent cases triturations up to the sixth are most suitable.

Natrum muriaticum is very seldom indicated in recent, but so much more so in inveterate cases. The stages are very unequal, the chill continuous, the heat moderate, but accompanied by all sorts of accessory symptoms, among which headache occupies the most prominent rank; the perspiration is either wanting, or else it is excessive and debilitating. At the same time the patient is troubled with chronic catarrh of the mouth and stomach, constant constipation, renal catarrh, palpitations of the heart. The patient has a grayish-yellow look; the spleen and liver are very much enlarged.

Arnica is adapted to recent as well as inveterate cases if the chill is preceded by violent thirst which abates almost entirely after the heat breaks out; if during the hot stage every little current of air causes the patient to feel chilly, and if, during this stage he seems to be listless but at the same time very restless.

To these remedies we add a few from Hartmann, concerning which we do not possess any personal experience.

Belladonna in quotidian fever, with horrid headache, vertigo, hallucinations, injected eyes, nausea, vomiting, constant constipation; or in fevers where each paroxysm is associated with a severe neuralgic attack.

Cina, if the fever commences with vomiting of food followed by canine hunger; the attacks come on every day.

Pulsatilla; vomiting of mucus at the commencement of the chill, heat and sweat without thirst; mucous diarrhœa during the apyrexia, with loathing of food and nausea.

Antimonium crudum; heat and sweat break out at the same time, the sweat being only transitory; loss of appetite, eructations, nausea, vomiting, thickly-coated tongue, bitter taste, tension and pressure at the stomach, pain in the chest.

Bryonia; the fever sets in early in the morning; the attack is ushered in with vertigo, pressure and a gnawing sensation in the sinciput; at the same time a dry cough with stinging pains in the chest, dyspnœa, vomiturition.

Sabadilla; the attacks set in with great regularity, neither postpone nor anticipate; short chill, followed by thirst and lastly heat; or only chill without heat or sweat; apyrexia with frequent chilly creeping, pressure and distention at the stomach, with loss of appetite, nocturnal, dry cough, pain in the chest, dyspnœa.

Ignatia; the chill is removed by external covering; some parts feel cold, others hot; heat only on the outside, without thirst; dulness of the head during the hot stage, bruising pain in the occiput, right side, pressure at the pit of the stomach, great lassitude, paleness of the face, etc. Thirst only after the paroxysm.

Carbo vegetabilis; the attack is preceded by a beating in the temples, tearing in the teeth and extremities, stretching, cold feet. Thirst and great lassitude during the chill. During the hot stage, without thirst: headache, vertigo, flushed face, obscuration of vision, nausea, pain in the stomach, abdomen, chest, dyspnœa; the fever is succeeded by severe headache.

Capsicum; the chill prevails, attended with intense thirst which is wanting or only very moderate during the hot stage; sweat during the heat. During the chill: anxiety, restlessness, inability to collect one's-self, sensitiveness to noise; headache, ptyalism, vomiting of mucus, splenetalgia, backache, tearing and contracting sensation in the extremities. During the heat: stinging in the head, fetor from the mouth, colic with ineffectual urging to stool, pain in the chest and back, tearing in the lower limbs.

Tartarus emeticus; drowsiness during the attack; *Opium* is to be given if real sopor is present.

We might increase this list, if we would name all the different remedies that might possibly be indicated. But we do not even regard most of the above-mentioned remedies as real fever and ague remedies; their choice depends upon the nature of the accompanying symptoms which, if a cure takes place, would have proved to be the cause, not the consequence of the fever. If we wish to be certain of selecting the right remedy, we have to inquire with great care whether the intermittent character of the attack only constitutes an accidental, although very prominent symptom, or whether the other symptoms emanate from the intermittent paroxysm as their fountain-head. In the latter case the remedies that have been named first, deserve a preference over any other; in the former case the symptoms which are most prominent during the apyrexia, decide a choice of the remedy.

In congestive chills as well as in the febres comitatæ the threatening accessory symptoms are the main indications. The most suitable remedies cannot be indicated *a priori*.

A fever and ague cachexia is always such a complicated affection, that it is impossible to indicate therapeutic rules for its management applicable to every case. The whole organism is involved, at times the spleen being more severely affected, at other times the liver, or the stomach and intestines, then again the lungs: sometimes the greatest danger emanates from the anæmic condition of the patient, so that it is often very difficult to hit upon the right remedy. If *China* had not been abused, it will meet most of the symptoms, and will prove the best remedy in the case. If *Quinine* had been taken to excess, *Arsen.* will help in the large majority of cases; this remedy should not be given up all at once, if the improvement is not very speedy; in such a case it is much better to change the dose than the remedy. *Ferrum* is adapted to all cases where the anæmia and debility are highly developed, but no œdema has yet set in; the patients complain somewhat of congestion of the chest and heart, nor is the stomach disposed to retain any nourishment. *Natrum muriaticum* and *Lycopodium* are indicated if the digestive organs are chiefly affected, and the derangement is characterized by symptoms peculiar to these two drugs. Other remedies may be required for extraordinary symptoms. We doubt, however, whether *Belladonna* and *Staphysagria*, recommended by Hartmann, are ever of any use in this cachexia.

There is no special diet that can be recommended for fever and ague. It depends in every case upon the state of the digestive organs and the necessity of guarding the stomach against every pernicious influence, for it is upon the normal functions of the stomach that depends the possibility of the patient's sinking strength being restored to its natural tone. If possible, the patient had better leave the malarious district, and remove to the mountains where recovery takes place most rapidly.

2. Typhus.

Typhus occurs in two forms that do not differ much from each other, namely: typhus abdominalis and typhus exanthematicus. More recently this last-named form has become much less frequent than the former. In spite of these differences the etiology of both forms is pretty much the same; up to this period we have not succeeded in discovering the reasons for the appearance of either one or the other form.

Typhus originates in some infectious agent; all that is known of this agent is that it is caused by the decomposition of animal substances. Hence typhus occurs most frequently where the decomposition of animal matter is most favored by circumstances, namely in large cities and hospitals; likewise in localities which are least favorably situated for carrying away the products of decomposition, such as cities built in a flat country and with imperfect drainage. The infectious principle at times seems to act with great intensity, at other times very mildly, so that typhus in crowded localities sometimes breaks out with an extraordinary virulence, and at other times with comparative mildness. According to all probability, a graduated difference of this kind is chiefly owing to the quantity of the infectious agent that acts upon the organism, not to its quality. The contagium is reproduced by the patient. We cannot share the views which prevail concerning the formation of a contagium. We do not consider any form of typhus contagious. An apparently contagious transmission of typhus only takes place among those who have been for some time exposed to the emanations from the infected individual, not among those who have only been in contact with the patient for a short period of time. These remarks likewise apply to exanthematic typhus which is considered as decidedly contagious, but which only appears so for the reason that it produces a larger quantity and a more infectious quality of contagious matter. Physicians in private practice are seldom attacked, notwithstanding they are brought in closest contact with the patients when exploring their chests; hospital-physicians and nurses, on the contrary, are taken down very often. More recently the level of the surface-water has been more particularly examined with reference to typhus and cholera; a high level is supposed to favor the breaking out of these plagues. We are still without any reliable data in this respect. In large cities the construction of wells and water-closets deserves great attention; where both are so close together that the well-water can be contaminated by the contents of the closets, typhus is very likely to occur. This subject is without doubt worthy the most serious attention of the Board of Health, for typhus is not only one of the most dangerous, but likewise one of the most frequent diseases.

A few points can easily be inferred from what we have said, such as: epidemic and endemic, slightly endemic and sporadic type of typhus; breaking out of typhus in very damp and hot years, during the hot months of the summer and in the fall; likewise in crowded hospitals, more particularly if they are full of wounded soldiers; or in densely populated streets, tenement-houses, on shipboard, etc. Typhus occasioned by an insufficient supply of food, or by unwholesome and deteriorated food, is less easily accounted for.

One attack of typhus does not always, but very generally, protect against a second attack. There are certain other circumstances that almost positively preclude the possibility of typhus, especially abdominal typhus; these are: Intermittent fever, tuberculosis, carcinoma, heart-disease of the higher grade. Age does not establish any positive lines of demarcation; except infants, persons of any age may be attacked, but more particularly young people and individuals up to the age of fifty. Vigorous constitutions are more easily attacked and likewise more severely.

Exciting causes are: Fear and anxiety; a sudden change of diet, when persons settle in a locality where typhus is endemic; catarrh of the intestines; mental depression, both by excessive mental labor as well as by care and grief.

Symptoms and Course. We deem it unnecessary to analyze the pathological anatomy of typhus, for the reason that the prominent post-mortem phenomena scarcely ever correspond with definite groups of symptoms in the phenomenal totality of the disease. Hence, we confine ourselves to a few more important data. In abdominal typhus the ulcers in the intestines act the most important part; they have even given rise to the name of this form of the disease. However, it behooves us to premise the statement that in their various phases these ulcers do not correspond with definite phases in the total course of the disease. The ulcers form as follows: At first the mucous lining of the ileum is strikingly hyperæmic, more particularly in its lower half; gradually this venous hyperæmia becomes centered in Peyer's and Brunner's glands, which swell up considerably together with the mesenteric glands. In the former the inflammatory infiltration may be reabsorbed, or else, which happens much more frequently, the infiltration is decomposed, destroying the super-incumbent mucous lining, and giving rise to an ulcer, the enteric or typhous ulcer. This ulcer is most commonly located in the inferior extremity of the ileum and, according as it arises from a solitary or a conglomerate gland, may be round and small, or enlarge to the size of half a dollar, with irregular, undermined borders. The healing takes place very slowly; the destructive process may likewise penetrate to the deeper tissues, perforating the intestine. The subsequent cicatrix never causes stricture of the intestine. The intestinal ulceration very seldom assumes a chronic form, resulting in a slow, hectic fever. Beside the intestinal ulcers, the spleen shows tolerably constant alterations; in the first weeks it enlarges even to six times its normal size, the capsule is very tense, the substance of the spleen exceedingly vascular and crumbling, its color is very dark; afterwards the swelling goes down again almost to the natural proportions of the organ, the capsule is relaxed, the parenchyma pale and anæmic. Except these two almost constant phenomena, typhus does not offer any permanent, certainly no characteristic signs. The brain, especially, remains unaltered; the lungs, on the contrary, show at first symptoms of pulmonary irritation; afterwards hypostatic, less frequently lobular or lobar pneumonia. During the first weeks of the disease the muscles have a somewhat characteristically dark color, and the internal surface of the arteries has likewise a dark-red appearance. In exanthematic typhus the intestinal ulceration does not exist, whereas in this form likewise the spleen is considerably hypertrophied and softened, and the vessels also have a bright appearance as if injected. Other constantly present anatomical alterations are not perceived.

Abdominal typhus very rarely breaks out suddenly; it is generally preceded for a few days or even a week by indefinite symptoms, such as lassitude, indisposition to work, loss of spirits, impaired appetite, very seldom hunger almost bordering upon a voracious desire for food; wandering rheumatoid pains in the limbs, especially in the back, headache of an indeterminate type, sleep full of dreams.

The disease is generally ushered in by a chill of moderate violence, or by a marked fainting sensation which is soon followed by the characteristic feeling of illness, namely: an inability to stand erect or move about, and a desire to lie down. Very seldom one of these conditions is entirely wanting, so that it is difficult to point out the real beginning of the disease; instead of one severe chill we often meet with a succession of very feeble chills. The disease now develops itself in the following manner: The patients feel weak, have neither the strength nor the desire to rise from their beds; headache, at times more frontal, and at other times, in the more violent cases, in the occiput, throbbing and very distressing; complete loss of appetite; altered, generally pasty taste; vomiting not very frequent; bowels quite torpid in the first week; restless sleep; when waking early in the morning, the patients commence very soon to complain of phantasms which they cannot avoid; yet they talk very rationally and are perfectly conscious of seeing phantasms. The pulse is generally full, very seldom exceeding one hundred beats, very often dicrotic; the temperature is high, the skin feels burning-hot. The breathing is almost constantly hurried, anxious, the patient talks hurriedly, yet, if desired, he is able to take a long breath. The spleen is generally swollen, the swelling increasing rapidly in size, and is not unfrequently painful. The abdomen does not show any constant alterations, but when the iliocœcal region is pressed upon, the patients complain of pain in this region, and a gurgling sensation is communicated to the finger, with which the pressure is made. The tongue is at times coated very thickly, at other times it only has a whitish coating, and again it looks quite clean, but the coating changes as the disease progresses. Sometimes the patients complain of a little hacking cough, and exhibit symptoms of a slight bronchial catarrh. The urine is less in quantity, saturated, notwithstanding that the patients often experience a very violent thirst. All these symptoms remain in force only in very violent cases; most generally a sensible remission of these symptoms takes place towards the end of the first week.

In the second week the symptoms of the disease undergo a marked change, unless the morbid process takes a turn towards recovery, which is very seldom the case. For the present we only speak of typhus of a moderately severe type. In this stage the patients lose their consciousness more and more; they are either lying in a state of lethargic apathy, or else, it is only with great difficulty that they are able to reply to questions or to give utterance to their own ideas. In the evening and during the night this soporous prostration is generally interrupted by a state of nervous exaltation, during which the patients manifest their internal nervousness by animated talking or by a constant endeavor to escape from their beds. Sensations of pain now cease entirely; when asked how they feel, they answer: "Quite well;" they express no desire for drink, but they swallow the offered beverage hurriedly and greedily; when repeatedly asked to do so, they put out their tongues slowly and tremulously, and forget to draw them in again. Another evidence that the influence of the brain is almost entirely suspended is, that the patients persevere for a long time in an uncomfortable position, and that they allow the urine and fæces to escape into their beds. At the beginning of the second, and very frequently already at the end of the first week, the patients complain of a violent buzzing in the ears, afterwards they are evidently hard of hearing. Corresponding with these changes the countenances of the patients become altered. Although the complexion seems to shine, yet it has a livid hue; the eyes stare, or they have a vague and unsteady expression; when raised in their beds, the patients at once turn pale and look as if they would faint. The various functions show the following deviations from their normal condition: The fever is intense, the temperature rises in the evening to 100° or 102° Fahr., with slight morning-remissions; the pulse is seldom below 100, nor is it often above 120, it is weaker than usual and sometimes dicrotic. The tongue, which already showed a good deal of dryness in the first week, now is constantly dry; the streaked coating, which had marked it hitherto, now vanishes; it shows a peculiarly red color, and the papillæ seem to have become effaced; towards the end of the second week the tongue appears covered with a brownish incrustation. The appetite is entirely wanting, yet the patients will taste of what they are offered to eat. They do not seem thirsty, yet they drink greedily the proffered beverage. At this stage the abdomen begins to bloat quite considerably; when the ilio-cœcal region is pressed upon very hard, the patients distort the corners of their mouths. Diarrhœa now usually sets in, from four to eight passages taking place involuntarily every day. They have a yellowish color, deposit a sediment of thick consistence over which floats a watery, opalescent substance. The urine is secreted in smaller quantities, it is dark and is frequently voided involuntarily; sometimes it is retained altogether, so that the bladder becomes very much distended. The respiration is still accelerated, yet the peculiar hurried breathing of the first week is scarcely yet perceived; posteriorly the lungs generally return hypostatic dulness; catarrhal symptoms are likewise discovered, although the patients scarcely ever cough and only rarely bring up a tenacious, yellowish mucus. The spleen continues to enlarge, although, owing to the distention of the bowels and the consequent displacement of the spleen upwards, the enlargement cannot well be discovered by a physical exploration. Upon the abdomen, thorax and back roseola-spots break out in greater or less number, some of which are usually present already at the end of the first week.

About the middle of the second week all these symptoms generally show an increase, less frequently a remission; both the increase and the remission are, however, of short duration.

In the third week, especially at the commencement, the symptoms continue to increase in intensity. The patients are now lying in a state of complete apathy; in the day-time they are only slightly delirious, but during the night the nervous exaltation is much worse, attended with subsultus tendinum and grasping at flocks. The prostration is so great that the patients are no longer able to sit erect; they are constantly lying on their backs, and the body, yielding to the law of gravitation, settles from the pillow downwards towards the middle of the bed. The tongue is only slowly protruded after loud and repeated requests; it is quite dry, with a fuliginous coating which is likewise exhibited on the teeth and at the nostrils. Deglutition is very difficult, and it is only with a great effort that the patient is able to swallow very small quantities of liquid at one time. The diarrhœa continues, but the passages are generally less copious, and not unfrequently tinged with blood. The urinary secretions continue to decrease and paralysis of the bladder is not an unfrequent occurrence. The abdomen is greatly distended and is no longer sensitive to pressure. The other symptoms continue unchanged, except that the roseola-spots pale off and become complicated with miliaria and sometimes with ecchymoses. Bedsores are now very apt to torment the patient. Emaciation proceeds very rapidly and his whole appearance is that of a general collapse. Up to the middle of the third week, the fever maintains its intensity. In cases where the disease continues during the fourth week, no remission of the fever is perceptible. In most cases, however, the seventeenth day is characterized by a sudden abatement of the fever and of most of the other derangements of the functions. This improvement at times is only apparent, inasmuch as in a few hours already the symptoms again exacerbate; but at other times it is a real improvement marking the beginning of recovery. If the patients die, it is most generally at this period; the remission just alluded to, when followed by an exacerbation of the symptoms, is generally looked upon as a fatal change. Death takes place with symptoms of paralysis of the heart and lungs. In favorable cases the fever remits every morning on the last days of the third week, whereas the evening-exacerbations decrease in violence, the consciousness returns gradually and with it a desire for food and drink. At this stage the fever scarcely ever shows a sudden and considerable decrease, with a correspondingly sudden beginning of convalescence.

With the third week typhus of a medium grade has reached its intensity in so far as signs of convalescence now begin to show themselves, although very slowly. Every case of typhus out-lasting the third week, may be safely regarded as very severe. Except complications take place, no new symptoms develop themselves during the fourth and fifth weeks. The remissions of the fever are very distinct and grow more decided in character; the pulse, on the contrary, increases in weakness and frequency. The patient looks as if he were in a state of terrible collapse; occasionally threatening paroxysms of collapse really take place, more particularly in the night; in the later course of the disease, such paroxysms are, however, not as dangerous as they seem. In the case of adults the consciousness usually returns towards the end of the fourth week; but, if the fever continues, delirium is still very frequent towards evening. The diarrhœa is at times less than it was, and at other times more profuse; in some cases it now ceases altogether. The skin looks clean, with the exception of miliaria here and there. The bed-sores which are never wanting during such a protracted course of the disease, grow rapidly in extent and malignancy.

If the fever runs a course of four weeks, recovery takes place very slowly. In very fortunate cases recovery goes on uninterruptedly, but most frequently its course is disturbed by all sorts of accidental inconveniences, such as vomiting after certain kinds of food, or even after any kind; sudden disappearance of the appetite that had just begun to return; return or protracted continuance of the diarrhœa; exacerbations of the fever. The decubitus, the nature and conduct of which afford an excellent criterium by which the amount of progress in the recovery of the patient can be measured, sometimes causes a great deal of serious trouble, provided the final cure of the fever is very much delayed. Death either takes place in consequence of the utter prostration of the patient, or else is caused by the complications and sequelæ that will be mentioned hereafter. Before, however, dwelling upon them, we have to mention various frequently occurring deviations from the general course of the disease. It ought to be observed, however, that typhus varies in its manifestations more than any other disease, sometimes to such an extent that it is only with great difficulty that the attack can be diagnosed as typhus.

Abortive typhus may terminate in convalescence in the first or second week. In both cases the phenomena of typhus may present a character of great gravity, and may cease quite suddenly; it even generally happens that in typhus running a very short course, the outbreak of the disease is characterized by very violent symptoms. The complete cessation of the pathological process at the end of the first week, including a sudden decrease of the temperature, is a very rare event. It has been doubted whether such cases ought to be regarded as typhus; but these doubts are unfounded. That typhus can abort, is most indubitably witnessed in families where this process of abortion takes place side by side with the most intense forms of the disease. More commonly the fever aborts in the second week. In such cases all the symptoms still continue to increase at the commencement of the second week, even to a very high degree; the somnolence, however, is not very marked; in its stead we notice more frequently great nervous exaltation; the diarrhœa is never very profuse. On the eleventh day the fever distinctly remits, the remission being sometimes preceded by a severe exacerbation. Every day the remission becomes more distinct and more considerable; the appetite returns at the same time and the tongue loses its dryness. The diarrhœa generally ceases as soon as the fever begins to abate. If no striking disturbance takes place, the patient enters on the twenty-first day upon his full and rapidly-progressing convalescence. But if the patient is exposed to severe emotional excitements, or commits serious dietetic transgressions by over-eating and the like, a relapse may readily take place in precisely such cases, and the patient may expose himself to great danger.

A precipitated course of typhus is not a very frequent occurrence. The disease which, at the onset, broke out in its fiercest intensity, increases within the first week or even within the first three days to such a degree that life becomes extinct even without the supervention of any special complications; it seems as though the organism sank exhausted and paralyzed under its excessive efforts to react. This course is only met with among individuals with exceedingly robust and plethoric constitutions.

A protracted course of typhus, or the so-called febris nervosa lenta, is likewise only rarely met with in comparison with other forms of this disease. It occurs more particularly among feeble, nervous individuals, hence more especially among females. There are two modifications of this disease. In the first place the disease may creep along imperceptibly, without a chill or any evident sign of serious illness. The patients lose their strength more and more, their appetite leaves them all at once, they are not tormented by thirst. There is no great rise of temperature, the skin feels even remarkably cool; the pulse is at times very quick and small, upwards of one hundred and twenty, at other times strikingly slow. Diarrhœa may be entirely absent, or is very inconsiderable. The patients look pallid, or else their cheeks show a hectic, circumscribed, easily changing redness. The tongue is seldom coated, never fuliginous, generally of a bright-red color, smooth as a mirror, and greatly disposed to become dry. The spleen is evidently enlarged. In this way the patients may remain six, eight or more weeks without the least change in the symptoms taking place. Recovery almost always takes place imperceptibly. Death either takes place in consequence of slow and intense exhaustion or else by the supervention of acute complications. In the other case the disease sets in like typhus of a middle grade, continues this course during the first three weeks, but in the fourth week it assumes the lentescent type with the previously-described symptoms of the first variety, except that the prostration is still greater and the diarrhœa is much more common. This form is most easily succeeded by sequelæ.

Typhus of a more intense type runs a very characteristic course among children during the first period of dentition. The disease begins with the symptoms of a severe catarrhal fever, with intense heat, passing sweats, occasional vomiting, constipation; the pulse, instead of exceeding one hundred and twenty beats which it frequently does in catarrhal fever, usually ranges from one hundred to one hundred and twenty. Towards the end of the first week the somnolence changes to sopor, and in the second week to a deep coma; diarrhœa sets in, the passages as well as the urinary secretions taking place involuntarily; the face assumes an appearance of collapse at an early period, the pupils are almost always considerably dilated; deglutition is difficult, only small quantities can be swallowed at a time. The little patients most commonly signify the presence of a severe headache by moving a hand or a forearm over their foreheads at short intervals, and uttering every now and then the characteristic "*cri encéphalique.*" One side of the body is generally completely paralyzed. The patients remain in this condition which looks very much like meningitis, for weeks without showing the least sign of a change. To judge from the four cases that we have met with in the last two years, it seems to us as though the end of the sixth week were the decisive term of this fever; for on the first day of the seventh week these four children were again restored to consciousness. In such cases the diagnosis has to depend entirely upon the pulse which, in contra-distinction to an inflammatory cerebral affection, especially to acute hydrocephalus, constantly remains at one hundred and twenty; likewise upon the presence of diarrhœa, upon the hypertrophy of the spleen which is seldom very considerable; and finally upon the fetid odor with which the sick-chamber is filled and which strikes one invariably on entering the room from the open air, even if the apartment is ventilated with ever so much care. Sequelæ are not very common in such cases; nor is, in spite of the worst apparent signs, the prognosis so very bad, provided the eighteenth day is safely passed.

In conclusion we have to make mention of pneumo-typhus, a modification which occurs very frequently at times, whereas it is not met with at all in other epidemics. The supposition that in such a case the typhoid process runs its course upon the pulmonary, instead of upon the intestinal lining membrane, is not correct; for the affection of the intestinal lining membrane is not entirely wanting, although it may be inconsiderable. In pneumo-typhus the inflammatory irritation of the bronchia which we meet with in every case of typhus, increases to a more marked degree of intensity; real pneumonia supervenes, and the additional advent of hypostasis occasions a very threatening combination utterly overshadowing the abdominal phenomena. Pneumo-typhus may exist from the beginning of the disease, or it may break out in the course of the first, second, and even third week, most generally in a very insidious manner. Beside the physical signs, pneumo-typhus is not revealed by any other reliable sign, although the presence of a very hurried, superficial respiration, a frequent and painful cough, fan-like motion of the alæ nasi during respiration, circumscribed redness of one or both cheeks ought to excite suspicion, and awaken our attention to the disease. The course of the disease is not retarded by this form of typhus, but the critical days are very commonly missed. The danger is very great. Very often pneumo-typhus is followed by the development of florid phthisis, probably owing to the circumstance that the typhoid process in the lungs causes existing tubercles to suppurate.

The number of complications that may break out during the course of typhus is very great; for this reason we only mention the following which are most common and most important: Hemorrhages from the bowels and nose; the latter occur more frequently at the beginning than during the subsequent course of the disease; they are of very little importance, provided the loss of blood is not excessive; as a rule, the patients feel relieved after the bleeding: Intestinal hemorrhage, on the contrary, occurs during the later period of the disease, and becomes very dangerous either on account of its copiousness, or on account of its exceedingly debilitating influence. If the blood is not discharged from the anus, the hemorrhage may superinduce a sudden and complete collapse. Petechiæ and extensive ecchymoses are ominous symptoms which indicate a bad composition of the blood. The frequently-occurring and excessive cerebral exaltation is of importance in so far as it induces the necessity of constantly watching the patient; it manifests itself more frequently in the first and second week than in the subsequent course of the disease, and, since it may break out at any time, typhus-patients should never be left alone for one instant. A sudden collapse, with paralysis of the heart, is not generally met with until after the second week, very often while the fever seems to pursue an apparently mild course; one attack of this kind seldom terminates fatally; but a repetition of the attack, which generally takes place in the evening or during the night, is very apt to end in death. Parotitis has already been spoken of before; it is neither a good nor an absolutely bad symptom. Ulcers in the larynx may lead to ulceration of the cartilages, and by this means endanger life; if inconsiderable, they may likewise endanger life by superinducing œdema glottidis. The worst changes are those occasioned by ulcers in the intestines, namely consecutive peritonitis, and perforation of the intestines with peritoneal inflammation. Both these changes are exceedingly dangerous to life; peritonitis is more apt to set in previous to the intestinal ulceration, the latter may take place at any time after the second week, even after convalescence is already very far advanced. If no adhesion had previously taken place between the intestines and the peritoneum, the inflammation of this membrane soon becomes diffuse and ends fatally in a few hours.

Meteorism is a common symptom in typhus; when excessive, and when it threatens paralysis, the meteorism becomes a very dangerous condition.

Among the numerous sequelæ of typhus we distinguish intestinal phthisis, occasioned by the number, and continued ulceration of the infiltrated glands of Peyer, and the solitary glands of Brunner; this ulceration is a very common cause of a protracted convalescence, and may finally terminate in fatal ascites. It is a curable condition. Inflammations of serous membranes are not unfrequent, but they do not, properly speaking, belong to the sequelæ. Ulcers of the larynx may lead to stenosis and to obstinate, generally incurable hoarseness. Paralysis of the extremities, especially the lower, and paralysis of single organs of sense, are often met with, but as a rule, they gradually disappear again without any treatment. It is only in rare cases that the mind remains impaired for life. Decubitus may even penetrate to the bones, and may cause death long after the typhus had ceased. Although typhus scarcely ever attacks individuals with decided, especially florid tuberculosis, we often see patients who had been convalescent for weeks, suddenly relapse into a fever, and, in a very short period of time, perish by tubercular phthisis. Whether typhus causes the slumbering germ to grow, or, by its own inherent agency, implants the tubercular disease, has to remain an open question for the present. The former is the more probable of the two.

Exanthematic typhus runs a much more decidedly typical course than typhus abdominalis; in this respect it bears the greatest resemblance to acute exanthems.

It sets in with very uncharacteristic precursory symptoms, lassitude, want of spirits, a feeling of illness, slight catarrhal symptoms, headache, anxious dreams disturbing his sleep, etc. These symptoms precede the real outbreak by two to seven days.

The invasion of the disease is generally marked by a violent chill, less frequently by alternate chilliness and heat. The chill is almost immediately succeeded by intense heat, at the same time as the patients are unable to keep themselves erect. Amid the symptoms that have been described as pathognomonic of abdominal typhus, and which are generally much more intense when occurring as phenomenal manifestations of exanthematic typhus, more particularly the dulness and cloudiness of the sensorium, the roseola-spots make their appearance between the fifth and seventh day, first in small numbers on the trunk, but rapidly multiplying and covering the whole body except the face. In size, shape and color these spots resemble measles, except that they are never strikingly raised above the skin. The enlargement of the spleen and the continued violent fever enable us to distinguish this exanthem from measles; it remits about the seventh day, but breaks out so much worse again afterwards.

In the second week, all the symptoms reach their highest degree of intensity, and may continue unchanged during the whole of the following week; the cerebral symptoms and the excessive prostration are particularly prominent. The abdomen retains its normal shape; no meteorism takes place as in abdominal typhus, nor is the diarrhœa which is very often wanting, of the same character as the diarrhœa of typhus abdominalis. In cases of a moderate degree of intensity, the fever commonly abates in the second half of the second, less frequently at the commencement of the third week; such an abatement is immediately preceded by an exacerbation. The temperature falls considerably in a very short period of time, the pulse likewise falls to ninety, to hundred, and even a smaller number of beats. At the same time, a considerable change takes place in the whole condition of the patient. The sensorium is still clouded, but he commences to enjoy a quiet sleep, he is more quiet in his waking condition: a desire for food is felt, and in a few days convalescence is under full headway, so that at the beginning of the fourth week the patient is able to leave his bed, although he still feels weak for a long time. Up to the middle of the second week, the exanthem continues to increase, the spots assume a darker color; but as soon as the fever abates, the spots show a livid tint, and pale off rapidly without even leaving a vestige of their existence. Not unfrequently the spots, some of them at least, change to real petechiæ; altogether this form of typhus is distinguished by a tendency to hemorrhagic effusions, and to hemorrhages from every possible organ. Among the complications, inflammatory affections of the respiratory organs are the most striking; in general, a severe bronchial catarrh is very apt to be present at the first outbreak of the disease. A fatal termination most commonly takes place towards the end of the second week, amid the same symptoms as those that characterize a fatal termination of abdominal typhus. If the disease lasts beyond this period, it is generally owing to these complications; but such a more protracted course is a rare occurrence. With the exception of a long continuance of the cerebral functions, no other sequelæ are apt to occur.

The prognosis of abdominal typhus is very uncertain; a tumultuous outbreak of the disease does not justify the conclusion that the course of the disease will be one of great danger, nor does a mild beginning prognosticate an equally mild ending. Life may become suddenly endangered at any period of the disease. According to Wunderlich, those cases are the most serious where the fever does not distinctly remit at the end of the first week. A slow pulse ought to be regarded as a favorable rather than as an unfavorable symptom. The absence of diarrhœa, more especially if an obstinate constipation exists in its place, is a very favorable symptom. A girl of fourteen years who had a most violent attack of typhus, had no passage from her bowels for twenty-one days; on the twenty-second day recovery commenced and progressed very rapidly. No greater folly can be perpetrated than to administer cathartics in typhus. Symptoms denoting a rapid and deep-seated decomposition of the blood, and likewise a rapid increase of the decubitus, render the prognosis more dubious; so do extensive complications when affecting important organs. For the exanthematic form of typhus, when running an uncomplicated course, the prognosis is, upon the whole, favorable, notwithstanding the phenomena of the disease have a very threatening look. Complications of exanthematic typhus are likewise overcome much more readily than those occurring during the course of abdominal typhus, for the reason that exanthematic typhus does not consume the patient's strength as rapidly and thoroughly as the latter.

Treatment. Among all possible diseases there is no disease of which it is so difficult to decide whether the treatment that has been pursued hitherto has been of any, or of how much use. Our opponents cannot be blamed for doubting our successes; the expectant method often furnishes equally favorable results; at no period during the course of typhus can a positive prognosis be set up, and the diagnosis is likewise exposed to a good many uncertainties. After all, the superiority of the two methods of treating typhus can only be decided by comparing the number of deaths in the same epidemic, and in a number of epidemics. In this respect, Homœopathy has a decided advantage, for the number of deaths under homœopathic treatment never exceeds seven to eight per cent., whereas under other methods of treatment this number amounts to twenty and more per cent. These figures cannot be impeached by accusing us of errors in diagnosis, which our opponents are just as capable of committing as we are.

We omit casting an inquiring glance at the manner in which typhus is treated by the Old School, and by the adherents of the New and Newest School of Homœopathy; an inquiry of this kind would not be very profitable; we cannot help wondering, however, that the rational physicians who consider typhus inaccessible to remedial agents, should combat it with such a mass of heterogeneous medicines. However, we must dwell upon two points that are of importance to us homœopathic physicians who are so often called upon for aid in the later stages of typhus. In the first place we wish to point out the consequences of a revulsive or derivative treatment. Sanguineous depletions which are so often resorted to even now, have a bad effect, not only immediately but likewise at a later period; the patients lapse more speedily into sopor, their prostration becomes more excessive, they perish in larger numbers, or, if convalescence sets in, it takes place more slowly and incompletely. Cathartics have likewise a permanently bad effect, and we feel prompted to regard venesection and the use of purgatives in typhus as acts of wickedness. In the second place, we generally notice that patients who have been fed on large doses of Chlorates or Quinine, have the functional power of their stomachs impaired for weeks, and that the integrity of their cerebral functions is restored very slowly.

Regarding the homœopathic treatment of typhus, we do not share the views of all our Colleagues in this respect. They quote a large number of remedies for typhus with the most minute and delicate indications, whereas it is our belief that we as yet possess only a small number of real remedies for typhus, by which we mean remedies that have it in their power to modify the course of the disease, and that most of the other remedies that have been recommended for this disease, only correspond with a few prominent symptoms. Our opinion is based upon the proposition that typhus owes its existence to some definite toxical agent that penetrates the organism from without, as is the case with acute exanthems. It is for this reason that in no epidemic disease the curative virtue of one or more remedies as genuine epidemic-remedies, has been so thoroughly tested as in typhus; and in our opinion the most important task which a physician has to fulfil in every epidemic is, to find out the general remedies adapted to each. A second, still more important circumstance resulting from this previous opinion is, that the remedy should never be changed unless distinctly new, unexpected morbid phenomena manifest themselves that are not in harmony with the normal course of the disease. If this course of treatment had been pursued before, and if the natural course of typhus had been watched and regarded with more care, our knowledge of treating typhus would most likely be much further advanced than it really is. How much, for instance, can be claimed for the efficacy of a remedy that was administered on the fifteenth or sixteenth day of the disease, if the fever suddenly moderates on the seventeenth?

We wish to call attention to another mistake that very much impairs the physician's professional usefulness. In treating typhus or other typical diseases, we are very apt to proceed as we do in treating other diseases; we forget the typical character. We want to break the fever at any price, and the rage of bringing this about induces us to administer a new remedy every day. But typhus cannot be cut short, except within the above-stated, definite boundaries; typhus never disappears before the seventh day; no typhus terminates critically on the eighth, ninth, fifteenth or sixteenth day, any more than a measle or scarlatina-eruption can be altered by medicines.

The real typhus-remedies corresponding with the whole course of this disease, are: *Bryonia alba, Rhus toxicodendron, Arsenicum, Phosphorus, Acidum phosphoricum* and *muriaticum*.

Bryonia alba corresponds to those forms of typhus that run a mild or moderately-intense course. The initial symptoms are sometimes so indefinite that both the selection of a remedy and the diagnosis are uncertain, and our choice would properly not fall upon Bryonia. But as soon as the typhoid character of the disease has become fully established, Bryonia is indicated by the following symptoms: Violent, pressive headache, buzzing in the ears, dulness of the sensorium, yet the patient does not yet lose his consciousness; yellowish and thick, white coating on the tongue whose edges are bright-red, without great tendency to dryness; acute pains in the ileo-cœcal and splenetic regions; nausea or even vomiting after every meal; constipation; torpor of the bowels or occasional diarrhœa; pulse full and not very rapid. *Bryonia* corresponds fully with these initial symptoms, and generally with the whole course of the disease which seldom outlasts the seventeenth day. We have often seen typhus cut short at the end of the second week by simply confining the treatment to the use of Bryonia. In febris nervosa lenta Bryonia is likewise one of our best remedies; its use in this disease is of course more restricted, owing to the variable nature of the symptoms. In exanthematic typhus *Bryonia* is a distinguished remedy as long as the brain is not altogether deprived of its functional power. We do not point out single groups of symptoms for the reason that the symptoms of the disease as well as those of the remedy are too manifold.

Rhus toxicodendron differs in its indications so essentially from those of Bryonia that it is scarcely possible to confound the two remedies with each other. *Rhus tox.* corresponds to typhus of very intense character; it begins with a chill, followed immediately after by burning heat and, even on the first few days, by all the symptoms that render the diagnosis certain. We may lay it down as a rule that *Rhus* is indicated the more specifically the more speedily the true character of typhus can be diagnosed. *Rhus* is especially indicated by active delirium and great prostration, a dark and livid redness of the cheeks, injected eyes, early dryness and redness of the tongue, and a copious diarrhœa which sets in soon after the fever has fairly shown its true character. Cases adapted to *Rhus*, never run a speedy course, nor will the crisis have to be expected previous to the seventeenth day; until then the medicine may be continued without fear unless some other medicine should be indicated by particular symptoms; the symptoms of *Rhus* correspond to all the stages of a most intense typhus, even to the third week. An alleviating epistaxis, stools tinged with blood, a severe bronchial affection with a dirty-looking, sanguinolent expectoration are special indications for *Rhus*, which may likewise prove efficacious in pneumotyphus. In exanthematic typhus *Rhus* generally has the advantage over Bryonia not only on account of the greater intensity of the fever, but of the whole course of the disease. Rhus is generally indicated by excessive reactive endeavors with insufficiency of reactive power, and an excessive irritability of the nervous system. There is scarcely another remedy that has shown its good effects in so many cases, although we must never expect to cut the fever short with this remedy.

Arsenicum album is the most prominent remedy in typhus; it will even cure cases that seemed utterly hopeless. The cases adapted to *Arsen.* resemble those indicating Rhus, at least in the beginning. The fever is intense, the patients are very restless and show by their behavior that they are in great distress; the least pressure on the ileocœcal region and the region of the spleen causes pain. Symptoms of decomposition of the blood set in at an early period, such as nose-bleed, bloody diarrhœa, badly-colored, bloody sputa, petechiæ on the skin; the stools have a foul odor, the exhalations emanating from the patient generally, are very fetid. Instead of perfect sopor we have a change between great nervous excitement and complete prostration. Bedsores break out at an early period of the disease, forming gangrenous scurfs with dark-red borders. The pulse is very frequent, hard and tense. The patients are tormented by an unquenchable thirst. Generally *Arsenicum* is recommended for the second half of the second, and for the third week; but we doubt whether this is practically correct; in our opinion we should accomplish a great deal more by means of Arsenicum, if the remedy were more frequently administered from the commencement or at least in the first week of the disease, for in such a case it might show its effect upon the whole course of typhus. Since Arsenicum is more than any other medicine adapted to the worst forms of all infectious diseases, it seems wrong to delay its administration until the symptoms indicating Arsenicum, are developed in their most malignant intensity. Years ago Fleischmann showed that typhus generally runs a favorable course under the influence of Arsenicum, and we should think that several hundred cures ought to be something in its favor. Fleischmann, however, generalizes too much, whereas Wurmb, on the other hand, errs in individualizing beyond necessity. After all, the balance inclines in Fleischmann's favor, for *Arsen.* produces the symptoms of lentescent as well as of inflammatory and putrid typhus. Our advice therefore is that *Arsen.* should be given more frequently than has been customary, from the very beginning of the attack, and that we should not wait until the disease has fully developed its pernicious character. A few special indications for *Arsen.* are the following: Striking and typical remission of the fever, having the appearance of an actual intermission. Marked meteorism of the bowels, with gurgling in the bowels, but no diarrhœa. Extensive hypostasis of the lungs, with bronchitis and considerable hoarseness. Irregular action of the heart, absence of the second sound of the heart. Paroxysms of sudden collapse towards midnight. Fetid breath. Frequent retching and even vomiting, immediately after drinking, in the second and the subsequent weeks or during convalescence. Considerable enlargement of the spleen. In exanthematic typhus *Arsen.* is indicated much less frequently, and is chiefly adapted only to the putrid form, the so-called putrid typhus. In lentescent typhus *Arsen.* is an excellent remedy, if the symptoms exacerbate every other day; if the patients are tormented by anxiety; if every little meal causes retching and vomiting, although the tongue is clean. *Arsen.* is so much more extensively applicable the more typhus assumes the epidemic form; likewise in endemic typhus. Most observers advocate repeated doses of the second to the fourth trituration. [We remember a case of exanthematic typhus where the putrid stage had fully set in; the patient was emaciated and extremely prostrated; the teeth looked black; the tongue was swollen, blackish and bleeding; blood oozed from the gums; the skin was covered with petechiæ, from many of which a black, foul, decomposed blood was constantly oozing; involuntary, bloody, horridly-smelling stools. A few globules of *Arsen.* 18th excited a reaction which ended in perfect recovery in one week. H.]

Phosphorus is one of the most important remedies in typhus; its curative action is, however, limited to certain sharply defined cases; it cannot be regarded as a general remedy for typhus, in the same sense as *Arsen.* or *Bryon.*—Above all, *Phosphorus* is indicated in pneumo-typhus with violent bronchitis, hepatization, together with hypostasis and laryngitis. It is a sovereign remedy for this condition, unsurpassed by any other medicine. It is indicated by the following abdominal symptoms: Frequent diarrhœic stools at an early period of the disease, coming on after every meal, of a dark-dingy, blackish-gray color, or mixed with decomposed blood and containing shreds of intestinal mucous lining. Extreme prostration after every discharge. Numerous roseola-spots, with ecchymoses and sudamina. Burning heat of the trunk, with cold sweat about the head and on the extremities. Pulse frequent, small and feeble. Sensitiveness of the region of the liver and stomach; considerable meteorism. A characteristic indication for *Phosphorus* is vomiting in the first, and at the commencement of the second week; the vomiting contains watery-bilious and slimy masses which are brought up with great distress. In exanthematic typhus, *Phosphorus* is one of the first remedies, for the reason that the pulmonary symptoms are generally very prominent and involve the most danger.—Among the sequelæ, *Phosphorus* is indicated by diarrhœa when it acts like colliquative diarrhœa. Hartmann points to sexual excitement as a not unfrequent indication for *Phosphorus*.

Acidum phosphoricum renders eminent service in typhus; even the Rational School acknowledges its power in this disease without, of course, mentioning the source where this knowledge was obtained. Phosphoric acid is a truly specific remedy in lentescent typhus, and is never indicated, if the fever is high and the nerves greatly excited. The patients are lying in a state of excessive prostration and apathy, without being exactly in a state of sopor; the face is rather pallid, not turgescent, the pulse very frequent, feeble and small; the tongue is not very dry; it is smooth as a mirror, red. The thirst is inconsiderable; diarrhœa moderate, the discharges occurring only now and then; the meteorism is not very marked. The disease does not show any tendency to a speedy change; perceptible remissions do not take place. The whole process has the appearance of a gradual extinction of the vital powers, without any decided reactive efforts being perceptible on the part of the organism. Beside the cases where *Acidum phosphor.* is indicated from the beginning, sometimes after Bryonia, but never, properly speaking, after Rhus or Arsenicum, *Phosphori acidum* can likewise come into play, if, at the end of the fourth week, convalescence seems to remain stationary, more particularly if a moderate diarrhœa is frequent.

Of the other mineral acids, **Acidum muriaticum** is sometimes used; the forms of typhus requiring this acid are, upon the whole, very rare. Muriatic acid is more particularly adapted to lentescent putrid typhus where the decomposition of the fluids is slow and extensive, but does not set in suddenly. The general symptoms resemble those of Phosphoric acid, only the fever is more severe, the restlessness is more marked and the following local symptoms are present: Frequent diarrhœic stools, but scanty; the characteristic fæcal discharges are mingled with shreds of intestinal mucous lining and with lumps of whitish mucus. The discharges are most commonly involuntary; the meteorism is very great. The mucous lining of the mouth is ulcerated here and there, the ulcerations being covered with a dirty-white coating. The bedsores have an indolent, pale look; they are painless and extend very rapidly. The patients' breath is very offensive; they have an aversion to any kind of food, but they crave fresh cold water. [Settling down in the bed, is characteristic of this acid. H.]

So far as our present experience goes, these remedies conclude the number of our typhus-remedies; it remains for us now to indicate a number of other remedies that are more or less useful for various phenomena, but do not correspond with the whole character and course of the disease. We will mention them as briefly as possible.

If **Aconitum** is prescribed for the violent fever at the beginning of typhus, it is probably for no other reason than because the diagnosis is not yet satisfactorily cleared up; we do not believe that Aconitum is capable of either exerting a curative or palliative effect in typhus.

Belladonna, which undoubtedly seems to be indicated in the first week of the fever, may sometimes moderate its violence at that period, especially the excessive cerebral hyperæmia, but it will scarcely ever produce a striking and incontrovertible effect. It renders most efficient aid against the severe bronchitis of the first week. In the later course of the disease, it is scarcely ever indicated. [We think Bæhr underrates the great virtues of *Belladonna* as a specific remedy for typhus. We have cured many cases of typhus where no other remedy was used except Belladonna. We will mention a few of them.

A girl of thirteen years, of a healthy constitution and very mild temperament, was attacked with a severe angina fancium. Next day she was slightly delirious, complained of seeing people in the room, strange-looking faces, dogs, etc. Pulse about one hundred and ten; cheeks scarlet-red, eyes sparkling, tongue dry, like sole-leather, skin dry and hot, urine red, without any sediment; bowels constipated; great prostration and rapid emaciation. I gave her *Belladonna* 1st attenuation. On the seventh day she left her bed fully recovered.

A lady of about forty years was attacked with pleuro-pneumonia; on the third day of the disease, the symptoms of typhus were fully developed. Severe headache; eyes sparkling; cheeks pale, with occasional deep flushes; tongue parched, and of a deep-brown color like sole-leather; skin dry and hot; pulse about one hundred and twenty; bowels constipated, urine of a deep-yellow color with a reddish tint; grasping at flocks, picking at the bedclothes; furious delirium; intense thirst, but the least attempt to swallow a drop of liquid caused the patient to utter a piercing cry and threw her into violent spasms, with foam at the mouth. The patient took nothing but *Belladonna*. She improved very gradually every week; sometimes no improvement became perceptible under a fortnight. The whole course of the disease extended during a period of three months, I mean from the first outbreak of the fever to the day when the patient took her first ride out in a carriage

A young lady of twenty-three years was attacked with lentescent typhus; the leading symptoms were: headache, somnolence, dry and hot skin, pulse one hundred and twenty; tongue of a deep-brown color, very dry but smooth as a mirror; urine of a deep-yellow color; prostration, utter loss of appetite, emaciation; bronchial irritation. The disease ran a course of twenty-one days. The patient took nothing but Belladonna, middle and lower potencies. H.]

Arnica in its whole pathogenesis shows so much resemblance to typhus that it must astonish everybody that this remedy should not have been employed in this disease more frequently than it has. The characteristic indications result from a merely superficial view of the symptoms. The disease is more like an inflammatory fever, the cheeks are pale, with flushes of redness, the pulse is not very much accelerated, the heat is unequally distributed. The patients show an extraordinary sensitiveness of the organs of sense, together with a distressing headache; nose-bleed, bloody expectoration; active delirium without great bodily restlessness. It is questionable whether Arnica can do anything for bedsores. As regards the kind and intensity of the cases to which *Arnica* is homœopathic, this medicine occupies a middle rank beween *Rhus* and *Bryonia*.

Carbo vegetabilis is regarded by many as an exquisite remedy for typhus. We do not share this opinion, and simply believe Carbo adapted to certain anomalous manifestations in the course of the disease. Carbo may be exhibited if the patients are sunk in a state of apathy without any marked symptoms of reaction; if the body is burning-hot and the extremities are icy-cold; if the functional power of the heart fails very speedily; if petechiæ break out in large numbers, with extensive hypostasis of the lungs, foul and decomposed diarrhœic stools, frequent attacks of an ominous collapse, wide-spread decubitus, with burning pain of the sores. *Carbo* is rather suitable in cases that seem to be adapted to *Bryonia* or *Acidum phosphoricum*. In the subsequent course of the disease, *Carbo* is more particularly indicated by the bronchial catarrh, if there is a good deal of tenacious mucus that can only be expectorated with a great deal of difficulty; during the convalescence, this remedy may sometimes be required by the characteristic diarrhœa.

Digitalis can only be exhibited in lentescent typhus, if constipation is associated with great irritability of the stomach and painfulness of the region of the liver; the pulse is at times rapid, at other times slow and feeble, and is very much accelerated by every motion, especially by rising from a recumbent position; the sensorium is clouded but consciousness is never entirely lost, and although there is no diarrhœa, yet the strength and the flesh waste away very rapidly. Digitalis is undoubtedly deserving of great consideration in typhus, were it only for the reason that its sphere of action is limited and distinctly circumscribed.

Closely related to the former remedy is **Cuprum**, concerning whose faculty of producing a connected series of typhoid symptoms Frerichs' observation in Mengershausen (see Frank's Archiv. vol. IV.) furnishes the most conclusive testimony. Without reproducing the facts related in that publication, we recommend them to the careful study of all homœopathic practitioners. The copper-typhus sets in and runs its course without any violent fever, but an extraordinary prostration at once makes its appearance, which increases so rapidly amid symptoms of sanguineous decomposition (nose-bleed, petechiæ) that in a short time death takes place with all the symptoms of general paralysis.

Secale cornutum is indicated if the attack sets in with convulsions, paralysis of the extremities, gangrenous ulcers especially on the extremities, extensive ecchymoses on the skin.

Kreosotum corresponds to putrid typhus if copious atonic hemorrhages exist.

Stramonium, Hyoscyamus, Helleborus are only suitable for corresponding cerebral symptoms. In our opinion they will seldom accomplish any real good, nor will they be required for the reason that a delirium of the most varied forms does not constitute any essential deviation from the normal course of typhus. [We do not agree with Bæhr so far as *Hyoscyamus* is concerned. We know from experience that an acute outbreak of typhus may yield to Hyoscyamus. A robust merchant of about forty years came home with a terrible headache. He had had a heavy chill in his counting-room which was very soon followed by fever. The cephalic distress was principally located in one side of the head. *Bryonia* was given. Next day delirium set in, with picking at the bedclothes; the patient was constantly talking about his business, and wanted to leave his bed; the prostration was very great, and he lost flesh visibly; the bowels were loose, the discharges having an offensive smell. The patient was constantly troubled with the paintings on the wall falling to one side. A drop of the tincture of *Hyoscyamus* was mixed in half a tumbler of water, of which mixture a dessertspoonful was given him every two hours. After the second dose he dropped to sleep, and woke after a refreshing sleep in full tide of recovery. H.]

The same remarks apply to **Opium**; this remedy is said to frequently have removed the deep sopor of typhus-patients; we have never been able to accomplish such a result by means of Opium. [A man had an attack of exanthematic typhus; the fever had run six weeks, and the patient seemed irretrievably lost. Towards the end of the sixth week the following symptoms had developed themselves: The patient was constantly settling down in his bed; the eyes were half closed, with the eye-balls turned upwards in their sockets; depression of the lower jaw; strings of a ropy saliva were hanging out at the corners of the mouth; tongue thick and tremulous; involuntary stools; miliaria; excessive emaciation, complete lethargy. A few drops of Muriatic Acid in half a tumbler of water re-awakened the sinking reaction. The paralytic symptoms were followed by a deep sopor. This was on the evening of the forty-first day. A drop of *Opium* was mixed in half a tumbler of water, of which mixture the patient took a dessertspoonful every two hours. Next morning, instead of the usual exacerbation a sound sleep set in, which lasted with short interruptions, for a whole week. No further medicine was given. The patient drove out in a fortnight, perfectly well. In my opinion the *Opium* had a curative effect in this case. H.]

Camphora acts well for a short time when given as an intermediate remedy for sudden paroxysms of severe collapse coming on the heel of great exaltation of the cerebral functions.

A few other, most unimportant remedies will be found indicated under catarrh of the stomach which very often bears a deceptive similarity to the lighter grades of typhus.

The general management and the diet to be observed in typhus are of more importance than in any other disease. It is unfortunately true that in this respect physicians are often guilty of the most unpardonable delinquencies. In managing typhus-patients we observe the following rules, the usefulness of which has been abundantly established, and which we have never known to result in any mischief to the patient. The patients should lie on a mattress, never on feather-beds which promote the development of bedsores. A woollen blanket with a linen sheet is sufficient covering. The windows in the sick-room should never be shut entirely, no matter in what season of the year; if possible, the room should always be kept properly ventilated by securing a current of air along the ceiling. If possible, the patients should often be changed to another bed, and even to another room. Once every day, and, if the disease has reached its height, several times a day, the patient should be washed with cold water over the largest part of his body; an ablution of this kind affords an immense amount of comfort to the patient.

The passages from the bowels and bladder have to be removed as soon as possible. If possible, the same person should never be in constant attendance on the patient, lest he should become too much impregnated with the typhus-contagium. Only the most indispensable conversation should be held with the patient, and all mental excitement should be strictly avoided. As long as the violence of the fever continues, no great supply of nourishment is required; the patient does not desire anything, nor should he be persuaded to partake of anything substantial. Liquid nourishment is best adapted to his condition. If the patient desires, he may have: beef-tea, broth (no veal-broth), chicken-broth, milk diluted with one-third water, malt-beer cooked with sago or gruel, which should be allowed to cool before it is used; mucilaginous soups, but not exclusively. The best beverage is fresh water; this should be given the patient quite often, even if he does not call for it, for it is the best means of repairing the waste of moisture caused by the fever. Sugar-water is hurtful; water with the juice of fruit dissolved in it, may be partaken of in very moderate quantities. Soda-water very soon becomes offensive to the patient. Water with a little wine is perfectly appropriate in the later course of the disease. Malt-beer with a little sugar is perfectly admissible; it imparts more than any other beverage the sensation that the thirst is quenched, and the patients crave it even when they are lying in a state of sopor. We have never seen it do any harm. Many patients manifest a strong desire for fruit, which they may partake of stewed, but moderately, not too often; stewed prunes without the skin are the best kind.

The diet during the period of convalescence is very difficult to manage properly. Either a real canine hunger is experienced by the patients, or else the stomach craves food without being able to digest it. The former is the more common result under homœopathic treatment, the latter is often the result of the abuse of drugs. In the former case the patient's craving for food may be gratified every two hours, but the quantity ought to be small each time, and the food ought moreover to be substantial. Beef, chickens, venison, but very little farinaceous food which, by the deposition of quantities of fæcal matter, might irritate ulcers in the intestines that are not entirely healed. Good vegetables are decidedly beneficial. Individuals recovering from typhus have to be treated like persons that were near starving to death. If the stomach is weak, the food has to be selected with so much more care, nor should the patient be too often persuaded to eat. Good wine after a meal sometimes has a marvelously good effect, whereas, if the patient is tormented by canine hunger, it is rather hurtful than beneficial. A resumption of our habitual stimulants, such as coffee, tea, tobacco, should be postponed as long as possible. The patients may be allowed the use of fresh air as soon as expedient; no apprehension need be entertained of their taking cold.

[Among the recent additions to our Materia Medica, *Baptisia tinctoria* or the wild Indigo is recommended for typhoid fever. This drug was first brought to the notice of the homœopathic profession by Dr. Hoyt in the sixth volume of the North American Journal. The following interesting cases were published by him:

Mrs. C. was taken with typhus-fever and treated allopathically. She became so reduced that her life was despaired of. After the continuation of the fever for thirty-one days, as a last resort, Mr. C. prepared a decoction of the Baptisia; taking a piece of the root about three inches long and three-eighths of an inch thick, steeping it in half a pint of water. He commenced by giving her five or six drops of the decoction once in fifteen minutes, increasing till he gave nearly a teaspoonful at a dose. In about one hour and a half the surface of the patient presented an appearance as though she had been literally scalded, so red was the skin, accompanied with a most intense superficial heat; at the same time noticing large drops of sweat standing on her forehead, the medicine was discontinued. In a few minutes a profuse perspiration appeared all over her body which continued for nearly twelve hours, or till she was bathed freely with brandy and water. From this time she began to improve, and with the occasional administration of a drop or two of the remedy, got well, without any febrile symptoms. It is worthy of remark that immediately upon the administration of the remedy she became quiet and fell asleep; she had been restless and delirious for three weeks previous.

Mr. and Mrs. S. being very unwell, I was called and found them suffering with continued fever. After prescribing Aconite, Rhus, etc., without much effect, and my patients growing rapidly worse, I was induced to use the Baptisia in decoction as in the former case. I remained to watch the operation of the remedy. To my great surprise, in about an hour the perspiration appeared upon the foreheads of my patients, and it gradually covered the entire surface. In about six hours they were thoroughly bathed with tepid water; the next morning scarce a vestige of the fever remained, and a rapid recovery followed.

Mr. R. was taken with typhus fever, and had the usual homœopathic remedies for several days. An unfavorable prognosis was given and the Baptisia decided upon. It was administered and its effects watched. In this case drop-doses of an alcoholic tincture were used. The fever was reduced more than one half in a few hours, and by a continuation of the remedy he was saved. A fierce delirium was present in this case, but it rapidly gave way under the action of the medicine.

English practitioners, Drs. Hughes, Kidd, and others, speak of this medicine very favorably in the incipient stages of typhus, and more particularly when gastric fevers show a tendency to lapse into the typhoid type. According to Dr. Edwin M. Hale, the following are the characteristic indications for its use: Chilliness all day, heat at night; chilliness with soreness of the whole body; heavy, dull, bruised sensation in the head, stupefying headache, confusion of ideas, delirium at night, heavy sleep with frightful dreams, dry and red tongue, or brown coated tongue, sticky mouth, fetid breath, fetid sweat, and great fetor of the discharges (urine and stool), great debility and nervous prostration, with erethism; ulcerations of a bad character, etc.

According to my own experience, Baptisia is not so much indicated in fully developed typhus as in intermediate forms of gastrointestinal fever and abdominal typhus. My experience in the use of this drug is limited, but I doubt whether any good can be expected from it after the ulcerative process in abdominal typhus has fully set in. In the first stages of exanthematic typhus, when no other medicines are indicated by characteristic symptoms, Baptisia may have a good effect in kindling a decided reaction. H.]

3. Febris Icterodes.
Yellow Fever.

This is an epidemic fever of a specific nature and a continuous type, so called because the skin and conjunctiva look yellow, although cases have been known to occur where this yellowness is almost entirely absent. Such patients complain of severe supra-orbital headache, and soon become delirious. In the subsequent course of the disease the urinary secretions become suspended, interstitial hemorrhages take place, the patient passes black stools and vomits a black substance; this is the stage of black vomit, which generally terminates fatally.

This fever is endemic in low districts on the sea-coast, more particularly on some of the West India Islands, Cuba, and in some of our Southern cities, New Orleans, Mobile, Savannah, Charleston, and even higher North, Wilmington, Norfolk, Baltimore, and occasionally is brought even to Philadelphia and New York. It has likewise been imported into European ports, Lisbon, Southampton, and St. Nazaire, in the Department of the Lower Loire, in France; but the fever has never been known to propagate beyond the 48° North latitude, nor without a temperature of 72° Fahr. It has a period of incubation of from three to eight, ten and even more days.

It is generally supposed that yellow fever attacks a person only once during his lifetime, but I have known individuals in New Orleans who had two, and one person who had three attacks of the fever during different epidemics. That this fever is a specific fever, owing its existence to some specific contagium by which it is propagated, and which may adhere to such fomites as woollens, feathers, cotton, letters, etc., is not only no longer doubted, but is a fact established beyond the shadow of a doubt by the Lisbon epidemic of 1857, and by the importation of the disease from Havana into the port of St. Nazaire by the "Anne Marie," in 1861, and by the Royal mail-steamer "La Plata" into the port of Southampton, in the month of November, 1852.

That yellow fever is a contagious disease, is likewise shown by Dr. Holcombe's interesting report of the yellow fever epidemic, which visited Natchez and the surrounding neighborhood in 1853. "The first cases of the fever," writes the Doctor in the twelfth number of the North American Journal of Homœopathy, "appeared in families some members of which had come from New Orleans within a few weeks. The houses were pleasantly situated in the central part of the city, and the tenants all in comfortable circumstances. There were four distinct centres of emanation whence the disease spread in every direction, not reaching the suburbs until after several weeks. Many of the inhabitants who fled into the country, carried the disease with them. One gentleman sickened on the road, and stopped at the house of a friend, twelve miles from town, where he died of yellow fever. One of the family speedily exhibited the same disease and died. Another fled into an adjoining county, where he also sickened and communicated the disease to those around him.

"In this manner neighborhoods were scourged by yellow fever where the disease was utterly unknown.

"In several cases which came under my observation, the families were carefully isolated, with the exception of one messenger, who was permitted to visit the town on necessary business, and uniformly that messenger was the first attacked. This epidemic was undoubtedly contagious."

The yellow fever epidemic which visited Lisbon in 1857, was carefully investigated by Dr. Lyons, of Dublin, who describes five distinct forms of the disease: 1st, the algid form; 2d, the sthenic form; 3d, the hemorrhagic form; 4th, the purpuric form; and 5th, the typhous form.

The algid type is the most suddenly fatal form of the disease. "The patient, while in the enjoyment of his usual health, and in the midst of his usual occupation, feels suddenly the effects, as it were, of a sudden blow from a heavy bar on the back, falls down while walking or standing, and dies within a few hours in profound collapse, and after exhibiting more or less of the other symptoms of this fever." The countenance became sunken, the eyes looked dull and filmy, the face and trunk presented a dirty livid hue, and the surface was dotted with points of venous congestion, and hemorrhagic spots or patches like purpura broke out here and there. In severe cases the tongue and breath were cold.

In the sthenic form the symptoms of an inflammatory condition of the system, severe headache, a high, full and hard pulse, flushed face and throbbing in the temples, were present.

The hemorrhagic type was characterized by effusions of blood from various organs and tissues, "the hemorrhage never being single, nor from any one source or organ only."

In the purpuric form the distinctive signs are purpuric patches of various tints and colors, caused by subcutaneous effusions of the coloring matter of the blood.

The typhous form is most generally a sequela of the other types; in some cases the disease presents the character of typhus, with stupor, nervous prostration and other typhoid symptoms, from the outset of the attack.

In reference to the course and characteristics of yellow fever, Dr. Holcombe imparts the following interesting information in his interesting paper:

"Yellow fever, like scarlatina, presents a wide range of manifestation, from an ephemeral mildness to the most malignant severity. The impending attack is sometimes foreshadowed for a few hours by languor, restlessness, and malaise, most commonly a chill comes on, without premonition. Sometimes heat, shiverings, headache and nausea, are all confusedly mingled in the onset. When the febrile reaction is complete, the pain in the head, back and limbs is sometimes exceedingly severe; the skin is hot and dry; the pulse full and hard, from 100 to 130; urine scanty and high colored; eyes injected, watery, brilliant; tongue covered with a pasty, white coat, with red edges and apex; there is sometimes a good deal of mucous and bilious vomiting. This paroxysm, scarcely distinguishable from the incipient stage of bilious remittent, lasts from twelve to thirty-six hours, terminating in a general or partial perspiration with great diminution, but seldom with the disappearance of the symptoms. This remission is the rule, but the exceptions are numerous, and I have repeatedly seen the fever continue uninterruptedly four or five days. In a few hours the patient declares himself worse, and another train of symptoms arises. The pain in the head, back and limbs is not so poignant, frequently is entirely absent. The pulse, tongue and skin may remain natural, whilst in fact the patient is verging into a most critical state. The febrile irritation is rather of the typhoid than of the sthenic type, the pulse being soft, rapid and sometimes irregular. Pain more frequently exists in the epigastric, occasionally in the umbilical or hypochondriac regions. It is sometimes intolerable, while in cases of imminent danger the symptom may be entirely wanting. Diarrhœa, or dysentery, may accompany this stage, but constipation is more common. Burning in the pit of the stomach, acid and acrid eructations, flatulence, thirst, nausea, all combine to produce a remarkable sense of prostration, and a great degree of tossing and sleeplessness. The skin and conjunctiva assume a light lemon-hue, which deepens into a deep orange or gamboge color, although this symptom is by no means universal. The urine is of a sulphur or saffron yellow, and stains linen. Sometimes there is slight strangury, and in bad cases the secretion of urine is totally suppressed. Hemorrhage from the gums and fauces or other mucous membranes is now common. Vomiting becomes a distressing and an alarming symptom. The matters ejected pass from a greenish-yellow into a brownish or claret-colored hue; sometimes blood, red, dark, or brown, is thrown up. The appearance of coffee-ground vomit leaves but a ray of hope. Still the patient may recover through a tardy convalescence, very liable to relapse. If the disease be not arrested, the temperature of the skin falls, the hemorrhage becomes more profuse or ominous, the circulation fails, extreme jactitation comes on, delirium or coma supervenes, and dissolution is occasionally preceded by general convulsions. The patients seemed generally to be worst on the first, third, and fifth days. Death appeared to be more common on the sixth, but some few died as early as the third day, and many lingered beyond a week. Several cases terminated in dysentery and a good number in common intermittent fever.

"The above sketch is purely typical, the symptoms of which would not be presented by any one single case.

"I will now mention some local features of importance which have come under my own observation.

"*Head.* The headache was severe during the first paroxysm, but abated during the remission, seldom to return and never to resume its prior intensity. It was throbbing, boring, with a sensation of undulation in the cranium. There was commonly soreness of the eye-balls in motion, sometimes photophobia, and in one case violent earache. There was sometimes a sensation as if the head was very much enlarged. In a few cases the headache was general, but was mostly referred to the supra-orbital region. I believe it will usually be found that, when the organic functions bear the brunt of the disease, the headache will be referred to the anterior part of the cranium, while the derangements of animal life are rather displayed by vertical and occipital headache.

"*Eyes.* The redness, brilliancy, and watery suffusion of the eye is more marked in the first stage of yellow fever than in any of its allied diseases.

"*Mouth.* Spontaneous ptyalism sometimes occurred, one or two cases of which were ascribed by the unscrupulous malice of our opponents to the secret use of Calomel.

"*Stomach.* Positive pain in the epigastrium sometimes occurred, but there was more frequently only soreness, and sense of weakness and oppression. Thirst, burning in the pit of the stomach, and an indescribable, empty, gnawing, sinking feeling, preceded and accompanied the nausea and vomiting, which were the most troublesome and distressing of the yellow fever symptoms. An insensibility to external pressure stood occasionally in strange discordance with the gastric irritability, and other symptoms of gastro-enteritis. Acid and acrid eructations were very common. Every thing, even cold water, was said by the patient to 'turn sour on the stomach.' Conjoined with these symptoms, there was sometimes a morbid, canine hunger which made the patient forget every thing else and think that, could he only eat something, he would feel perfectly well. The nausea was provoked by eating, by motion, and, in some cases, by lying on the left side. Hiccough, which Dr. Stokes considers a strong sign of inflammation about the cardiac orifice of the stomach, occurred in some bad cases. The matters ejected varied in their nature. Black vomit likewise occurred, sometimes in great quantities, and when the patient was much prostrated, the fluid was merely gulped up, running out at the corners of the mouth. It is said to be distinctly acid, reddening litmus paper, and effervescing with carbonates. It is not always a fatal symptom.

"*Genito-urinary Apparatus.* The uterus and vagina were by no means exempted from the hemorrhagic tendencies of the other mucous membranes. In a few cases the urine was at first limpid, then yellow, and, occasionally, turbid and brownish like porter. This last was sometimes largely excreted, without proving critical. Suppression of urine is perhaps more frequent in this disease than in any other, excepting Asiatic cholera. It was always a symptom of formidable character, and, when conjoined with black vomit and delirium, presaged too certainly the approach of death.

"*Chest.* The thoracic organs were not principally deranged. A soft, full, compressible pulse, averaging hundred, was very common throughout the disease, whether mild or severe. In one case the wrist was pulseless for some hours, as in Asiatic cholera, the pulsation returning during a partial, but transitory reaction.

"*Nervous System.* In all points of view, as the medium of the mind and of the senses, as an excito-motory apparatus, both voluntary and involuntary, the nervous system was both primarily and secondarily implicated. The subjective phenomena were numerous and distressing: pains, nausea, vertigo, numbness, bad taste, thirst, hunger, coldness, burning heat, frightful dreams, etc. The abdominal pains of the second stage, and even the thirst, heartburn, nausea, etc., were sometimes distinctly, but irregularly intermittent, like the pains of colic, which is explained by the fact that all the functions of the ganglionic plexus are rhythmical in their character. According to Volkmann, even a current of electricity is not transmitted continuously through them, but is broken up into a number of successive shocks. Delirium occurring in the first stage, was of little importance. Later in the disease, it was in some cases furious, the patient struggling desperately to get out of bed, but generally it was of the mild, incoherent typhoid type. In an old drunkard it was precisely the delirium of *mania a potu.* Stupor, even to profound coma, often marked the last stages.

"*Skin.* The temperature of the skin after the febrile paroxysm was commonly natural. In a few cases there was the calor mordax of typhus.

"The perspirations were very irregular, often partial, sometimes offensive, and never, that I could discern, of the least prognostic value. The yellowness came on generally by the third or fourth day, seldom earlier, sometimes not until convalescence was established. Petechiæ were sometimes observed in protracted cases. The eruption was sometimes vesicular, sometimes like what is known as prickly heat, sometimes like nettle-rash, and again the skin presented the lobster-like redness of scarlatina."

Prognosis. Aitken arranges the data to judge from, into symptoms which are favorable, and those which are not so. Favorable symptoms: "A slow pulse and moderate temperature of the body, and quiet stomach. Streaks of blood during the stage of black vomit, or after acid elimination has set in, are favorable, if the corpuscles are found entire. If the urinary secretion continue, and the black vomit be scanty from the first, or is afterwards suppressed, the patient may yet survive. Urine simply albuminous is a less serious sign than when it also contains tube-casts. Free, copious urine, no matter how dark or bilious, is the most favorable of any sign. Prognostics may be derived from the effects of treatment." Under homœopathic treatment the prognosis is infinitely more favorable than under the Old School treatment with their murderous doses of Calomel and Quinine.

Dr. Holcombe treated one hundred and forty cases of yellow fever between the 13th of August and the 15th of December, 1853. None of them were cases of ephemeral sickness, nothing but unequivocal, strongly marked yellow fever was admitted into the list. Of this number seventy-one were white, and sixty-nine colored; of the colored thirty-nine were blacks, and thirty mulattoes. The adults were ninety-three; children forty-seven; cases in town one hundred and eleven; cases in the country twenty-nine. Males sixty, females eighty. At least one-half of the cases were very severe, the patients being for several days in a critical and dangerous situation. Of the one hundred and forty cases, nine died. Of these six were treated homœopathically from the beginning, one case was complicated with abortion and profuse hemorrhage; another, a cachectic negro, died six weeks after the day of attack in a typhoid condition, the sequel of the fever. Three came into the doctor's hands on the fourth and fifth day of the fever, two of them having employed allopathic measures.

Doctor Davis, the pioneer of Homœopathy in that region, treated four hundred and fifteen cases, with twenty-four deaths. — "The unfavorable signs are: The more fiery crimson the tip and edge of the tongue, the more irritable the stomach, the severer the headache, the worse the prognosis of the first stage, and vice versa; but a streak of blood in the early vomit indicates much danger from the attack. In the second stage the earlier or more complete the suppression of urine, and the more copious the ejection of black vomit, the more imminent the danger. If the urine be scanty, and loaded with tube-casts, entangled in epithelial and coagulable matter, a light buff-colored curdy sediment indicates a complex lesion of the secreting structure of the kidneys. It is the urine symptom in its maximum of severity, and is as fatal as if the suppression had already occurred. A faltering of the articulation is a bad prognostic, and a difficulty of protruding the tongue, enhances it. The danger of the case is enhanced by inflammatory complications, and by hypertrophy of the heart. A recent residence in a temperate climate; the race or complexion of the individual; the fact of his previously having suffered from an attack, will enter into an estimate of his chances of recovery."

Treatment. Doctor Holcombe reports: "If the chill was violent, or persisted long, I ordered the *tincture of Camphor* in drop doses every ten minutes, a procedure eminently successful in Asiatic cholera, and in the cold stage of malignant intermittents. I met, not long since, in Cullen's Materia Medica, some interesting facts in proof of the last substantiated view, namely, that its primary effect is a great reduction of animal temperature. The operation of Camphor is so evanescent, that it in no wise interferes with the efficacy of subsequent remedies. *Aconite* and *Belladonna* were used in alternation in the first stage. To run a parallel between the symptoms of yellow fever and these drugs, would be to abstract whole pages from the Materia Medica. I need not speculate on the pathology of Aconite and Belladonna poisonings. They evidently show that profound lesion of innervation, subsequent nervous and vascular erethism, and local determination to the cutaneous and nervous membranes so strongly characteristic of the yellow-fever poisoning. They are complements of each other in making out the whole morbid picture, and were therefore used in alternation, every half hour at first, the interval being afterwards lengthened to one, and in mild cases, to two hours. In a few cases I used a drop of pure tincture in half a tumbler of water; but I generally contented myself with five or six drops of the first centesimal dilution prepared in the same manner, of which one teaspoonful was given at a time. A similar preparation of *Ipecacuanha* was commonly left, to be administered after each act of vomiting. In very mild cases these remedies alone sufficed.

"When the second stage came on, the cerebro-spinal symptoms disappearing, or being much ameliorated, while the patient complained of nausea, prostration, acid or burning sensations, pain in the abdomen, thirst, restlessness, etc., a change of remedies was demanded.

"On studying the symptoms of this stage, ninety-nine homœopaths out of a hundred would suggest *Arsenicum* as one of the main remedies. But lest my allopathic reader should distrust Hahnemann's Materia Medica, or Jahr's Manual, I will collate from the nearest allopathic authority, which happens to be Taylor on Poisons, some of the prominent symptoms of the Arsenical pathogenesis.

"Faintness, depression, nausea, with intense burning in the region of the stomach, increased by pressure. Violent vomiting of a brown turbid matter, mixed with mucus, and sometimes stained with blood. Sense of constriction, with a feeling of burning in the throat, often accompanied by intense thirst. Pulse small, frequent and irregular. Skin cold and clammy in the stage of collapse, at other times it is very hot. Respiration feeble, and accompanied with sighing. Inflammation of the conjunctiva with suffusion of the eyes, and intolerance of light. Irritation of the skin, accompanied by an eruption. Exfoliation of the cuticle. Great nervous irritability. Intolerable pain in the bowels, with bloody stools. Great emaciation, want of sleep, urine scanty, high-colored, and passed with an effort. Suppression of urine. Strangury and jaundice have been also noticed among the secondary symptoms. Delirium, jactitation, coma, convulsions.

"Finally the anatomical lesions of Arsenic are also remarkably similar to those of yellow fever. They are the pure dynamic effects of the drug acting through the nervous system; for it is well known that its specific effects on the stomach will be produced by injecting the veins or inserting it into a wound. Mr. Taylor says: "Arsenic is not an irritant poison; it does not seem to possess any corrosive properties, that is, it has no chemical action on the animal tissues, and the changes met with in the alimentary canal of a person poisoned by it, are referrible to the effects of the inflammation excited by the poison, and not to any chemical action.""

"In looking for a complemental medicine to alternate with Arsenic, in order to fill up the morbid picture, we keep in view that it must be capable, chemically or otherwise, of deteriorating and devitalizing the blood, so as to give rise to hemorrhage and extravasation, and render it unfit for the nutritive demands of the nervous system. No poisons, animal, vegetable or mineral, do this more uniformly and effectually than the virus of serpents. Crotalus and Lachesis are remarkably similar in their action, like the isomorphous substances in Dr. Blake's interesting experiments. We chose *Lachesis* in the fifth dilution, alternating it with the fourth trituration of *Arsenicum*, at intervals of an hour. When *Belladonna* and *Arsenicum* produced no amelioration, a change to *Arsen.* and *Lachesis* brought about the desired amendment.

"These remedies were sufficient for very many severe cases of yellow fever, but occasional symptoms arose from the idiosyncrasy of the individual, or the peculiarity of the case, which called for other remedies. *Veratrum* was very useful in allaying the vomiting and abdominal pains. *Tartar emetic* succeeded promptly in some cases of prolonged and distressing nausea. *Chamomilla* did more for this gastric irritability than its rather mild pathogenesis would lead us to expect, particularly in the cases of women and children. Mustard plasters to the epigastrium, and cold enemata were also used as palliatives for the nausea and vomiting. Very hot fomentations frequently diminished the excruciating pains in the bowels. When diarrhœa or dysenteric symptoms supervened, *Mercurius*, *Phosphorus* or Colocynth relieved them readily. *Cantharides* scarcely ever failed to remove strangury, and restore the venal secretions, in conjunction with Arsenic. *Nux vomica* was frequently employed as an adjuvant in persons much addicted to alcoholic liquors. *Chamomilla*, *Sabina* or *Secale* generally caused the symptoms of threatened abortion to disappear. When the strong characteristics of yellow fever gradually subsided, leaving the system prostrated and torpid, *Rhus* and *Bryonia* were used with good effect. *Belladonna*, *Coffea* and *Hyoscyamus* were sometimes indicated at night for nervous sleeplessness. *Millefolium* was used in one case of abundant hemorrhage from the mouth, and whether it was a coincidence or a cure, it was almost immediately checked. Some of our ultra-Hahnemannian brethren may find fault with us for using such low dilutions, repeating them so frequently, and sometimes employing three remedies in quick succession. But the malignity and rapidity of the disease, the diversity and frequent incongruity of the symptoms, their Protean forms and treacherous character, warranted us in active and decisive measures. Homœopathic aggravation, under such circumstances, is very little to be apprehended, foreshadowing as it does a curative result. A resort to the higher dilutions, 6th, 12th or 30th after the lower had failed, was attended, in some cases, with the happiest effect.

"If the above remedies proved inefficacious, if the patient sank, if the vomiting became worse, with brownish stains in the matter ejected, or any of those various hues which indicated hemorrhage from the gastric mucous membrane, *Nitrate of Silver* was the remedy, conjoined with *Arsenicum* and *Lachesis*. We made a first and second centesimal trituration, and as the latter did just as well as the former, perhaps better, I infer that the action, like that of Arsenicum, was not topically stimulant, but dynamic. Indeed, what stimulus, in the allopathic sense of the word, can the one ten-thousandth of a grain of *Nitrate of Silver*, dissolved in half a tumbler of water, administered in teaspoonful doses, give to the whole gastric mucous membrane? A much more *curative* one, I venture to say, than the same remedy would have made in larger doses. As it was, the medicine frequently aggravated; and one patient complained bitterly of the nausea it produced. In this case, all the dangerous symptoms were arrested by Lachesis. One negro woman lived a week after black vomit had set in, apparently, but not permanently, rallied by *Nitrate of Silver*, *Carbo vegetabilis* and *Hydrocyanic acid*.

"Strict attention was paid to diet; a point of vast importance in managing the diseases of the blood-making apparatus. Arrowroot, rice-water and black tea with a little sugar and milk in it, were the standard articles for the first stage. During the second stage, the canine hunger was sometimes distressing; but besides the above nutriment, we seldom permitted anything but a teaspoonful of pure cream at regular intervals. Ice was allowed, in moderate quantities, for the thirst. During convalescence, the slightest imprudence in eating was apt to induce relapse. I have seen toasted bread, chicken broth, soft boiled eggs, etc., decidedly injurious. When the patient is able to pass from the farinaceous articles to something more nutritive, he may be permitted at once to chew pieces of good beef-steak. This is much better than beef-tea, because the act of mastication extracts the saliva, and incorporates it with the animal juice, thereby facilitating its digestion. Alcoholic stimulants were seldom given during the disease, or recommended to promote recovery. Confirmed topers, however, were permitted to use small quantities of their favorite beverages during the latter stages of the disease." H.]

4. Cholera Asiatica.
Asiatic Cholera.

Asiatic cholera is an intensely epidemic disease; sporadic cases, even if they bear the greatest resemblance to cholera, cannot be regarded as such, but must be set down as very violent cases of cholerine. We will not inquire where and how cholera first originated. The important point with us is to be acquainted with the manner in which this epidemic spreads. Cholera is caused by a special contagium which is multiplied by the disease and is contained in the excrements; its presence anywhere else is very doubtful. Hence the infection is principally spread by contact with the excrementitious matter of cholera-patients. This proposition which was first started by Pettenkofer is the only one among the multitude of hypotheses bearing on this point, by which the various bizarre modifications in the spread of the epidemic can be accounted for in a natural manner. This involves a second point, namely: that the development of the contagium does not take place within the body of the patient, but in the excrements after their removal out of the body, and that this development takes place so much more rapidly and intensely the more the conditions for a rapid decomposition of the excrements are accumulated. The infection is promoted by all kinds of affections affiliated to cholera, hence chiefly by gastro-intestinal catarrh, by circumstances exerting a depressing effect upon the mind, by a cold, by dietetic transgressions. Neither age nor sex shows either a greater or a less susceptibility to the disease. The epidemic now raging in Egypt furnishes a striking example of the origin and spread of cholera. Hence cholera is not contagious properly speaking.

Symptoms and Course. It cannot be stated with perfect certainty how soon, after the infection has taken place, the first symptoms of the disease show themselves, but all circumstances tend to show that the period of incubation only lasts three days. It has no characteristic symptoms; the alterations caused by the dread of the fearful malady must not be mistaken for manifestations of the disease itself.

A preliminary stage in reality does not exist. The first sign that infection has taken place, is a painless diarrhœa which is very thin, but is still somewhat tinged with bile; the patient has from three to six discharges every day. On a careful examination, a number of shreds of epithelium are discovered in the excrements. The diarrhœa is not always associated with a marked feeling of malaise; sometimes the only symptoms present are a disproportionate feeling of lassitude, an increase of thirst and an impaired appetite. That this premonitory diarrhœa is real cholera, is shown by the circumstance that it is capable of spreading the infection. At any rate, every diarrhœa which sets in at the time of epidemic cholera ought to be regarded as a premonitory symptom of the disease. At times the diarrhœa only lasts a few hours, at other times a few days, scarcely ever beyond a week. It may terminate the attack, or else the disease may pass into the more malignant and more characteristic forms of the epidemic.

This passage to the more malignant type generally takes place quite suddenly. A copious evacuation takes place resembling rice-water, simultaneously with which the debility increases very rapidly. These evacuations succeed each other with more or less rapidity, an agonizing thirst supervenes, and very soon the patient is attacked with vomiting of substances resembling the alvine evacuations, but having a little more color. At the same time the patients are no longer able to preserve the erect posture; they are tormented by a peculiar anguish which they point out as being located in the præcordia; the urinary secretions are scanty or entirely suppressed, the patients have a cadaverous appearance, the eyes are sunken, surrounded by dark margins, the skin is cool, the head is bathed in a cool perspiration; the pulse is small; at this stage cramps of the glutei muscles and of other muscular bundles make their appearance. The affection may persist for some time at this height, very seldom longer than twelve hours, after which recovery takes place, the passages gradually resuming a bilious tinge, becoming less copious and less frequent, and the skin warming up again. Convalescence from this milder form of the disease always proceeds rapidly, without being disturbed by consecutive diseases. Usually, however, this mild form sooner or later passes into the most violent form of the disease.

This type of cholera, designated as cholera asphyctica or algida, very seldom breaks out all at once at the outset, but very often succeeds the premonitory diarrhœa with the suddenness of a flash of lightness. The quantity of matter evacuated by the anus and mouth, is enormous; it is colorless and inodorous, contains shreds of epithelium and a few flocks of mucus. These evacuations often succeed each other without the least intermission. The thirst now becomes agonizing; the vomiting is excited every time after the patient swallows a drink of water. His anxiety is excessive; at times he complains of violent pains in the pit of the stomach, and he is likewise tormented by severe cramps in the calves. The urinary secretion is entirely suppressed. The consequences of the immense losses of fluids show themselves very speedily. The skin becomes cold, very soon it assumes a cyanotic color, loses its elasticity to such a degree that a fold of integument on the hands, if pinched up, remains in this condition for a long time; the face has a cadaverous appearance, the eyes are deeply sunken in their sockets, the nose is pointed, the lips blue. The temperature is like that of ice. The radial pulse can no longer be felt, not even that of the larger arteries; the sounds of the heart are very feeble, the second sound is often wanting; respiration is labored, the breath is cold; the voice is extinct. After this condition has lasted for twelve hours at most, death takes place, previous to which the evacuations upwards and downwards generally cease and the extreme prostration changes to a complete stupor, without any real death-struggle, and without the râle which usually precedes death. The disease may change for the better even after it has reached the acme of the stage of asphyxia, although recovery from this stage is an event of rare occurrence.

The stage of reaction shows the most remarkable differences. The disease may uniformly but slowly progress towards convalescence. This change as well as the beginning of reaction generally is indicated by the circumstance that the patients are able to retain liquids on their stomachs, and that the radial pulse returns. Gradually the temperature of the skin is restored, the alvine discharges diminish in number and are more and more colored; at first they are generally mixed with shreds of intestinal mucous membrane, and have a foul smell. The prostration continues for a few days, the urine is at first turbid and shows traces of an inflammatory process going on in the kidneys. Such a simple convalescence from cholera algida is always an exception, not the rule. In other cases the icy coldness is suddenly succeeded by a febrile excitement, a rapid and full pulse, cerebral hyperæmia; this change is either speedily followed by convalescence, or else, typhoid phenomena make their appearance. The more malignant forms of cholera are very generally followed by typhoid symptoms. After the cessation of the vomiting and a return of the pulse, the pulse becomes hard, full and frequent; the turgescence of the skin is very marked. The brain seems blunted, the patients are lying in a state of sopor and delirium, very much prostrated; the temperature rises considerably; the thirst continues and the patient has even occasional attacks of vomiting, the diarrhœic stools are decomposed and have a foul smell; the tongue is dry and has a fuliginous coating. Every symptom points to the supervention of an intense typhus, with which the symptoms of an intense nephritis are generally associated. The transition from this typhoid condition to health always takes place very slowly, although more rapidly than in cases of true typhus. A favorable turn generally takes place already in the second week. Death is a very common termination of this condition. Cholera has no positive sequelæ, although the most diversified derangements remain after an attack of cholera, which generally result from the circumstance that the circulation in the various organs had almost been arrested during the frigid stage to the point of inflammatory infiltration. We do not give a detailed statement of the anatomical changes in cholera, because they are almost generally without any characteristic significance. Beside the excessive but perfectly explicable dryness of the tissues, we constantly meet with an extensive destruction of the epithelium of the mucous membrane of the ileum; the gall-bladder is found distended with bile. At all events, the anatomical lesions are not sufficient to account for the frightful rapidity of the development of cholera; the lesions of the intestinal epithelium certainly cannot be the only cause of the profuse watery evacuations.

Treatment. We will in the first place call attention in a few remarks to the prophylactic treatment which can be arranged in cholera more easily than in any other epidemic. We know that the excrements of the patients are by far the most active vehicles of the contagium. Hence, it behooves us either to destroy this contagium in the excrements, or else, to remove it. For this reason the discharges should at once be mixed with Sulphate of Iron, and should not be thrown into water-closets, but into deep ditches remote from inhabited dwellings. The soiled bed-linen is best cleansed by boiling it. In order to protect uninfected persons, they must be forbidden to visit the houses of the sick, and above all, the use of the water-closets must be absolutely prohibited. Nurses should never remain with the patient too long at a time. The enactment of further measures is the business of the health-authorities; all sanitary measures must aim at this one object, to keep the excrements of cholera-patients remote from all contact with healthy persons. On the other hand, it is unnecessary and useless to try to prevent the spread of cholera by placing all cholera-patients in strict quarantine. If cholera were contagious, every physician would have an attack of it. Among the precautionary measures which it behooves each individual to observe, the following are the most important: As much as possible a regular mode of living; the use of simple and substantial nourishment; the slightest possible deviation from one's regular mode of living; avoidance of all debilitating influences, such as excessive mental exertions, depressing emotions, etc., more particularly avoidance of the excessive use of spirits. Whatever tends to excite diarrhœa, must be discarded. Persons must take care not to get chilled or overheated. Every diarrhœa with which a person may be attacked, or with which he may already be affected during an epidemic, should be carefully attended to. The observance of these preventive rules is at all events a much more efficient prophylactic than all the other vaunted preservatives which are almost always made up of spirits. Good claret is the only kind of wine that can be safely allowed as unhurtful. No reasonable person will deny the usefulness of suitable prophylactic means which everybody should employ in his own, and likewise advise in other families under the direction of an enlightened physician.

The medicines which a good deal of clinical experience has pointed out as our best remedies for cholera, are not numerous; in view of the great uniformity which the leading symptoms present in all epidemics, no great variety of remedial agents can be expected; from the practical stand-point, this must be looked upon as a great boon to the physician. Our remedies the efficacy of which has been corroborated by trials, are: *Ipecacuanha, Camphora, Veratrum album, Cuprum,* and *Arsenicum;* this list does not include the remedies for the typhoid condition remaining after cholera.

Ipecacuanha is less indicated for real cholera than for the premonitory diarrhœa; its efficacy in this diarrhœa is certainly great, and an attenuated tincture of Ipecacuanha can be safely recommended as the best domestic remedy during epidemic cholera. Real cholera requires *Ipecacuanha*, if the vomiting is much worse than the diarrhœa. *Ipecacuanha* is, moreover, an important remedy in the cholera of little children.

Camphora is recommended by Hahnemann himself for an incipient attack. This recommendation has not been very extensively verified by experience; nevertheless, if the attack is not too violent, the tincture of Camphor had better be tried; likewise, if the attack is preceded by unequivocal, premonitory symptoms, in the so-called cholera sicca. Hahnemann announces the following symptoms for which Camphor has been used in many cases with great success: Sudden and rapid failing of strength, so that the person attacked cannot stand on his legs; alteration of the features, sunken eyes, bluish and icy-cold face, coolness of the rest of the body; hopeless despondency and anxiety as if he would be asphyxiated; stupefaction, insensibility; constant and unintelligible moaning; burning in the stomach and fauces; crampy pains in the calves; painfulness of the pit of the stomach to contact; thirst, nausea, vomiting and diarrhœa have not yet set in. After taking Camphor, sweat soon breaks out as a sure sign that an improvement has commenced. As soon as this takes place, the remedy must be given less frequently and in smaller quantities, otherwise it might give rise to a troublesome cerebral hyperæmia. For the typhoid symptoms remaining after cholera, *Camphor* has likewise been given; the exhibition of Camphor in this condition is, indeed, justified by the similarity of its pathogenesis to the symptoms characterizing uræmia. The results, however, are not as yet very numerous.

Veratrum album is, without doubt, our most important remedy for cholera. If we wish to derive good effects from its use, we have to begin its administration in good season, and give it at once for the premonitory diarrhœa, especially if it is colorless. *Veratrum* is indicated still more, if the attack commences with vomiting and diarrhœa; this remedy often stays the further progress of the disease. *Veratrum* is less reliable if the symptoms of cholera are fully developed, although even then it surpasses all other remedies in efficacy. Of course, no remedy acts as favorably after the disease has made considerable headway; it is for this reason that *Veratrum* should be given at as early a period as possible. If the restlessness of the patient has given way to a dull apathy and insensibility; if the skin is cold as marble and the pulse has become perfectly extinct, *Veratrum* is no longer indicated. In general, it is proper to say that *Veratrum album* ceases to exert a favorable effect after the symptoms of reaction have become extinct.

Cuprum is highly commended by some, and entirely rejected by other physicians. An investigation will show that the latter class reject Cuprum because they have not given the proper dose; *Cuprum* 30 cannot be expected to have any effect in such a very acute disease. *Cuprum* is not only indicated when the evacuations are still unchecked, but likewise in the stage of asphyxia. This medicine is not endowed with much power to check the diarrhœa, but it is a valuable remedy in preventing the general paralysis of the organism. For this reason, as long as vomiting and diarrhœa are still present, *Cuprum* had better be given in alternation with *Veratrum*, more particularly if the spasms are very general and rather of the clonic form. In the frigid stage *Cuprum* alone is indicated, if the following symptoms are present: Loss of consciousness; spasmodic twitching of the fingers and toes; trismus; audible gurgling of the beverage down the œsophagus; no vomiting, in its place distressing, ineffectual efforts to vomit; the diarrhœa has ceased, but on pressing on the bowels a loud gurgling is heard, giving rise to the suspicion that the stools are not expelled, because paralysis of the intestines has set in. *Cuprum* is likewise indicated if the pulse not only becomes feeble, but intermittent at an early period of the disease. It is of great importance what preparation is used. We doubt whether metallic Copper can ever act with great promptness; we prefer the *Acetate* and *Sulphate* of *Copper*.

Arsenicum album displays its curative action in those terribly rapid cases where cholera algida at once sets in without any premonitory symptoms. The most essential indications for Arsenicum are: Sudden and complete exhaustion, vanishing of the pulse together with violent palpitations of the heart, great dyspnœa, inexpressible anguish, constant tossing about, horrid thirst, yet the least quantity of liquid is vomited up again immediately; burning distress in the region of the stomach and upper portion of the bowels; complete suppression of urine. In such cases *Arsenicum* should be given at once, without any other medicine being resorted to in the first place. After the exhibition of Arsenic the urine is often secreted in large quantity, a very favorable change.

Beside these most important remedies we mention the following, accompanying some of them with brief indications or giving only their names. It is not an easy thing to introduce new cholera-remedies to the favorable notice of the Profession, for the reason that the above-named remedies have proven themselves reliable in this fearful epidemic to such a degree that they must necessarily cast all other medicines that are recommended for cholera, into the shade. Who would want to experiment with untried remedies in such a rapidly and terribly fatal plague?

Carbo vegetabilis has not unfrequently been found useful at a period in the course of the disease when no special medicine is decidedly indicated. *Carbo* may be administered in the asphyctic stage, if the diarrhœa and vomiting have ceased, if every spasmodic movement has disappeared, and the patient lies as if dead. *Carbo* is frequently indicated after *Arsenicum*, and is particularly in its place in cases where every sign of reaction had seemed extinct from the beginning.

Acidum hydrocyanum has similar indications as *Carbo*, but differs from this medicine in the succession of its symptoms. It is indicated if the attack at once assumes the highest degree of intensity, so that but a few hours intervene between the commencement of the attack and the moment when death seems to be lurking on the threshold; *Carbo* may be sufficient if the failing of the strength is less rapid.

Opium deserves attention in the cholera of little children; it is seldom suitable for adults.

Colchicum cannot be regarded as a remedy for cholera, for the reason that it has not the colorless stools.

We name moreover: *Jatropha curcas*, *Iris versicolor*, *Cicuta virosa*, *Conium*, *Secale cornutum*; these remedies, however, are either unreliable as similia, or because they have not been sufficiently proved.

As regards dose, almost all observers agree in recommending the lower preparations, even the strong tinctures, frequently repeated.

We have to devote a few lines to the management and diet of cholera-patients. Warm external applications are generally of very little use; they are apt to increase the patients' restlessness, and have to be resorted to very guardedly. Continued but gentle frictions with cold wet clothes are much more beneficial. At the onset of the attack, food is utterly out of the question. The best beverage is fresh well-water; this will moderate the thirst for a moment at any rate. Small lumps of ice in the mouth likewise refresh the patient a good deal. If Champagne can be had, it may be administered in tablespoonful doses with great advantage.

The typhoid symptoms after cholera are so changeable that it is next to impossible to recommend a positive course of treatment for them. The most important remedies are: *Belladonna*, *Bryonia*, *Phosphorus*, *Opium*, *Acidum phosphoricum* and *muriaticum; Cantharides* and *Terebinthina* may be chiefly relied upon as remedies for the often prominently developed nephritis. As a rule, the treatment should be conducted upon the same principles as the treatment of typhus. The returning appetite has to be gratified with great caution. In cholera, as in typhus, the intestinal canal recovers its normal integrity very slowly.

[During the epidemic cholera of 1849 I recommended the saturated tincture of Aconite-root as a specific for cholera. This recommendation was laughed at by some, and very coolly received by others. In the May number of the North American Journal of Homœopathy, 1867, we find an article by Doctor Cramoity, translated from the Bulletin de la Société Médicale homœopathique de France, by Doctor John Davies of Chicago. In this article Doctor Cramoity claims for the *tincture* of Aconite the rank of a Cholera-specific. He claims that from a therapeutic point of view the characteristic feature in cholera is the *acceleration* or the augmentation of the pulsations. "This," says the Doctor, "is not a hypothesis; for we can well remember in the cholera-cases we examined when under our supervisiso in the Charity-hospital, in 1854, and in our private Clinic in 1865, that the increase of the pulse more or less coincided with the degree of the disease, and not with the anguish or suffering; because the pulse frequently disappeared at this moment.

"At the commencement of the epidemic of 1865 we did not appreciate these symptoms, and had the misfortune to lose four cases, two women and two children; to these we had given the remedies prescribed in the books for similar cases, which remedies were said to be the most efficacious in such circumstances.

"This is therefore the reason for our presenting this theory of the treatment of cholera: our experience and observation establish the fact that the *tincture of Aconite* is the grand curative agent of inflammatory diseases, and the regulator of the circulation.

"We have prescribed from fifteen to twenty drops of the *tincture of Aconite* in six to eight ounces of distilled water, a teaspoonful of the same to be taken every ten, twenty or thirty minutes, according to the intensity of the symptoms. Under its influence, the patient begins to revive, the circulation of the blood returns to its normal condition; the pulse rises, the internal heat ceases; the thirst is allayed, and the vomiting and diarrhœa arrested. At the same time the bluish cast of countenance disappears, the cadaverous expression changes to a natural one, the agitation of mind and body is replaced by a tranquil condition; the dread of death is transformed to joy and hope, and the patient recovers in three to four hours."

Several cases are mentioned where the patients, after having been fruitlessly treated with the usual cholera-remedies, such as: *Camphor*, *Veratrum*, *Arsenicum*, *Cuprum*, and sinking very fast into the last stage of collapse, were speedily and completely cured with large doses of the concentrated tincture of Aconite.

Indeed, why should Aconite be overlooked as a great and specific remedy for cholera? If there is any truth in the homœopathic law, the effects of Aconite upon the normal human organism point to it as a remedy for cholera. We do not think that it supersedes the use of other valuable specifics for this terrible epidemic, nor do they, on the other hand, supersede the use of Aconite. A few cases of poisoning will conclusively demonstrate the homœopathicity of Aconite to Asiatic cholera. With high potencies we must, of course, not expect to accomplish anything; large doses of the concentrated tincture are required to produce a curative effect.

The following case of poisoning is reported by Doctor Jacob Reed, Jr., of this place: A man, forty-five years of age, under treatment of rheumatism, swallowed a teaspoonful of liniment composed of equal parts of the tincture of Aconite-root and water. This was followed by pain in the epigastrium, numbness of the hands and feet, and a sense of formication over the whole body. One hour after, the dose was repeated. At the time of my visit, an hour and a half after the first dose, the man had swallowed over a drachm of the strongest tincture of the root. I found him in a complete state of collapse; after the second dose he had vomited repeatedly, first bilious matter changing into copious watery discharges; he had also had several very large rice-water discharges from the bowels; he complained of terrible pain and anxiety about the heart, was pulseless, skin cold and clammy, face indicative of great suffering and fear, breath cold to the hand; occasional paroxysms of general opisthotonic spasms would leave him in a prostrated condition in which it would seem that his constantly expressed fear that he should die, was about to be realized.

Before I questioned the family, from my first examination of the case, I judged it to be cholera; indeed, if there had been cases of cholera in town, I would have thought it unnecessary to investigate the case further. I discovered the mistake that had been made, and under the free use of stimulants, Coffee and Opium, he recovered, but not until after three or four hours continuance of the above severe symptoms."

The following case of poisoning from the tincture of Aconite-root is reported in the October number, 1868, of the Medical and Surgical Reporter, published in Philadelphia. By mistake a child was given a teaspoonful of the strong tincture of Aconite-root. The patient was a boy, six years of age. Doctor Hays of Covington, Ky., where the poisoning occurred, reports as follows: I found the patient so much prostrated that, had there been an epidemic of cholera, and had I no examination to aid me, or any previous history, but had to depend upon the appearance of the patient, I would undoubtedly have pronounced it a collapsed state of cholera. The skin was cold, clammy and livid, with a profuse perspiration, there was no pulse to be felt at the wrist, the action of the heart was quite feeble and irregular, the capillaries were scarcely able to be refilled when their contents were poured out. The head was cold, the eyes were natural in appearance, except the dilatation of the pupils which was extreme and not at all sensitive to the effects of light. The facial expression was haggard, the nose pinched, the breathing extremely labored, the lungs were filled with mucus, the rattle of which could be distinctly heard in any part of the room. The patient's bowels moved several times involuntarily. Under proper treatment the boy recovered."

The eleventh case of poisoning by Aconite in my Materia Medica was regarded by Dr. Pereyra of Bordeaux as such an exact representation of the symptoms of cholera that the doctor concluded to antidote the symptoms with Guaco which he had found efficacious during the paralytic stage of cholera. The poisoning was caused by a large dose of Aconite taken by a rheumatic patient in the hospital of Bordeaux, France. All the pathognomic cholera-symptoms were reproduced in this case.

Doctor Richard Hughes, in his Manual of Pharmaco-dynamics urges the claims of Aconite as a remedy for Asiatic cholera. Page 38, Vol. I. he writes: "Some very striking phenomena are observed in the sphere of the circulation. In acute poisoning the dilated pupils, the pale face, the quick and contracted pulse, and the general coldness within and without speak of an excitation of the vaso-motor nerves throughout the body, analogous to that of the musculo-motor centres which results in tetanus. In other words, we have a condition answering to the chill of fever, the cold stage of ague, the *collapse of cholera.*" Page 44 he writes: "Lastly in the collapse of Asiatic cholera, where the chill is so deadly that, were it not for the 'consecutive fever,' its true nature would be hardly recognizable, Aconite will still assert its power. I venture to predict that it will some day be recognized as superior even to Arsenic in those terrible cases where vomiting and purging are well nigh absent, and death seems eminent from the arrest of the circulation."

If the Doctor will turn to the pages of the British Journal some twenty years back, he will find that I made the same prediction at that time, and was laughed at for my pains. H.]

C. CONSTITUTIONAL DISEASES WITHOUT DEFINITE INFECTION.

1. Chlorosis.

Green-sickness.

Chlorosis as an idiopathic disease occurs exclusively among females, and is connected with the sexual functions in a manner that we are as yet unable to account for by a precise and logical process of reasoning. Chlorosis occurs chiefly between the ages of thirteen and twenty-four years, seldom at a later period; if it does, it can be traced to secondary disturbances, such as: confinements of young women coming rapidly one after another, more especially if the women nurse their own children. Hence the real cause of chlorosis has to be traced to the sexual sphere; but it is easily perceived that unconquerable obstacles stand in the way of a thorough investigation. The disease sometimes breaks out previous to the first appearance of the menses, more frequently after several menstrual periods; as an entirely primary disease it only breaks out among unmarried women. It appears to be hereditary; females of a pale complexion are more liable to be attacked with it; no constitution is exempt from the disease, although delicate individuals with irritable nerves are more susceptible to it. Among other causes we may mention: Insufficient exercise, mental exertions without corresponding muscular activity; excitement of the fancy, especially when caused by novel-reading; excitement of the sexual instinct by onanism, improper converse with the other sex; deprivation of open air, and interference with the free expansion of the chest by tight dresses. In a given case it is extremely difficult to find out the proper cause; for this reason, close attention in watching the symptoms is indispensable, as for instance in the case of robust young country-girls. Chlorosis is very commonly met with among the daughters of a tuberculous mother.

Symptoms and Course. A number of observations have established the fact that the number of blood-corpuscles is very much less in the blood of chlorotic patients; in very deep-seated cases this number is diminished by four-fifths of the normal quantity. We do not know what the cause of this deficiency is, but this deficiency accounts for most of the symptoms of the disease. It generally commences very slowly. The patients become more irritable, they are apt to get tired after every little effort; they are liable to changes of color; the skin soon loses its bright lustre, and the patients complain of feeling chilly at an early period of the disease. Inasmuch as the pathological picture which now develops itself, may be characterized by a variety of symptoms, we prefer describing the derangements as they appear in each special organ and system.

The skin at times has the color of wax; at other times it is rather yellowish or of a dingy-white, the veins being either not at all or but indistinctly perceptible. The color of the cheeks may change quite often within a very brief period of time. The visible mucous membranes are more or less without color. Œdematous symptoms only occur in the highest grades of the disease, and excite a suspicion that some other disease is at the bottom of these symptoms. The following symptoms occur in the digestive range: Impaired appetite, aversion to meat, longing for strange articles of diet, such as vinegar, chalk, coffee-beans; bloating of the stomach after every meal, acidity of the stomach, generally the bowels are very torpid. In the nervous system we discover excessive irritability, neuralgia, hysteric symptoms, fitful mood. — The breathing is accelerated; the least physical effort causes an attack of dyspnœa, sometimes to a very high degree. The circulation is accelerated, very seldom retarded; disposition to transitory palpitations of the heart which are easily excited by a physical effort; anæmic murmur in the large veins of the neck. The menses are irregular, sometimes entirely suppressed or very tardy, sometimes more profuse than usual, but always of a lighter color or even quite colorless. Accompanying these symptoms are pains of the most diversified kind, very generally uterine catarrh. The urine has a strikingly pale color. The patients generally sleep very soundly and have to sleep a long time; sleep never refreshes them.

One or the other of these derangements is generally wanting; at other times one of them is very prominent, whereas another is inconsiderable; thus it happens that the most varied groups of symptoms often develop themselves which, however, have essentially the same meaning. The one characteristic symptom is never absent: dyspnœa and palpitation of the heart from the least unusual effort, especially after going up stairs.

The course of chlorosis is always more or less protracted, sometimes very chronic. This, however, must be expected, since the disorder is depending upon anomalies of nutrition that come on very gradually and which can, no more than their consequences, be extirpated very suddenly. If no particular disturbances take place, the affection can sometimes be cured in a few weeks, whereas, if the usual mode of living which had acted as the exciting cause, is persevered in, the trouble may continue for years. In such cases the disease has remissions and exacerbations, and is most commonly more violent in the summer than in the winter-season. Uncomplicated chlorosis always terminates in recovery; it is only when circumstances favor the disease that disturbances of the nervous system and the sexual sphere, but less frequently of the heart, remain. Among the complications, the simultaneous presence of tuberculosis and scrofulosis is most threatening. We generally find that scrofulous girls who are attacked with chlorosis, recover their health to some extent for a year or two, after which they die of consumption, or phthisis may set in as a direct development of a protracted chlorosis.

Treatment. This has to be directed with a view of meeting the cause as well as the symptoms of the case. To meet the symptoms, medicines have to be used; but before prescribing our remedy, we ought to find out what the remedy is given for, what we intend to accomplish with it, and what we can legitimally expect from its operation. Most generally, physicians aim at bringing back the menses; if this is accomplished, they fancy that they have gained the battle. This view, however, is not only totally erroneous, but may result in a good deal of mischief. The menses are neither the cause of chlorosis nor do they indicate the grade of its importance. They are often absent, or, if present, they are generally irregular, pale, watery, but may likewise be profuse and occur too frequently. This shows that they have no characteristic significance in this disease. This is so true that after the menses cease, the cure of the disease sometimes commences, as we see in the case of young girls who are sent from the city into the country where they gain every day in health and strength without seeing any catamenial discharge for months. Of course, chlorosis cannot be said to be entirely cured unless menstruation has resumed its regular course, the more so the older the patients are.

The true remedies for chlorosis are: *Ferrum, Arsenicum, Calcarea carbonica, Plumbum, Sepia, Pulsatilla;* many other remedies may be required for intermediate conditions.

Ferrum. This medicine is a real specific for simple, uncomplicated chlorosis; every simple case of this disease yields to the curative action of *Iron.* If physicians complain of the inefficiency of this medicine, it is most probably their own fault; for, if given at the proper time and in the right quantity, *Iron* always acts beneficently, nor need any evil effects be apprehended from this agent if the stomach is weak and irritable. It is for such gastric symptoms that *Iron* is more particularly suitable. The sooner the remedy is administered the more speedily it will act; the longer its exhibition is delayed, the less reliable it becomes. It is impossible to determine the proper dose *a priori;* all we can say is that beyond the third trituration the medicine has no effect and that it is very often necessary to resort to the crude substance. This has to be found out by careful trials. Of the numerous ferrugineous preparations one praises one, and another another preparation; each may be useful, because each may effect a cure. We are still without any criterium by which the usefulness of any particular preparation could be determined; we prefer that which is least liable to change. Among these preparations the simple *Ferrum redactum* of the Pharmacopœa is undoubtedly the most appropriate. It may be used with excellent success in the first or second trituration and is at all events preferable to iron-filings. Among the salts of Iron we generally prefer the *Acetate* on account of its ready solubility; only the salt has to be frequently prepared fresh, because it is easily decomposed. The *Sulphate* and *Muriate* may be used, but they have no special advantages. Chalybeate waters do not enjoy any special superiority; their administration requires some caution and care. In inveterate cases of a high degree of intensity, they are undoubtedly preferable; their use renders it absolutely necessary that the patient should change her mode of living, which she might otherwise be indisposed to do. The use of *Ferrum* is contra-indicated by the following symptoms: Previous employment of the drug in enormous doses; even small doses cause a marked hyperæmia about the heart and lungs. The last-mentioned effect is apt to occur when tubercles are present in the lungs.

Arsenicum is less frequently indicated, but, when indicated, it has an eminently curative effect. It is suitable in all cases of chlorosis that have been mismanaged with *Ferrum* and which are generally characterized by a high degree of debility, with excessive irritability, œdematous paleness, cardiac phenomena even during rest, and complete gastro-ataxia. *Arsenicum* is likewise important, if the previously mentioned symptoms are associated with a disposition to adiposis, paroxysms of dyspnœa or else continued shortness of breath, profuse menstruation, liver-complaint, violent cardialgia, sleeplessness at night, drowsiness in the day-time. It is remarkable how soon after the administration of *Arsenicum* the normal appetite returns and the sickly complexion is replaced by a brighter hue.

Calcarea carbonica, unaided by other remedies, scarcely ever effects a cure of chlorosis; generally *Ferrum* has to be given afterwards. It is indicated by a disposition to congestions of the head and chest; constant and abrupt changes of color; a lively and irritable temperament; the menses are too profuse and premature; acidity of the stomach with complete loathing of animal diet, craving for farinaceous and indigestible food. In such cases Ferrum often agrees best after Calcarea. As a general rule this remedy is only suitable to chlorotic persons during the period of pubescence.

Plumbum aceticum is recommended by Winter in accordance with sound reasoning; we have no personal experience with this drug. It is indicated by the following circumstances and symptoms. Severe orthopnœa and dyspnœa, inconquerable constipation, extreme muscular debility, œdema of the feet. If, in addition to these symptoms, we take the numerous cardiac phenomena, the gastric difficulties and the cough, we obtain a striking picture of an intense, inveterate chlorosis. Beside Winter's, we are not acquainted with any trials that other physicians have made with Lead.

Sepia may be regarded as an excellent remedy for the paroxysms of hemicrania which constitute a source of distress to chlorotic females with brown hair and lively temperaments. *Sepia* is likewise adapted to chlorosis emanating from the sexual organs as secondary affections.

Pulsatilla has been long regarded as a remedy for chlorosis; however, we are of opinion that most of the cures of chlorosis that are attributed to the exclusive use of *Pulsatilla*, are questionable. *Pulsatilla* is no remedy for primary chlorosis, although we cheerfully admit that, like Sepia, it is a very excellent remedy in secondary chlorosis. *Pulsatilla* is likewise excellent for special symptoms, such as: pain in the stomach, headache, toothache; but chlorosis is scarcely ever acted upon by this medicine.

The removal of the cause, including a certain preventive treatment up to a certain degree, is scarcely ever heeded with sufficient attention. We are not able to determine all the special causes of chlorosis, but the general causes can be clearly made out, and this is sufficient both to guard against the disease and to promote the cure. Let our young ladies be properly educated, and let all premature excitement of the fancy be carefully avoided; let all fashions interfering with the respiration and the digestion be discarded; let our girls have an abundance of very active exercise in the open air; let the mothers' attention be directed to the deleterious practice of onanism and to all premature sexual excitement; and above all, let all novel-reading be strictly prohibited. If the disease has once broken out, a radical change in the mode of living is eminently advisable; city-girls ought to be sent into the country, and country-girls to town. A change of this kind alone is often sufficient to effect a cure. Of course, the deleterious influences to which we have alluded, have to be strictly avoided. The patients had better confine themselves to the use of milk, leaving off both tea and coffee. A moderate amount of bodily exercise is necessary, continued and fatiguing exercise is hurtful. Cheerful company promotes the cure very much. Sleep should not be limited to a fixed number of hours; on the other hand, constant somnolence should not be yielded to.

[Bæhr has left out three remedies that may render efficient service in the treatment of chlorosis; they are: *Aconite*, if chlorosis is complicated with tuberculosis; such patients are apt to have a dark sallow complexion sometimes with a greenish tint and deep flushes on the cheeks; they are troubled with palpitations, dyspnœa, stitching pains in the chest.—*Digitalis;* in some chlorotic patients the pulse is irregular and intermittent and the heart's action is characterized by similar changes; such symptoms indicate Digitalis. *Belladonna* is indicated by frequent paroxysms of headache in the forepart of the head; the headache is accompanied by bright flushes on the cheeks, deep sparkling looks, heat in the head; such patients are apt to be of a lymphatic disposition and passive turn of mind. H.]

2. Rheuma.

Rheumatism.

Under this heading we comprehend a group of morbid conditions concerning whose essence our knowledge is very defective; all they have in common is, that they are localized in the fibrous tissues, the muscles, tendons, joints, aponeuroses, etc. We may add that all rheumatic affections are very much aggravated by the influence of cold.

Their etiology is no less uncertain and vague than their nomenclature. Whereas the acute forms occur chiefly between the years of fourteen and thirty-five, the chronic forms are principally met with after the fortieth year of age. The former are principally occasioned by exposure to colds and wet, the latter more particularly by damp and cold dwellings, and by continued exposure to wet weather and permanently dwelling in wet localities. There are atmospheric conditions which frequently cause epidemic rheumatism, generally in company with extensive catarrhal diseases. One attack of rheumatism begets a tendency to new attacks. In the case of females, chronic rheumatism is decidedly favored by the influences of the critical age.

The rheumatic process shows itself in four distinct forms which we shall describe separately, although their treatment will be condensed in one, in order to avoid unnecessary repetitions.

a. *Acute Articular Rheumatism.*

This form of rheumatism often arises from a cold and from exposure to atmospheric influences; it not unfrequently assumes an epidemic type and, in such a case, breaks out most commonly in the fall and winter.

The disease commences very gradually with a vague feeling of malaise, accompanied with slight catarrhal symptoms; it may break out after severe attacks of angina, very seldom suddenly, and scarcely ever with a chill, but with alternate chills and heat. Simultaneously with the fever, very seldom after, and still less seldom before, one or more joints become painful; the pain rapidly increases, and the joint swells, sometimes with, and at other times without redness; at this period the least motion and the least pressure cause pain, so that the patients remain perfectly quiet for fear of hurting themselves. Generally several joints are attacked at once, very seldom only one at a time, never all the joints at once from the start. The disease progresses in a very characteristic manner. While the joint that was first attacked, is getting better in three to five days, sometimes with a complete cessation of the pain as well as the swelling, other joints are attacked in the same manner; in this manner most of the other joints are invaded, after which the rheumatism frequently breaks out again in the joint whence it had originally proceeded. At times the swelling is quite considerable, at other times scarcely perceptible; sometimes it is confined to the joint alone, at other times the surrounding parts are very extensively involved; not unfrequently the articular extremities feel enlarged. The constitutional symptoms are at times very violent, at other times very slight; this depends a good deal upon the number of joints involved. The fever runs pretty high, remitting very irregularly; the temperature is not much raised above the normal level; pulse about hundred, in very acute cases increasing very seldom to one hundred and twenty and upwards, small and changeable; a copious perspiration, having a musty-sour smell, continues during the whole course of the disease, corresponding with which the patients are tormented by a distressing thirst. The urine is very scanty, saturated, and, on cooling, deposits a copious sediment. The digestion is slow, the appetite impaired, but very seldom entirely suspended.

The course of uncomplicated rheumatism is never very rapid, generally more or less wavering; recovery takes place gradually; single joints may remain painful and swollen for a long time, the pulse remains obstinately accelerated, the perspiration continues, the weakness abates very slowly. A favorable change takes place very seldom after the first week, a little more frequently after the second, but most commonly only after the third and fourth week. Very often we have noticed that, before the disease terminates, every joint is attacked twice, and that the second attack only lasts half as long as the first. In violent cases all the joints are affected together at the termination of the attack, some, however, are more acutely inflamed than others.

Complications generally occasion a more protracted course of the disease, and determine the amount of danger involved in the attack. Among these complications we seldom meet with pneumonia, pleu ritis, peritonitis; endo- and pericarditis, on the contrary, are very common occurrences. Such complications must be expected so much more certainly the larger the number of joints that are simultaneously involved, and the more fiercely they are attacked. In a majority of cases the cardiac inflammation develops itself so imperceptibly that it is scarcely betrayed by a single symptom; it very seldom sets in with a chill or with acute pain. A symptom that ought always to excite our suspicion, is the hurried breathing and the abrupt talking of the patient. If this symptom becomes manifest, the heart must be explored forthwith. This, however, should be done every day during an attack of acute rheumatism.

The disease generally terminates in recovery, although very slowly, and leaving various inconveniences and discomforts, more particularly a peculiar laming weakness. Death is a very rare termination, except when such complications supervene as generally terminate fatally. Very seldom the rheumatic inflammation increases to such an extent that suppuration takes place; if this happens, the suppurative process always involves a good deal of danger. Among the consecutive diseases, structural alterations of the heart, with their distressing consequences, occur most frequently; paralytic conditions are less frequent, and, moreover, disappear again very speedily. Almost all patients retain a great tendency to relapses.

b. *Acute Muscular Rheumatism.*

This rheumatism owes its existence almost exclusively to a heavy cold; such muscles are most easily attacked as were engaged in active work when the exposure took place.

This form of rheumatism is one of the milder sort. In rare cases only, it sets in with an acute fever and a continual perspiration, the same as acute articular rheumatism; however, it is of shorter duration and much less dangerous, leaving of course a marked disposition to chronic muscular rheumatism. Most generally muscular rheumatism develops itself very rapidly, even suddenly, in company with more or less severe catarrhal complaints. In the invaded muscles, the number of which is seldom very great, and which are almost always in close relationship with each other, violent, drawing-tearing pains are experienced during every motion; these pains are likewise felt, if the muscles remain for a long time in the same position, as at night, in bed; the pains are increased by cold, and likewise by humid warmth; dry warmth relieves them.

The character of the pathological group depends of course upon the muscular bundles that are invaded, and the violent pain sometimes suggests the thought that internal organs are inflamed. This idea may be suggested by rheumatism of the thoracic and intercostal muscles, where the respiration, cough, sneezing, turning about, cause an intense pain; likewise by rheumatism of the abdominal muscles where peritonitis is so easily suspected. With proper management and care this form of rheumatism ends in recovery in one week at latest. However, by neglecting to guard against relapses, an acute attack may very easily terminate in a chronic form, and contractions and paralytic conditions may arise which can only be removed with great difficulty.

c. *Chronic Articular Rheumatism.*

It most frequently develops itself out of the acute form of which it constitutes a rest as it were; it likewise arises from the continued action of damp and cold places.

Chronic rheumatism is less frequently located in the external integuments of the joints where acute articular rheumatism is generally seated, than in the synovial lining, the ligaments and articular cartilages. Little by little these grow thicker and rough, which is the reason that, after a time, crepitation is heard in the articulation. The disease seldom involves a number of joints; generally it is limited to one or a few only. Neither the swelling nor the pain is very considerable; to some extent the power of motion remains, yet the patients may be entirely deprived of the use of the affected limb, whereas the rest of the body is perfectly sound. The rheumatism has remissions followed by exacerbations each of which leaves the condition of the joints somewhat worse, and may even lead to anchylosis. These exacerbations often look like an attack of acute rheumatism with fever and slight inflammation of the affected part; sometimes, however, they are without fever, and distinguished only by pain and loss of mobility. Chronic rheumatism sometimes remains after repeated attacks of acute rheumatism of which it seems to constitute an ultimate stage. The joint is not greatly distorted by the disease. A complete cure is very much impeded by the extreme obstinacy of the trouble, and likewise by the impossibility of preventing the joint from being acted upon by influences that never cease, by their presence, to perpetuate the disease.

d. *Arthritis Deformans*, *Arthritic Rheumatism*.

This form of articular rheumatism always runs an exceedingly chronic course; it does not develop itself out of the acute form, occurs very rarely previous to the thirty-fifth year of age, and is most frequent after the fortieth year. It breaks out among all classes, especially, however, the lower; on this account it is very difficult to determine the degree of influence exerted by bad food or damp dwellings over this disease. Arthritic rheumatism affects more particularly the female sex; the critical age undoubtedly favors an outbreak of this disease, for we meet with it most frequently about this time.

The disease may attack any joint in the body, but it is mostly limited to the joints of the hands and feet, affecting both sides of the body at the same time. It generally commences in the hand, whose joints become more or less painful, especially when they are moved or pressed upon laterally. Sometimes the pain is principally felt in bed; crepitation is very soon heard in the joint. The joint swells very slowly; at times long intervals occur in the further continuance of the swelling, after which the arthritic process resumes its course amid renewed paroxysms of pain. Towards the end the shape of the joints is very much altered, especially the shape of the phalangeal articulations. The articular extremities look bulbous, they are especially enlarged in breadth; they feel hard; their integumentous covering has a natural color; the articular surfaces are no longer in complete coaptation, giving the opposite bones the appearance of being dislocated, and imparting to the hands and feet a deformed shape. The power of motion is not entirely suspended, but motion is very painful; in the very highest grades of the disease the joints are entirely immovable. Life is not endangered by this condition, but its curability is very doubtful. The swelling never disappears entirely; all that can be properly aimed at by treatment, is to arrest the further progress of the disease.

Treatment. Owing to the peculiar vagueness and indefiniteness of the single forms of rheumatism, whether acute or chronic, we find it difficult to decide whether and what medicines have exerted a curative effect upon the disease. The consequence is that an unreasonably large number of medicines have been employed for this disease, all with more or less pretended effect, yet in similar cases the same remedy does not always produce the same curative result. The natural course of the disease is not taken into account, and a spontaneous cure is mistaken for the work of art.

Another reason why our remedies for rheumatism are not perfectly reliable, is the vagueness attaching to a definition of this term. Here we have a striking demonstration of the fact that it is injurious to treat diseases in accordance with pathological names, and that there is, on the other hand, great advantage in individualizing cases according to the rules of Homœopathy, without troubling ourselves whether the morbid condition is called rheumatism or something else, provided the abnormal process ceases. No disease embarrasses the Rational School more than rheumatism which makes a laughing-stock of all hypothetical speculations.

Although we have no very exalted opinion of the power of homœopathic medicines over rheumatism, yet we assert without hesitation that the homœopathic treatment of rheumatism is more effectual than any other; at the same time we admit that it is desirable that we should be able to accomplish a great deal more. In our opinion, one of the principal reasons why we so often fail in curing rheumatism is the dread homœopathic physicians seem to entertain, in administering large doses, which rheumatism often requires, as is evidenced in the case of Sulphur.

In the following paragraphs we only mention the leading remedies more fully; of the other less important remedies we only give the names, for we believe that too large a number of drugs is prejudicial.

Aconitum is the main remedy in acute articular rheumatism if the pulse is not only frequent but likewise full and hard, the temperature is considerably higher, the joint is red and exceedingly sensitive to contact; it is suitable for nervous, irritable, plethoric individuals; or when pericarditis or endocarditis has supervened. Further indications may be gathered from the Materia Medica Pura. Aconite has been less frequently used in chronic cases where it sometimes acts with great efficacy. Aconite is less adapted to chronic articular than to muscular rheumatism, especially when the disease is located in the upper extremities. [Aconite is a specific remedy for rheumatism of the deltoid muscle. H.]

Bryonia alba is a leading remedy for acute and chronic rheumatism, except the arthritic form. The symptoms of this medicine are so numerous that we have to content ourselves with furnishing a few general indications. *Bryonia* is most suitable for rheumatism caused by exposure to cold and dampness after a severe muscular effort; the violent fever soon adopts an adynamic form; the articular swelling is dark-red and exceedingly painful; the respiratory organs show symptoms of inflammation; the perspiration has a sour smell. In muscular rheumatism, *Bryonia* is indicated by the following symptoms: The muscles of the trunk are the seat of the disease, especially the thoracic muscles; the patient feels much better during rest; the pains are severe tearing pains, and incline to shift from one place to another.

Mercurius. That Mercury possesses a remarkable power to cause a variety of rheumatic pains, is shown by syphilitic patients whose cases are mismanaged by large doses of Mercury. Mercurius is not so much adapted to chronic as to most forms of acute and subacute rheumatism, with the following general indications: The fever runs high; the pulse is remarkably quick and hard, the perspiration very copious and having a musty smell, the thirst is exceedingly tormenting. The local swelling is not very great, but painful, intensely red, giving rise to the apprehension of pus forming in the joint; it is not apt to shift about; even if other joints are affected, yet the original joint remains swollen and painful; the breath is foul, the tongue has a thick, yellow coating, the appetite is gone, every kind of food causes nausea. The skin is covered with copious sudamina. The pains are worse every night, towards midnight, aggravated by severe cold and ameliorated by external warmth. The more frequently relapses set in, the more specially is Mercurius indicated. In muscular rheumatism, Mercurius is indicated by the following circumstances: the pains exacerbate at night, they are deep-seated as if the periosteum were attacked, with great sensitiveness to gentle as well as firm pressure. In complicating inflammations of vital organs, *Mercurius* deserves a leading position, in cardiac inflammation as well as in pneumonia and pleuritis, likewise in meningitis.

Rhus toxicodendron is adapted to every form of rheumatism, except arthritic. In acute articular rheumatism, it is indicated by the following symptoms: Violent fever, with tendency to the adynamic type, delirium and excessive restlessness; the swelling is inconsiderable, admits of some motion, is intensely red and somewhat sensitive to contact. The perspiration is not considerable. The patients are constantly changing their position, for even after lying for a short time in the same position, the pains are very much increased Feather beds are intolerable, so is external artificial warmth. For muscular rheumatism, *Rhus tox.* is the best remedy, if the attack is caused by exposure to wet; if the above-mentioned circumstances either improve or aggravate the symptoms; if the pains at once become associated with paralysis and contraction; if the muscles of the lower extremities are the seat of the disease. Rheumatic paralysis particularly points to *Rhus.* In chronic articular rheumatism, Rhus is of little, if any use. [Rhus is generally recommended for rheumatism, if the patient contracted the disease in consequence of getting soaking wet. This indication is unreliable. Some time ago I was called to see a Catholic priest who, while visiting a man in the country, was overtaken by a thunder-storm and was drenched to the skin. In this condition he had to travel eight miles on horseback. Next day he was attacked with neuralgic rheumatism in the upper third of the left upper arm. The pain was as if the bone and marrow were being ground into a thousand fragments. After having been treated allopathically for a whole week, with large doses of Morphia, Quinine, etc., the patient was reduced to a shadow by the pain, deprivation of sleep, etc. Being sent for, I found the arm apparently natural, but the sensitiveness so great that the least attempt to touch the affected limb, caused the patient to exclaim and shudder. The pain extorted agonizing cries. I made up my mind that *Mercury* was his remedy, of which he took the first centesimal trituration, a powder every hour. Already after the first powder the pain began to abate, and next morning he was completely relieved and went out again, two days after my first visit. H.]

Pulsatilla, according to Hartmann and others, is indicated in mild, subacute rheumatism of the joints and muscles; the affection shifts about frequently and speedily; the pains exacerbate in the evening and at night; they are violent tearing, drawing and jerking pains, increased by warmth, improved by cold, at least for a short time. Pulsatilla is seldom appropriate in chronic rheumatism, more so in the rheumatism of muscles and of the joints. It is neither a reliable remedy, nor one that can be often used for the reason that the rheumatism to which *Pulsatilla* corresponds, is not of frequent occurrence. [For rheumatism of the dorsum of the foot, *Pulsatilla* is an excellent specific. A lady, seventy years of age, of a yielding and rather phlegmatic temperament, had an attack of acute rheumatism of the dorsum of the right foot. It was very much swollen, red, excessively painful, and very sensitive to contact. The swelling had a shining appearance. The pain was much worse at night, and deprived her of sleep; the fever ran high. She had been suffering in this way for three nights. I gave her six globules of *Pulsatilla* 18, dissolved in half a tumbler of water, to be taken in dessert-spoonful doses every two hours. After the first dose already the pain moderated, she very soon fell asleep, perspired a little during the night, and next morning was entirely free from pain, fever and swelling. H.]

Colchicum is not exactly a remedy for acute rheumatism, but is excellent in subacute affections of the joints and muscles, the external parts of the former being chiefly affected. The fever is not violent, mingled with constant chills, either without or with very little perspiration, the urine is saturated and deposits a copious sediment. The painful joints are neither red nor swollen; the pains increase considerably at night or by motion and contact. The attack comes on in damp and cold weather.

Tartarus emeticus deserves to be used more than it so far has been; it is one of those remedies that have a good effect in exceedingly painful local muscular rheumatism, for instance, rheumatism of the dorsal muscles contracted after a cold during the performance of a fatiguing muscular effort. In such a case, Tartar emetic very soon brings relief. In acute articular rheumatism Tartar emetic is indicated by the following symptoms: Marked swelling of a number of joints, the pains are not very great during rest, but this rest is frequently interrupted by spontaneous, spasmodic, very painful contractions of single bundles of muscles. There is not much fever; the symptoms of digestive derangement, on the contrary, are very prominent. A condition marked by such symptoms, sometimes occurs during the subsequent course of articular rheumatism, scarcely ever at the commencement.

Digitalis purpurea is, in our opinion, a most important remedy in acute articular rheumatism; in the last few years we have often seen this remedy produce a striking effect and shorten the course of the disease. We do not deem it necessary to demonstrate the similarity of Digitalis to rheumatism; the physiological action of this drug as recorded in the Materia Medica, explains this similarity beyond the possibility of cavil. We do not, however, feel able, to give the special indications of Digitalis in every particular case, for the simple reason that we have not had sufficient opportunities to test it in practice. So far we have been guided in the exhibition of Digitalis by the following points: Hurried, small pulse easily affected by motion; increased strength of the beating of the heart, but the sounds are muffled and indistinct, mingled with arterial murmurs; hurried respiration, with ability to draw a long breath; hurried, abrupt speech; almost complete suspension of the urinary secretion; shining-white swelling of the joints, not very sensitive to pressure; a number of joints are attacked at once; the whole body is very pale. During the whole course of the disease we have given this medicine without any other drug, and in spite of the violence of the symptoms, we have never been able to discover any symptoms of cardiac inflammation, for which Digitalis might, however, likewise be indicated. In conclusion we desire to state that Digitalis holds a high rank as a remedy for rheumatism among the Rational physicians; there is undoubtedly a reason for this.

Sulphur bears almost the same specific relation to the rheumatic process that Mercury does to syphilis. In an acute attack we would not think of giving *Sulphur;* on the other hand, Sulphur is indispensable to remove the remaining traces of acute rheumatism, upon which the extraordinary disposition to relapses generally depends. What this remedy is capable of accomplishing in chronic rheumatism, is shown by the numerous cures which are every year wrought by the use of Sulphur-springs, and which it is impossible to doubt. We doubt, however, whether similar results can be obtained by giving Sulphur internally in small doses; at any rate, we have never been able to accomplish such a task. All we have been able to do has been to improve the case, but we have never yet achieved a perfect cure with these small doses. This shows that there must be a something, a higher curative power in Sulphur-springs, which small doses of Sulphur do not possess. Sulphur exerts a curative power over arthritic rheumatism; it arrests the progress of the disease, and materially reduces the swelling of the joints.

Ferrum is applicable in primary chronic rheumatism as well as after an acute attack, if the patient has been very much reduced in flesh. It never shows its favorable effects all at once; on this account the remedy must not be discontinued too soon.

[**Caulophyllum thalictroides,** the blue cohosh, is highly recommended for rheumatism of the smaller joints. Dr. R. Ludlam, of Chicago, prescribed it for a case of inveterate rheumatism of the metacarpal joints of the left hand, in doses of two grains of the second decimal trituration every two hours, until relief was obtained. The patient was a servant-girl; she had not slept for two or more nights. After the second dose she fell asleep, and her pain vanished from that time forward. There was no metastasis of the complaint, and in two days she was down stairs at work. While she remained in the family, two years, she had no return of the disease. The Doctor writes: "Since the above result was obtained, I have frequently prescribed the *Caulophyllin* for articular rheumatism affecting the *smaller* joints, and several times with a signal success. It has, however, appeared more effectual in case of females than of males, who were ill with this painful disease." H.]

Beside these remedies the following deserve being mentioned. In acute cases: *Arnica, Belladonna, Nitrum, Spigelia;* in sub-acute and more chronic affections: *Ledum, Sabina, Cocculus, Mezereum, Clematis, Rhododendron, Ruta, Oleander* (especially in cases of rheumatic paralysis); finally, in inveterate cases: *Iodium, Causticum, Calcarea carbonica, Silicea.* [In arthritic rheumatism, grafted upon a scrofulous basis, *Aconite* and *Iodine* are indispensable. H.]

Although Sulphur-springs are the most effectual remedy for constitutional rheumatism, yet there are other means calculated either to heal or prevent new attacks; some of these means are often sufficient to perform a cure. In this class we rank the cold-water treatment, sea-bathing, the Turkish and Russian baths. The two last-mentioned have to be employed with great care; if they help at all, the favorable effect is seen already after a few baths.

It is a matter of course that the cause should be removed as much as may be.

The diet in acute rheumatism is easily managed; the patients either do not crave any nourishment, or their appetite is very much impaired. Fat and greasy articles of diet are decidedly injurious; acid substances, especially stewed fruit, have a very good effect; raw fruit may be partaken of, but moderately.

3. Arthritis.
Gout.

The cause of gout is involved in a great deal of obscurity; speculations on this subject have led to the most one-sided hypotheses. All that we know positively is, that gout is not only an hereditary, but in the majority of the cases that come under our notice, an inherited disease; however, it may likewise originate as a primary malady.

We likewise know positively that, if the body receives a larger supply of animal food than can be assimilated either by bodily or mental labor, or that, if quantities of heavy or sour wines or heavy

Arthritis.

beer are drank, the outbreak of the disease is very much facilitated; but whether such causes can occasion the disease primarily, is very questionable. A large majority of cases occur among the male sex; the disease breaks out between the ages of thirty-five and seventy years; if it attacks persons before this time, the disease is inherited. In accordance with these statements we find that gout chiefly attacks the higher strata of society.

Symptoms and Course. Gout is a decidedly chronic disease the course of which is interrupted by acute attacks. It originates very gradually, with a train of symptoms that do not enable us to draw reliable conclusions regarding the nature of the disease. Shortly after a period, during which a good many dietetic transgressions had been committed, the patients feel out of sorts, irritable, ill-humored, they complain of pain in the stomach, heartburn, vomiting of a sour liquid, pressure and repletion in the abdomen, hemorrhoids, gastric headache, and the urine is saturated. After these preliminary symptoms have lasted for a longer or shorter period, the first

Paroxysm of Gout sets in, in the vast majority of cases during sleep, at night. The patient is roused from sleep by a violent, boring-burning pain, with a sensation as if the part were in a vice; at the first attack this pain is almost without an exception seated in the first articulation of the big toe of one or the other foot, increasing very rapidly to such a degree of intensity, that the patients are almost beside themselves. Very soon the painful spot shows a vivid redness and is more or less swollen; but neither redness nor swelling ever spreads over the adjoining parts. Motion is impossible, and external pressure causes such an intense pain that the patients cannot even bear the least touch of the blanket. This pain is often accompanied by a high fever which sometimes remits so fully on the following morning, amid a profuse perspiration, that the day is spent with scarcely any pain. The next night, however, the pain returns, showing that the disease is still there. This change goes on between one and two weeks, until the painfulness and redness, and soon after the swelling, disappear pretty suddenly, and the patients feel well again, even better than before the attack. The only striking change after the attack is the great quantity of urates which never fail to be deposited in the urine.

This first attack may terminate the whole disease, especially if the patient changes his present mode of living with determined firmness and consistency. If this is not done, a new attack takes place after a certain lapse of time; this second attack chiefly breaks out during the period from February to April. This circumstance is in some respects accounted for by the patient's more luxurious mode of living during the winter-season, when he takes at the same time less active exercise than usual. The interval is entirely free from ailments until shortly previous to the new attack, when the former premonitory symptoms again make their appearance.

With every new attack the free intervals are more and more obscured and shortened, the local disorder leaves calculous deposits on the diseased joint, with more or less permanent pains and a higher or less degree of immobility. The paroxysms are less acute, but instead of at most two, they last eight or twelve weeks; other joints, especially those of the feet, knees, hands and shoulders, likewise become involved. The so-called *chronic* or *atonic gout* now is an established infirmity. The more numerous the changes that remain after the attack, the more joints are affected, the longer the attack lasts, the more prominently the chronic affection shows its characteristic features during the interval. The digestion is permanently deranged, the patients complain of pains in the stomach, which sometimes increase to severe paroxysms of cardialgia; they complain, moreover, of acidity of the stomach, pressure, fulness and flatulence after every meal, torpor of the bowels and hemorrhoidal distress; they are very irritable and out of humor. Nutrition is more and more impaired, the complexion assumes a yellow-grayish appearance. The circulation is disturbed in various ways. Such disturbances are very significant in so far as they generally point to a degeneration of the valves and arteries; they commence with frequent, but short-lasting congestions, palpitations, attacks of angina pectoris, asthmatic complaints. The affected joints become more and more deformed and anchylosed.

At a more advanced age and by observing a strict diet, this chronic gout may terminate in recovery; of course, the concretions in the joints remain. This form of gout may likewise assume the character of the so-called *anomalous gout*, which sometimes ushers in the whole disease; in such a case it becomes exceedingly difficult to establish a reliable diagnosis. Anomalous gout may likewise succeed the first attack of gout in the place of chronic gout. The patients suffer with the complaints of chronic gout; above all, the urine looks very cloudy depositing large quantities of urates; but in the place of acute pains in the joints, we have short-lasting pains shifting about from place to place frequently and speedily, without swelling or redness, but very frequently with gradual impairment of the mobility of the joints. Of particular importance are the intermediate affections of internal organs that have been designated as retrograde or metastatic gout. Sometimes they, indeed, depend upon material changes, products of a permanently established arthritic process; sometimes, however, the organs are attacked in a manner corresponding perfectly with the invasion of the tarsal articulation. The internal organs that are principally attacked, are the heart and stomach, less frequently the brain; the attack consists in a sudden violent inflammation with horrid pains, and, as far as the brain is concerned, with considerable danger, for the attack may terminate fatally in a few days.

Arthritis scarcely ever terminates directly fatally; it is still less frequently succeeded by perfect recovery. Death results mostly from alterations in the organs of the circulation, very seldom from a gradual prostration of strength. Recovery being generally imperfect, the prognosis is only conditionally favorable.

Treatment. It has to be directed against the single paroxysm, in which case it is necessarily symptomatic; and likewise against the chronic disease, in which case it aims at removing the cause.

The treatment of the single paroxysm leads us to the remedies that have been indicated for rheumatism; this is a necessary consequence of the pathological vagueness of both affections and of the insufficiency of our physiological provings. Many remedies are recommended for gout, the value of which is very questionable; in recommending them, their authors probably overlooked the fact that an attack of gout sometimes terminates spontaneously in one week. At the same time we are bound to admit that we are not acquainted with any complete cures of gout under homœopathic treatment. In selecting a remedy, a characteristic phenomenon of the gout, namely the deposition of urates in the urine, must not be lost sight of. Unfortunately the sediments in the urine have not been tested chemically by our provers.

For the single paroxysm which is accompanied by violent fever, *Aconite* renders the most eminent service, but it has to be given in large and frequently repeated doses. *Arnica* has often done good service, if the attack had been caused by mechanical injuries, or if it sets in after great physical exertions; if the inflamed joint was intensely red, and the patients were very restless in spite of their pains. *Arnica* is likewise excellent in cases of metastasis to the brain. According to Hartmann, *Pulsatilla* is indicated by the following symptoms: The pains abate in cool air; the local affection shifts its locality very rapidly; the affection of the knee is characterized by shooting, drawing-stitching pains. Such symptoms may scarcely ever occur in reality. *Sabina* is, like Pulsatilla, indicated if the affection inclines to rapidly change its locality, but more particularly if the change takes place from the big toe-joint to the hand, and *vice versa;* the pains are alleviated in the cool air, and the patient is constantly obliged to change the position of the affected part. We have observed all these symptoms in the case of a girl who had swallowed a quantity of Sabina for the purpose of producing a miscarriage; these symptoms convey an exact image of an attack of gout. *Staphysagria,* if the paroxysms of gout of the tarsal joint gradually assume the form of anomalous gout. *Nux vomica* is evidently recommended on account of the exciting cause; its pathogenesis does not show any homœopathicity to gout. *Digitalis* is eminently useful if the attacks are gradually changing in character, and have lasted a good while; in such transitions to chronic gout *Digitalis* is scarcely ever surpassed by any other remedy; but it must not be given in too small a dose. The first favorable change effected by *Digitalis* is the supervention of a short sleep. *Ledum* responds to the imperfect, long-lasting paroxysms involving the carpal and shoulder-joints. *Baryta* is adapted to affections of the knee.

The treatment of the whole disease is more important than that of a single attack, which is always somewhat precarious. The former treatment must be limited in its main features, especially at the beginning of the disease when the intervals are still unclouded, to the enforcement of an appropriate mode of living. What sort of regimen arthritic patients should follow, is evident from what we have said when speaking of the etiology of the disease. In the subsequent course of the disease when the derangements have already become more permanent, it may be difficult to get along without medicines, but they cannot be indicated *a priori* for the reason that the symptoms are too diversified. The following remedies are very often suitable: *Nux vomica, Lycopodium, Ferrum, Arsenicum, Sulphur, Acidum sulphuricum,* [also *Acidum benzoicum.* H.] In the case of persons of a more advanced age, they must not be altogether deprived of their usual supply of substantial nourishment; nor should the use of wine be entirely prohibited. Sometimes a great deal of good is accomplished, if we substitute a weak grog in the place of the wine, or one kind of wine for another;

light claret is the least injurious to such patients. Arthritic patients being so readily disposed to forget the strict rules laid down for them by their physicians, it is necessary that these rules should be repeatedly impressed upon their memory.

Among the mineral springs, the use of which is sometimes unavoidable in such cases, Carlsbad-springs occupy the first rank, provided the constitution has not yet suffered too much; next to Carlsbad, we recommend Vichy, if the patients have already a leaden complexion, the cautious use of Pyrmont-water does everything that can be expected, to raise the sinking power of the organism, whereas feeble chalybeate springs have no perceptible effect. Many other mineral waters are recommended, and the patients improve by the use of all of them, but no more, generally speaking, than they would have done without drinking the water, provided they had strictly adhered to the severe regimen enforced at the springs.

4. Hydropsia.

Dropsy.

We have assigned this place to this class of diseases because the treatment of dropsy is so uniformly the same that a separate description of the disease as developed in special organs or systems would have led to many useless repetitions.

Dropsy is never an idiopathic disease, but always secondary, although it sometimes appears to be of a primary character. In general, all conditions which, in the long run, interfere with the circulation, or retain the water in the blood, lead to dropsy; likewise any other conditions that result in the production of a high grade of hyperæmia or anæmia. In most cases, however, something else has to become associated with these conditions, otherwise it would be difficult to comprehend why many anomalies should be able to continue so long before resulting in the development of dropsy. We are unacquainted with the nature of this something; whether it is a relaxation of the coats of the vessels, or a more copious supply of water in the blood, or whatever else, we have not yet been able to find out. Most likely it is from this unknown cause that dropsy, consequent upon a general marasmus, without any special, mechanical cause results. In accordance with the above-mentioned three categories, dropsy sets in, if the flow of the venous blood into the right heart is interfered with; if the circulation is obstructed by thrombi in the larger venous trunks (as for instance in consequence of phlebitis in the lower extremity, in the case of lying-in women; ascites arising from inflammation of the vena portarum); in the case of pulmonary affections impeding the reflux of the blood, such as emphysema, hydro-thorax, pneumo-thorax; in consequence of affections of the liver resulting from obstructions of the portal circulation. — In the case of renal affections, if the function of the kidneys is very much interfered with ; in chlorosis, affections of the spleen with hydræmia, after copious losses of blood, or after severe, debilitating diseases, in general in conditions of debility of a high order.

Symptoms. At the onset dropsy is more or less local; as a rule, it commences with a swelling round the ankles, less frequently in the face; ascites takes place only when the liver is diseased. In this case it may remain localized as ascites; in the former case it gradually spreads throughout the whole of the subcutaneous cellular tissue, unites with ascites, and finally with œdema of the lungs or brain, in which case death soon results.

Dropsical effusions are generally accompanied and sometimes preceded by prostration, and by decrease of the urinary secretions. The urine is dark, saturated, becoming cloudy in a short time; the quantity is sometimes very scanty. All the other watery secretions are likewise less, or they are entirely suspended; the stools are very dry, the skin is dry and cracks easily, incapable of perspiration, the mucous membranes are likewise dry, on which account the patient is often tormented by a distressing thirst.

Dropsy at times develops itself very speedily and universally, sometimes slowly and progressing very gradually. It is especially after nephritis that water accumulates very rapidly; it collects most slowly in company with affections of the lungs. It is unnecessary for us to describe the special forms of dropsy; these forms and the constitutional symptoms accompanying them, can easily be determined without any further description.

The *Course* of the disease is at times uninterrupted, leading speedily to death, or else it makes pauses, a portion of the serum that had been poured out into the cellular tissue or the cavities, being reabsorbed. This may result from a transitory cessation or diminution of the obstruction in the circulation, or from copious excretions of urine, watery discharges from the bowels, oozing through cracks in the skin, or from a general invigoration of the whole organism. Death generally takes place by œdema of the

Hydropsia.

lungs or brain. Recovery is attended with copious discharges of urine, very rarely with diarrhœa alone.

The **Prognosis** depends upon the chances of removing or neutralizing the primary obstruction or derangement.

The **Treatment** has to be chiefly directed against removing the cause; if this is not possible, it has to be almost purely symptomatic or palliative. The causal indication is met by the remedies that have been indicated when the affections of the various organs were treated of; we need not repeat them in this place. Symptomatically we shall have to select remedies capable of stimulating the diminished action of the kidneys, or of the circulatory organs, and, by this means, of promoting indirectly the absorption of the fluid. We possess a tolerable number of such remedies which sometimes help to diminish dropsy depending upon some incurable disease, and by which means Homœopathy enjoys a striking advantage over any other method of treatment. In mentioning these remedies, we will accompany them with short statements, for there are so many possible groups of symptoms, that it is impossible to furnish special indications upon an extensive scale. Moreover, the chronic nature of the disease enables us to compare the remedies in our Materia Medica with all proper attention.

Arsenicum album is our most important diuretic. It is suitable in all forms of dropsy, more particularly in dropsy depending upon heart-disease, and œdema of the lungs. After giving *Arsenicum*, a copious diuresis will sometimes set in with astonishing rapidity, after which the dropsical swelling speedily disappears. The result is most doubtful, if we have only ascites to contend against. Inasmuch as the medicine shows its good effect in a few days already, after a few doses had been taken, it is useless to continue it for a longer period, in the vain hope of eliciting good effects from it by persisting in its use.

Digitalis purpurea is much less reliable than Arsenicum, although it is much easier to determine the indications for its use. It is particularly useful in dropsy depending upon, or accompanied by a high degree of general debility; the dropsy is caused by pulmonary or cardiac disease. Digitalis is never indicated for ascites alone, but so much more specifically for œdema of the lungs. The nature of the exciting causes is such that *Digitalis* can only act as a palliative; if small doses remain ineffectual, larger doses should be resorted to before the medicine is discontinued.

China is particularly useful in dropsy setting in after debilitating diseases, great losses of blood, and when the liver is affected. Upon the whole, however, we have to place China among the less reliable medicines.

Helleborus niger is not adapted to slowly developing cases of dropsy, but it is an excellent remedy in acute dropsy, probably because this form of the disease generally arises from an affection of the kidneys which comes within the curative range of this drug.

Apis at one time was greatly extolled as a remedy for dropsy, but practical trials have disappointed us; we have never been able to obtain any decided results by means of Apis. It is recommended for every form of dropsy.

Acidum fluoricum has been used by Haubold with success for the anasarca of a drunkard. We are not aware that this medicine has been often used, but we urgently recommend it for trial.

Prunus spinosa is so urgently recommended for general dropsy that it is undoubtedly advisable to try it. Hartmann has seen good effects from this medicine in dropsy depending upon heart-disease.

Aurum muriaticum is recommended for general dropsy as well as for dropsy depending upon derangement of the liver, or for ascites alone, especially in the case of cachectic individuals.

[**Apocynum cannabinum** in various doses, but principally in larger quantities, has frequently cured dropsy, general dropsy as well as hydrothorax.

Helonin is recommended for dropsy arising from renal difficulties, such as albuminuria, Bright's disease, etc.

Cochineal is useful in dropsy from the same cause. H.]

The following remedies are indicated by the nature of the exciting cause rather than by the presence of the serous effusion: *Cantharis, Terebinthina* (for renal affections); *Tart. stib., Carbo veget., Squilla, Sulphur* (for pulmonary affections); *Ferrum, Kali carbonicum, Phosphorus, Iodium, Mercurius* (for affections of the liver); *Lycopodium, Sulphur* (for chronic catarrh of the bladder).

In no disease it is more difficult to select a suitable remedy than in dropsy; nor are we in any disease more frequently disappointed by the medicine employed, very often on account of some cause hidden from observation. These disappointments are very often owing to the circumstance that we do not give a sufficiently large dose; it is well known, however, that dropsy requires to be treated with larger doses than almost any other disease, although there may be exceptions to this rule.

Paracentesis is only to be resorted to as a last resort; it scarcely ever heightens the susceptibility to medicinal action, and very generally leads so much more speedily to a fatal termination, for the reason that the water accumulates again so much more rapidly. On this account the operation had better be deferred as long as possible.

[5. Scorbutus.
Scurvy.

Aitken defines scurvy as follows: "A morbid state ushered in by debility, lassitude, lowness of spirits, attended by fetor of the breath, sponginess of the gums, which swell by irritation, till they overhang the teeth in palmated excrescences. Livid, subcutaneous patches and spots appear upon the skin, especially on the lower extremities among the roots of the hair. Spontaneous hemorrhages may take place from the mucous canals; contractions of the muscles and tendons of the limbs occur, with pains, and sometimes superficial ulcerations. An altered state of the albumen of the blood is associated with this condition, and the phenomena are brought about by a deficient supply of the organic vegetable acids or of the salts of fresh vegetables."

Scurvy has been the scourge of armies and navies from the earliest periods of human history. The Roman army under Germanicus was decimated by it after a long encampment in Germany beyond the Rhine. The French army under Louis IX. in Palestine was almost wholly destroyed by this plague. Thousands of sailors and soldiers became its victims until Cook finally succeeded in conquering it; on his return home in 1775, after a three years' cruise, he brought back a crew of one hundred and twelve men in a sound condition, having only lost one man by disease.

Post-mortem Appearances. Poupart and Lind inform us that the "principal effects of the disease were observed in all cases in the cellular tissue of the extremities." Lind says that "effused blood often lay in large concrete masses on the periosteum, while the bellies of the muscles of the legs and thighs seemed quite stuffed with it, often an inch in thickness." Water and blood were often found effused into the cavities of the chest and abdomen. Poupart found that "on examining the joints, the epiphyses had entirely separated from the bones; and in other cases that the cartilages of the sternum had separated from their bones; and bones that had united after being broken, very often separated again at the site of fracture." The spleen was found very much enlarged, soft and engorged with coagulated blood.

The phenomena of scurvy point to the blood as the seat of some essential alterations in this disease. All the leading constituents of the blood seem to be present, but their normal proportion is disturbed and one or the other essential ingredient is found altered in quantity and quality. Various opinions have been advanced by Christison, Garrod, and others, regarding the causes of scurvy; but it is sufficient briefly to state, that "one of the most evident changes from the healthy condition is seated in the blood, which is altered in composition either by the addition to it of some ingredient or ingredients, or by the absence of such, which ought to exist in it; and the deficient ingredient may be one of the ordinary constituents of the blood, or it may be some principle or element entering into their composition. This deficiency is due to the absence of certain articles of diet; and the disease is known by experience to be at once cured by supplying those articles." (Aitken.)

Symptoms. The first manifestation of the disease is a change of color in the face. The countenance looks bloated, and has a livid, jaundiced hue. A bad symptom is when the disease sets in with a puffiness of the skin around the orbits; the sclerotic conjunctiva is tumid and gives the cornea an appearance as if seen at the bottom of a well. Wandering, rheumatoid pains in the limbs are complained of; the patients feel weary, yet the pulse remains soft; there is no fever, on the contrary, the animal temperature seems depressed. A very high grade of stomatitis develops itself. The gums look spongy and hang over the teeth in flesh-like, palmated excrescences; they bleed readily; in bad cases the inside of the cheeks sloughs off in shreds, the tongue looks broad, flabby and indented; the odor from the mouth is very fetid. At the same time an eruption like flea-bites breaks out on the lower extremities, it has a purple-hue and may ulcerate if the disease becomes very severe. The muscles of the legs become indurated and painful, and the skin is discolored in large patches and sometimes over the larger part of the leg. In the higher grades of scurvy, these patches may break out in ulcerations which are generally located on the calves of the legs, buttocks, hams, shoulders and arms. The skin is exceedingly irritable, the merest rub causing an hemorrhagic effusion under the skin. Deprivation of sleep constitutes one of the keenest sufferings of scorbutic patients. Their strength may be so completely exhausted that death may result from the most trifling bodily effort. Scurvy at the present time is a very rare disease, and with our present means of treatment and our perfect knowledge of the nature of the disease, it scarcely ever runs to a fatal termination.

Etiology and Treatment. At one time, the excessive or exclusive use of salt-provisions was supposed to be the cause of scurvy, but we know now that scurvy may likewise result from the exclusive use of fresh as well as salt meat. The real cause of scurvy is a deprivation of fresh vegetables. By supplying this want, the disease is readily and effectually cured. " The disease," writes Dr. Parkes, " so fatal when left to itself, is cured with the greatest facility. Symptoms, apparently the most grave and serious, vanish as if by magic, and without leaving behind them any very serious injury to the constitution. The sanious discharge from scorbutic sores has been known to change color and to become healthy in a few hours after the commencement of treatment. In pure cases of scurvy, the blood, and the blood only, is at fault." " Lemon-juice," writes Dr. Watson, " is really a specific against scurvy, whether it be employed as a preventive or as a remedy. It supplies something to the blood which is essential to its healthy properties." According to Budd, the potato seems to be no less efficacious as a remedy and preventive. Parkes observes that " good lemon-juice seems to be more effectual than pure citric acid." The absence of fresh vegetables deprives the system of the acids which are necessary to the nutrition of the organism; these are citric, tartaric, acetic, lactic and malic acids which form carbonates in the system by entering into combination with alkalies. " When we inquire," says Dr. Parkes, " whether there is any proof of the deficiency of these particular acids and salts from the diets which cause scurvy, we find the strongest evidence not only that this is the case, but that their addition to the diet cures scurvy with great certainty. Tartaric, and especially citric acid, when combined with alkalies, have always been considered the anti-scorbutic remedies, *par excellence*, and the evidence on this point seems very complete. " Of the vegetable anti-scorbutics," writes Clymer in his American edition of Aitken, "the potato enjoys, and probably deservedly, the highest reputation; sailors cut it in slices, which they pack in molasses; next to it are onions, sliced and eaten raw; which are greedily devoured by scurvy-patients. Cabbage in the form of sourkrout, sorrel, the wild artichoke, the maguey or American aloë, the prickly pear, the dandelion, lamb's-quarter, green corn, the yam, apples, have all been found excellent anti-scorbutics. Uncooked fruits and vegetables are more efficient than cooked in the prevention and cure of scurvy."

Dr. Parkes recommends Citrates, Tartrates, Lactates, and Malates of Potash, as drinks, or as additions to the food.

Most of the above statements have been taken from Aitken, Watson, and from Parkes' work on the pathology and treatment of scurvy, to which we therefore refer for more extensive information. H.]

6. Scrofulosis.

This is a constitutional anomaly which it is as difficult to define as rheumatism, perhaps more so. At any rate we do not desire to present an imperfect definition of the disease, and we therefore content ourselves with stating that scrofulosis is a disease of the first period of development, the presence of which is manifested by morbid conditions of a peculiar character, more particularly in the glands, skin and bones.

Scrofulosis may be inherited from scrofulous parents, whose disease is not necessarily, but in a majority of cases, reproduced in the children. It may likewise be regarded as an inherited disease, if the parents were affected with some chronic disorder (more especially the mother during pregnancy), such as tuberculosis, constitutional syphilis, malarial cachexia, mercurialism. Finally there is every reason why scrofulosis should be regarded as inherited, when the disease breaks out among the offspring of marriages between near relatives, and after such marriages had been continued for several generations.

Scrofulosis may likewise be acquired by exposure to influences that continually impair the process of nutrition. Above all, it is a deficient supply of food, or improper food generally, that develops scrofulosis in children the more certainly the sooner the child was exposed to such an influence. This is the reason why children that are chiefly fed on farinaceous soups, bread, potatoes, easily become scrofulous, the more certainly the smaller the quantity of milk they were allowed at the same time. Potatoes, and next to them farinaceous food, are the articles of diet to which scrofulosis is chiefly attributed. Children who are nursed by healthy mothers, can likewise become scrofulous if they are fed too often, or if they are kept too long at the breast, which is so often done in the country by women who are anxious to prevent another conception. Moreover, scrofulosis is not perhaps directly caused, but decidedly promoted, not only by improper food, but likewise by an insufficient supply of fresh air, want of exercise, living in damp dwellings, inattention to the skin.

If hereditary scrofulosis and the last-mentioned circumstances meet, scrofulosis reaches the acme of its development. In our opinion, improper nutrition is a much more frequent cause of scrofulosis than hereditary descent. Parents generally bring up their children as they had been brought up themselves; the absurdities of their own parents have become engrafted upon them with the mother's milk, and the grandmother generally stands by the cradle as a faithful watch-dog to prevent the old routine from being departed from in the least particular. In this point of view it is often proper to say, not that scrofulosis has been inherited, but that absurd views concerning the bringing up of children have been transmitted from one generation to another. As an evidence of the truth of this statement, we mention the circumstance that the first-born in a family is apt to have a feeble and sickly constitution, whereas children born at a subsequent period, are healthy; or that some children who were brought up on improper food, become scrofulous, whereas no sign of scrofula is manifested in children with whom more rational maxims are pursued.

Scrofulosis always breaks out in childhood. It seldom manifests itself before the second year. Children that are very large and bloated in the first two years, almost always become scrofulous at a later period; children with firm muscles and slender forms are scarcely ever attacked with the disease. Scrofulosis scarcely ever breaks out after the second dentition, still less frequently after the age of pubescence.

Symptoms and Course. It is very difficult to furnish a complete picture of the scrofulous disease, for the reason that it manifests itself in so many different localities and diversified forms; hence a few general statements will have to suffice. Scrofula chiefly localizes itself in the

Lymphatic Glandular System. Either we find a more or less extensive hypertrophied degeneration, or else an exudation tending to suppuration, the surrounding cellular tissue being more or less involved in this process. In the former case the swollen glands may remain unchanged for many years until they gradually disappear, most commonly at the age of pubescence, leaving only a few trifling remnants of diseased structure. The inflammatory exudation is seldom deposited in an acute form; generally the glands swell slowly and without pain, the swelling sometimes even remains stationary, or else retrogrades, until gradually one portion of the gland becomes injected, fluctuates and breaks. The suppuration generally takes place very slowly, because the decomposition of the pus goes forward step by step. In other cases, especially in individuals with sickly constitutions, a complete decomposition of the exudation takes place before the swelling discharges; in such a case the discharge indeed takes place very rapidly, but other glands are attacked so much more speedily one after the other, and the patient's strength is undermined by hectic fever. The cervical and posterior cervical glands are generally attacked first and most extensively; but the morbid process may likewise be transmitted to every other part of the body. It becomes most threatening, if the mesenteric or bronchial glands are invaded; in such a case obstinate and severe catarrhal irritations may set in, which are often enough followed by hectic fever and death. If scrofulosis can be suspected, every chronic intestinal catarrh, every chronic bronchitis, must necessarily be traceable to a scrofulous origin.

The skin is very often the first organ that shows symptoms of the scrofulous taint. It is but too often the case that children who, up to the time when they were weaned, looked fleshy and solid, after they are weaned, are attacked by cutaneous eruptions that almost always look like eczema and impetigo, less frequently like ecthyma or pemphigus; the incrustations are generally accompanied by obstinate ulcers which constitute characteristic symptoms of scrofula. While the exanthem, which is most commonly confined to the head, is still out, or soon after its disappearance, the glands become affected.

The localization in the bones and joints is one of the most dangerous signs of scrofulosis. We refer to what we have said concerning the bones and articulations in a former chapter; we wish to observe, moreover, that the inflammatory forms run a very protracted course, and that it is only when the patient's constitution is in a very bad state, that those forms terminate in hectic fever and death, but, on the other hand, leave the affected joints with an impaired mobility, anchylosed and deformed. Scrofulous inflammation of the vertebræ is the most threatening, for it either leads to curvature of the spine or develops hectic fever by the origination of congestive abscesses.

Another symptom of scrofula is the ophthalmia which we have already described in a previous chapter. It is either confined to the margins of the lids, or involves the whole conjunctiva. The ears of scrofulous children have a peculiar inclination to discharge, with eczema breaking out at the same time round the ears; very seldom only, and then only if the affection is very deep-seated, the inflammatory process communicates itself to the ossicula and the mastoid bone.

The mucous membranes do not show any particular morbid symptoms, but an extraordinary susceptibility to catarrhs, especially the nasal and buccal mucous membrane. In the nose the copious secretion is associated with soreness and ulceration, and a swelling of the whole nose, in which the upper lip generally participates in a manner that is exclusively peculiar to scrofulosis. In the mouth we notice frequent attacks of angina, with disposition to hypertrophy of the tonsils.

It is only the highest grades of scrofulosis that are accompanied by peculiar affections of internal organs, such as fatty liver, acute hydrocephalus, etc.

These various localizations manifest themselves in the most diversified combinations and successions, sometimes one at a time, and at other times all together. Their course is always slow and dragging, subject to many oscillations between remissions and exacerbations, but generally terminates in recovery, as long as the vital organs remain unaffected by the disease, always, however, leaving some remnants of the disease behind. Even suppuration of the vertebræ sometimes terminates in recovery with surprising rapidity.

The general state of the organism is of importance both to the course of the disease as well as to the treatment. Pathologists have adopted two kinds of scrofulous constitution, the erethic and torpid; they are indeed sharply separated from each other in practice. The erethic scrofulous constitution is distinguished by a lively circulation and a marked tendency to febrile affections. Such children have a fine, transparent skin, flushed cheeks with great tendency to sudden changes of color in the face, an extreme nervous irritability, increased mental activity, melting, languishing eyes, delicate bones, and slightly-developed muscles. The torpid scrofulous constitution, on the contrary, is characterized by a diminished activity of the circulation and reproduction, and great tendency to adiposis. The whole body of such a person looks bloated, especially the face, the features are coarse, the nose and upper lip are swollen, the bones, especially the skull, are large, and the limbs coarsely-shaped; other characteristics are: a distended abdomen, flabby muscles, mental and bodily indolence, a dingy-looking, yellowish-gray skin, disposition to canine voracity. From such general symptoms the speedy outbreak of local scrofulous affections can be predicted with tolerable certainty; frequently, however, especially if a proper mode of living is pursued from an early period, the scrofulous habit disappears entirely, sometimes at the age of seven years, without having occasioned any local diseases.

Treatment. The treatment of the various local scrofulous diseases has already been discussed in former chapters, and all that remains for us to do here, is to consider the disease in its totality. According to what we have said when treating of the etiology of the disease, it is evident that the causal indication in scrofulosis occupies the first rank. Before any medical treatment can be thought of, the mode of living has to be thoroughly changed. This change refers mostly to diet, habitation, exercise in the open air, attention to the skin, etc.; in cases of erethic scrofulosis it has likewise to take into special account the mental development of the patient, which should never be forced, and premature, and should always go hand in hand with an abundance of bodily exercise. In this respect it is difficult to lay down specific rules which might be adapted to one child, and decidedly contrary to the constitution of another. The physician should carefully investigate, and afterwards remedy the defects of education, but definite laws cannot be laid down to reach such a result. The causal indication likewise includes measures having reference to a true and useful prophylactic treatment; hence, a physician should make it his duty to watch over the education of the children confided to his care, in every possible direction and aspect of the case. How much trouble will a physician save himself by such a course, and how much care and anxiety to others!

Except in local affections, the medicine that may be regarded as the chief remedy for scrofulosis, is *Calcarea carbonica*. It never corresponds with a torpid, but so much more decidedly with an erethic habit. This remedy is not sufficient to alter the habit, a correct mode of living is indispensable to accomplish this purpose; but Calcarea is a most important adjuvans in the treatment. Inasmuch as the effect of this or any of the following remedies is always slow and never very striking, the medicines prescribed for scrofula will have to be given at long intervals. Side by side with this remedy, and equally efficacious for the scrofula of torpid constitutions, we mention *Arsenicum* which we recommend upon our own responsibility rather than the recommendations of other physicians, since very little is said about this medicine in homœopathic literature as a remedy for scrofula. We have to observe, however, that *Arsen.*

is only indicated by the general symptoms, and only by a few, indeed very few local lesions. *Ferrum* holds the mean between these two remedies; it is adapted to the erethic as well as the torpid constitution, provided the process of sanguification is decidedly deficient or imperfect, as may be seen from a disposition to congestions, hemorrhages, palpitation of the heart, ataxia of the stomach, and a deficient secretion of bile. *Ferrum* is chiefly suitable, if scrofula is most strikingly developed during the age of pubescence, it is much less adapted to the scrofula of childhood. *Sulphur* must not be forgotten in this place; it is, however, better adapted to the localized forms of the disease than to its general and vaguely expressed symptoms. Sulphur is a distinguished remedy, if the digestion is very irregular; if a disposition to constipation is very marked; if the abdomen is very much distended, the mesenteric glands can be distinctly felt, the cervical and posterior cervical glands are swollen, but painless, the nose and upper lip are swollen, but not inflamed. Sulphur is likewise indicated in chronic bronchial catarrh depending upon infiltration of the bronchial glands.

These four remedies are the only ones that we can designate as generally anti-scrofulous. Other remedies require special indications. We will mention the leading remedies of this class, referring for particulars to our former chapters on conjunctivitis, lymphadenitis, ostitis, chronic intestinal catarrh, etc.; they are: *China, Iodium, Silicea, Aurum muriaticum, Baryta carbonica, Hepar sulphuris, Magnesia carbon., Conium maculatum, Mercurius, Graphites, Spongia.*

We cannot help mentioning two preparations that are used a great deal by lay-persons, even without a physician's order. One is *Oleum jecoris aselli*, cod-liver oil. We shall revert to this medicine in the next chapter; a few words on the subject will suffice in this place. Cod-liver oil is decidedly useful if the digestion is impaired, if the stomach seems disinclined to retain food, and if frequent diarrhœic discharges set in; if, moreover, nutrition is impaired, the body is emaciated and destitute of animal juices. If the appetite is good, the digestion regular, and there is a marked disposition to adiposis, cod-liver oil is decidedly hurtful; in such a case it is apt to derange digestion and impair the appetite. However, in view of the high reputation which cod-liver oil enjoys, neither physician nor patient cares about the harm it may possibly do, imagining as they do that good results must be got out of the oil by sheer force. A proceeding of this kind is, of course, prejudicial. The second remedy are saltwater-baths, with or without an addition of malt. That they have a good effect, is evidenced by the numerous baths prepared of the mother-lye of salt-works. When used at home the favorable effect of the baths may be charged to the benefit which the skin derives from the operation. In the case of children attention to the skin is too often and disgracefully neglected.

7. Tuberculosis.

Tuberculosis is not only the most frequent of all constitutional diseases, but likewise the most common of all diseases. According to Wunderlich it is characterized by deposits into all sorts of tissues and organs, of a pale, yellowish or gray color, of a soft cheesy, and sometimes a harder or softer consistence, of the size of small granulations to the size of larger bodies, in which the organic elements (molecular granules and a few imperfect nucleated bodies) persevere in a low state, without any organic connection with each other or with the adjoining tissue; do not show themselves capable of any further development, and either dry up, or else, become decomposed and melt.

The formation of these deposits or tubercles depends in most cases upon peculiar conditions of the organism with which we are almost unacquainted; it is very questionable whether tubercles can ever be formed without some constitutional anomaly, hence, whether they constitute a purely local affection from which the constitutional disease emanates at a later period. This seems to us just as improbable as the formation of carcinoma without a previous constitutional anomaly. We will designate the radical disease in tuberculosis as the tubercular diathesis. In almost every case tuberculosis can be demonstrated as developing itself under the following circumstances: It may result from a deficient supply or the bad quality of the food in the same manner as has been indicated for scrofulosis; in this manner tuberculosis often succeeds the latter so that when, at the age of pubescence, scrofulosis disappears, tubercles take the place of the former. It may likewise be occasioned by a deficient activity of the respiratory organs, as may occur during certain trades, which will be named by and by, or as may result from tight dressing, or from a sedentary mode of life. Whether a pre-existing germ is excited or created by such causes, is uncertain; the former, however, seems to us more probable. It may likewise be inherited like scrofula.

The tubercular diathesis does not manifest itself by any positive symptoms, and the so-called tubercular habit consists of nothing else than the symptoms of general debility and imperfect assimilation. There die as many men without as with this habit. The only point that enables us to be tolerably sure of the existence of a tubercular diathesis, is the fact that the person was affected with scrofula when young.

Tuberculosis is found equally distributed in both sexes, perhaps a little more among women. It breaks out chiefly between the ages of eighteen and thirty years.

The deposition of tubercles, and hence the tubercular disease generally; perhaps likewise, in many cases, the origin of the peculiar tubercular diathesis, are founded in the following circumstances.

A scanty supply and a bad quality of food, damp dwellings, deficient exercise in the open air. On this account the disease is chiefly met with in the lower walks of life, and likewise occurs more frequently in cities than in the country; among individuals whose business confines them to a room; among prisoners.

Too rapid growth, more particularly if the growing persons are fed on improper nourishment, for this will occasion a condition of great debility.

Continued depressing emotions, especially sorrow and grief, homesickness. The connection of cause and effect between these influences and the disease is not clearly made out; but that this connection exists, can be shown by a number of cases; tubercles are often very properly designated as tears shed inwardly.

Circumstances incident to pregnancy, confinement, lactation, the more certainly, the more rapidly one confinement follows another, and the longer the infant is nursed at the breast. Women with tuberculous dispositions generally pass very well through their first confinement; they keep up the nursing business for a year, without losing much strength, but after that, they complain of feeling exhausted. During the next pregnancy they apparently feel better in every respect, but immediately after confinement the symptoms of an approaching tuberculosis multiply; while nursing her child, the mother experiences all sorts of inconveniences; the next pregnancy again brings an improvement, until phthisis suddenly breaks out in all its might, usually during the first weeks after a new confinement, and very often runs a very rapid course to a fatal termination.

A sudden change in the mode of living; if an occupation requiring constant exercise in the open air, is exchanged for a sedentary business; a luxurious mode of living is suddenly replaced by a mode of living full of privations; if the climate is suddenly changed, if persons move all at once from a warm into a cold climate.

Circumstances and conditions that permanently interfere with the breathing; tight dresses preventing a free expansion of the chest; occupations that render constant stooping necessary, as in the carpenters' and tailors' trade, etc.; or trades in consequence of which the lungs become filled with fine dust.

Diseases of the respiratory organs. Frequent attacks of acute bronchial catarrh, pneumonia, pleuritis; above all, measles, whooping-cough and influenza are very common exciting causes of tubercular deposits.

Most diseases that cause a rapid decline in the assimilative functions, such as: Typhus, dysentery, cholera, chlorosis, diabetes, inveterate syphilis, chronic exanthems, especially prurigo.

Influences which greatly debilitate the nervous system, such as long continued mental labor, venereal excess, self-abuse.

What causes are chiefly instrumental in exciting the first outbreak of the disease, is hard to decide. If the germ is present, the most trivial event may kindle the spark into a flame.

Certain conditions of system afford a certain immunity from tuberculosis; among these conditions we distinguish: an extensive pulmonary emphysema, malformation of the thorax, considerable cardiac defects, carcinoma. It is likewise certain that mid-mountain air diminishes the chances of tuberculosis becoming a fully-developed disease. In the following pages we shall only give a description of pulmonary tuberculosis, furnishing now and then a hint concerning the tuberculosis of other organs.

In order to understand the meaning of the perceptible symptoms of the disease, a knowledge of the pathologico-anatomical changes is more indispensable than in most other diseases. We meet with three essentially distinct forms of tuberculosis. namely: chronic miliary tuberculosis, infiltrated tuberculosis, and acute miliary tuberculosis.

In chronic miliary tuberculosis, the single tubercular granules are found irregularly scattered in the lungs, sometimes singly, and at other times in large clusters, always chiefly occupying the apex of the lungs, and very often limited to the upper lobes. The single granulation is at first of a grayish color, tolerably firm, after which it assumes a yellowish tint and acquires a cheesy consistence, and, at this point, may dry up to a calcareous little body which is like a rough little stone to the feel; or else, it may soften and be transformed into pus. These suppurating granulations may give rise in the lungs to vomicæ or cavities filled with pus, and of a greater or less size in proportion as the number of granulations is greater or smaller. The vomicæ may be present in large numbers; they may either remain isolated, or else unite, forming caverns of the size of a goose-egg. The vomica enlarges either by the dissolution of the tubercles that are still embedded in its walls, or else, the deposition of tubercles in the walls of the vomica goes forward uninterruptedly, the latter process being the one that is most common. The walls of the vomica are excavated, permeated by obliterated vessels and bronchia, or, if the bronchia are destroyed, their irregularly corroded orifices open into the cavity. The blood-vessels resist the destructive process longer than the bronchia, and most commonly shrivel up; but if they are destroyed while blood is still circulating through them, they may give rise to extensive hemorrhages. The vomica may be entirely isolated, or else, it may be in communication with one or more bronchial ramifications. In its growth it may penetrate the pleura and even the chest-wall. The parts surrounding the vomica show bronchial catarrh, interstitial pneumonia in some localities, with subsequent atrophy, bronchiectasia, emphysema. The vomica may empty itself and cicatrize, or else, it may become closed and, without being entirely empty, its contents may become transformed into calcareous matter. The pleura, even if not touched by the tuberculous process, is generally thickened and the two pleuras adhere. Inasmuch as in miliary tuberculosis the deposition of tubercles takes place in successive groups or clusters, tubercles are not generally found uniformly altered, but are met with in all the stages of their course.

Infiltrated tuberculosis is distinguished from the former class by the circumstance that a pneumonic exudation is transformed into tubercular matter, while the organism had either been in a state of apparently sound health, or during the presence of tubercles in other parts. The infiltrated substance passes through the same changes that have been described above, but it usually dissolves much more rapidly, causes much more radical destructions and its transformation into calcareous matter takes place more tardily.

In acute miliary tuberculosis we meet with an extensive deposition of granulations not merely in the whole pulmonary parenchyma, but likewise in the pleura, the pia mater, the peritoneum, and the abdominal viscera. The homogeneous uniformity of the granulations shows their simultaneous origin; in the chronic form this does not occur very extensively.

Tuberculosis of the intestines, which is scarcely ever absent during the course of pulmonary tuberculosis, reveals at the commencement of the disease granulations in Peyer's and Brunner's glands. These tubercles change to separate round ulcers which unite as they increase in size, and spread in the ileum in a circular form.

The most common alterations co-existing with pulmonary tuberculosis, are: Tubercular ulcers in the larynx, resembling those in the intestines; fatty degeneration of the liver, dilatation of the right heart, or atrophy of the heart, slight degree of Bright's disease of the kidneys.

Symptoms and Course. In describing this disease we shall adhere to the most common form, namely: chronic miliary tuberculosis.

It is very difficult to say, with any thing like certainty, when the disease really commences. The deposition of the first tubercles, especially if not very numerous, is accompanied by symptoms that seem too insignificant to a patient to complain of to a physician. When a physician is consulted, the disease is already sufficiently advanced to be discoverable by the usual means of exploration; at its first beginning no such result can be obtained. That the disease is beginning to set in, can almost positively be inferred if individuals who were afflicted with scrofula when young, or persons with a tubercular habit, show the following symptoms: Disposition to pulmonary hyperæmia, with palpitation of the heart; disposition to bronchial, tracheal and laryngeal catarrh, the attacks being very obstinate, with bloody sputa, long-lasting hoarseness; general nervous irritability, irritability and increased frequency of the pulse. Repeated attacks of catarrh ought especially to excite suspicion, for they evidently indicate the period when the first tubercles are deposited. Very often, however, the deposition may be going on for a long time without any apparent symptoms, in which case the supervention of a severe bronchial catarrh which gets worse all the time, shows the sudden outbreak of phthisis or, in other words, of the purulent dissolution of the tubercles. In young women the disease not unfrequently sets in with all the symptoms of chlorosis, which may lead to very injurious mistakes. The older the patients, the less distinctly is the beginning of the disease recognizable. Very seldom, however, the disease breaks out suddenly in such a manner that an apparent fulness of health is suddenly followed by a state of illness with all the characteristics of tuberculosis; a more or less sickly condition almost always precedes the outbreak. It would be of great importance if the first deposition of tubercles could be clearly made out by a physical exploration of the lungs. We only know of two tolerably reliable indications, early attention to which may be of the most decided importance to the treatment. One is a prolonged, although not very much louder expiratory murmur, which is particularly important if it is heard during a slow expiration with closed mouth. The second is the so-called "*respiration saccadée*," jerking, wavy, cogged-wheeled respiration, which is most distinctly perceived during an inspiration. In the place of an uniform blowing murmur we hear an inspiratory murmur at intervals, but not otherwise altered in any respect. Another reliable sign is if, during a slight catarrhal attack, the apices of the lungs exhibit symptoms of catarrhal irritation. Another sign is, when the expectoration looks like soaked sago, or is transparent, having the shape of fine, firm threads; this is a symptom of chronic catarrh of the finest bronchial ramifications.

The existence of a tolerably severe, protracted, acute bronchial catarrh, or a more or less violent hæmoptysis generally, is an evident and very seldom doubtful sign that the phthisis has set in. At the same time the patients complain of unusual debility, stitches, or a peculiar drawing pain in the upper lobes of the lungs, peculiar rheumatoid pains in the arm of the affected side; the respiration is accelerated, the pulse very frequent; this acceleration is very much increased by the least motion; the existing fever very soon shows typical exacerbations setting in in the morning between nine and eleven, or in the evening between five and seven o'clock, or at both these periods, and sometimes attended with such complete remissions that the fever has very much the appearance of an intermittent disease.

From this beginning, the symptoms can easily be observed further in their character of phenomena of tubercular phthisis, with various modifications during their course to which we will first call attention before describing the various local symptoms.

The course of the disease, especially among individuals of a more advanced age, is marked by stages. After the first evidently tubercular catarrh has slowly disappeared, a feeling of almost perfect health is again enjoyed by the patient, who is at most reminded of the slumbering danger by a dry cough or a disposition to shortness of breath after an unusual bodily exertion or after talking. In the course of months, and sometimes not till years have elapsed, another catarrh breaks out which likewise ends without any untoward symptoms, and these changes continue until finally an acute attack of marked intensity terminates in fully developed phthisis. At the same time, nutrition may remain perfect for years, the patient may retain his flesh and healthy complexion, or else he may lose his flesh gradually, and acquire a more or less anæmic appearance.

A chronic, uniform course of phthisis occurs much less frequently after an acute catarrh. On the contrary it sets in with very trifling symptoms, a slight, hacking cough, loss of flesh, palpitation of the heart, shortness of breath, etc., and the patient already presents a complete picture of phthisis when all at once an acute catarrh sets in which is suddenly transformed into the actual disease. Or else no acute catarrh ever takes place, the patients continue to fail almost imperceptibly, hectic fever supervenes, a tuberculous diarrhœa and œdema make their appearance, and death takes place amid symptoms of complete exhaustion.

A subacute course of the disease, phthisis florida, succeeds the initial catarrh sometimes immediately, especially in the case of young individuals and after confinement, likewise after severe acute diseases; very frequently it forms the conclusion of the more chronic forms of phthisis. This subacute course is particularly distinguished by intense hectic fever, tuberculous diarrhœa, disposition to pulmonary hemorrhage. The most vigorous patients fail within eight or ten weeks, nor is it at all possible to arrest the course of the disease in the least degree.

In reviewing the most important local alterations caused by tubercular phthisis, we have in the first place to attend to the physical symptoms.

Except perhaps in very acute cases, the form of the thorax is plainly and characteristically altered. The thorax is flattened, pressed in and descends lower down, so that the shoulders form a very obtuse angle with the longitudinal axis of the thorax, and the neck appears to be elongated. The intercostal spaces are sunken, more particularly the jugular fossa, the clavicles are very prominent; the sternum is much depressed, its upper portion often stands out, so as to form an angle with the rest; the shoulder-blades stand out very prominently. These changes are most striking, if they only exist in one side of the thorax; it is true that in such a case not all these changes are so decidedly marked, but they are more striking to the eye. The movements of the thorax are very much changed; respiration is carried on with the lower portion of the thorax, and still more with the diaphragm and the abdomen, whereas the upper ribs are scarcely moved. On palpation, increased vibrations are often perceived from the voice in the upper portion of the lungs.

In the beginning of chronic miliary tuberculosis, percussion sometimes does not reveal the least change; as the depositions increase, the sound becomes less full, tympanitic, and finally completely empty. Percussion only yields truly valuable results at the apices of the lungs and in the infraclavicular region; if dulness is plainly returned in these parts, an empty sound in other portions of the lungs authorizes the conclusion that tubercles are deposited. If caverns have formed close to the thoracic wall, percussion sometimes returns a metallic ring or the sound of a cracked pot.

Auscultation returns the most reliable results, because they are most commonly present. In a previous paragraph we have shown the value of the prolonged expiratory murmur and of the "*respiration saccadée*" in the apices of the lungs. If these symptoms become associated with sub-crepitant râles, the diagnosis becomes so much more certain. In proportion as the infiltration increases, the respiratory murmur becomes more and more bronchial, and remains so, even if caverns form, or else amphoric sounds and the metallic ring supervene during the râle. It is often of importance to auscultate during a paroxysm of cough, because at such a time certain sounds, especially the râle, are heard more distinctly. If the tubercular deposits are very extensive, pectoriloquy has often a very high pitch.

The cough of tuberculous persons varies exceedingly. At the beginning a constant short and hacking cough is very usually present, sometimes interrupted by severe paroxysms, resulting in the expectoration of a light-colored, scanty mucus; or else, the cough sets in in irregular paroxysms which are generally excited by marked changes in the temperature and by pulmonary efforts; these paroxysms often last for several hours, and end with retching; the sago-like expectoration follows in a few hours. A cough that at once sets in, with a copious expectoration, is a rare occurrence. After suppuration has taken place, the cough becomes much less wearing and spasmodic; the coughing fit readily results in copious expectoration. Between the more violent paroxysms, a constant hacking takes place, during which the mucous râle is distinctly heard. In very rare cases there is no cough during the whole course of the disease, although the infiltration may be extensive and numerous caverns may exist.

Previous to the deposition of numerous tubercles and their purulent dissolution, the expectoration is without any characteristic features. Nevertheless a continual expectoration of clear mucus is always a suspicious symptom; but such an expectoration acquires significance when it is traversed by fine streaks of a yellowish color, and when, moreover, it frequently appears streaked with blood. Still more characteristic is the presence of sago-like firm little lumps and fibres. Much less frequently hard, yellow or greenish, cheesy little lumps are coughed up at an early period; they generally taste very badly, and frequently have an offensive odor. Sometimes the expectoration contains small lumps of calcareous matter, chalk-like tubercles, seldom, however, previous to suppuration having fully set in; usually after caverns have formed. The cavernous expectoration has a yellow-gray color, less frequently a greenish color, is firmly coherent; in the water it forms irregular, shaggy balls which slowly sink to the bottom; it is surrounded by a quantity of clear bronchial mucus with which, however, it does not mix. The microscope discovers elastic fibres in this expectoration, a sure sign of existing phthisis.

The larynx and trachea seldom remain intact during the whole course of the disease; they show more or less marked symptoms of catarrhal irritation. At an early period of the disease, the voice becomes husky or loses its resonnance and firmness of tone; at a later period, these organs become painful, according as the above-described ulcers are located, and not unfrequently complete aphonia sets in.

The phenomena of the circulatory organs are not by any means constant, but at the beginning of tuberculosis we generally find dilatation of the right heart, disposition to a tumultuous action of the heart, blowing murmurs under the clavicle, anæmic murmurs in the jugulars, continuation of the sounds of the heart as far as both apices of the lungs. Afterwards the heart becomes more and more atrophied. The tendency to sudden changes of color is a striking phenomenon only at the commencement of the disease. Very soon the pulse becomes frequent and feebler than usual, it is accelerated by every movement. In the stage of phthisis it almost always exceeds 100, sometimes rising to 140. It is only exceptionally that the pulse of phthisicky patients is retarded, and then only occasionally and alternating with a frequent pulse. As a rule, the pulse affords the best means of judging how far the patient's strength has already been consumed by the disease.

The digestive functions are generally very much impaired. Usually at an early period of the disease the appetite grows poorly, or cardialgic pains are experienced after eating, which are not unfrequently followed by distressing vomiting. The appetite seldom remains natural; sometimes, generally shortly previous to the patient's death, he experiences a morbidly increased hunger. Except in phthisis florida, the stools generally remain natural for a long time; diarrhœa only sets in after the symptoms of extensive suppuration of intestinal tubercles have become manifest. These diarrhœic stools are peculiar, partly papescent and partly watery, resembling mustard in color and appearance; most commonly the passages are accompanied by a quantity of gas, they frequently contain blood and pus, and are seldom colorless. They are not frequent, from three to six a day, generally two in the morning in quick succession, in the day-time they occur after the patient has partaken of nourishment. Sometimes they are preceded by slight colicky pains, at other times they are quite painless. They are always a bad symptom, for the longer the diarrhœa postpones, the longer is the patient's strength preserved. In the first period of the disease, the patient is sometimes troubled with diarrhœic stools, but they generally abate in proportion as the pulmonary symptoms decrease in intensity; if the tendency to diarrhœa has once become established, the course of the disease is generally very rapid. The liver sometimes becomes very troublesome to phthisicky patients in consequence of frequent paroxysms of hyperæmia.

The skin does not show any special symptoms; it is pale and sometimes exhibits a yellowish tint. The fatal termination is sometimes preceded by a painful decubitus. At an early period of the disease the muscles begin to show symptoms of atrophy. A characteristic sign of phthisis is the bulbous thickening of the first phalanges; most likely this change takes place because the ends of the fingers do not participate in the general emaciation.

What is peculiar is, that in most consumptives the sexual passion is very much excited, especially in the case of men, and that the virile power continues so long unimpaired in spite of the general emaciation. The menses remain natural for a long time; if they cease, death may positively be expected within a few months. The urinary secretions do not undergo any abnormal changes; if colliquative sweats break out, the urine is of course diminished.

Infiltrated tubercles are seldom met with, except in the lungs. This form of tuberculosis develops itself from pneumonia, seldom from pleuritis with firm exudation. The inflammatory exudation is not reabsorbed, but transformed into tubercular matter which shows an extraordinary tendency to suppurate; the course of the disease is very seldom protracted. The transformation into tubercular matter generally takes place while tubercular deposits already exist; but it may likewise take place in the case of individuals who had never shown any signs of constitutional tuberculosis.

A pneumonia setting in with such peculiar symptoms, may run a perfectly normal course at first; or else, symptoms of adynamia may show themselves at the outset, more particularly a very rapid pulse which does not show any change on the critical days, and an exceedingly exhausting diarrhœa. Not unfrequently the infiltration is observed to take place at intervals. Most usually tubercular pneumonia is met with in the upper lobes of the lungs. It tends to rapid destruction of the parenchyma, to pneumothorax, and to fistulous openings through the chest-walls. In other respects it develops the same phenomena as chronic miliary tuberculosis while rapidly running its course.

Acute miliary tuberculosis attacks simultaneously every noble organ in the body. It rarely ever breaks out in individuals who so far had enjoyed a seemingly perfect health, more commonly after acute, debilitating diseases, but most generally it sets in as a termination of chronic miliary tuberculosis.

The symptoms of this form are entirely like those of a violent attack of typhus, with which the disease might be confounded so much more easily as it likewise runs its course by stages of seven days. It generally sets in with violent vomiting; after the cessation of the vomiting there is loss of consciousness, and the other symptoms characterizing hydrocephalus to which we therefore refer.

Treatment and Prognosis. Although the prognosis in tubercular diseases is absolutely unfavorable; although the prospect of a tubercular disease that had been diagnosed with positive certainty, is very slim, yet the labor of a physician in this direction is not without reward, since it may be in his power to postpone the fatal termination. Professional aid becomes still more important, if it is tendered at a period when the tubercular disease was still hidden, or had emerged into light with sufficient distinctness to be recognized in its true character with a tolerably reliable degree of certainty. Although success cannot be positively promised at this period, yet it is our opinion that the formation of tubercles can either be prevented, or that their further development can be stayed. After all, the case may perhaps be the same as that of other acute or chronic diseases which only become incurable after they are too far advanced. Unfortunately the aid of the physician is not sought until the suppurative process has already set in, in other words, in the stage of phthisis, when help is exceedingly doubtful.

It cannot be denied that tuberculosis is curable at any period during its course, although such a result happens very seldom after hectic fever has set in, and more particularly after the tuberculous process has invaded the intestines and the larynx. For this reason no case should at once be abandoned as beyond the reach of successful treatment. A complete cure, that is, a complete reabsorption of the tubercular deposits, indeed cannot be expected; remnants of the disease will remain, and a new outbreak may take place at any time.

What we have said shows that the treatment must aim at three objects: preventive treatment, the treatment of tuberculosis as a constitutional disease, and the treatment of the acute intercurrent exacerbations and their most prominent symptoms.

The preventive treatment has to embrace a vast range, if it is to be of any use. Inasmuch as mistakes in the first education and care of children may promote, if not originate, scrofulosis, and inasmuch as scrofulosis may easily terminate in tuberculosis, the means of prevention must necessarily go back to the first years of childhood. A correct mode of living from the earliest infancy is an excellent preventive against the dreaded disease; every physician should see to it that physical laws are properly obeyed in the rearing of children, for this will at the same time prevent a legion of other diseases. A physician's duties in this respect are so much more sacred as so many false customs and wrong maxims have been grafted upon the education of the young by the present age. Unfortunately it cannot be denied that physicians pay too little attention to the first development of childhood, and that they confine their solicitude much more to the treatment of existing diseases than to their prevention. Of course, preventing diseases does not pay. We have not space to exhaust the whole subject of prevention; hence we have to limit ourselves to a statement of the most essential points. The diet should be regulated in accordance with the principles which are more and more universally recognized as correct. Above all, during the first two years the nourishment should principally be milk; afterwards other easily digested articles of diet may be added in suitable quantity and order. Potatoes should not by any means constitute the chief nourishment of children, nor should they be fed, as has been the custom, with milk and farinaceous preparations. But not only the quality, also the quantity of the food, which should moreover be supplied at regular intervals, should have our careful attention. It may seem a small matter for a physician to bother about such trifles, when the children are robust and healthy, but it is not a small matter; on the contrary, it is a subject of great importance. Beside proper diet, a salubrious home, fresh air, exercise and cleanliness must likewise be provided for the little ones. The mental culture is likewise of the utmost importance. Daily experience shows that precocious development and continued mental exertions render children irritable, make them look pale, deprive them of their appetite, and predispose them for all sorts of bodily sufferings. These symptoms show themselves, already in the seventh year, but still more at the age of pubescence, particularly among females. How many individuals fall victims at an early age to an unreasonable and precocious mania for acquiring knowledge! The only means of counteracting the absurd claims of our schools is gymnastics in all its forms, especially if it lays particular stress upon the cultivation of the respiratory muscles, but not by imitating the modern plan of practising neck-breaking tours-de-force, and straining the muscles to the outermost limits. A proper system of hardening children should likewise be pursued with a view of rendering them capable at an early period of bearing abrupt changes of temperature without being made sick by the exposure.

If it is proper that all these rules should be enforced in the education of every child, it is still more important that they should be strictly carried out in the case of scrofulous children or children born of tuberculous parents.

At the age of pubescence all the signs denoting the accession of tuberculosis, become more apparent, and the tuberculous habit frequently shows its peculiar characteristics at an early age. To the above-stated rules a few other important rules may be added. In the first place the young people must be taught to breathe properly, not merely with one portion of the respiratory muscles. Nothing is more conducive to this end than early singing lessons taking care to pay particular attention to a correct practice of the middle notes. It is less important that young people should be invited to perform frequent and deep inspirations, and slow expirations; such instructions are too easily forgotten. It is during this period of development that gymnastics perform real miracles; chamber-gymnastics in particular becomes an invaluable aid in the harmonious development of the muscles. However, in practising with the arms, heavy weights must not be used. The dress, likewise, deserves our attention; it should be of such a style as not to interfere with the freedom of respiration. If a catarrh occurs, it must not be neglected; chlorosis should likewise be carefully attended to. In selecting a trade or a profession, male individuals should avoid such as are known to favor the development of tuberculosis. Women should be cautioned against reckless dancing and the continued application to work that requires constant sitting.

A rigid prophylactic treatment is likewise necessary if symptoms of tubercles have broken out, and if the tendency to catarrh has at the same time become very prominent. Whatever involves an increased activity on the part of the lungs, such as running, dancing, continued talking in large crowds, hurried going upstairs or ascending an eminence, should be strictly avoided at this stage; so should anything that interferes with the action of the lungs, such as continued stooping in a sitting posture, tight clothing, etc. The patient now ought to practice deep inspirations; a substantial, but simple diet, without any artificial stimulants, is likewise indispensable. It being of essential importance that the patient should avoid all opportunities of being attacked with acute catarrh, he will have to avoid keen and cold winds, and provide himself with a respirator, the usefulness of which has not yet been sufficiently recognized. The damper the atmosphere of the place where the patient resides, the more important it is that he should wear flannel undershirts; this rule applies more particularly to the female sex. A sojourn in crowded rooms that are lighted with gas, and in damp and musty churches is exceedingly prejudicial. Proper ventilation and a moderate heating of the rooms should not escape our attention. At this period the food should be more simple and of a more digestible quality than ever; animal food deserves a decided preference. Milk now commends itself as an excellent nourishment, provided the patients are able to bear it, which is unfortunately not always the case. We should be led too far if we would enumerate all the particulars concerning diet and hygiene; indeed, strict rules cannot always be enforced, the physician has to accommodate himself to the circumstances of the patient, and has to blink at a good many omissions. We must insist, however, that a woman suspected of tuberculosis, should never nurse her children at the breast. It behooves us likewise to direct attention to the circumstance that the mental labor and the mood and disposition of the patient are of the utmost importance to the course of the disease. We doubt whether grief and care can cause tubercles, but what is absolutely certain is, that depression of spirits, sorrow and care, and continued chagrin accelerate the course of tuberculosis, and that a good deal of mental excitement likewise exerts a pernicious influence. Even a change for a few weeks only from their usual surroundings to a quiet and pleasant retreat, affects the patients beneficiently.

What we have said shows how much importance we attach to a correctly-understood preventive treatment. Various medicines are likewise of importance during the course of occult tuberculosis; however, they need not be mentioned in this place, since the indications correspond to the most ordinary precursors of tuberculosis, namely chlorosis and scrofulosis, under which respective heads the medicines and their special indications will be found named.

We have now reached the treatment of the fully developed tubercular disease. This treatment, of course, has to be chiefly medicinal, although the above stated dietetic rules should be continued in all their force. It is difficult to furnish full and precise information in this direction; in the first place the groups of symptoms are too manifold, and in the second place it is next to impossible to draw positive conclusions from clinical cases, for the reason that the same remedy which helped in one case and effected a brilliant cure, showed itself perfectly ineffectual in another, apparently similar case. We do not intend to supersede the Materia Medica by furnishing symptomatic groups, and therefore prefer giving mere names, referring to the Materia Medica for the symptomatic detail.

Bronchial catarrhs that break out as an acute disease, and afterwards assume a chronic form, first claim our attention. Their rapid cure is of immense importance to the course of the whole disease. As soon as we have ascertained that a person attacked with catarrh has tubercles, we must in the first place insist upon the patient remaining confined to his room, the temperature of which should be uniformly kept at about 60° F. On the other hand, such patients should not be all at once confined to their beds. *Aconitum* which is suitable in catarrh generally, is still more adapted to tubercular bronchial catarrh commencing with a violent fever which is characterized by great heat without much perspiration. Upon the whole, however, we prefer *Belladonna* in this form of bronchial catarrh as well as in simple bronchitis; for particular indications we refer to our remarks in the chapter on acute bronchitis. *Belladonna* is not only adapted to cases with high fever, but likewise to cases without much fever; no remedy is as effectual in moderating the constantly tormenting cough as Belladonna. *Bryonia* is an excellent remedy, if the patient complains of much lassitude without a great deal of high fever; the drawing-stitching pains in one apex of the lungs and the pains in the arm corresponding with this part of the lungs, or tearing through all the limbs, are likewise complained of; Bryonia is seldom of any use in the subsequent course of the catarrh. *Digitalis* has rendered us excellent service for some years past in similar cases as those for which Bryonia is indicated; only if Digitalis is to help, the cough must not be dry. It has seemed to us that this remedy arrests, or else reduces the cough very greatly more speedily than any other remedy. *Spongia* is an excellent remedy if the catarrh commences with obstinate hoarseness, the cough remains for a long time dry and barking, spasmodic, attended with congestive sensations in the chest and asthmatic complaints. *Bromine* is symptomatically very similar to tubercular catarrh; however, the clinical results that have so far been obtained with Bromine, are not yet very numerous. *Pulsatilla* is indicated if nothing remains of the catarrh but a racking cough with scanty expectoration of mucus. For other remedies we refer to diseases of the lungs.

If, instead of breaking out with acute catarrh, tuberculosis breaks out with bloody cough, we have to depend particularly upon three remedies, namely *Aconite*, *Arnica* and *Digitalis*, the symptomatic indications of which can easily be studied in the Materia Medica.

If the treatment of these initial affections has left no doubt in our minds that we have to deal with tuberculosis, it then behooves us to treat the disease as a whole, without, however, neglecting the symptomatic appearances. It would be a great mistake, however, if after the catarrh is fortunately subdued, we were now to pursue an exclusively symptomatic treatment.

The patient may seem ever so well, yet he must still be treated as if he were sick. His whole mode of living must be strictly conformable to the rules which we have laid down; a consistent and persevering enforcement of these rules is the surest guarantee for the prevention of new and the calcification of existing tubercular deposits. The only medicines that can now come to the support of the hygienic means, are *Ferrum* and *Calcarea carbonica*. *Ferrum*, whether it is used as a medicinal preparation or as mineral water, has to be administered with a good deal of caution. If the patients show an extreme disposition to pulmonary hyperæmia, they are very sensitive to the action of Iron; any dose of unusual size excites their circulation and makes them cough up blood. Since this result is principally owing to the dose, we have a ready explanation why the Old School has been so averse to prescribing Iron in tuberculosis. If it is given in small doses, not below the second trituration, we shall very speedily notice good effects from the drug, if it is administered for the following symptoms and conditions: Pale complexion with disposition to a change of color, or with a yellowish tint; deficient appetite, or perverse cravings, with disposition to pain in the stomach, and constipation; frequent palpitations of the heart and transitory congestions of the lungs; disproportionate muscular debility; lassitude from the least unusual motion; irritability of temper excited by the least unpleasant impressions. The indications for *Calcarea* do not differ much from those of *Iron*. The patients have a florid appearance, their cheeks are very much flushed, the skin being at the same time very delicate; they are apt to complain of congestive headache; they have an excitable disposition and sanguine temperament; at times they digest their food very regularly, at other times they are troubled with diarrhœa; unless they are under some special excitement, the patients complain of weakness, although, when in pleasant company, no sign of weakness is perceptible; the sexual system is very active, the menses are profuse and set in prematurely and with acute pains.

Under the operation of these two drugs, the use of which ought to be discontinued sometimes for a week at a time, we sometimes see the whole disease arrested or even retrograde; of course, the patients have to be very particular in observing the strictest diet. We need not suppose that these two remedies produce their favorable effect simply by promoting the general nutrition, since they often effect a favorable change even at a later stage of the disease.

China and **Arsenicum** are two remedies that can likewise be used at the beginning of the tuberculous process, although they are less reliable than the former. *China* is indicated if the pulmonary affection seems to constitute the whole difficulty, but still more, if it commences with the symptoms of a severe hyperæmia of the liver, and if the patients very soon show a cachectic appearance. It is well known how often pains in the liver constitute symptoms of tuberculosis, and how often such patients were formerly sent to Carlsbad to return home again in a dying condition. *Arsenicum album* has only been employed by us for tuberculosis in the last few years; the cases where *Arsenicum* is indicated, are too few to enable us to express a positive opinion on its therapeutic value at this time. So far we have found the remedy of use in cases of tuberculosis with almost typical, long-lasting paroxysms of cough attended with retching, and vomiting of small quantities of tenacious mucus, succeeded in a few days by an easy expectoration of the above-mentioned sago-like little lumps. The paroxysms of cough are ushered in with a sensation like violent asthma and are accompanied by severe dyspnœa. The general health is not as much impaired as the violent cough might lead one to expect.

This so-called first stage of tuberculosis, that is, the period when the tubercular deposits have not yet commenced to suppurate, is the time when a cure of the disease can be hoped for with some certainty. Unfortunately this stage is too often overlooked by the patient as well as by the physician. To the above-mentioned remedies which have to be exhibited for months, a number of other remedies have to be added that we require to use for the removal of all the trifling inconveniences inherent in the disease. This is of the highest importance lest the nutrition of the organism should be impaired beyond what it necessarily will be by the tubercular process. We cannot go into details in this particular. Cod-liver oil, a change of climate, and other methods of cure will be treated of by and by.

After the supervention of the suppurative stage, the medicinal treatment has to be considerably modified. We now have to meet two indications, the necessity of preventing the further deposition of tubercular matter, and, secondly, of circumscribing its purulent dissolution. We need hardly state that the prognosis now is much more unfavorable than previously. To the remedies that have just been named, we now have to add a number of others acting directly upon the local process. The use of *Ferrum*, at this stage, requires still more caution than before. Other remedies are: *Iodium*, *Phosphorus*, *Kali carbon.*, *Hepar sulphuris calc.*, *Silicea*, *Digitalis*, *Plumbum*, *Cuprum* and *Natrum muriaticum*. All these remedies seem to have a marvelous effect in some cases, whereas in apparently similar cases they leave us in the lurch, so that it is exceedingly difficult to establish positive indications from clinical results. We omit them so much more readily as the slow course of the disease affords plenty of time to consult the Materia Medica for special symptoms. A few hints will, therefore, prove sufficient.

Iodium is undoubtedly one of our most important remedies in confirmed phthisis; it only suits, however, after the expectoration has become purulent. This remedy effects, more frequently than any other, curative results, provided we do not obstinately insist upon giving only small doses. *Iodine* 6 sometimes has a good effect, but *Iodine* 1 is often indispensable, nor need any unpleasant effects be apprehended from the use of such large doses. *Iodium* is more particularly indicated if tuberculosis is the result of scrofulosis, in the case of young and robust individuals; if diarrhœa is present, *Iodine* does not act favorably as a rule.

Kali carbonicum has, beside the general symptoms of phthisis, a characteristically persistent, sharp-stitching pain at a circumscribed spot in the chest. Unfortunately this remedy often disappoints our expectations.

Hepar sulphuris calc. is particularly suitable if the disease threatens to run rapidly to a fatal termination; a severe fever sets in at the onset, the cough is rather dry, although the patients themselves hear a rattling and wheezing in the lungs; scrofulosis had preceded the tuberculosis. Violent diarrhœa contra-indicates Hepar.

Silicea is only suitable for the slow phthisis of old people; its effect is questionable.

Phosphorus, according to our own experience, is less adapted to phthisis as a whole than to single symptoms. It has to be used with caution, for no other medicine causes hæmoptoë as easily as Phosphorus; no other medicine disagrees so completely in the long run. The chief indications for *Phosphorus* are: Continued hoarseness, with a distressing, dry cough, sore feeling in the larynx and trachea; pain in the stomach after every meal, also retching and vomiting of mucus; continual diarrhœa, which is excited by eating, after every meal; excessive excitement of the sexual passion.

Plumbum ought to be used more frequently than has yet been the case; the dose must neither be too weak, nor too strong. It sometimes has a good effect after every other remedy has disappointed us, more particularly if there are considerable vomicæ, and the patient is tormented by copious, watery diarrhœic stools accompanied by severe pain.

Cuprum deserves our commendation in florid or galloping phthisis;

its symptoms are so striking that we limit ourselves to referring the reader to the Materia Medica.

Digitalis purpurea is, like Cuprum, particularly adapted to galloping phthisis with intense hectic fever from the commencement; the patient complains of palpitation of the heart, coughs up blood frequently, has no appetite; the bowels are constipated and the pulse is exceedingly quick. *Digitalis* is the most reliable remedy to moderate the hectic fever, but the dose must not be too small. Nor should the dose be excessively large, because large doses are apt to excite the patient.

Natrum muriaticum is only useful in chronic cases, attended with severe disturbances of the cardiac functions.

Millefolium is an important domestic remedy for tuberculosis. Our provings point to it as such, but clinical results are still wanting.

Sulphur, which is too often mentioned as a remedy for phthisis, is not, in our opinion, adapted to a single case of this disease; we have used it frequently, but have never seen it do any good; where it is said to have produced a good effect, chronic pneumonia has probably been confounded with tuberculosis.

Concerning the best method of applying all these drugs in practice, views differ considerably. The more striking these differences are, the more earnestly we recommend the golden mean not only in respect to the size, but likewise in respect to the repetition of the dose. The attenuations from the third to the sixth are generally sufficient; lower attenuations are scarcely ever necessary, higher ones are unreliable. We do not like to give more than one dose a day of the appropriate remedy, sometimes only one dose every two or three days. If a remedy has once been selected, it should not be given up too soon; if the improvement under it seems to stand still, a lower attenuation had better be used before the medicine is entirely abandoned. If this should have been found necessary, and the remedy that is chosen after the former, likewise proves ineffectual, it may be well to return once more to the last remedy that seemed to improve the case. A change of this kind sometimes has a very good effect. We would likewise warn against a medicine being given for every little symptom and a strictly symptomatic treatment being indulged in. This is decidedly injurious and may defeat all chances of a successful termination.

This now leads us to mention a few remedies that are not contained in our Materia Medica Pura. As regards *Cod-liver oil*, even the Physiological School admits that it acts well in phthisis. The Iodine it contains being present only in a very small quantity, the boldest conclusions were resorted to for the purpose of substantiating the theory that the oil alone is the curative agent. That this theory is erroneous, can easily be shown by some other oil being substituted for cod-liver oil; the same effect will not be obtained. The small quantity of Iodine is sufficient for the homœopath to account for the action of the oil. That it should be used with caution, has already been stated at the conclusion of our chapter on scrofulosis; the same maxims that were laid down on that occasion, are likewise applicable to phthisis, so much more as it is decidedly injurious to phthisicky patients to have their appetite disturbed and their normal digestion interfered with. The dose should likewise be carefully measured; a tablespoonful in the morning is sufficient, two spoonfuls at a time are a very big dose. It is decidedly improper to prescribe a spoonful morning and evening. A morning-dose is sufficient; in the evening the oil disagrees with most persons. No other medicine should be given with cod-liver oil.

Whey-cures which have found great favor with many, have a great deal against them in cases of perfectly developed phthisis; they render the stomach very sensitive. For our own part, we prefer the therapeutic use of milk, provided the same rigid diet is pursued in connection with a milk-cure that is indispensable when a whey-cure is pursued. Milk does not agree, if the patients indulge at the same time in a luxurious mode of living, and a highly seasoned diet. Nor should it be overlooked that milk is a very substantial kind of nourishment, and that hence it should not be used as a mere beverage, but should be taken in the place of other food, as a regular meal.

Mineral-waters are highly recommended for tuberculosis, but we must confess that we are not acquainted with a single kind that effects only a tolerably favorable change. The weak chalybeate springs sometimes render good service in the same manner as medicinal preparations of Iron; only they have to be used with great caution. In other respects spas are not more beneficial than a sojourn in a beautiful country, accompanied by a suitable mode of living generally.

A prolonged stay in an elevated region of country has undoubtedly a directly healing influence over phthisis, although the cure is seldom complete. We believe that living in a mid-mountain atmosphere is better than all climatic cure-places; it facilitates respiration, increases the capacity of the lungs, and hardens the organism generally. The unusual results obtained by Dr. Brehmer in Görbersdorf abundantly testify to the excellence of his curative method which is entirely based upon the action of attenuated atmospheric air. No physician should leave these results unnoticed, since it may be possible to send the patient into a high region of country without changing the climate to which he is habituated.

We do not think much of systematic cure-places, such as Cairo, Madeira, Algiers, Pisa, Venice, Nice, Meran, etc.; they never exert a directly curative influence, but are only useful by preventing the frequent return of acute catarrhs. Madeira, on account of the sea-air, and Meran, on account of its high situation, deserve most commendation. As a rule, climatic cure-places act the less favorably the more their climate differs from that to which the patient has been accustomed. After his return home, he is so much more susceptible to colds; a Southern climate could only be preferred, provided the patient intends to make it his permanent residence. Unfortunately this is impossible for a large majority of tuberculous patients. Above all, patients already far gone in consumption, should not be sent away far from home.

The remedies and general measures which we have proposed for a direct cure of tuberculosis and phthisis, even though it is so often impossible to employ them, or though they can only be employed on a limited scale, should never be omitted even in apparently hopeless cases. We can point to three patients who seemed to be on the point of death, and who suddenly improved and lived for a number of years in tolerable health.

It remains for us to devote a few words to the symptomatic treatment of a few straggling symptoms. Leaving a direct cure out of the question, it is so much more important to speedily remove single disturbances the less they are connected with the usual course of tuberculosis; moreover, the duty of rendering the patient's exit from life as easy as possible, imposes upon us the other duty of sometimes resorting to a purely symptomatic treatment. In the following paragraphs we will give a few hints with reference to this subject.

The cough generally causes the greatest distress to the patients, leaving them no rest. At the beginning of phthisis, when the patient is constantly teased with a dry cough and dyspnœa, *Belladonna* usually has a very excellent effect. In the later course of the disease, after suppuration had really set in, we have obtained speedy and real relief by means of small doses of *Morphine*, one-twentieth or one-fiftieth of a grain at a dose, nor have we ever hesitated to avail ourselves of the narcotic properties of this agent. *Cannabis* is exceedingly unreliable. For a cough with a copious, fetid expectoration, *Carbo veget.* often proves a most excellent remedy.

Hectic fever never requires special remedies; it is a necessary attribute of florid phthisis.

Hæmoptysis has to be stopped as soon as possible, not only on account of the anxiety of the patient, but of the loss of blood. *Aconitum, Arnica, Digitalis, Ipecacuanha, Belladonna* sometimes arrest it very speedily; if they do not, and the loss of blood is great and threatening, a small teaspoonful of table-salt may be administered; this will sometimes effect an immediate stoppage of the hemorrhage.

The laryngeal difficulties are purely symptomatic; they do not yield to any medicine.

For violent headache which deprives the patient of sleep, *Digitalis* and *Arsenicum* are excellent remedies.

The gastric derangements are manifold; they are most distressing, if every time the patient partakes of a little nourishment, he experiences pain in the stomach, nausea, retching, vomiting. For such symptoms *Ferrum* generally acts as a specific remedy. *Arsenicum, Iodine, Kreosotum* likewise deserve our attention.

Diarrhœa, when not occasioned by intestinal tubercles, is treated according to the usual rules. If it assumes a tuberculous character, *Phosphorus* and *Phosphori acidum, Ipecac., Calcarea acetica* and *phosphorica* are the proper remedies.

Pulmonary hyperæmia generally yields to *Aconite; Belladonna* and *Kali nitricum,* likewise *Arnica* may prove useful for such a condition.

Infiltrated tuberculosis is treated according to the same principles as miliary tuberculosis; *Iodium* is a very important remedy in this disease, likewise *Lycopodium* and *Sulphur*, together with *Phosphorus*.

Acute miliary tuberculosis generally defies every attempt to cure it, so much more as it is generally very difficult to diagnose it with certainty. *Verat. alb., Digitalis, Cuprum, Tartarus stibiatus, Phosphorus* may be tried, but the experiment will generally prove fruitless.

In conclusion we will mention a few remedies that are variously recommended for tuberculosis; at times for the disease in its totality, and sometimes for single symptoms; these remedies are: *Kreosotum, Kali hydriodicum, Stannum, Ledum, Manganum, Baryta, Alumina, Causticum.* This number might still be increased, if we could imagine every possible change in advance, and every occurrence that might complicate or interrupt the course of tuberculosis. In view of so many changeable and diversified groups of symptoms, all that we could well be expected to do was, to explain the general principles upon which the treatment of the disease should be conducted.

As regards diet, we need not dwell upon it any further; it results from what we have said when speaking of the prophylactic treatment and the etiological causes of the disease.

The following chapters, referring more particularly to the blood and the sphere of nutrition, are taken from the last number of Kafka's second volume.

8. Constitutional Plethora, Polyæmia, Hyperæmia.

[The volume of blood is increased; this increase of the volume of the blood involves a proportionate increase of the number of blood-corpuscles and of the albumen. It is true that many modern pathologists deny the existence of plethora; they maintain that nobody has too much blood and that plethora most commonly depends upon an augmentation of the red corpuscles or upon an increased quantity of the fibrin in the blood. But daily experience teaches us that a constitutional hyperæmia does occur, although not very frequently, and that it represents a derangement which occasions morbid symptoms.

A constitutional plethora most frequently occurs in the case of young people who, having a good and active digestion, consume a quantity of meat and other protein material, without taking much exercise. It is likewise observed in the case of older persons who, while appropriating a large supply of food, lead a sedentary or indolent mode of life. It is not unfrequently the consequence of a suppressed flow of blood, such as the menstrual or hemorrhoidal flow, etc., and is frequently coincident with a peculiar plethoric constitution, the influence of climate or the seasons.

A general hyperæmia may be occasioned by circumstances which, by momentarily increasing the action of the heart, may lead to congestions in various parts of the body, whereby a rupture of the vessels and consequent hemorrhage may be occasioned. The most common causes of general hyperæmia are: excessive bodily and mental exertions, such as running, dancing, going upstairs, ascending eminences, etc., too long continued thinking, committing to memory, studying at night, sedentary habits; violent excitement of the feelings, as may be caused by anger, love, jealousy, etc.; the immoderate indulgence of spirits, heating beverages, stimulating food, exciting and stimulating medicines. Colds, cold winds, stormy weather, a sudden cooling off, sudden changes of temperature, an unexpected supervention of hot weather as in spring; or the supervention of some acute disease, may give rise to general hyperæmia.

The blood of plethoric individuals is dark and viscid, and is generally distributed irregularly: it is most commonly the lungs, liver, spleen and muscles that are the seat of hyperæmia; after death copious coagula are met with in the heart and vessels, most generally sanguineous deposits and exudations. The muscles have a darker color and tear more readily; the heart is dilated, and when sawed through, the bones look dark-red.

The general characteristic signs of plethora consist in the fulness and volume of the radial pulse, turgescence of the veins, a vivid and mostly florid color of the skin, increased turgor of this organ, a more elevated temperature of the body and a constant disposition to perspire. In the majority of cases, the size and weight of the body, and the deposition of fat are considerably increased.

This condition may exist without a disturbance of the general health being perceptible. However, the presence of the above-mentioned exciting causes may lead to abnormal phenomena of the highest importance. The rapid increase of the action of the heart may give rise to rush of blood to the head, or to the chest, liver, kidneys, pelvic viscera, etc., and the more immediate consequences of these congestions frequently are inflammations or hemorrhages, or a relaxation of some portion of the vascular system and consequent dilatation of the vessels.

The degrees of true plethora vary; sometimes they are very slight, scarcely perceptible; at other times they are quite striking, and even so intense that highly characteristic constitutional changes may be determined by the plethora. The so-called apoplectic habit or the square constitution (constitutio quadrata) represent the highest grade of true plethora; the face is cherry or blue-red, the neck is thick and short, the shoulders are broad, the body is large and fat; on stooping, the face turns dark-red, the least bodily exertion, such as running, going upstairs or ascending an eminence, causes dyspnœa or palpitation of the heart, or determination of blood to the head, lungs, etc.

Individuals of this description generally feel very uncomfortable in hot weather, in heated or close rooms, in a horizontal posture or when the head is too low, after the use of spirituous or heating beverages; whereas they generally feel a great deal better in cool weather, after exercise in the open air, when observing a rigid diet and drinking cold water, after bleeding at the nose and copious stool. All these circumstances together in former times induced the belief that such individuals are principally predisposed to cerebral apoplexy. Pathological anatomy, however, has shown us that a predisposition to apoplexy does not so much depend upon the constitutio quadrata as upon a peculiar morbid condition of the blood-vessels which are either abnormally rigid or liable to being torn; it has likewise shown us that such persons are disposed to hemorrhages of any kind and that it is more especially to plastic exudations that they are most frequently liable.

A genuine constitutional plethora either terminates in a reduction of the volume of blood to a normal quantity, or in an abnormal deposition of fat and a fatty degeneration of the heart and bloodvessels, in consequence of which hemorrhages occur quite frequently, or varicose conditions of the veins may take place, or the heart may become suddenly paralyzed.

In slight degrees of plethora, the prognosis is generally favorable. In higher grades of this disease, it is necessary to establish our prognosis with great caution, for the reason that trivial causes may sometimes give rise to important changes, involving the possibility of a fatal termination.

Treatment. The homœopathic treatment of general plethora constitutes a most memorable epoch in the history of Homœopathy. At a time when general and local depletions were most shamefully abused in all the clinics and hospitals of the civilized world; when the most celebrated teachers of medicine taught the doctrine that a general hyperæmia must be met by artificially reducing the quantity of blood, Hahnemann had the courage to protest against this absurd method of treatment, and to assert that in most cases sanguineous depletions were not only unnecessary but positively hurtful. For years his views were sought to be refuted by argument and ridicule, until, finally, calm observations in the clinics of Vienna and Prague, which were more particularly conducted with great discretion and impartiality during the treatment of pneumonia, resulted in establishing the fact, that venesections and local depletions are unnecessary in most, and hurtful in many cases. This conviction which was proclaimed by Hahnemann thirty or forty years previous, has now been adopted as a ruling principle in all medical clinics. Venesection has almost entirely fallen into disuse; leeching is very rarely resorted to, and cupping is known only by name. Impartial and enlightened professors of clinical medicine admit unreservedly that this revolutionary change is primarily due to Homœopathy, and secondarily to the results obtained by post-mortem observations, and to the observations instituted by unprejudiced practitioners at the sick-bed.

In order to overcome a plethoric condition of the system, the homœopathic method of treatment not only dispenses with sanguineous depletions, but it likewise rejects the abuse of cathartics which are still in vogue and are still regarded and recommended as means of derivation from more important organs. Nor does Homœopathy resort to vesicatories, since they not only fail of accomplishing the purpose of derivation, but are in most cases employed without any benefit.

In treating plethora homœopathically, we do not merely regard the fact of an excess of blood, but likewise the phenomena connected with it, the exciting causes and the constitutional condition of the patient generally.

We have stated in a previous paragraph that the increased action of the heart most commonly determines a rush of blood to various internal or external organs or systems, and that this determination of blood may superinduce hyperæmia, inflammatory conditions, hemorrhages, dilatations of vessels. It is upon these conditions and a simultaneous consideration of the anamnestic circumstances that the selection of a homœopathic remedy is based. It is not by any means immaterial whether we have to deal with congestions to the head, or to the chest, liver, etc.; whether they have resulted in simple hyperæmia, or in inflammatory processes, hemorrhages, etc.; whether the plethoric condition was caused by a cold, by an emotion, by excessive bodily exertions, by the unfavorable influences of climate, temperature, etc., whether the patient's organization is of a vigorous or delicate kind. All these circumstances have to be considered in selecting a remedy from among the large number of those whose effects upon the normal organism have been carefully determined by provings and which will secure for us the speediest, best and most certain results.

If a cold has taken place by exposure to a current of air, by a sudden change of temperature, by the action of a keen North or East-wind; or if the patient has been exposed to a severe fit of mortification, to fright, or has undergone excessive bodily exertions by running, dancing, going upstairs or ascending an eminence, walking too great a distance, etc.; if, in consequence, the impulse of the heart has become much stronger, the skin has assumed a tinge of vivid redness, the bodily temperature has been considerably raised, the pulse has become full and large: we at once resort to *Aconite* 3 in solution, every hour, even if local congestive or inflammatory processes have already set in. Already in a few hours the patient begins to transpire, especially if the morbid condition is the result of a cold; or even, without perspiration the impulse of the heart becomes quieter and the vascular tumult is appeased without venesection or local depletions having been resorted to. We obtain the same success if the above-mentioned causes have induced a collapsed appearance of the patients, the pulse is contracted and the bodily temperature is diminished, yet the impulse of the heart continues vigorous and the head is hot. In such cases the peripheral vessels are generally contracted, and the congestion of the internal organs is so much more marked; upon a condition of this kind, Aconite likewise acts with the most striking effect. A fact of this kind, which has been verified in thousands of instances, shows that Aconite, in homœopathic doses, has a decidedly calming influence over the morbidly excited action of the heart, and that it is by this means alone that true plethora can be subdued.

Physicians who do not dispense their own medicines, can easily satisfy themselves of the truth of this statement by prescribing one drop of the tincture in an ounce of water, and ordering a teaspoonful of this mixture every hour or even every half hour.

If the symptoms of general plethora are accompanied with distinct symptoms of cerebral congestions, the treatment indicated for cerebral hyperæmia will have to be pursued.

For marked congestions of the chest, we give *Bryon.* 3, if the shortness of breath is attended with pleuritic stitches and a dry cough; or *Phosph.* 3, both remedies in solution, every hour, if dyspnœa, oppression of the chest, a dry and tight cough, and danger of pneumonia or hæmoptoë are present.

If the patients have become very much excited by mental labor, committing to memory, by anger or vexation, abuse of spirits, or have indulged in over-eating or luxurious living; if they complain of pressure in the frontal region, with nausea or actual saburral vomiting; if the tongue has a yellowish coating, the taste is sour or pasty; if the patients are troubled with frequent eructations and distention of the abdomen; if they are irritable, irascible, and the bowels are torpid, *Nux vom.* 3 in solution, every hour, will not only remove the hyperæmia but likewise the gastric disturbance.

Under similar circumstances and for similar symptoms, *Carbo veg.* 6 or *Calc. carb.* 6 may likewise prove useful.

The last-named remedies, to which we add *Sulphur* 6, render good service for general plethora superinduced by the suppression of habitual hemorrhoids; if arising from menstrual suppression, we resort to *Conium, Digitalis* or *Crocus* 3.

These statements, which are suggested by daily practice, are simply intended to show the manner in which we avail ourselves of the results of our physiological provings. These statements do not by any means present an exhaustive discussion of the subject, and do not obviate the necessity, in extraordinary cases, of studying the Materia Medica with special reference to a given case, since we have many other remedies, such as *Mercur., Hepar sulph., Rhus tox., Lycop., Sepia, Tart. emet., Iodium,* etc., which are capable of removing a general plethora.

Regarding the diet, we recommend to plethoric individuals the use of vegetables, abstinence from spirits and heating beverages, daily exercise in the open air for a couple of hours, avoidance of exciting or depressing emotions, of sedentary habits and protracted sleeping.

A spurious sort of plethora accompanying emphysema of the lungs, hypertrophy of the left ventricle, insufficiency or stenosis of the bicuspid valve, goitre, stenosis of the larynx, has been fully described in the chapters where these diseases are treated of.

Kafka relates the case of a lady, seventy years old, with a large and indurated goitre, in consequence of which she became cyanotic, short-breathed, dyspeptic, very feeble and somnolent. Iodine proving ineffectual for these symptoms, *Arsen.* 3, three doses a day, was resorted to. In a few days already a decided improvement set in. H.]

9. Anæmia, Oligæmia.

Deficiency or rather Paleness of the Blood.

[It is only true anæmia, or deficiency of blood consequent upon excessive losses of this fluid, that consists in a diminution of the quantity of the blood without any simultaneous alteration in the normal composition of this fluid. Spurious anæmia with which we shall principally deal in this chapter, constitutes a disease of the blood where the number of the red corpuscles is more or less diminished, in consequence of which the blood becomes paler and appears variously altered both quantitatively and qualitatively.

Hence it is with a qualitative rather than with a quantitative disease of the blood that we have to deal with, where the deficiency of red blood-disks constitutes a characteristic phenomenon, on which account it would be more appropriate, according to Vogel, to denominate the disease *oligocythæmia*.

In a normal condition of the organism, the reproduction of red corpuscles equilibrates their decay, so that, within certain limits, the percentage amount of blood-disks in the blood, and their total quantity remains unchanged.

In diseases, however, this relative proportion is disturbed, so that more blood-disks decay than are reproduced; hence arises the condition which Vogel denominates *oligocythæmia*.

The results of our pathological and anatomical investigations show that the blood of anæmic individuals is deficient in red corpuscles; it contains less hæmatin and fibrin, but on the other hand an excess of serum.

The anæmic blood is fluid, pale, the clot is small, soft, floats in a quantity of serum, its specific gravity is diminished; the crassamentum which is sometimes entirely wanting, is less dense and easily disintegrated.

Anæmia is either a primary or secondary morbid process.

A constitutional anæmia depends upon certain ante-natal influences or conditions of development; its causes are either unknown or not satisfactorily accounted for.

It is either congenital, or inherent in the process of development, or in the period of involution.

Congenital anæmia occurs among children of sickly, debilitated parents or of parents afflicted with anæmia, tuberculosis, constitutional syphilis, carcinoma or other exhausting diseases; it occurs among children born before their full term, among children born feeble, or whose mothers were suffering with uterine diseases or hemorrhages.

Anæmia inherent in the period of development either occurs during the first, less frequently during the second dentition, or after the children are weaned, or in consequence of a too rapid growth or at the period of pubescence, more particularly if this period delays or is unduly protracted, or if the sexual instinct is awakened prematurely and is attended with frequent excitement of the fancy and the sexual organs (chlorosis).

The anæmia of involution most commonly occurs during the critical period of females, or during old age, or if marasmus sets in prematurely.

Consecutive anæmia sets in simultaneously with, or in consequence of derangements the causes of which are generally known and directly diminish the quantity and deteriorate the quality of the blood.

The quantity of the blood is diminished by acute losses of this fluid, such as bloodletting, hemorrhages, operations, wounds, and likewise by frequent attacks of chronic hemorrhage.

The quantity and quality of the blood are impaired by losses of fluids, as in consequence of catharsis and diarrhœa, continued or frequent vomiting, profuse suppuration, excessive or too long continued nursing, profuse blennorrhœa and perspiration, ptyalism, copious nocturnal emissions, onanism and other sexual excesses.

A loss of strength, such as may arise from excessive muscular exertions, long marches, running, etc., or from hard work, after severe febrile or inflammatory diseases, especially when attended with copious serous, plastic, purulent or hemorrhagic exudations; after various acute exanthems, such as measles, scarlatina, variola, etc.; after frequent pregnancies occurring at short intervals, and after frequent miscarriages, etc., may likewise induce a greater consumption of red corpuscles than the organism is capable of reproducing, and may consequently bring about a condition of anæmia.

Consecutive anæmia may likewise occur in consequence of an insufficient production of blood-disks and hæmatin owing to a deficient supply of food or a total deprivation of nourishment by fasting, starvation-cures, or a scanty supply of, or vitiated food; bad or stagnant water, unfavorable climatic or atmospher influences, excessive cold or heat, damp or vitiated air without a sufficient supply of oxygen, in damp valleys or malarious districts, on the borders of large rivers where frequent inundations occur; or in consequence of the inhalation, in mines, of air impregnated with carbo-hydrogen or carbonic acid; or likewise in consequence of a deficient supply of light in damp cellars serving as human habitations, or in consequence of deprivation of sleep, long watching, continued and long-lasting pains and spasms, depressing emotions, such as grief, care, sorrow, mortification, home-sickness, disappointed love, etc.; or in consequence of the working of such passions, as envy, pride, ambition, etc.; likewise from excessive mental exertions, abuse of the sexual organs, etc.; or in consequence of diseases of such organs as are physiologically important to the production and propulsion of the blood, such as: diseases of the lungs, heart, arteries, veins, lymphatic glands, liver, spleen, kidneys, uterus, intestinal canal, etc.; it may likewise result from the inhalation of dust or metallic vapors of chemical substances exerting a hurtful influence upon the formation of the sanguineous fluid, such as: Arsen., lead, copper, phosphorus, mercury, silex, zinc, etc. The abuse of Opium, Belladonna, tobacco, alcohol, etc., and the abuse of certain kinds of nutrient substances, such as: potatoes, tea, etc., may likewise lead to anæmia.

Secondary anæmia only occurs as an accompaniment of other morbid processes, upon which it depends. It occurs in the course of tuberculosis, constitutional syphilis, carcinoma, scurvy, scrofulosis, rhachitis, diabetes, puerperal fever, etc., likewise in the course of chronic articular rheumatism, helminthiasis, diseases of the brain and spinal marrow, in the course of chronic exudations, such as: hydrothorax, hydropericardia, ascites, anasarca, ovarian dropsy, etc.

Having dwelt with sufficient detail upon the general and etiological part of anæmia, we now give a description of its symptomatic manifestations.

The skin is pallid in various degrees, sometimes yellowish or of a grayish white, at other times livid; the paleness of the lips, gums, palpebral conjunctiva and ears is particularly striking. The cutaneous veins appear delicate, bluish, thin and empty. The sclerotic most commonly exhibits a bluish-gray appearance. The temperature of the skin, especially that of the extremities, is in most cases diminished; even the temperature of the axillæ not unfrequently falls below the normal standard. Anæmic persons exhibit a characteristic sensitiveness to cold, a fondness for warmth, and frequent shiverings increasing even to violent shaking chills. The muscles of anæmic persons are very often soft and flabby; in many cases the bodily weight becomes less, more particularly in anæmia of a higher grade, which is frequently combined with atrophy, subcutaneous œdema or hydræmia. The muscular strength is always less; after the least bodily exertion, the patients experience great lassitude in the extremities. When ascending an eminence, going upstairs, dancing, or making the least attempt to run, anæmic individuals turn remarkably pale, become short-breathed, the heart palpitates, and, if the anæmia is of a high grade, syncope may set in. The pulse is mostly small, feeble, short and accelerated. The increase of the frequency of the pulse from slight exertions, walking about, and even from sitting up in bed, is a characteristic symptom. If we are in doubt concerning the degree of anæmia, we may direct the patient to walk about; if the pulse increases in frequency after such a trifling effort, we may rest assured that the anæmia has reached a high degree.

The palpitations of the heart, with which such patients are frequently troubled, are often attended with systolic blowing murmurs in the region of the heart and in the larger vessels. The more fully developed the anæmia, the feebler the impulse of the heart, so that in the highest grades of the disease, as in cholera, the second sound of the heart and that of the arteries disappears entirely.

The cerebral functions are generally depressed; anæmic individuals are sad, low-spirited, monosyllabic, melancholy; they sleep a good deal, are sleepy even in the day-time, whereas at night they sometimes lie awake for hours.

On making a slight bodily effort, their sight becomes obscured, they are attacked with buzzing in the ears and vertigo, phenomena which, in high grades of anæmia, may even increase unto syncope. Such patients are frequently attacked by periodical paroxysms of headache, prosopalgia, cardialgia, coxalgia, sometimes by toothache (neuralgia of anæmic persons).

The spinal nerves likewise become frequently involved in the anæmic condition, so that either disturbances of the sentient system take place in the shape of frequent attacks of pain, or of the motor system in the shape of spasms.

Respiration only becomes impeded after excessive bodily exertions; owing to the deficient oxydation of the blood, the patient has to yawn or sigh quite frequently.

The appetite is frequently impaired, or the patient experiences a desire for uncommon things, such as charcoal, chalk, lime, roast coffee, acids, bitter substances, etc.; the digestion is weak, the appetite is speedily satisfied, and, after eating, such patients are frequently attacked with oppression of the stomach or flatulence. The thirst is often very much increased, sometimes quite normal, the bowels are generally torpid, the urine is pale, watery, generally quite copious and has an alkaline reaction. In the case of male patients, the sexual functions remain unaffected; in the case of women, however, the menses often become irregular, or very scanty, or they are entirely suspended. Profuse menses are of much less frequent occurrence; they exert a very prejudicial influence upon the general organism. Anæmic women are very frequently attacked with leucorrhœa and sterility. The secretion of milk is impaired, the milk is watery, thin, not nourishing, hence anæmic women are unfit for the business of nursing and the children who are fed on such milk, generally become anæmic.

Most anæmic persons feel better in a state of rest and in a horizontal posture, whereas they soon feel tired when standing, walking, or when performing bodily labor. Hence they generally feel lazy, are not disposed to work, and soon have to desist from their labor. We are acquainted with patients who become exhausted even after doing the lightest kind of work, such as knitting, crocheting, embroidering, etc., and even become shortbreathed, experience an oppression on the chest, palpitation of the heart, sometimes even pains in the muscles of the arms, chest and back, or after standing or walking for some time, pains in the muscles of the calves or thighs.

As a general rule, anæmic persons feel most uncomfortable in the morning-hours; their sleep is not refreshing or strengthening; the feeling of lassitude does not leave them, on which account they remain sad and depressed in spirits until, in the course of the day, they become artificially stimulated by the use of coffee, tea, wine, beer, broth, etc. This circumstance is very important in a diagnostic point of view; whereas anæmic persons look pale and feel languid while their stomachs are empty, and at such times either yawn or complain of headache and are generally morose: they commonly feel much better after using the above-mentioned stimulants or immediately after eating, their complexion looks much better, they are more active and cheerful. Very seldom anæmic individuals experience an oppression at the stomach, cardialgia or rush of blood to the head after eating or drinking, or feel otherwise uncomfortable and languid.

Diarrhœa, hemorrhages of every kind, even if very slight, nocturnal emissions, sexual intercourse and nursing aggravate the symptoms of anæmia. Depressing emotions and mental exertions likewise cause aggravations, whereas moderate bodily and mental exercise, cheerful company and surroundings affect anæmic persons very favorably.

An anæmic condition is most strikingly increased by the supervention of some acute disease. An occurrence of this kind is apt to bring on an adynamic condition, prostration and sopor; such an acute attack is often attended with fibrinous or serous exudations, drags along very slowly, and convalescence is in most cases very protracted.

All the above-mentioned circumstances are of great importance to the homœopathic physician, on which account we have dwelt upon them very minutely.

It is only anæmic conditions consequent upon acute losses of blood and other animal fluids that run an acute course; other forms of anæmia run a chronic course and, while the exciting cause continues, may last weeks, months and even years.

The more speedily anæmia develops itself, the more rapidly the phenomena characteristic of anæmia set in.

If anæmia runs a protracted course, the greatest attention is often required on the part of the physician in order to accurately observe the pathognomonic symptoms of anæmia. A deficiency of the colored corpuscles causes a more or less vitiated nutrition, a gradual vanishing of the fat and of the vital turgor, a decrease of the natural temperature and of the muscular strength, a high degree of lassitude, indolence and ill-humor, increased beating of the heart after slight bodily exertions, disorders of the nervous system resulting in attacks of pain or spasm of the most diversified kind.

The termination in recovery frequently occurs spontaneously, if the exciting causes cease of themselves, as is often the case in constitutional or consecutive anæmia. Very frequently a complete cure is effected by artificial means.

After acute losses of blood or other fluids, the water and salts of the blood are often speedily restored, without the reproduction of the red corpuscles taking place with equal rapidity. In consequence of this, a hyperæmic condition is apt to set in, which is described under the name of serous plethora and is often accompanied with congestions of the head, febrile irritation, violent palpitations of the heart, sleeplessness, etc.

The more complete the anæmia, the more the fat and muscular strength disappear, the viscera and tissues likewise become impoverished; the watery constituents of the blood increase more and more, and the red corpuscles decrease in proportion; this is the reason why certain parts of the body gradually become œdematous and why serous transudations into the different cavities of the body occur at a later period. This hydræmic condition is most commonly observed after copious losses of blood and other animal fluids, after continued derangements of the digestive system, in consequence of cardiac and valvular anomalies, of Bright's disease, after severe acute diseases and exanthems, during long-continued attacks of fever and ague, chlorosis, during a highly developed tuberculosis, carcinoma, caries and other wasting diseases.

If an improvement or cure cannot be obtained, marasmus and exhaustion set in.

It may likewise happen that the blood is deficient in red corpuscles and so much richer in colorless blood-globules. A condition of this kind is generally connected with diseases of the lymphatic glands, the liver, spleen or uterus, and is designated by the name of *leucæmia*.

If the blood is deficient in red blood-disks, but has an excess of pigment which is likewise deposited in the tissues, a condition of this kind is denominated *melanæmia;* it occurs most frequently after old and violent intermittent fevers.

After rapid alvine evacuations, as in cholera, the highest grade of anæmia is complicated with inspissation of the blood which is characterized by the highest degree of debility and coldness of the extremities and attended with fainting-like paroxysms and absence of the second cardiac and arterial sound. If this condition cannot be removed, it leads to paralysis of the heart.

In treating anæmia, the prognosis depends, above all, upon the various forms and degrees of the disease. The better the exciting causes are known and the more easily they can be removed; the more easily and certainly the loss of the red corpuscles can be repaired and the harmony between their consumption and regeneration can be effected, the more favorable is the prognosis.

Among the forms of constitutional anæmia, those inherent in the period of evolution admit of a favorable prognosis; in congenital anæmia, and in the anæmia of the critical age, the prognosis is less favorable; it is least favorable in the anæmia of old people.

In consecutive anæmia, that which is consequent on loss of blood, animal fluids generally and of strength, admits of a more favorable prognosis than anæmia depending upon climate, atmosphere, local circumstances, or the nature of one's business. Anæmia arising from scanty or unwholesome nourishment, vitiated air, unhealthy habitations, bad water, abuse of spirits or certain kinds of drugs, likewise admits of a more favorable prognosis than anæmia arising from the effects of passions whose impressions are lasting and cannot be effaced.

The prognosis is most unfavorable in consecutive anæmia where the consumption and reproduction of the red corpuscles are simultaneously invaded by disease, as is the case in diarrhœa or hemorrhages with simultaneous catarrh of the stomach, or when during extreme bodily exertions, the supply of food is deficient; or when the process of nursing is disordered by grief; or when frequent nocturnal emissions are accompanied with disappointment in love.

Secondary anæmia can only be cured in case the primary disease can be removed.

Age has no decided influence upon the prognosis; old people may recover very speedily after severe diseases, hemorrhages, diarrhœa, etc., whereas children and robust adults often require a long time for their restoration. This depends chiefly upon the consumption of the blood; in youth and robust manhood this consumption goes on very rapidly and often outweighs the process of restoration, whereas in old age much less blood is consumed, the regenerative process being carried on at an equal ratio.

Intercurrent diseases of any kind during the course of anæmia render the prognosis more uncertain, since the number of blood-disks which is anyhow scanty, decreases with more or less rapidity, more particularly in acute febrile and inflammatory diseases, and most seriously during typhus and intermittent fevers. The prognosis is doubtful for the additional reason that a rapid destruction of the red blood-disks is attended with a rapid sinking of the vital energy, and a high grade of adynamia, or destructive suppurations or gangrenous disorganizations may be the consequence.

Treatment. In our opinion anæmia is a most important pathological condition developed in the depths of the various morbid processes; it frequently becomes an object of observation and hence claims our most serious attention.

The homœopathic treatment of anæmia comprehends three divisions of equal importance: the removal of the causes, diet, and the use of remedial agents.

If the causes are known and can be removed, the first step towards a cure is frequently made. Hence all losses of blood and other fluids, the waste of strength, have to be arrested as speedily as possible; anomalies depending upon birth, constitution, age, sex, development, etc., have to be regulated; excessive bodily or mental exertions, depressing emotions, sexual excesses have to be rigidly avoided; the unfavorable influences of climate and atmosphere have to give way to more favorable surroundings; the supply has to be of the right quality and quantity; errors of nutrition and assimilation have to be corrected; the circumstances of education, mode of living, occupation, habit, etc., have to be considered; diseases of single organs and systems, and constitutional anomalies by which anæmic conditions are so often engendered, have to be carefully observed, and the bad effects of sudden changes of temperature, weather, a sudden rise or fall of the barometer or thermometer, or unfavorable influences of the season, have to be counteracted by appropriate measures.

In cases where the causes of anæmia are unknown, where they are not sufficiently accounted for and cannot be investigated, as is most commonly the case in regard to the various forms of constitutional anæmia, we adhere to our previous statement that the diminution of the red corpuscles, and the consequent anæmia, is either occasioned by a too rapid consumption, or by a deficient reproduction of these bodies, or by both these causes at once. If one or the other of these causes prevails, the homœopathic treatment is regulated accordingly, and the true nature of anæmia is reached and modified by these means.

The dietetic treatment of anæmia has for its object to so regulate the circumstances of the patient as to secure the normal restoration of the blood. The diet is so important that our opponents attribute to it exclusively the good effects of our treatment. Although we do not deny that many forms of anæmia, especially of the consecutive kind, are cured by a suitable diet after the removal of the causes, there are many other forms of anæmia, especially constitutional and secondary, where the best dietetic measures are insufficient, and where the interference of art is indispensable to a cure.

General dietetic rules adapted to all forms of anæmia cannot be established for the reason that every special case requires a dietetic management of its own. For the present we content ourselves with mentioning the general dietetic arrangements that deserve attention in most cases. Special dietetic rules will be indicated when treating of the special forms of anæmia.

If the process of sanguification and nutrition is to be improved, the condition of the digestive organs has to be carefully attended to above everything else.

If anæmic individuals digest very rapidly; if, soon after a copious meal, they again feel hungry; if they do not experience any trouble after eating; if they feel comfortable after a meal and have no fever, the most nourishing diet may be indulged in by such patients. They may use strong soups with the concentrated extract of beef, roast-beef, steak, à-la-mode beef, various kinds of roast without much fat, venison, eggs, farinaceous food, light vegetables which are not of the flatulent kind, cake prepared with sugar, but not fat and without yeast; fish which is not too fat, is likewise allowable, such as trout, salmon, cod, pike, pickerel, etc.

Fat food, salad seasoned with sharp vinegar, husks, fresh bread, etc., should be rigidly avoided.

Stewed fruit is generally more easily digested than raw fruit.

Eggs, almonds, cottage-cheese may be partaken of in moderate quantities.

A well fermented beer is the best beverage for anæmic persons; during a meal light wines may be indulged in. A little Champaigne may be used with the dessert.

If there is a good deal of vascular excitement, disposition to headache and congestions, with sleeplessness, affections of the heart or lungs, hemorrhage, etc., the use of wine has to be strictly avoided; beer, if partaken of discretly or diluted with water and sweetened with sugar, generally agrees with most patients.

Anæmic persons had better eat frequently, every few hours, than too much at once. If a sensation of hunger, or of a so-called "empty stomach" is hurtful, and may give rise to frequent yawning, cardialgia, headache, a disagreeable and audible rumbling in the bowels, weakness of the extremities and even attacks resembling syncope; on the other hand, overloading the stomach is frequently attended with oppression of this organ, flatulence, nausea or even vomiting and diarrhœa, by which conditions the patients are weakened and the anæmia is made worse.

If the digestion is prostrated, our main object must be to restore this important function as speedily as possible to its normal state; for without it no restoration of tissue, and hence no amelioration of the blood can be thought of. The management of the digestive apparatus will be indicated when we give the medicinal treatment. For the present, it may suffice to state that the sick stomach must not be loaded with heavy nourishment; the least excess causes the patient serious distress and increases the gastric disorder.

As long as the appetite is wanting, the patient had better eat nothing but weak soups; under certain circumstances he may be allowed a dish of milk, or some farinaceous preparation or stewed fruit. Beer or wine, whether pure or diluted, can only be allowed, if not counter-indicated by any of the above-mentioned circumstances.

If the appetite improves, more nourishing soups, light white meat, soft-boiled eggs and a light farinaceous diet may be allowed; as the digestion continues to improve, beef, venison and a strengthening diet may be resorted to.

Cooling things, such as: ice, lemonade, orangeade, raspberry-juice, soda-water with wine or syrups, are only permitted by us, if the patients do not cough, are not troubled with diarrhœa or cardialgia, and are not inclined to abdominal pains.

We give these dietetic rules in detail for the reason that we have often seen practitioners urge upon anæmic patients the most substantial diet without regard to their digestive capacities. Being unable, for want of appetite, to comply with the demands of their physicians, the poor patients, instead of gaining in health and strength, continued to fail and were finally obliged to seek help elsewhere.

Exercise and rest are of great importance to the process of sanguification. It is just as important to regulate the amount of exercise with reference to the existing amount of bodily strength, as it is important to measure the amount of supply proportionally to the strength of the digestive powers.

As a rule, anæmic patients have pale and flabby muscles deprived of their normal energy, elasticity and powers of perseverence. All their muscles and muscular bodies exhibit a certain degree of functional debility; the muscles of the trunk and extremities betray this weakness by a feeling of languor and lassitude; those of the thorax by shortness of breath, those of the heart by an accelerated beating of this organ, those of the stomach by weakness of digestion, those of the intestinal canal by indolence of the secretions and by flatulence, those of the uterus by dysmenorrhœa or sterility, etc. This is the reason why anæmic individuals, when exercising too rapidly or too much, are apt to be attacked with dyspnœa, palpitation of the heart, an increase of temperature, in consequence of which abnormal cerebral irritations in the shape of hemicrania or headache occur. An increased frequency of the pulse is not unfrequently accompanied by such a high degree of weariness that, unless the patients rest, syncope may take place. The after-effects of excessive muscular exertions consist in a high degree of weariness and weakness, in muscular pains, spasms and cramps, especially in the chest and calves, in loss of appetite and sleep.

On the contrary, muscular movements adapted to the patient's strength, and followed by timely rest, produce a gradual invigoration of the muscular fibre, a more active circulation, a proportionate waste and supply, an improvement in all the functions, and a higher activity in the process of nutrition.

It is an etablished fact that a great deal of strength is lost by an excess of active exercise, and that it is restored again by subsequent rest; exercise is to rest as consumption to restoration, waste to supply. This shows the importance of subjecting the conduct of anæmic persons in regard to these two factors to a more particular examination.

Anæmic persons should not take any long walks; as soon as they feel exhausted, experience dyspnœa or palpitation of the heart, or commence to perspire, they ought to rest and not resume their walk until they feel able and disposed to do so. Their muscular strength is best ascertained by the condition of the pulse during a walk. If the pulse becomes hurried during such exercise, it is a sure sign that their strength is not very great and that much exercise is hurtful to them.

Walking rapidly and up hill, in a damp and cold air, or against currents of air, on damp soil, have to be carefully avoided, lest other diseases should set in in consequence of such exposure.

Short rides in the country, or excursions on the water, are the most appropriate exercise; these may be followed by short walks on a level, in a shady alley, garden, forest, or meadow, to be followed by adequate rest.

Running, jumping, climbing, ascending a hill, journeys on foot, heavy work, wrestling, fencing, etc., should be rigorously avoided by anæmic persons.

Dancing is an entertainment which, in pleasant company, contributes a good deal to cheering up the spirits; on this account we do not prohibit it entirely, except, however, waltzing which we positively interdict. In cases of pulmonary, cardiac and cerebral diseases, dancing is prejudicial under all circumstances.

We permit riding on horseback if the patients feel strong enough for this kind of exercise and, while riding, do not experience any palpitation of the heart or dyspnœa. Long rides, galloping, and a sharp trot, do not agree as a rule.

The well known indolence of anæmic persons, their disposition to sit or lie down, should not be encouraged by their physician; a protracted rest or a total deprivation of exercise diminishes the functional energy of the muscles and may even result in their atrophy and paralysis.

Sleep and waking likewise exert a powerful influence upon the life of the blood.

Anæmic persons who sleep too much, generally become indolent, peevish, complain of dulness of the head, inability to think; they yawn, look bloated, the blood becomes paler, the muscular fibre more relaxed, and the formation of fat and the serosity of the blood become very marked.

The want of regular sleep as well as complete sleeplessness make the anæmia worse, and frequently result in nervous erethism, hyperæsthesia, debility, digestive derangements, and emaciation.

A natural sleep of six, seven or eight hours is refreshing, strengthening, promotes the restoration of the muscular fibre, improves the process of sanguification, and invigorates the cerebral functions.

Voluntary watching when the hours which should be devoted to sleep, are spent in a state of intentional wakefulness, is very prejudicial to anæmic individuals. The will acting in opposition to the natural want, an effort takes place both of a physical and psychical nature and equal to the sleeplessness added to an excess of bodily and mental exertion, in consequence of which the anæmia becomes more deep-seated.

On this account, anæmic persons should neither watch with the sick, nor for purposes of manual or other work; they should not read, study or travel at night. Even social entertainments should not be indulged in after midnight, so that the remainder of the night can be devoted to rest.

Depressing emotions, such as grief, sorrow, mortified feelings, fear, homesickness, disappointed love, etc., and excessive passions, such as envy, hatred, jealousy, ambition, wounded pride, etc., affect anæmic patients equally badly as sleeplessness. Hence it is necessary in the case of anæmic persons that this morbid direction of the thoughts and feelings should be moderated or entirely subdued by an appeal to their reason as well as by the personal influence of the physician.

The atmospheric air is likewise of great importance as a means of improving the quality of the blood; the purity of the air and the quantity of oxygen it contains contribute greatly to the increase of the red corpuscles. If the digestion is at the same time active, and a sufficient supply of proper nourishment is introduced into the organism, bad cases of anæmia are sometimes cured by these simple means without medicine. It is more particularly the anæmia of convalescent patients that can be removed in this manner.

Anæmic persons residing in crowded cities or in damp and close districts where the air is rendered impure by frequent inundations, coal-vapors, decaying vegetable matter, etc., should, if their circumstances permit, be sent during the warm season into regions of country where the air is pure and rich in oxygen.

The dwellings of anæmic persons must be dry, spacious, with facilities for being easily heated, accessible to sunlight. We know from experience that damp and chilly dwellings give rise to a variety of diseases.

The clothing of anæmic individuals has to be adapted to the season and the weather; the want of animal heat and an extreme sensitiveness to changes of temperature make it desirable that anæmic persons should be warmly clad or, at any rate, that they should at all times and places be provided with a supply of thick clothing, so as to be protected against the bad effects of sudden changes of temperature or of a sudden access of bad weather. They must be cautioned against leaving off their winter-clothing too soon, or against throwing off their cloaks, coats or shawls in cool places or while covered with perspiration.

Anæmic persons who are disposed to sadness and to keep away from company, must be cheered up by pleasant surroundings, quiet games, entertaining books, theatrical representations, frequent but not too long walks or rides, short journeys, etc.

Baths are only useful to anæmic persons if their temperature is pleasant to them. Experience has shown that baths with a temperature of over 88° F. cause a loss of muscular power and bodily weight in the case of anæmic patients, whereas baths below 50° F. cause chilliness, a loss of animal heat, followed by an excess of reaction. For this reason the best plan to be adopted for such patients is to give them tepid baths between 65 and 85° F. only two or three times a week, and only fifteen to twenty minutes to each bath.

Swimming may be allowed, provided the patients are sufficiently strong, and neither are troubled with cough, nor dyspnœa, nor diarrhœa; the temperature of the river or sea-water must at least be 57 to 60° F., that of the air at least 64; there must be no cool or keen wind, nor must the air be damp or chilly. Hydræmic patients should not bathe under any circumstances.

In high grades of anæmia sexual intercourse is hurtful to persons of either sex; however, if they improve in looks, if they feel more vigorous and frequently experience sexual desires or nocturnal emissions, moderate sexual intercourse is admissible.

The medicinal treatment of anæmia requires a good deal of discretion and judgment on the part of the physician. In selecting a remedy, it is not only of importance that the exciting causes should be carefully investigated, but that the physician should understand whether the anæmia he is called upon to treat, is of a primary or secondary character. A primary anæmia generally admits of a direct treatment and is curable, whereas a secondary anæmia always requires a careful consideration of the primary pathological process, and can only be reached indirectly by homœopathic remedial agents, and not unfrequently resists the most rational and judicious treatment.

A direct anti-anæmic treatment requires, beside the removal of the cause and a suitable diet, the use of such remedies as have it in their power to correct the process of sanguification by their direct influence. We have no universal specific for anæmia. After investigating the various forms of anæmia, their causes and the morbid processes upon which they depend, we are able to avail ourselves of a considerable number of remedies whose effects upon the human organism have been carefully studied, and by their means to obtain favorable results with surprising rapidity even in severe cases where medicinal aid seemed all but useless.

Since the selection of homœopathic remedies for anæmia is principally determined by the nature of the exciting causes and by the resemblance between the remedies and the disease, we have deemed it proper to present the various forms of anæmia and to indicate the special treatment of each of them. By this means we obtain a clearer perception of the various morbid processes, and greater facilities in surveying the list of specially adapted remedial agents.

10. Congenital Anæmia.

Owing to hemorrhages of the mother during pregnancy or during the act of parturition, children are often born anæmic. If they arrive at full term, they generally look fleshy, but in the place of the natural bright flesh-color, the skin has a pale-yellow appearance; the nails and lips likewise look pale, and the sclerotica has a bluish color. Their movements are not very vigorous, their voice is feeble, they do not sleep much, moan a good deal, and nurse very feebly.

Such infants very soon pick up strength at the breast of a healthy wet-nurse whose milk, rendered more nourishing by a good meat-diet and the use of beer, easily and speedily accomplishes the restoration of the red blood-disks.

If anæmic children are at the same time born feeble, they are generally emaciated, look old, wrinkled; they are sometimes so feeble that their moans can scarcely be heard; their weakness is so great that they find it very difficult to take the breast, and sometimes decline doing so.

Such children have to be fed on the nurse's milk by means of a little spoon; otherwise, being too feeble to draw the milk from the breast, they would soon perish of exhaustion; in order to support the deficient nutrition, it is likewise proper to bathe the little ones once a day in tepid cow's-milk. As soon as they have become somewhat more lively and vigorous, we introduce every day the little finger into their mouths for the purpose of ascertaining whether they are able to nurse. If they are strong enough to draw the milk, they may then be put to the breast; by pursuing this course, they generally gain very rapidly.

If anæmic children are born before their full term, they generally sleep a great deal, have a wrinkled skin which is covered with a fine downy hair; they look old, their little nails are soft, the hair on their heads is short, their heads are disproportionately large, their fontanels are far apart, etc.

Such children have to be roused from their sleep quite often, in order to feed them a little nurse's milk by means of a spoon; this should be done at least once every two or three hours, if their vital energy is to be preserved and sufficiently strengthened. The nutrition is likewise sustained by tepid milk-baths and injections of tepid milk or soup; the injections should only be given in small quantities, about half an ounce, in order to secure their retention in the intestinal canal and subsequent absorption.

For purposes of nutrition, the milk of healthy and robust nurses is much better than that of mothers whose milk has become watery in consequence of copious hemorrhages or exhausting diseases, or which has become greatly deprived of its protein constituents.

Congenital anæmia occasioned by diseases of the parents or of the mother alone, is generally very obstinate, frequently continuing during the whole period of dentition and even beyond the period of pubescence. Such children generally cut their teeth at a late period and with difficulty, are frequently attacked with derangements of the digestive functions and of the nervous system, among the nervous disorders are subject to frequent attacks of eclampsia; they begin to run about, and they acquire the use of speech at a late period, generally have a pale and bloated appearance, have weak and thin extremities, a bloated belly; enlargements of the spleen, liver and mesenteric glands are frequent occurrences which are moreover often accompanied by leucæmia; they show great liability to softening of the bones and to scrofulosis, to nasal, bronchial and intestinal catarrhs, to croupous processes and basilar meningitis. The most common results of congenital and protracted anæmia are tuberculosis, scrofulosis, rhachitis and atrophy.

Children afflicted with congenital anæmia should have healthy wet-nurses during the first months, they should be taken out into the open air as often as the weather permits, the use of sugar-tits should be strictly prohibited, nor should they be fed on thick gruel or pap, lest the digestive functions should become disordered; they should never be fed to excess, they should be kept clean and frequently bathed in tepid water. Acute or chronic gastric, intestinal or bronchial catarrhs have to be treated in the manner indicated in their respective chapters; they favor more than anything else the diminution of the red corpuscles.

Sleep is likewise a function of great importance to such children. If they will not sleep at all, or can only be got to sleep with great difficulty, we administer *Calc.* 6, or *Nux vom.* 3, or *Puls.* 3, or *Merc. sol.* 3, a dose every two or three hours.

If the children become exceedingly restless, so that they will not remain in their beds and have to be carried about all the time, the most approved remedies for such a trouble are *Arsen.* 3, *Bellad.* 3, *Ignat.* 3, *Nux vom.* 3, or *Calc.* 6, or *Sulph.* 6.

If, especially during the period of dentition, they frequently start from their sleep and afterwards remain wakeful, we resort to *Chamom.* 3, *Coffea* 3, *Nux vom.* 3, or *Natrum mur.* 6, or *Silic.* 6.

The slow dentition of such children is attended with great delay in the process of ossification; the fontanels remain open for a long time, the skull-bones are thin and fragile, the articular cartilages grow thick and rickety; the vertebral column and the long bones are liable to become curved.

In such cases *Calc.* 6 to 30, two doses a day, is a splendid remedy which speedily regulates the digestive and assimilative functions, thus improving the quality of the blood and visibly promoting the process of ossification. What *Iron* is to chlorosis, *Arsen.* to hydræmia, that *Lime* is to delaying ossification. This remedy is likewise of great value where the skin is bloated, the abdomen meteoristically distended, the extremities are thin, the mesenteric glands swollen and where the patients are at the same time suffering with gastric, nasal or intestinal catarrhs. The continued use of this remedy for several weeks, in increasingly large doses, accompanied by a proper dietetic management, may lead to favorable results even in cases where an hereditary disposition to tuberculosis is present.

If the delay in the process of ossification has already resulted in actual curvatures; if single bones have become hypertrophied, if the angular edges of the long bones have become rounded off like cylinders, if the articular extremities become disproportionately large and the broad bones thick, we may be sure that osteomalacia has set in. In such cases a gelatinous substance is found exuded into the cells of the friable and interstitially distended osseous tissue, in consequence of which the bones not only become distorted, but osteoporosis takes place, or a dilatation of the medullary canals and cells.

Such phenomena find a sovereign remedy in *Silicea* 6 to 30, two doses a day. What *Lime* is to a delaying ossification, that *Silicea* is to osteomalacia. Silicea, by first regulating the digestive and assimilative functions, corrects the composition of the blood and not only secures a reabsorption of the gelatinous mass, but even a perfect ossification.

This remedy likewise renders efficient service in cases of hereditary disposition and, like *Calcarea*, is often administered with advantage in alternation with *Sulphur* 6 to 30.

If *Silicea* is not sufficient, we resort to *Phosphorus* 3 to 6, with which we have obtained the most satisfactory results in the case of feeble and exhausted children who did not acquire the use of their legs until very late. (See the article "Meningitis Spinalis, Spondylitis.")

Children who learn to walk with difficulty or at a late period, must not be made to stand upon their feet; every attempt at making them walk, is an injury to them. It is better for them to lie down as much as possible. Carrying them in a sitting posture or without changing from one arm to another, frequently gives rise to spinal curvatures. To afford them the enjoyment of fresh air, they have to be dragged about lying on their backs in a little carriage.

In all cases of congenital anæmia, country-air and a meat diet are very beneficial.

We have already cautioned parents against overfeeding. In order to keep the children quiet, some parents and nurses are in the habit of keeping them at the breast the whole night. As soon as the children cry a little, they are put to the breast, or tits are put into their mouths, or they are stuffed with farinaceous paps or thick gruels. Even after weaning them, this system of overfeeding is continued; children are constantly eating bread, pieces of boiled potato, cake, etc. These vicious habits are the beginning of imperfect chylification. The habit of keeping the digestive organs constantly employed, leads afterwards to an insatiable voracity. The digestive organs, being constantly excited to an uninterrupted activity, become weak; the children have to vomit frequently, they are suffering from acidity of the stomach, accumulations of phlegm, gastric disorders, painful diarrhœa or flatulent colic, bloated bellies, weakness and thinness of the extremities and other disorders resulting in the final development of scrofulosis, rickets and preparing the road for the invasion of tuberculosis.

Nurselings may be put to the breast every two or three hours; and after they are weaned, children should have their meals at regular periods; between meals they may be allowed to run out and play in the open air. Atmospheric oxygen is as necessary to an improvement of the quality of the blood as adequate nourishment is to sound nutrition. Digestion, says Moleschott, transforms the food into constituents of the blood, atmospheric oxygen transforms the blood-disks into tissue-making substances.

Good food and an abundant supply of pure air are often sufficient to impart to feeble and rickety children an appearance of health and strength.

Exercise in the open air, and more particularly the various juvenile games, throwing the ball, trundling the hoop, jumping the rope, etc., are very much to be commended. Of course, children must be warned against getting heated, or cooling themselves by throwing off some of their clothing, or drinking cold water while heated.

Under similar precautions fishing, hunting, berrying, etc., **may** likewise be permitted, because a moderate exercise of this kind promotes the metamorphosis of the tissues.

Children born of tuberculous parents, or born feeble and sickly, should not be sent to school before they are seven years old; generally such children have bright intellects, but their minds should not be developed at the expense of their bodily health. They had better be taught only a few hours a day; the rest of the day may be devoted to invigorating their constitutions.

As has been said before, congenital anæmia very frequently depends upon some hereditary disposition which, owing to some tuberculous, syphilitic, carcinomatous or other exhausting disease of the parents, or to some chronic uterine disease of the mother, continues far beyond the period of dentition and growth, and, in cases of the sudden invasion of some acute disease, plays an important part. In such cases a single acute local affection frequently constitutes the beginning of a series of changes in adjoining or affiliated organs or systems. A simple nasal catarrh, for instance, may be seen followed by palpebral blennorrhœa, or an inflammation of the conjunctiva of the bulbus may be seen accompanied by the most violent photophobia and by ulcers of the cornea, sometimes by otorrhœa and bronchial catarrh, or diarrhœa, etc.; in short, a whole series of disorders of the mucous lining may break out.

In another case a simple tonsillitis is succeeded by hypertrophy of the tonsils; at the same time the submaxillary, cervical, posterior cervical, axillary and even parotid glands may be seen infiltrated and even erysipelatous, presenting a series of glandular diseases.

A simple pleuritis, pneumonia or bronchitis is often the beginning of a deposition of tubercles in the pleura or lungs; a simple intestinal catarrh is not unfrequently the beginning of subsequent tuberculosis of the intestines and mesenteric glands; a sun-stroke often occasions the outbreak of basilar meningitis.

A simple cold, or excessive fatigue may give rise to spontaneous limping, a fall on the knee to white swelling, a fall or blow on the tibia to periostitis or exostosis, an injury of the nose to ozæna, etc.

For this reason it is of the utmost importance that a physician should observe and appreciate such hereditary dispositions with all the attention they are entitled to. Unfortunately it is often the case that anæmic or feeble children are neglected by their parents; their sickly condition is attributed to dentition, the fact of growth, development, and a physician is only applied to after an acute disease has actually broken out. In such a case the actual disease has to be treated with great discretion, nor ought the hereditary disposition to be left unconsidered. If it should appear to the physician that an acute disease is struggling but imperfectly into a full manifestation, that the disease threatens to assume a chronic form or to pass through a series of other pathological forms, he will have to investigate at once the anamnestic circumstances of the parents and will have to employ such remedies as will weaken or counteract this tendency. Thus the judicious and methodical use of the *Iodide of Potassium* or of the *Muriate of Gold* will correct the syphilitic tendency, that of *Calc.*, *Iodine*, *Sulphur* or Cod-liver oil the tuberculous tendency, that of *Conium* or *Aurum mur. natr.* the tendency to carcinoma. *Ars.* or *Silic.* will remove or correct the sickly disposition of children consequent upon chronic suppurations, blennorrhœas or colliquations of the parents, and will prevent the development of chronic diseases which it may be either difficult or impossible to cure.

It sometimes happens that children who look healthy and plump at birth, in a few days already look pallid and flabby, they cry or moan a good deal, do not sleep well, the lips lose their vermilion hue, the sclerotica assumes a bluish appearance, the features are sharply delineated, the palpebral conjunctiva and the ears look pale, and the muscles lose their tone. In a more advanced stage of this form of anæmia the children look like old people, the muscles grow perceptibly thinner, and on the neck and extremities visible signs of atrophy make their appearance.

An anæmic condition of this kind is most frequently caused by an insufficient supply of milk on the part of the mother or nurse. If the children pass little urine and not as often as they ought to; if they do not go to sleep while nursing; if, after nursing, they grow restless and moan a good deal, let the mother or nurse insert her finger into the child's mouth. If the finger is taken hold of greedily and sucked at, this is a sure sign that the child is hungry and craves more nourishment.

In such a case the breasts should be examined at once. If, on making pressure around the nipple, the milk does not spirt out readily; if the mother is pale and feeble; if she had lost a good deal of blood during parturition or had been sick for a long time during her pregnancy, it becomes at once evident from such circumstances that she cannot possibly afford her infant a sufficient supply of nourishment.

Sometimes there is an abundance of milk in the breasts, but it is watery, like curd, and, when collected in a tumbler with tepid water, it soon mixes up with the water without forming undulating threads or clouds. If the mother had previously lost a good deal of blood or had been afflicted with some severe disease; or if she is subject to paroxysms of mental depression from grief, care, jealousy, anger, etc., the milk loses its nutritive quality, becomes watery, is destitute of protein, and consequently does not nourish the child. In all such cases the child should at once be placed in the care of a sound and strong wet-nurse.

If anæmia sets in notwithstanding the quantity and quality of the milk are perfectly satisfactory, the cause of the trouble must be sought for somewhere else; it may be overfeeding, catarrhal irritations of the stomach, bowels, bronchia, etc., for which we refer the reader to the respective chapters where these diseases are treated of.

For the anæmia and convulsions arising from teething, and the consequent sleeplessness and ptyalism (driveling, drooling), we refer the reader to the chapter on Eclampsia infantum.

The excessive ptyalism is not unfrequently attended with chronic stomatitis or gingivitis. In either case *Merc. solub.* 3 is an excellent remedy; likewise *Calc. carb.* 3 to 6, if the gums are pale, and the children are very nervous, fretful and wakeful.

A too rapid growth sometimes superinduces an anæmic condition attended with muscular debility and sometimes with a liability of the capillary vessels to rupture.

If such children, as they approach the period of puberty, exert themselves beyond their strength, or are exposed to high degrees of temperature, or perform unusual mental efforts, they are often attacked with nosebleed or even hæmoptysis. These symptoms are of special importance in the case of children born of tuberculous parents.

For the treatment of tuberculosis we refer the reader to the chapter on tuberculosis. For the anæmia without great muscular debility or other complications, we generally give two or three daily doses of *Ferr.* 1 with much success. More recently we have made use in many cases of the *syrup of Iron*, of which we give two or three tablespoonfuls a day. This preparation agrees with children who seem to be quite fond of it.

If the muscular debility is not very prominent, we find the above-mentioned preparations of Iron sufficient. If the muscles are very weak, we resort to *Quinine* 1, two or three doses a day. If this remedy is not sufficient to remove the anæmia, we give Quinine and *Ferrum* in alternation, giving *Quinine* one day and *Ferr.* the next; or a dose of *Ferrum* in the morning after breakfast, shortly before dinner a dose of Quinine, another dose of *Ferr.* in the afternoon, and a dose of *Quinine* at night. Either method leads very speedily to a successful result.

For the nosebleed of anæmic individuals, two or three doses of *Crocus* 3 a day proves very efficient. If debility is a prominent symptom, *China* 1 or *Phosphor.* 3 are important remedies which will arrest severe hemorrhages. After the nosebleed ceases, the general treatment of anæmia has to be continued.

For hæmoptysis from excessive walking, dancing, running, ascending eminences, etc., attended with vascular erethism, *Acon.* 3 in solution, a dose every fifteen or thirty minutes, in connection with cold applications to the chest, renders most excellent service.

If, under similar circumstances, the lungs have become wearied by much talking or loud reading, blowing on wind-instruments, etc., and an oppression is felt on the chest, and symptoms of pneumonia threaten, we at once resort to *Phosph.* 3 in solution, a dose every hour or half hour; at the same time we employ cold applications to the chest. We likewise refer the reader to the chapter on hæmoptysis or hemorrhage from the lungs.

Nux vom. 3 may prove a good remedy for the hæmoptysis of anæmic persons, when caused by excessive mental labor or by the abuse of spirits.

For the best means of invigorating the constitution, diet, exercise, occupation, etc., we refer the reader to the chapter on tuberculosis.

For the anæmia of chlorotic persons, the reader is referred to the chapter on Chlorosis.

11. Consecutive Anæmia.

Consecutive anæmia is in every particular case attended with a diminution of fat, decrease of strength and loss of bodily weight. These conditions, together with their exciting causes and consequences, are of great importance for the selection of the right remedy. Among the phenomena which accompany or follow this form of anæmia, we distinguish paroxysms of syncope, spasms, neuralgia, hyperæsthesia, anæsthesia, debility, emaciation, hydræmia.

The treatment of acute anæmia consequent upon severe hemorrhages from the lungs, stomach, bowels, womb, etc., has been indicated in the chapters where these accidents are treated of.

Chronic anæmia, consequent upon repeated losses of blood, even when complicated with hydræmic symptoms, requires *China* 1, from three to four doses a day, if debility is the prominent symptom; and *Ferr. met.* 1, one to three doses a day, if the anæmic symptoms are the most prominent. A strengthening diet, rest and fresh air are likewise indispensable. If both these conditions exist at the same time, we prescribe *China* and *Ferrum* in alternate doses.

For the debility superinduced by sexual excesses we give *Phosphor.* 3 or *China* 1; for anæmia *Phosphori ac.* 1, or *Calc. carb.* 6, or *Puls.* 3; for a disposition to hypochondria or melancholy or habitual constipation or excited sexual passion, *Nux vom.* 3, or *Plat.* 6; for dyspepsia *Nux vom.* 3, or *Puls.* 3, or *Sepia* 6, two or three doses a day. The cure is hastened by complete abstemiousness and cold bathing.

For debility from excessive nursing we give *China* 1, or *Phosphori ac.* 1; for anæmia, *Calc.* 6 or *Puls.* 3; for oppression on the chest, *Phos.* 3; for vaginal blennorrhœa, *Sep.* 6; for a high degree of anæmia, *Ferr. lact.* or *met.* 1. Of course the nursing must be at once discontinued and a strengthening diet be pursued.

For anæmia after profuse suppurations, with debility, emaciation or hydræmic symptoms, we give *Ars.* 3, with fistulous ulcers *Silic.* 6, with suppurations of glands *Hep. sulph.* 3 or *Iodine* 3 or *Silic.* 6, with chronic caries *Silic.* 6 or *Asaf.* 3, or *Lycop.* 6; with cutaneous suppurations *Hep.* 3 or *Silic.* 6.

Anæmia, consequent upon profuse perspiration, yields to *China* 1, or *Phosp.* 3, and sometimes to *Calc.* 6. At the same time we have the body rubbed twice a day with dilute brandy or a very weak solution of Phosphorus, one drachm of the first dilution to six ounces of distilled water.

For anæmia from excessive diarrhœa, with rapid emaciation, debility, disposition to relapses, we give *Ars.* 3; and if the pulse is small, quick, with audible purring through the veins, we resort to two or three daily doses of the *Acetate* or *Sulphate* of *Iron*.

Anæmia after excessive vomiting is met by *Ars.* 3.

Anæmia after profuse ptyalism generally yields to *China* 1 or *Quinine* 1, two or three daily doses.

Anæmia after excessive walking, running, dancing, etc., is met by *Arnica* 1, a few doses a day, together with frictions with a solution of Arnica. *Ruta* may be employed in a similar manner. *Rhus tox.* is indicated if the weary limbs feel lamed and they can only be moved with difficulty.

For anæmia caused by excessive mental exertions we depend upon *Calc.* 6 or *Nux vom.* 3; in obstinate cases upon *Sepia* 6.

Anæmia from nervous sleeplessness is generally attended with cerebral erethism, for which we give *Cocc.* 3, *Nux vom.* 3, and chiefly *Ignat.* 3, two or three doses a day.

12. Secondary Anæmia.

Secondary anæmia may occur as an accompaniment of various constitutional diseases, such as tuberculosis, chlorosis, syphilis, carcinoma, glandular diseases, diabetes melitus, Bright's disease, round ulcer of the stomach, etc. Such forms of anæmia require no special treatment; they disappear together with the constitutional malady upon which they depend. H.]

13. Marasmus, Tabes.

[This anomaly of the functions of nutrition consists in a perceptible decrease of the normal roundness and fulness of the body.

Primarily marasmus arises in consequence of congenital debility, a deficient supply of nourishment, excessive bodily or mental labor, continued mental depression, sexual excesses, self-abuse, continued sitting, too frequent confinements. Very often the cause is unknown.

Secondarily this disease may be superinduced by excessive secretion, seminal losses, excessive perspiration, ptyalism, excessive nursing, long-lasting diarrhœa, blennorrhœa, diabetes melitus, continued losses of blood, chronic suppurations or discharges of ichor, exhausting diseases, pyæmia, cancer, syphilis, tuberculosis, long-lasting intermittents, etc.

Marasmus likewise arises in consequence of chronic blood-poisoning, by *Arsen.*, *Lead*, *Mercury*, etc., or in consequence of exhausted strength, most frequently in childhood and old age; it may likewise occur in consequence of continued nervous irritability, sleeplessness, chronic febrile conditions, etc.

Marasmus is chiefly characterized by a gradual or rapid emaciation, disappearance of the adipose tissue, a wrinkled skin, flabbiness of the muscles. The skin is mostly dry, extenuated, wrinkled, rough and scaly, without turgor or elasticity; at times it is yellowish, at other times strikingly pale, or cachectic; at times it is covered with local or colliquative perspiration; the hair on the head falls out more and more, the nails become curved and brittle, the extremities are mostly cool, the patients frequently complain of a feeling of coldness and cannot get warm.

At times the appetite is great, increasing even to canine hunger, but the hunger is soon appeased and digestion takes place very slowly. At other times the patients experience an irresistible aversion to meat or certain kinds of food. In most cases the thirst is increased.

The breath is often fetid, the gums are atrophied, the teeth are denuded, and gradually become loose and fall out.

The voice is feeble and without resonnance, the respiration is frequently normal, but often oppressed, and after the least bodily exertion dyspnœa and palpitation of the heart set in. The breasts become pendulous and flabby, the abdomen is at times sunken, at other times distended; the bowels are at times loose, at other times constipated, and again dysenteric; the urine is mostly secreted in small quantities and saturated, the genital organs become atrophied and the sexual instinct is either diminished or becomes entirely extinct. The pulse is small and feeble, sleep fatiguing rather than refreshing, sometimes it is very much disturbed; the patients are either hypochondriac or irascible; sometimes they show much apathy or obstinacy, their memory is weakened, their behavior is often childish and vacillating. The muscles are flabby and atrophied, and the strength becomes less and less.

The disease may last months or years; in some cases marasmus progresses at a rapid rate to a fatal termination.

Recovery can only be obtained if the exciting causes can be removed; however, it takes place very slowly, sometimes with frequent interruptions and disposition to relapses.

Wounds, ulcers, abscesses, etc., heal slowly and with difficulty; accidental diseases run a slow course which inclines to become chronic. If the patients are compelled to remain in a recumbent posture, hypostatic inflammations are very apt to set in.

According to the nature of the cause and of existing complications, death may take place by anæmia, hydræmia, dropsy, pyæmia, embolism, gangrene, etc.

The prognosis is favorable only if the disease remains after severe diseases, losses of blood and other animal fluids, excessive exertions, etc. The marasmus of children is likewise a curable disease, provided the causes can be removed.

In marasmus senilis, and in the marasmus consequent upon incurable diseases, such as tuberculosis, carcinoma, diabetes, caries, diseases of the brain or spinal marrow, etc., the prognosis is unfavorable.

Treatment. Marasmus scarcely ever sets in without anæmia to which we refer the reader for further details, more particularly consecutive anæmia and the anæmia inherent in the period of involution.

The marasmus consequent upon intermittent fevers is always accompanied with malarial cachexia, the treatment of which has been indicated in the chapter on intermittent fever.

Marasmus senilis is almost always complicated with anæmia. It occurs either between the years of forty and fifty (marasmus præcox, premature old age), or after the age of sixty or seventy years. For the treatment of marasmus præcox we refer the reader to the treatment of the anæmia of involution; as regards the marasmus of old people, we treat it according to its symptomatic indications.

If the anæmia is not very considerable; if the loss of muscular or adipose tissue is attended with great debility, disposition to sleep in the day-time, feeble impulse and sounds of the heart, with oppression on the chest, dyspnœa after slight exertions, disposition to painful diarrhœa, we recommend *Phosphor.* 3, a dose every two hours.

This admirable remedy acts much better upon such symptoms than Quinine; it quickens the circulation, invigorates the digestive functions, regulates the alvine evacuations, and is likewise indicated if the patients are attacked with vertigo when walking, stooping, closing their eyes, turning the head, with a sensation as if they had to tumble over to one side or the other.

If the patients are weak and anæmic, dyspeptic with disposition to constipation, hypochondriac, irascible; if they are subject to vertigo and nausea; if their gait is unsteady and dragging, we give *Nux vom.* 3 every two hours, until these symptoms improve, after which we give *Quinine* with excellent effect. *Ferrum carbon.* or *metal.* may likewise be given after Nux. In such a case we give these remedies in daily alternation with excellent effect.

For obstinate dyspeptic symptoms without any symptoms of gastric or intestinal catarrh, we have sometimes given *Pepsin*, in doses of three to five grains.

Arsen. 3, a dose every two or three hours, may be employed in cases of anæmia if the patients are very feeble, faint frequently, are dyspeptic and thirsty, restless at night, so that they have to get up and walk about; this remedy is eminently proper if hectic fever has set in, with fetor from the mouth and large ecchymoses on the lower extremities. A small and feeble pulse, cold extremities, painless and cadaverously smelling diarrhœic stools, œdema of the lower extremities are further indications for *Ars.* which may still afford help in the most desperate cases.

If this remedy is not sufficient, we resort to *Chininum arsenicosum* 1, three to four doses a day, and order small quantities of pure old wine to be taken during the intervals.

In all cases of incipient or far advanced marasmus, a strengthening diet is of the utmost importance. We recommend broth, extract of beef, old wine, if possible old claret, Malaga, Port or Tokay in small quantities either pure or diluted with water; good porter is likewise appropriate. The patients must be kept warm, especially the feet, lest other diseases should supervene. Country and mid-mountain air, the use of strengthening springs and, if the lower extremities are very weak, the use of electricity by induction, are powerful adjuvants during the treatment and promote a cure. H.]

14. Obesitas, Adiposis, Polysarcia, Obesity.

An excessive accumulation of fat is a morbid condition that may be attended with a variety of important derangements.

A disposition to obesity is at times congenital, at other times hereditary; it frequently occurs already in childhood; it is much less frequent after the period of pubescence is passed and is most frequently noticed in advanced manhood. As a rule, women are more frequently subject to fatness than men.

An accumulation of fat in the subcutaneous cellular tissue is often so excessive that the skin is an inch in thickness and the circumference of the body becomes monstrous. The thickest layers of fat are found on the breasts, abdomen and thighs. There are fat persons weighing from four to six hundred pounds.

Adiposis presupposes a peculiar disposition; many persons can eat and drink as much as they please, they remain thin nevertheless; many, on the contrary, eat scantily, are a prey to depressing emotions, and yet grow or remain fat.

Excessive fatness may be caused by a too copious supply of food, or too much fat or substantial food, and a simultaneous deficiency of exercise in the open air; drinking beer and spirits to excess; sleeping too long; mental indolence; abstemiousness from sexual intercourse, want of active labor, disposition to idleness, a phlegmatic temperament.

An excessive deposition of fat may likewise be occasioned by castration, or at the critical age, after severe diseases, etc.

An accumulation of fat in the subcutaneous cellular tissue generally takes place very gradually: single parts of the body grow fuller and rounder, the white or yellowish skin becomes smooth and, in consequence of the increased secretion of sebum, glistens like fat and has a fatty feel. The more the body increases in volume, the more numerous become the semi-circular furrows in various parts of the body, for instance in the umbilical region, in the middle of the thighs, at the nape of the neck, under the chin. If the accumulation of fat becomes excessive, the neck vanishes more and more, the abdomen bulges very strikingly, and the gluteal region expands more and more in breadth and becomes more and more repulsive. In consequence of the excessive fulness of the abdomen, the diaphragm is pushed up more and more, and the cavity of the thorax being encroached upon, the lungs are compressed. The natural consequence of this condition is a striking dyspnœa with which very fat persons are more or less afflicted. This dyspnœa embarrasses them in walking, going upstairs, ascending an eminence or performing the slightest bodily labor. Fat persons generally have to lie on their backs, in which position they snore, have frightful dreams which often cause them to cry out suddenly as if tormented by anxiety. The compression of the lungs, the encroachment upon the thoracic cavity and the consequent dyspnœa cause disturbances in the circulation characterized by palpitation of the heart, syncope, determination of blood to the head or liver, stomach, kidneys, uterus, etc.

At the commencement of the disease, the digestion is generally very active and frequently degenerates in canine hunger; after the fatness has acquired a high degree, the patients often become dyspeptic, are tormented by flatulence, acidity of the stomach, eructations. In consequence of the resulting congestion of the stomach and liver, the slightest meal leads to oppression of the stomach and nausea which frequently increases to sour or bilious vomiting. Such patients are not troubled with costiveness, and frequently have two or three papescent evacuations in the course of the day. The urine is frequently cloudy, opalescent; after bodily work, the emission of urine is attended with a burning sensation in the urethra, and a quantity of uric acid is deposited.

The perspiration has a peculiar, sometimes a rancid smell, or like the odor of a goat. In the above-mentioned semi-circular furrows or folds the frequent sweating causes an erythema which afterwards changes to a moist and exceedingly fetid intertrigo. This may likewise take place under the breasts, between the thighs and pudendum, and even at the anus.

The pulse is mostly feeble, small and easily compressible, the sensitiveness to cold is much less, the menses are scanty, the sexual instinct frigid or even extinct; women are often sterile.

As a rule, fat persons are indolent, apathetic; they dread bodily exercise, even a little mental labor; their muscles are deficient in tone, their senses are dull, their intellect is torpid, and they are inclined to sleep.

These phenomena are not, however, without exception; a great many fat persons remain quick, of active mind and body; we have known a fat old gentleman who danced more vigorously than his young associates and, not feeling tired, at the same time entertained his company with the most piquant anecdotes.

Polysarcia is frequently attended with a disposition to parasitical growths, such as lipoma, cancerous depositions, or with a tendency to scurvy or dropsy.

While teething, fat children are in danger from congestions of the head. It is very seldom that they live to an old age. Fat persons are often suddenly struck down with apoplexy and paralysis of the heart. Intercurrent diseases often assume a dangerous character on account of the existing disturbances in the respiration and circulation. Fat persons are frequently anæmic; in such a case, especially after severe diseases, hydræmic conditions frequently develop themselves which it is difficult to distinguish from morbid fatness. Fat persons are frequently attacked with boils and carbuncles; the latter frequently run a dangerous course, causing vast destructions in the subcutaneous cellular tissue. Acute diseases are often succeeded by dropsy or marasmus.

On this account a good deal of cautious reserve should be used in establishing a prognosis in high grades of polysarcia, more especially if an atheromatous degeneration of the blood-vessels or a fatty degeneration of the heart may be suspected.

Treatment. An excessive deposition of fat is an anomaly in the sphere of nutrition which, in our opinion, depends upon a weakness of the assimilative functions. In the case of children it is frequently caused by over-feeding, and in the case of adults an excessive supply of nourishment is likewise the frequent cause of fatness. In either case the overloading of the digestive organs weakens them, the food is not adequately transformed into firm constituents, such as muscular fibre, osseous tissue, but, remaining at a low stage of assimilation, is transformed into carbo-hydrates.

Starting from this point of view, the treatment of adiposis should, in our judgment, aim at invigorating the assimilative energy of the organism and at the same time preventing an excessive supply of fat-making food.

It is a well-known fact that adiposis cannot be arrested by any known method of treatment. For, independently of the weakness of the assimilative functions, we frequently have to contend against other congenital, hereditary or individual, known or unknown tendencies which favor the excessive deposition of fat and which it is either difficult or impossible to control.

For this reason, when treating polysarcia, we confine ourselves to such dietetic and hygienic measures as will quicken the metamorphosis of the tissues and invigorate the assimilative functions; at the same time we resort to such internal remedies as will correct constitutional tendencies and promote nutrition.

In order to accomplish this object with as much speed and certainty as possible, we prescribe regular meals and a moderate diet, but sufficient to satisfy the appetite; such patients had better confine themselves to lean and young meat, with fresh vegetables and salad, and abstain from rich soups, fat gravies, fat farinaceous food, fat fish, potatoes, beans and peas, quantities of bread, beer, spirits; they must likewise avoid coffee, tea and tobacco, for these substances retard digestion and interfere with the metamorphosis of the tissues. The best beverage for such patients is fresh water, or wine and water, acidulated alkaline beverages with or without wine, water mixed with acidulated jellies. For breakfast we recommend weak beef-broth or vegetable soups without fat, or skimmed milk with a little sugar; eggs and chocolate have to be avoided, they contain too much fatty matter. For dessert we permit fresh or stewed fruit, and for supper a light soup and stewed fruit. Food spiced with a little pepper agrees with such patients, provided it is not fat. Water-ices are likewise allowable, ice-cream is too rich and must be avoided.

Together with these dietetic arrangements which have to be strictly obeyed if they are to do any good, the following rules are of special importance. In order to stimulate the metamorphosis of the tissues and secure the introduction of as much oxygen as possible into the organism, fat persons should walk or ride on horseback whenever their time and circumstances will permit; riding in a carriage is of no use to them; active exercise in the open air, especially in the morning and evening, promotes in a high degree the assimilation of food and the metamorphosis of the tissues. It is well if, during their walk, they frequently drink cold water, rest a little when tired and then continue their walk. The more exercise they take in the open air, the more healthy the blood becomes and the more the fat disappears. They had better sleep as little as possible, and avoid inaction as much as they can. Active exercise at home, while attending to their domestic affairs, is advisable; idleness promotes the deposition of fat. Swimming, riding on horseback, hunting, cold ablutions, cold baths, in bad weather walking up and down in the room at a rapid rate; gymnastic exercises, if resorted to in systematic order, impart great activity to the metamorphosis of the tissues.

These measures, if carried out strictly, are often alone sufficient to arrest the tendency to fatness and diminish the amount of fat. The so-called panting-cure, which has been frequently resorted to in modern times, rests almost upon the same principles and has produced good results in some cases. In pursuing a strict diet, the main point is for the patients to persevere until the mass of fat has considerably decreased and they have gained in agility and ease of motion. In pursuing a dietetic treatment, the bodily strength increases instead of diminishing, the blood does not grow paler but it attains a higher degree of oxygenation, and the weight and circumference of the body decrease, whereas all the physical and psychical functions become more animated.

In conducting the internal treatment, we pay particular attention to the disturbances in the respiration and circulation, the functions of the stomach and intestinal canal, the quality of the blood and the other coexisting abnormal symptoms.

Fat persons are often short-breathed, especially when going upstairs or performing the slightest bodily work, or walking a little faster than usual. In such cases a careful exploration of the thorax and abdomen becomes indispensable. If, on percussing the region of the heart, we discover a dulness over a larger surface, the impulse of the heart remaining vigorous and the sounds of the heart loud and distinct, we infer the existence of a larger abnormal deposition of fat about the heart or in the mediastinum, in consequence of which the thoracic cavity becomes contracted and the normal expansion of the lungs is interfered with. For these symptoms we give *Arnica* 2, from six to ten drops in half a pint of water, a dessertspoonful every two or three hours. At the same time we recommend the diet that has already been pointed out as most conducive to persons suffering with adiposis. By continuing this treatment for weeks, at intervals of two or three days, we have restored patients to an apparently perfect state of health. Whether the Arnica acts by diminishing the pressure of the fat upon the heart, or bringing about a reabsorption of the fat-molecules, remains an open question.

If the dulness in the cardiac region is attended with feebleness of the impulse, and if the sounds of the heart are likewise less distinct, we infer a fatty metamorphosis of the heart, for the treatment of which we refer the reader to the article on fatty degeneration of the heart.

If the fatty degeneration is accompanied by dilatation of the heart and pulmonary emphysema, we pursue the treatment recommended for emphysema.

If the patient is dyspeptic, the abdomen meteoristically distended, the region of the stomach bulges, the liver, spleen and the heart are pressed upwards; if the stomach is acid, and nausea and vomiting are complained of, the first thing to be done is that a strict diet should be rigidly enforced. Such derangements generally arise from luxurious living or the abuse of spirits. Persons who are in the habit of using spirits, may gradually be weaned from this indulgence by diluting their drinks. A sudden and total deprivation often superinduces an injurious weakness. Internally we give *Nux vom.* 3, or *Natr. mur.* 6, or *Carbo veg.* 6, two or three doses a day, until the abdomen becomes softer, the breathing easier, the appetite keener and the diaphragm has resumed its natural position.

If the abdomen is not meteoristically distended, the region of the stomach does not bulge, and the other symptoms continue the same, the abdominal integuments are very thick, the bowels are torpid and the hemorrhoidal veins somewhat swollen, it is simply the mass of fat accumulated in the abdominal integuments, in the mesentery and in the omentum, which contracts the abdominal cavity and, by pushing up the diaphragm, causes the above-mentioned difficulties. These can be remedied by strictly following the dietetic measures suggested in a previous paragraph. Internally we persevere in the systematic use of *Capsicum* 2 or 3, and have obtained handsome results by this means.

Attention has likewise to be paid to the liver. This viscus is likewise liable to fatty degeneration giving rise to digestive derangements, dyspnœa, pressure in the epigastrium. The treatment for fatty liver has been indicated in the chapter on diseases of the liver.

Other conditions which sometimes accompany fatty degenerations of internal viscera, or adiposis generally, such as: hyperæmia of the liver, palpitation of the heart, fainting fits, sudden rush of blood to the head or chest and other symptoms of plethora; anæmia, dyspepsia, intertrigo, etc., require the same treatment as is found indicated in the respective chapters where these conditions are spoken of.

Adiposis is sometimes benefitted by the use of mineral springs. Patients of this kind should never visit spas for purposes of health without the advice and consent of their family-physician. Chalybeate springs may be advisable in some cases; in others Sulphur springs, in others effervescent waters, and in others again Iodine springs. In all cases let the diet and general hygiene of the patient be regulated by his physician. H.]

15. Uræmia.

[*Anatomical Characteristics.* The cadavers of uræmic patients do not exhibit any striking alterations by which the grave symptoms during the course of the disease could be satisfactorily accounted for. The brain and spinal marrow do not show any pathological alterations of tissue, nor any constantly occurring anomalies in the condition of their blood and vessels. The lungs are sometimes infiltrated as in pneumonia, the bowels are injected, sometimes covered with follicular ulcerations, the kidneys are frequently hyperæmic, or inflamed, or degenerated. The serous effusions which not unfrequently occur in the extremities, as well as the mucus of the stomach and the secretions in the lungs have been found to produce an alkaline reaction and to contain ammonia.

The blood sometimes has a violet color and, in many cases, shows greater coagulability and an increase of fibrin.

According to Frerichs, the blood contains in all cases where the characteristic symptoms of uræmia are present, carbonate of ammonia in varying quantities, sometimes manifesting its presence by its disagreeable odor and at other times effervescing by the addition of muriatic acid.

Uræmia.

Etiology. Uræmia is only observed in the course of other diseases. It may be caused by obstructions in the secretion of urine, as may occur during an intense hyperæmia of the kidneys, nephritis, extensive infiltration of the renal canaliculi in Bright's disease, in the course of scarlatina, etc.; or in degeneration of the kidneys by renal calculi, carcinoma, atrophy, etc., or during the shrinking of the substance of the kidneys in old people; or it may be caused by obstructions in the excretion of the urine, in consequence of pressure upon both ureters, or in consequence of obstacles at the sphincter of the bladder or in the urethra, as in the case of stone or gravel, or from hypertrophy of the prostate, strictures of the urethra, etc.

Uræmia may likewise occur during the last months of pregnancy, during or after parturition, in the course of scarlatina, cholera, etc., or from effusion of the urine between the tissues as during operations, wounds, injuries, perforations, etc.

Symptoms. According to the course and intensity of the symptoms we distinguish acute and chronic uræmia.

Acute uræmia is almost always preceded by a diminished secretion of urine, or the secretion of urine meets with difficulties or is obstructed; at times there is only a reabsorption of the urine in consequence of effusion of urine into the cellular tissue. The first signs of uræmic intoxication of the blood often consist in vomiting and diarrhœa, or only in vomiting, sometimes in apathy and drowsiness, or in headache with vomiting, weakness of sight and bland delirium; or convulsions and amaurosis set in all at once, and are commonly followed by uræmia of the highest degree of intensity. At other times the invasion of uræmia takes place with a violent chill followed by intense fever with typhoid symptoms. If cerebral symptoms set in, they generally point to the presence of adynamia; we notice a dulness of perception, a difficulty of collecting one's mind, stupefaction, somnolence or a deep sopor; the delirium is generally of the bland or moaning kind. In rare cases only there is great restlessness, an excited state of the mind, loud delirium, desire to escape, etc. The cerebral symptoms are frequently associated with amblyopia, vertigo, mistiness of sight, or even real amaurosis, deficient irritability of the pupil with hardness of hearing and buzzing in the ears, gritting of the teeth or trismus. The buccal cavity and teeth are generally dry, the thirst is very moderate, the appetite is entirely gone, the voice is rough or husky, the respiration accelerated, dyspnœic or stertorous. The expired air has often the smell of urea or contains traces of ammonia.

The abdomen is distended, at times the distention is but trifling, at other times meteoristic, the alvine evacuations are frequently diarrhœic, the skin is either dry or covered with a perspiration that has the smell of urea, or with a fine dust consisting of urea; in some cases petechiæ or miliary vesicles make their appearance. The pulse is always very hurried and small, some times irregular and filiform. Towards the end of the disease, spasmodic tremors, muscular jactitations, subsultus tendinum and an automatic grasping and feeling around, with continued coma, tracheal rattling and finally paralysis of the sphincters set in.

Chronic uræmia develops itself gradually during continued derangements or obstructions in the secretion of urine, or in consequence of a continued decomposition of the urine that had remained behind in the urinary ducts. Chronic uræmia is characterized by such phenomena as the following: Sickly, anæmic appearance; continued loss of appetite, generally with a thickly-coated tongue; aversion to meat, dryness of the mouth; an increase of thirst, generally with a desire for sour or cooling things; increasing lassitude, drowsiness; slowness of speech and thought, apathy and forgetfulness; constantly increasing dyspnœa, muscular debility and emaciation; costiveness or serous diarrhœa; dryness and sometimes violent itching of the skin which not unfrequently appears studded with eczema, lichen, ecthyma, etc.; asthmatic difficulties, serous catarrh, œdema of the lungs, finally anasarca and general dropsy in consequence of the constantly increasing marasmus.

Course, Terminations, Prognosis. Acute uræmia sometimes runs a very rapid course, striking the patient down with the suddenness of lightning: if, in the course of Bright's disease, scarlatina, in the last days of pregnancy, previous to or subsequent to confinement, etc., the urine is suddenly retained or is reabsorbed in consequence of an effusion of urine into the cellular tissue; or if the urine remains stagnant, and an ammoniacal decomposition of this fluid takes place: vomiting, eclampsia or amaurosis set in, phenomena which are so speedily followed by a deep sopor, continued convulsions or symptoms of paralysis of the brain, that death may result in a few hours or only at the expiration of one or two days.

In the majority of cases the disease runs a less rapid course. The symptoms manifest themselves gradually, sometimes diminish and then increase again in intensity, according as the disturbance in the secretion and excretion of the urine improves or gets worse.

Severe cases are characterized by a constantly increasing stupor or sopor, or by an increase of the typhoid symptoms. Cases which set in with symptoms of cerebral irritation and bear some resemblance to meningitis, occur much less frequently. The existing disturbances in the urinary secretions and excretions shed light on the diagnosis. The more violent the symptoms of uræmia, the shorter the course of the disease; the milder the symptoms, the more chronic its course.

The worst cases occur if, in consequence of retention, stagnation or effusion of urine into the cellular tissue, the urine is decomposed and the blood is poisoned with carbonate of ammonia; this infection is designated by Treitz as *ammoniæmia*.

Considerable quantities of urea and carbonate of ammonia are not only found in the blood, but likewise in the stomach, intestinal canal and other secretory organs. The presence of carbonate of ammonia in the stomach is manifested by copious vomiting of substances that have an ammoniacal odor.

If the uræmic blood is decomposed in the intestinal canal or is decomposed already when entering the circulation: watery diarrhœic stools take place having the odor of ammonia; or else a dysenteric process sets in, attended with a diphtheritic or gangrenous destruction of the mucous membrane of the large intestine and of imminent peril to the preservation of vitality. The buccal mucous membrane frequently exhibits scurfy exfoliations spreading down into the throat, in consequence of which the voice becomes husky and sometimes extinct as in the case of cholera-patients. The saliva, the milk in the breasts, the perspiration contain carbonate of ammonia and have the odor of ammonia. The expired air likewise spreads an odor of urine and ammonia. The skin is frequently seen covered with a whitish ammoniacal dust, crystals of urea and the chloride of sodium.

The irritating action of Ammonia upon the various organs frequently causes a momentary hyperæmia of the brain which very soon results in sopor; in the lungs an intense catarrh or croupous inflammation develops itself; effusions rapidly set in in the pleura, pericardium, peritoneum and in the ventricles of the brain: the stagnation and decomposition of the urine in the bladder frequently lead to inflammations and suppurations of the vesical lining membrane, or to depositions of pus between the different layers of the bladder, in consequence of which the symptoms of ammoniæmia and pyæmia may appear together. If renal dropsy is at the same time present, the accumulations of serum under the skin and the various transudations contain urea and carbonate of ammonia.

The course of ammoniæmia is either acute or chronic; its symptoms bear the greatest resemblance to uræmia with which it is frequently confounded. The above-mentioned pathognomonic symptoms give the exact diagnostic distinctions between these two conditions. Uræmic symptoms frequently occur without any symptoms of ammoniæmia; but the latter never exist without the former.

Acute ammoniæmia likewise sometimes runs its course with the suddenness of lightning, especially in the case of anæmic and exceedingly debilitated patients. Vomiting sets in, or vomiting and diarrhœa, or diarrhœa without vomiting, or else a sudden dysentery followed by a rapidly increasing sopor and death in twelve, twenty-four or forty-eight hours. In most cases acute ammoniæmia, if it runs a moderate course, lasts a few weeks; but the possibility of sudden effusions into the pleura, pericardium, cerebral ventricles, etc.: the possible supervention of croupous pneumonia or acute œdema of the lungs, etc., impart a high degree of danger to the disease. Chills frequently occur during the course of acute ammoniæmia, frequently with typical regularity and bearing a highly deceptive resemblance to intermittent fever.

Chronic uræmia as well as chronic ammoniæmia may last months and even years; they may get better and worse again according as the determining causes decrease or increase in virulence. The worst cases generally occur in consequence of ischuria or anuria. If the desire to urinate can be restored, the danger is momentarily removed.

Dryness of the mucous membrane of the mouth and fauces, " as though every atom of moisture had been absorbed by blotting paper, the mucous membrane appearing dry and glistening;" hoarseness or even aphonia; the plainly ammoniacal odor of the expired air; a constant aversion to meat; livid color of the skin, a progressive emaciation and muscular debility constitute, according to Professor Jaksch, reliable diagnostic signs of ammoniæmia which are very seldom observed in cases of uræmia. Convulsions, amaurosis and dropsy have never been seen by Jaksch in the course of ammoniæmia. However, since this condition never occurs except in the course of uræmia, we hold that the above-described phenomena may likewise characterize a condition of uræmia.

Light and moderate, even severe and very acute cases of uræmia and ammoniæmia frequently terminate in recovery, provided the obstacles which impede the excretion of urine, can be removed. These diseases, however, are peculiarly liable to relapses in which case very serious accidents may occur.

Cases setting in with a sudden and crushing violence, almost always terminate fatally.

Paralysis of the brain, croupous pneumonia or dysentery with gangrenous destruction of the intestinal mucous membrane, or serous effusions into the various cavities of the body, or a high degree of marasmus and general dropsy frequently lead to a fatal termination.

In cases of great intensity the prognosis is most commonly unfavorable.

In mild cases of uræmia and ammoniæmia the prognosis depends upon the possibility of removing the disturbance of the urinary secretion and excretion either totally or partially. This condition likewise applies to the chronic form of uræmia or ammoniæmia.

The access of convulsions or amaurosis is generally a very bad prognostic.

Vomiting and serous diarrhœa sometimes constitute a favorable prognostic symptom in the course of ammoniæmia, for the reason that quantities of the carbonate of ammonia are often excreted by this means. If croupous pneumonia, œdema of the lungs, dysentery and a deep sopor set in, the prognosis is doubtful.

Treatment. Whenever the secretion and excretion of urine is interfered with or entirely obstructed, the cautious physician will at once be reminded of the possibility of a sudden or gradual development of uræmic symptoms. These can only be prevented by the speediest possible restoration of the excretion of urine either by the use of internal remedies or by mechanical means or by an operation.

In very acute cases where the disease develops its symptoms with extraordinary rapidity; where the vomiting, or a paroxysm of eclampsia, or the sudden invasion of amaurosis is speedily followed by deep sopor, any kind of treatment is in the majority of cases utterly powerless. If we do not soon succeed in securing an outlet to the stagnant urine and, by means of an appropriate medicine which has to be repeated again and again at short intervals, removing the sopor and the accompanying paralytic condition of the brain, the patients are irretrievably doomed.

If such symptoms make their appearance during the act of parturition or in the last period of pregnancy, they are caused by the obstructed excretion of urine consequent upon the pressure of the gravid uterus upon the ureters and bladder. In such very acute cases the patient can only be saved by bold measures: artificial delivery should at once be resorted to, after which the urine is drawn off with the catheter. A dose of *Hyosc.* 3, or *Opium* 3, or *Hydrocyan. ac.* 3, or *Lactuca virosa* 3, may be given every five, ten or fifteen minutes. In a case of this kind, occurring immediately after confinement, where the symptoms of acute uræmia developed themselves with fearful rapidity, the patient was at once relieved by the application of cold compresses to the region of the distended bladder. The organ contracted and the urine was expelled with the fierceness of a torrent. The case occurred in Dr. Hempel's practice.

If the jaws are locked, the medicine may be administered subcutaneously. If no improvement sets in in one hour, a second, and a third remedy, etc., may be injected, etc. This is the only way of preventing a fatal issue.

In the course of scarlatina, uræmic symptoms may set in with sudden violence in consequence of croupous nephritis resulting in a sudden obstruction of the urinary canal, with plastic exudation. Here, help can only be afforded by the speedy removal of the inflammatory process in the kidneys. For this purpose we give every ten minutes a dose of *Hepar sulph. calc.* 3 or *Kali hydriod.* 1. If the exhibition of these remedies for two or three hours results in a more copious diuresis with numerous fibrinous casts, life may be saved.

If symptoms of cerebral hyperæmia prevail, we give *Bellad.* or *Atropin.*, *Apis*, *Stramon.* or *Conium* 3.

If sopor is most prominent, we resort to *Bellad.*, *Lact. vir.*, *Agar.*, or *Anac.* 3.

For anæmic and paralytic symptoms we give *Arsen.* 3, *China* 1 or *Chinin. arsen.* 1, or *Phosph.* 3, *Phosph.* 1 or 2, or *Camphor.* 3.

For very acute strangury, with scanty and hot urine, or discharges of the urine drop by drop, and if the urine is mixed with albumen or blood, *Cantharis* 3 is appropriate.

Chronic uræmia generally occurs with vomiting, constant loss of appetite, coated tongue and aversion to certain kinds of food; it is generally mistaken for catarrh of the stomach and treated accordingly. In atony of the urinary bladder, hypertrophy of the walls of this viscus or of the prostate; in strictures of the urethra, etc., the excretion of urine, according to the statement of the patients, not unfrequently takes place without much difficulty. The apparently gastric phenomena continue, however, in spite of the most careful medicinal treatment, and gradually increase in intensity. In such cases the statements of the patients must not be depended upon, but the bladder must be carefully explored immediately after an emission of urine. Almost in every case of this kind a larger or smaller quantity of urine will be found left in the bladder; as long as this urine is pure and undecomposed, it only causes uræmic symptoms; but as soon as ammonia develops itself in this urine, and the fluid becomes cloudy, acrid and spreads a fetid odor, ammoniæmic symptoms make their appearance.

In such cases it is absolutely necessary to draw off the urine at least twice a day with the catheter in order that all stagnation of urine may be prevented. At the same time the difficulty causing the retention of urine, such as the torpor of the detrusor urinæ muscle, the hypertrophy of the prostate, urethral strictures, etc., has to be treated with appropriate homœopathic or surgical means, for which we refer to the chapter on diseases of the Urinary Organs.

We have already stated that, if the cerebral symptoms are very prominent, such as headache with vomiting, dryness of the mouth, bland delirium and somnolence, we either administer *Bellad.* or *Atropin.* or likewise *Hyosc.* 3.

If the gastric symptoms prevail, with aversion to meat, we give *Sulph.* 6, *Sepia* 6, *Natrum carb.* 6, or *Puls.* 3.

If the anæmia and muscular debility are far advanced, with dryness in the mouth, extensive anasarca, incipient effusion into the pleural cavity or pericardium, etc., we use *Arsen.* 3, or *Chinin. arsen.* 1 to 2, or *Lachesis* 6.

If there is a particular tendency to serous diarrhœa, we resort to *Phosph.* 3, or *Arsen.* 3, or *Argent. nitr.* 3.

Dysenteric symptoms yield very rapidly to *Corr. subl.* 2 to 3, *Hepar s.* 3, or *Sulph.* 6.

If the dysentery is attended with septic symptoms, we administer *Arsen.* 3, or *Carbo veg.* 6, or *China* 3, or *Mur. ac.* 1 to 2.

Intercurrent pneumonias are almost always of the croupous kind, and require to be treated with *Iodine. Phosph.* has never done us any good in such cases.

Ammoniæmic phenomena are treated by us in accordance with the same maxims; so far, however, we are not acquainted with a single reliable remedy for this species of blood-poisoning. *Phosph.* has seemed to produce some improvement; *Lycop., Phosph. ac.,*

Nitri ac. have been tried by us with some good results. *Arsen.* and *Hep. sulph.* proved useless. *Asafœt.* 3 may perhaps do some good. We likewise recommend *Kreos.* and *Petrol.* 3 by way of experiment. Such conditions, as a general pruritus, pneumonia, bronchial catarrh, œdema of the lungs, the various exanthemata, etc., have to be treated according to the rules laid down in the chapters where these diseases are specially discussed.

In acute uræmia the diet has to be very much restricted. Patients afflicted with chronic uræmia might partake of some meat if they had not an irresistible aversion to meat-diet of every description. In such cases eggs, milk, vegetables, fish, a light farinaceous diet and beer have to be the main articles of food.

Patients who are very much debilitated, may likewise partake of a little old wine.

If such patients are tormented by itching of the skin, relief is obtained by washing the body with dilute vinegar and brandy, or by taking a tepid bran-bath two or three times a week. H.]

16. Pyæmia.
Purulent Decomposition of the Blood.

[***Anatomical Characteristics.*** Collections of pus are always found in the cadavers of pyæmic persons, most frequently in the lungs, less frequently in the liver, spleen, kidneys, in the subcutaneous cellular tissue, in the muscles and sometimes in the brain. They form abscesses which are generally located at the periphery of organs and have a cuneiform shape. Their apex is always turned inwards, their base outwards. When first forming they represent circumscribed hemorrhagic infarctions of a dark-red or even blackish-red color and a dense consistence. Under the microscope the vessels look turgid and are filled with red corpuscles. These firm spots afterwards assume a gray sickly appearance, soften from the centre outwards and form abscesses which never consist of normal pus but always of decayed fibrin, the detritus of tissue and decomposed serous pus.

Formerly these abscesses were regarded by Rokitansky as pyæmic metastases and attributed to an infection of the blood by purulent matter. Virchow has however shown by numerous experiments that these abscesses are the result of embolia; in other words that they are caused by the transfer of particles of tissue from one place to another; that pure pus never engenders pyæmia, but that it must be in a state of decomposition and contain decayed fibrin and that it is the entrance of the latter into the circulation which causes the obstructions in the bloodvessels that are afterward transformed into abscesses.

Etiology. Most frequently pyæmia arises from suppurations in the interior of organs, from the downward burrowing of abscesses, purulent inflammations of joints, gangrenous localizations, during the course of phlebitis, periphlebitis, metrophlebitis, lymphangioitis, endocarditis; in the course of puerperal fever, typhus, variola; in consequence of suppurations after surgical operations, wounds, etc. Decomposition of the pus is an indispensable condition for the development of pyæmia. This decomposition is occasioned by a want of cleanliness, vitiated air, crowding of sick-rooms with wounded men, effusion of urine into the cellular tissue, access of air into open wounds or ulcers.

The infection of the blood is supposed to emanate from the decayed purulent serum.

Symptoms. The pyæmic process almost always commences with a chill followed by intense heat. Sometimes the chills recur in such a manner that the heat is mingled with chilly creepings or even severe paroxysms of chills. The pulse at once becomes hurried as soon as the pyæmia sets in; it is seldom below one hundred, small and easily compressible. In most cases delirium sets in during the heat, with restlessness, heat of the head, dulness of the sensorium and tendency to sopor. The patients feel very much exhausted, the appetite is entirely gone, thirst intense, the tongue becomes dry, cracks, the teeth are covered with brown sordes, the nostrils look sooty. Sometimes aphthæ form on the mucous membrane of the mouth and fauces. Very often bronchial catarrh, pneumonia and pleuritis supervene. The bowels are generally constipated, the skin is hot and dry, sometimes icteric or livid or else profuse sweats break out, with sudamina or numerous pustules. Subcutaneous abscesses are very frequently accompanied by erysipelas of the skin, inflammations of internal organs by violent paroxysms of fever and local pains, purulent effusions into articular cavities by painfulness and swelling of the joints.

Very frequently the abscesses become flabby and lax, and their contents change to ichor; the wounds assume a sickly appearance and become diphtheritic. In such cases profuse diarrhœic stools often set in, or hemorrhages from internal organs, bedsores or partial paralysis.

Course, Terminations, Prognosis. The course of the

disease is sometimes very rapid, This is most frequently the case in puerperal fever; the patients are attacked with chills and intense fever-heat which does not remit; they become delirious, lose their consciousness, lapse into a deep sopor and die in forty-eight or sixty hours. In such cases pyæmic localizations are frequently met with in the brain or lungs.

A milder course of the disease is marked by distinct remissions lasting from ten to sixteen hours in benignant and only three to four hours in malignant cases. The shorter the remission the more dangerous the course of the disease. The more violent the fever: the more imminent the danger of internal or external inflammations, the shorter the course of the disease and the more frequent a fatal termination.

In moderate forms of the disease it may last four, five or six weeks and terminate in recovery. Convalescence is however in all cases a slow process, slower even than after typhus.

In cases running a rapid course the prognosis is generally fatal.

In a mild form of the disease a good deal depends upon the circumstance whether the various manifestations of the pathological process can be improved. If we succeed in moderating the inflammatory symptoms and sustaining the strength of the patient, the prognosis is usually favorable.

Sopor, constant diarrhœa, hemorrhages, decubitus, paralysis of the sphincters do not admit of a favorable prognosis. A diphtheritic change in existing wounds is likewise a symptom of very bad omen.

Treatment. If we deal with morbid processes in the course of which pyæmia may be apprehended (see etiology), we must take care to prevent this result. To this end existing abscesses have to be opened in due season, wounds have to be kept clean and the access of air into such cavities has to be carefully guarded against. At the same time the sick-room has to be frequently ventilated, over-crowding with patients has to be avoided, cleanliness and good nursing have to be seen to.

If, in the course of the above-mentioned diseases repeated shiverings or chills set in, they always denote the beginning of pyæmia; the symptoms are evidently of a typhoid character, associated with great debility and dissolution of the blood.

For this reason, with a view of preventing as speedily as possible the great loss of strength or correcting the fluids, we resort at once to *Quinine* 1, a dose every two hours, and continue this remedy until the chills cease and the violence of the fever abates.

If a high grade of anæmia and great prostration manifest themselves during the chills, it is well to substitute *Chinin. arsenicosum* 1, a dose every two hours.

The further course of the pyæmic process resembles that of typhus and the subsequent treatment is likewise like that of typhus.

The more violent the paroxysms of fever and the longer the exacerbations last, the more imminent becomes the danger of inflammation. On this account the physician should be unremitting in his attention; he should frequently examine the surface of the body, and especially the abdomen; a physical exploration of the thorax is likewise indispensable. If the sensorium is depressed, it is important that, during such explorations, the frequency of the respirations or any impediments to the act of breathing, or a distortion of the features when pressure is made upon the abdomen or muscles, should be carefully noted. Inflammations in the subcutaneous cellular tissue, or in the muscles, in internal viscera, in the joints, never fail to occur, and they have to be removed as speedily as possible. For the treatment to be pursued in such cases we refer the reader to the chapters on meningitis, parotitis, arthrocace, pneumonia, puerperal fever, typhus.

Of excellent effect in the course of pyæmia are ablutions of the body with dilute vinegar, two or three times a day. If pustules show themselves on different parts of the body, they can be destroyed and their increase in number prevented by rubbing the parts with coarse, wet cloths. Larger pustules have to be opened with a lancet.

For the aphthæ or diphtheritic exudations in the mouth and fauces we have in vain used *Iodine*, *Merc.*, *Borax* and *Hepar sulph*. The much vaunted *Kali chloricum* and *Arg. nitr.* likewise proved fruitless. Generally these processes only cease with the cessation of pyæmia. In the case of aphthæ the frequent rinsing or washing of the mouth with cold water; and in the case of diphtheritic exudations frictions of the buccal and pharyngeal mucous membrane with dry linen rags, or which have been dipped in cold water, render excellent service.

Abscesses have to be sought for with great care and, even if deep-seated, have to be emptied as speedily as possible.

The dietetic and general precautionary measures to be adopted during convalescence are the same as those that have been recommended for abdominal typhus.

After the termination of the disease a high degree of anæmia and muscular debility generally remains. For the former we give *Ferr. metall.*, *carbon.*, or *lacticum* 1; for the latter *China* 1 or *Quinine* 1, two or three doses a day, together with a strengthening diet.

Country-air is well calculated to promote convalescence.

In the British Journal Vol. 26, page 480, Lachesis is recommended for pyæmia. This agent may be adapted to some cases. In our hands a case of pyæmic phlebitis of the left lower extremity promptly yielded to *Belladonna* preceded by a few doses of Aconite; and a case of pneumonic pyæmia to *Tartar emetic*. H.]

17. Septicæmia.
Putrid Decomposition of the Blood.

[Anatomical Characteristics. The blood is of dark color, and does not turn red when exposed to the air; it loses its coagulibility either totally or only partially, putrefies more rapidly and, in many cases, has an acid reaction. The serum has frequently a bloody color, the blood-corpuscles are partially dissolved and the blood-vessels are penetrated by their contents. In the interior of the tissues we frequently discover infiltrations with dissolved hæmatin.

Etiology. In most cases septicæmia proceeds from gangrened localities or is occasioned by local processes of decomposition or transformation into ichor. Not unfrequently it is the consequence of contagious or miasmatic influences, as in the plague, dysentery, etc. Or it may arise by the decomposition of substances that ought to have been excreted but remain behind in the organism, as in acute gastric and intestinal catarrhs, ichorous exudations, etc. In many cases the etiological origin of the disease remains unknown, in which case the septic infection of the blood has to be exclusively ascribed to the genius epidemicus or to endemic influences with which we are unacquainted.

Symptoms. The septic condition sets in with or without precursory symptoms. The precursory symptoms consist in weariness and heaviness of the body; in dull headache accompanied by a sense of dreariness, dulness and apathetic indifference; in restless and unrefreshing sleep; in dull, wandering pains in the limbs; in pressure at the stomach and in the loins; in loss of appetite with a sensation of repletion, and with an insipid, bitter or foul taste; in frequent chills with fugitive heat and occasional outbreak of sweat; in the secretion of strong-smelling urine and in alvine evacuations having a foul odor. These symptoms having continued for a shorter or longer period, and sometimes without any preliminary symptoms, a violent chill sets in followed by a moderate or intense fever-heat. This heat has the peculiarity of imparting to the hand a stinging or biting sensation (calor mordax). The symptoms of adynamia which now develop themselves resemble those that characterize the higher and highest grades of ileo-typhus and plague. Most generally the septic symptoms only make their appearance after the patients have become debilitated and apathetic to such an extent that they faint away when the least attempt is made to raise them or change their position. The first sign of septic decomposition is the fetor of the mouth; the breath and the bodily exhalations likewise spread a putrid odor, so that, whenever the patient raises the bed-cover by his motion, a sickening stench affects the nostrils. Stool and urine likewise have a cadaverous smell. The dissolution of the blood is made manifest by the following symptoms: readily-bleeding gums in consequence of which the mouth, tongue, teeth and lips acquire a black-brown appearance; frequent nose-bleed, vomiting of blood, bloody and foul-smelling diarrhœic stools, hæmaturia, hemorrhages from the vagina and uterus. Blood has even been known to exude from the canthi and ears. At the same time petechiæ make their appearance, either in the shape of ecchymotic spots or of streaks of suffused blood in various parts of the body; on parts of the body which are exposed to continued pressure, bedsores break out which generally become gangrenous. At the height of the disease inflammations of the meningæ, pleura or peritoneum frequently show themselves, with sanguineo-serous exudations, occasional swellings of the parotid glands that soon become ichorous, aphthæ in the mouth and throat or pains in the joints, with effusion of bloody serum into the articular cavities.

If the disease reaches the highest degree of intensity, a continued sopor sets in, with trembling of extremities, subsultus tendinum, grasping at flocks, involuntary evacuations, cold perspiration and fainting fits, and the patients die from exhaustion.

Course, Terminations, Prognosis. Cases consequent upon gangrene or the reabsorption of ichor, are very seldom preceded by preliminary symptoms; most commonly a chill occurs very suddenly, after which the typhoid symptoms develop themselves with intensity and more or less rapidity. Such cases generally run a very acute course, the adynamic and septic symptoms set in with overwhelming virulence, so that a fatal termination takes place already in two or three days. Some cases run a milder course for two, three or four weeks and upwards, and sometimes recover.

Cases arising in consequence of a contagium or miasm or from unknown causes, generally set in with precursory symptoms; the intensity of the pathognomonic phenomena mostly depends upon the violence of the exciting cause or upon constitutional tendencies. If the prevailing type of disease is of a malignant character, and the individual has a feeble, sickly or debilitated constitution, the phenomena of septicæmia are generally very violent and the disease runs a rapid course. The most dangerous cases are, if the fever remits but little or not at all, the prostration is excessive, and the septic phenomena make their appearance at an early period. Nevertheless, even the most threatening symptoms should not be sufficient to discourage the physician: as in typhus, so in septicæmia, the disease may have reached the acme of its intensity, when all at once the fever abates while copious fetid sweats break out, or frequent discharges of urine take place, or bloody, also ash-colored and fetid stools are passed, after which the disease progresses slowly towards final recovery.

In most cases death takes place by exhaustion, or in consequence of intense and frequent hemorrhages, or by paralysis, gangrenous decubitus, gangrene in other parts of the body, or by effusions of a bloody serum into the various cavities of the body.

As after-diseases we notice a long-lasting weakness of the whole organism, obstinate derangements of the digestive functions or in the composition of the blood, a high degree of anæmia, hectic fever, a cachectic appearance followed by dropsy or marasmus.

As a rule the prognosis is doubtful. Very acute cases with trifling or no remissions are almost always fatal. Frequent hemorrhages; foul-smelling excretions, a fetid breath and perspiration, soporous conditions, the access of gangrenous decubitus, partial paralysis, rapid prostration with collapse of the features, discoloration of the petechiæ, subsultus tendinum and grasping at flocks, a vitiated constitution and depressing social circumstances are unfavorable prognostic signs.

Treatment. When treating ichorous abscesses, ulcers or ichorous wounds, or any other pathological processes where gangrene has supervened, we must always be prepared for the supervention of septic phenomena. In many cases septicæmia can be prevented by diligent washing of the abscesses, ulcers, wounds or gangrenous

Septicæmia.

places with chlorine-water or with a solution of Kreosote, by frequently and carefully ventilating and fumigating the sick-chamber, and by observing the most scrupulous cleanliness and attending to the most careful nursing of the sick.

As soon as chills or shiverings set in, we at once administer *Quinine* 1, or *Chinin. arsenicos.* 1 for the reasons that we have stated when treating of pyæmia.

In cases with precursory symptoms we likewise have chills which are generally succeeded by a more or less intense fever, as in other acute diseases. From the beginning to the end the treatment is the same as that for typhus.

In great prostration with fetor of the mouth, fetid breath and sweat, we give *Ars.* 3 every hour.

This remedy not only moderates the burning fever and prevents the rapid prostration, but it has likewise a decided effect upon the decomposition of organic material, by which means the further progress of the septicæmia is arrested and hemorrhages, petechiæ, decubitus are prevented.

Even if all reasonable ground for hope had disappeared, *Arsen.* may still prove an efficient remedy if the skin is cool, the features are collapsed, the patient is exceedingly prostrated, in a soporous condition with muttering delirium, grasping at flocks, subsultus tendinum, petechiæ, ecchymoses, involuntary, bloody and cadaverously-smelling stools and even gangrenous decubitus.

Carbo veg. 6 in solution, a dose every hour or two hours may prove serviceable in similar circumstances.

If the symptoms of adynamia prevail; if the patients are sunk in apathy or sopor; if they faint when trying to raise themselves in bed; if, on trying to hold a thing, their hands tremble; if, on trying to put out their tongue, it trembles; if, when lying on their backs they settle down in the bed, and if they pass bloody, cadaverously-smelling stools, we give *China* 1, or *Chinin. arsenicos.* 1, or *Phosph.* 3, every hour or two hours (also *Muriatic acid*).

In many cases, especially if the septic condition has to be attributed to a contagium, the adynamia is accompanied by symptoms of extreme nervous irritation; the patients have a dry or burning heat, are tormented with loquacious or noisy delirium, their cheeks show a circumscribed redness, their thirst is very great, their pulse is hurried and feeble, with grasping at flocks, subsultus tendinum, catching at imaginary objects, constant desire to get up and dress, etc. For such symptoms we give *Rhus tox.* 3 every hour, even if petechiæ, bloody stools, meteorism and clammy sweats are present.

If a high degree of stupor prevails, if the skin is cool, the perspiration clammy, the features collapsed, the pulse small and filiform, and if the petechiæ or ecchymoses are at the same time of a bluish-gray color, *Camphora* 1, in hourly doses, has power to raise the sunken vitality and bring about a favorable reaction.

For violent nosebleed, vomiting of blood, septic hæmaturia or hemorrhages from the vagina we administer with good success *Ergotin* 1, every two hours.

For excessive hemorrhages and their consequences we administer doses of *Sulphuric* or *Nitric ac.* 1, or *Ferr. mur.* 1, at rapid intervals.

For long-lasting syncope with rapid prostration we alternate the previously-mentioned remedies with *Moschus* 1; at the same time we feed the patient on broth in order to repair the waste by the loss of blood as speedily as possible.

Gangrenous decubitus or gangrene of other parts is treated as under typhus.

During the burning fever we have the skin bathed with dilute vinegar or aromatic vinegar, or, if the prostration is very great, with wine and water.

As a beverage during the fever we resort to water with current jelly or syrups. If the skin is cool and the patient very feeble, dilute wine is preferable. If the patient threatens to faint from exhaustion, a spoonful of good wine may be given.

During convalescence the rules indicated for typhus have to be followed.

which had been hot hitherto, and the extremities gradually cool off, whereas the trunk and especially the abdomen feel hot; very soon the little patients become apathetic and, with their eyes half closed, lie in a soporous condition, from which, however, they are easily roused when spoken to. They hurriedly grasp the tumbler, hold on to it with both hands and are unwilling to relinquish their hold. Very often they start from their slumber with a cry, and, after looking about wildly, they relapse into their sopor. At the same time the children become rapidly emaciated, especially about the neck; the pulse becomes smaller and more hurried, the alvine evacuations acquire a foul odor, become watery, are destitute of fæcal matter and distinguished from the urine only by their cadaverous smell; the respiration becomes short and labored, and is often accompanied by a tormenting cough. Finally there is complete loss of consciousness and sensibility, the eyeballs are distorted, spasms or convulsions set in, with symptoms of the most profound exhaustion.

This hydrocephaloid condition is distinguished from true hydrocephalus by the absence of the pathognomonic signs of the latter, namely: rigidity of the nape of the neck, the piercing cri encéphalique, boring with the head into the pillow backwards, the diminished frequency of the pulse and respiration, the retraction of the abdomen, the dilatation of the pupils and the automatic grasping at the head.

If the above-mentioned precursory symptoms usher in a typhoid condition, the children have frequent attacks of vomiting and diarrhœa while the supervening fever very soon reaches a high degree of intensity; they do not sleep, the tongue and lips become dry, the nostrils have a sooty appearance; there is an expression of suffering and anxiety in the countenance; the little patients become rapidly emaciated, the skin looks pallid, they are very restless, want to be carried all the time and moan unceasingly. At last they quiet down, become cooler, and, owing to the anæmia of the brain, lapse into a soporous condition which is generally a precursor of approaching death.

In some cases the symptoms are less striking and the disease runs a chronic course; the diarrhœa and vomiting, the intense thirst, the bloating and painfulness of the abdomen, the rapid emaciation and the gradual prostration most commonly set in without fever, and, unless the disease is arrested, the patients slowly die of exhaustion.

The gastromalacia of adults is not characterized by such striking pathognomonic symptoms; in the case of old people who have died of gastromalacia, derangements of the digestive functions are said to have slowly manifested themselves, with oppression and pain in the region of the stomach, dryness of the tongue and rapidly developing marasmus are said to have been noticed without it having been possible to localize the disease in any particular spot.

Course, Termination, Prognosis. The course of gastromalacia is either acute, as when the disease breaks out suddenly in the form of cholera or gastritis, in which case it often terminates in twenty-four, thirty-six or forty-eight hours; or most commonly it is less acute, as when the disease assumes an hydrocephaloid or typhoid form, in which case it may run a course of several weeks including the precursory spmptoms; the disease may likewise run a chronic course, during which the morbid phenomena develop themselves slowly and may continue weeks and even months.

The disease either terminates in complete recovery, most generally in its most acute or chronic form, or in death. Death either takes place at the height of the acute process, amid convulsions, or, in case the disease runs a slow course, by exhaustion of the vital powers or in consequence of cerebral anæmia.

In the case of children, the prognosis is always doubtful; it is most favorable in the very acute or in the chronic form. Badly fed, weakly, neglected and impoverished children are chiefly liable to succumb to the disease.

Treatment. The treatment is to be conducted in accordance with the form under which the disease happens to manifest itself. If it assumes the symptoms of cholera, we resort to *Ars.* 3, *Veratr. alb.* 3, or *Tart. emet.* 3.

If the vomiting is chiefly sour and the stools have a sour smell, are watery and corrosive, attended with violent colicky pains; if the thirst is excessive, the extremities are icy-cold, and the children are covered with a cold and clammy perspiration and lying in a state of torpor bordering upon insensibility, we give *Ars.* in solution, a teaspoonful every fifteen minutes.

If the vomiting is greenish and sour, and the act of vomiting is preceded by paroxysms of nausea and fainting, the watery and inodorous alvine discharges are very copious and attended with severe colicky pains; and if the extreme collapse is accompanied by convulsions, we give *Veratrum* in the same manner.

If these symptoms are accompanied by sopor instead of convulsions, we resort to *Tart. emet.*, same dose. These three remedies are perfectly reliable and sometimes effect an improvement after the first dose.

If the disease breaks out in the form of gastritis, *Bellad.* 3 is a sovereign remedy which speedily moderates both the pains and the fever and arrests the vomiting and diarrhœa. We give this remedy in solution, a teaspoonful every fifteen minutes, extending the intervals as soon as an improvement becomes apparent. If no improvement sets in in two or three hours, we resort to the *Sulphate of Atropine* 3 same dose and form, with which we have often succeeded in subduing the most dangerous symptoms. At the same time we apply cold water compresses to the region of the stomach, and if the abdomen is painful and bloated, likewise to the latter. If the whole body is very hot, we resort to general ablutions with dilute vinegar.

If, after the termination of the acute stage, the patients are collapsed, with cold extremities, frequent diarrhœic stools, sopor or convulsions, *Ars.* 3 or *Laches.* 6 may be resorted to, a few drops of wine or brandy and water may be administered, the cold extremities may be rubbed with warm wine or brandy and enveloped in warm cloths, after which a favorable reaction and a general improvement will sometimes set in even in cases that had seemed hopeless.

If the disease breaks out in the form of an hydrocephaloid, we are guided in the selection of a remedy by the febrile phenomena, the evacuations, the strength of the patient and the cerebral symptoms.

As long as there is fever and the evacuations continue frequent, the children retain their strength, the brain is free, but the head is hot and heavy, we give *Bellad.* 3 in solution, every hour.

If the extremities are cool, the children are pale and languid, the trunk is hot, the alvine evacuations are copious and symptoms of sopor set in, we give *Verat. alb.* 3 in the same dose and form.

If collapse and signs of insensibility show themselves, with sudden cries and starting from the deep sopor, or even convulsions, we depend chiefly upon *Arsen.* 3 in solution, every half hour or hour. *Tart. emet.* 3, and *Laches.* 6, may likewise prove useful in such cases.

For typhoid gastromalacia we recommend *Phosphor acid.* 3 **or** *Rhus tox.* 3 in solution, every hour.

If cerebral anæmia supervenes, we give *Ars.* 3, and *Laches.* 6, wine and water, etc., as for the gastric form of gastromalacia.

The chronic form of gastromalacia requires *Arsen.* 3. *Kreosot.* 3, and *Argent. nitr.* 3.

Kreosote is excellent, if the sour vomiting and rapid emaciation are prominent symptoms, the alvine discharges are not very frequent.

Secale cornutum 3 is indicated by sub-acute attacks, with sour and foul smelling vomiting, sensitiveness, heat and bloating of the region of the stomach, expression of distress in the countenance, sinking pulse, clammy and cold skin, prostration, fetid, sero-mucous discharges from the bowels.

Arg. nitr. 3 is indicated by a semi-paralytic condition of the intestinal canal, the beverage is at once discharged again by the rectum with a rumbling noise, the stools are watery and colorless and are only distinguished from the urine by their cadaverous odor. A cure of such a case of this kind is reported by Kafka in the second volume of the Hom. Vierteljahrsschrift, number 4, page 405.

The convalescence is generally very slow. Convalescent children have to be fed on good beef- or chicken-broth, milk, barley-coffee, dry rusk, arrow-root, etc.

Gastromalacia generally setting in after the children are weaned, we will here subjoin a few remarks about weaning.

Children should not be weaned until they are able to partake of other nourishment beside mother's milk.

Weakly or anæmic children who are troubled with acidity of the stomach, dyspepsia or diarrhœa, have to remain at the breast until these morbid conditions are removed and the little patients look better and are more vigorous. Experience has shown that such children do not digest the nourishment which is given them after they are weaned and that symptoms of gastromalacia are very apt to supervene in consequence of the increasing weakness of their digestive powers. If such children show symptoms of dyspepsia or of gastro-intestinal catarrh, they have to be attended to as soon as possible.

Children who are brought up on farinaceous diet, or with sugar-tits habitually in their mouths, are most commonly subject to such derangements. We have likewise observed the beginning of a long line of gastric and intestinal affections which afterward lead to gastromalacia, in the case of infants who are fed on cold nourishment in the night, when mothers or nurses are too indolent to first warm it before giving it to the little ones. For this reason the choice of food as well as its preparation and the time of giving it to the children, are of the utmost importance.

For children who have been weaned, the most suitable kinds of nourishment are barley-coffee, carefully-strained cocoa-shells boiled in milk, skimmed milk sweetened with a little sugar, beef- or chicken-broth without salt and at first mixed with a little milk and sweetened with a small quantity of sugar; after a while a little salt may be added and some wheat bread-crust may be grated in and boiled with the broth. All this kind of nourishment has to be given warm and in small quantities.

Children should be accustomed at an early age to a certain regularity in their meals; there should be an interval of two or three hours between one meal and the next in order to prevent overfeeding and give the food a chance to be properly assimilated. Fresh well-water, not too cold, is the best drink for children. If intestinal catarrh supervenes, a slimy decoction, such as rice-water, arrow-root or slippery elm may be substituted in the place of water.

By observing these rules, gastromalacia can be prevented, and a vigorous and healthful development of the infantile organism can be secured.

19. Goitre, Bronchocele.
Derbyshire Neck.

Goitre is a well-known enlargement of the thyroid body in front of the neck. Sometimes the enlargement involves only one lobe of the gland, but most commonly both lobes are hypertrophied.

This disease is endemic in many parts of the United States, especially in districts where limewater is habitually used for cooking and drinking purposes. It is remarkably prevalent in Derbyshire, England, and in some of the deep, damp valleys of Switzerland. The river Saskatchawan in British North-America is notorious for its goitre-producing qualities.

The structure of goitre varies; it may consist of a simple engorgement of the blood-vessels; or the capsules of the parenchyma of the gland may be distended by a gelatinous fluid. We have seen thyroid glands enormously enlarged and of an osseous hardness. Sometimes the enlargement chiefly takes place on the inside, impeding respiration and even threatening suffocation. If a sore throat often seems to defy all treatment it is because the soreness depends upon this internal enlargement of the thyroid body, which may be scarcely visible on the outside. We have known cases of goitre terminating in tubercular phthisis; in such cases the structure of the goitre, from the incipiency of the disorganization, was identical with that of the tubercular deposition.

Treatment. For all practical purposes it is sufficient to distinguish the simple vascular enlargement of goitre, and the hypertrophy of the thyroid parenchyma. The cartilaginous, schirrous and tubercular disorganization may resist all treatment, although not in all cases.

In unacclimated individuals first coming under the influence of lime water, we have sometimes succeeded in arresting an incipient goitre by causing the patient to consume quantities of lemon-juice, sour fruit, and to drink water acidulated with lemon-juice or vinegar.

A simple vascular enlargement of the thyroid gland often yields to Aconite alone; sometimes *Aconite* and *Iodine* have to be used in alternation internally and compresses of a weak solution of *Iodine* may have to be applied externally.

We sometimes employ with a good deal of success compresses of bay-rum with which the tincture of *Iodine* is mixed in the proportion of one drachm of *Iodine* to a quart-bottle of bay-rum; a weak solution of *Iodine* being at the same time used internally; even very hard, cartilaginous goitres sometimes yield to this treatment.

The tincture of *Iodine* rubbed upon the goitre, has been of comparatively little use in our hands. We have derived more benefit from the Iodide of Potassium-ointment and a solution of five grains of the salt used internally every day.

Another excellent application is an ointment of the *Iodide of Mercury*. Some persons are very sensitive to the action of this ointment, and it has therefore to be used with great care. Even one-sixteenth of a grain of the *Iodide* has been known to blister the skin most shockingly. We have succeeded in removing very large and rather soft goitres with an ointment containing only the one hundredth part of a grain of the Iodide.

There are cases of goitre where Spongia, or roast sponge, has to be given internally and an ointment of Spongia has at the same time to be applied externally. In other cases *Calcarea* and *Hepar sulphuris* may be required to act upon the constitutional disposition. Goitre is very apt to reappear even after it had seemed to have completely disappeared under the influence of appropriate treatment. H.]

ALPHABETICAL INDEX

OF THE

DISEASES TREATED OF IN THESE TWO VOLUMES.

(The Roman figure II refers to the diseases described in the second volume.)

	Page
Abscess, = Psoas, see Psoitis.	
Abscess, retropharyngeal	294
Acid stomach, see Catarrh of the stomach, acute and chronic	359 and 379
Acne II	478
—— rosacea II	482
Adiposis II	714
Adipósitas cordis II	382
Albuminuria, see Bright's disease.	
Amenorrhœa II	55
Ammoniæmia, see Uræmia.	
Amygdalitis	284
Amyloid liver	541
Anæmia II	687
—— of the brain	65
——, congenital, II	701
——, consecutive, II	709
——, secondary, II	711
Anasarca, see Dropsy.	
Aneurysms II	436
Angina catarrhalis	281
—— parotidea	314
—— pectoris II	405
—— tonsillaris	284
Anthrax II	503
Aphthæ	279
Apoplexy, cerebral	70
Arteries, inflammation of the, II	436
Arthritis II	640
—— deformons II	634
Ascarides	493
Ascites, see Dropsy.	
Asiatic cholera II	613
Asthma II	311
Ataxia, progressive locomotor II	425
Atrophy of the liver, acute yellow	542
Aurigo, see Jaundice.	
Barber's itch II	480
Biliari calculi	564
Bilious fever	422

	Page
Bladder, inflammation of the	625
——, paralysis of the	634
Blennorrhœa of the conjunctiva, acute	242
—— —— —— chronic	243
—— of the urethra II	1
—— of the vagina, see Gonorrhœa of the female and leucorrhæa.	
Blood, deficient, II	687
——, pale, II	687
Bloody urine	629
Bones, inflammation of, II	410
Bottle-nose II	482
Bowels, inflammation of the	435
——, occlusion. obstruction of the	479
——, stenosis of the	479
Brain, anæmia of the	65
——, concussion of the	92
——, congestion of the, see Brain, hyperæmia of the.	
——, dropsy of the, see Hydrocephalus	99
——, hyperæmia of the	57
——, Inflammation of the	86
——, yellow softening of the	99
Breasts, see Mammæ.	
Bright's disease of the kidneys	596
Bronchia, acute inflammation of the, II	164
——, chronic inflammation of the, II	210
——, dilatation of the, II	234
Bronchitis, acute, II	164
——, chronic, II	230
Bronchiectasia II	234
Bronchocele II	736
Calculi, biliari	564
——, renal	614
Cancer, see also Carcinoma.	
—— aquaticus	307
—— of the mammæ II	100
—— of the womb II	81

(745)

Alphabetical Index.

Capsular hepatitis............................ 531
Carbuncle II..................................... 503
Carcinoma of the liver.................... 569
—— of the stomach......................... 375
——, see also Cancer.
Cardialgia.. 391
Carditis II.. 347
Caries of the vertebræ, see Spondylitis..................................... 120
—— of vertebræ, see also Pott's disease.
Catalepsy.. 177
Catamenia, see Menses.
Cataract.. 256
Catarrh... 263
——, acute laryngotracheal, II........ 107
——, chronic laryngotracheal, II..... 129
——, chronic intestinal.................... 413
——, intestinal................................ 404
——, simple intestinal..................... 406
—— of the stomach, acute............. 359
—— —— —— chronic.................... 379
—— of the urethra II....................... 1
—— of the vagina II........................ 20
Catarrhus intestinalis...................... 404
—— ventriculi acutus...................... 359
—— ventriculi chronicus................. 379
Catarrhal fever............................... 422
Cellular tissue of the intestinal canal, inflammation of the........ 451
Cellulitis.. 451
Cephalalgia..................................... 220
Cephalæmatoma............................. 218
Cerebritis, (see also meningitis)....... 94
Cerebro-spinal meningitis............... 130
Chancre II....................................... 543
Change of life II.............................. 87
Chest, dropsy of the, II................... 342
Chicken-pox, see Variola.
Child-bed fever, see Puerperal fever.
Chlorosis II..................................... 624
Cholelithiasis.................................. 564
Cholera, Asiatic, II.......................... 613
—— infantum................................. 413
—— sporadica................................ 408
Cholerine.. 408
Chorea.. 170
Cirrhosis of the liver....................... 539
Clap, see Gonorrhœa.
Climacteric period II....................... 87
Climaxis II...................................... 87

Cœcum, inflammation of the......... 440
Cold in the head............................. 263
Colic.. 468
Concussion of the brain................. 92
Congestion of the brain, see Brain, hyperæmia of the.
—— of the lungs II........................ 150
Congestive chill, see Intermittent fever.
Conjunctiva, acute blennorrhœa of the.. 242
——, chronic blennorrhœa of the... 243
——, catarrhal inflammation of the 237
——, scrofulous inflammation of the 249
Conjunctivitis blennorrhoica.......... 242
—— catarrhalis.............................. 237
—— scrofulosa.............................. 249
Consumption, dorsal..................... 129
Convulsions of infants and parturient women, see Eclampsia infantum and parturientium.
Copper-nose II............................... 482
Cornea, inflammation of the......... 256
Corneitis.. 256
Coryza.. 263
Coxalgia II..................................... 427
Coxarthrocace II............................ 427
Critical Age II................................. 87
Croup, membranous, II................. 112
Cystitis... 625
Cystoplegia.................................... 634
Cystospasmus................................ 632
Dandriff II..................................... 470
Debility, see Anæmia.
Degeneration of the heart, fatty, II. 382
Delirium tremens II....................... 463
Dentition, see Eclampsia infantum.
Deranged stomach, see Catarrh of the stomach, acute and chronic....359, 379
Derbyshire neck II......................... 743
Diabetes melitus............................ 617
Diaphragm, hernia of the, II......... 324
——, inflammation of the, II......... 322
Diaphragmitis II............................ 322
Diarrhœa,—for the various forms of diarrhœa, see Catarrh, intestinal, 404 to 413
——, chronic, see also Catarrh, intestinal............................. 413
Dilatation of the heart II............... 381
—— of the veins II........................ 438

Alphabetical Index. 747

Entry	Page
Dilatation of the bronchia II.	234
Diphtheria	296
Diphtheritis	296
Dorsal consumption	129
Dropsy II., see also Anasarca, Ascites	645
—— of the brain, see Hydrocephalus	99
—— of the chest II., see also Hydrothorax	342
—— of the lungs II, see also Œdema of the lungs	307
Dysentery, catarrhal	455
——, epidemic	457
Dysmenorrhœa II.	60
Dyspepsia, acute, see Catarrh of the stomach, acute	359
——, chronic, see Catarrh of the stomach, chronic	379
Dysphagia inflammatoria	326
Ear, inflammation of the inner	258
——, inflammation of the outer	261
Eclampsia	154
—— infantum	154
—— parturientium	163
Ecthyma II.	499
Eczema II.	490
Emphysema of the lungs II.	235
Emprosthotonos, see Tetanus.	
Encephalitis, (see also Meningitis)	94
Encephalomacia	108
Enchondroma II.	420
Endocarditis II	347
Enlargement, see Hypertrophy.	
Enteralgia	468
Enteric fever, see Typhus.	
Enteritis	435
Enuresis nocturna	631
Epilepsy	139
Epistaxis	269
Erysipelas II	455
Erythema II	453
Eyes, inflammation of the, see ophthalmia.	
—— of newborn infants, inflammation of the	247
Face-ache	227
Falling, see Prolapsus.	
Fatness, see Obesitas.	
Fatty degeneration of the heart II.	382
—— liver	540
Favus II	506

Entry	Page
Febris gastrica catarrhalis, mucosa et biliosa	422
—— icterodes II.	602
Fever and ague II.	563
——, bilious	422
——, catarrhal	422
——, enteric, see Typhus.	
——, gastric	422
——, intermittent, II	563
——, mucous	422
——, puerperal, II.	34
——, spotted	130
——, typhoid, see Typhus.	
——, yellow, II	602
Fish-skin II	473
Fluor albus II	20
Fothergill's prosopalgia	227
Furuncle II	503
Gangrene of the lungs II.	303
Gastric fever	422
Gastritis	361
Gastrodynia, see Cardialgia.	
Gastromalacia, II.	737
Gland, inflammation of the parotid	314
Glossitis	311
Glottis, œdema of the, II	137
——, spasm of the, II	140
Glycosuria	617
Goitre II	736
Gonarthrocace II.	430
Gonitis II	430
Gonorrhœa of the female II	22
—— of the male II	1
Gout II.	640
Gravel	614
Green-sickness II.	624
Grippe II.	182
Gums, scurvy of the	322
Gutta rosacea II.	482
Hæmatemesis	383
Hæmaturia	629
Headache	220
Heart, dilatation of the, II.	381
——, fatty degeneration of the, II.	382
——, hypertrophy of the, II	372
——, inflammation of the, II	347
——, palpitation of the, II.	379, 399
Heartburn, see Catarrh of the stomach, acute and chronic	359 and 379
Helcosis II	145

Alphabetical Index.

	Page
Helminthiasis	492
Hemicrania	221
Hemiplegia, see Paralysis.	
Hemorrhage in the kidneys	609
—— from the lungs II	154
—— from the nose	269
—— from the stomach	383
—— from the womb II	66
Hemorrhoids	485
Hepatitis, acute	528
——, capsular	531
——, chronic	537
Hernia of the diaphragm II	324
Herpes II	486
—— circinnatus II	490
——, facial, II	487
—— Iris II	490
——, preputial, II	487
—— Zoster II	488
Hiccup II	323
Hip-disease	427
Hip-joint, inflammation of, II	427
Hives II	466
Honey-comb tetter II	506
Hydrocephalus, acute	99
—— (stricte sic dictus)	109
Hydrothorax II	342
Hyperæmia of the brain	57
——, constitutional, II	681
—— of the liver	522
—— of the lungs II	150
Hypertrophy of the heart II	372
—— of the liver	538
Hypochondria	207
Hypochondriasis, see Hypochondria	207
Hypopyon	256
Hysteria	190
Ichthyosis II	473
Icterus	554
Impetigo II	497
Indigestion, acute, see Catarrh of the stomach, acute	359
Inflammation of the arteries II	436
—— of the bladder	625
—— of bones II	410
—— of the bowels	435
—— of the brain	86
—— of the breasts II	95
—— of the bronchia, acute, II	164
—— —— —— chronic II	210
Inflammation of the cellular tissue of the intestinal canal	451
—— of the cæcum	440
—— of the conjunctiva, blennorrhœic	242
—— —— —— catarrhal	237
—— —— —— scrofulous	249
—— of the cornea	256
—— of the diaphragm II	322
—— of the inner ear	258
—— of the outer ear	261
—— of the heart II	347
—— of the hip-joint II	427
—— of the iris	256
—— of the joints II	426
—— of the kidneys	586
—— of the knee-joint II	430
—— of the larynx	107
—— of the liver, acute	529
—— —— chronic	537
—— of the capsules of the liver	531
—— of the lungs II	243
—— of lymphatic glands II	445
—— of lymphatic vessels & glands II	442
—— of the nose	268
—— of the œsophagus	326
—— of the ovaries II	45
—— of the pancreas	578
—— of the parotid gland	314
—— —— —— malignant	317
—— of the periosteum II	410
—— of the peritoneum	503
—— of the pleura II	325
—— of the psoas-muscle II	421
—— of the rectum, catarrhal	445
—— of the sclerotica	256
—— of the spinal cord	110
—— of the spleen	573
—— of the stomach	361
—— of the tarsus II	433
—— of the testes II	13
—— of the tongue	311
—— of the tonsils	284
—— of the trachea	107
—— of the urethra II	1
—— of the veins II	436
—— of the vena porta	532
—— of the vertebræ, see Spondylitis	120
—— of the womb II	27
—— —— puerperal, II	34
Influenza II	182
Insufficiency of aortic valves II	394

Alphabetical Index. 749

	Page		Page
Insufficiency of mitral valve II	388	Lymphadenitis chronica II	445
Intercostal neuralgia II	450	Lymphangioitis II	442
Intermittent fever II	563	Lymphatics, acute inflammation of, II	442
Iris, inflammation of the	256		
Iritis	256	Lymphatic vessels and glands, chronic inflammation of, II	445
Irregularities, menstrual	47		
Irritation, spinal	135	Malaria, see Intermittent fever.	
Ischias II	447	Mammæ, cancer of the, II	100
Itch II	507	——, inflammation of the, II	95
Jacob's ulcer II	483	Mania-a-potu, see Delirium tremens.	
Jaundice	554	Marasmus II	711
Joints, inflammation of, II	426	Mastitis II	95
Kidneys, diseases of the	580	Mastodynia II	99
——, hemorrhage in the	609	Measles II	513
——, inflammation of the	586	Megrim	221
Knee-joint, inflammation of, II	430	Melituria	617
Laryngitis submucosa II	137	Membranous croup II	112
Laryngotracheitis catarrhalis acuta II	107	Meningitis	86
		—— cerebro-spinalis	130
—— chronica II	129	—— spinalis, see Inflammation of the spinal cord	110
—— crouposa II	112		
Laryngotracheal catarrh, chronic, II	129	Meningitis, tubercular, granular, basilar	99
Larynx, inflammation of the, II	107		
——, ulcers of the, II	145	Menorrhagia, see Menses, profuse.	
Leucorrhœa II	20	Menostasia, see Amenorrhœa.	
Lichen II	474	Menses, difficult, II	60, 61
Liver, acute yellow atrophy of the	542	——, profuse, II	57
——, carcinoma of the	569	——, scanty, II	60
——, cirrhosis of the	538	——, suppression of the, II	55
——, fatty	540	Menstrual irregularities II	47
——, hyperæmia of the	522	Mentagra II	480
——, hypertrophy of the	538	Metritis II	27
——, acute inflammation of the	529	—— puerperalis II	34
——, nutmeg-	538	Metrorrhagia II	66
——, waxy or amyloid	541	Miliaria II	469
Lockjaw, see Tetanus	178	Morbilli II	513
Lumbago II	422	Mumps	314
Lumbrici, see Worms.		Myocarditis II	347
Lungs, congestion of the II	150	Myelitis, see Inflammation of the spinal cord	110
——, dropsy of the, II	307		
——, emphysema of the, II	235	Nasitis	268
——, gangrene of the, II	303	Nephritis	586
——, hemorrhage from the, II	154	Nerve, neuralgia of ischiadic, II	447
——, hyperæmia of the, II	150	Nettle-rash II	466
——, inflammation of the, II	243	Neuralgia Fothergilli, see Prosopalgia.	
——, œdema of the, II	307		
——, plethora of the, II	150	—— intercostalis II	450
Lupus II	483	—— of ischiadic nerve II	447
Luxation, spontaneous, see Hip-disease.		—— spinalis	135
		—— trigemini	227
Lymphadenitis acuta II	442	—— of the vagina II	92

	Page		Page
Neuralgia of the womb II	89	Phthisis, see Tuberculosis.	
Noma	307	Piles	485
Nose, hemorrhage from the	269	Pityriasis II	470
——, Inflammation of the	268	Plethora, constitutional, II	681
—— bleed	269	—— of the lungs II	150
Nutmeg-liver	538	Pleura, inflammation of the, II	325
Obesitas II	714	Pleurisy II	325
Occlusion, obstruction of the bowels	479	Pleuritis II	325
Odontalgia	328	Pleurothotonos, see Tetanus.	
Œsophagitis	326	Pneumonia II	243
Œsophagus, inflammation of the	326	Pneumorrhagia II	154
Œdema glottidis II	137	Pneumothorax II	343
—— of the lungs II	307	Polyæmia II	681
Oligæmia II	687	Polypi in the nose	267
Oophoritis II	45	—— of the rectum	450
Ophthalmia, see Conjunctivitis, Corneitis, Iritis, Sclerotitis.		Polysarcia II	714
		Pompholix II	501
—— neonatorum	247	Porcupine disease II	473
Opisthotonos, see Tetanus.		Pott's disease II	410
Orchitis II	13	—— —— see also Spondylitis	120
Orthotonos, see Tetanus.		Proctitis	445
Ostitis II	410	Progressive muscular paralysis II	424
Otitis externa	261	Prolapsus of the rectum	451
—— interna	258	—— of the womb II	88
Ovaries, inflammation of the, II	45	Prosopalgia	227
Ovaritis II	45	—— intermittent	233
Ozæna	264	Prurigo II	476
Pædarthrocace II	420	Pruritus vulvæ II	88
Palpitation of the heart II	379, 399	Psoas-abscess, see Psoitis.	
Palsy, see Paralysis.		Psoas-muscle, inflammation of the, II	421
Pancreas, inflammation of the	578	Psoitis II	421
Pancreatitis	578	Psoriasis II	472
Paralysis	183	Ptyalism	319
——, progressive muscular, II	424	Puerperal inflammation of the womb II	34
Paraplegia, see Paralysis.			
Paresis, see Paralysis.		—— fever II	34
Parotitis	314	Pulmonary hemorrhage II	154
—— maligna	317	Pyæmia II	728
Pemphigus II	501	Pylephlebitis	532
Perforating ulcer of the stomach	368	Pyrosis, see Heartburn.	
Pericarditis II	347	Quinsy	284
Pericardium, inflammation of the, II	347	Ramolissement, see Softening.	
Perihepatitis	531	Ranula	324
Periosteum, inflammation of, II	410	Rash II	469
Periostitis II	410	Rectum, catarrhal inflammation of the	445
Peritoneum, inflammation of the	503		
Peritonitis	503	——, polypi in the	450
Perityphlitis	440	——, prolapsus of the	451
Pertussis II	193	Renal calculi	614
Phlebitis II	436	Retina, inflammation of the	256
Phlebectasia II	438	Retinitis	257

Alphabetical Index. 751

	Page		Page
Retropharyngeal abscess	294	Spontaneous limping, see Hip-disease.	
Rhachitis II	416	—— luxation, see Hip-disease.	
Rheumatism II	630	Spotted fever	130
——, arthritic, II	634	Stenocardia	405
——, acute articular, II	630	Stenosis of the bowels	479
——, chronic articular, II	633	—— of cardiac orifices II	389, 396
——, acute muscular, II	632	Stomach, acid, see Catarrh of the stomach, acute and chronic, 359 and 379	
Rickets II	416		
Ring-worm, see Herpes Iris.			
Roseola II	465	——, derangement of the, see Catarrh of the stomach, acute and chronic	359 and 379
Round ulcer of the stomach	368		
Rubeolæ II	465		
Running from the urethra, see Gonorrhœa, Urethritis.		——, acute catarrh of the	359
		——, chronic catarrh of the	379
Rupia II	499	——, carcinoma of the	375
Salivation	319	——, hemorrhage from the	383
Scabies II	507	——. inflammation of the	361
Scald-head II	506	——, chronic or perforating or round ulcer of the	368
Scalp, bloody tumor of the	218		
Scarlatina II	522	——, softening of the, see Gastromalacia.	
Scarlet-fever II	522		
Sclerotica, inflammation of the	256	——, spasm of the	391
Sclorotitis	256	——, weak, see Dyspepsia.	
Sciatica, see Ischias.		Stomatitis	273
Scorbutus II	649	Stone-pock II	478
Scrofulosis II	652	Strophulus II	474
Scurvy II	649	Summer-complaint	413
—— of the gums	322	Suppression of the menses II	55
Seborrhœa II	505	Sycosis II	480
Septicæmia II	732	Syphilis II	542
Shingles II	488	——, secondary, II	548
Singultus II	323	——, tertiary, II	551
Smallpox II	532	Tabes II	711
Softening of the brain, yellow	99	—— dorsalis	129
—— of the stomach, see Gastromalacia.		Tænia solium, see Tape-worm.	
		Tape-worm	494
Sore throat	281	Tarsus, inflammation of the, II	433
Spasm of the bladder	632	Teething, see Dentition.	
—— of the facial nerve	234	Testicles, inflammation of the, II	13
—— of the glottis II	140	Tetanus	178
—— of the stomach	391	Tetter, scaly, II	472
Spasmus nervi facialis	234	—— II	486
Spermatorrhœa II	16	——, see also Herpes.	
Spina ventosa II	420	Throat, catarrhal inflammation of the	281
Spinal cord, inflammation of the	110		
—— irritation	135	——, sore	281
Spleen, see Hypochondria	207	Thrush, see Aphthæ	279
——, inflammation of the	573	Tic convulsif	234
Splenitis	573	—— douloureux, see Neuralgia Fothergilli.	
Spondurthrocace, see Spondylitis	120		
Spondylitis	120	Tinea capitis II	506

Tongue, inflammation of the 311	Varices II. 438
Tonsillitis. 284	Varicose veins II 438
Tonsils, inflammation of the........... 284	Varicella, see Variola.
Toothache 328	Variola II. 532
Tooth-rash II. 474	Varioloid, see Variola.
Trismus. 178	Veins, dilatation of, II. 438
Tuberculosis II. 658	—— inflammation of the, II. 436
Tumor albus genu II 430	Vena porta, inflammation of the...... 532
—— of the scalp, bloody 218	Venereal disease II 542
Tussis convulsiva II..... 193	Vertebræ, inflammation of the 120
Typhlitis 440	Vertigo 69
Typhoid fever, see Typhus.	St. Vitus' dance, see Chorea............ 170
Typhus II. 576	Wasting palsy, see Progressive muscular paralysis.
Ulcer, Jacob's 483	
—— of the stomach, chronic............ 368	Waterbrash, see Catarrh of the stomach, acute and chronic... 359 and 379
Ulcers of the larynx II. 145	
Ulcus perforans ventriculi seu rotundum 368	Waxy liver 541
	Weak stomach, see Dyspepsia.
Uræmia II 720	Wetting the bed. 631
Urethra, blennorrhœa of the, II...... 1	White swelling II. 430
——, catarrh of the, II. 1	Whites, II 20
——, inflammation of the, II 1	Whooping-cough II 193
Urethritis II 1	Wolf II 483
Urine, bloody 629	Womb, cancer of the, II. 81
Urticaria II. 466	——, hemorrhage from the, II. 66
Uterine hemorrhage II. 66	——, inflammation of the 27
Uterus, see Womb.	——, neuralgia of the, II 89
Vagina, catarrh of the, II. 20	——, prolapsus of the, II 88
——, neuralgia of the, II. 92	——, puerperal inflammation of the, II.. 34
Vaginismus II. 94	
Vaginitis II. 20	
Vaginodynia II 92	Worms. 492
Valve, insufficiency of mitral, II...... 388	Yellow atrophy of the liver, acute... 542
Valves, insufficiency of aortic, II..... 394	—— fever II 602
Valvular diseases II. 388, 399	Zona II. 488